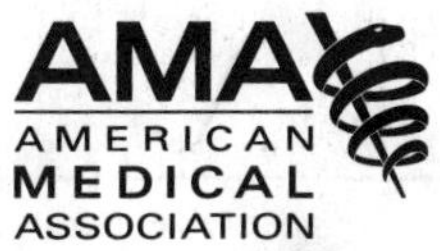

Dear *AMA Physician ICD-9-CM* Customer:

Thank you for your purchase of the American Medical Association *Physician ICD-9-CM 2006 Volumes 1 and 2* edition codebook. Your 2006 edition provides a complete and comprehensive approach to medical diagnosis coding.

The codes contained in this book are the official code set issued by the U.S. Department of Health and Human Services, effective October 1, 2005 through September 30, 2006.

Your AMA *Physician ICD-9-CM 2006 Volumes 1 and 2* edition features:

- Intuitive symbols and color coding that alerts users to critical coding and reimbursement issues.
- A comprehensive diagnosis coding tutorial.
- Anatomical illustrations to help relate diagnosis codes to organ system.
- Complete CMS guidelines.
- Medicare requirements and penalties for non-compliance.
- Rules on completing the CMS-1500 claim form.
- A tabular list of procedures, alphabetical index, and specifications for procedure classification.
- For more information on ICD-9-CM please visit www.ama-assn.org/go/cpt. Click on ICD-9-CM 2006 Special Reports and Regulatory Information.

Thank you for your commitment to the American Medical Association's line of coding and reimbursement products. If you have any questions or comments, please do not hesitate to call our customer service department at 800 621-8335.

Sincerely,

Erica Duke

Erica Duke
Marketing Manager

Other AMA Press Titles

Coding and Reimbursement:
CPT® 2006 Professional Edition
CPT® 2006 Standard Edition
CPT® 2006 Electronic Professional Edition
CPT® Changes 2006: An Insider's View
CPT® Changes Archives: An Insider's View Past and Present 2000-2006 CD-ROM
CPT® 2006 for Outpatient Services
Principles of CPT® Coding, Fourth Edition
Coding with Modifiers: A Guide to Correct CPT® and HCPCS Level II Modifier Usage
CPT® Assistant Newsletter
CPT® Express Reference Coding Cards

AMA Physician ICD-9-CM 2006, Volumes 1 and 2 Compact
AMA Hospital ICD-9-CM 2006, Volumes 1, 2, & 3 Full size Edition
AMA Hospital ICD-9-CM 2006, Volumes 1, 2, & 3 Compact
Principles of ICD-9-CM Coding, Third Edition
ICD-9-CM 2006 Express Reference Coding Cards

AMA HCPCS 2006 Level II
2006 HCPCS Level II ASCII Data Files on CD-ROM

Medicare RBRVS 2006: The Physician's Guide
RBRVS Payment Calculator CD-ROM, 2006

HIPAA Related Titles:
Coding for HIPAA: How to Report Professional Claims
HIPAA Transaction: A Non-Technical Business Guide for Health Care
HIPAA Plain and Simple
Handbook for HIPAA Security Implementation
Field Guide to HIPAA Implementation, Revised Edition
HIPAA Policies and Procedures Desk Reference

Practice Management:
Medical Practice Policies and Procedures
Handbook of Medical Office Communication
EHR Implementation

To see our complete line, please visit us at www.amapress.com or call
1 800-621-8335 for a free catalog.

International Classification of Diseases

9th Revision
Clinical Modification

Volumes 1 and 2

Physician

ICD-9-CM 2006

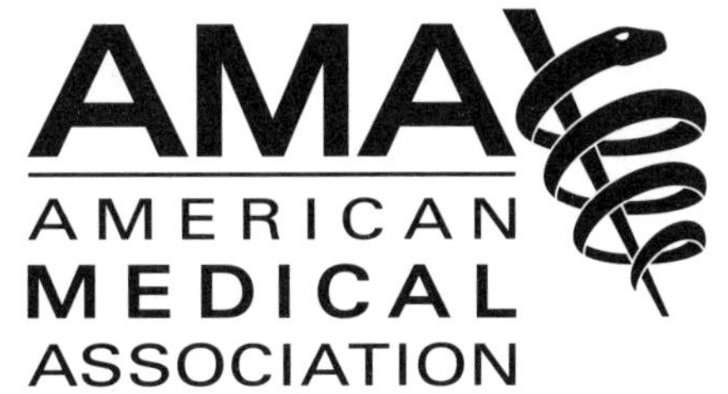

First Printing – July 2005

OP065306 (Softbound)
ISBN: 1-57947-691-0

OP065106 (Spiral)
ISBN 1-57947-692-9

Additional copies may be ordered by telephoning 800-621-8335

Special Reports and regulatory information can be found by visiting www.ama-assn.org/go/cpt. Click on ICD-9-CM 2006 Special Reports and Regulatory Information.

BP42:05-P-058:8/05

The AMA's official coding resource for procedural codes, descriptions, rules, and guidelines

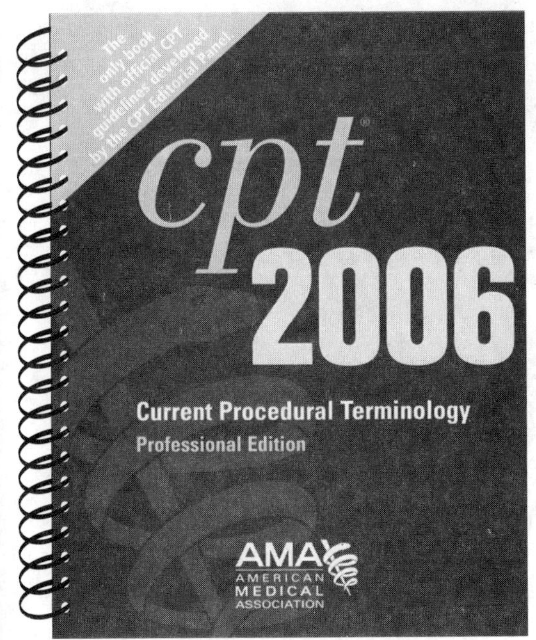

Spiralbound, 8.5" x 11", 700 pages
Available November 2005
Order #: EP054106
Price: **$91.95** AMA Member Price: **$70.95**

Changes to the CPT® 2006 procedural codes and descriptions affect almost every section, the guidelines, and appendixes. In addition to 281 new codes, 95 deleted codes, and 65 revised codes, major changes include moderate sedation, hydration, infusions, and chemotherapy, nursing facility & domiciliary care services, GI laparoscopy procedures, pathology and laboratory, skin replacement surgery, and electrophysiology.

Stay up-to-date on the new *CPT 2006* code changes that will impact code accuracy and claims submission. Rely on the *AMA CPT Professional* codebook to provide you with:

- **Color-coded symbols and highlights.** Locate code sections easier and identify the new and revised code and text changes with ease.
- **Summary of additions, deletions, and revisions in Appendix B.** Provides a quick reference to 2006 changes without having to refer to previous editions.
- **Procedural and anatomical illustrations.** Helps you interpret and report medical procedures and services.
- **Exclusive *CPT® Assistant* newsletter and *CPT® Changes* book citations.** Provides additional in-depth guidance needed to code accurately.

Understand the changes to CPT® 2006 in detail and code CPT accurately

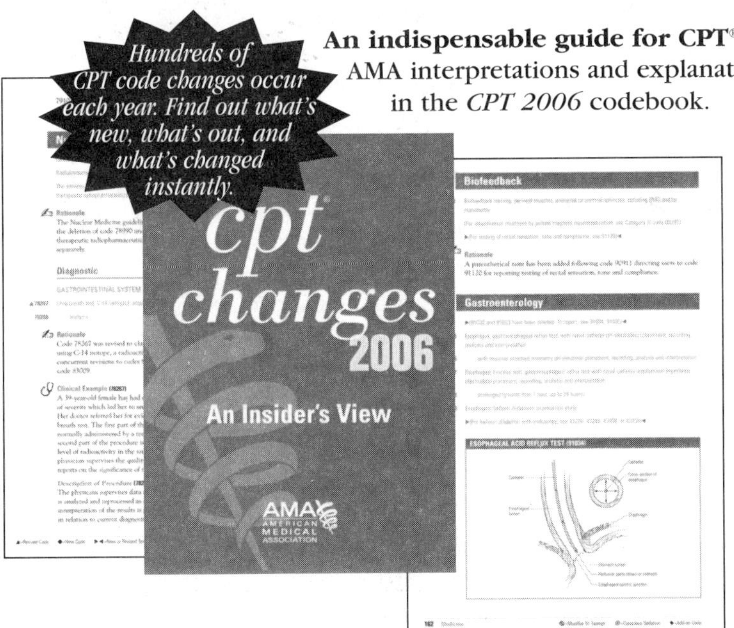

An indispensable guide for CPT® users! *CPT® Changes 2006* provides the official AMA interpretations and explanations for each CPT code, guideline, and text change in the *CPT 2006* codebook.

- Organized by CPT code section and code number, just like the CPT codebook.
- Detailed rationales provide an explanation as to why the code change occurred.
- Illustrations and useful clinical examples and procedural descriptions are presented to help you understand the practical application for that code.
- "At-a-glance" tabular review of 2006 code, text, and guideline changes.

Softbound, 7" x 10", 300 pages
Available November 2005
Order #: OP512906
Price: **$62.95** AMA Member Price: **$45.95**

Order Today! Call 800 621-8335 or order online at www.amapress.com.

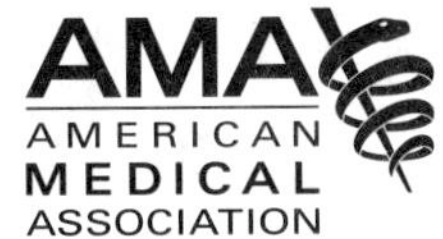

Introduction

HISTORY AND FUTURE OF ICD-9

The *International Classification of Diseases, Ninth Revision, Clinical Modification* (ICD-9-CM) is based on the official version of the World Health Organization's Ninth Revision, International Classification of Diseases (ICD-9). ICD-9 classifies morbidity and mortality information for statistical purposes and for the indexing of hospital records by disease and operations for data storage and retrieval.

This modification of ICD-9 supplants the Eighth Revision International Classification of Diseases, Adapted for Use in the United States (ICDA-8) and the Hospital Adaptation of ICDA (H-ICDA).

The concept of extending the International Classification of Diseases for use in hospital indexing was originally developed in response to a need for a more efficient basis for storage and retrieval of diagnostic data. In 1950, the U.S. Public Health Service and the Veterans Administration began independent tests of the International Classification of Diseases for hospital indexing purposes. The following year, the Columbia Presbyterian Medical Center in New York City adopted the International Classification of Diseases, Sixth Revision, with some modifications for use in its medical record department. A few years later, the Commission on Professional and Hospital Activities (CPHA) in Ann Arbor, Michigan, adopted the International Classification of Diseases with similar modifications for use in hospitals participating in the Professional Activity Study.

The problem of adapting ICD for indexing hospital records was taken up by the US National Committee on Vital and Health Statistics through its subcommittee on hospital statistics. The subcommittee reviewed the modifications made by the various users of ICD and proposed that uniform changes be made. This was done by a small working party.

In view of the growing interest in the use of the International Classification of Diseases for hospital indexing, a study was undertaken in 1956 by the American Hospital Association and the American Medical Record Association (then the American Association of Medical Record Librarians) of the relative efficiencies of coding systems for diagnostic indexing. This study indicated the International Classification of Diseases provided a suitable and efficient framework for indexing hospital records. The major users of the International Classification of Diseases for hospital indexing purposes then consolidated their experiences, and an adaptation was first published in December 1959. A revision was issued in 1962 and the first "Classification of Operations and Treatments" was included.

In 1966, the international conference for revising the International Classification of Diseases noted the eighth revision of ICD had been constructed with hospital indexing in mind and considered the revised classification suitable, in itself, for hospital use in some countries. However, it was recognized that the basic classification might provide inadequate detail for diagnostic indexing in other countries. A group of consultants was asked to study the eighth revision of ICD (ICD-8) for applicability to various users in the United States. This group recommended that further detail be provided for coding of hospital and morbidity data. The American Hospital Association was requested to develop the needed adaptation proposals. This was done by an advisory committee (the Advisory Committee to the Central Office on ICDA). In 1968 the United States Public Health Service published the product, Eighth Revision International Classification of Diseases, Adapted for Use in the United States. This became commonly known as ICDA-8, and beginning in 1968 it served as the basis for coding diagnostic data for both official morbidity and mortality statistics in the United States.

In 1968, the CPHA published the Hospital Adaptation of ICDA (H-ICDA) based on both the original ICD-8 and ICDA-8. In 1973, CPHA published a revision of H-ICDA, referred to as H-ICDA-2. Hospitals throughout the United States were divided in their use of these classifications until January 1979, when ICD-9-CM was made the single classification intended primarily for use in the United States, replacing these earlier related, but somewhat dissimilar, classifications.

Physicians have been required by law to submit diagnosis codes for Medicare reimbursement since the passage of the Medicare Catastrophic Coverage Act of 1988. This act requires physician offices to include the appropriate diagnosis codes when billing for services provided to Medicare beneficiaries on or after April 1, 1989. The Centers for Medicare and Medicaid Services (formerly known as Health Care Financing Administration) designated ICD-9-CM as the coding system physicians must use.

In 1993, the World Health Organization published the newest version. It is the International Classification of Diseases, 10th Revision, ICD-10. This version contains the greatest number of changes in the history of ICD. There are more codes (5,500 more than ICD-9) to allow more specific reporting of diseases and newly recognized conditions. ICD-10 consists of three volumes; tabular list (volume I), instructions (volume 2), and the alphabetic index (volume 3). It contains 21 chapters including two supplementary ones. The codes are alphanumeric (A00–T98, V01–Y98 and Z00–Z99). Currently ICD-10 is being used in some European countries with implementation expected after the year 2008 in the United States.

ICD-9-CM BACKGROUND

In February 1977, a steering committee was convened by the National Center for Health Statistics to provide advice and counsel in developing a clinical modification of ICD-9. The organizations represented on the steering committee included the following:

- American Association of Health Data Systems
- American Hospital Association
- American Medical Record Association
- Association for Health Records
- Council on Clinical Classifications
- Centers for Medicare and Medicaid Services, Department of Health and Human Services
- WHO Center for Classification of Diseases for North America, sponsored by the National Center for Health Statistics, Department of Health and Human Services

The Council on Clinical Classifications was sponsored by the following:

- American Academy of Pediatrics
- American College of Obstetricians and Gynecologists
- American College of Physicians
- American College of Surgeons
- American Psychiatric Association
- Commission on Professional and Hospital Activities

The steering committee met periodically in 1977. Clinical guidance and technical input were provided by task forces on classification from the Council on Clinical Classification's sponsoring organizations.

ICD-9-CM is a clinical modification of the World Health Organization's ICD-9. The term "clinical" is used to emphasize the modification's intent: to serve as a useful tool to classify morbidity data for indexing medical records, medical care review, and ambulatory and other medical care programs, as well as for basic health statistics. To describe the clinical picture of the patient, the codes must be more precise than those needed only for statistical groupings and trend analysis.

CHARACTERISTICS OF ICD-9-CM

ICD-9-CM far exceeds its predecessors in the number of codes provided. The disease classification has been expanded to include health-related conditions and to provide greater specificity at the fifth-digit level of detail. These fifth digits are not optional; they are intended for use in recording the information substantiated in the clinical record.

Volume I (tabular list) of ICD-9-CM contains four appendices:

Appendix A: Morphology of Neoplasms

Appendix B: Deleted effective October 1, 2004

Appendix C: Classification of Drugs by American Hospital Formulary Service List Number and Their ICD-9-CM Equivalents

Appendix D: Classification of Industrial Accidents According to Agency

Appendix E: List of Three-Digit Categories

These appendices are included as a reference to provide further information about the patient's clinical picture, to further define a diagnostic statement, to aid in classifying new drugs, or to reference three-digit categories.

Volume 2 (alphabetic index) of ICD-9-CM contains many diagnostic terms that do not appear in volume I since the index includes most diagnostic terms currently in use.

THE DISEASE CLASSIFICATION

ICD-9-CM is totally compatible with its parent system, ICD-9, thus meeting the need for comparability of morbidity and mortality statistics at the international level. A few fourth-digit codes were created in existing three-digit rubrics only when the necessary detail could not be accommodated by the use of a fifth-digit subclassification. To ensure that each rubric of ICD-9-CM collapses back to its ICD-9 counterpart the following specifications governed the ICD-9-CM disease classification:

Specifications for the tabular list:

1. Three-digit rubrics and their contents are unchanged from ICD-9.
2. The sequence of three-digit rubrics is unchanged from ICD-9.
3. Three-digit rubrics are not added to the main body of the classification.
4. Unsubdivided three-digit rubrics are subdivided where necessary to
   - add clinical detail
   - isolate terms for clinical accuracy
5. The modification in ICD-9-CM is accomplished by adding a fifth digit to existing ICD-9 rubrics, except as noted under #7 below.
6. The optional dual classification in ICD-9 is modified.
   - Duplicate rubrics are deleted:
     - four-digit manifestation categories duplicating etiology entries
     - manifestation inclusion terms duplicating etiology entries
   - Manifestations of disease are identified, to the extent possible, by creating five-digit codes in the etiology rubrics.
   - When the manifestation of a disease cannot be included in the etiology rubrics, provision for its identification is made by retaining the ICD-9 rubrics used for classifying manifestations of disease.
7. The format of ICD-9-CM is revised from that used in ICD-9.
   - American spelling of medical terms is used.
   - Inclusion terms are indented beneath the titles of codes.
   - Codes not to be used for primary tabulation of disease are printed in italics with the notation, "*code first underlying disease.*"

Specifications for the alphabetic index:

1. The format of the alphabetic index follows that of ICD-9.
2. When two codes are required to indicate etiology and manifestation, the manifestation code appears in brackets (eg, diabetic cataract 250.5 *[366.41]*).

How to Use *ICD-9-CM* Volumes 1 & 2

This AMA's *ICD-9-CM, Volumes 1 and 2,* is based on the official version of the *International Classification of Diseases, Ninth Revision, Clinical Modification, Sixth Edition,* issued by the U.S. Department of Health and Human Services. Annual code changes are implemented by the government and are effective October 1 and valid through September 30 of the following year.

To accommodate the coder's approach to coding, the alphabetic index (Volume 2) has been placed before the tabular list (Volume 1). This allows the user to locate the term in the index, then confirm the accuracy of the code in the tabular list.

10 STEPS TO CORRECT CODING

To code accurately, it is necessary to have a working knowledge of medical terminology and to understand the characteristics, terminology, and conventions of ICD-9-CM. Transforming descriptions of diseases, injuries, conditions and procedures into numerical designations (coding) is a complex activity and should not be undertaken without proper training.

Originally, coding allowed retrieval of medical information by diagnoses and operations for medical research, education, and administration. Coding today is used to describe the medical necessity of a procedure. This process facilitates payment of health services, evaluation of utilization patterns and the study of the appropriateness of health care costs. Coding provides the basis for epidemiological studies and research into the quality of health care being provided. Incorrect or inaccurate coding can lead to investigations of fraud and abuse. Therefore, coding must be performed correctly and consistently to produce meaningful statistics to aid in planning for the health needs of the nation.

Follow the steps below to code correctly:

Step 1: Identify the reason for the visit (eg, sign, symptom, diagnosis, condition to be coded).

Physicians describe the patient's condition using terminology that includes specific diagnoses as well as symptoms, problems or reasons for the encounter. If symptoms are present but a definitive diagnosis has not yet been determined, code the symptoms. Do not code conditions that are referred to as "rule out," "suspected," "probable" or "questionable."

Step 2: Always consult the Alphabetic Index, Volume 2, before turning to the Tabular List.

The most critical rule is to begin a code search in the index. Never turn first to the Tabular List (Volume 1), as this will lead to coding errors and less specificity in code assignments. To prevent coding errors, use both the Alphabetic Index and the Tabular List when locating and assigning a code.

Step 3: Locate the main entry term.

The Alphabetic Index is arranged by condition. Conditions may be expressed as nouns, adjectives and eponyms. Some conditions have multiple entries under their synonyms. Main terms are identified using boldface type.

Step 4: Read and interpret any notes listed with the main term

Notes are identified using italicized type.

Step 5: Review entries for modifiers

Nonessential modifiers are in parentheses. These parenthetical terms are supplementary words or explanatory information that may either be present or absent in the diagnostic statement and do not affect code assignment.

Step 6: Interpret abbreviations, cross-references, symbols and brackets

Cross-references used are "*see*," "*see* category" or "*see* also." The abbreviation NEC may follow main terms or subterms. NEC (not elsewhere classified) indicates that there is no specific code for the condition even though the medical documentation may be very specific. The ☑ box indicates the code requires an additional digit. If the appropriate digits are not found in the index, in a box beneath the main term, you MUST refer to the tabular list. Italicized brackets *[ ]*, are used to enclose a second code number that must be used with the code immediately preceding it and in that sequence.

Step 7: Choose a tentative code and locate it in the tabular list.

Be guided by any inclusion or exclusion terms, notes or other instructions, such as "*code first*" and "use additional code," that would direct the use of a different or additional code from that selected in the index for a particular diagnosis, condition or disease.

Step 8: Determine whether the code is at the highest level of specificity.

Assign three-digit codes (category codes) if there are no four-digit codes within the code category. Assign four-digit codes (subcategory codes) if there are no five-digit codes for that category. Assign five-digit codes (fifth-digit subclassification codes) for those categories where they are available.

Step 9: Consult the color coding and reimbursement prompts, including the age, sex, and Medicare as secondary payer edits. Refer to the key at the bottom of the page for definitions of colors and symbols.

Step 10: Assign the code.

ORGANIZATION

Introduction

The introductory material in this book includes the history and future of ICD-9-CM as well as an overview of the classification system.

Official ICD-9-CM Conventions

This section provides a full explanation of all the official footnotes, symbols, instructional notes, and conventions found in the official government version.

Additional Conventions

Exclusive color-coding, symbols, and notations have been included in the *AMA's ICD-9-CM, Volumes 1 and 2,* to alert coders to important coding and reimbursement issues. This section provides a full explanation of the additional conventions used throughout this book.

Summary of Code Changes

This section includes a complete listing of all code changes for the current year.

Valid Three-digit Code Table

ICD-9-CM is composed of codes with either 3, 4, or 5 digits. A code is invalid if it has not been coded to the full number of digits required for that code. There are a certain number codes that are valid for reporting as three digit codes. A list of these valid three-digit codes is included as a convenient reference when auditing claims.

Coding Guidelines

Included in this book are the official ICD-9-CM coding guidelines as approved by the four cooperating parties of the ICD-9-CM Coordination and Maintenance Committee. Failure to comply with these official coding guidelines may result in denied or delayed claims.

Disease Classification: Alphabetic Index to Diseases

The Alphabetic Index to Diseases is separated by tabs labeled with the letters of the alphabet, contains diagnostic terms for illnesses, injuries and reasons for encounters with health care professionals. Both the Table of Drugs and Chemicals and the Alphabetic Index to External Causes of Injury and Poisoning are easily located with the tabs in this section.

Disease Classification: Tabular List of Diseases

The Tabular List of Diseases arranges the ICD-9-CM codes and descriptors numerically. Color tabs divide this section into chapters, identified by the code range on the tab.

The tabular list includes two supplementary classifications:

- V Codes—Supplementary Classification of Factors Influencing Health Status and Contact with Health Services (V01–V85)
- E Codes—Supplementary Classification of External Causes of Injury and Poisoning (E800–E999)

ICD-9-CM includes four official appendixes.

- Appendix A — Morphology of Neoplasms
- Appendix B — Deleted effective October 1, 2004
- Appendix C — Classification of Drugs by AHFS List
- Appendix D — Classification of Industrial Accidents According to Agency
- Appendix E — List of Three-digit Categories

ICD-9-CM Official Conventions

ICD-9-CM FOOTNOTES, SYMBOLS, INSTRUCTIONAL NOTES AND CONVENTIONS

This AMA's *ICD-9-CM, Volumes 1 and 2* preserves all the footnotes, symbols, instructional notes and conventions found in the government's official version. Accurate coding depends on understanding the meaning of these elements.

The following appear in the disease tabular list, unless otherwise noted.

OFFICIAL GOVERNMENT SYMBOLS

§ The section mark preceding a code denotes a footnote on the page. This symbol is used only in the Tabular List of Diseases.

ICD-9-CM CONVENTIONS USED IN THE TABULAR LIST

In addition to the symbols and footnotes above, the ICD-9-CM disease tabular has certain abbreviations, punctuation, symbols, and other conventions. Our *AMA's ICD-9-CM, Volumes 1 and 2* preserves these conventions. Proper use of the conventions will lead to efficient and accurate coding.

Abbreviations

NEC Not elsewhere classifiable

This abbreviation is used when the ICD-9-CM system does not provide a code specific for the patient's condition.

NOS Not otherwise specified

This abbreviation is the equivalent of 'unspecified' and is used only when the coder lacks the information necessary to code to a more specific four-digit subcategory.

[ ] Brackets enclose synonyms, alternative terminology or explanatory phrases.

Brackets that appear beneath a code indicate the fifth digits that are considered valid fifth digits for the code. This convention is applied for those instances in ICD-9-CM where not all common fifth digits are considered valid for each subcategory within a category.

( ) Parentheses enclose supplementary words, called nonessential modifiers, that may be present in the narrative description of a disease without affecting the code assignment.

[ ] Slanted brackets that appear in the Alphabetic Indexes indicate mandatory multiple coding. Both codes must be assigned to fully describe the condition and are sequenced in the order listed.

: Colons are used in the tabular list after an incomplete term that needs one or more of the modifiers that follow in order to make it assignable to a given category.

} Braces enclose a series of terms, each of which is modified by the statement appearing to the right of the brace.

OTHER CONVENTIONS

Boldface Boldface type is used for all codes and titles in the Tabular List.

Italicized Italicized type is used for all exclusion notes and to identify codes that should not be used for describing the primary diagnosis.

INSTRUCTIONAL NOTES

These notes appear only in the Tabular List of Diseases

Includes An includes note further defines or clarifies the content of the chapter, subchapter, category, subcategory, or subclassification.

Excludes Terms following the word "*Excludes*" are not classified to the chapter, subchapter, category, subcategory, or specific subclassification code under which it is found. The note also may provide the location of the excluded diagnosis. Excludes notes are italicized.

Use additional code

This instruction signals the coder that an additional code should be used if the information is available to provide a more complete picture of that diagnosis.

Code first underlying disease

The *Code first underlying disease* instructional note found under certain codes is a sequencing rule. Most often this sequencing rule applies to the etiology/manifestation convention and is found under the manifestation code. The manifestation code may never be used alone or as a primary diagnosis (i.e., sequenced first). The instructional note, the code and its descriptor appear in italics in the tabular list.

Not all codes with a 'Code first underlying disease' instructional note are part of the etiology/manifestation convention. The 'Code first' note will appear, but the title of the code and the instructional note are not in italics. These codes may be reported alone or as the secondary diagnosis. Two codes are required and sequenced as listed in the index.

Code, if applicable, any causal condition first:

A code with this note indicates that this code may be assigned as a principal diagnosis when the causal condition is unknown or not applicable. If a causal condition is known, then the code for that condition should be sequenced as the principal or first-listed diagnosis.

Omit code

"*Omit code*" is used to instruct the coder that no code is to be assigned. When this instruction is found in the Alphabetic Index to Diseases the medical term should not be coded as a diagnosis.

***See* Condition:**

The "*see* condition" note found in the Alphabetic Index to Disease instructs the coder to refer to a main term for the condition. This note will follow index terms that are nouns for anatomical sites or adjectival forms of disease term.

Morphology Codes

For each neoplastic disease listed in the index, a morphology code is provided that identifies histological type and behavior.

The histology is identified by the first four digits and the behavior is identified by the digit following the slash. Appendix A of Volume 1 contains a listing of morphology codes. This appendix is helpful when the pathology report identifies the neoplasm by using an M code. The coder may refer to Appendix A to determine the nomenclature of the neoplasm that will be the main term to search in the Index.

Additional Conventions

SYMBOLS AND NOTATIONS

New and Revised Text Symbols

● A bullet at a code or line of text indicates that that the entry is new.

▲ A triangle in the Tabular List indicates that the code title is revised. In the Alphabetic Index, the triangle indicates that a code has changed.

▶◀ These symbols appear at the beginning and at the end of a section of new or revised text.

When these symbols appear on a page there will be a date on the lower outside corner of the page indicating the date of the change, (eg, October 2005).

Additional Digits Required

✓4th This symbol indicates that the code requires a fourth-digit.

✓5th This symbol indicates that a code requires a fifth-digit.

☑ This symbol found only in the alphabetic index sections and the Table of Drugs and Chemicals indicates that an additional digit is required. Referring to the tabular section is essential to locate the appropriate additional digit.

AHA'S *CODING CLINIC FOR ICD-9-CM* REFERENCES

The four cooperating parties have designated the AHA's *Coding Clinic for ICD-9-CM* as the official publication for coding guidelines. The references are identified by the notation AHA: followed by the issue, year and page number.

In the example below, AHA's *Coding Clinic for ICD-9-CM*, third quarter 1991, page 15, contains a discussion on code assignment for vitreous hemorrhage:

379.23 Vitreous hemorrhage
AHA: 3Q, '91, 15

The table below explains the abbreviations in the *Coding Clinic* references:

J-F	January/February
M-A	March/April
M-J	May/June
J-A	July/August
S-O	September/October
N-D	November/December
1Q	First quarter
2Q	Second quarter
3Q	Third quarter
4Q	Fourth quarter

Age and Sex Edit Symbols

The age edits below address OCE edits and are used to detect inconsistencies between the patient's age and diagnosis. They appear in the Tabular List of Diseases to the right of the code description.

Newborn Age: 0

These diagnoses are intended for newborns and neonates and the patient's age must be 0 years.

Pediatric Age: 0-17

These diagnoses are intended for children and the patient's age must between 0 and 17 years.

Maternity Age: 12-55

These diagnoses are intended for the patients between the age of 12 and 55 years.

Adult Age: 15-124

These diagnoses are intended for the patients between the age of 15 and 124 years.

The sex symbols below address OCE edits and are used to detect inconsistencies between the patient's sex and diagnosis. They appear in the Tabular List of Diseases to the right of the code description:

♂ **Male diagnosis only**

This symbol appears to the right of the code description. This reference appears in the disease tabular list.

♀ **Female diagnosis only**

This symbol appears to the right of the code description. This reference appears in the disease tabular list.

COLOR CODING

To alert the coder to Medicare outpatient code edits and other important reimbursement issues, color bars have been added over the code descriptors in the Tabular List. Some codes carry more than one color.

Carriers use the Medicare Outpatient Code Editor (OCE) to examine claims for coding and billing accuracy and completeness. Color codes in this book signify Medicare code edits for manifestation codes not to be reported as a primary diagnosis, and when a more specific diagnosis code should be used.

Manifestation Code

These codes will appear in italic type as well as with a blue color bar over the code title. A manifestation code is not allowed to be reported as a primary diagnosis because each describes a manifestation of some other underlying disease, not the disease itself. This is also referred to as mandatory multiple coding. Code the underlying disease first. A "*Code first underlying disease*" instructional note will appear with underlying disease codes identified. In the Alphabetic Index these codes are listed as the secondary code in slanted bracket with the code for the underlying disease listed first.

Other Specified Code

These codes will appear with a gray color bar over the code title. Use these codes when the documentation indicates a specified diagnosis, but the ICD-9-CM system does not have a specific code that describes the diagnosis. These codes are may be stated as "Other" or "Not elsewhere classified (NEC)."

Unspecified Code

These codes will have a yellow color bar over the code title. Use these codes when the neither the diagnostic statement nor the documentation provides enough information to assign a more specified diagnosis code. These codes may be stated as "Unspecified" or "Not otherwise specified (NOS)." Note: Do not assign these codes when a more specific diagnosis has been determined.

OTHER NOTATIONS

DEF: This symbol indicates a definition of disease term. The definition will appear in blue type in the Disease Tabular List.

MSP This identifies specific trauma codes that alert the carrier that another carrier should be billed first and Medicare billed second if payment from the first payer does not equal or exceed the amount Medicare would pay.

PDx This symbol identifies a V code that can only be used as a primary diagnosis.

SDx This symbol identifies a V code that can only be used as a secondary diagnosis.

Note: A V code without a symbol may be used as either a primary or secondary diagnosis.

Summary of Code Changes

DISEASE TABULAR LIST (VOLUME 1)

238.7	Includes term added
250.4	Use additional code note term added
250.5	Use additional code note term added
	Use additional code note terms revised
257.8	Includes terms deleted
	Excludes term added
● 259.5	Androgen insensitivity syndrome
	Includes terms added
276.5	Includes terms deleted
● 276.50	Volume depletion, unspecified
● 276.51	Dehydration
● 276.52	Hypovolemia
	Includes term added
▲ 278	▶Overweight,◀ obesity and other hyperalimentation
▲ 278.0	▶Overweight and◀ obesity
	Use additional code note added
● 278.02	Overweight
282.49	Includes term added
282.7	Includes term deleted
283.0	Excludes term revised
284.9	Includes term deleted
	Excludes note added
285.0	Includes term deleted
	Excludes note added
▲ 285.21	Anemia in ~~end stage renal disease~~ ▶chronic kidney disease◀
	Includes term added
287.0	Excludes term revised
287.3	Includes terms deleted
● 287.30	Primary thrombocytopenia, unspecified
	Includes term added
● 287.31	Immune thrombocytopenic purpura
	Includes terms added
● 287.32	Evans' syndrome
● 287.33	Congenital and hereditary thrombocytopenic purpura
	Includes terms added
	Excludes note added
● 287.39	Other primary thrombocytopenia
Chapter 5.	Mental Disorders (290-319)-Chapter introductory paragraphs deleted
● 291.82	Alcohol induced sleep disorders
	Includes terms added
291.89	Includes term deleted
● 292.85	Drug induced sleep disorders
	Includes terms added
292.89	Includes term deleted
307.4	Excludes terms added
307.41	Includes terms added
307.42	Includes terms added
307.44	Includes terms added
	Excludes term added
▲ 307.45	Circadian rhythm sleep disorder ▶of nonorganic origin◀
	Includes terms deleted
307.59	Includes term revised
323.6	Includes term added
323.8	Includes term added
● 327	Organic sleep disorders
● 327.0	Organic disorders of initiating and maintaining sleep [Organic insomnia]
	Excludes terms added
● 327.00	Organic insomnia, unspecified
● 327.01	Insomnia due to medical condition classified elsewhere
	Code first note added
	Excludes note added
● 327.02	Insomnia due to mental disorder
	Code first note added
	Excludes note added
● 327.09	Other organic insomnia
● 327.1	Organic disorders of excessive somnolence [Organic hypersomnia]
	Excludes note added
● 327.10	Organic hypersomnia, unspecified
● 327.11	Idiopathic hypersomnia with long sleep time
● 327.12	Idiopathic hypersomnia without long sleep time
● 327.13	Recurrent hypersomnia
	Includes terms added
● 327.14	Hypersomnia due to medical condition classified elsewhere
	Code first note added
	Excludes note added
● 327.15	Hypersomnia due to mental disorder
	Code first note added
	Excludes note added
● 327.19	Other organic hypersomnia
● 327.2	Organic sleep apnea
	Excludes note added
● 327.20	Organic sleep apnea, unspecified
● 327.21	Primary central sleep apnea
● 327.22	High altitude periodic breathing
● 327.23	Obstructive sleep apnea (adult) (pediatric)
● 327.24	Idiopathic sleep related nonobstructive alveolar hypoventilation
	Includes term added
● 327.25	Congenital central alveolar hypoventilation syndrome
● 327.26	Sleep related hypoventilation/hypoxemia in conditions classifiable elsewhere
	Code first note added
● 327.27	Central sleep apnea in conditions classified elsewhere
	Code first note added
● 327.29	Other organic sleep apnea
● 327.3	Circadian rhythm sleep disorder
	Includes terms added
	Excludes note added
● 327.30	Circadian rhythm sleep disorder, unspecified
● 327.31	Circadian rhythm sleep disorder, delayed sleep phase type
● 327.32	Circadian rhythm sleep disorder, advanced sleep phase type
● 327.33	Circadian rhythm sleep disorder, irregular sleep-wake type
● 327.34	Circadian rhythm sleep disorder, free-running type
● 327.35	Circadian rhythm sleep disorder, jet lag type
● 327.36	Circadian rhythm sleep disorder, shift work type
● 327.37	Circadian rhythm sleep disorder in conditions classified elsewhere
	Code first note added
● 327.39	Other circadian rhythm sleep disorder
● 327.4	Organic parasomnia
	Excludes note added
● 327.40	Organic parasomnia, unspecified
● 327.41	Confusional arousals
● 327.42	REM sleep behavior disorder
● 327.43	Recurrent isolated sleep paralysis
● 327.44	Parasomnia in conditions classified elsewhere
	Code first note added
● 327.49	Other organic parasomnia
● 327.5	Organic sleep related movement disorders
	Excludes note added
● 327.51	Periodic limb movement disorder
	Includes term added
● 327.52	Sleep related leg cramps
● 327.53	Sleep related bruxism
● 327.59	Other organic sleep related movement disorders
● 327.8	Other organic sleep disorders
332.1	Includes term added
333	Excludes term added
333.1	Includes term added
333.7	Includes term added
333.82	Includes term added
333.90	Includes term added
	Use additional code note added
333.99	Includes term added
	Use additional code note added
357.4	Code first note revised
362.01	Includes terms deleted
● 362.03	Nonproliferative diabetic retinopathy NOS
● 362.04	Mild nonproliferative diabetic retinopathy
● 362.05	Moderate nonproliferative diabetic retinopathy
● 362.06	Severe nonproliferative diabetic retinopathy
● 362.07	Diabetic macular edema
	Includes term added
	Instructional note added
402	Use additional code note revised
▲ 403	Hypertensive ~~renal~~ ▶kidney◀ disease
	Use additional code note added
▲ 403.0	Hypertensive ~~renal~~ ▶kidney◀ disease, Malignant
▲ 403.00	Hypertensive ~~renal~~ ▶kidney◀ disease, malignant, without ~~mention of renal failure~~ ▶chronic kidney disease◀
▲ 403.01	Hypertensive ~~renal~~ ▶kidney◀ disease, malignant, with ~~renal failure~~ ▶chronic kidney disease◀
▲ 403.1	Hypertensive ~~renal~~ ▶kidney◀ disease, Benign
▲ 403.10	Hypertensive ~~renal~~ ▶kidney◀ disease, benign, without ~~mention of renal failure~~ ▶chronic kidney disease◀
▲ 403.11	Hypertensive ~~renal~~ ▶kidney◀ disease, benign, with ~~renal failure~~ ▶chronic kidney disease◀
▲ 403.9	Hypertensive ~~renal~~ ▶kidney◀ disease, Unspecified
▲ 403.90	Hypertensive ~~renal~~ ▶kidney◀ disease, unspecified, without ~~mention of renal failure~~ ▶chronic kidney disease◀
▲ 403.91	Hypertensive ~~renal~~ ▶kidney◀ disease, unspecified, with ~~renal failure~~ ▶chronic kidney disease◀
▲ 404	Hypertensive heart and ~~renal~~ ▶kidney◀ disease
	Use additional code note revised
	Use additional code note added
▲ 404.0	Hypertensive heart and ~~renal~~ ▶kidney◀ disease, Malignant
▲ 404.00	Hypertensive heart and ~~renal~~ ▶kidney◀ disease, malignant, without ~~mention of~~ heart failure or ~~renal failure~~ ▶ chronic kidney disease◀
▲ 404.02	Hypertensive heart and ~~renal~~ ▶kidney◀ disease, malignant, with ~~renal failure~~ ▶chronic kidney disease◀
▲ 404.03	Hypertensive heart and ~~renal~~ ▶kidney◀ disease, malignant, with heart failure and ~~renal failure~~ ▶chronic kidney disease◀
▲ 404.1	Hypertensive heart and ~~renal~~ ▶kidney◀ disease, Benign
▲ 404.10	Hypertensive heart and ~~renal~~ ▶kidney◀ disease, benign, without ~~mention of~~ heart failure or ~~renal failure~~ ▶ chronic kidney disease◀
▲ 404.12	Hypertensive heart and ~~renal~~ ▶kidney◀ disease, benign, with ~~renal failure~~ ▶chronic kidney disease◀
▲ 404.13	Hypertensive heart and ~~renal~~ ▶kidney◀ disease, benign, with heart failure and ~~renal failure~~ ▶chronic kidney disease◀
▲ 404.9	Hypertensive heart and ~~renal~~ ▶kidney◀ disease, Unspecified
▲ 404.90	Hypertensive heart and ~~renal~~ ▶kidney◀ disease, unspecified, without ~~mention of~~ heart failure or ~~renal failure~~ ▶ chronic kidney disease◀
▲ 404.92	Hypertensive heart and ~~renal~~ ▶kidney◀ disease, unspecified, with ~~renal failure~~ ▶chronic kidney disease◀
▲ 404.93	Hypertensive heart and ~~renal~~ ▶kidney◀ disease, unspecified, with heart failure and ~~renal failure~~ ▶chronic kidney disease◀
410	Includes term added
410.0	Includes term added
410.1	Includes term added

▶◀ Revised Text ● New Code ▲ Revised Code Title

410.2 Includes term added
410.3 Includes term added
410.4 Includes term added
410.5 Includes term added
410.6 Includes term added
410.7 Includes term added
410.8 Includes term added
410.9 Includes term added
420.0 Code first note revised
● 426.82 Long QT syndrome
● 443.82 Erythromelalgia
443.89 Includes term deleted
Section PNEUMONIA AND INFLUENZA (480-487)
Excludes term revised
487 Excludes term deleted
487.0 Use additional code note added
507 Excludes term revised
524.51 Includes term deleted
525.1 Code first note added
525.10 Includes term deleted
● 525.4 Complete edentulism
Use additional code note added
● 525.40 Complete edentulism, unspecified
Includes term added
● 525.41 Complete edentulism, class I
● 525.42 Complete edentulism, class II
● 525.43 Complete edentulism, class III
● 525.44 Complete edentulism, class IV
● 525.5 Partial edentulism
Use additional code note added
● 525.50 Partial edentulism, unspecified
● 525.51 Partial edentulism, class I
● 525.52 Partial edentulism, class II
● 525.53 Partial edentulism, class III
● 525.54 Partial edentulism, class IV
552.8 Excludes note added
▲ 567 Peritonitis ▶and retroperitoneal infections◀
567.2 Includes terms deleted
● 567.21 Peritonitis (acute) generalized
Includes term added
● 567.22 Peritoneal abscess
Includes terms added
● 567.23 Spontaneous bacterial peritonitis
● 567.29 Other suppurative peritonitis
Includes term added
● 567.3 Retroperitoneal infections
● 567.31 Psoas muscle abscess
● 567.38 Other retroperitoneal abscess
● 567.39 Other retroperitoneal infections
567.8 Includes terms deleted
● 567.81 Choleperitonitis
Includes term added
● 567.82 Sclerosing mesenteritis
Includes terms added
● 567.89 Other specified peritonitis
Includes terms added
▲ 585 Chronic ~~renal failure~~ ▶kidney disease (CKD)◀
Use additional code note added
● 585.1 Chronic kidney disease, Stage I
● 585.2 Chronic kidney disease, Stage II (mild)
● 585.3 Chronic kidney disease, Stage III (moderate)
● 585.4 Chronic kidney disease, Stage IV (severe)
● 585.5 Chronic kidney disease, Stage V
● 585.6 End stage renal disease
● 585.9 Chronic kidney disease, unspecified
Includes terms added
593.9 Includes term added
Includes terms revised
Excludes term added
Excludes terms deleted
▲ 599.6 Urinary obstruction, ~~unspecified~~
Includes terms deleted
Excludes term added
● 599.60 Urinary obstruction, unspecified
Includes terms added
● 599.69 Urinary obstruction, not elsewhere classified
607.84 Excludes term revised
648.8 Instructional note revised
Use additional code note added
● 651.7 Multiple gestation following (elective) fetal reduction
Includes term added
● 651.70 Multiple gestation following (elective) fetal reduction, unspecified as to episode of care or not applicable
● 651.71 Multiple gestation following (elective) fetal reduction, delivered, with or without mention of antepartum condition
● 651.73 Multiple gestation following (elective) fetal reduction, antepartum condition or complication
660.8 Use additional code note added
▲ 728.87 Muscle weakness ▶(generalized)◀
742 Excludes note added
748 Excludes term added
752 Excludes term revised
752.11 Includes term deleted
752.41 Includes term added
752.7 Excludes term revised
Chapter 15. CERTAIN CONDITIONS ORIGINATING IN THE PERINATAL PERIOD (760-779)
Includes note revised
760.74 Includes term added
● 760.77 Noxious influences affecting fetus or newborn via placenta or breast milk, Anticonvulsants
Includes terms added
● 760.78 Noxious influences affecting fetus or newborn via placenta or breast milk, Antimetabolic agents
Includes terms added
● 763.84 Meconium passage during delivery
Excludes note added
▲ 770.1 ~~Meconium~~ ▶Fetal and newborn◀ aspiration ~~syndrome~~
Includes terms deleted
Excludes terms added
● 770.10 Fetal and newborn aspiration, unspecified
● 770.11 Meconium aspiration without respiratory symptoms
Includes term added
● 770.12 Meconium aspiration with respiratory symptoms
Includes terms added
Use additional code note added
● 770.13 Aspiration of clear amniotic fluid without respiratory symptoms
Includes term added
● 770.14 Aspiration of clear amniotic fluid with respiratory symptoms
Includes terms added
Use additional code note added
● 770.15 Aspiration of blood without respiratory symptoms
Includes term added
● 770.16 Aspiration of blood with respiratory symptoms
Includes terms added
Use additional code note added
● 770.17 Other fetal and newborn aspiration without respiratory symptoms
● 770.18 Other fetal and newborn aspiration with respiratory symptoms
Includes terms added
Use additional code note added
● 770.85 Aspiration of postnatal stomach contents without respiratory symptoms
Includes term added
● 770.86 Aspiration of postnatal stomach contents with respiratory symptoms
Includes terms added
Use additional code note added
771 Includes note revised
● 779.84 Meconium staining
Excludes terms added
779.89 Use additional code note added
780.5 Excludes terms added
▲ 780.51 Insomnia with sleep apnea, ▶unspecified◀
▲ 780.52 ~~Other~~ Insomnia, ▶unspecified◀
Includes term deleted
▲ 780.53 Hypersomnia with sleep apnea, ▶unspecified◀
▲ 780.54 ~~Other~~ Hypersomnia, ▶unspecified◀
Includes term deleted
▲ 780.55 Disruption of 24 hour sleep wake cycle, ▶unspecified◀
Includes terms deleted
▲ 780.57 ~~Other and~~ Unspecified sleep apnea
▲ 780.58 Sleep related movement disorder, ▶unspecified◀
Includes term deleted
780.92 Excludes note added
● 780.95 Other excessive crying
Excludes note added
783.2 Use additional code note added
783.9 Excludes term revised
788.2 Excludes note added
794.31 Excludes note added
795.09 Includes term added
▲ 799.0 Asphyxia ▶and hypoxemia◀
Excludes term revised
Excludes term added
● 799.01 Asphyxia
● 799.02 Hypoxemia
996 Excludes term added
996.4 Use additional code note added
● 996.40 Unspecified mechanical complication of internal orthopedic device, implant, and graft
● 996.41 Mechanical loosening of prosthetic joint
Includes term added
● 996.42 Dislocation of prosthetic joint
Includes terms added
● 996.43 Prosthetic joint implant failure
Includes term added
● 996.44 Peri-prosthetic fracture around prosthetic joint
● 996.45 Peri-prosthetic osteolysis
● 996.46 Articular bearing surface wear of prosthetic joint
● 996.47 Other mechanical complication of prosthetic joint implant
Includes term added
● 996.49 Other mechanical complication of other internal orthopedic device, implant, and graft
Excludes term added
996.66 Use additional code note added
SUPPLEMENTARY CLASSIFICATION OF FACTORS INFLUENCING HEALTH STATUS AND CONTACT WITH HEALTH SERVICES ▶(V01-V85)◀
V03 Excludes term revised
V07.39 Excludes term revised
V12.0 Excludes note added
● V12.42 Personal history of, Infections of the central nervous system
Includes terms added
V12.6 Excludes term added
● V12.60 Personal history of, Unspecified disease of respiratory system
● V12.61 Personal history of, Pneumonia (recurrent)
● V12.69 Personal history of, Other diseases of respiratory system
● V13.02 Personal history of, Urinary (tract) infection
● V13.03 Personal history of, Nephrotic syndrome
● V15.88 Personal history of, History of fall
Includes term added
● V17.81 Family history of, Osteoporosis
● V17.89 Family history of, Other musculoskeletal diseases
● V18.9 Family history of, Genetic disease carrier
V26.21 Excludes term revised
● V26.31 Testing for genetic disease carrier status
● V26.32 Other genetic testing
● V26.33 Genetic counseling
V45.1 Includes terms added
▲ 46.1 Other dependence on machines, Respirator ▶[Ventilator]◀
● V46.13 Encounter for weaning from respirator [ventilator]
● V46.14 Mechanical complication of respirator [ventilator]
Includes term added
● V49.84 Bed confinement status
V54 Excludes term revised
V54.0 Excludes term revised
▲ V58.1 ▶Encounter for antineoplastic◀ chemotherapy ▶and immunotherapy◀
Excludes term added
● V58.11 Encounter for antineoplastic chemotherapy
● V58.12 Encounter for antineoplastic immunotherapy

▶◀ Revised Text ● New Code ▲ Revised Code Title

● V59.7 Donors, Egg (oocyte) (ovum)
● V59.70 Egg (oocyte) (ovum) donor, unspecified
● V59.71 Egg (oocyte) (ovum) donor, under age 35, anonymous recipient
Includes term added
● V59.72 Egg (oocyte) (ovum) donor, under age 35, designated recipient
● V59.73 Egg (oocyte) (ovum) donor, age 35 and over, anonymous recipient
Includes term added
● V59.74 Egg (oocyte) (ovum) donor, age 35 and over, designated recipient
V61.10 Includes terms added
V61.20 Includes term added
V61.8 Includes term added
V62.2 Includes term added
V62.3 Includes term added
V62.4 Includes term added
V62.81 Includes term added
● V62.84 Suicidal ideation
Excludes term added
V62.89 Includes terms added
▲ V64.0 Vaccination not carried out ~~because of contraindication~~
● V64.00 Vaccination not carried out, unspecified reason
● V64.01 Vaccination not carried out because of acute illness
● V64.02 Vaccination not carried out because of chronic illness or condition
● V64.03 Vaccination not carried out because of immune compromised state
● V64.04 Vaccination not carried out because of allergy to vaccine or component
● V64.05 Vaccination not carried out because of caregiver refusal
● V64.06 Vaccination not carried out because of patient refusal
● V64.07 Vaccination not carried out for religious reasons
● V64.08 Vaccination not carried out because patient had disease being vaccinated against
● V64.09 Vaccination not carried out for other reason
V65.4 Excludes term revised
● V69.5 Behavioral insomnia of childhood
PERSONS WITHOUT REPORTED DIAGNOSIS ENCOUNTERED DURING EXAMINATION AND INVESTIGATION OF INDIVIDUALS AND POPULATIONS ▶(V70-V85)◀
V70.0 Excludes term added
V72.4 Excludes term deleted
● V72.42 Pregnancy examination or test, positive result
V72.81 Includes term added
V72.82 Includes term added
V72.83 Includes terms added
Excludes term added
V72.84 Includes term added
● V72.86 Encounter for blood typing
● V85 Body Mass Index
Includes term added
Instructional note added
● V85.0 Body Mass Index less than 19, adult
● V85.1 Body Mass Index between 19-24, adult
● V85.2 Body Mass Index between 25-29, adult
● V85.21 Body Mass Index 25.0-25.9, adult
● V85.22 Body Mass Index 26.0-26.9, adult
● V85.23 Body Mass Index 27.0-27.9, adult
● V85.24 Body Mass Index 28.0-28.9, adult
● V85.25 Body Mass Index 29.0-29.9, adult
● V85.3 Body Mass Index between 30-39, adult
● V85.30 Body Mass Index 30.0-30.9, adult
● V85.31 Body Mass Index 31.0-31.9, adult
● V85.32 Body Mass Index 32.0-32.9, adult
● V85.33 Body Mass Index 33.0-33.9, adult
● V85.34 Body Mass Index 34.0-34.9, adult
● V85.35 Body Mass Index 35.0-35.9, adult
● V85.36 Body Mass Index 36.0-36.9, adult
● V85.37 Body Mass Index 37.0-37.9, adult
● V85.38 Body Mass Index 38.0-38.9, adult
● V85.39 Body Mass Index 39.0-39.9, adult
● V85.4 Body Mass Index 40 and over, adult
E904.2 Excludes term revised

▶◀ Revised Text ● New Code ▲ Revised Code Title

Valid Three-digit ICD-9-CM Codes

Three-digit ICD-9-CM codes are used to identify a condition or disease only when a fourth or fifth digit is not available. The following are the only ICD-9-CM codes that are valid without further specificity.

024 Glanders

025 Melioidosis

035 Erysipelas

037 Tetanus

042 Human Immunodeficiency Virus (HIV) Infection

048 Other enterovirus diseases of central nervous system

061 Dengue

064 Viral encephalitis transmitted by other and unspecified arthropods

071 Rabies

075 Infectious mononucleosis

080 Louse-borne [epidemic] typhus

096 Late syphilis, latent

101 Vincent's angina

118 Opportunistic mycoses

124 Trichinosis

129 Intestinal parasitism, unspecified

135 Sarcoidosis

138 Late effects of acute poliomyelitis

179 Malignant neoplasm of uterus, part unspecified

181 Malignant neoplasm of placenta

185 Malignant neoplasm of prostate

193 Malignant neoplasm of thyroid gland

217 Benign neoplasm of breast

220 Benign neoplasm of ovary

226 Benign neoplasm of thyroid gland

243 Congenital hypothyroidism

260 Kwashiorkor

261 Nutritional marasmus

262 Other severe protein-calorie malnutrition

267 Ascorbic acid deficiency

311 Depressive disorder, not elsewhere classified

316 Psychic factors associated with diseases classified elsewhere

317 Mild mental retardation

319 Unspecified mental retardation

325 Phlebitis and thrombophlebitis of intracranial venous sinuses

326 Late effects of intracranial abscess or pyogenic infection

340 Multiple sclerosis

390 Rheumatic fever without mention of heart involvement

393 Chronic rheumatic pericarditis

412 Old myocardial infarction

430 Subarachnoid hemorrhage

431 Intracerebral hemorrhage

436 Acute, but ill-defined, cerebrovascular disease

452 Portal vein thrombosis

460 Acute nasopharyngitis [common cold]

462 Acute pharyngitis

463 Acute tonsillitis

470 Deviated nasal septum

475 Peritonsillar abscess

481 Pneumococcal pneumonia

485 Bronchopneumonia, organism unspecified

486 Pneumonia, organism unspecified

490 Bronchitis, not specified as acute or chronic

496 Chronic airway obstruction, not elsewhere classified

500 Coal workers' pneumoconiosis

501 Asbestosis

502 Pneumoconiosis due to other silica or silicates

503 Pneumoconiosis due to other inorganic dust

504 Pneumoconopathy due to inhalation of other dust

505 Pneumoconiosis, unspecified

514 Pulmonary congestion and hypostasis

515 Postinflammatory pulmonary fibrosis

541 Appendicitis, unqualified

542 Other appendicitis

566 Abscess of anal and rectal regions

570 Acute and subacute necrosis of liver

586 Renal failure, unspecified

587 Renal sclerosis, unspecified

591 Hydronephrosis

605 Redundant prepuce and phimosis

630 Hydatidiform mole

631 Other abnormal product of conception

632 Missed abortion

650 Delivery in a completely normal case

677 Late effect of complication of pregnancy, childbirth, and the puerperium

683 Acute lymphadenitis

684 Impetigo

700 Corns and callosities

725 Polymyalgia rheumatica

734 Flat foot

769 Respiratory distress syndrome

797 Senility without mention of psychosis

920 Contusion of face, scalp, and neck except eye(s)

931 Foreign body in ear

932 Foreign body in nose

936 Foreign body in intestine and colon

937 Foreign body in anus and rectum

938 Foreign body in digestive system, unspecified

981 Toxic effect of petroleum products

986 Toxic effect of carbon monoxide

990 Effects of radiation, unspecified

V08 Asymptomatic HIV infection status

V51 Aftercare involving the use of plastic surgery

Coding Guidelines

ICD-9-CM OFFICIAL GUIDELINES FOR CODING AND REPORTING

Effective April 1, 2005
Narrative changes appear in bold text
The guidelines have been updated to include the V Code Table.

The Centers for Medicare and Medicaid Services (CMS) and the National Center for Health Statistics (NCHS), two departments within the U.S. Federal Government's Department of Health and Human Services (DHHS) provide the following guidelines for coding and reporting using the International Classification of Diseases, 9th Revision, Clinical Modification (ICD-9-CM). These guidelines should be used as a companion document to the official version of the ICD-9-CM as published on CD-ROM by the U.S. Government Printing Office (GPO).

These guidelines have been approved by the four organizations that make up the Cooperating Parties for the ICD-9-CM: the American Hospital Association (AHA), the American Health Information Management Association (AHIMA), CMS, and NCHS. These guidelines are included in the official government version of the ICD-9-CM and also appear in *Coding Clinic for ICD-9-CM*, published by the AHA.

These guidelines are a set of rules that have been developed to accompany and complement the official conventions and instructions provided within the ICD-9-CM itself. These guidelines are based on the coding and sequencing instructions in Volumes 1, 2, and 3 of ICD-9-CM, but provide additional instruction. **Adherence to these guidelines when assigning ICD-9-CM diagnosis and procedure codes is required under the Health Insurance Portability and Accountability Act (HIPAA). The diagnosis codes (Volumes 1-2) have been adopted under HIPAA for all health care settings. Volume 3 procedure codes have been adopted for inpatient procedures reported by hospitals.** A joint effort between the health care provider and the coder is essential to achieve complete and accurate documentation, code assignment, and reporting of diagnoses and procedures. These guidelines have been developed to assist both the health care provider and the coder in identifying those diagnoses and procedures that are to be reported. The importance of consistent, complete documentation in the medical record cannot be overemphasized. Without such documentation accurate coding cannot be achieved. **The entire record should be reviewed to determine the specific reason for the encounter and the conditions treated.**

The term "encounter" is used for all settings, including hospital admissions. In the context of these guidelines, the term "provider" is used throughout the guidelines to mean physician or any qualified health care practitioner who is legally accountable for establishing the patient's diagnosis. Only this set of guidelines, approved by the cooperating parties, is official.

The guidelines are organized into sections. Section I includes the structure and conventions of the classification and general guidelines that apply to the entire classification, and chapter-specific guidelines that correspond to the chapters as they are arranged in the classification. Section II includes guidelines for selection of principal diagnosis for non-outpatient settings. Section III includes guidelines for reporting additional diagnoses in non-outpatient settings. Section IV is for outpatient coding and reporting.

Section I. Conventions, general coding guidelines and chapter-specific guidelines

i. **The postpartum and peripartum eriods**
j. **Code 677 Late effect of complication of pregnancy**
k. **Abortions**

12. Chapter 12: Diseases Skin and Subcutaneous Tissue (680–709)
Reserved for future guideline expansion
13. Chapter 13: Diseases of Musculoskeletal and Connective Tissue (710–739)
Reserved for future guideline expansion
14. Chapter 14: Congenital Anomalies (740–759)
    a. **Codes in categories 740-759, Congenital anomalies**
15. Chapter 15: Newborn (Perinatal) Guidelines (760-779)
    a. **General perinatal rules**
    b. **Use of codes V30-V39**
    c. **Newborn transfers**
    d. **Use of category V29**
    e. **Use of other V codes on perinatal records**
    f. **Maternal causes of perinatal morbidity**
    g. **Congenital anomalies in newborns**
    h. **Coding additional perinatal diagnoses**
    i. **Prematurity and fetal growth retardation**
    j. **Newborn sepsis**
16. Chapter 16: Signs, Symptoms and Ill-Defined Conditions (780–799)
17. Chapter 17: Injury and Poisoning (800-999)
    a. **Coding of injuries**
    b. **Coding of fractures**
    c. **Coding of burns**
    d. **Coding of debridement of wound, infection, or burn**
    e. **Adverse effects, poisoning and toxic effects**
18. Classification of Factors Influencing Health Status and Contact with Health Service (Supplemental V01-V85)
    a. **Introduction**
    b. **V codes use in any health care setting**
    c. **V codes indicate a reason for an encounter**
    d. **Categories of V codes**
19. Supplemental Classification of External Causes of Injury and Poisoning (E codes, E800–E999)
    a. **General E code coding guideline**
    b. **Place of occurrence guideline**
    c. **Adverse effects of drugs, medicinal and biological substances guidelines**
    d. **Multiple cause E code coding guidelines**
    e. **Child and adult abuse guideline**
    f. **Unknown or suspected intent guideline**
    g. **Undetermined cause**
    h. **Late effects of external cause guidelines**
    i. **Misadventures and complications of care guidelines**
    j. **Terrorism guidelines**

Section II. Selection of Principal Diagnosis

A. Codes for symptoms, signs, and ill-defined conditions
B. Two or more interrelated conditions, each potentially meeting the definition for principal diagnosis
C. Two or more diagnoses that equally meet the definition for principal diagnosis
D. Two or more comparative or contrasting conditions
E. A symptom(s) followed by contrasting/comparative diagnoses
F. Original treatment plan not carried out
G. Complications of surgery and other medical care
H. Uncertain diagnosis

Section III. Reporting Additional Diagnoses

A. Previous conditions
B. Abnormal findings
C. Uncertain diagnosis

Section IV. Diagnostic Coding and Reporting Guidelines for Outpatient Services

A. Selection of first-listed condition
B. Codes from 001.0 through V85.4
C. Accurate reporting of ICD-9-CM diagnosis codes
D. Selection of codes 001.0 through 999.9
E. Codes that describe symptoms and signs
F. Encounters for circumstances other than a disease or injury
G. Level of detail in coding
   1. ICD-9-CM codes with three, four, or five digits
   2. Use of full number of digits required for a code
H. ICD-9-CM code for the diagnosis, condition, problem, or other reason for encounter/visit
I. "Probable," "suspected," "questionable," "rule out," or "working diagnosis"
J. Chronic diseases
K. Code all documented conditions that coexist
L. Patients receiving diagnostic services only
M. Patients receiving therapeutic services only
N. Patients receiving preoperative evaluations only
O. Ambulatory surgery
P. Routine outpatient prenatal visits

Section I. Conventions, general coding guidelines and chapter-specific guidelines

The conventions, general guidelines, and chapter-specific guidelines are applicable to all health care settings unless otherwise indicated.

A. Conventions for the ICD-9-CM

The conventions for the ICD-9-CM are the general rules for use of the classification independent of the guidelines. These conventions are incorporated within the index and tabular of the ICD-9-CM as instructional notes. The conventions are as follows:

1. Format:
The ICD-9-CM uses an indented format for ease in reference

2. Abbreviations

a. Index abbreviations
NEC "Not elsewhere classifiable"—This abbreviation in the index represents "other specified." When a specific code is not available for a condition, the index directs the coder to the "other specified" code in the tabular.

b. Tabular abbreviations
NEC "Not elsewhere classifiable"—This abbreviation in the tabular represents "other specified." When a specific code is not available for a condition, the tabular includes an NEC entry under a code to identify the code as the "other specified" code (See section I.A.5.a.,"Other" codes).

NOS "Not otherwise specified"—This abbreviation is the equivalent of unspecified. (See section I.A.5.b., "Unspecified" codes)

3. Punctuation

[ ] Brackets are used in the Tabular List to enclose synonyms, alternative wording, or explanatory phrases. Brackets are used in the index to identify manifestation codes. (See section I.A.6., Etiology/manifestations)

( ) Parentheses are used in both the index and tabular to enclose supplementary words that may be present or absent in the statement of a disease or procedure without affecting the code number to which it is assigned. The terms within the parentheses are referred to as nonessential modifiers.

: Colons are used in the Tabular List after an incomplete term needs one or more of the modifiers following the colon to make it assignable to a given category.

4. Includes and excludes notes and inclusion terms

Includes: This note appears immediately under a three-digit code title to further define, or give examples of, the content of the category.

Excludes: An excludes note under a code indicates that the terms excluded from the code are to be coded elsewhere. In some cases the codes for the excluded terms should not be used in conjunction with the code from which they are excluded. An example of this is a congenital condition excluded from an acquired form of the same condition. The congenital and acquired codes should not be used together. In other cases, the excluded terms may be used together with an excluded code. An example of this is when fractures of different bones are coded to different codes. Both codes may be used together if both types of fractures are present.

Inclusion terms: List of terms included under certain four- and five-digit codes. These terms are the conditions for which that code number is to be used. The terms may be synonyms of the code title, or, in the case of "other specified" codes, the terms are a list of the various conditions assigned to that code. The inclusion terms are not necessarily exhaustive. Additional terms found only in the index may also be assigned to a code.

5. **Other and unspecified codes**

   a. "Other" codes—Codes titled "other" or "other specified" (usually a code with a fourth digit of 8 or fifth digit of 9 for diagnosis codes) are for use when the information in the medical record provides detail for which a specific code does not exist. Index entries with NEC in the line designate "other" codes in the tabular. These index entries represent specific disease entities for which no specific code exists so the term is included within an "other" code.

   b. "Unspecified" codes—Codes (usually a code with a fourth digit of 9 or fifth of 0 for diagnosis codes) titled "unspecified" are for use when the information in the medical record is insufficient to assign a more specific code.

6. **Etiology/manifestation convention ("code first," "use additional code," and "in diseases classified elsewhere" notes)**—Certain conditions have both an underlying etiology and multiple body system manifestations due to the underlying etiology. For such conditions, the ICD-9-CM has a coding convention that requires the underlying condition to be sequenced first followed by the manifestation. Wherever such a combination exists, there is a "use additional code" note at the etiology code, and a "code first" note at the manifestation code. These instructional notes indicate the proper sequencing order of the codes, etiology followed by manifestation.

   In most cases the manifestation codes will have in the code title, "in diseases classified elsewhere." Codes with this title are a component of the etiology/manifestation convention. The code title indicates that it is a manifestation code. "In diseases classified elsewhere," codes are never permitted to be used as first listed or principal diagnosis codes. They must be used in conjunction with an underlying condition code, and they must be listed following the underlying condition.

   There are manifestation codes that do not have "in diseases classified elsewhere" in the title. For such codes a "use additional code" note will still be present and the rules for sequencing apply.

   In addition to the notes in the tabular, these conditions also have a specific index entry structure. In the index both conditions are listed together with the etiology code first followed by the manifestation codes in brackets. The code in brackets is always to be sequenced second.

   The most commonly used etiology/manifestation combinations are the codes for diabetes mellitus, category 250. For each code under category 250 there is a use additional code note for the manifestation that is specific for that particular diabetic manifestation. Should a patient have more than one manifestation of diabetes, more than one code from category 250 may be used with as many manifestation codes as are needed to fully describe the patient's complete diabetic condition. The category 250 diabetes codes should be sequenced first, followed by the manifestation codes.

   "Code first" and "use additional code" notes are also used as sequencing rules in the classification for certain codes that are not part of an etiology/manifestation combination. See section I.B.9., "Multiple coding for a single condition."

7. **"And"**
   The word "and" should be interpreted to mean either "and" or "or" when it appears in a title.

8. **"With"**
   The word "with" in the Alphabetic Index is sequenced immediately following the main term, not in alphabetical order.

9. **"See" and "see also"**
   The "see" instruction following a main term in the index indicates that another term should be referenced. It is necessary to go to the main term referenced with the "see" note to locate the correct code.

   A "see also" instruction following a main term in the index instructs that there is another main term that may also be referenced that may provide additional index entries that may be useful. It is not necessary to follow the "see also" note when the original main term provides the necessary code.

B. General coding guidelines

1. **Use of both Alphabetic Index and Tabular List**—Use both the Alphabetic Index and the Tabular List when locating and assigning a code. Reliance on only the Alphabetic Index or the Tabular List leads to errors in code assignments and less specificity in code selection.

2. **Locate each term in the alphabetic index**—Locate each term in the Alphabetic Index and verify the code selected in the Tabular List. Read and be guided by instructional notations that appear in both the Alphabetic Index and the Tabular List.

3. **Level of detail in coding**—Diagnosis and procedure codes are to be used at their highest number of digits available.

   ICD-9-CM diagnosis codes are composed of codes with either three, four, or five digits. Codes with three digits are included in ICD-9-CM as the heading of a category of codes that may be further subdivided by the use of four and/or fifth digits, which provide greater detail.

   A three-digit code is to be used only if it is not further subdivided. Where fourth-digit subcategories and/or fifth-digit subclassifications are provided, they must be assigned. A code is invalid if it has not been coded to the full number of digits required for that code. For example, acute myocardial infarction, code 410, has fourth digits that describe the location of the infarction (e.g., 410.2 Of inferolateral wall), and fifth digits that identify the episode of care. It would be incorrect to report a code in category 410 without a fourth and fifth digit.

   ICD-9-CM Volume 3 procedure codes are composed of codes with either three or four digits. Codes with two digits are included in ICD-9-CM as the heading of a category of codes that may be further subdivided by the use of third and/or fourth digits, which provide greater detail.

4. **Code or codes from 001.0 through V85.4**—The appropriate code or codes from 001.0 through V85.4 must be used to identify diagnoses, symptoms, conditions, problems, complaints, or other reason(s) for the encounter/visit.

5. **Selection of codes 001.0 through 999.9**—The selection of codes 001.0 through 999.9 will frequently be used to describe the reason for the admission/encounter. These codes are from the section of ICD-9-CM for the classification of diseases and injuries (e.g., infectious and parasitic diseases; neoplasms; symptoms, signs, and ill-defined conditions, etc.).

6. **Signs and symptoms**—Codes that describe symptoms and signs, as opposed to diagnoses, are acceptable for reporting purposes when a related definitive diagnosis has not been established (confirmed) by the provider. Chapter 16 of ICD-9-CM, "Symptoms, Signs, and Ill-defined Conditions" (codes 780.0-799.9) contain many, but not all, codes for symptoms.

7. **Conditions that are an integral part of a disease process**—Signs and symptoms that are integral to the disease process should not be assigned as additional codes.

8. **Conditions that are not an integral part of a disease process**—Additional signs and symptoms that may not be associated routinely with a disease process should be coded when present.

9. **Multiple coding for a single condition**—In addition to the etiology/manifestation convention that requires two codes to fully describe a single condition that affects multiple body systems, there are other single conditions that also require more than one code. "Use additional code" notes are found in the tabular at codes that are not part of an etiology/manifestation pair where a secondary code is useful to fully describe a condition. The sequencing rule is the same as the etiology/manifestation pair where a secondary code is useful to fully describe a condition. The sequencing rule is the same; "use additional code" indicates that a secondary code should be added.

   For example, for infections that are not included in chapter 1, a secondary code from category 041 Bacterial infection in conditions classified elsewhere and of unspecified site, may be required to identify the bacterial organism causing the infection. A "use additional code" note will normally be found at the infectious disease code, indicating a need for the organism code to be added as a secondary code.

   "Code first" notes are also under certain codes that are not specifically manifestation codes but may be due to an underlying cause. When a "code first" note is present and an underlying condition is present, the underlying condition should be sequenced first.

   "Code, if applicable, any causal condition first" notes indicate that this code may be assigned as a principal diagnosis when the causal condition is unknown or not applicable. If a causal condition is known, then the code for that condition should be sequenced as the principal or first-listed diagnosis.

Multiple codes may be needed for late effects, complication codes, and obstetric codes to more fully describe a condition. See the specific guidelines for these conditions for further instruction.

10. **Acute and chronic conditions**—If the same condition is described as both acute (subacute) and chronic, and separate subentries exist in the Alphabetic Index at the same indentation level, code both and sequence the acute (subacute) code first.

11. **Combination code**—A combination code is a single code used to classify:
    - Two diagnoses
    - A diagnosis with an associated secondary process (manifestation)
    - A diagnosis with an associated complication

    Combination codes are identified by referring to subterm entries in the Alphabetic Index and by reading the inclusion and exclusion notes in the Tabular List.

    Assign only the combination code when that code fully identifies the diagnostic conditions involved or when the Alphabetic Index so directs. Multiple coding should not be used when the classification provides a combination code that clearly identifies all of the elements documented in the diagnosis. When the combination code lacks necessary specificity in describing the manifestation or complication, an additional code should be used as a secondary code.

12. **Late effects**—A late effect is the residual effect (condition produced) after the acute phase of an illness or injury has terminated. There is no time limit on when a late effect code can be used. The residual may be apparent early, such as in cerebrovascular accident cases, or it may occur months or years later, such as that due to a previous injury. Coding of late effects generally requires two codes sequenced in the following order: The condition or nature of the late effect is sequenced first... The late effect code is sequenced second.

    An exception to the above guidelines are those instances where the code for late effect is followed by a manifestation code identified in the Tabular List and title, or the late effect code has been expanded (at the fourth- and fifth-digit levels) to include the manifestation(s). The code for the acute phase of an illness or injury that led to the late effect is never used with a code for the late effect.

13. **Impending or threatened condition**—Code any condition described at the time of discharge as "impending" or "threatened" as follows:

    If it did occur, code as confirmed diagnosis. If it did not occur, reference the Alphabetic Index to determine if the condition has a subentry term for "impending" or "threatened" and also reference main term entries for "Impending" and for "Threatened." If the subterms are listed, assign the given code. If the subterms are not listed, code the existing underlying condition(s) and not the condition described as impending or threatened.

C. Chapter-specific coding guidelines

In addition to general coding guidelines, there are guidelines for specific diagnoses and/or conditions in the classification. Unless otherwise indicated, these guidelines apply to all health care settings. Please refer to section II for guidelines on the selection of principal diagnosis.

1. Chapter 1: Infectious and Parasitic Diseases (001-139)

a. Human immunodeficiency virus (HIV) infections

1) Code only confirmed cases—Code only confirmed cases of HIV infection/illness. This is an exception to the hospital inpatient guideline section II, H.

In this context, "confirmation" does not require documentation of positive serology or culture for HIV; the provider's diagnostic statement that the patient is HIV positive or has an HIV-related illness is sufficient.

2) Selection and sequencing of HIV codes

(a) Patient admitted for HIV-related condition—If a patient is admitted for an HIV-related condition, the principal diagnosis should be 042, followed by additional diagnosis codes for all reported HIV-related conditions.

(b) Patient with HIV disease admitted for unrelated condition—If a patient with HIV disease is admitted for an unrelated condition (such as a traumatic injury), the code for the unrelated condition (e.g., the nature of injury code) should be the principal diagnosis. Other diagnoses would be 042 followed by additional diagnosis codes for all reported HIV-related conditions.

(c) Whether the patient is newly diagnosed—Whether the patient is newly diagnosed or has had previous admissions/encounters for HIV conditions is irrelevant to the sequencing decision.

(d) Asymptomatic human immunodeficiency virus—V08 Asymptomatic human immunodeficiency virus [HIV] infection, is to be applied when the patient without any documentation of symptoms is listed as being "HIV positive," "known HIV," "HIV test positive," or similar terminology. Do not use this code if the term "AIDS" is used or if the patient is treated for any HIV-related illness or is described as having any condition(s) resulting from his/her HIV positive status; use 042 in these cases.

(e) Patients with inconclusive HIV serology—Patients with inconclusive HIV serology, but no definitive diagnosis or manifestations of the illness, may be assigned code 795.71 Inconclusive serologic test for human immunodeficiency virus [HIV].

(f) Previously diagnosed HIV-related illness—Patients with any known prior diagnosis of an HIV-related illness should be coded to 042. Once a patient has developed an HIV-related illness, the patient should always be assigned code 042 on every subsequent admission/encounter. Patients previously diagnosed with any HIV illness (042) should never be assigned to 795.71 or V08.

(g) HIV infection in pregnancy, childbirth and the puerperium—During pregnancy, childbirth, or the puerperium, a patient admitted (or presenting for a health care encounter) because of an HIV-related illness should receive a principal diagnosis code of 647.6x Other specified infectious and parasitic diseases in the mother classifiable elsewhere but complicating the pregnancy, childbirth or the puerperium, followed by 042 and the code(s) for the HIV-related illness(es). Codes from chapter 15 always take sequencing priority.

Patients with asymptomatic HIV infection status admitted (or presenting for a health care encounter) during pregnancy, childbirth, or the puerperium should receive codes of 647.6x and V08.

(h) Encounters for testing for HIV—If a patient is being seen to determine his/her HIV status, use code V73.89 Screening for other specified viral disease. Use code V69.8 Other problems related to lifestyle, as a secondary code if an asymptomatic patient is in a known high risk group for HIV. Should a patient with signs or symptoms or illness, or a confirmed HIV related diagnosis be tested for HIV, code the signs and symptoms or the diagnosis. An additional counseling code V65.44 may be used if counseling is provided during the encounter for the test.

When a patient returns to be informed of his/her HIV test results, use code V65.44 HIV counseling, if the results of the test are negative.

If the results are positive but the patient is asymptomatic, use code V08 Asymptomatic HIV infection. If the results are positive and the patient is symptomatic, use code 042 HIV infection, with codes for the HIV-related symptoms or diagnosis. The HIV counseling code may also be used if counseling is provided for patients with positive test results.

b. Septicemia, systemic inflammatory response syndrome (SIRS), sepsis, severe sepsis, and septic shock

1) Sepsis as principal diagnosis or secondary diagnosis

(a) Sepsis as principal diagnosis—If sepsis is present on admission and meets the definition of principal diagnosis, the underlying systemic infection code (e.g., 038.xx, 112.5, etc.) should be assigned as the principal diagnosis, followed by code 995.91 Systemic inflammatory response syndrome due to infectious process without organ dysfunction, as required by the sequencing rules in the Tabular List. Codes from subcategory 995.9 can never be assigned as a principal diagnosis.

(b) Sepsis as secondary diagnoses—When sepsis develops during the encounter (it was not present on admission), the sepsis codes may be assigned as secondary diagnoses, following the sequencing rules provided in the Tabular List.

(c) Documentation unclear as to whether sepsis present on admission—If the documentation is not clear whether the sepsis was present on admission, the provider should be queried. After provider query, if sepsis is determined at that point to have met the definition of principal diagnosis, the underlying systemic infection (038.xx, 112.5, etc.) may be used as the principal diagnosis along with code 995.91 Systemic inflammatory response syndrome due to infectious process without organ dysfunction.

2) Septicemia/sepsis—In most cases, it will be a code from category 038 Septicemia, that will be used in conjunction with a code from subcategory 995.9 such as the following:

(a) **Streptococcal sepsis**—If the documentation in the record states streptococcal sepsis, codes 038.0 and code 995.91 should be used, in that sequence.

(b) **Streptococcal septicemia**—If the documentation states streptococcal septicemia, only code 038.0 should be assigned; however, the provider should be queried whether the patient has sepsis, an infection with SIRS.

(c) **Sepsis or SIRS must be documented**—Either the term sepsis or SIRS must be documented to assign a code from subcategory 995.9.

3) **Terms "sepsis," " severe sepsis," or "SIRS"**—If the terms sepsis, severe sepsis, or SIRS are used with an underlying infection other than septicemia, such as pneumonia, cellulitis, or a nonspecified urinary tract infection, a code from category 038 should be assigned first, then code 995.91, followed by the code for the initial infection. The use of the terms sepsis or SIRS indicates that the patient's infection has advanced to the point of a systemic infection so the systemic infection should be sequenced before the localized infection. The instructional note under subcategory 995.9 instructs to assign the underlying systemic infection first.

Note: The term "urosepsis" is a nonspecific term. If that is the only term documented then only code 599.0 should be assigned based on the default for the term in the ICD-9-CM index, in addition to the code for the causal organism if known.

4) **Severe sepsis**—For patients with severe sepsis, the code for the systemic infection (e.g., 038.xx, 112.5, etc) or trauma should be sequenced first, followed by either code 995.92 Systemic inflammatory response syndrome due to infectious process with organ dysfunction, or code 995.94 Systemic inflammatory response syndrome due to noninfectious process with organ dysfunction. Codes for the specific organ dysfunctions should also be assigned.

5) **Septic shock**

(a) Sequencing of septic shock—Septic shock is a form of organ dysfunction associated with severe sepsis. A code for the initiating underlying systemic infection followed by a code for SIRS (code 995.92) must be assigned before the code for septic shock. As noted in the sequencing instructions in the Tabular List, the code for septic shock cannot be assigned as a principal diagnosis.

(b) Septic shock without documentation of severe sepsis—Septic shock cannot occur in the absence of severe sepsis. A code from subcategory 995.9 must be sequenced before the code for septic shock. The use additional code notes and the code first note provide sequencing instructions.

6) **Sepsis and septic shock associated with abortion**—Sepsis and septic shock associated with abortion, ectopic pregnancy, and molar pregnancy are classified to category codes in chapter 11 (630-639).

7) **Negative or inconclusive blood cultures**—Negative or inconclusive blood cultures do not preclude a diagnosis of septicemia or sepsis in patients with clinical evidence of the condition; however, the provider should be queried.

8) **Newborn sepsis—See section I.C.15.j for information on the coding of newborn sepsis.**

9) **Sepsis due to a postprocedural infection—Sepsis resulting from a postprocedural infection is a complication of care. For such cases code 998.59 Other postoperative infections, should be coded first followed by the appropriate codes for the sepsis. The other guidelines for coding sepsis should then be followed for the assignment of additional codes.**

10) **External cause of injury codes with SIRS—An external cause code is not needed with codes 995.91 Systemic inflammatory response syndrome due to infectious process without organ dysfunction, or 995.92 Systemic inflammatory response syndrome due to infectious process with organ dysfunction.**

Refer to section I.C.19.a.7 for instruction on the use of external cause of injury codes with codes for SIRS resulting from trauma.

2. Chapter 2: Neoplasms (140-239)

General guidelines

Chapter 2 of the ICD-9-CM contains the codes for most benign and all malignant neoplasms. Certain benign neoplasms, such as prostatic adenomas, may be found in the specific body system chapters. To properly code a neoplasm it is necessary to determine from the record if the neoplasm is benign, in situ, malignant, or of uncertain histologic behavior. If malignant, any secondary (metastatic) sites should also be determined.

The neoplasm table in the Alphabetic Index should be referenced first. However, if the histological term is documented, that term should be referenced first, rather than going immediately to the neoplasm table, in order to determine which column in the neoplasm table is appropriate. For example, if the documentation indicates "adenoma," refer to the term in the Alphabetic Index to review the entries under this term and the instructional note to "see also neoplasm, by site, benign." The table provides the proper code based on the type of neoplasm and the site. It is important to select the proper column in the table that corresponds to the type of neoplasm. The tabular should then be referenced to verify that the correct code has been selected from the table and that a more specific site code does not exist.

See section I. C. 18.d.4. for information regarding V codes for genetic susceptibility to cancer.

a. **Treatment directed at the malignancy**—If the treatment is directed at the malignancy, designate the malignancy as the principal diagnosis.

b. **Treatment of secondary site**—When a patient is admitted because of a primary neoplasm with metastasis and treatment is directed toward the secondary site only, the secondary neoplasm is designated as the principal diagnosis even though the primary malignancy is still present.

c. **Coding and sequencing of complications**—Coding and sequencing of complications associated with the malignancies or with the therapy thereof are subject to the following guidelines:

1) **Anemia associated with malignancy**—When admission/encounter is for management of an anemia associated with the malignancy, and the treatment is only for anemia, the anemia is designated at the principal diagnosis and is followed by the appropriate code(s) for the malignancy.

2) **Anemia associated with chemotherapy**—When the admission/encounter is for management of an anemia associated with chemotherapy or radiotherapy and the only treatment is for the anemia, the anemia is sequenced first followed by the appropriate code(s) for the malignancy.

3) **Management of dehydration due to the malignancy**—When the admission/encounter is for management of dehydration due to the malignancy or the therapy, or a combination of both, and only the dehydration is being treated (intravenous rehydration), the dehydration is sequenced first, followed by the code(s) for the malignancy.

4) **Treatment of a complication resulting from a surgical procedure**—When the admission/encounter is for treatment of a complication resulting from a surgical procedure, designate the complication as the principal or first-listed diagnosis if treatment is directed at resolving the complication.

d. **Primary malignancy previously excised**—When a primary malignancy has been previously excised or eradicated from its site and there is no further treatment directed to that site and there is no evidence of any existing primary malignancy, a code from category V10 Personal history of malignant neoplasm, should be used to indicate the former site of the malignancy. Any mention of extension, invasion, or metastasis to another site is coded as a secondary malignant neoplasm to that site. The secondary site may be the principal or first-listed with the V10 code used as a secondary code.

e. **Admissions/encounters involving chemotherapy and radiation therapy**

1) **Episode of care involves surgical removal of neoplasm**—When an episode of care involves the surgical removal of a neoplasm, primary or secondary site, followed by adjunct chemotherapy or radiation treatment, the neoplasm code should be assigned as principal or first-listed diagnosis, using codes in the 140–198 series or where appropriate in the 200–203 series.

2) **Patient admission/encounter solely for administration of chemotherapy**—If a patient admission/encounter is solely for the administration of chemotherapy or radiation therapy code V58.0 Encounter for radiation therapy, or V58.1 Encounter for chemotherapy, should be the first-listed or principal diagnosis. If a patient receives both chemotherapy and radiation therapy both codes should be listed, in either order of sequence.

3) **Patient admitted for radiotherapy/chemotherapy and develops complications**—When a patient is admitted for the purpose of radiotherapy or chemotherapy and develops complications such as uncontrolled nausea and vomiting or dehydration, the principal or first-listed diagnosis is V58.0 Encounter for radiotherapy, or V58.1

Encounter for chemotherapy, followed by any codes for the complications.

See section I.C.18.d.8. for additional information regarding aftercare V codes.

f. **Admission/encounter to determine extent of malignancy**—When the reason for admission/encounter is to determine the extent of the malignancy, or for a procedure such as paracentesis or thoracentesis, the primary malignancy or appropriate metastatic site is designated as the principal or first-listed diagnosis, even though chemotherapy or radiotherapy is administered.

g. **Symptoms, signs, and ill-defined conditions listed in chapter 16**—Symptoms, signs, and ill-defined conditions listed in chapter 16 characteristic of, or associated with, an existing primary or secondary site malignancy cannot be used to replace the malignancy as principal or first-listed diagnosis, regardless of the number of admissions or encounters for treatment and care of the neoplasm.

h. **Encounter for prophylactic organ removal—For encounters specifically for prophylactic removal of breasts, ovaries, or another organ due to a genetic susceptibility to cancer or a family history of cancer, the principal or first-listed code should be a code from subcategory V50.4 Prophylactic organ removal, followed by the appropriate genetic susceptibility code and the appropriate family history code.**

If the patient has a malignancy of one site and is having prophylactic removal of another site to prevent either a new primary malignancy or metastatic disease, a code for the malignancy should also be assigned in addition to a code from subcategory V50.4. A V50.4 code should not be assigned if the patient is having organ removal for treatment of a malignancy, such as the removal of the testes for the treatment of prostate cancer.

3. Chapter 3: Endocrine, Nutritional, and Metabolic Diseases and Immunity Disorders (240-279)

a. **Diabetes mellitus—Codes under category 250 Diabetes mellitus, identify complications/manifestations associated with diabetes mellitus. A fifth-digit is required for all category 250 codes to identify the type of diabetes mellitus and whether the diabetes is controlled or uncontrolled.**

1) Fifth digits for category 250: The following are the fifth digits for the codes under category 250:

0 type II or unspecified type, not stated as uncontrolled

1 type I, [juvenile type], not stated as uncontrolled

2 type II or unspecified type, uncontrolled

3 type I, [juvenile type], uncontrolled

The age of a patient is not the sole determining factor, though most type I diabetics develop the condition before reaching puberty. For this reason type I diabetes mellitus is also referred to as juvenile diabetes.

2) Type of diabetes mellitus not documented—If the type of diabetes mellitus is not documented in the medical record the default is type II.

3) Diabetes mellitus and the use of insulin—All type I diabetics must use insulin to replace what their bodies do not produce. However, the use of insulin does not mean that a patient is a type I diabetic. Some patients with type II diabetes mellitus are unable to control their blood sugar through diet and oral medication alone and do require insulin. If the documentation in a medical record does not indicate the type of diabetes but does indicate that the patient uses insulin, the appropriate fifth digit for type II must be used. For type II patients who routinely use insulin, code V58.67 Long-term (current) use of insulin, should also be assigned to indicate that the patient uses insulin. Code V58.67 should not be assigned if insulin is given temporarily to bring a type II patient's blood sugar under control during an encounter.

4) Assigning and sequencing diabetes codes and associated conditions—When assigning codes for diabetes and its associated conditions, the code(s) from category 250 must be sequenced before the codes for the associated conditions. The diabetes codes and the secondary codes that correspond to them are paired codes that follow the etiology/manifestation convention of the classification (See section I.A.6., Etiology/manifestation convention). Assign as many codes from category 250 as needed to identify all of the associated conditions that the patient has. The corresponding secondary codes are listed under each of the diabetes codes.

5) Diabetes mellitus in pregnancy and gestational diabetes

(a) For diabetes mellitus complicating pregnancy, see aection I.C.11.f., Diabetes mellitus in pregnancy.

(b) For gestational diabetes, see section I.C.11, g., Gestational diabetes.

6) Insulin pump malfunction

(a) Underdose of insulin due to insulin pump failure An underdose of insulin due to an insulin pump failure should be assigned 996.57 Mechanical complication due to insulin pump, as the principal or first listed code, followed by the appropriate diabetes mellitus code based on documentation.

(b) Overdose of insulin due to insulin pump failure The principal or first-listed code for an encounter due to an insulin pump malfunction resulting in an overdose of insulin should also be 996.57 Mechanical complication due to insulin pump, followed by code 962.3 Poisoning by insulins and antidiabetic agents, and the appropriate diabetes mellitus code based on documentation.

4. Chapter 4: Diseases of Blood and Blood Forming Organs (280-289)

Reserved for future guideline expansion

5. Chapter 5: Mental Disorders (290-319)

Reserved for future guideline expansion

6. Chapter 6: Diseases of Nervous System and Sense Organs (320-389)

Reserved for future guideline expansion

7. Chapter 7: Diseases of Circulatory System (390-459)

a. Hypertension

Hypertension Table

The hypertension table, found under the main term, "Hypertension," in the Alphabetic Index, contains a complete listing of all conditions due to or associated with hypertension and classifies them according to malignant, benign, and unspecified.

1) **Hypertension, essential, or NOS**—Assign hypertension (arterial) (essential) (primary) (systemic) (NOS) to category code 401 with the appropriate fourth digit to indicate malignant (.0), benign (.1), or unspecified (.9). Do not use either .0 malignant or .1 benign unless medical record documentation supports such a designation.

2) **Hypertension with heart disease**—Heart conditions (425.8, 429.0–429.3, 429.8, 429.9) are assigned to a code from category 402 when a causal relationship is stated (due to hypertension) or implied (hypertensive). Use an additional code from category 428 to identify the type of heart failure in those patients with heart failure. More than one code from category 428 may be assigned if the patient has systolic or diastolic failure and congestive heart failure.

The same heart conditions (425.8, 429.0–429.3, 429.8, 429.9) with hypertension, but without a stated casual relationship, are coded separately. Sequence according to the circumstances of the admission/encounter.

3) **Hypertensive renal disease with chronic renal failure**—Assign codes from category 403, Hypertensive renal disease, when conditions classified to categories 585-587 are present. Unlike hypertension with heart disease, ICD-9-CM presumes a cause-and-effect relationship and classifies renal failure with hypertension as hypertensive renal disease.

4) **Hypertensive heart and renal disease**—Assign codes from combination category 404, Hypertensive heart and renal disease, when both hypertensive renal disease and hypertensive heart disease are stated in the diagnosis. Assume a relationship between the hypertension and the renal disease, whether or not the condition is so designated. Assign an additional code from category 428 to identify the type of heart failure. More than one code from category 428 may be assigned if the patient has systolic or diastolic failure and congestive heart failure.

5) **Hypertensive cerebrovascular disease**—First assign codes from 430–438 Cerebrovascular disease, then the appropriate hypertension code from categories 401–405.

6) **Hypertensive retinopathy**—Two codes are necessary to identify the condition. First assign the code from subcategory 362.11 Hypertensive retinopathy, then the appropriate code from categories 401–405 to indicate the type of hypertension.

7) **Hypertension, secondary**—Two codes are required: one to identify the underlying etiology and one from category 405 to identify the hypertension. Sequencing of codes is determined by the reason for admission/encounter.

8) **Hypertension, transient**—Assign code 796.2 Elevated blood pressure reading without diagnosis of hypertension, unless patient has an established diagnosis of hypertension. Assign code 642.3x for transient hypertension of pregnancy.

9) **Hypertension, controlled**—Assign appropriate code from categories 401–405. This diagnostic statement usually refers to an existing state of hypertension under control by therapy.

10) **Hypertension, uncontrolled**—Uncontrolled hypertension may refer to untreated hypertension or hypertension not responding to current therapeutic regimen. In either case, assign the appropriate code from categories 401-405 to designate the stage and type of hypertension. Code to the type of hypertension.

11) **Elevated blood pressure**—For a statement of elevated blood pressure without further specificity, assign code 796.2, Elevated blood pressure reading without diagnosis of hypertension, rather than a code from category 401.

b. **Cerebral infarction/stroke/cerebrovascular accident (CVA)—The terms stroke and CVA are often used interchangeably to refer to a cerebral infarction. The terms stroke, CVA, and cerebral infarction NOS are all indexed to the default code 434.91, Cerebral artery occlusion, unspecified, with infarction. Code 436, Acute, but ill-defined, cerebrovascular disease, should not be used when the documentation states stroke or CVA.**

c. **Postoperative cerebrovascular accident—A cerebrovascular hemorrhage or infarction that occurs as a result of medical intervention is coded to 997.02, Iatrogenic cerebrovascular infarction or hemorrhage. Medical record documentation should clearly specify the cause- and-effect relationship between the medical intervention and the cerebrovascular accident in order to assign this code. A secondary code from the code range 430-432 or from a code from subcategories 433 or 434 with a fifth digit of "1" should also be used to identify the type of hemorrhage or infarct.**

This guideline conforms to the use additional code note instruction at category 997. Code 436, Acute, but ill-defined, cerebrovascular disease, should not be used as a secondary code with code 997.02.

d. **Late effects of cerebrovascular disease**

1) **Category 438, late effects of cerebrovascular disease**—Category 438 is used to indicate conditions classifiable to categories 430–437 as the causes of late effects (neurologic deficits), themselves classified elsewhere. These "late effects" include neurologic deficits that persist after initial onset of conditions classifiable to 430–437. The neurologic deficits caused by cerebrovascular disease may be present from the onset or may arise at any time after the onset of the condition classifiable to 430-437.

2) **Codes from category 438 with codes from 430–437**—Codes from category 438 may be assigned on a health care record with codes from 430–437, if the patient has a current cerebrovascular accident (CVA) and deficits from an old CVA.

3) **Code V12.59**—Assign code V12.59 (and not a code from category 438) as an additional code for history of cerebrovascular disease when no neurologic deficits are present.

8. Chapter 8: Diseases of Respiratory System (460-519)

a. **Chronic obstructive pulmonary disease [COPD] and asthma**

1) **Conditions that comprise COPD and asthma—The conditions that comprise COPD are obstructive chronic bronchitis, subcategory 491.2, and emphysema, category 492. All asthma codes are under category 493 Asthma. Code 496 Chronic airway obstruction, not elsewhere classified, is a nonspecific code that should be used only when the documentation in a medical record does not specify the type of COPD being treated.**

2) **Acute exacerbation of chronic obstructive bronchitis and asthma—The codes for chronic obstructive bronchitis and asthma distinguish between uncomplicated cases and those in acute exacerbation. An acute exacerbation is a worsening or a decompensation of a chronic condition. An acute exacerbation is not equivalent to an infection superimposed on a chronic condition, though an exacerbation may be triggered by an infection.**

3) **Overlapping nature of the conditions that comprise COPD and asthma—Due to the overlapping nature of the conditions that make up COPD and asthma, there are many variations in the way these conditions are documented. Code selection must be based on the terms as documented. When selecting the correct code for the documented type of COPD and asthma, it is essential to first review the index and then verify the code in the Tabular List. There are many instructional notes under the different COPD subcategories and codes. It is important that all such notes be reviewed to ensure correct code assignment.**

4) **Acute exacerbation of asthma and status asthmaticus—An acute exacerbation of asthma is an increased severity of the asthma symptoms, such as wheezing and shortness of breath. Status asthmaticus refers to a patient's failure to respond to therapy administered during an asthmatic episode and is a life-threatening complication that requires emergency care. If status asthmaticus is documented by the provider with any type of COPD or with acute bronchitis, the status asthmaticus should be sequenced first. It supersedes any type of COPD, including that with acute exacerbation or acute bronchitis. It is inappropriate to assign an asthma code with fifth-digit 2, with acute exacerbation, together with an asthma code with fifth-digit 1, with status asthmaticus. Only the fifth-digit 1 should be assigned.**

b. **Chronic obstructive pulmonary disease [COPD] and bronchitis**

1) **Acute bronchitis with COPD—Acute bronchitis, code 466.0, is due to an infectious organism. When acute bronchitis is documented with COPD, code 491.22 Obstructive chronic bronchitis with acute bronchitis, should be assigned. It is not necessary to also assign code 466.0. If a medical record documents acute bronchitis with COPD with acute exacerbation, only code 491.22 should be assigned. The acute bronchitis included in code 491.22 supersedes the acute exacerbation. If a medical record documents COPD with acute exacerbation without mention of acute bronchitis, only code 491.21 should be assigned.**

9. Chapter 9: Diseases of Digestive System (520-579)

Reserved for future guideline expansion

10. Chapter 10: Diseases of Genitourinary System (580-629)

Reserved for future guideline expansion

11. Chapter 11: Complications of Pregnancy, Childbirth, and the Puerperium (630-677)

a. **General rules for obstetric cases**

1) **Codes from chapter 11 and sequencing priority**—Obstetric cases require codes from chapter 11, codes in the range 630-677 Complications of pregnancy, childbirth, and the puerperium. Chapter 11 codes have sequencing priority over codes from other chapters. Additional codes from other chapters may be used in conjunction with chapter 11 codes to further specify conditions. Should the provider document that the pregnancy is incidental to the encounter, then code V22.2 should be used in place of any chapter 11 codes. It is the provider's responsibility to state that the condition being treated is not affecting the pregnancy.

2) **Chapter 11 codes used only on the maternal record**—Chapter 11 codes are to be used only on the maternal record, never on the record of the newborn.

3) **Chapter 11 fifth digits**—Categories 640-648, 651-676 have required fifth-digits, which indicate whether the encounter is antepartum, postpartum and whether a delivery has also occurred.

4) **Fifth digits, appropriate for each code**—The fifth digits, which are appropriate for each code number, are listed in brackets under each code. The fifth digits on each code should all be consistent with each other. That is, should a delivery occur all of the fifth digits should indicate the delivery.

b. Selection of OB principal or first-listed diagnosis

1) **Routine outpatient prenatal visits**—For routine outpatient prenatal visits when no complications are present, codes V22.0 Supervision of normal first pregnancy, and V22.1 Supervision of other normal pregnancy, should be used as the first-listed diagnoses. These codes should not be used in conjunction with chapter 11 codes.

2) **Prenatal outpatient visits for high-risk patients**—For prenatal outpatient visits for patients with high-risk pregnancies, a code from category V23 Supervision of high-risk pregnancy, should be used as the principal or first-listed diagnosis. Secondary chapter 11 codes may be used in conjunction with these codes if appropriate.

3) **Episodes when no delivery occurs**—In episodes when no delivery occurs, the principal diagnosis should correspond to the principal complication of the pregnancy, which necessitated the encounter. Should more than one complication exist, all of which are treated or monitored, any of the complication codes may be sequenced first.

4) **When a delivery occurs**—When a delivery occurs, the principal diagnosis should correspond to the main circumstances or complication of the delivery. In cases of cesarean delivery, the selection of the principal diagnosis should correspond to the reason the cesarean delivery was performed unless the reason for admission/encounter was unrelated to the condition resulting in the cesarean delivery.

5) **Outcome of delivery**—An outcome of delivery code, V27.0-V27.9, should be included on every maternal record when a delivery has occurred. These codes are not to be used on subsequent records or on the newborn record.

c. Fetal conditions affecting the management of the mother

1) **Fetal condition responsible for modifying the management of the mother**—Codes from category 655 Known or suspected fetal abnormality affecting management of the mother, and category 656 Other fetal and placental problems affecting the management of the mother, are assigned only when the fetal condition is actually responsible for modifying the management of the mother, i.e., by requiring diagnostic studies, additional observation, special care, or termination of pregnancy. The fact that the fetal condition exists does not justify assigning a code from this series to the mother's record.

2) **In utero surgery—In cases when surgery is performed on the fetus, a diagnosis code from category 655 Known or suspected fetal abnormalities affecting management of the mother, should be assigned identifying the fetal condition. Procedure code 75.36 Correction of fetal defect, should be assigned on the hospital inpatient record.**

No code from chapter 15, the perinatal codes, should be used on the mother's record to identify fetal conditions. Surgery performed in utero on a fetus is still to be coded as an obstetric encounter.

d. HIV infection in pregnancy, childbirth and the puerperium
During pregnancy, childbirth, or the puerperium, a patient admitted because of an HIV-related illness should receive a principal diagnosis of 647.6X Other specified infectious and parasitic diseases in the mother classifiable elsewhere, but complicating the pregnancy, childbirth, or the puerperium, followed by 042 and the code(s) for the HIV-related illness(es).

Patients with asymptomatic HIV infection status admitted during pregnancy, childbirth, or the puerperium should receive codes of 647.6X and V08.

e. Current conditions complicating pregnancy—Assign a code from subcategory 648.x for patients that have current conditions when the condition affects the management of the pregnancy, childbirth, or the puerperium. Use additional secondary codes from other chapters to identify the conditions, as appropriate.

f. Diabetes mellitus in pregnancy—Diabetes mellitus is a significant complicating factor in pregnancy. Pregnant women who are diabetic should be assigned code 648.0x Diabetes mellitus complicating pregnancy, and a secondary code from category 250 Diabetes mellitus, to identify the type of diabetes.

Code V58.67 Long-term (current) use of insulin, should also be assigned if the diabetes mellitus is being treated with insulin.

g. Gestational diabetes—Gestational diabetes can occur during the second and third trimester of pregnancy in women who were not diabetic prior to pregnancy. Gestational diabetes can cause complications in the pregnancy similar to those of pre-existing diabetes mellitus. It also puts the woman at greater risk of developing diabetes after the pregnancy. Gestational diabetes is coded to 648.8x Abnormal glucose tolerance. Codes 648.0x and 648.8x should never be used together on the same record.

Code V58.67 Long-term (current) use of insulin, should also be assigned if the gestational diabetes is being treated with insulin.

h. Normal delivery, code 650

1) **Normal delivery**—Code 650 is for use in cases when a woman is admitted for a full-term normal delivery and delivers a single, healthy infant without any complications antepartum, during the delivery, or postpartum during the delivery episode. **Code 650 is always a principal diagnosis. It is not to be used if any other code from chapter 11 is needed to describe a current complication of the antenatal, delivery, or perinatal period. Additional codes from other chapters may be used with code 650 if they are not related to or are in any way complicating the pregnancy.**

2) **Normal delivery with resolved antepartum complication**—Code 650 may be used if the patient had a complication at some point during her pregnancy, but the complication is not present at the time of the admission for delivery.

3) **V27.0 Single liveborn, outcome of delivery**—V27.0 Single liveborn, is the only outcome of the delivery code appropriate for use with 650.

i. The postpartum and peripartum periods

1) **Postpartum and peripartum periods**—The postpartum period begins immediately after delivery and continues for six weeks following delivery. The peripartum period is defined as the last month of pregnancy to five months postpartum.

2) **Postpartum complication**—A postpartum complication is any complication occurring within the six-week period.

3) **Pregnancy-related complications after six-week period**—Chapter 11 codes may also be used to describe pregnancy-related complications after the six-week period should the provider document that a condition is pregnancy related.

4) **Postpartum complications occurring during the same admission as delivery**—Postpartum complications that occur during the same admission as the delivery are identified with a fifth digit of 2. Subsequent admissions/encounters for postpartum complications should be identified with a fifth digit of 4.

5) **Admission for routine postpartum care following delivery outside hospital**—When the mother delivers outside the hospital prior to admission and is admitted for routine postpartum care and no complications are noted, code V24.0 Postpartum care and examination immediately after delivery, should be assigned as the principal diagnosis.

6) **Admission following delivery outside hospital with postpartum conditions**—A delivery diagnosis code should not be used for a woman who has delivered prior to admission to the hospital. Any postpartum conditions and/or postpartum procedures should be coded.

j. Code 677 Late effect of complication of pregnancy

1) **Code 677**—Code 677 Late effect of complication of pregnancy, childbirth, and the puerperium is for use in those cases when an initial complication of a pregnancy develops a sequelae requiring care or treatment at a future date.

2) **After the initial postpartum period**—This code may be used at any time after the initial postpartum period.

3) **Sequencing of code 677**—This code, like all late effect codes, is to be sequenced following the code describing the sequelae of the complication.

k. Abortions

1) **Fifth digits required for abortion categories**—Fifth digits are required for abortion categories 634-637. Fifth-digit 1, incomplete, indicates that all of the products of conception have not been expelled from the uterus. Fifth-digit 2, complete, indicates that all

products of conception have been expelled from the uterus prior to the episode of care.

2) **Code from categories 640-648 and 651-659**—A code from categories 640-648 and 651-659 may be used as additional codes with an abortion code to indicate the complication leading to the abortion.

Fifth-digit 3 is assigned with codes from these categories when used with an abortion code because the other fifth digits will not apply. Codes from the 660-669 series are not to be used for complications of abortion.

3) **Code 639 for complications**—Code 639 is to be used for all complications following abortion. Code 639 cannot be assigned with codes from categories 634-638.

4) **Abortion with liveborn fetus**—When an attempted termination of pregnancy results in a liveborn fetus assign code 644.21 Early onset of delivery, with an appropriate code from category V27 Outcome of delivery. The procedure code for the attempted termination of pregnancy should also be assigned.

5) **Retained products of conception following an abortion**—Subsequent admissions for retained products of conception following a spontaneous or legally induced abortion are assigned the appropriate code from category 634 Spontaneous abortion, or 635 Legally induced abortion, with a fifth digit of 1 (incomplete). This advice is appropriate even when the patient was discharged previously with a discharge diagnosis of complete abortion.

12. Chapter 12: Diseases of Skin and Subcutaneous Tissue (680-709)

Reserved for future guideline expansion

13. Chapter 13: Diseases of Musculoskeletal and Connective Tissue (710-739)

Reserved for future guideline expansion

14. Chapter 14: Congenital Anomalies (740-759)

a. **Codes in categories 740-759 Congenital anomalies—Assign an appropriate code(s) from categories 740-759, Congenital anomalies, when an anomaly is documented. A congenital anomaly may be the principal/first-listed diagnosis on a record or a secondary diagnosis. Use additional secondary codes from other chapters to specify conditions associated with the anomaly, if applicable. Codes from chapter 14 may be used throughout the life of the patient. If a congenital anomaly has been corrected, a personal history code should be used to identify the history of the anomaly.**

For the birth admission, the appropriate code from category V30 Liveborn infants, according to type of birth should be sequenced as the principal diagnosis, followed by any congenital anomaly codes, 740-759.

15. Chapter 15: Newborn (Perinatal) Guidelines (760-779)

For coding and reporting purposes the perinatal period is defined as birth through the 28th day following birth. The following guidelines are provided for reporting purposes. Hospitals may record other diagnoses as needed for internal data use.

a. **General perinatal rules**

1) **Chapter 15 codes—They are never for use on the maternal record. Codes from chapter 11, the obstetric chapter, are never permitted on the newborn record. Chapter 15 code may be used throughout the life of the patient if the condition is still present.**

2) **Sequencing of perinatal codes—Generally, codes from chapter 15 should be sequenced as the principal/first-listed diagnosis on the newborn record, with the exception of the appropriate V30 code for the birth episode, followed by codes from any other chapter that provide additional detail. The "use additional code" note at the beginning of the chapter supports this guideline. If the index does not provide a specific code for a perinatal condition, assign code 779.89 Other specified conditions originating in the perinatal period, followed by the code from another chapter that specifies the condition. Codes for signs and symptoms may be assigned when a definitive diagnosis has not been established.**

3) **Birth process or community acquired conditions—If a newborn has a condition that may be either due to the birth process or community acquired and the documentation does not indicate which it is, the default is due to the birth process and the code from chapter 15 should be used. If the condition is community acquired, a code from chapter 15 should not be assigned.**

4) **Code all clinically significant conditions**—All clinically significant conditions noted on routine newborn examination should be coded. A condition is clinically significant if it requires:

- Clinical evaluation; or
- Therapeutic treatment; or
- Diagnostic procedures; or
- Extended length of hospital stay; or
- Increased nursing care and/or monitoring; or
- Has implications for future health care needs

Note: The perinatal guidelines listed above are the same as the general coding guidelines for "additional diagnoses," except for the final point regarding implications for future health care needs. **Codes should be assigned for conditions that have been specified by the provider as having implications for future health care needs. Codes from the perinatal chapter should not be assigned unless the provider has established a definitive diagnosis.**

b. **Use of codes V30-V39**—When coding the birth of an infant, assign a code from categories V30-V39, according to the type of birth. A code from this series is assigned as a principal diagnosis and assigned only once to a newborn at the time of birth.

c. **Newborn transfers**—If the newborn is transferred to another institution, the V30 series is not used at the receiving hospital.

d. **Use of category V29**

1) **Assigning a code from category V29**—Assign a code from category V29 Observation and evaluation of newborns and infants for suspected conditions not found, to identify those instances when a healthy newborn is evaluated for a suspected condition that is determined after study not to be present. Do not use a code from category V29 when the patient has identified signs or symptoms of a suspected problem; in such cases, code the sign or symptom.

A code from category V29 may also be assigned as a principal diagnosis for readmissions or encounters when the V30 code no longer applies. Codes from category V29 are for use only for healthy newborns and infants for which no condition after study is found to be present.

2) **V29 code on a birth record**—A V29 code is to be used as a secondary code after the V30 Outcome of delivery, code.

e. **Use of other V codes on perinatal records—V codes other than V30 and V29 may be assigned on a perinatal or newborn record code. The codes may be used as a principal or first-listed diagnosis for specific types of encounters or for readmissions or encounters when the V30 code no longer applies.**

See section I.C.18 for information regarding the assignment of V codes.

f. **Maternal causes of perinatal morbidity**—Codes from categories 760-763 Maternal causes of perinatal morbidity and mortality, are assigned only when the maternal condition has actually affected the fetus or newborn. The fact that the mother has an associated medical condition or experiences some complication of pregnancy, labor, or delivery does not justify the routine assignment of codes from these categories to the newborn record.

g. **Congenital anomalies in newborns**—For the birth admission, the appropriate code from category V30 Liveborn infants according to type of birth, should be used, followed by any congenital anomaly codes, categories 740-759. **Use additional secondary codes from other chapters to specify conditions associated with the anomaly, if applicable.**

Also, see section I.C.14 for information on the coding of congenital anomalies.

h. **Coding additional perinatal diagnoses**

1) **Assigning codes for conditions that require treatment**—Assign codes for conditions that require treatment or further investigation, prolong the length of stay, or require resource utilization.

2) **Codes for conditions specified as having implications for future health care needs**—Assign codes for conditions that have been specified by the provider as having implications for future health care needs.

Note: This guideline should not be used for adult patients.

3) **Codes for newborn conditions originating in the perinatal period**—Assign a code for newborn conditions originating in the perinatal period (categories 760-779), as well as complications arising during the current episode of care classified in other chapters, only if the diagnoses have been documented by the responsible provider at the time of transfer or discharge as having affected the fetus or newborn.

i. **Prematurity and fetal growth retardation**—Providers utilize different criteria in determining prematurity. A code for prematurity should not be assigned unless it is documented. The fift-digit assignment for codes from category 764 and subcategories 765.0 and 765.1 should be based on the recorded birth weight and estimated gestational age.

A code from subcategory 765.2 Weeks of gestation, should be assigned as an additional code with category 764 and codes from 765.0 and 765.1 to specify weeks of gestation as documented by the provider in the record.

j. **Newborn sepsis—Code 771.81 Septicemia [sepsis] of newborn, should be assigned with a secondary code from category 041 Bacterial infections in conditions classified elsewhere and of unspecified site, to identify the organism. It is not necessary to use a code from subcategory 995.9 Systemic inflammatory response syndrome (SIRS), on a newborn record. A code from category 038 Septicemia, should not be used on a newborn record. Code 771.81 describes the sepsis.**

16. Chapter 16: Signs, Symptoms and Ill-Defined Conditions (780-799)

Reserved for future guideline expansion

17. Chapter 17: Injury and Poisoning (800-999)

a. **Coding of injuries**—When coding injuries, assign separate codes for each injury unless a combination code is provided, in which case the combination code is assigned. Multiple injury codes are provided in ICD-9-CM but should not be assigned unless information for a more specific code is not available. These codes are not to be used for normal, healing surgical wounds or to identify complications of surgical wounds.

The code for the most serious injury, as determined by the provider and the focus of treatment, is sequenced first.

1) **Superficial injuries**—Superficial injuries such as abrasions or contusions are not coded when associated with more severe injuries of the same site.

2) **Primary injury with damage to nerves/blood vessels**—When a primary injury results in minor damage to peripheral nerves or blood vessels, the primary injury is sequenced first with additional code(s) from categories 950-957 Injury to nerves and spinal cord, and/or 900-904 Injury to blood vessels. When the primary injury is to the blood vessels or nerves, that injury should be sequenced first.

b. **Coding of fractures**—The principles of multiple coding of injuries should be followed in coding fractures. Fractures of specified sites are coded individually by site in accordance with both the provisions within categories 800-829 and the level of detail furnished by medical record content. Combination categories for multiple fractures are provided for use when there is insufficient detail in the medical record (such as trauma cases transferred to another hospital), when the reporting form limits the number of codes that can be used in reporting pertinent clinical data, or when there is insufficient specificity at the fourth-digit or fifth-digit level. More specific guidelines are as follows:

1) **Multiple fractures of same limb**—Multiple fractures of same limb classifiable to the same three-digit or four-digit category are coded to that category.

2) **Multiple unilateral or bilateral fractures of same bone**—Multiple unilateral or bilateral fractures of same bone(s) but classified to different fourth-digit subdivisions (bone part) within the same three-digit category are coded individually by site.

3) **Multiple fracture categories 819 and 828**—Multiple fracture categories 819 and 828 classify bilateral fractures of both upper limbs (819) and both lower limbs (828), but without any detail at the fourth-digit level other than open and closed type of fractures.

4) **Multiple fractures sequencing**—Multiple fractures are sequenced in accordance with the severity of the fracture. The provider should be asked to list the fracture diagnoses in the order of severity.

c. **Coding of burns**—Current burns (940-948) are classified by depth, extent, and by agent (E code). Burns are classified by depth as first degree (erythema), second degree (blistering), and third degree (full-thickness involvement).

1) **Sequencing of burn codes**—Sequence first the code that reflects the highest degree of burn when more than one burn is present.

2) **Burns of the same local site**—Classify burns of the same local site (three-digit category level, 940-947) but of different degrees to the subcategory identifying the highest degree recorded in the diagnosis.

3) **Non-healing burns**—Non-healing burns are coded as acute burns. Necrosis of burned skin should be coded as a non-healed burn.

4) **Code 958.3 Posttraumatic wound infection**—Assign code 958.3 Posttraumatic wound infection, not elsewhere classified, as an additional code for any documented infected burn site.

5) **Assign separate codes for each burn site**—When coding burns, assign separate codes for each burn site. Category 946 Burns of multiple specified sites, should only be used if the locations of the burns are not documented. Category 949 Burn, unspecified, is extremely vague and should rarely be used.

6) **Burns classified according to extent of body surface involved**—Assign codes from category 948 Burns, when the site of the burn is not specified or when there is a need for additional data. It is advisable to use category 948 as additional coding when needed to provide data for evaluating burn mortality, such as that needed by burn units. It is also advisable to use category 948 as an additional code for reporting purposes when there is mention of a third-degree burn involving 20 percent or more of the body surface.

In assigning a code from category 948:

- Fourth-digit codes are used to identify the percentage of total body surface involved in a burn (all degree).
- Fifth digits are assigned to identify the percentage of body surface involved in third-degree burn.
- Fifth-digit zero (0) is assigned when less than 10 percent or when no body surface is involved in a third-degree burn.
- Category 948 is based on the classic "rule of nines" in estimating body surface involved: head and neck are assigned 9 percent, each arm 9 percent, each leg 18 percent, the anterior trunk 18 percent, posterior trunk 18 percent, and genitalia 1 percent. Providers may change these percentage assignments where necessary to accommodate infants and children who have proportionately larger heads than adults and patients who have large buttocks, thighs, or abdomen that involve burns.

7) **Encounters for treatment of late effects of burns**—Encounters for the treatment of the late effects of burns (i.e., scars or joint contractures) should be coded to the residual condition (sequelae) followed by the appropriate late effect code (906.5-906.9). A late effect E code may also be used, if desired.

8) **Sequelae with a late effect code and current burn**—When appropriate, both a sequelae with a late effect code, and a current burn code may be assigned on the same record **(when both a current burn and sequelae of an old burn exist).**

d. **Coding of debridement of wound, infection, or burn**—Excisional debridement involves an excisional debridement (surgical removal or cutting away), as opposed to a mechanical (brushing, scrubbing, washing) debridement.

For coding purposes, excisional debridement **is assigned to code** 86.22.

Nonexcisional debridement is assigned to **code** 86.28.

e. **Adverse effects, poisoning and toxic effects**—The properties of certain drugs, medicinal and biological substances, or combinations of such substances, may cause toxic reactions. The occurrence of drug toxicity is classified in ICD-9-CM as follows:

1) **Adverse effect**—When the drug was correctly prescribed and properly administered, code the reaction plus the appropriate code from the E930-E949 series. Codes from the E930-E949 series must be used to identify the causative substance for an adverse effect of drug, medicinal and biological substances, correctly prescribed and properly administered. The effect, such as tachycardia, delirium, gastrointestinal hemorrhaging, vomiting, hypokalemia, hepatitis, renal failure, or respiratory failure, is coded and followed by the appropriate code from the E930-E949 series.

Adverse effects of therapeutic substances correctly prescribed and properly administered (toxicity, synergistic reaction, side effect, and idiosyncratic reaction) may be due to (1) differences among patients, such as age, sex, disease, and genetic factors, and (2) drug-related factors, such as type of drug, route of administration, duration of therapy, dosage, and bioavailability.

2) Poisoning

(a) Error was made in drug prescription—Errors made in drug prescription or in the administration of the drug by provider, nurse, patient, or other person, use the appropriate poisoning code from the 960-979 series.

(b) Overdose of a drug intentionally taken—If an overdose of a drug was intentionally taken or administered and resulted in drug toxicity, it would be coded as a poisoning (960-979 series).

(c) Nonprescribed drug taken with correctly prescribed and properly administered drug—If a nonprescribed drug or medicinal agent was taken in combination with a correctly prescribed and properly administered drug, any drug toxicity or other reaction resulting from the interaction of the two drugs would be classified as a poisoning.

(d) Sequencing of poisoning—When coding a poisoning or reaction to the improper use of a medication (e.g., wrong dose, wrong substance, wrong route of administration) the poisoning code is sequenced first, followed by a code for the manifestation. If there is also a diagnosis of drug abuse or dependence to the substance, the abuse or dependence is coded as an additional code.

See section I.C.3.a.6.b. if poisoning is the result of insulin pump malfunctions and section I.C.19 for general use of E codes.

3) Toxic effects

(a) Toxic effect codes—When a harmful substance is ingested or comes in contact with a person, this is classified as a toxic effect. The toxic effect codes are in categories 980-989.

(b) Sequencing toxic effect codes—A toxic effect code should be sequenced first, followed by the codes that identify the result of the toxic effect.

(c) External cause codes for toxic effects—An external cause code from categories E860-E869 for accidental exposure, code E950.6 or E950.7 for intentional self-harm, category E962 for assault, or categories E980-E982 for undetermined, should also be assigned to indicate intent.

18. Classification of Factors Influencing Health Status and Contact with Health Service (Supplemental V01-V85)

Note: The chapter-specific guidelines provide additional information about the use of V codes for specified encounters.

a. Introduction—ICD-9-CM provides codes to deal with encounters for circumstances other than a disease or injury. The Supplementary Classification of Factors Influencing Health Status and Contact with Health Services (V01-V85) is provided to deal with occasions when circumstances other than a disease or injury (codes 001-999) are recorded as a diagnosis or problem.

There are four primary circumstances for the use of V codes:

1) A person who is not currently sick encounters the health services for some specific reason, such as to act as an organ donor, to receive prophylactic care, such as inoculations or health screenings, or to receive counseling on health related issues.

2) A person with a resolving disease or injury, or a chronic, long-term condition requiring continuous care, encounters the health care system for specific aftercare of that disease or injury (e.g., dialysis for renal disease; chemotherapy for malignancy; cast change). A diagnosis/symptom code should be used whenever a current, acute diagnosis is being treated or a sign or symptom is being studied.

3) Circumstances or problems influence a person's health status but are not in themselves a current illness or injury.

4) Newborns, to indicate birth status

b. V codes use in any health care setting—V codes are for use in any healthcare setting. V codes may be used as either a first-listed (principal diagnosis code in the inpatient setting) or secondary code, depending on the circumstances of the encounter. Certain V codes may only be used as first listed, others only as secondary codes. See section I.C.18.e, V code table.

c. V codes indicate a reason for an encounter—They are not procedure codes. A corresponding procedure code must accompany a V code to describe the procedure performed.

d. Categories of V codes

1) Contact/exposure—Category V01 indicates contact with or exposure to communicable diseases. These codes are for patients who do not show any sign or symptom of a disease but have been exposed to it by close personal contact with an infected individual or are in an area where a disease is epidemic. These codes may be used as a first-listed code to explain an encounter for testing, or, more commonly, as a secondary code to identify a potential risk.

2) Inoculations and vaccinations—Categories V03-V06 are for encounters for inoculations and vaccinations. They indicate that a patient is being seen to receive a prophylactic inoculation against a disease. The injection itself must be represented by the appropriate procedure code. A code from V03-V06 may be used as a secondary code if the inoculation is given as a routine part of preventive health care, such as a well-baby visit.

3) Status—Status codes indicate that a patient is either a carrier of a disease or has the sequelae or residual of a past disease or condition. This includes such things as the presence of prosthetic or mechanical devices resulting from past treatment.

A status code is informative, because the status may affect the course of treatment and its outcome. A status code is distinct from a history code. The history code indicates that the patient no longer has the condition.

A status code should not be used with a diagnosis code from one of the body system chapters, if the diagnosis code includes the information provided by the status code. For example, code V42.1 Heart transplant status, should not be used with code 996.83 Complications of transplanted heart. The status code does not provide additional information. The complication code indicates that the patient is a heart transplant patient.

The status V codes/categories are:

V02 Carrier or suspected carrier of infectious diseases—Carrier status indicates that a person harbors the specific organisms of a disease without manifest symptoms and is capable of transmitting the infection.

V08 Asymptomatic HIV infection status—This code indicates that a patient has tested positive for HIV but has manifested no signs or symptoms of the disease.

V09 Infection with drug-resistant microorganisms—This category indicates that a patient has an infection that is resistant to drug treatment. Sequence the infection code first.

V21 Constitutional states in development

V22.2 Pregnant state, incidental—This code is a secondary code only for use when the pregnancy is in no way complicating the reason for visit. Otherwise, a code from the obstetric chapter is required.

V26.5x Sterilization status

V42 Organ or tissue replaced by transplant

V43 Organ or tissue replaced by other means

V44 Artificial opening status

V45 Other postsurgical states

V46 Other dependence on machines

V49.6 Upper limb amputation status

V49.7 Lower limb amputation status

V49.81 Postmenopausal status

V49.82 Dental sealant status

V49.83 Awaiting organ transplant status

V58.6 Long-term (current) drug use—This subcategory indicates a patient's continuous use of a prescribed drug (including such things as aspirin therapy) for the long-term treatment of a condition or for prophylactic use. It is not for use for patients who have addictions to drugs.

V83 Genetic carrier status—**Genetic carrier status indicates that a person carries a gene, associated with a particular disease, which may be passed to offspring who may develop that disease. The person does not have the disease and is not at risk of developing the disease.**

V84 Genetic susceptibility status—Genetic susceptibility indicates that a person has a gene that increases the risk of that person developing the disease.

Note: Categories V42-V46, and subcategories V49.6, V49.7 are for use only if there are no complications or malfunctions of the organ or tissue replaced, the amputation site, or the equipment on which the patient is dependent. These are always secondary codes.

4) **History (of)**—There are two types of history V codes, personal and family. Personal history codes explain a patient's past medical condition that no longer exists and is not receiving any treatment but that has the potential for recurrence, and therefore may require continued monitoring. The exceptions to this general rule are category V14 Personal history of allergy to medicinal agents, and subcategory V15.0 Allergy, other than to medicinal agents. A person who has had an allergic episode to a substance or food in the past should always be considered allergic to the substance.

Family history codes are for use when a patient has a family member(s) who has had a particular disease that causes the patient to be at higher risk of also contracting the disease.

Personal history codes may be used in conjunction with follow-up codes and family history codes may be used in conjunction with screening codes to explain the need for a test or procedure. History codes are also acceptable on any medical record regardless of the reason for visit. A history of an illness, even if no longer present, is important information that may alter the type of treatment ordered.

The history V code categories are:

V10 Personal history of malignant neoplasm
V12 Personal history of certain other diseases
V13 Personal history of other diseases
Except: V13.4 Personal history of arthritis, and V13.6 Personal history of congenital malformations. These conditions are life-long so are not true history codes.
V14 Personal history of allergy to medicinal agents
V15 Other personal history presenting hazards to health
Except: V15.7 Personal history of contraception
V16 Family history of malignant neoplasm
V17 Family history of certain chronic disabling diseases
V18 Family history of certain other specific diseases
V19 Family history of other conditions

5) **Screening**—Screening is the testing for disease or disease precursors in seemingly well individuals so that early detection and treatment can be provided for those who test positive for the disease. Screenings that are recommended for many subgroups in a population include routine mammograms for women over 40, a fecal occult blood test for everyone over 50, an amniocentesis to rule out a fetal anomaly for pregnant women over 35, because the incidence of breast cancer and colon cancer in these subgroups is higher than in the general population, as is the incidence of Down's syndrome in older mothers.

The testing of a person to rule out or confirm a suspected diagnosis because the patient has some sign or symptom is a diagnostic examination, not a screening. In these cases, the sign or symptom is used to explain the reason for the test.

A screening code may be a first-listed code if the reason for the visit is specifically the screening exam. It may also be used as an additional code if the screening is done during an office visit for other health problems. A screening code is not necessary if the screening is inherent to a routine examination, such as a Pap smear done during a routine pelvic examination.

Should a condition be discovered during the screening then the code for the condition may be assigned as an additional diagnosis.

The V code indicates that a screening exam is planned. A procedure code is required to confirm that the screening was performed.

The screening V code categories:

V28 Antenatal screening
V73-V82 Special screening examinations

6) **Observation**—There are two observation V code categories. They are for use in very limited circumstances when a person is being observed for a suspected condition that is ruled out. The observation codes are not for use if an injury or illness or any signs or symptoms related to the suspected condition are present. In such cases the diagnosis/symptom code is used with the corresponding E code to identify any external cause.

The observation codes are to be used as principal diagnosis only. The only exception to this is when the principal diagnosis is required to be a code from the V30 Live born infant, category. Then the V29 observation code is sequenced after the V30 code. Additional codes may be used in addition to the observation code but only if they are unrelated to the suspected condition being observed.

The observation V code categories:

V29 Observation and evaluation of newborns for suspected condition not found
For the birth encounter, a code from category V30 should be sequenced before the V29 code.
V71 Observation and evaluation for suspected condition not found

7) **Aftercare**—Aftercare visit codes cover situations when the initial treatment of a disease or injury has been performed and the patient requires continued care during the healing or recovery phase, or for the long-term consequences of the disease. The aftercare V code should not be used if treatment is directed at a current, acute disease or injury, the diagnosis code is to be used in these cases. Exceptions to this rule are codes V58.0 Radiotherapy, and V58.1 Chemotherapy. These codes are to be first listed, followed by the diagnosis code when a patient's encounter is solely to receive radiation therapy or chemotherapy for the treatment of a neoplasm. Should a patient receive both chemotherapy and radiation therapy during the same encounter, codes V58.0 and V58.1 may be used together on a record with either one being sequenced first.

The aftercare codes are generally first listed to explain the specific reason for the encounter. An aftercare code may be used as an additional code when some type of aftercare is provided in addition to the reason for admission and no diagnosis code is applicable. An example of this would be the closure of a colostomy during an encounter for treatment of another condition.

Certain aftercare V code categories need a secondary diagnosis code to describe the resolving condition or sequelae, for others, the condition is inherent in the code title.

Additional V code aftercare category terms include fitting and adjustment, and attention to artificial openings.

Status V codes may be used with aftercare V codes to indicate the nature of the aftercare. For example code V45.81 Aortocoronary bypass status, may be used with code V58.73 Aftercare following surgery of the circulatory system, NEC, to indicate the surgery for which the aftercare is being performed. Also, a transplant status code may be used following code V58.44 Aftercare following organ transplant, to identify the organ transplanted. A status code should not be used when the aftercare code indicates the type of status, such as using V55.0 Attention to tracheostomy with V44.0 Tracheostomy status.

The aftercare V category/codes:

V52 Fitting and adjustment of prosthetic device and implant
V53 Fitting and adjustment of other device
V54 Other orthopedic aftercare
V55 Attention to artificial openings
V56 Encounter for dialysis and dialysis catheter care
V57 Care involving the use of rehabilitation procedures
V58.0 Radiotherapy
V58.1 Chemotherapy
V58.3 Attention to surgical dressings and sutures
V58.41 Encounter for planned post-operative wound closure
V58.42 Aftercare, surgery, neoplasm
V58.43 Aftercare, surgery, trauma
V58.44 Aftercare involving organ transplant
V58.49 Other specified aftercare following surgery
V58.7x Aftercare following surgery
V58.81 Fitting and adjustment of vascular catheter
V58.82 Fitting and adjustment of non-vascular catheter
V58.83 Monitoring therapeutic drug
V58.89 Other specified aftercare

8) **Follow-up**—The follow-up codes are used to explain continuing surveillance following completed treatment of a disease, condition, or injury. They imply that the condition has been fully treated and no longer exists. They should not be confused with aftercare codes that explain current treatment for a healing condition or its sequelae. Follow-up codes may be used in conjunction with history codes to provide the full picture of the healed condition and its treatment. The follow-up code is sequenced first, followed by the history code.

A follow-up code may be used to explain repeated visits. Should a condition be found to have recurred on the follow-up visit, then the diagnosis code should be used in place of the follow-up code.

The follow-up V code categories:

V24 Postpartum care and evaluation

V67 Follow-up examination

9) **Donor**—Category V59 is the donor codes. They are used for living individuals who are donating blood or other body tissue. These codes are only for individuals donating for others, not for self-donations. They are not for use to identify cadaveric donations.

10) **Counseling**—Counseling V codes are used when a patient or family member receives assistance in the aftermath of an illness or injury, or when support is required in coping with family or social problems. They are not necessary for use in conjunction with a diagnosis code when the counseling component of care is considered integral to standard treatment.

The counseling V categories/codes:

V25.0 General counseling and advice for contraceptive management

V26.3 Genetic counseling

V26.4 General counseling and advice for procreative management

V61 Other family circumstances

V65.1 Person consulted on behalf of another person

V65.3 Dietary surveillance and counseling

V65.4 Other counseling, not elsewhere classified

11) **Obstetrics and related conditions**—See section I.C.11., the obstetrics guidelines for further instruction on the use of these codes.

V codes for pregnancy are for use in those circumstances when none of the problems or complications included in the codes from the obstetrics chapter exist (a routine prenatal visit or postpartum care). Codes V22.0 Supervision of normal first pregnancy, and V22.1 Supervision of other normal pregnancy, are always first listed and are not to be used with any other code from the OB chapter.

The outcome of delivery, category V27, should be included on all maternal delivery records. It is always a secondary code.

V codes for family planning (contraceptive) or procreative management and counseling should be included on an obstetric record either during the pregnancy or the postpartum stage, if applicable.

Obstetrics and related conditions V code categories:

V22 Normal pregnancy

V23 Supervision of high-risk pregnancy
Except: V23.2 Pregnancy with history of abortion. Code 646.3 Habitual aborter, from the OB chapter is required to indicate a history of abortion during a pregnancy.

V24 Postpartum care and evaluation

V25 Encounter for contraceptive management
Except V25.0x (See section I.C.18.d.11, Counseling)

V26 Procreative management
Except V26.5x Sterilization status, V26.3 and V26.4 (See section I.C.18.d.11., Counseling)

V27 Outcome of delivery

V28 Antenatal screening (See section I.C.18.d.6., Screening)

12) **Newborn, infant and child**—See section I.C.15, the newborn guidelines, for further instruction on the use of these codes.

Newborn V code categories:

V20 Health supervision of infant or child

V29 Observation and evaluation of newborns for suspected condition not found (See section I.C.18.d.7, Observation).

V30-V39 Liveborn infant according to type of birth

13) **Routine and administrative examinations**—The V codes allow for the description of encounters for routine examinations, such as a general check-up or, examinations for administrative purposes, such as a pre-employment physical. The codes are for use as first-listed codes only, and are not to be used if the examination is for diagnosis of a suspected condition or for treatment purposes. In such cases the diagnosis code is used. During a routine exam, should a diagnosis or condition be discovered, it should be coded as an additional code. Pre-existing and chronic conditions and history codes may also be included as additional codes as long as the examination is for administrative purposes and not focused on any particular condition.

Preoperative examination V codes are for use only in those situations when a patient is being cleared for surgery and no treatment is given.

The V code categories/code for routine and administrative examinations:

V20.2 Routine infant or child health check Any injections given should have a corresponding procedure code.

V70 General medical examination

V72 Special investigations and examinations
Except V72.5 and V72.6

14) **Miscellaneous V codes**—The miscellaneous V codes capture a number of other health care encounters that do not fall into one of the other categories.

Certain of these codes identify the reason for the encounter, others are for use as additional codes that provide useful information on circumstances that may affect a patient's care and treatment.

Miscellaneous V code categories/codes:

V07 Need for isolation and other prophylactic measures

V50 Elective surgery for purposes other than remedying health states

V58.5 Orthodontics

V60 Housing, household, and economic circumstances

V62 Other psychosocial circumstances

V63 Unavailability of other medical facilities for care

V64 Persons encountering health services for specific procedures, not carried out

V66 Convalescence and palliative care

V68 Encounters for administrative purposes

V69 Problems related to lifestyle

15) **Nonspecific V codes**—Certain V codes are so nonspecific, or potentially redundant with other codes in the classification, that there can be little justification for their use in the inpatient setting. Their use in the outpatient setting should be limited to those instances when there is no further documentation to permit more precise coding. Otherwise, any sign or symptom or any other reason for a visit that is captured in another code should be used.

Nonspecific V code categories/codes:

V11 Personal history of mental disorder—A code from the mental disorders chapter, with an in remission fifth digit, should be used.

V13.4 Personal history of arthritis

V13.6 Personal history of congenital malformations

V15.7 Personal history of contraception

V23.2 Pregnancy with history of abortion

V40 Mental and behavioral problems

V41 Problems with special senses and other special functions

V47 Other problems with internal organs

V48 Problems with head, neck, and trunk

V49 Problems with limbs and other problems

Exceptions:

V49.6 Upper limb amputation status

V49.7 Lower limb amputation status

V49.81 Postmenopausal status

V49.82 Dental sealant status

V49.83 Awaiting organ transplant status

V51 Aftercare involving the use of plastic surgery

V58.2 Blood transfusion, without reported diagnosis

V58.9 Unspecified aftercare

V72.5 Radiological examination, NEC

V72.6 Laboratory examination
Codes V72.5 and V72.6 are not to be used if any sign or symptoms, or reason for a test is documented. See section IV.K. and section IV.L. of the outpatient guidelines.

V Code Table

Items in bold indicate a change from the October 2003 table. Items underlined have been moved within the table since October 2003.

FIRST LISTED: V codes/categories/subcategories which are only acceptable as principal/first listed.

Codes:

V22.0 Supervision of normal first pregnancy
V22.1 Supervision of other normal pregnancy
V46.12 Encounter for respirator dependence during power failure
V56.0 Extracorporeal dialysis
V58.0 Radiotherapy
V58.1 Chemotherapy
V58.0 and V58.1 may be used together on a record with either one being sequenced first, when a patient receives both chemotherapy and radiation therapy during the same encounter.

Categories/Subcategories:

V20 Health supervision of infant or child
V24 Postpartum care and examination
V29 Observation and evaluation of newborns for suspected condition not found
Exception: A code from the V30-V39 may be sequenced before the V29 if it is the newborn record.
V30-V39 Liveborn infants according to type of birth
V59 Donors
V66 Convalescence and palliative care
Exception: V66.7 Palliative care
V68 Encounters for administrative purposes
V70 General medical examination
Exception: V70.7 Examination of participant in clinical trial
V71 Observation and evaluation for suspected conditions not found
V72 Special investigations and examinations
Exceptions:
V72.5 Radiological examination, NEC
V72.6 Laboratory examination

FIRST OR ADDITIONAL: V code categories/subcategories which may be either principal/first-listed, or additional codes.

Codes:

V43.22 Fully implantable artificial heart status
V49.81 Asymptomatic postmenopausal status (age-related) (natural)
V70.7 Examination of participant in clinical trial

Categories/Subcategories:

V01 Contact with or exposure to communicable diseases
V02 Carrier or suspected carrier of infectious diseases
V03-V06 Need for prophylactic vaccination and inoculations
V07 Need for isolation and other prophylactic measures
V08 Asymptomatic HIV infection status
V10 Personal history of malignant neoplasm
V12 Personal history of certain other diseases
V13 Personal history of other diseases
Exception:
V13.4 Personal history of arthritis
V13.69 Personal history of other congenital malformations
V16-V19 Family history of disease
V23 Supervision of high-risk pregnancy
V25 Encounter for contraceptive management
V26 Procreative management
Exception: V26.5 Sterilization status
V28 Antenatal screening
V45.7 Acquired absence of organ
V50 Elective surgery for purposes other than remedying health states
V52 Fitting and adjustment of prosthetic device and implant
V53 Fitting and adjustment of other device
V54 Other orthopedic aftercare
V55 Attention to artificial openings
V56 Encounter for dialysis and dialysis catheter care
Exception: V56.0 Extracorporeal dialysis
V57 Care involving use of rehabilitation procedures
V58.3 Attention to surgical dressings and sutures
V58.4 Other aftercare following surgery
V58.6 Long-term (current) drug use
V58.7 Aftercare following surgery to specified body systems, not elsewhere classified
V58.8 Other specified procedures and aftercare
V61 Other family circumstances
V63 Unavailability of other medical facilities for care
V65 Other persons seeking consultation without complaint or sickness
V67 Follow-up examination
V69 Problems related to lifestyle
V73-V82 Special screening examinations
V83 Genetic carrier status

ADDITIONAL ONLY: V code categories/subcategories which may only be used as additional codes, not principal/first listed.

Codes:

V13.61 Personal history of hypospadias
V22.2 Pregnancy state, incidental
V49.82 Dental sealant status
V49.83 Awaiting organ transplant status
V66.7 Palliative care
V85 Body mass index

Categories/Subcategories:

V09 Infection with drug-resistant microorganisms
V14 Personal history of allergy to medicinal agents
V15 Other personal history presenting hazards to health
Exception: V15.7 Personal history of contraception
V21 Constitutional states in development
V26.5 Sterilization status
V27 Outcome of delivery
V42 Organ or tissue replaced by transplant
V43 Organ or tissue replaced by other means
Exception: V43.22 Fully implantable artificial heart status
V44 Artificial opening status
V45 Other postsurgical states
Exception: Subcategory V45.7 Acquired absence of organ
V46 Other dependence on machines
Exception: V46.12 Encounter for respirator dependence during power failure
V49.6x Upper limb amputation status
V49.7x Lower limb amputation status
V60 Housing, household, and economic circumstances
V62 Other psychosocial circumstances
V64 Persons encountering health services for specified procedure, not carried out
V84 Genetic susceptibility to disease

NONSPECIFIC CODES AND CATEGORIES:

V11 Personal history of mental disorder
V13.4 Personal history of arthritis
V13.69 Personal history of congenital malformations
V15.7 Personal history of contraception
V40 Mental and behavioral problems
V41 Problems with special senses and other special functions
V47 Other problems with internal organs
V48 Problems with head, neck, and trunk
V49 Problems with limbs and other problems
Exceptions:
V49.6 Upper limb amputation status
V49.7 Lower limb amputation status
V49.81 Postmenopausal status (age-related) (natural)
V49.82 Dental sealant status
V49.83 Awaiting organ transplant status
V51 Aftercare involving the use of plastic surgery
V58.2 Blood transfusion, without reported diagnosis
V58.5 Orthodontics
V58.9 Unspecified aftercare
V72.5 Radiological examination, NEC
V72.6 Laboratory examination

19. Supplemental Classification of External Causes of Injury and Poisoning (E-codes, E800-E999)

Introduction: These guidelines are provided for those who are currently collecting E codes in order that there will be standardization in the process. If your institution plans to begin collecting E codes, these guidelines are to be applied. The use of E codes is supplemental to the application of ICD-9-CM diagnosis codes. E codes are never to be recorded as principal diagnoses (first-listed in non-inpatient setting) and are not required for reporting to CMS.

External causes of injury and poisoning codes (E codes) are intended to provide data for injury research and evaluation of injury prevention strategies. E codes capture how the injury or poisoning happened (cause), the intent (unintentional or accidental; or intentional, such as suicide or assault), and the place where the event occurred.

Some major categories of E codes include:

- Transport accidents
- Poisoning and adverse effects of drugs, medicinal substances and biologicals
- Accidental falls
- Accidents caused by fire and flames
- Accidents due to natural and environmental factors
- Late effects of accidents, assaults or self injury
- Assaults or purposely inflicted injury
- Suicide or self inflicted injury

These guidelines apply to the coding and collection of E codes from records in hospitals, outpatient clinics, emergency departments, other ambulatory care settings and provider offices, and nonacute care settings, except when other specific guidelines apply.

a. General E code coding guidelines

1) **Used with any code in the range of 001-V85.4**—An E code may be used with any code in the range of 001-V85.4, which indicates an injury, poisoning, or adverse effect due to an external cause.

2) **Assign the appropriate E code for all initial treatments**—Assign the appropriate E code for the initial encounter of an injury, poisoning, or adverse effect of drugs, **not for subsequent treatment.**

3) **Use the full range of E codes**—Use the full range of E codes to completely describe the cause, the intent and the place of occurrence, if applicable, for all injuries, poisonings, and adverse effects of drugs.

4) **Assign as many E codes as necessary**
Assign as many E codes as necessary to fully explain each cause. If only one E code can be recorded, assign the E code most related to the principal diagnosis.

5) **The selection of the appropriate E code**—The selection of the appropriate E code is guided by the Index to External Causes, which is located after the Alphabetical Index to Diseases and by inclusion and exclusion notes in the Tabular List.

6) **E code can never be a principal diagnosis**—An E code can never be a principal (first-listed) diagnosis.

7) **External cause code(s) with systemic inflammatory response syndrome (SIRS)—An external cause code(s) may be used with codes 995.93 Systemic inflammatory response syndrome due to noninfectious process without organ dysfunction, and 995.94 Systemic inflammatory response syndrome due to noninfectious process with organ dysfunction, if trauma was the initiating insult that precipitated the SIRS. The external cause(s) code should correspond to the most serious injury resulting from the trauma. The external cause code(s) should only be assigned if the trauma necessitated the admission in which the patient also developed SIRS. If a patient is admitted with SIRS but the trauma has been treated previously, the external cause codes should not be used.**

b. Place of occurrence guideline—Use an additional code from category E849 to indicate the place of occurrence for injuries and poisonings. The place of occurrence describes the place where the event occurred and not the patient's activity at the time of the event.

Do not use E849.9 if the place of occurrence is not stated.

c. Adverse effects of drugs, medicinal and biological substances guidelines

1) **Do not code directly from the Table of Drugs**—Do not code directly from the Table of Drugs and Chemicals. Always refer back to the Tabular List.

2) **Use as many codes as necessary to describe**—Use as many codes as necessary to describe completely all drugs, medicinal or biological substances.

3) **If the same E code would describe the causative agent**—If the same E code would describe the causative agent for more than one adverse reaction, assign the code only once.

4) **If two or more drugs, medicinal or biological substances**—If two or more drugs, medicinal or biological substances are reported, code each individually unless the combination code is listed in the Table of Drugs and Chemicals. In that case, assign the E code for the combination.

5) **When a reaction results from the interaction of a drug(s)**—When a reaction results from the interaction of a drug(s) and alcohol, use poisoning codes and E codes for both.

6) **If the reporting format limits the number of E codes**—If the reporting format limits the number of E codes that can be used in reporting clinical data, code the one most related to the principal diagnosis. Include at least one from each category (cause, intent, place) if possible.

If there are different fourth-digit codes in the same three-digit category, use the code for "other specified" of that category. If there is no "other specified" code in that category, use the appropriate "unspecified" code in that category.

If the codes are in different three-digit categories, assign the appropriate E code for other multiple drugs and medicinal substances.

7) **Codes from the E930-E949 series**—Codes from the E930-E949 series must be used to identify the causative substance for an adverse effect of drug, medicinal and biological substances, correctly prescribed and properly administered. The effect, such as tachycardia, delirium, gastrointestinal hemorrhaging, vomiting, hypokalemia, hepatitis, renal failure, or respiratory failure, is coded and followed by the appropriate code from the E930-E949 series.

d. Multiple cause E code coding guidelines—If two or more events cause separate injuries, an E code should be assigned for each cause. The first listed E code will be selected in the following order:

E codes for child and adult abuse take priority over all other E codes. See section I.C.19.e., Child and adult abuse guidelines.

E codes for terrorism events take priority over all other E codes except child and adult abuse.

E codes for cataclysmic events take priority over all other E codes except child and adult abuse and terrorism.

E codes for transport accidents take priority over all other E codes except cataclysmic events and child and adult abuse and terrorism.

The first-listed E code should correspond to the cause of the most serious diagnosis due to an assault, accident, or self-harm, following the order of hierarchy listed above.

e. Child and adult abuse guideline

1) **Intentional injury**—When the cause of an injury or neglect is intentional child or adult abuse, the first-listed E code should be assigned from categories E960-E968 Homicide and injury purposely inflicted by other persons, (except category E967). An E code from category E967 Child and adult battering and other maltreatment, should be added as an additional code to identify the perpetrator, if known.

2) **Accidental intent**—In cases of neglect when the intent is determined to be accidental E code E904.0 Abandonment or neglect of infant and helpless person, should be the first-listed E code.

f. Unknown or suspected intent guideline

1) **If the intent (accident, self-harm, assault) of the cause of an injury or poisoning is unknown**—If the intent (accident, self-harm, assault) of the cause of an injury or poisoning is unknown or unspecified, code the intent as undetermined, E980-E989.

2) **If the intent (accident, self-harm, assault) of the cause of an injury or poisoning is questionable**—If the intent (accident, self-harm, assault) of the cause of an injury or poisoning is questionable, probable or suspected, code the intent as undetermined, E980-E989.

g. Undetermined cause—When the intent of an injury or poisoning is known, but the cause is unknown, use codes E928.9 Unspecified accident, E958.9 Suicide and self-inflicted injury by unspecified means, and E968.9 Assault by unspecified means.

These E codes should rarely be used, as the documentation in the medical record, in both the inpatient outpatient and other settings, should normally provide sufficient detail to determine the cause of the injury.

h. Late effects of external cause guidelines

1) Late effect E codes—Late effect E codes exist for injuries and poisonings but not for adverse effects of drugs, misadventures, and surgical complications.

2) Late effect E codes (E929, E959, E969, E977, E989, or E999.1)—A late effect E code (E929, E959, E969, E977, E989, or E999.1) should be used with any report of a late effect or sequela resulting from a previous injury or poisoning (905-909).

3) Late effect E code with a related current injury—A late effect E code should never be used with a related current nature of injury code.

4) Use of late effect E codes for subsequent visits—Use a late effect E code for subsequent visits when a late effect of the initial injury or poisoning is being treated. There is no late effect E code for adverse effects of drugs. Do not use a late effect E code for subsequent visits for follow-up care (e.g., to assess healing, to receive rehabilitative therapy) of the injury or poisoning when no late effect of the injury has been documented.

i. Misadventures and complications of care guidelines

1) Code range E870-E876—Assign a code in the range of E870-E876 if misadventures are stated by the provider.

2) Code range E878-E879—Assign a code in the range of E878-E879 if the provider attributes an abnormal reaction or later complication to a surgical or medical procedure, but does not mention misadventure at the time of the procedure as the cause of the reaction.

j. Terrorism guidelines

1) Cause of injury identified by the federal government (FBI) as terrorism—When the cause of an injury is identified by the federal government (FBI) as terrorism, the first-listed E code should be a code from category E979 Terrorism. The definition of terrorism employed by the FBI is found at the inclusion note at E979. The terrorism E code is the only E code that should be assigned. Additional E codes from the assault categories should not be assigned.

2) Cause of an injury is suspected to be the result of terrorism—When the cause of an injury is suspected to be the result of terrorism a code from category E979 should not be assigned. Assign a code in the range of E codes based on the documentation of intent and mechanism.

3) Code E979.9 Terrorism, secondary effects—Assign code E979.9 Terrorism, secondary effects, for conditions occurring subsequent to the terrorist event. This code should not be assigned for conditions that are due to the initial terrorist act.

4) Statistical tabulation of terrorism codes—For statistical purposes these codes will be tabulated within the category for assault, expanding the current category from E960-E969 to include E979 and E999.1.

Section II. Selection of Principal Diagnosis

The circumstances of inpatient admission always govern the selection of principal diagnosis. The principal diagnosis is defined in the Uniform Hospital Discharge Data Set (UHDDS) as "that condition established after study to be chiefly responsible for occasioning the admission of the patient to the hospital for care."

The UHDDS definitions are used by hospitals to report inpatient data elements in a standardized manner. These data elements and their definitions can be found in the July 31, 1985, *Federal Register* (vol. 50, no. 147), pp. 31038-40.

Since that time the application of the UHDDS definitions has been expanded to include all non-outpatient settings (acute care, short-term, long-term care and psychiatric hospitals; home health agencies; rehab facilities; nursing homes, etc.).

In determining principal diagnosis the coding conventions in the ICD-9-CM, Volumes 1 and 2 take precedence over these official coding guidelines. (See section I.A., Conventions, for the ICD-9-CM).

The importance of consistent, complete documentation in the medical record cannot be overemphasized. Without such documentation the application of all coding guidelines is a difficult, if not impossible, task.

A. Codes for symptoms, signs, and ill-defined conditions

Codes for symptoms, signs, and ill-defined conditions from chapter 16 are not to be used as principal diagnosis when a related definitive diagnosis has been established.

B. Two or more interrelated conditions, each potentially meeting the definition for principal diagnosis.

When there are two or more interrelated conditions (such as diseases in the same ICD-9-CM chapter or manifestations characteristically associated with a certain disease) potentially meeting the definition of principal diagnosis, either condition may be sequenced first, unless the circumstances of the admission, the therapy provided, the Tabular List, or the Alphabetic Index indicate otherwise.

C. Two or more diagnoses that equally meet the definition for principal diagnosis

In the unusual instance when two or more diagnoses equally meet the criteria for principal diagnosis as determined by the circumstances of admission, diagnostic workup and/or therapy provided, and the Alphabetic Index, Tabular List, or another coding guidelines do not provide sequencing direction, any one of the diagnoses may be sequenced first.

D. Two or more comparative or contrasting conditions.

In those rare instances when two or more contrasting or comparative diagnoses are documented as "either/or" (or similar terminology), they are coded as if the diagnoses were confirmed and the diagnoses are sequenced according to the circumstances of the admission. If no further determination can be made as to which diagnosis should be principal, either diagnosis may be sequenced first.

E. A symptom(s) followed by contrasting/comparative diagnoses

When a symptom(s) is followed by contrasting/comparative diagnoses, the symptom code is sequenced first. All the contrasting/comparative diagnoses should be coded as additional diagnoses.

F. Original treatment plan not carried out

Sequence as the principal diagnosis the condition, which after study occasioned the admission to the hospital, even though treatment may not have been carried out due to unforeseen circumstances.

G. Complications of surgery and other medical care

When the admission is for treatment of a complication resulting from surgery or other medical care, the complication code is sequenced as the principal diagnosis. If the complication is classified to the 996-999 series and the code lacks the necessary specificity in describing the complication, an additional code for the specific complication should be assigned.

H. Uncertain diagnosis

If the diagnosis documented at the time of discharge is qualified as "probable," "suspected," "likely," "questionable," "possible," or "still to be ruled out," code the condition as if it existed or was established. The bases for these guidelines are the diagnostic workup, arrangements for further workup or observation, and initial therapeutic approach that correspond most closely with the established diagnosis.

Note: This guideline is applicable only to short-term, acute, long-term care and psychiatric hospitals.

Section III. Reporting Additional Diagnoses

GENERAL RULES FOR OTHER (ADDITIONAL) DIAGNOSES

For reporting purposes the definition for "other diagnoses" is interpreted as additional conditions that affect patient care in terms of requiring:

- Clinical evaluation; or
- Therapeutic treatment; or
- Diagnostic procedures; or
- Extended length of hospital stay; or
- Increased nursing care and/or monitoring.

The UHDDS item #11-b defines other diagnoses as "all conditions that coexist at the time of admission, that develop subsequently, or that affect the treatment received and/or the length of stay. Diagnoses that relate to an earlier episode which have no bearing on the current hospital stay are to be excluded." UHDDS definitions apply to inpatients in acute care, short-term, long-term care and psychiatric hospital settings. The UHDDS definitions are used by acute care short-term hospitals to report inpatient data elements in a standardized manner. These data elements and their definitions can be found in the July 31, 1985, *Federal Register* (vol. 50, no. 147), pp. 31038-40.

Since that time the application of the UHDDS definitions has been expanded to include all non-outpatient settings (acute care, short-term,

long-term care and psychiatric hospitals; home health agencies; rehab facilities; nursing homes, etc.).

The following guidelines are to be applied in designating other diagnoses when neither the Alphabetic Index nor the Tabular List in ICD-9-CM provides direction. The listing of the diagnoses in the patient record is the responsibility of the attending provider.

A. Previous conditions
If the provider has included a diagnosis in the final diagnostic statement, such as the discharge summary or the face sheet, it should ordinarily be coded. Some providers include in the diagnostic statement resolved conditions or diagnoses and status-post procedures from previous admission that have no bearing on the current stay. Such conditions are not to be reported and are coded only if required by hospital policy.

However, history codes (V10-V19) may be used as secondary codes if the historical condition or family history has an impact on current care or influences treatment.

B. Abnormal findings
Abnormal findings (laboratory, x-ray, pathologic, and other diagnostic results) are not coded and reported unless the provider indicates their clinical significance. If the findings are outside the normal range and the **attending** provider has ordered other tests to evaluate the condition or prescribed treatment, it is appropriate to ask the provider whether the abnormal finding should be added.

Please note: This differs from the coding practices in the outpatient setting for coding encounters for diagnostic tests that have been interpreted by a provider.

C. Uncertain Diagnosis
If the diagnosis documented at the time of discharge is qualified as "probable," "suspected," "likely," "questionable," "possible," or "still to be ruled out," code the condition as if it existed or was established. The bases for these guidelines are the diagnostic workup, arrangements for further workup or observation, and initial therapeutic approach that correspond most closely with the established diagnosis.

Note: This guideline is applicable only to short-term, acute, long-term care and psychiatric hospitals.

Section IV. Diagnostic Coding and Reporting Guidelines for Outpatient Services

These coding guidelines for outpatient diagnoses have been approved for use by hospitals/providers in coding and reporting hospital-based outpatient services and provider-based office visits.

Information about the use of certain abbreviations, punctuation, symbols, and other conventions used in the ICD-9-CM Tabular List (code numbers and titles), can be found in section IA of these guidelines, under "Conventions for the ICD-9-CM." Information about the correct sequence to use in finding a code is also described in section I.

The terms "encounter" and "visit" are often used interchangeably in describing outpatient service contacts and, therefore, appear together in these guidelines without distinguishing one from the other.

Though the conventions and general guidelines apply to all settings, coding guidelines for outpatient and provider reporting of diagnoses will vary in a number of instances from those for inpatient diagnoses, recognizing that:

- The Uniform Hospital Discharge Data Set (UHDDS) definition of principal diagnosis applies only to inpatients in acute, short-term, long-term care **and psychiatric** hospitals.
- Coding guidelines for inconclusive diagnoses (probable, suspected, rule out, etc.) were developed for inpatient reporting and do not apply to outpatients.

A. Selection of first-listed condition
In the outpatient setting, the term "first-listed diagnosis" is used in lieu of principal diagnosis.

In determining the first-listed diagnosis the coding conventions of ICD-9-CM, as well as the general and disease-specific guidelines take precedence over the outpatient guidelines.

Diagnoses often are not established at the time of the initial encounter/visit. It may take two or more visits before the diagnosis is confirmed.

The most critical rule involves beginning the search for the correct code assignment through the Alphabetic Index. Never begin searching initially in the Tabular List as this will lead to coding errors.

B. Codes from 001.0 through V85.4
The appropriate code or codes from 001.0 through V84.8 must be used to identify diagnoses, symptoms, conditions, problems, complaints, or other reason(s) for the encounter/visit.

C. Accurate reporting of ICD-9-CM diagnosis codes
For accurate reporting of ICD-9-CM diagnosis codes, the documentation should describe the patient's condition, using terminology which includes specific diagnoses as well as symptoms, problems, or reasons for the encounter. There are ICD-9-CM codes to describe all of these.

D. Selection of codes 001.0 through 999.9
The selection of codes 001.0 through 999.9 will frequently be used to describe the reason for the encounter. These codes are from the section of ICD-9-CM for the classification of diseases and injuries (e.g. infectious and parasitic diseases; neoplasms; symptoms, signs, and ill-defined conditions, etc.).

E. Codes that describe symptoms and signs
Codes that describe symptoms and signs, as opposed to diagnoses, are acceptable for reporting purposes when a diagnosis has not been established (confirmed) by the provider. Chapter 16 of ICD-9-CM, Symptoms, Signs, and Ill-defined Conditions (codes 780.0-799.9) contain many, but not all, codes for symptoms.

F. Encounters for circumstances other than a disease or injury
ICD-9-CM provides codes to deal with encounters for circumstances other than a disease or injury. The Supplementary Classification of Factors Influencing Health Status and Contact with Health Services (V01.0-V84.8) is provided to deal with occasions when circumstances other than a disease or injury are recorded as diagnosis or problems.

G. Level of Detail in Coding

1. **ICD-9-CM codes with three, four, or five digits—**ICD-9-CM is composed of codes with either three, four, or five digits. Codes with three digits are included in ICD-9-CM as the heading of a category of codes that may be further subdivided by the use of fourth and/or fifth digits, which provide greater specificity.
2. **Use of full number of digits required for a code—**A three-digit code is to be used only if it is not further subdivided. Where fourth-digit subcategories and/or fifth-digit subclassifications are provided, they must be assigned. A code is invalid if it has not been coded to the full number of digits required for that code. See also discussion under section I.b.3., General coding guidelines, Level of detail in coding.

H. ICD-9-CM code for the diagnosis, condition, problem, or other reason for encounter/visit
List first the ICD-9-CM code for the diagnosis, condition, problem, or other reason for encounter/visit shown in the medical record to be chiefly responsible for the services provided. List additional codes that describe any coexisting conditions. **In some cases the first-listed diagnosis may be a symptom when a diagnosis has not been established (confirmed) by the physician.**

I. "Probable," "suspected," "questionable," "rule out," or "working diagnosis"
Do not code diagnoses documented as "probable," "suspected," "questionable," "rule out," or "working diagnosis." Rather, code the condition(s) to the highest degree of certainty for that encounter/visit, such as symptoms, signs, abnormal test results, or other reason for the visit. **Please note:** This differs from the coding practices used by **short-term, acute care, long-term care, and psychiatric** hospitals.

J. Chronic diseases
Chronic diseases treated on an ongoing basis may be coded and reported as many times as the patient receives treatment and care for the condition(s).

K. Code all documented conditions that coexist
Code all documented conditions that coexist at the time of the encounter/visit, and require or affect patient care treatment or management. Do not code conditions that were previously treated and no longer exist. However, history codes (V10-V19) may be used as secondary codes if the historical condition or family history has an impact on current care or influences treatment.

L. Patients receiving diagnostic services only
For patients receiving diagnostic services only during an encounter/visit, sequence first the diagnosis, condition, problem, or other reason for encounter/visit shown in the medical record to be chiefly responsible for the outpatient services provided during the encounter/visit. Codes for other diagnoses (e.g., chronic conditions) may be sequenced as additional diagnoses.

For outpatient encounters for diagnostic tests that have been interpreted by a physician and the final report is available at the time of coding, code any confirmed or definitive diagnosis(es) documented in the interpretation. Do not code related signs and symptoms as additional diagnoses.

Please note: This differs from the coding practice in the hospital inpatient setting regarding abnormal findings on test results.

M. Patients receiving therapeutic services only

For patients receiving therapeutic services only during an encounter/visit, sequence first the diagnosis, condition, problem, or other reason for encounter/visit shown in the medical record to be chiefly responsible for the outpatient services provided during the encounter/visit. Codes for other diagnoses (e.g., chronic conditions) may be sequenced as additional diagnoses.

The only exception to this rule is that when the primary reason for the admission/encounter is chemotherapy, radiation therapy, or rehabilitation, the appropriate V code for the service is listed first, and the diagnosis or problem for which the service is being performed is listed second.

N. Patients receiving preoperative evaluations only

For patients receiving preoperative evaluations only, sequence **first** a code from category V72.8 Other specified examinations, to describe the pre-op consultations. Assign a code for the condition to describe the reason for the surgery as an additional diagnosis. Code also any findings related to the pre-op evaluation.

O. Ambulatory surgery

For ambulatory surgery, code the diagnosis for which the surgery was performed. If the postoperative diagnosis is known to be different from the preoperative diagnosis at the time the diagnosis is confirmed, select the postoperative diagnosis for coding, since it is the most definitive.

P. Routine outpatient prenatal visits

For routine outpatient prenatal visits when no complications are present, code V22.0 Supervision of normal first pregnancy, **or** V22.1 Supervision of other normal pregnancy, should be used as **the** principal diagnosis. These codes should not be used in conjunction with chapter 11 codes.

A

Note — Use the following fifth-digit subclassification with categories 634–637:

0	*unspecified*
1	*incomplete*
2	*complete*

☑ Additional Digit Required — Refer to the Tabular List (Numeric Code Section) for Additional Digit Selection
▶◀ Revised Text ● New Line ▲ Revised Code

Abortion — *continued*
with — *continued*
embolism (air) (amniotic fluid) (blood clot) (pulmonary) (pyemic) (septic) (soap) 637.6 ☑
genital tract and pelvic infection 637.0 ☑
hemorrhage, delayed or excessive 637.1 ☑
metabolic disorder 637.4 ☑
renal failure (acute) 637.3 ☑
sepsis (genital tract) (pelvic organ) 637.0 ☑
urinary tract 637.7 ☑
shock (postoperative) (septic) 637.5 ☑
specified complication NEC 637.7 ☑
toxemia 637.3 ☑
unspecified complication(s) 637.8 ☑
urinary tract infection 637.7 ☑
accidental — *see* Abortion, spontaneous
artificial — *see* Abortion, induced
attempted (failed) — *see* Abortion, failed
criminal — *see* Abortion, illegal
early — *see* Abortion, spontaneous
elective — *see* Abortion, legal
failed (legal) 638.9
with
damage to pelvic organ (laceration) (rupture) (tear) 638.2
embolism (air) (amniotic fluid) (blood clot) (pulmonary) (pyemic) (septic) (soap) 638.6
genital tract and pelvic infection 638.0
hemorrhage, delayed or excessive 638.1
metabolic disorder 638.4
renal failure (acute) 638.3
sepsis (genital tract) (pelvic organ) 638.0
urinary tract 638.7
shock (postoperative) (septic) 638.5
specified complication NEC 638.7
toxemia 638.3
unspecified complication(s) 638.8
urinary tract infection 638.7
fetal indication — *see* Abortion, legal
fetus 779.6
following threatened abortion — *see* Abortion, by type
habitual or recurrent (care during pregnancy) 646.3 ☑
with current abortion (*see also* Abortion, spontaneous) 634.9 ☑
affecting fetus or newborn 761.8
without current pregnancy 629.9
homicidal — *see* Abortion, illegal
illegal 636.9 ☑
with
damage to pelvic organ (laceration) (rupture) (tear) 636.2 ☑
embolism (air) (amniotic fluid) (blood clot) (pulmonary) (pyemic) (septic) (soap) 636.6 ☑
genital tract and pelvic infection 636.0 ☑
hemorrhage, delayed or excessive 636.1 ☑
metabolic disorder 636.4 ☑
renal failure 636.3 ☑
sepsis (genital tract) (pelvic organ) 636.0 ☑
urinary tract 636.7 ☑
shock (postoperative) (septic) 636.5 ☑
specified complication NEC 636.7 ☑
toxemia 636.3 ☑
unspecified complication(s) 636.8 ☑
urinary tract infection 636.7 ☑
fetus 779.6
induced 637.9 ☑
illegal — *see* Abortion, illegal
legal indications — *see* Abortion, legal
medical indications — *see* Abortion, legal
therapeutic — *see* Abortion, legal
late — *see* Abortion, spontaneous
legal (legal indication) (medical indication) (under medical supervision) 635.9 ☑
with
damage to pelvic organ (laceration) (rupture) (tear) 635.2 ☑
embolism (air) (amniotic fluid) (blood clot) (pulmonary) (pyemic) (septic) (soap) 635.6 ☑
genital tract and pelvic infection 635.0 ☑

Abortion — *continued*
legal — *continued*
with — *continued*
hemorrhage, delayed or excessive 635.1 ☑
metabolic disorder 635.4 ☑
renal failure (acute) 635.3 ☑
sepsis (genital tract) (pelvic organ) 635.0 ☑
urinary tract 635.7 ☑
shock (postoperative) (septic) 635.5 ☑
specified complication NEC 635.7 ☑
toxemia 635.3 ☑
unspecified complication(s) 635.8 ☑
urinary tract infection 635.7 ☑
fetus 779.6
medical indication — *see* Abortion, legal
mental hygiene problem — *see* Abortion, legal
missed 632
operative — *see* Abortion, legal
psychiatric indication — *see* Abortion, legal
recurrent — *see* Abortion, spontaneous
self-induced — *see* Abortion, illegal
septic — *see* Abortion, by type, with sepsis
spontaneous 634.9 ☑
with
damage to pelvic organ (laceration) (rupture) (tear) 634.2 ☑
embolism (air) (amniotic fluid) (blood clot) (pulmonary) (pyemic) (septic) (soap) 634.6 ☑
genital tract and pelvic infection 634.0 ☑
hemorrhage, delayed or excessive 634.1 ☑
metabolic disorder 634.4 ☑
renal failure 634.3 ☑
sepsis (genital tract) (pelvic organ) 634.0 ☑
urinary tract 634.7 ☑
shock (postoperative) (septic) 634.5 ☑
specified complication NEC 634.7 ☑
toxemia 634.3 ☑
unspecified complication(s) 634.8 ☑
urinary tract infection 634.7 ☑
fetus 761.8
threatened 640.0 ☑
affecting fetus or newborn 762.1
surgical — *see* Abortion, legal
therapeutic — *see* Abortion, legal
threatened 640.0 ☑
affecting fetus or newborn 762.1
tubal — *see* Pregnancy, tubal
voluntary — *see* Abortion, legal
Abortus fever 023.9
Aboulomania 301.6
Abrachia 755.20
Abrachiatism 755.20
Abrachiocephalia 759.89
Abrachiocephalus 759.89
Abrami's disease (acquired hemolytic jaundice) 283.9
Abramov-Fiedler myocarditis (acute isolated myocarditis) 422.91
Abrasion — *see also* Injury, superficial, by site
cornea 918.1
dental 521.20
extending into
dentine 521.22
pulp 521.23
generalized 521.25
limited to enamel 521.21
localized 521.24
teeth, tooth (dentifrice) (habitual) (hard tissues) (occupational) (ritual) (traditional) (wedge defect) (*see also* Abrasion, dental) 521.20
Abrikossov's tumor (M9580/0) — *see also* Neoplasm, connective tissue, benign
malignant (M9580/3) — *see* Neoplasm, connective tissue, malignant
Abrism 988.8
Abruption, placenta — *see* Placenta, abruptio
Abruptio placentae — *see* Placenta, abruptio

Abscess (acute) (chronic) (infectional) (lymphangitic) (metastatic) (multiple) (pyogenic) (septic) (with lymphangitis) (*see also* Cellulitis) 682.9
abdomen, abdominal
cavity 567.22 ▲
wall 682.2
abdominopelvic 567.22 ▲
accessory sinus (chronic) (*see also* Sinusitis) 473.9
adrenal (capsule) (gland) 255.8
alveolar 522.5
with sinus 522.7
amebic 006.3
bladder 006.8
brain (with liver or lung abscess) 006.5
liver (without mention of brain or lung abscess) 006.3
with
brain abscess (and lung abscess) 006.5
lung abscess 006.4
lung (with liver abscess) 006.4
with brain abscess 006.5
seminal vesicle 006.8
specified site NEC 006.8
spleen 006.8
anaerobic 040.0
ankle 682.6
anorectal 566
antecubital space 682.3
antrum (chronic) (Highmore) (*see also* Sinusitis, maxillary) 473.0
anus 566
apical (tooth) 522.5
with sinus (alveolar) 522.7
appendix 540.1
areola (acute) (chronic) (nonpuerperal) 611.0
puerperal, postpartum 675.1 ☑
arm (any part, above wrist) 682.3
artery (wall) 447.2
atheromatous 447.2
auditory canal (external) 380.10
auricle (ear) (staphylococcal) (streptococcal) 380.10
axilla, axillary (region) 682.3
lymph gland or node 683
back (any part) 682.2
Bartholin's gland 616.3
with
abortion — *see* Abortion, by type, with sepsis
ectopic pregnancy (*see also* categories 633.0-633.9) 639.0
molar pregnancy (*see also* categories 630-632) 639.0
complicating pregnancy or puerperium 646.6 ☑
following
abortion 639.0
ectopic or molar pregnancy 639.0
bartholinian 616.3
Bezold's 383.01
bile, biliary, duct or tract (*see also* Cholecystitis) 576.8
bilharziasis 120.1
bladder (wall) 595.89
amebic 006.8
bone (subperiosteal) (*see also* Osteomyelitis) 730.0 ☑
accessory sinus (chronic) (*see also* Sinusitis) 473.9
acute 730.0 ☑
chronic or old 730.1 ☑
jaw (lower) (upper) 526.4
mastoid — *see* Mastoiditis, acute
petrous (*see also* Petrositis) 383.20
spinal (tuberculous) (*see also* Tuberculosis) 015.0 ☑ *[730.88]*
nontuberculous 730.08
bowel 569.5
brain (any part) 324.0
amebic (with liver or lung abscess) 006.5
cystic 324.0
late effect — *see* category 326
otogenic 324.0
tuberculous (*see also* Tuberculosis) 013.3 ☑

☑ Additional Digit Required — Refer to the Tabular List (Numeric Code Section) for Additional Digit Selection

▶◀ Revised Text ● New Line ▲ Revised Code

Abscess (*see also* Cellulitis) — *continued*
- mesentery, mesenteric 567.22 ▲
- mesosalpinx (*see also* Salpingo-oophoritis) 614.2
- milk 675.1 ☑
- Monro's (psoriasis) 696.1
- mons pubis 682.2
- mouth (floor) 528.3
- multiple sites NEC 682.9
- mural 682.2
- muscle 728.89
  - psoas 567.31 ●
- myocardium 422.92
- nabothian (follicle) (*see also* Cervicitis) 616.0
- nail (chronic) (with lymphangitis) 681.9
  - finger 681.02
  - toe 681.11
- nasal (fossa) (septum) 478.1
  - sinus (chronic) (*see also* Sinusitis) 473.9
- nasopharyngeal 478.29
- nates 682.5
- navel 682.2
  - newborn NEC 771.4
- neck (region) 682.1
  - lymph gland or node 683
- nephritic (*see also* Abscess, kidney) 590.2
- nipple 611.0
  - puerperal, postpartum 675.0 ☑
- nose (septum) 478.1
  - external 682.0
- omentum 567.22 ▲
- operative wound 998.59
- orbit, orbital 376.01
- ossifluent — *see* Abscess, bone
- ovary, ovarian (corpus luteum) (*see also* Salpingo-oophoritis) 614.2
- oviduct (*see also* Salpingo-oophoritis) 614.2
- palate (soft) 528.3
  - hard 526.4
- palmar (space) 682.4
- pancreas (duct) 577.0
- paradontal 523.3
- parafrenal 607.2
- parametric, parametrium (chronic) (*see* also Disease, pelvis, inflammatory) 614.4
  - acute 614.3
- paranephric 590.2
- parapancreatic 577.0
- parapharyngeal 478.22
- pararectal 566
- parasinus (*see also* Sinusitis) 473.9
- parauterine (*see also* Disease, pelvis, inflammatory) 614.4
  - acute 614.3
- paravaginal (*see also* Vaginitis) 616.10
- parietal region 682.8
- parodontal 523.3
- parotid (duct) (gland) 527.3
  - region 528.3
- parumbilical 682.2
  - newborn 771.4
- pectoral (region) 682.2
- pelvirectal 567.22 ▲
- pelvis, pelvic
  - female (chronic) (*see also* Disease, pelvis, inflammatory) 614.4
    - acute 614.3
  - male, peritoneal (cellular tissue) — *see* Abscess, peritoneum
  - tuberculous (*see also* Tuberculosis) 016.9 ☑
- penis 607.2
  - gonococcal (acute) 098.0
    - chronic or duration of 2 months or over 098.2
- perianal 566
- periapical 522.5
  - with sinus (alveolar) 522.7
- periappendiceal 540.1
- pericardial 420.99
- pericecal 540.1
- pericemental 523.3
- pericholecystic (*see also* Cholecystitis, acute) 575.0
- pericoronal 523.3
- peridental 523.3
- perigastric 535.0 ☑

Abscess (*see also* Cellulitis) — *continued*
- perimetric (*see also* Disease, pelvis, inflammatory) 614.4
  - acute 614.3
- perinephric, perinephritic (*see also* Abscess, kidney) 590.2
- perineum, perineal (superficial) 682.2
  - deep (with urethral involvement) 597.0
  - urethra 597.0
- periodontal (parietal) 523.3
  - apical 522.5
- periosteum, periosteal (*see also* Periostitis) 730.3 ☑
  - with osteomyelitis (*see also* Osteomyelitis) 730.2 ☑
    - acute or subacute 730.0 ☑
    - chronic or old 730.1 ☑
- peripleuritic 510.9
  - with fistula 510.0
- periproctic 566
- periprostatic 601.2
- perirectal (staphylococcal) 566
- perirenal (tissue) (*see also* Abscess, kidney) 590.2
- perisinuous (nose) (*see also* Sinusitis) 473.9
- peritoneum, peritoneal (perforated) (ruptured) 567.22 ▲
  - with
    - abortion — *see* Abortion, by type, with sepsis
    - appendicitis 540.1
    - ectopic pregnancy (*see also* categories 633.0-633.9) 639.0
    - molar pregnancy (*see also* categories 630-632) 639.0
  - following
    - abortion 639.0
    - ectopic or molar pregnancy 639.0
  - pelvic, female (*see also* Disease, pelvis, inflammatory) 614.4
    - acute 614.3
  - postoperative 998.59
  - puerperal, postpartum, childbirth 670.0 ☑
  - tuberculous (*see also* Tuberculosis) 014.0 ☑
- peritonsillar 475
- perityphlic 540.1
- periureteral 593.89
- periurethral 597.0
  - gonococcal (acute) 098.0
    - chronic or duration of 2 months or over 098.2
- periuterine (*see also* Disease, pelvis, inflammatory) 614.4
  - acute 614.3
- perivesical 595.89
- pernicious NEC 682.9
- petrous bone — *see* Petrositis
- phagedenic NEC 682.9
  - chancroid 099.0
- pharynx, pharyngeal (lateral) 478.29
- phlegmonous NEC 682.9
- pilonidal 685.0
- pituitary (gland) 253.8
- pleura 510.9
  - with fistula 510.0
- popliteal 682.6
- postanal 566
- postcecal 540.1
- postlaryngeal 478.79
- postnasal 478.1
- postpharyngeal 478.24
- posttonsillar 475
- posttyphoid 002.0
- Pott's (*see also* Tuberculosis) 015.0 ☑ *[730.88]*
- pouch of Douglas (chronic) (*see also* Disease, pelvis, inflammatory) 614.4
- premammary — *see* Abscess, breast
- prepatellar 682.6
- prostate (*see also* Prostatitis) 601.2
  - gonococcal (acute) 098.12
    - chronic or duration of 2 months or over 098.32
- psoas 567.31 ▲
  - tuberculous (*see also* Tuberculosis) ● 015.0 ☑ *[730.88]* ●
- pterygopalatine fossa 682.8
- pubis 682.2

Abscess (*see also* Cellulitis) — *continued*
- puerperal — *see* Puerperal, abscess, by site
- pulmonary — *see* Abscess, lung
- pulp, pulpal (dental) 522.0
  - finger 681.01
  - toe 681.10
- pyemic — *see* Septicemia
- pyloric valve 535.0 ☑
- rectovaginal septum 569.5
- rectovesical 595.89
- rectum 566
- regional NEC 682.9
- renal (*see also* Abscess, kidney) 590.2
- retina 363.00
- retrobulbar 376.01
- retrocecal 567.22 ▲
- retrolaryngeal 478.79
- retromammary — *see* Abscess, breast
- retroperineal 682.2
- retroperitoneal 567.38 ▲
- retropharyngeal 478.24
  - tuberculous (*see also* Tuberculosis) 012.8 ☑
- retrorectal 566
- retrouterine (*see also* Disease, pelvis, inflammatory) 614.4
  - acute 614.3
- retrovesical 595.89
- root, tooth 522.5
  - with sinus (alveolar) 522.7
- round ligament (*see also* Disease, pelvis, inflammatory) 614.4
  - acute 614.3
- rupture (spontaneous) NEC 682.9
- sacrum (tuberculous) (*see also* Tuberculosis) 015.0 ☑ *[730.88]*
  - nontuberculous 730.08
- salivary duct or gland 527.3
- scalp (any part) 682.8
- scapular 730.01
- sclera 379.09
- scrofulous (*see also* Tuberculosis) 017.2 ☑
- scrotum 608.4
- seminal vesicle 608.0
  - amebic 006.8
- septal, dental 522.5
  - with sinus (alveolar) 522.7
- septum (nasal) 478.1
- serous (*see also* Periostitis) 730.3 ☑
- shoulder 682.3
- side 682.2
- sigmoid 569.5
- sinus (accessory) (chronic) (nasal) (*see also* Sinusitis) 473.9
  - intracranial venous (any) 324.0
    - late effect — *see* category 326
- Skene's duct or gland 597.0
- skin NEC 682.9
  - tuberculous (primary) (*see also* Tuberculosis) 017.0 ☑
- sloughing NEC 682.9
- specified site NEC 682.8
  - amebic 006.8
- spermatic cord 608.4
- sphenoidal (sinus) (*see also* Sinusitis, sphenoidal) 473.3
- spinal
  - cord (any part) (staphylococcal) 324.1
    - tuberculous (*see also* Tuberculosis) 013.5 ☑
  - epidural 324.1
- spine (column) (tuberculous) (*see also* Tuberculosis) 015.0 ☑ *[730.88]*
  - nontuberculous 730.08
- spleen 289.59
  - amebic 006.8
- staphylococcal NEC 682.9
- stitch 998.59
- stomach (wall) 535.0 ☑
- strumous (tuberculous) (*see also* Tuberculosis) 017.2 ☑
- subarachnoid 324.9
  - brain 324.0
  - cerebral 324.0
  - late effect — *see* category 326
  - spinal cord 324.1
- subareolar — *see also* Abscess, breast
  - puerperal, postpartum 675.1 ☑

Absence — *continued*
- fibula, congenital (*see also* Deformity, reduction, lower limb) — *continued*
  - with
    - complete absence of distal elements 755.31
    - tibia 755.35
      - with
        - complete absence of distal elements 755.31
        - femur (incomplete) 755.33
          - with complete absence of distal elements 755.31
- finger (acquired) V49.62
  - congenital (complete) (partial) (*see also* Deformity, reduction, upper limb) 755.29
    - meaning all fingers (complete) (partial) 755.21
    - transverse 755.21
- fissures of lungs (congenital) 748.5
- foot (acquired) V49.73
  - congenital (complete) 755.31
- forearm (acquired) V49.65
  - congenital (complete) (partial) (with absence of distal elements, incomplete) (*see also* Deformity, reduction, upper limb) 755.25
    - with
      - complete absence of distal elements (hand and fingers) 755.21
      - humerus (incomplete) 755.23
- fovea centralis 743.55
- fucosidase 271.8
- gallbladder (acquired) V45.79
  - congenital 751.69
- gamma globulin (blood) 279.00
- genital organs
  - acquired V45.77
  - congenital
    - female 752.89
      - external 752.49
      - internal NEC 752.89
    - male 752.89
      - penis 752.69
- genitourinary organs, congenital NEC 752.89
- glottis 748.3
- gonadal, congenital NEC 758.6
- hair (congenital) 757.4
  - acquired — *see* Alopecia
- hand (acquired) V49.63
  - congenital (complete) (*see also* Deformity, reduction, upper limb) 755.21
- heart (congenital) 759.89
  - acquired — *see* Status, organ replacement
- heat sense (*see also* Disturbance, sensation) 782.0
- humerus, congenital (complete) (partial) (with absence of distal elements, incomplete) (*see also* Deformity, reduction, upper limb) 755.24
  - with
    - complete absence of distal elements 755.21
    - radius and ulna (incomplete) 755.23
- hymen (congenital) 752.49
- ileum (acquired) (postoperative) (posttraumatic) V45.72
  - congenital 751.1
- immunoglobulin, isolated NEC 279.03
  - IgA 279.01
  - IgG 279.03
  - IgM 279.02
- incus (acquired) 385.24
  - congenital 744.04
- internal ear (congenital) 744.05
- intestine (acquired) (small) V45.72
  - congenital 751.1
    - large 751.2
  - large V45.72
    - congenital 751.2
- iris (congenital) 743.45
- jaw — *see* Absence, mandible
- jejunum (acquired) V45.72
  - congenital 751.1
- joint, congenital NEC 755.8
- kidney(s) (acquired) V45.73
  - congenital 753.0

Absence — *continued*
- labium (congenital) (majus) (minus) 752.49
- labyrinth, membranous 744.05
- lacrimal apparatus (congenital) 743.65
- larynx (congenital) 748.3
- leg (acquired) V49.70
  - above knee V49.76
  - below knee V49.75
  - congenital (partial) (unilateral) (*see also* Deformity, reduction, lower limb) 755.31
    - lower (complete) (partial) (with absence of distal elements, incomplete) 755.35
      - with
        - complete absence of distal elements (foot and toes) 755.31
        - thigh (incomplete) 755.33
          - with complete absence of distal elements 755.31
    - upper — *see* Absence, femur
- lens (congenital) 743.35
  - acquired 379.31
- ligament, broad (congenital) 752.19
- limb (acquired)
  - congenital (complete) (partial) (*see also* Deformity, reduction) 755.4
    - lower 755.30
      - complete 755.31
      - incomplete 755.32
      - longitudinal — *see* Deficiency, lower limb, longitudinal
      - transverse 755.31
    - upper 755.20
      - complete 755.21
      - incomplete 755.22
      - longitudinal — *see* Deficiency, upper limb, longitudinal
      - transverse 755.21
  - lower NEC V49.70
  - upper NEC V49.60
- lip 750.26
- liver (congenital) (lobe) 751.69
- lumbar (congenital) (vertebra) 756.13
  - isthmus 756.11
  - pars articularis 756.11
- lumen — *see* Atresia
- lung (bilateral) (congenital) (fissure) (lobe) (unilateral) 748.5
  - acquired (any part) V45.76
- mandible (congenital) 524.09
- maxilla (congenital) 524.09
- menstruation 626.0
- metacarpal(s), congenital (complete) (partial) (with absence of distal elements, incomplete) (*see also* Deformity, reduction, upper limb) 755.28
  - with all fingers, complete 755.21
- metatarsal(s), congenital (complete) (partial) (with absence of distal elements, incomplete) (*see also* Deformity, reduction, lower limb) 755.38
  - with complete absence of distal elements 755.31
- muscle (congenital) (pectoral) 756.81
  - ocular 743.69
- musculoskeletal system (congenital) NEC 756.9
- nail(s) (congenital) 757.5
- neck, part 744.89
- nerve 742.8
- nervous system, part NEC 742.8
- neutrophil 288.0
- nipple (congenital) 757.6
- nose (congenital) 748.1
  - acquired 738.0
- nuclear 742.8
- ocular muscle (congenital) 743.69
- organ
  - of Corti (congenital) 744.05
  - or site
    - acquired V45.79
    - congenital NEC 759.89
- osseous meatus (ear) 744.03
- ovary (acquired) V45.77
  - congenital 752.0
- oviduct (acquired) V45.77
  - congenital 752.19

Absence — *continued*
- pancreas (congenital) 751.7
  - acquired (postoperative) (posttraumatic) V45.79
- parathyroid gland (congenital) 759.2
- parotid gland(s) (congenital) 750.21
- patella, congenital 755.64
- pelvic girdle (congenital) 755.69
- penis (congenital) 752.69
  - acquired V45.77
- pericardium (congenital) 746.89
- perineal body (congenital) 756.81
- phalange(s), congenital 755.4
  - lower limb (complete) (intercalary) (partial) (terminal) (*see also* Deformity, reduction, lower limb) 755.39
    - meaning all toes (complete) (partial) 755.31
    - transverse 755.31
  - upper limb (complete) (intercalary) (partial) (terminal) (*see also* Deformity, reduction, upper limb) 755.29
    - meaning all digits (complete) (partial) 755.21
    - transverse 755.21
- pituitary gland (congenital) 759.2
- postoperative — *see* Absence, by site, acquired
- prostate (congenital) 752.89
  - acquired V45.77
- pulmonary
  - artery 747.3
  - trunk 747.3
  - valve (congenital) 746.01
  - vein 747.49
- punctum lacrimale (congenital) 743.65
- radius, congenital (complete) (partial) (with absence of distal elements, incomplete) 755.26
  - with
    - complete absence of distal elements 755.21
    - ulna 755.25
      - with
        - complete absence of distal elements 755.21
        - humerus (incomplete) 755.23
- ray, congenital 755.4
  - lower limb (complete) (partial) (*see also* Deformity, reduction, lower limb) 755.38
    - meaning all rays 755.31
    - transverse 755.31
  - upper limb (complete) (partial) (*see also* Deformity, reduction, upper limb) 755.28
    - meaning all rays 755.21
    - transverse 755.21
- rectum (congenital) 751.2
  - acquired V45.79
- red cell 284.9
  - acquired (secondary) 284.8
  - congenital 284.0
  - hereditary 284.0
  - idiopathic 284.9
- respiratory organ (congenital) NEC 748.9
- rib (acquired) 738.3
  - congenital 756.3
- roof of orbit (congenital) 742.0
- round ligament (congenital) 752.89
- sacrum, congenital 756.13
- salivary gland(s) (congenital) 750.21
- scapula 755.59
- scrotum, congenital 752.89
- seminal tract or duct (congenital) 752.89
  - acquired V45.77
- septum (congenital) — *see also* Imperfect, closure, septum
  - atrial 745.69
    - and ventricular 745.7
  - between aorta and pulmonary artery 745.0
  - ventricular 745.3
    - and atrial 745.7
- sex chromosomes 758.81
- shoulder girdle, congenital (complete) (partial) 755.59
- skin (congenital) 757.39

Note — Use the following fifth-digit subclassification with the following codes: 305.0, 305.2-305.9:

0	*unspecified*	*2*	*episodic*
1	*continuous*	*3*	*in remission*

☑ Additional Digit Required — Refer to the Tabular List (Numeric Code Section) for Additional Digit Selection

- **Acholuric jaundice** (familial) (splenomegalic) (*see also* Spherocytosis) 282.0
  - acquired 283.9
- **Achondroplasia** 756.4
- **Achrestic anemia** 281.8
- **Achroacytosis, lacrimal gland** 375.00
  - tuberculous (*see also* Tuberculosis) 017.3 ☑
- **Achroma, cutis** 709.00
- **Achromate** (congenital) 368.54
- **Achromatopia** 368.54
- **Achromatopsia** (congenital) 368.54
- **Achromia**
  - congenital 270.2
  - parasitica 111.0
  - unguium 703.8
- **Achylia**
  - gastrica 536.8
    - neurogenic 536.3
    - psychogenic 306.4
  - pancreatica 577.1
- **Achylosis** 536.8
- **Acid**
  - burn — *see also* Burn, by site
    - from swallowing acid — *see* Burn, internal organs
  - deficiency
    - amide nicotinic 265.2
    - amino 270.9
    - ascorbic 267
    - folic 266.2
    - nicotinic (amide) 265.2
    - pantothenic 266.2
  - intoxication 276.2
  - peptic disease 536.8
  - stomach 536.8
    - psychogenic 306.4
- **Acidemia** 276.2
  - arginosuccinic 270.6
  - fetal
    - affecting management of pregnancy 656.3 ☑
    - before onset of labor, in liveborn infant 768.2
    - during labor, in liveborn infant 768.3
    - intrauterine 656.3 ☑
    - unspecified as to time of onset, in liveborn infant 768.4
  - pipecolic 270.7
- **Acidity, gastric** (high) (low) 536.8
  - psychogenic 306.4
- **Acidocytopenia** 288.0
- **Acidocytosis** 288.3
- **Acidopenia** 288.0
- **Acidosis** 276.2
  - diabetic 250.1 ☑
  - fetal, affecting management of pregnancy 756.8 ☑
  - fetal, affecting newborn 768.9
  - kidney tubular 588.89
  - lactic 276.2
  - metabolic NEC 276.2
    - with respiratory acidosis 276.4
    - late, of newborn 775.7
  - renal
    - hyperchloremic 588.89
    - tubular (distal) (proximal) 588.89
  - respiratory 276.2
    - complicated by
      - metabolic acidosis 276.4
      - metabolic alkalosis 276.4
- **Aciduria** 791.9
  - arginosuccinic 270.6
  - beta-aminoisobutyric (BAIB) 277.2
  - glutaric
    - type I 270.7
    - type II (type IIA, IIB, IIC) 277.85
    - type III 277.86
  - glycolic 271.8
  - methylmalonic 270.3
    - with glycinemia 270.7
  - organic 270.9
  - orotic (congenital) (hereditary) (pyrimidine deficiency) 281.4
- **Acladiosis** 111.8
  - skin 111.8
- **Aclasis**
  - diaphyseal 756.4
  - tarsoepiphyseal 756.59
- **Acleistocardia** 745.5
- **Aclusion** 524.4
- **Acmesthesia** 782.0
- **Acne** (pustular) (vulgaris) 706.1
  - agminata (*see also* Tuberculosis) 017.0 ☑
  - artificialis 706.1
  - atrophica 706.0
  - cachecticorum (Hebra) 706.1
  - conglobata 706.1
  - conjunctiva 706.1
  - cystic 706.1
  - decalvans 704.09
  - erythematosa 695.3
  - eyelid 706.1
  - frontalis 706.0
  - indurata 706.1
  - keloid 706.1
  - lupoid 706.0
  - necrotic, necrotica 706.0
    - miliaris 704.8
  - neonatal 706.1 ●
  - nodular 706.1
  - occupational 706.1
  - papulosa 706.1
  - rodens 706.0
  - rosacea 695.3
  - scorbutica 267
  - scrofulosorum (Bazin) (*see also* Tuberculosis) 017.0 ☑
  - summer 692.72
  - tropical 706.1
  - varioliformis 706.0
- **Acneiform drug eruptions** 692.3
- **Acnitis** (primary) (*see also* Tuberculosis) 017.0 ☑
- **Acomia** 704.00
- **Acontractile bladder** 344.61
- **Aconuresis** (*see also* Incontinence) 788.30
- **Acosta's disease** 993.2
- **Acousma** 780.1
- **Acoustic** — *see* condition
- **Acousticophobia** 300.29
- **Acquired** — *see* condition
- **Acquired immune deficiency syndrome** — *see* Human immunodeficiency virus (disease) (illness) (infection)
- **Acquired immunodeficiency syndrome** — *see* Human immunodeficiency virus (disease) (illness) (infection)
- **Acragnosis** 781.99
- **Acrania** 740.0
- **Acroagnosis** 781.99
- **Acroasphyxia, chronic** 443.89
- **Acrobrachycephaly** 756.0
- **Acrobystiolith** 608.89
- **Acrobystitis** 607.2
- **Acrocephalopolysyndactyly** 755.55
- **Acrocephalosyndactyly** 755.55
- **Acrocephaly** 756.0
- **Acrochondrohyperplasia** 759.82
- **Acrocyanosis** 443.89
  - newborn 770.83
    - meaning transient blue hands and feet — *omit code* ●
- **Acrodermatitis** 686.8
  - atrophicans (chronica) 701.8
  - continua (Hallopeau) 696.1
  - enteropathica 686.8
  - Hallopeau's 696.1
  - perstans 696.1
  - pustulosa continua 696.1
  - recalcitrant pustular 696.1
- **Acrodynia** 985.0
- **Acrodysplasia** 755.55
- **Acrohyperhidrosis** (*see also* Hyperhidrosis) 780.8
- **Acrokeratosis verruciformis** 757.39
- **Acromastitis** 611.0
- **Acromegaly, acromegalia** (skin) 253.0
- **Acromelalgia** 443.82 ▲
- **Acromicria, acromikria** 756.59
- **Acronyx** 703.0
- **Acropachy, thyroid** (*see also* Thyrotoxicosis) 242.9 ☑
- **Acropachyderma** 757.39
- **Acroparesthesia** 443.89
  - simple (Schultz's type) 443.89
  - vasomotor (Nothnagel's type) 443.89
- **Acropathy thyroid** (*see also* Thyrotoxicosis) 242.9 ☑
- **Acrophobia** 300.29
- **Acroposthitis** 607.2
- **Acroscleriasis** (*see also* Scleroderma) 710.1
- **Acroscleroderma** (*see also* Scleroderma) 710.1
- **Acrosclerosis** (*see also* Scleroderma) 710.1
- **Acrosphacelus** 785.4
- **Acrosphenosyndactylia** 755.55
- **Acrospiroma, eccrine** (M8402/0) — *see* Neoplasm, skin, benign
- **Acrostealgia** 732.9
- **Acrosyndactyly** (*see also* Syndactylism) 755.10
- **Acrotrophodynia** 991.4
- **Actinic** — *see also* condition
  - cheilitis (due to sun) 692.72
    - chronic NEC 692.74
    - due to radiation, except from sun 692.82
  - conjunctivitis 370.24
  - dermatitis (due to sun) (*see also* Dermatitis, actinic) 692.70
    - due to
      - roentgen rays or radioactive substance 692.82
      - ultraviolet radiation, except from sun 692.82
        - sun NEC 692.70
  - elastosis solare 692.74
  - granuloma 692.73
  - keratitis 370.24
  - ophthalmia 370.24
  - reticuloid 692.73
- **Actinobacillosis, general** 027.8
- **Actinobacillus**
  - lignieresii 027.8
  - mallei 024
  - muris 026.1
- **Actinocutitis** NEC (*see also* Dermatitis, actinic) 692.70
- **Actinodermatitis** NEC (*see also* Dermatitis, actinic) 692.70
- **Actinomyces**
  - israelii (infection) — *see* Actinomycosis
  - muris-ratti (infection) 026.1
- **Actinomycosis, actinomycotic** 039.9
  - with
    - pneumonia 039.1
  - abdominal 039.2
  - cervicofacial 039.3
  - cutaneous 039.0
  - pulmonary 039.1
  - specified site NEC 039.8
  - thoracic 039.1
- **Actinoneuritis** 357.89
- **Action, heart**
  - disorder 427.9
    - postoperative 997.1
  - irregular 427.9
    - postoperative 997.1
    - psychogenic 306.2
- **Active** — *see* condition
- **Activity decrease, functional** 780.99
- **Acute** — *see also* condition
  - abdomen NEC 789.0 ☑
  - gallbladder (*see also* Cholecystitis, acute) 575.0
- **Acyanoblepsia** 368.53
- **Acyanopsia** 368.53
- **Acystia** 753.8
- **Acystinervia** — *see* Neurogenic, bladder
- **Acystineuria** — *see* Neurogenic, bladder

☑ Additional Digit Required — Refer to the Tabular List (Numeric Code Section) for Additional Digit Selection

▶◀ Revised Text ● New Line ▲ Revised Code

Adactylia, adactyly (congenital) 755.4
lower limb (complete) (intercalary) (partial) (terminal) (*see also* Deformity, reduction, lower limb) 755.39
meaning all digits (complete) (partial) 755.31
transverse (complete) (partial) 755.31
upper limb (complete) (intercalary) (partial) (terminal) (*see also* Deformity, reduction, upper limb) 755.29
meaning all digits (complete) (partial) 755.21
transverse (complete) (partial) 755.21
Adair-Dighton syndrome (brittle bones and blue sclera, deafness) 756.51
Adamantinoblastoma (M9310/0) — *see* Ameloblastoma
Adamantinoma (M9310/0) — *see* Ameloblastoma
Adamantoblastoma (M9310/0) — *see* Ameloblastoma
Adams-Stokes (-Morgagni) disease or syndrome (syncope with heart block) 426.9
Adaptation reaction (*see also* Reaction, adjustment) 309.9
Addiction — *see also* Dependence
absinthe 304.6 ☑
alcoholic (ethyl) (methyl) (wood) 303.9 ☑
complicating pregnancy, childbirth, or puerperium 648.4 ☑
affecting fetus or newborn 760.71
suspected damage to fetus affecting management of pregnancy 655.4 ☑
drug (*see also* Dependence) 304.9 ☑
ethyl alcohol 303.9 ☑
heroin 304.0 ☑
hospital 301.51
methyl alcohol 303.9 ☑
methylated spirit 303.9 ☑
morphine (-like substances) 304.0 ☑
nicotine 305.1
opium 304.0 ☑
tobacco 305.1
wine 303.9 ☑
Addison's
anemia (pernicious) 281.0
disease (bronze) (primary adrenal insufficiency) 255.4
tuberculous (*see also* Tuberculosis) 017.6 ☑
keloid (morphea) 701.0
melanoderma (adrenal cortical hypofunction) 255.4
Addison-Biermer anemia (pernicious) 281.0
Addison-Gull disease — *see* Xanthoma
Addisonian crisis or melanosis (acute adrenocortical insufficiency) 255.4
Additional — *see also* Accessory
chromosome(s) 758.5
13-15 758.1
16-18 758.2
21 758.0
autosome(s) NEC 758.5
sex 758.81
Adduction contracture, hip or other joint — *see* Contraction, joint
ADEM (acute disseminated encephalomyelitis) (postinfectious) 136.9 *[323.6]* ●
infectious 323.6 ●
noninfectious 323.8 ●
Adenasthenia gastrica 536.0
Aden fever 061
Adenitis (*see also* Lymphadenitis) 289.3
acute, unspecified site 683
epidemic infectious 075
axillary 289.3
acute 683
chronic or subacute 289.1
Bartholin's gland 616.8
bulbourethral gland (*see also* Urethritis) 597.89
cervical 289.3
acute 683
chronic or subacute 289.1
chancroid (Ducrey's bacillus) 099.0
chronic (any lymph node, except mesenteric) 289.1
mesenteric 289.2
Cowper's gland (*see also* Urethritis) 597.89

Adenitis — *continued*
epidemic, acute 075
gangrenous 683
gonorrheal NEC 098.89
groin 289.3
acute 683
chronic or subacute 289.1
infectious 075
inguinal (region) 289.3
acute 683
chronic or subacute 289.1
lymph gland or node, except mesenteric 289.3
acute 683
chronic or subacute 289.1
mesenteric (acute) (chronic) (nonspecific) (subacute) 289.2
mesenteric (acute) (chronic) (nonspecific) (subacute) 289.2
due to Pasteurella multocida (P. septica) 027.2
parotid gland (suppurative) 527.2
phlegmonous 683
salivary duct or gland (any) (recurring) (suppurative) 527.2
scrofulous (*see also* Tuberculosis) 017.2 ☑
septic 289.3
Skene's duct or gland (*see also* Urethritis) 597.89
strumous, tuberculous (*see also* Tuberculosis) 017.2 ☑
subacute, unspecified site 289.1
sublingual gland (suppurative) 527.2
submandibular gland (suppurative) 527.2
submaxillary gland (suppurative) 527.2
suppurative 683
tuberculous — *see* Tuberculosis, lymph gland
urethral gland (*see also* Urethritis) 597.89
venereal NEC 099.8
Wharton's duct (suppurative) 527.2
Adenoacanthoma (M8570/3) — *see* Neoplasm, by site, malignant
Adenoameloblastoma (M9300/0) 213.1
upper jaw (bone) 213.0
Adenocarcinoma (M8140/3) — *see also* Neoplasm, by site, malignant

Note — The list of adjectival modifiers below is not exhaustive. A description of adenocarcinoma that does not appear in this list should be coded in the same manner as carcinoma with that description. Thus, "mixed acidophil-basophil adenocarcinoma," should be coded in the same manner as "mixed acidophil-basophil carcinoma," which appears in the list under "Carcinoma."

Except where otherwise indicated, the morphological varieties of adenocarcinoma in the list below should be coded by site as for "Neoplasm, malignant."

with
apocrine metaplasia (M8573/3)
cartilaginous (and osseous) metaplasia (M8571/3)
osseous (and cartilaginous) metaplasia (M8571/3)
spindle cell metaplasia (M8572/3)
squamous metaplasia (M8570/3)
acidophil (M8280/3)
specified site — *see* Neoplasm, by site, malignant
unspecified site 194.3
acinar (M8550/3)
acinic cell (M8550/3)
adrenal cortical (M8370/3) 194.0
alveolar (M8251/3)
and
epidermoid carcinoma, mixed (M8560/3)
squamous cell carcinoma, mixed (M8560/3)
apocrine (M8401/3)
breast — *see* Neoplasm, breast, malignant
specified site NEC — *see* Neoplasm, skin, malignant
unspecified site 173.9

Adenocarcinoma (M8140/3) — *continued*
basophil (M8300/3)
specified site — *see* Neoplasm, by site, malignant
unspecified site 194.3
bile duct type (M8160/3)
liver 155.1
specified site NEC — *see* Neoplasm, by site, malignant
unspecified site 155.1
bronchiolar (M8250/3) — *see* Neoplasm, lung, malignant
ceruminous (M8420/3) 173.2
chromophobe (M8270/3)
specified site — *see* Neoplasm, by site, malignant
unspecified site 194.3
clear cell (mesonephroid type) (M8310/3)
colloid (M8480/3)
cylindroid type (M8200/3)
diffuse type (M8145/3)
specified site — *see* Neoplasm, by site, malignant
unspecified site 151.9
duct (infiltrating) (M8500/3)
with Paget's disease (M8541/3) — *see* Neoplasm, breast, malignant
specified site — *see* Neoplasm, by site, malignant
unspecified site 174.9
embryonal (M9070/3)
endometrioid (M8380/3) — *see* Neoplasm, by site, malignant
eosinophil (M8280/3)
specified site — *see* Neoplasm, by site, malignant
unspecified site 194.3
follicular (M8330/3)
and papillary (M8340/3) 193
moderately differentiated type (M8332/3) 193
pure follicle type (M8331/3) 193
specified site — *see* Neoplasm, by site, malignant
trabecular type (M8332/3) 193
unspecified type 193
well differentiated type (M8331/3) 193
gelatinous (M8480/3)
granular cell (M8320/3)
Hürthle cell (M8290/3) 193
in
adenomatous
polyp (M8210/3)
polyposis coli (M8220/3) 153.9
polypoid adenoma (M8210/3)
tubular adenoma (M8210/3)
villous adenoma (M8261/3)
infiltrating duct (M8500/3)
with Paget's disease (M8541/3) — *see* Neoplasm, breast, malignant
specified site — *see* Neoplasm, by site, malignant
unspecified site 174.9
inflammatory (M8530/3)
specified site — *see* Neoplasm, by site, malignant
unspecified site 174.9
in situ (M8140/2) — *see* Neoplasm, by site, in situ
intestinal type (M8144/3)
specified site — *see* Neoplasm, by site, malignant
unspecified site 151.9
intraductal (noninfiltrating) (M8500/2)
papillary (M8503/2)
specified site — *see* Neoplasm, by site, in situ
unspecified site 233.0
specified site — *see* Neoplasm, by site, in situ
unspecified site 233.0
islet cell (M8150/3)
and exocrine, mixed (M8154/3)
specified site — *see* Neoplasm, by site, malignant
unspecified site 157.9
pancreas 157.4

Adenocarcinoma (M8140/3) — *continued*
- islet cell — *continued*
  - specified site NEC — *see* Neoplasm, by site, malignant
  - unspecified site 157.4
- lobular (M8520/3)
  - specified site — *see* Neoplasm, by site, malignant
  - unspecified site 174.9
- medullary (M8510/3)
- mesonephric (M9110/3)
- mixed cell (M8323/3)
- mucinous (M8480/3)
- mucin-producing (M8481/3)
- mucoid (M8480/3) — *see* also Neoplasm, by site, malignant
  - cell (M8300/3)
    - specified site — *see* Neoplasm, by site, malignant
    - unspecified site 194.3
- nonencapsulated sclerosing (M8350/3) 193
- oncocytic (M8290/3)
- oxyphilic (M8290/3)
- papillary (M8260/3)
  - and follicular (M8340/3) 193
  - intraductal (noninfiltrating) (M8503/2)
    - specified site — *see* Neoplasm, by site, in situ
    - unspecified site 233.0
  - serous (M8460/3)
    - specified site — *see* Neoplasm, by site, malignant
    - unspecified site 183.0
- papillocystic (M8450/3)
  - specified site — *see* Neoplasm, by site, malignant
  - unspecified site 183.0
- pseudomucinous (M8470/3)
  - specified site — *see* Neoplasm, by site, malignant
  - unspecified site 183.0
- renal cell (M8312/3) 189.0
- sebaceous (M8410/3)
- serous (M8441/3) — *see also* Neoplasm, by site, malignant
  - papillary
    - specified site — *see* Neoplasm, by site, malignant
    - unspecified site 183.0
- signet ring cell (M8490/3)
- superficial spreading (M8143/3)
- sweat gland (M8400/3) — *see* Neoplasm, skin, malignant
- trabecular (M8190/3)
- tubular (M8211/3)
- villous (M8262/3)
- water-clear cell (M8322/3) 194.1

Adenofibroma (M9013/0)
- clear cell (M8313/0) — *see* Neoplasm, by site, benign
- endometrioid (M8381/0) 220
  - borderline malignancy (M8381/1) 236.2
  - malignant (M8381/3) 183.0
- mucinous (M9015/0)
  - specified site — *see* Neoplasm, by site, benign
  - unspecified site 220
- prostate 600.20
  - with urinary retention 600.21
- serous (M9014/0)
  - specified site — *see* Neoplasm, by site, benign
  - unspecified site 220
- specified site — *see* Neoplasm, by site, benign
- unspecified site 220

Adenofibrosis
- breast 610.2
- endometrioid 617.0

Adenoiditis 474.01
- acute 463
- chronic 474.01
  - with chronic tonsillitis 474.02

Adenoids (congenital) (of nasal fossa) 474.9
- hypertrophy 474.12
- vegetations 474.2

Adenolipomatosis (symmetrical) 272.8

Adenolymphoma (M8561/0)
- specified site — *see* Neoplasm, by site, benign
- unspecified 210.2

Adenoma (sessile) (M8140/0) — *see* also Neoplasm, by site, benign

> *Note — Except where otherwise indicated, the morphological varieties of adenoma in the list below should be coded by site as for "Neoplasm, benign."*

- acidophil (M8280/0)
  - specified site — *see* Neoplasm, by site, benign
  - unspecified site 227.3
- acinar (cell) (M8550/0)
- acinic cell (M8550/0)
- adrenal (cortex) (cortical) (functioning) (M8370/0) 227.0
  - clear cell type (M8373/0) 227.0
  - compact cell type (M8371/0) 227.0
  - glomerulosa cell type (M8374/0) 227.0
  - heavily pigmented variant (M8372/0) 227.0
  - mixed cell type (M8375/0) 227.0
- alpha cell (M8152/0)
  - pancreas 211.7
  - specified site NEC — *see* Neoplasm, by site, benign
  - unspecified site 211.7
- alveolar (M8251/0)
- apocrine (M8401/0)
  - breast 217
  - specified site NEC — *see* Neoplasm, skin, benign
  - unspecified site 216.9
- basal cell (M8147/0)
- basophil (M8300/0)
  - specified site — *see* Neoplasm, by site, benign
  - unspecified site 227.3
- beta cell (M8151/0)
  - pancreas 211.7
  - specified site NEC — *see* Neoplasm, by site, benign
  - unspecified site 211.7
- bile duct (M8160/0) 211.5
- black (M8372/0) 227.0
- bronchial (M8140/1) 235.7
  - carcinoid type (M8240/3) — *see* Neoplasm, lung, malignant
  - cylindroid type (M8200/3) — *see* Neoplasm, lung, malignant
- ceruminous (M8420/0) 216.2
- chief cell (M8321/0) 227.1
- chromophobe (M8270/0)
  - specified site — *see* Neoplasm, by site, benign
  - unspecified site 227.3
- clear cell (M8310/0)
- colloid (M8334/0)
  - specified site — *see* Neoplasm, by site, benign
  - unspecified site 226
- cylindroid type, bronchus (M8200/3) — *see* Neoplasm, lung, malignant
- duct (M8503/0)
- embryonal (M8191/0)
- endocrine, multiple (M8360/1)
  - single specified site — *see* Neoplasm, by site, uncertain behavior
  - two or more specified sites 237.4
  - unspecified site 237.4
- endometrioid (M8380/0) — *see* also Neoplasm, by site, benign
  - borderline malignancy (M8380/1) — *see* Neoplasm, by site, uncertain behavior
- eosinophil (M8280/0)
  - specified site — *see* Neoplasm, by site, benign
  - unspecified site 227.3
- fetal (M8333/0)
  - specified site — *see* Neoplasm, by site, benign
  - unspecified site 226
- follicular (M8330/0)
  - specified site — *see* Neoplasm, by site, benign
  - unspecified site 226

Adenoma (M8140/0) — *see also* Neoplasm, by site, benign — *continued*
- hepatocellular (M8170/0) 211.5
- Hürthle cell (M8290/0) 226
- intracystic papillary (M8504/0)
- islet cell (functioning) (M8150/0)
  - pancreas 211.7
  - specified site NEC — *see* Neoplasm, by site, benign
  - unspecified site 211.7
- liver cell (M8170/0) 211.5
- macrofollicular (M8334/0)
  - specified site NEC — *see* Neoplasm, by site, benign
  - unspecified site 226
- malignant, malignum (M8140/3) — *see* Neoplasm, by site, malignant
- mesonephric (M9110/0)
- microfollicular (M8333/0)
  - specified site — *see* Neoplasm, by site, benign
  - unspecified site 226
- mixed cell (M8323/0)
- monomorphic (M8146/0)
- mucinous (M8480/0)
- mucoid cell (M8300/0)
  - specified site — *see* Neoplasm, by site, benign
  - unspecified site 227.3
- multiple endocrine (M8360/1)
  - single specified site — *see* Neoplasm, by site, uncertain behavior
  - two or more specified sites 237.4
  - unspecified site 237.4
- nipple (M8506/0) 217
- oncocytic (M8290/0)
- oxyphilic (M8290/0)
- papillary (M8260/0) — *see* also Neoplasm, by site, benign
  - intracystic (M8504/0)
- papillotubular (M8263/0)
- Pick's tubular (M8640/0)
  - specified site — *see* Neoplasm, by site, benign
  - unspecified site
    - female 220
    - male 222.0
- pleomorphic (M8940/0)
- polypoid (M8210/0)
- prostate (benign) 600.20
  - with urinary retention 600.21
- rete cell 222.0
- sebaceous, sebaceum (gland) (senile) (M8410/0) — *see* also Neoplasm, skin, benign
  - disseminata 759.5
- Sertoli cell (M8640/0)
  - specified site — *see* Neoplasm, by site, benign
  - unspecified site
    - female 220
    - male 222.0
- skin appendage (M8390/0) — *see* Neoplasm, skin, benign
- sudoriferous gland (M8400/0) — *see* Neoplasm, skin, benign
- sweat gland or duct (M8400/0) — *see* Neoplasm, skin, benign
- testicular (M8640/0)
  - specified site — *see* Neoplasm, by site, benign
  - unspecified site
    - female 220
    - male 222.0
- thyroid 226
- trabecular (M8190/0)
- tubular (M8211/0) — *see* also Neoplasm, by site, benign
  - papillary (M8460/3)
  - Pick's (M8640/0)
    - specified site — *see* Neoplasm, by site, benign
    - unspecified site
      - female 220
      - male 222.0
- tubulovillous (M8263/0)
- villoglandular (M8263/0)
- villous (M8261/1) — *see* Neoplasm, by site, uncertain behavior

☑ Additional Digit Required — Refer to the Tabular List (Numeric Code Section) for Additional Digit Selection

▶◀ Revised Text ● New Line ▲ Revised Code

☑ Additional Digit Required — Refer to the Tabular List (Numeric Code Section) for Additional Digit Selection
▶◀ Revised Text ● New Line ▲ Revised Code

- **Admission** — *continued*
  - for — *continued*
    - vaccination, prophylactic — *continued*
      - plague V03.3
      - pneumonia V03.82
      - poliomyelitis V04.0
        - with diphtheria-tetanus-pertussis (DTP+ polio) V06.3
      - rabies V04.5
      - respiratory syncytial virus (RSV) V04.82
      - rubella alone V04.3
        - with measles and mumps (MMR) V06.4
      - smallpox V04.1
      - specified type NEC V05.8
      - Streptococcus pneumoniae [pneumococcus] V03.82
        - with
          - influenza V06.6
      - tetanus toxoid alone V03.7
        - with diphtheria [Td] [DT] V06.5
          - and pertussis (DTP) (DTaP) V06.1
      - tuberculosis (BCG) V03.2
      - tularemia V03.4
      - typhoid alone V03.1
        - with diphtheria-tetanus-pertussis (TAB + DTP) V06.2
      - typhoid-paratyphoid alone (TAB) V03.1
      - typhus V05.8
      - varicella (chicken pox) V05.4
      - viral encephalitis, arthropod-borne V05.0
      - viral hepatitis V05.3
      - yellow fever V04.4
    - vasectomy V25.2
    - vasoplasty for previous sterilization V26.0
    - vision examination V72.0
    - vocational therapy V57.22
    - waiting period for admission to other facility V63.2
      - undergoing social agency investigation V63.8
    - well baby and child care V20.2
    - x-ray of chest
      - for suspected tuberculosis V71.2
      - routine V72.5
- **Adnexitis** (suppurative) (*see also* Salpingo-oophoritis) 614.2
- **Adolescence** NEC V21.2
- **Adoption**
  - agency referral V68.89
  - examination V70.3
  - held for V68.89
- **Adrenal gland** — *see* condition
- **Adrenalism** 255.9
  - tuberculous (*see also* Tuberculosis) 017.6 ☑
- **Adrenalitis, adrenitis** 255.8
  - meningococcal hemorrhagic 036.3
- **Adrenarche, precocious** 259.1
- **Adrenocortical syndrome** 255.2
- **Adrenogenital syndrome** (acquired) (congenital) 255.2
  - iatrogenic, fetus or newborn 760.79
- **Adrenoleukodystrophy** 277.86
  - neonatal 277.86
  - x-linked 277.86
- **Adrenomyeloneuropathy** 277.86
- **Adventitious bursa** — *see* Bursitis
- **Adynamia** (episodica) (hereditary) (periodic) 359.3
- **Adynamic**
  - ileus or intestine (*see also* Ileus) 560.1
  - ureter 753.22
- **Aeration lung, imperfect, newborn** 770.5
- **Aerobullosis** 993.3
- **Aerocele** — *see* Embolism, air
- **Aerodermectasia**
  - subcutaneous (traumatic) 958.7
    - surgical 998.81
  - surgical 998.81
- **Aerodontalgia** 993.2
- **Aeroembolism** 993.3
- **Aerogenes capsulatus infection** (*see also* Gangrene, gas) 040.0
- **Aero-otitis media** 993.0
- **Aerophagy, aerophagia** 306.4
  - psychogenic 306.4
- **Aerosinusitis** 993.1
- **Aerotitis** 993.0
- **Affection, affections** — *see also* Disease
  - sacroiliac (joint), old 724.6
  - shoulder region NEC 726.2
- **Afibrinogenemia** 286.3
  - acquired 286.6
  - congenital 286.3
  - postpartum 666.3 ☑
- **African**
  - sleeping sickness 086.5
  - tick fever 087.1
  - trypanosomiasis 086.5
    - Gambian 086.3
    - Rhodesian 086.4
- **Aftercare** V58.9
  - artificial openings — *see* Attention to, artificial, opening
  - blood transfusion without reported diagnosis V58.2
  - breathing exercise V57.0
  - cardiac device V53.39
    - defibrillator, automatic implantable V53.32
    - pacemaker V53.31
      - carotid sinus V53.39
  - carotid sinus pacemaker V53.39
  - cerebral ventricle (communicating) shunt V53.01
  - chemotherapy session (adjunctive) (maintenance) V58.11 ▲
  - defibrillator, automatic implantable cardiac V53.32
  - exercise (remedial) (therapeutic) V57.1
    - breathing V57.0
  - extracorporeal dialysis (intermittent) (treatment) V56.0
  - following surgery NEC V58.49
    - for
      - injury V58.43
      - neoplasm V58.42
      - organ transplant V58.44
      - trauma V58.43
    - joint replacement V54.81
    - of
      - circulatory system V58.73
      - digestive system V58.75
      - genital organs V58.76
      - genitourinary system V58.76
      - musculoskeletal system V58.78
      - nervous system V58.72
      - oral cavity V58.75
      - respiratory system V58.74
      - sense organs V58.71
      - skin V58.77
      - subcutaneous tissue V58.77
      - teeth V58.75
      - urinary system V58.76
    - wound closure, planned V58.41
  - fracture V54.9
    - healing V54.89
      - pathologic
        - ankle V54.29
        - arm V54.20
          - lower V54.22
          - upper V54.21
        - finger V54.29
        - foot V54.29
        - hand V54.29
        - hip V54.23
        - leg V54.24
          - lower V54.26
          - upper V54.25
        - pelvis V54.29
        - specified site NEC V54.29
        - toe(s) V54.29
        - vertebrae V54.27
        - wrist V54.29
      - traumatic
        - ankle V54.19
        - arm V54.10
          - lower V54.12
          - upper V54.11
        - finger V54.19
        - foot V54.19
- **Aftercare** — *continued*
  - fracture — *continued*
    - healing — *continued*
      - traumatic — *continued*
        - hand V54.19
        - hip V54.13
        - leg V54.14
          - lower V54.16
          - upper V54.15
        - pelvis V54.19
        - specified site NEC V54.19
        - toe(s) V54.19
        - vertebrae V54.17
        - wrist V54.19
    - removal of
      - external fixation device V54.89
      - internal fixation device V54.01
    - specified care NEC V54.89
  - gait training V57.1
    - for use of artificial limb(s) V57.81
  - internal fixation device V54.09
  - involving
    - dialysis (intermittent) (treatment)
      - extracorporeal V56.0
      - peritoneal V56.8
      - renal V56.0
    - gait training V57.1
      - for use of artificial limb(s) V57.81
    - growth rod
      - adjustment V54.02
      - lengthening V54.02
    - internal fixation device V54.09
    - orthoptic training V57.4
    - orthotic training V57.81
    - radiotherapy session V58.0
    - removal of
      - dressings V58.3
      - fixation device
        - external V54.89
        - internal V54.01
      - fracture plate V54.01
      - pins V54.01
      - plaster cast V54.89
      - rods V54.01
      - screws V54.01
      - surgical dressings V58.3
      - sutures V58.3
      - traction device, external V54.89
  - neuropacemaker (brain) (peripheral nerve) (spinal cord) V53.02
  - occupational therapy V57.21
  - orthodontic V58.5
  - orthopedic V54.9
    - change of external fixation or traction device V54.89
    - following joint replacement V54.81
    - internal fixation device V54.09
    - removal of fixation device
      - external V54.89
      - internal V54.01
    - specified care NEC V54.89
  - orthoptic training V57.4
  - orthotic training V57.81
  - pacemaker
    - brain V53.02
    - cardiac V53.31
    - carotid sinus V53.39
    - peripheral nerve V53.02
    - spinal cord V53.02
  - peritoneal dialysis (intermittent) (treatment) V56.8
  - physical therapy NEC V57.1
    - breathing exercises V57.0
  - radiotherapy session V58.0
  - rehabilitation procedure V57.9
    - breathing exercises V57.0
    - multiple types V57.89
    - occupational V57.21
    - orthoptic V57.4
    - orthotic V57.81
    - physical therapy NEC V57.1
    - remedial exercises V57.1
    - specified type NEC V57.89
    - speech V57.3
    - therapeutic exercises V57.1
    - vocational V57.22
  - renal dialysis (intermittent) (treatment) V56.0

☑ Additional Digit Required — Refer to the Tabular List (Numeric Code Section) for Additional Digit Selection

▶◀ Revised Text ● New Line ▲ Revised Code

☑ Additional Digit Required — Refer to the Tabular List (Numeric Code Section) for Additional Digit Selection
▶◀ Revised Text ● New Line ▲ Revised Code

Aleukia — *continued*
  hemorrhagica 284.9
    acquired (secondary) 284.8
    congenital 284.0
    idiopathic 284.9
  splenica 289.4
Alexia (congenital) (developmental) 315.01
  secondary to organic lesion 784.61
Algoneurodystrophy 733.7
Algophobia 300.29
Alibert's disease (mycosis fungoides) (M9700/3) 202.1 ☑
Alibert-Bazin disease (M9700/3) 202.1 ☑
Alice in Wonderland syndrome 293.89
Alienation, mental (*see also* Psychosis) 298.9
Alkalemia 276.3
Alkalosis 276.3
  metabolic 276.3
    with respiratory acidosis 276.4
  respiratory 276.3
Alkaptonuria 270.2
Allen-Masters syndrome 620.6
Allergic bronchopulmonary aspergillosis 518.6
Allergy, allergic (reaction) 995.3
  air-borne substance (*see* also Fever, hay) 477.9
    specified allergen NEC 477.8
  alveolitis (extrinsic) 495.9
    due to
      Aspergillus clavatus 495.4
      cryptostroma corticale 495.6
      organisms (fungal, thermophilic actinomycete, other) growing in ventilation (air conditioning systems) 495.7
    specified type NEC 495.8
  anaphylactic shock 999.4
    due to food — *see* Anaphylactic shock, due to, food
  angioneurotic edema 995.1
  animal (cat) (dog) (epidermal) 477.8
    dander 477.2
    hair 477.2
  arthritis (*see also* Arthritis, allergic) 716.2 ☑
  asthma — *see* Asthma
  bee sting (anaphylactic shock) 989.5
  biological — *see* Allergy, drug
  bronchial asthma — *see* Asthma
  conjunctivitis (eczematous) 372.14
  dander, animal (cat) (dog) 477.2
  dandruff 477.8
  dermatitis (venenata) — *see* Dermatitis
  diathesis V15.09
  drug, medicinal substance, and biological (any) (correct medicinal substance properly administered) (external) (internal) 995.2
    wrong substance given or taken NEC 977.9
      specified drug or substance — *see* Table of Drugs and Chemicals
  dust (house) (stock) 477.8
  eczema — *see* Eczema
  endophthalmitis 360.19
  epidermal (animal) 477.8
  feathers 477.8
  food (any) (ingested) 693.1
    atopic 691.8
    in contact with skin 692.5
  gastritis 535.4 ☑
  gastroenteritis 558.3
  gastrointestinal 558.3
  grain 477.0
  grass (pollen) 477.0
    asthma (*see also* Asthma) 493.0 ☑
    hay fever 477.0
  hair, animal (cat) (dog) 477.2
  hay fever (grass) (pollen) (ragweed) (tree) (*see also* Fever, hay) 477.9
  history (of) V15.09
    to
      eggs V15.03
      food additives V15.05
      insect bite V15.06
      latex V15.07
      milk products V15.02

Allergy, allergic — *continued*
  history — *continued*
    to — *continued*
      nuts V15.05
        peanuts V15.01
      radiographic dye V15.08
      seafood V15.04
      specified food NEC V15.05
      spider bite V15.06
  horse serum — see Allergy, serum
  inhalant 477.9
    dust 477.8
    pollen 477.0
    specified allergen other than pollen 477.8
  kapok 477.8
  medicine — *see* Allergy, drug
  migraine 346.2 ☑
  milk protein 558.3
  pannus 370.62
  pneumonia 518.3
  pollen (any) (hay fever) 477.0
    asthma (*see also* Asthma) 493.0 ☑
  primrose 477.0
  primula 477.0
  purpura 287.0
  ragweed (pollen) (Senecio jacobae) 477.0
    asthma (*see also* Asthma) 493.0 ☑
    hay fever 477.0
  respiratory (*see also* Allergy, inhalant) 477.9
    due to
      drug — *see* Allergy, drug
      food — *see* Allergy, food
  rhinitis (*see also* Fever, hay) 477.9
    due to food 477.1
  rose 477.0
  Senecio jacobae 477.0
  serum (prophylactic) (therapeutic) 999.5
    anaphylactic shock 999.4
  shock (anaphylactic) (due to adverse effect of correct medicinal substance properly administered) 995.0
    food — *see* Anaphylactic shock, due to, food
    from serum or immunization 999.5
      anaphylactic 999.4
  sinusitis (*see also* Fever, hay) 477.9
  skin reaction 692.9
    specified substance — *see* Dermatitis, due to
  tree (any) (hay fever) (pollen) 477.0
    asthma (*see also* Asthma) 493.0 ☑
  upper respiratory (*see also* Fever, hay) 477.9
  urethritis 597.89
  urticaria 708.0
  vaccine — *see* Allergy, serum
Allescheriosis 117.6
Alligator skin disease (ichthyosis congenita) 757.1
  acquired 701.1
Allocheiria, allochiria (*see also* Disturbance, sensation) 782.0
Almeida's disease (Brazilian blastomycosis) 116.1
Alopecia (atrophicans) (pregnancy) (premature) (senile) 704.00
  adnata 757.4
  areata 704.01
  celsi 704.01
  cicatrisata 704.09
  circumscripta 704.01
  congenital, congenitalis 757.4
  disseminata 704.01
  effluvium (telogen) 704.02
  febrile 704.09
  generalisata 704.09
  hereditaria 704.09
  marginalis 704.01
  mucinosa 704.09
  postinfectional 704.09
  seborrheica 704.09
  specific 091.82
  syphilitic (secondary) 091.82
  telogen effluvium 704.02
  totalis 704.09
  toxica 704.09
  universalis 704.09
  x-ray 704.09
Alpers' disease 330.8

Alpha-lipoproteinemia 272.4
Alpha thalassemia 282.49
Alphos 696.1
Alpine sickness 993.2
Alport's syndrome (hereditary hematurianephropathy-deafness) 759.89
Alteration (of), **altered**
  awareness 780.09
    transient 780.02
  consciousness 780.09
    persistent vegetative state 780.03
    transient 780.02
  mental status 780.99
    amnesia (retrograde) 780.93
    memory loss 780.93
Alternaria (infection) 118
Alternating — *see* condition
Altitude, high (effects) — *see* Effect, adverse, high altitude
Aluminosis (of lung) 503
Alvarez syndrome (transient cerebral ischemia) 435.9
Alveolar capillary block syndrome 516.3
Alveolitis
  allergic (extrinsic) 495.9
    due to organisms (fungal, thermophilic actinomycete, other) growing in ventilation (air conditioning systems) 495.7
    specified type NEC 495.8
  due to
    Aspergillus clavatus 495.4
    Cryptostroma corticale 495.6
  fibrosing (chronic) (cryptogenic) (lung) 516.3
    idiopathic 516.3
    rheumatoid 714.81
  jaw 526.5
  sicca dolorosa 526.5
Alveolus, alveolar — *see* condition
Alymphocytosis (pure) 279.2
Alymphoplasia, thymic 279.2
Alzheimer's
  dementia (senile)
    with behavioral disturbance 331.0 *[294.11]*
    without behavioral disturbance 331.0 *[294.10]*
  disease or sclerosis 331.0
    with dementia — *see* Alzheimer's, dementia
Amastia (*see also* Absence, breast) 611.8
Amaurosis (acquired) (congenital) (*see also* Blindness) 369.00
  fugax 362.34
  hysterical 300.11
  Leber's (congenital) 362.76
  tobacco 377.34
  uremic — *see* Uremia
Amaurotic familial idiocy (infantile) (juvenile) (late) 330.1
Ambisexual 752.7
Amblyopia (acquired) (congenital) (partial) 368.00
  color 368.59
    acquired 368.55
  deprivation 368.02
  ex anopsia 368.00
  hysterical 300.11
  nocturnal 368.60
    vitamin A deficiency 264.5
  refractive 368.03
  strabismic 368.01
  suppression 368.01
  tobacco 377.34
  toxic NEC 377.34
  uremic — *see* Uremia
Ameba, amebic (histolytica) — *see also* Amebiasis
  abscess 006.3
    bladder 006.8
    brain (with liver and lung abscess) 006.5
    liver 006.3
      with
        brain abscess (and lung abscess) 006.5
        lung abscess 006.4

☑ Additional Digit Required — Refer to the Tabular List (Numeric Code Section) for Additional Digit Selection
▶◀ Revised Text ● New Line ▲ Revised Code

- **Ameba, amebic** (histolytica) — *see also* Amebiasis — *continued*
  - abscess — *continued*
    - lung (with liver abscess) 006.4
      - with brain abscess 006.5
    - seminal vesicle 006.8
    - spleen 006.8
  - carrier (suspected of) V02.2
  - meningoencephalitis
    - due to Naegleria (gruberi) 136.2
    - primary 136.2
- **Amebiasis** NEC 006.9
  - with
    - brain abscess (with liver or lung abscess) 006.5
    - liver abscess (without mention of brain or lung abscess) 006.3
    - lung abscess (with liver abscess) 006.4
      - with brain abscess 006.5
  - acute 006.0
  - bladder 006.8
  - chronic 006.1
  - cutaneous 006.6
  - cutis 006.6
  - due to organism other than Entamoeba histolytica 007.8
  - hepatic (*see also* Abscess, liver, amebic) 006.3
  - nondysenteric 006.2
  - seminal vesicle 006.8
  - specified
    - organism NEC 007.8
    - site NEC 006.8
- **Ameboma** 006.8
- **Amelia** 755.4
  - lower limb 755.31
  - upper limb 755.21
- **Ameloblastoma** (M9310/0) 213.1
  - jaw (bone) (lower) 213.1
    - upper 213.0
  - long bones (M9261/3) — *see* Neoplasm, bone, malignant
  - malignant (M9310/3) 170.1
    - jaw (bone) (lower) 170.1
      - upper 170.0
  - mandible 213.1
  - tibial (M9261/3) 170.7
- **Amelogenesis imperfecta** 520.5
  - nonhereditaria (segmentalis) 520.4
- **Amenorrhea** (primary) (secondary) 626.0
  - due to ovarian dysfunction 256.8
  - hyperhormonal 256.8
- **Amentia** (*see also* Retardation, mental) 319
  - Meynert's (nonalcoholic) 294.0
    - alcoholic 291.1
  - nevoid 759.6
- **American**
  - leishmaniasis 085.5
  - mountain tick fever 066.1
  - trypanosomiasis — *see* Trypanosomiasis, American
- **Ametropia** (*see also* Disorder, accommodation) 367.9
- **Amianthosis** 501
- **Amimia** 784.69
- **Amino acid**
  - deficiency 270.9
    - anemia 281.4
  - metabolic disorder (*see also* Disorder, amino acid) 270.9
- **Aminoaciduria** 270.9
  - imidazole 270.5
- **Amnesia** (retrograde) 780.93
  - auditory 784.69
    - developmental 315.31
    - secondary to organic lesion 784.69
  - dissociative 300.12
  - hysterical or dissociative type 300.12
  - psychogenic 300.12
  - transient global 437.7
- **Amnestic** (confabulatory) **syndrome** 294.0
  - alcohol-induced persisting 291.1
  - drug-induced persisting 292.83
  - posttraumatic 294.0
- **Amniocentesis screening** (for) V28.2
  - alphafetoprotein level, raised V28.1
  - chromosomal anomalies V28.0
- **Amnion, amniotic** — *see also* condition
  - nodosum 658.8 ☑
- **Amnionitis** (complicating pregnancy) 658.4 ☑
  - affecting fetus or newborn 762.7
- **Amoral trends** 301.7
- **Amotio retinae** (*see also* Detachment, retina) 361.9
- **Ampulla**
  - lower esophagus 530.89
  - phrenic 530.89
- **Amputation**
  - any part of fetus, to facilitate delivery 763.89
  - cervix (supravaginal) (uteri) 622.8
    - in pregnancy or childbirth 654.6 ☑
      - affecting fetus or newborn 763.89
  - clitoris — *see* Wound, open, clitoris
  - congenital
    - lower limb 755.31
    - upper limb 755.21
  - neuroma (traumatic) — *see also* Injury, nerve, by site
    - surgical complication (late) 997.61
  - penis — *see* Amputation, traumatic, penis
  - status (without complication) — *see* Absence, by site, acquired
  - stump (surgical) (posttraumatic)
    - abnormal, painful, or with complication (late) 997.60
    - healed or old NEC — *see also* Absence, by site, acquired
      - lower V49.70
      - upper V49.60
  - traumatic (complete) (partial)

> *Note — "Complicated" includes traumatic amputation with delayed healing, delayed treatment, foreign body, or infection.*

  - arm 887.4
    - at or above elbow 887.2
      - complicated 887.3
    - below elbow 887.0
      - complicated 887.1
    - both (bilateral) (any level(s)) 887.6
      - complicated 887.7
    - complicated 887.5
  - finger(s) (one or both hands) 886.0
    - with thumb(s) 885.0
      - complicated 885.1
    - complicated 886.1
  - foot (except toe(s) only) 896.0
    - and other leg 897.6
      - complicated 897.7
    - both (bilateral) 896.2
      - complicated 896.3
    - complicated 896.1
    - toe(s) only (one or both feet) 895.0
      - complicated 895.1
  - genital organ(s) (external) NEC 878.8
    - complicated 878.9
  - hand (except finger(s) only) 887.0
    - and other arm 887.6
      - complicated 887.7
    - both (bilateral) 887.6
      - complicated 887.7
    - complicated 887.1
    - finger(s) (one or both hands) 886.0
      - with thumb(s) 885.0
        - complicated 885.1
      - complicated 886.1
    - thumb(s) (with fingers of either hand) 885.0
      - complicated 885.1
  - head 874.9
  - late effect — *see* Late, effects (of), amputation
  - leg 897.4
    - and other foot 897.6
      - complicated 897.7
    - at or above knee 897.2
      - complicated 897.3
    - below knee 897.0
      - complicated 897.1
- **Amputation** — *continued*
  - traumatic — *continued*
    - leg — *continued*
      - both (bilateral) 897.6
        - complicated 897.7
      - complicated 897.5
    - lower limb(s) except toe(s) — *see* Amputation, traumatic, leg
    - nose — *see* Wound, open, nose
    - penis 878.0
      - complicated 878.1
    - sites other than limbs — *see* Wound, open, by site
    - thumb(s) (with finger(s) of either hand) 885.0
      - complicated 885.1
    - toe(s) (one or both feet) 895.0
      - complicated 895.1
    - upper limb(s) — *see* Amputation, traumatic, arm
- **Amputee** (bilateral) (old) — *see also* Absence, by site, acquired V49.70
- **Amusia** 784.69
  - developmental 315.39
  - secondary to organic lesion 784.69
- **Amyelencephalus** 740.0
- **Amyelia** 742.59
- **Amygdalitis** — *see* Tonsillitis
- **Amygdalolith** 474.8
- **Amyloid disease or degeneration** 277.3
  - heart 277.3 *[425.7]*
- **Amyloidosis** (familial) (general) (generalized) (genetic) (primary) (secondary) 277.3
  - with lung involvement 277.3 *[517.8]*
  - heart 277.3 *[425.7]*
  - nephropathic 277.3 *[583.81]*
  - neuropathic (Portuguese) (Swiss) 277.3 *[357.4]*
  - pulmonary 277.3 *[517.8]*
  - systemic, inherited 277.3
- **Amylopectinosis** (brancher enzyme deficiency) 271.0
- **Amylophagia** 307.52
- **Amyoplasia, congenita** 756.89
- **Amyotonia** 728.2
  - congenita 358.8
- **Amyotrophia, amyotrophy, amyotrophic** 728.2
  - congenita 756.89
  - diabetic 250.6 ☑ *[358.1]*
  - lateral sclerosis (syndrome) 335.20
  - neuralgic 353.5
  - sclerosis (lateral) 335.20
  - spinal progressive 335.21
- **Anacidity, gastric** 536.0
  - psychogenic 306.4
- **Anaerosis of newborn** 768.9
- **Analbuminemia** 273.8
- **Analgesia** (*see also* Anesthesia) 782.0
- **Analphalipoproteinemia** 272.5
- **Anaphylactic shock or reaction** (correct substance properly administered) 995.0
  - due to
    - food 995.60
      - additives 995.66
      - crustaceans 995.62
      - eggs 995.68
      - fish 995.65
      - fruits 995.63
      - milk products 995.67
      - nuts (tree) 995.64
      - peanuts 995.61
      - seeds 995.64
      - specified NEC 995.69
      - tree nuts 995.64
      - vegetables 995.63
    - immunization 999.4
    - overdose or wrong substance given or taken 977.9
      - specified drug — *see* Table of Drugs and Chemicals
    - serum 999.4
  - following sting(s) 989.5
  - purpura 287.0
  - serum 999.4

☑ Additional Digit Required — Refer to the Tabular List (Numeric Code Section) for Additional Digit Selection

▶◀ Revised Text ● New Line ▲ Revised Code

- **Anemia** — *continued*
  - septic 285.9
  - sickle-cell (*see also* Disease, sickle-cell) 282.60
  - sideroachrestic 285.0
  - sideroblastic (acquired) (any type) (congenital) (drug-induced) (due to disease) (hereditary) (primary) (secondary) (sex-linked hypochromic) (vitamin B_6 responsive) 285.0
    - refractory 238.7 ●
  - sideropenic (refractory) 280.9
    - due to blood loss (chronic) 280.0
      - acute 285.1
  - simple chronic 281.9
  - specified type NEC 285.8
  - spherocytic (hereditary) (*see also* Spherocytosis) 282.0
  - splenic 285.8
    - familial (Gaucher's) 272.7
  - splenomegalic 285.8
  - stomatocytosis 282.8
  - syphilitic 095.8
  - target cell (oval) 282.49
  - thalassemia 282.49
  - thrombocytopenic (*see also* Thrombocytopenia) 287.5
  - toxic 284.8
  - triosephosphate isomerase deficiency 282.3
  - tropical, macrocytic 281.2
  - tuberculous (*see also* Tuberculosis) 017.9 ☑
  - vegan's 281.1
  - vitamin
    - B_6-responsive 285.0
    - B_{12} deficiency (dietary) 281.1
      - pernicious 281.0
  - von Jaksch's (pseudoleukemia infantum) 285.8
  - Witts' (achlorhydric anemia) 280.9
  - Zuelzer (-Ogden) (nutritional megaloblastic anemia) 281.2
- **Anencephalus, anencephaly** 740.0
  - fetal, affecting management of pregnancy 655.0 ☑
- **Anergasia** (*see also* Psychosis, organic) 294.9
  - senile 290.0
- **Anesthesia, anesthetic** 782.0
  - complication or reaction NEC 995.2
    - due to
      - correct substance properly administered 995.2
      - overdose or wrong substance given 968.4
        - specified anesthetic — *see* Table of Drugs and Chemicals
  - cornea 371.81
  - death from
    - correct substance properly administered 995.4
    - during delivery 668.9 ☑
    - overdose or wrong substance given 968.4
    - specified anesthetic — *see* Table of Drugs and Chemicals
  - eye 371.81
  - functional 300.11
  - hyperesthetic, thalamic 348.8
  - hysterical 300.11
  - local skin lesion 782.0
  - olfactory 781.1
  - sexual (psychogenic) 302.72
  - shock
    - due to
      - correct substance properly administered 995.4
      - overdose or wrong substance given 968.4
      - specified anesthetic — *see* Table of Drugs and Chemicals
  - skin 782.0
  - tactile 782.0
  - testicular 608.9
  - thermal 782.0
- **Anetoderma** (maculosum) 701.3
- **Aneuploidy** NEC 758.5
- **Aneurin deficiency** 265.1
- **Aneurysm** (anastomotic) (artery) (cirsoid) (diffuse) (false) (fusiform) (multiple) (ruptured) (saccular) (varicose) 442.9
  - abdominal (aorta) 441.4
    - ruptured 441.3

- **Aneurysm** — *continued*
  - abdominal — *continued*
    - syphilitic 093.0
  - aorta, aortic (nonsyphilitic) 441.9
    - abdominal 441.4
      - dissecting 441.02
      - ruptured 441.3
      - syphilitic 093.0
    - arch 441.2
      - ruptured 441.1
    - arteriosclerotic NEC 441.9
      - ruptured 441.5
    - ascending 441.2
      - ruptured 441.1
    - congenital 747.29
    - descending 441.9
      - abdominal 441.4
        - ruptured 441.3
      - ruptured 441.5
      - thoracic 441.2
        - ruptured 441.1
    - dissecting 441.00
      - abdominal 441.02
      - thoracic 441.01
      - thoracoabdominal 441.03
    - due to coarctation (aorta) 747.10
    - ruptured 441.5
    - sinus, right 747.29
    - syphilitic 093.0
    - thoracoabdominal 441.7
      - ruptured 441.6
    - thorax, thoracic (arch) (nonsyphilitic) 441.2
      - dissecting 441.01
      - ruptured 441.1
      - syphilitic 093.0
    - transverse 441.2
      - ruptured 441.1
    - valve (heart) (*see also* Endocarditis, aortic) 424.1
  - arteriosclerotic NEC 442.9
    - cerebral 437.3
      - ruptured (*see also* Hemorrhage, subarachnoid) 430
  - arteriovenous (congenital) (peripheral) NEC (*see also* Anomaly, arteriovenous) 747.60
    - acquired NEC 447.0
      - brain 437.3
        - ruptured (*see also* Hemorrhage, subarachnoid) 430
      - coronary 414.11
      - pulmonary 417.0
    - brain (cerebral) 747.81
      - ruptured (*see also* Hemorrhage, subarachnoid) 430
    - coronary 746.85
    - pulmonary 747.3
    - retina 743.58
    - specified site NEC 747.89
      - acquired 447.0
    - traumatic (*see also* Injury, blood vessel, by site) 904.9
  - basal — *see* Aneurysm, brain
  - berry (congenital) (ruptured) (*see also* Hemorrhage, subarachnoid) 430
  - brain 437.3
    - arteriosclerotic 437.3
      - ruptured (*see also* Hemorrhage, subarachnoid) 430
    - arteriovenous 747.81
      - acquired 437.3
        - ruptured (*see also* Hemorrhage, subarachnoid) 430
      - ruptured (*see also* Hemorrhage, subarachnoid) 430
    - berry (congenital) (ruptured) (*see also* Hemorrhage, subarachnoid) 430
    - congenital 747.81
      - ruptured (*see also* Hemorrhage, subarachnoid) 430
    - meninges 437.3
      - ruptured (*see also* Hemorrhage, subarachnoid) 430
    - miliary (congenital) (ruptured) (*see also* Hemorrhage, subarachnoid) 430

- **Aneurysm** — *continued*
  - brain — *continued*
    - mycotic 421.0
      - ruptured (*see also* Hemorrhage, subarachnoid) 430
    - nonruptured 437.3
    - ruptured (*see also* Hemorrhage, subarachnoid) 430
      - syphilitic 094.87
    - syphilitic (hemorrhage) 094.87
    - traumatic — *see* Injury, intracranial
  - cardiac (false) (*see also* Aneurysm, heart) 414.10
  - carotid artery (common) (external) 442.81
    - internal (intracranial portion) 437.3
      - extracranial portion 442.81
      - ruptured into brain (*see also* Hemorrhage, subarachnoid) 430
    - syphilitic 093.89
      - intracranial 094.87
  - cavernous sinus (*see also* Aneurysm, brain) 437.3
    - arteriovenous 747.81
      - ruptured (*see also* Hemorrhage, subarachnoid) 430
    - congenital 747.81
      - ruptured (*see also* Hemorrhage, subarachnoid) 430
  - celiac 442.84
  - central nervous system, syphilitic 094.89
  - cerebral — *see* Aneurysm, brain
  - chest — *see* Aneurysm, thorax
  - circle of Willis (*see also* Aneurysm, brain) 437.3
    - congenital 747.81
      - ruptured (*see also* Hemorrhage, subarachnoid) 430
    - ruptured (*see also* Hemorrhage, subarachnoid) 430
  - common iliac artery 442.2
  - congenital (peripheral) NEC 747.60
    - brain 747.81
      - ruptured (*see also* Hemorrhage, subarachnoid) 430
    - cerebral — *see* Aneurysm, brain, congenital
    - coronary 746.85
    - gastrointestinal 747.61
    - lower limb 747.64
    - pulmonary 747.3
    - renal 747.62
    - retina 743.58
    - specified site NEC 747.89
    - spinal 747.82
    - upper limb 747.63
  - conjunctiva 372.74
  - conus arteriosus (*see also* Aneurysm, heart) 414.10
  - coronary (arteriosclerotic) (artery) (vein) (*see also* Aneurysm, heart) 414.11
    - arteriovenous 746.85
    - congenital 746.85
    - syphilitic 093.89
  - cylindrical 441.9
    - ruptured 441.5
    - syphilitic 093.9
  - dissecting 442.9
    - aorta 441.00
      - abdominal 441.02
      - thoracic 441.01
      - thoracoabdominal 441.03
    - syphilitic 093.9
  - ductus arteriosus 747.0
  - embolic — *see* Embolism, artery
  - endocardial, infective (any valve) 421.0
  - femoral 442.3
  - gastroduodenal 442.84
  - gastroepiploic 442.84
  - heart (chronic or with a stated duration of over 8 weeks) (infectional) (wall) 414.10
    - acute or with a stated duration of 8 weeks or less (*see also* Infarct, myocardium) 410.9 ☑
    - congenital 746.89
    - valve — *see* Endocarditis
  - hepatic 442.84
  - iliac (common) 442.2
  - infective (any valve) 421.0

- **Angiospasm** — *continued*
  - cerebral 435.9
  - cervical plexus 353.2
  - nerve
    - arm 354.9
      - axillary 353.0
      - median 354.1
      - ulnar 354.2
    - autonomic (*see also* Neuropathy, peripheral, autonomic) 337.9
    - axillary 353.0
    - leg 355.8
      - plantar 355.6
    - lower extremity — *see* Angiospasm, nerve, leg
    - median 354.1
    - peripheral NEC 355.9
    - spinal NEC 355.9
    - sympathetic (*see also* Neuropathy, peripheral, autonomic) 337.9
    - ulnar 354.2
    - upper extremity — *see* Angiospasm, nerve, arm
  - peripheral NEC 443.9
  - traumatic 443.9
    - foot 443.9
    - leg 443.9
  - vessel 443.9
- **Angiospastic disease or edema** 443.9
- **Angle's**
  - class I 524.21
  - class II 524.22
  - class III 524.23
- **Anguillulosis** 127.2
- **Angulation**
  - cecum (*see also* Obstruction, intestine) 560.9
  - coccyx (acquired) 738.6
    - congenital 756.19
  - femur (acquired) 736.39
    - congenital 755.69
  - intestine (large) (small) (*see also* Obstruction, intestine) 560.9
  - sacrum (acquired) 738.5
    - congenital 756.19
  - sigmoid (flexure) (*see also* Obstruction, intestine) 560.9
  - spine (*see also* Curvature, spine) 737.9
  - tibia (acquired) 736.89
    - congenital 755.69
  - ureter 593.3
  - wrist (acquired) 736.09
    - congenital 755.59
- **Angulus infectiosus** 686.8
- **Anhedonia** 302.72
- **Anhidrosis** (lid) (neurogenic) (thermogenic) 705.0
- **Anhydration** 276.51 ▲
  - with
    - hypernatremia 276.0
    - hyponatremia 276.1
- **Anhydremia** 276.52 ▲
  - with
    - hypernatremia 276.0
    - hyponatremia 276.1
- **Anidrosis** 705.0
- **Aniridia** (congenital) 743.45
- **Anisakiasis** (infection) (infestation) 127.1
- **Anisakis larva infestation** 127.1
- **Aniseikonia** 367.32
- **Anisocoria** (pupil) 379.41
  - congenital 743.46
- **Anisocytosis** 790.09
- **Anisometropia** (congenital) 367.31
- **Ankle** — *see* condition
- **Ankyloblepharon** (acquired) (eyelid) 374.46
  - filiforme (adnatum) (congenital) 743.62
  - total 743.62
- **Ankylodactly** (*see also* Syndactylism) 755.10
- **Ankyloglossia** 750.0
- **Ankylosis** (fibrous) (osseous) 718.50
  - ankle 718.57
  - any joint, produced by surgical fusion V45.4
  - cricoarytenoid (cartilage) (joint) (larynx) 478.79
  - dental 521.6
- **Ankylosis** — *continued*
  - ear ossicle NEC 385.22
    - malleus 385.21
  - elbow 718.52
  - finger 718.54
  - hip 718.55
  - incostapedial joint (infectional) 385.22
  - joint, produced by surgical fusion NEC V45.4
  - knee 718.56
  - lumbosacral (joint) 724.6
  - malleus 385.21
  - multiple sites 718.59
  - postoperative (status) V45.4
  - sacroiliac (joint) 724.6
  - shoulder 718.51
  - specified site NEC 718.58
  - spine NEC 724.9
  - surgical V45.4
  - teeth, tooth (hard tissues) 521.6
  - temporomandibular joint 524.61
  - wrist 718.53
- **Ankylostoma** — *see* Ancylostoma
- **Ankylostomiasis** (intestinal) — *see* Ancylostomiasis
- **Ankylurethria** (*see also* Stricture, urethra) 598.9
- **Annular** — *see also* condition
  - detachment, cervix 622.8
  - organ or site, congenital NEC — *see* Distortion
  - pancreas (congenital) 751.7
- **Anodontia** (complete) (partial) (vera) 520.0
  - with abnormal spacing 524.30
  - acquired 525.10
    - causing malocclusion 524.30
    - due to
      - caries 525.13
      - extraction 525.10
      - periodontal disease 525.12
      - trauma 525.11
- **Anomaly, anomalous** (congenital) (unspecified type) 759.9
  - abdomen 759.9
  - abdominal wall 756.70
  - acoustic nerve 742.9
  - adrenal (gland) 759.1
  - Alder (-Reilly) (leukocyte granulation) 288.2
  - alimentary tract 751.9
    - lower 751.5
    - specified type NEC 751.8
    - upper (any part, except tongue) 750.9
      - tongue 750.10
        - specified type NEC 750.19
  - alveolar 524.70
    - ridge (process) 525.8
    - specified NEC 524.79
  - ankle (joint) 755.69
  - anus, anal (canal) 751.5
  - aorta, aortic 747.20
    - arch 747.21
    - coarctation (postductal) (preductal) 747.10
    - cusp or valve NEC 746.9
    - septum 745.0
    - specified type NEC 747.29
  - aorticopulmonary septum 745.0
  - apertures, diaphragm 756.6
  - appendix 751.5
  - aqueduct of Sylvius 742.3
    - with spina bifida (*see also* Spina bifida) 741.0 ☑
  - arm 755.50
    - reduction (*see also* Deformity, reduction, upper limb) 755.20
  - arteriovenous (congenital) (peripheral) NEC 747.60
    - brain 747.81
    - cerebral 747.81
    - coronary 746.85
    - gastrointestinal 747.61
      - acquired — *see* Angiodysplasia ●
    - lower limb 747.64
    - renal 747.62
    - specified site NEC 747.69
    - spinal 747.82
    - upper limb 747.63
  - artery (*see also* Anomaly, peripheral vascular system) NEC 747.60
    - brain 747.81
- **Anomaly, anomalous** — *continued*
  - artery (*see also* Anomaly, peripheral vascular system) — *continued*
    - cerebral 747.81
    - coronary 746.85
    - eye 743.9
    - pulmonary 747.3
    - renal 747.62
    - retina 743.9
    - umbilical 747.5
  - arytenoepiglottic folds 748.3
  - atrial
    - bands 746.9
    - folds 746.9
    - septa 745.5
  - atrioventricular
    - canal 745.69
    - common 745.69
    - conduction 426.7
    - excitation 426.7
    - septum 745.4
  - atrium — *see* Anomaly, atrial
  - auditory canal 744.3
    - specified type NEC 744.29
      - with hearing impairment 744.02
  - auricle
    - ear 744.3
      - causing impairment of hearing 744.02
    - heart 746.9
      - septum 745.5
  - autosomes, autosomal NEC 758.5
  - Axenfeld's 743.44
  - back 759.9
  - band
    - atrial 746.9
    - heart 746.9
    - ventricular 746.9
  - Bartholin's duct 750.9
  - biliary duct or passage 751.60
    - atresia 751.61
  - bladder (neck) (sphincter) (trigone) 753.9
    - specified type NEC 753.8
  - blood vessel 747.9
    - artery — *see* Anomaly, artery
    - peripheral vascular — *see* Anomaly, peripheral vascular system
    - vein — *see* Anomaly, vein
  - bone NEC 756.9
    - ankle 755.69
    - arm 755.50
    - chest 756.3
    - cranium 756.0
    - face 756.0
    - finger 755.50
    - foot 755.67
    - forearm 755.50
    - frontal 756.0
    - head 756.0
    - hip 755.63
    - leg 755.60
    - lumbosacral 756.10
    - nose 748.1
    - pelvic girdle 755.60
    - rachitic 756.4
    - rib 756.3
    - shoulder girdle 755.50
    - skull 756.0
      - with
        - anencephalus 740.0
        - encephalocele 742.0
        - hydrocephalus 742.3
          - with spina bifida (*see also* Spina bifida) 741.0 ☑
        - microcephalus 742.1
    - toe 755.66
  - brain 742.9
    - multiple 742.4
    - reduction 742.2
    - specified type NEC 742.4
    - vessel 747.81
  - branchial cleft NEC 744.49
    - cyst 744.42
    - fistula 744.41
    - persistent 744.41
    - sinus (external) (internal) 744.41
  - breast 757.9

☑ Additional Digit Required — Refer to the Tabular List (Numeric Code Section) for Additional Digit Selection
▶◀ Revised Text ● New Line ▲ Revised Code

☑ Additional Digit Required — Refer to the Tabular List (Numeric Code Section) for Additional Digit Selection
▶◀ Revised Text ● New Line ▲ Revised Code

☑ Additional Digit Required — Refer to the Tabular List (Numeric Code Section) for Additional Digit Selection

▶◀ Revised Text ● New Line ▲ Revised Code

☑ Additional Digit Required — Refer to the Tabular List (Numeric Code Section) for Additional Digit Selection
▶◀ Revised Text ● New Line ▲ Revised Code

Arhinencephaly 742.2
Arias-Stella phenomenon 621.30
Ariboflavinosis 266.0
Arizona enteritis 008.1
Arm — *see* condition
Armenian disease 277.3
Arnold-Chiari obstruction or syndrome (*see also* Spina bifida) 741.0 ☑
- type I 348.4
- type II (*see also* Spina bifida) 741.0 ☑
- type III 742.0
- type IV 742.2

Arousals ●
- confusional 327.41 ●

Arrest, arrested
- active phase of labor 661.1 ☑
  - affecting fetus or newborn 763.7
- any plane in pelvis
  - complicating delivery 660.1 ☑
    - affecting fetus or newborn 763.1
- bone marrow (*see also* Anemia, aplastic) 284.9
- cardiac 427.5
  - with
    - abortion — *see* Abortion, by type, with specified complication NEC
    - ectopic pregnancy (*see also* categories 633.0-633.9) 639.8
    - molar pregnancy (*see also* categories 630-632) 639.8
  - complicating
    - anesthesia
      - correct substance properly administered 427.5
      - obstetric 668.1 ☑
      - overdose or wrong substance given 968.4
        - specified anesthetic — *see* Table of Drugs and Chemicals
    - delivery (cesarean) (instrumental) 669.4 ☑
    - ectopic or molar pregnancy 639.8
    - surgery (nontherapeutic) (therapeutic) 997.1
  - fetus or newborn 779.89
  - following
    - abortion 639.8
    - ectopic or molar pregnancy 639.8
  - postoperative (immediate) 997.1
    - long-term effect of cardiac surgery 429.4
- cardiorespiratory (*see also* Arrest, cardiac) 427.5
- deep transverse 660.3 ☑
  - affecting fetus or newborn 763.1
- development or growth
  - bone 733.91
  - child 783.40
  - fetus 764.9 ☑
    - affecting management of pregnancy 656.5 ☑
  - tracheal rings 748.3
- epiphyseal 733.91
- granulopoiesis 288.0
- heart — *see* Arrest, cardiac
- respiratory 799.1
  - newborn 770.89
- sinus 426.6
- transverse (deep) 660.3 ☑
  - affecting fetus or newborn 763.1

Arrhenoblastoma (M8630/1)
- benign (M8630/0)
  - specified site — *see* Neoplasm, by site, benign
  - unspecified site
    - female 220
    - male 222.0
- malignant (M8630/3)
  - specified site — *see* Neoplasm, by site, malignant
  - unspecified site
    - female 183.0
    - male 186.9
- specified site — *see* Neoplasm, by site, uncertain behavior
- unspecified site
  - female 236.2
  - male 236.4

Arrhinencephaly 742.2
- due to
  - trisomy 13 (13-15) 758.1
  - trisomy 18 (16-18) 758.2

Arrhythmia (auricle) (cardiac) (cordis) (gallop rhythm) (juvenile) (nodal) (reflex) (sinus) (supraventricular) (transitory) (ventricle) 427.9
- bigeminal rhythm 427.89
- block 426.9
- bradycardia 427.89
- contractions, premature 427.60
- coronary sinus 427.89
- ectopic 427.89
- extrasystolic 427.60
- postoperative 997.1
- psychogenic 306.2
- vagal 780.2

Arrillaga-Ayerza syndrome (pulmonary artery sclerosis with pulmonary hypertension) 416.0
Arsenical
- dermatitis 692.4
- keratosis 692.4
- pigmentation 985.1
  - from drug or medicinal agent
    - correct substance properly administered 709.09
    - overdose or wrong substance given or taken 961.1

Arsenism 985.1
- from drug or medicinal agent
  - correct substance properly administered 692.4
  - overdose or wrong substance given or taken 961.1

Arterial — *see* condition
Arteriectasis 447.8
Arteriofibrosis — *see* Arteriosclerosis
Arteriolar sclerosis — *see* Arteriosclerosis
Arteriolith — *see* Arteriosclerosis
Arteriolitis 447.6
- necrotizing, kidney 447.5
- renal — *see* Hypertension, kidney

Arteriolosclerosis — *see* Arteriosclerosis
Arterionephrosclerosis (*see also* Hypertension, kidney) 403.90
Arteriopathy 447.9
Arteriosclerosis, arteriosclerotic (artery) (deformans) (diffuse) (disease) (endarteritis) (general) (obliterans) (obliterative) (occlusive) (senile) (with calcification) 440.9
- with
  - gangrene 440.24
  - psychosis (*see also* Psychosis, arteriosclerotic) 290.40
  - ulceration 440.23
- aorta 440.0
- arteries of extremities — *see* Arteriosclerosis, extremities
- basilar (artery) (*see also* Occlusion, artery, basilar) 433.0 ☑
- brain 437.0
- bypass graft
  - coronary artery 414.05
    - autologous artery (gastroepiploic) (internal mammary) 414.04
    - autologous vein 414.02
    - nonautologous biological 414.03
    - of transplanted heart 414.07
  - extremity 440.30
    - autologous vein 440.31
    - nonautologous biological 440.32
- cardiac — *see* Arteriosclerosis, coronary
- cardiopathy — *see* Arteriosclerosis, coronary
- cardiorenal (*see also* Hypertension, cardiorenal) 404.90
- cardiovascular (*see also* Disease, cardiovascular) 429.2
- carotid (artery) (common) (internal) (*see also* Occlusion, artery, carotid) 433.1 ☑
- central nervous system 437.0
- cerebral 437.0
  - late effect — *see* Late effect(s) (of) cerebrovascular disease

Arteriosclerosis, arteriosclerotic — *continued*
- cerebrospinal 437.0
- cerebrovascular 437.0
- coronary (artery) 414.00
  - graft — *see* Arteriosclerosis, bypass graft
  - native artery 414.01
    - of transplanted heart 414.06
- extremities (native artery) NEC 440.20
  - bypass graft 440.30
    - autologous vein 440.31
    - nonautologous biological 440.32
  - claudication (intermittent) 440.21
    - and
      - gangrene 440.24
      - rest pain 440.22
        - and
          - gangrene 440.24
          - ulceration 440.23
            - and gangrene 440.24
      - ulceration 440.23
        - and gangrene 440.24
  - gangrene 440.24
  - rest pain 440.22
    - and
      - gangrene 440.24
      - ulceration 440.23
        - and gangrene 440.24
  - specified site NEC 440.29
  - ulceration 440.23
    - and gangrene 440.24
- heart (disease) — *see also* Arteriosclerosis, coronary
  - valve 424.99
    - aortic 424.1
    - mitral 424.0
    - pulmonary 424.3
    - tricuspid 424.2
- kidney (*see also* Hypertension, kidney) 403.90
- labyrinth, labyrinthine 388.00
- medial NEC (*see also* Arteriosclerosis, extremities) 440.20
- mesentery (artery) 557.1
- Mönckeberg's (*see also* Arteriosclerosis, extremities) 440.20
- myocarditis 429.0
- nephrosclerosis (*see also* Hypertension, kidney) 403.90
- peripheral (of extremities) — *see* Arteriosclerosis, extremities
- precerebral 433.9 ☑
  - specified artery NEC 433.8 ☑
- pulmonary (idiopathic) 416.0
- renal (*see also* Hypertension, kidney) 403.90
  - arterioles (*see also* Hypertension, kidney) 403.90
  - artery 440.1
- retinal (vascular) 440.8 *[362.13]*
- specified artery NEC 440.8
  - with gangrene 440.8 *[785.4]*
- spinal (cord) 437.0
- vertebral (artery) (*see also* Occlusion, artery, vertebral) 433.2 ☑

Arteriospasm 443.9
Arteriovenous — *see* condition
Arteritis 447.6
- allergic (*see also* Angiitis, hypersensitivity) 446.20
- aorta (nonsyphilitic) 447.6
  - syphilitic 093.1
- aortic arch 446.7
- brachiocephalica 446.7
- brain 437.4
  - syphilitic 094.89
- branchial 446.7
- cerebral 437.4
  - late effect — *see* Late effect(s) (of) cerebrovascular disease
  - syphilitic 094.89
- coronary (artery) — *see also* Arteriosclerosis, coronary
  - rheumatic 391.9
    - chronic 398.99
  - syphilitic 093.89
- cranial (left) (right) 446.5
- deformans — *see* Arteriosclerosis
- giant cell 446.5

☑ Additional Digit Required — Refer to the Tabular List (Numeric Code Section) for Additional Digit Selection

▶◀ Revised Text ● New Line ▲ Revised Code

Arteritis — *continued*
necrosing or necrotizing 446.0
nodosa 446.0
obliterans — *see also* Arteriosclerosis
subclaviocarotica 446.7
pulmonary 417.8
retina 362.18
rheumatic — *see* Fever, rheumatic
senile — *see* Arteriosclerosis
suppurative 447.2
syphilitic (general) 093.89
brain 094.89
coronary 093.89
spinal 094.89
temporal 446.5
young female, syndrome 446.7
Artery, arterial — *see* condition
Arthralgia (*see also* Pain, joint) 719.4 ☑
allergic (*see also* Pain, joint) 719.4 ☑
in caisson disease 993.3
psychogenic 307.89
rubella 056.71
Salmonella 003.23
temporomandibular joint 524.62
Arthritis, arthritic (acute) (chronic) (subacute) 716.9 ☑
meaning Osteoarthritis — *see* Osteoarthrosis

Note — Use the following fifth-digit subclassification with categories 711-712, 715-716:

0	*site unspecified*
1	*shoulder region*
2	*upper arm*
3	*forearm*
4	*hand*
5	*pelvic region and thigh*
6	*lower leg*
7	*ankle and foot*
8	*other specified sites*
9	*multiple sites*

allergic 716.2 ☑
ankylosing (crippling) (spine) 720.0
sites other than spine 716.9 ☑
atrophic 714.0
spine 720.9
back (*see also* Arthritis, spine) 721.90
Bechterew's (ankylosing spondylitis) 720.0
blennorrhagic 098.50
cervical, cervicodorsal (*see also* Spondylosis, cervical) 721.0
Charcôt's 094.0 *[713.5]*
diabetic 250.6 ☑ *[713.5]*
syringomyelic 336.0 *[713.5]*
tabetic 094.0 *[713.5]*
chylous (*see also* Filariasis) 125.9 *[711.7]* ☑
climacteric NEC 716.3 ☑
coccyx 721.8
cricoarytenoid 478.79
crystal (-induced) — *see* Arthritis, due to crystals
deformans (*see also* Osteoarthrosis) 715.9 ☑
spine 721.90
with myelopathy 721.91
degenerative (*see also* Osteoarthrosis) 715.9 ☑
idiopathic 715.09
polyarticular 715.09
spine 721.90
with myelopathy 721.91
dermatoarthritis, lipoid 272.8 *[713.0]*
due to or associated with
acromegaly 253.0 *[713.0]*
actinomycosis 039.8 *[711.4]* ☑
amyloidosis 277.3 *[713.7]*
bacterial disease NEC 040.89 *[711.4]* ☑
Behçet's syndrome 136.1 *[711.2]* ☑
blastomycosis 116.0 *[711.6]* ☑
brucellosis (*see also* Brucellosis) 023.9 *[711.4]* ☑
caisson disease 993.3
coccidioidomycosis 114.3 *[711.6]* ☑
coliform (Escherichia coli) 711.0 ☑

Arthritis, arthritic — *continued*
due to or associated with — *continued*
colitis, ulcerative (*see also* Colitis, ulcerative) 556.9 *[713.1]*
cowpox 051.0 *[711.5]* ☑
crystals (*see also* Gout)
dicalcium phosphate 275.49 *[712.1]* ☑
pyrophosphate 275.49 *[712.2]* ☑
specified NEC 275.49 *[712.8]* ☑
dermatoarthritis, lipoid 272.8 *[713.0]*
dermatological disorder NEC 709.9 *[713.3]*
diabetes 250.6 ☑ *[713.5]*
diphtheria 032.89 *[711.4]* ☑
dracontiasis 125.7 *[711.7]* ☑
dysentery 009.0 *[711.3]* ☑
endocrine disorder NEC 259.9 *[713.0]*
enteritis NEC 009.1 *[711.3]* ☑
infectious (*see also* Enteritis, infectious) 009.0 *[711.3]* ☑
specified organism NEC 008.8 *[711.3]* ☑
regional (*see also* Enteritis, regional) 555.9 *[713.1]*
specified organism NEC 008.8 *[711.3]* ☑
epiphyseal slip, nontraumatic (old) 716.8 ☑
erysipelas 035 *[711.4]* ☑
erythema
epidemic 026.1
multiforme 695.1 *[713.3]*
nodosum 695.2 *[713.3]*
Escherichia coli 711.0 ☑
filariasis NEC 125.9 *[711.7]* ☑
gastrointestinal condition NEC 569.9 *[713.1]*
glanders 024 *[711.4]* ☑
Gonococcus 098.50
gout 274.0
H. influenzae 711.0 ☑
helminthiasis NEC 128.9 *[711.7]* ☑
hematological disorder NEC 289.9 *[713.2]*
hemochromatosis 275.0 *[713.0]*
hemoglobinopathy NEC (*see also* Disease, hemoglobin) 282.7 *[713.2]*
hemophilia (*see also* Hemophilia) 286.0 *[713.2]*
Hemophilus influenzae (H. influenzae) 711.0 ☑
Henoch (-Schönlein) purpura 287.0 *[713.6]*
histoplasmosis NEC (*see also* Histoplasmosis) 115.99 *[711.6]* ☑
hyperparathyroidism 252.00 *[713.0]*
hypersensitivity reaction NEC 995.3 *[713.6]*
hypogammaglobulinemia (*see also* Hypogamma-globulinemia) 279.00 *[713.0]*
hypothyroidism NEC 244.9 *[713.0]*
infection (*see also* Arthritis, infectious) 711.9 ☑
infectious disease NEC 136.9 *[711.8]* ☑
leprosy (*see also* Leprosy) 030.9 *[711.4]* ☑
leukemia NEC (M9800/3) 208.9 ☑ *[713.2]*
lipoid dermatoarthritis 272.8 *[713.0]*
Lyme disease 088.81 *[711.8]* ☑
Mediterranean fever, familial 277.3 *[713.7]*
meningococcal infection 036.82
metabolic disorder NEC 277.9 *[713.0]*
multiple myelomatosis (M9730/3) 203.0 ☑ *[713.2]*
mumps 072.79 *[711.5]* ☑
mycobacteria 031.8 *[711.4]* ☑
mycosis NEC 117.9 *[711.6]* ☑
neurological disorder NEC 349.9 *[713.5]*
ochronosis 270.2 *[713.0]*
O'Nyong Nyong 066.3 *[711.5]* ☑
parasitic disease NEC 136.9 *[711.8]* ☑
paratyphoid fever (*see also* Fever, paratyphoid) 002.9 *[711.3]* ☑
Pneumococcus 711.0 ☑
poliomyelitis (*see also* Poliomyelitis) 045.9 ☑ *[711.5]* ☑
Pseudomonas 711.0 ☑
psoriasis 696.0
pyogenic organism (E. coli) (H. influenzae) (Pseudomonas) (Streptococcus) 711.0 ☑
rat-bite fever 026.1 *[711.4]* ☑
regional enteritis (*see also* Enteritis, regional) 555.9 *[713.1]*

Arthritis, arthritic — *continued*
due to or associated with — *continued*
Reiter's disease 099.3 *[711.1]* ☑
respiratory disorder NEC 519.9 *[713.4]*
reticulosis, malignant (M9720/3) 202.3 ☑ *[713.2]*
rubella 056.71
salmonellosis 003.23
sarcoidosis 135 *[713.7]*
serum sickness 999.5 *[713.6]*
Staphylococcus 711.0 ☑
Streptococcus 711.0 ☑
syphilis (*see also* Syphilis) 094.0 *[711.4]* ☑
syringomyelia 336.0 *[713.5]*
thalassemia 282.49 *[713.2]*
tuberculosis (*see also* Tuberculosis, arthritis) 015.9 ☑ *[711.4]* ☑
typhoid fever 002.0 *[711.3]* ☑
ulcerative colitis (*see also* Colitis, ulcerative) 556.9 *[713.1]*
urethritis
nongonococcal (*see also* Urethritis, nongonococcal) 099.40 *[711.1]* ☑
nonspecific (*see also* Urethritis, nongonococcal) 099.40 *[711.1]* ☑
Reiter's 099.3 *[711.1]* ☑
viral disease NEC 079.99 *[711.5]* ☑
erythema epidemic 026.1
gonococcal 098.50
gouty (acute) 274.0
hypertrophic (*see also* Osteoarthrosis) 715.9 ☑
spine 721.90
with myelopathy 721.91
idiopathic, blennorrheal 099.3
in caisson disease 993.3 *[713.8]*
infectious or infective (acute) (chronic) (subacute) NEC 711.9 ☑
nonpyogenic 711.9 ☑
spine 720.9
inflammatory NEC 714.9
juvenile rheumatoid (chronic) (polyarticular) 714.30
acute 714.31
monoarticular 714.33
pauciarticular 714.32
lumbar (*see also* Spondylosis, lumbar) 721.3
meningococcal 036.82
menopausal NEC 716.3 ☑
migratory — *see* Fever, rheumatic
neuropathic (Charcôt's) 094.0 *[713.5]*
diabetic 250.6 ☑ *[713.5]*
nonsyphilitic NEC 349.9 *[713.5]*
syringomyelic 336.0 *[713.5]*
tabetic 094.0 *[713.5]*
nodosa (*see also* Osteoarthrosis) 715.9 ☑
spine 721.90
with myelopathy 721.91
nonpyogenic NEC 716.9 ☑
spine 721.90
with myelopathy 721.91
ochronotic 270.2 *[713.0]*
palindromic (see also Rheumatism, palindromic) 719.3 ☑
pneumococcal 711.0 ☑
postdysenteric 009.0 *[711.3]* ☑
postrheumatic, chronic (Jaccoud's) 714.4
primary progressive 714.0
spine 720.9
proliferative 714.0
spine 720.0
psoriatic 696.0
purulent 711.0 ☑
pyogenic or pyemic 711.0 ☑
rheumatic 714.0
acute or subacute — *see* Fever, rheumatic
chronic 714.0
spine 720.9
rheumatoid (nodular) 714.0
with
splenoadenomegaly and leukopenia 714.1
visceral or systemic involvement 714.2
aortitis 714.89
carditis 714.2
heart disease 714.2
juvenile (chronic) (polyarticular) 714.30
acute 714.31
monoarticular 714.33

Arthritis, arthritic — *continued*
  rheumatoid — *continued*
    juvenile — *continued*
      pauciarticular 714.32
    spine 720.0
  rubella 056.71
  sacral, sacroiliac, sacrococcygeal (*see also* Spondylosis, sacral) 721.3
  scorbutic 267
  senile or senescent (*see also* Osteoarthrosis) 715.9 ☑
    spine 721.90
      with myelopathy 721.91
  septic 711.0 ☑
  serum (nontherapeutic) (therapeutic) 999.5 *[713.6]*
  specified form NEC 716.8 ☑
  spine 721.90
    with myelopathy 721.91
    atrophic 720.9
    degenerative 721.90
      with myelopathy 721.91
    hypertrophic (with deformity) 721.90
      with myelopathy 721.91
    infectious or infective NEC 720.9
    Marie-Strümpell 720.0
    nonpyogenic 721.90
      with myelopathy 721.91
    pyogenic 720.9
    rheumatoid 720.0
    traumatic (old) 721.7
    tuberculous (*see* also Tuberculosis) 015.0 ☑ *[720.81]*
  staphylococcal 711.0 ☑
  streptococcal 711.0 ☑
  suppurative 711.0 ☑
  syphilitic 094.0 *[713.5]*
    congenital 090.49 *[713.5]*
  syphilitica deformans (Charcôt) 094.0 *[713.5]*
  temporomandibular joint 524.69
  thoracic (*see also* Spondylosis, thoracic) 721.2
  toxic of menopause 716.3 ☑
  transient 716.4 ☑
  traumatic (chronic) (old) (post) 716.1 ☑
    current injury — *see* nature of injury
  tuberculous (*see also* Tuberculosis, arthritis) 015.9 ☑ *[711.4]* ☑
  urethritica 099.3 *[711.1]* ☑
  urica, uratic 274.0
  venereal 099.3 *[711.1]* ☑
  vertebral (*see also* Arthritis, spine) 721.90
  villous 716.8 ☑
  von Bechterew's 720.0
Arthrocele (*see also* Effusion, joint) 719.0 ☑
Arthrochondritis — *see* Arthritis
Arthrodesis status V45.4
Arthrodynia (*see also* Pain, joint) 719.4 ☑
  psychogenic 307.89
Arthrodysplasia 755.9
Arthrofibrosis, joint (*see also* Ankylosis) 718.5 ☑
Arthrogryposis 728.3
  multiplex, congenita 754.89
Arthrokatadysis 715.35
Arthrolithiasis 274.0
Arthro-onychodysplasia 756.89
Arthro-osteo-onychodysplasia 756.89
Arthropathy (*see also* Arthritis) 716.9 ☑

Note — Use the following fifth-digit subclassification with categories 711-712, 716:

0	*site unspecified*
1	*shoulder region*
2	*upper arm*
3	*forearm*
4	*hand*
5	*pelvic region and thigh*
6	*lower leg*
7	*ankle and foot*
8	*other specified sites*
9	*multiple sites*

  Behçet's 136.1 *[711.2]* ☑

Arthropathy (*see also* Arthritis) — *continued*
  Charcôt's 094.0 *[713.5]*
    diabetic 250.6 ☑ *[713.5]*
    syringomyelic 336.0 *[713.5]*
    tabetic 094.0 *[713.5]*
  crystal (-induced) — *see* Arthritis, due to crystals
  gouty 274.0
  neurogenic, neuropathic (Charcôt's) (tabetic) 094.0 *[713.5]*
    diabetic 250.6 ☑ *[713.5]*
    nonsyphilitic NEC 349.9 *[713.5]*
    syringomyelic 336.0 *[713.5]*
  postdysenteric NEC 009.0 *[711.3]* ☑
  postrheumatic, chronic (Jaccoud's) 714.4
  psoriatic 696.0
  pulmonary 731.2
  specified NEC 716.8 ☑
  syringomyelia 336.0 *[713.5]*
  tabes dorsalis 094.0 *[713.5]*
  tabetic 094.0 *[713.5]*
  transient 716.4 ☑
  traumatic 716.1 ☑
  uric acid 274.0
Arthrophyte (*see also* Loose, body, joint) 718.1 ☑
Arthrophytis 719.80
  ankle 719.87
  elbow 719.82
  foot 719.87
  hand 719.84
  hip 719.85
  knee 719.86
  multiple sites 719.89
  pelvic region 719.85
  shoulder (region) 719.81
  specified site NEC 719.88
  wrist 719.83
Arthropyosis (*see also* Arthritis, pyogenic) 711.0 ☑
Arthroscopic surgical procedure converted to open procedure V64.43
Arthrosis (deformans) (degenerative) (*see also* Osteoarthrosis) 715.9 ☑
  Charcôt's 094.0 *[713.5]*
  polyarticular 715.09
  spine (*see also* Spondylosis) 721.90
Arthus' phenomenon 995.2
  due to
    correct substance properly administered 995.2
    overdose or wrong substance given or taken 977.9
      specified drug — *see* Table of Drugs and Chemicals
    serum 999.5
Articular — *see also* condition
  disc disorder (reducing or non-reducing) 524.63
  spondylolisthesis 756.12
Articulation
  anterior 524.27
  posterior 524.27
  reverse 524.27
Artificial
  device (prosthetic) — *see* Fitting, device
  insemination V26.1
  menopause (states) (symptoms) (syndrome) 627.4
  opening status (functioning) (without complication) V44.9
    anus (colostomy) V44.3
    colostomy V44.3
    cystostomy V44.50
      appendico-vesicostomy V44.52
      cutaneous-vesicostomy V44.51
      specified type NEC V44.59
    enterostomy V44.4
    gastrostomy V44.1
    ileostomy V44.2
    intestinal tract NEC V44.4
    jejunostomy V44.4
    nephrostomy V44.6
    specified site NEC V44.8
    tracheostomy V44.0
    ureterostomy V44.6

Artificial — *continued*
  opening status — *continued*
    urethrostomy V44.6
    urinary tract NEC V44.6
    vagina V44.7
  vagina status V44.7
ARV (disease) (illness) (infection) — *see* Human immunodeficiency virus (disease) (illness) (infection)
Arytenoid — *see* condition
Asbestosis (occupational) 501
Asboe-Hansen's disease (incontinentia pigmenti) 757.33
Ascariasis (intestinal) (lung) 127.0
Ascaridiasis 127.0
Ascaridosis 127.0
Ascaris 127.0
  lumbricoides (infestation) 127.0
  pneumonia 127.0
Ascending — *see* condition
Aschoff's bodies (*see also* Myocarditis, rheumatic) 398.0
Ascites 789.5
  abdominal NEC 789.5
  cancerous (M8000/6) 197.6
  cardiac 428.0
  chylous (nonfilarial) 457.8
    filarial (*see also* Infestation, filarial) 125.9
  congenital 778.0
  due to S. japonicum 120.2
  fetal, causing fetopelvic disproportion 653.7 ☑
  heart 428.0
  joint (*see also* Effusion, joint) 719.0 ☑
  malignant (M8000/6) 197.6
  pseudochylous 789.5
  syphilitic 095.2
  tuberculous (*see also* Tuberculosis) 014.0 ☑
Ascorbic acid (vitamin C) **deficiency** (scurvy) 267
ASC-US (atypical squamous cells of undetermined significance) 795.01
ASC-H (atypical squamous cells cannot exclude high grade squamous intraepithelial lesion) 795.02
ASCVD (arteriosclerotic cardiovascular disease) 429.2
Aseptic — *see* condition
Asherman's syndrome 621.5
Asialia 527.7
Asiatic cholera (*see also* Cholera) 001.9
Asocial personality or trends 301.7
Asomatognosia 781.8
Aspergillosis 117.3
  with pneumonia 117.3 *[484.6]*
  allergic bronchopulmonary 518.6
  nonsyphilitic NEC 117.3
Aspergillus (flavus) (fumigatus) (infection) (terreus) 117.3
Aspermatogenesis 606.0
Aspermia (testis) 606.0
Asphyxia, asphyxiation (by) 799.01 ▲
  antenatal — *see* Distress, fetal
  bedclothes 994.7
  birth (*see also* Asphyxia, newborn) 768.9
  bunny bag 994.7
  carbon monoxide 986
  caul (*see also* Asphyxia, newborn) 768.9
  cave-in 994.7
    crushing — *see* Injury, internal, intrathoracic organs
  constriction 994.7
  crushing — *see* Injury, internal, intrathoracic organs
  drowning 994.1
  fetal, affecting newborn 768.9
  food or foreign body (in larynx) 933.1
    bronchioles 934.8
    bronchus (main) 934.1
    lung 934.8
    nasopharynx 933.0
    nose, nasal passages 932
    pharynx 933.0

- **Asphyxia, asphyxiation** — *continued*
  - food or foreign body — *continued*
    - respiratory tract 934.9
      - specified part NEC 934.8
    - throat 933.0
    - trachea 934.0
  - gas, fumes, or vapor NEC 987.9
    - specified — *see* Table of Drugs and Chemicals
  - gravitational changes 994.7
  - hanging 994.7
  - inhalation — *see* Inhalation
  - intrauterine
    - fetal death (before onset of labor) 768.0
      - during labor 768.1
    - liveborn infant — *see* Distress, fetal, liveborn infant
  - local 443.0
  - mechanical 994.7
    - during birth (*see also* Distress, fetal) 768.9
  - mucus 933.1
    - bronchus (main) 934.1
    - larynx 933.1
    - lung 934.8
    - nasal passages 932
    - newborn 770.18 ▲
    - pharynx 933.0
    - respiratory tract 934.9
      - specified part NEC 934.8
    - throat 933.0
    - trachea 934.0
    - vaginal (fetus or newborn) 770.18 ▲
  - newborn 768.9
    - with neurologic involvement 768.5
    - blue 768.6
    - livida 768.6
    - mild or moderate 768.6
    - pallida 768.5
    - severe 768.5
    - white 768.5
  - pathological 799.01 ▲
  - plastic bag 994.7
  - postnatal (*see also* Asphyxia, newborn) 768.9
    - mechanical 994.7
  - pressure 994.7
  - reticularis 782.61
  - strangulation 994.7
  - submersion 994.1
  - traumatic NEC — *see* Injury, internal, intrathoracic organs
  - vomiting, vomitus — *see* Asphyxia, food or foreign body
- **Aspiration**
  - acid pulmonary (syndrome) 997.3
    - obstetric 668.0 ☑
  - amniotic fluid 770.13 ▲
    - with respiratory symptoms 770.14 ●
  - bronchitis 507.0
  - clear amniotic fluid 770.13 ●
    - with ●
      - pneumonia 770.14 ●
      - pneumonitis 770.14 ●
      - respiratory symptoms 770.14 ●
  - contents of birth canal 770.17 ▲
    - with respiratory symptoms 770.18 ●
  - fetal 770.10 ▲
    - blood 770.15 ●
      - with ●
        - pneumonia 770.16 ●
        - pneumonitis 770.16 ●
    - pneumonitis 770.18 ●
  - food, foreign body, or gasoline (with asphyxiation) — *see* Asphyxia, food or foreign body
  - meconium 770.11 ▲
    - with ●
      - pneumonia 770.12 ●
      - pneumonitis 770.12 ●
      - respiratory symptoms 770.12 ●
    - below vocal cords 770.11 ●
      - with respiratory symptoms 770.12 ●
  - mucus 933.1
    - into
      - bronchus (main) 934.1
      - lung 934.8
      - respiratory tract 934.9
        - specified part NEC 934.8
- **Aspiration** — *continued*
  - mucus — *continued*
    - into — *continued*
      - trachea 934.0
    - newborn 770.17 ▲
    - vaginal (fetus or newborn) 770.17 ▲
  - newborn 770.10 ▲
    - with respiratory symptoms 770.18 ●
    - blood 770.15 ●
      - with ●
        - pneumonia 770.16 ●
        - pneumonitis 770.16 ●
        - respiratory symptoms 770.16 ●
  - pneumonia 507.0
    - fetus or newborn 770.18 ●
      - meconium 770.12 ●
  - pneumonitis 507.0
    - fetus or newborn 770.18 ▲
      - meconium 770.12 ●
    - obstetric 668.0 ☑
  - postnatal stomach contents 770.85 ●
    - with ●
      - pneumonia 770.86 ●
      - pneumonitis 770.86 ●
      - respiratory symptoms 770.86 ●
  - syndrome of newborn (massive) 770.18 ▲
    - meconium 770.12 ●
  - vernix caseosa 770.17 ▲
- **Asplenia** 759.0
  - with mesocardia 746.87
- **Assam fever** 085.0
- **Assimilation, pelvis**
  - with disproportion 653.2 ☑
    - affecting fetus or newborn 763.1
    - causing obstructed labor 660.1 ☑
      - affecting fetus or newborn 763.1
- **Assmann's focus** (*see also* Tuberculosis) 011.0 ☑
- **Astasia** (-abasia) 307.9
  - hysterical 300.11
- **Asteatosis** 706.8
  - cutis 706.8
- **Astereognosis** 780.99
- **Asterixis** 781.3
  - in liver disease 572.8
- **Asteroid hyalitis** 379.22
- **Asthenia, asthenic** 780.79
  - cardiac (*see also* Failure, heart) 428.9
    - psychogenic 306.2
  - cardiovascular (*see also* Failure, heart) 428.9
    - psychogenic 306.2
  - heart (*see also* Failure, heart) 428.9
    - psychogenic 306.2
  - hysterical 300.11
  - myocardial (*see also* Failure, heart) 428.9
    - psychogenic 306.2
  - nervous 300.5
  - neurocirculatory 306.2
  - neurotic 300.5
  - psychogenic 300.5
  - psychoneurotic 300.5
  - psychophysiologic 300.5
  - reaction, psychoneurotic 300.5
  - senile 797
  - Stiller's 780.79
  - tropical anhidrotic 705.1
- **Asthenopia** 368.13
  - accommodative 367.4
  - hysterical (muscular) 300.11
  - psychogenic 306.7
- **Asthenospermia** 792.2
- **Asthma, asthmatic** (bronchial) (catarrh) (spasmodic) 493.9 ☑

> *Note — The following fifth-digit subclassification is for use with codes 493.0-493.2, 493.9:*
>
> 0 *unspecified*
> 1 *with status asthmaticus*
> 2 *with (acute) exacerbation*

  - with
    - chronic obstructive pulmonary disease (COPD) 493.2 ☑
    - hay fever 493.0 ☑
    - rhinitis, allergic 493.0 ☑
- **Asthma, asthmatic** — *continued*
  - allergic 493.9 ☑
    - stated cause (external allergen) 493.0 ☑
  - atopic 493.0 ☑
  - cardiac (*see also* Failure, ventricular, left) 428.1
  - cardiobronchial (*see also* Failure, ventricular, left) 428.1
  - cardiorenal (*see also* Hypertension, cardiorenal) 404.90
  - childhood 493.0 ☑
  - Colliers' 500
  - cough variant 493.82
  - croup 493.9 ☑
  - detergent 507.8
  - due to
    - detergent 507.8
    - inhalation of fumes 506.3
    - internal immunological process 493.0 ☑
  - endogenous (intrinsic) 493.1 ☑
  - eosinophilic 518.3
  - exercise induced bronchospasm 493.81
  - exogenous (cosmetics) (dander or dust) (drugs) (dust) (feathers) (food) (hay) (platinum) (pollen) 493.0 ☑
  - extrinsic 493.0 ☑
  - grinders' 502
  - hay 493.0 ☑
  - heart (*see also* Failure, ventricular, left) 428.1
  - IgE 493.0 ☑
  - infective 493.1 ☑
  - intrinsic 493.1 ☑
  - Kopp's 254.8
  - late-onset 493.1 ☑
  - meat-wrappers' 506.9
  - Millar's (laryngismus stridulus) 478.75
  - millstone makers' 502
  - miners' 500
  - Monday morning 504
  - New Orleans (epidemic) 493.0 ☑
  - platinum 493.0 ☑
  - pneumoconiotic (occupational) NEC 505
  - potters' 502
  - psychogenic 316 *[493.9]* ☑
  - pulmonary eosinophilic 518.3
  - red cedar 495.8
  - Rostan's (*see also* Failure, ventricular, left) 428.1
  - sandblasters' 502
  - sequoiosis 495.8
  - stonemasons' 502
  - thymic 254.8
  - tuberculous (*see also* Tuberculosis, pulmonary) 011.9 ☑
  - Wichmann's (laryngismus stridulus) 478.75
  - wood 495.8
- **Astigmatism** (compound) (congenital) 367.20
  - irregular 367.22
  - regular 367.21
- **Astroblastoma** (M9430/3)
  - nose 748.1
  - specified site — *see* Neoplasm, by site, malignant
  - unspecified site 191.9
- **Astrocytoma** (cystic) (M9400/3)
  - anaplastic type (M9401/3)
    - specified site — *see* Neoplasm, by site, malignant
    - unspecified site 191.9
  - fibrillary (M9420/3)
    - specified site — *see* Neoplasm, by site, malignant
    - unspecified site 191.9
  - fibrous (M9420/3)
    - specified site — *see* Neoplasm, by site, malignant
    - unspecified site 191.9
  - gemistocytic (M9411/3)
    - specified site — *see* Neoplasm, by site, malignant
    - unspecified site 191.9
  - juvenile (M9421/3)
    - specified site — *see* Neoplasm, by site, malignant
    - unspecified site 191.9
  - nose 748.1
  - pilocytic (M9421/3)
    - specified site — *see* Neoplasm, by site, malignant

☑ Additional Digit Required — Refer to the Tabular List (Numeric Code Section) for Additional Digit Selection

▶◀ Revised Text ● New Line ▲ Revised Code

☑ Additional Digit Required — Refer to the Tabular List (Numeric Code Section) for Additional Digit Selection

▶◀ Revised Text ● New Line ▲ Revised Code

B

- **Baker's**
  - cyst (knee) 727.51
    - tuberculous (*see also* Tuberculosis) 015.2 ☑
  - itch 692.89
- **Bakwin-Krida syndrome** (craniometaphyseal dysplasia) 756.89
- **Balanitis** (circinata) (gangraenosa) (infectious) (vulgaris) 607.1
  - amebic 006.8
  - candidal 112.2
  - chlamydial 099.53
  - due to Ducrey's bacillus 099.0
  - erosiva circinata et gangraenosa 607.1
  - gangrenous 607.1
  - gonococcal (acute) 098.0
    - chronic or duration of 2 months or over 098.2
  - nongonococcal 607.1
  - phagedenic 607.1
  - venereal NEC 099.8
  - xerotica obliterans 607.81
- **Balanoposthitis** 607.1
  - chlamydial 099.53
  - gonococcal (acute) 098.0
    - chronic or duration of 2 months or over 098.2
  - ulcerative NEC 099.8
- **Balanorrhagia** — *see* Balanitis
- **Balantidiasis** 007.0
- **Balantidiosis** 007.0
- **Balbuties, balbutio** 307.0
- **Bald**
  - patches on scalp 704.00
  - tongue 529.4
- **Baldness** (*see also* Alopecia) 704.00
- **Balfour's disease** (chloroma) 205.3 ☑
- **Balint's syndrome** (psychic paralysis of visual fixation) 368.16
- **Balkan grippe** 083.0
- **Ball**
  - food 938
  - hair 938
- **Ballantyne (-Runge) syndrome** (postmaturity) 766.22
- **Balloon disease** (*see also* Effect, adverse, high altitude) 993.2
- **Ballooning posterior leaflet syndrome** 424.0
- **Baló's disease or concentric sclerosis** 341.1
- **Bamberger's disease** (hypertrophic pulmonary osteoarthropathy) 731.2
- **Bamberger-Marie disease** (hypertrophic pulmonary osteoarthropathy) 731.2
- **Bamboo spine** 720.0
- **Bancroft's filariasis** 125.0
- **Band(s)**
  - adhesive (*see also* Adhesions, peritoneum) 568.0
  - amniotic 658.8 ☑
    - affecting fetus or newborn 762.8
  - anomalous or congenital — *see also* Anomaly, specified type NEC
    - atrial 746.9
    - heart 746.9
    - intestine 751.4
    - omentum 751.4
    - ventricular 746.9
  - cervix 622.3
  - gallbladder (congenital) 751.69
  - intestinal (adhesive) (*see also* Adhesions, peritoneum) 568.0
    - congenital 751.4
  - obstructive (*see also* Obstruction, intestine) 560.81
  - periappendiceal (congenital) 751.4
  - peritoneal (adhesive) (*see also* Adhesions, peritoneum) 568.0
    - with intestinal obstruction 560.81
    - congenital 751.4
  - uterus 621,5
  - vagina 623.2
- **Bandl's ring** (contraction)
  - complicating delivery 661.4 ☑
    - affecting fetus or newborn 763.7
- **Bang's disease** (Brucella abortus) 023.1
- **Bangkok hemorrhagic fever** 065.4
- **Bannister's disease** 995.1
- **Bantam-Albright-Martin disease** (pseudohypoparathyroidism) 275.49
- **Banti's disease or syndrome** (with cirrhosis) (with portal hypertension) — *see* Cirrhosis, liver
- **Bar**
  - calcaneocuboid 755.67
  - calcaneonavicular 755.67
  - cubonavicular 755.67
  - prostate 600.90
    - with urinary retention 600.91
  - talocalcaneal 755.67
- **Baragnosis** 780.99
- **Barasheh, barashek** 266.2
- **Barcoo disease or rot** (*see also* Ulcer, skin) 707.9
- **Bard-Pic syndrome** (carcinoma, head of pancreas) 157.0
- **Bärensprung's disease** (eczema marginatum) 110.3
- **Baritosis** 503
- **Barium lung disease** 503
- **Barlow's syndrome** (meaning mitral valve prolapse) 424.0
- **Barlow (-Möller) disease or syndrome** (meaning infantile scurvy) 267
- **Barodontalgia** 993.2
- **Baron Münchausen syndrome** 301.51
- **Barosinusitis** 993.1
- **Barotitis** 993.0
- **Barotrauma** 993.2
  - odontalgia 993.2
  - otitic 993.0
  - sinus 993.1
- **Barraquer's disease or syndrome** (progressive lipodystrophy) 272.6
- **Barré-Guillain syndrome** 357.0
- **Barré-Liéou syndrome** (posterior cervical sympathetic) 723.2
- **Barrel chest** 738.3
- **Barrett's esophagus** 530.85
- **Barrett's syndrome or ulcer** (chronic peptic ulcer of esophagus) 530.85
- **Bársony-Polgár syndrome** (corkscrew esophagus) 530.5
- **Bársony-Teschendorf syndrome** (corkscrew esophagus) 530.5
- **Bartholin's**
  - adenitis (*see also* Bartholinitis) 616.8
  - gland — *see* condition
- **Bartholinitis** (suppurating) 616.8
  - gonococcal (acute) 098.0
    - chronic or duration of 2 months or over 098.2
- **Barth syndrome** 759.89 ●
- **Bartonellosis** 088.0
- **Bartter's syndrome** (secondary hyperaldosteronism with juxtaglomerular hyperplasia) 255.13
- **Basal** — *see* condition
- **Basan's** (hidrotic) **ectodermal dysplasia** 757.31
- **Baseball finger** 842.13
- **Basedow's disease or syndrome** (exophthalmic goiter) 242.0 ☑
- **Basic** — *see* condition
- **Basilar** — *see* condition
- **Bason's** (hidrotic) **ectodermal dysplasia** 757.31
- **Basopenia** 288.0
- **Basophilia** 288.8
- **Basophilism** (corticoadrenal) (Cushing's) (pituitary) (thymic) 255.0
- **Bassen-Kornzweig syndrome** (abetalipoproteinemia) 272.5
- **Bat ear** 744.29
- **Bateman's**
  - disease 078.0
  - purpura (senile) 287.2
- **Bathing cramp** 994.1
- **Bathophobia** 300.23
- **Batten's disease, retina** 330.1 *[362.71]*
- **Batten-Mayou disease** 330.1 *[362.71]*
- **Batten-Steinert syndrome** 359.2
- **Battered**
  - adult (syndrome) 995.81
  - baby or child (syndrome) 995.54
  - spouse (syndrome) 995.81
- **Battey mycobacterium infection** 031.0
- **Battledore placenta** — *see* Placenta, abnormal
- **Battle exhaustion** (*see also* Reaction, stress, acute) 308.9
- **Baumgarten-Cruveilhier** (cirrhosis) **disease, or syndrome** 571.5
- **Bauxite**
  - fibrosis (of lung) 503
  - workers' disease 503
- **Bayle's disease** (dementia paralytica) 094.1
- **Bazin's disease** (primary) (*see also* Tuberculosis) 017.1 ☑
- **Beach ear** 380.12
- **Beaded hair** (congenital) 757.4
- **Beals syndrome** 759.82
- **Beard's disease** (neurasthenia) 300.5
- **Bearn-Kunkel (-Slater) syndrome** (lupoid hepatitis) 571.49
- **Beat**
  - elbow 727.2
  - hand 727.2
  - knee 727.2
- **Beats**
  - ectopic 427.60
  - escaped, heart 427.60
    - postoperative 997.1
  - premature (nodal) 427.60
    - atrial 427.61
    - auricular 427.61
    - postoperative 997.1
    - specified type NEC 427.69
    - supraventricular 427.61
    - ventricular 427.69
- **Beau's**
  - disease or syndrome (*see also* Degeneration, myocardial) 429.1
  - lines (transverse furrows on fingernails) 703.8
- **Bechterew's disease** (ankylosing spondylitis) 720.0
- **Bechterew-Strümpell-Marie syndrome** (ankylosing spondylitis) 720.0
- **Beck's syndrome** (anterior spinal artery occlusion) 433.8 ☑
- **Becker's**
  - disease (idiopathic mural endomyocardial disease) 425.2
  - dystrophy 359.1
- **Beckwith (-Wiedemann) syndrome** 759.89
- **Bedclothes, asphyxiation or suffocation by** 994.7
- **Bed confinement status** V49.84 ●
- **Bednar's aphthae** 528.2
- **Bedsore** 707.00
  - with gangrene 707.00 *[785.4]*
- **Bedwetting** (*see also* Enuresis) 788.36
- **Beer-drinkers' heart** (disease) 425.5
- **Bee sting** (with allergic or anaphylactic shock) 989.5
- **Begbie's disease** (exophthalmic goiter) 242.0 ☑
- **Behavior disorder, disturbance** — *see also* Disturbance, conduct
  - antisocial, without manifest psychiatric disorder
    - adolescent V71.02
    - adult V71.01
    - child V71.02
  - dyssocial, without manifest psychiatric disorder
    - adolescent V71.02
    - adult V71.01
    - child V71.02
  - high risk — *see* Problem

☑ Additional Digit Required — Refer to the Tabular List (Numeric Code Section) for Additional Digit Selection

▶◀ Revised Text ● New Line ▲ Revised Code

Index — Birth — Blindness

☑ Additional Digit Required — Refer to the Tabular List (Numeric Code Section) for Additional Digit Selection

▶◀ Revised Text ● New Line ▲ Revised Code

Blindness — *continued*
- legal — *continued*
  - with impairment of better eye — *continued*
    - severe — *continued*
      - with — *continued*
        - lesser eye impairment — *continued*
          - near-total 369.13
          - profound 369.14
          - severe 369.22
          - total 369.12
    - total
      - with lesser eye impairment
        - total 369.01
- mind 784.69
- moderate
  - both eyes 369.25
    - with impairment of lesser eye (specified as)
      - blind, not further specified 369.15
      - low vision, not further specified 369.23
      - near-total 369.17
      - profound 369.18
      - severe 369.24
      - total 369.16
  - one eye 369.74
    - with vision of other eye (specified as)
      - near-normal 369.75
      - normal 369.76
- near-total
  - both eyes 369.04
    - with impairment of lesser eye (specified as)
      - blind, not further specified 369.02
      - total 369.03
  - one eye 369.64
    - with vision of other eye (specified as)
      - near-normal 369.65
      - normal 369.66
- night 368.60
  - acquired 368.62
  - congenital (Japanese) 368.61
  - hereditary 368.61
  - specified type NEC 368.69
  - vitamin A deficiency 264.5
- nocturnal — *see* Blindness, night
- one eye 369.60
  - with low vision of other eye 369.10
- profound
  - both eyes 369.08
    - with impairment of lesser eye (specified as)
      - blind, not further specified 369.05
      - near-total 369.07
      - total 369.06
  - one eye 369.67
    - with vision of other eye (specified as)
      - near-normal 369.68
      - normal 369.69
- psychic 784.69
- severe
  - both eyes 369.22
    - with impairment of lesser eye (specified as)
      - blind, not further specified 369.11
      - low vision, not further specified 369.21
      - near-total 369.13
      - profound 369.14
      - total 369.12
  - one eye 369.71
    - with vision of other eye (specified as)
      - near-normal 369.72
      - normal 369.73
- snow 370.24
- sun 363.31
- temporary 368.12
- total
  - both eyes 369.01
  - one eye 369.61
    - with vision of other eye (specified as)
      - near-normal 369.62
      - normal 369.63
- transient 368.12
- traumatic NEC 950.9
- word (developmental) 315.01
  - acquired 784.61
  - secondary to organic lesion 784.61

Blister — *see also* Injury, superficial, by site
- beetle dermatitis 692.89
- due to burn — *see* Burn, by site, second degree
- fever 054.9
- multiple, skin, nontraumatic 709.8

Bloating 787.3

Bloch-Siemens syndrome (incontinentia pigmenti) 757.33

Bloch-Stauffer dyshormonal dermatosis 757.33

Bloch-Sulzberger disease or syndrome (incontinentia pigmenti) (melanoblastosis) 757.33

Block
- alveolar capillary 516.3
- arborization (heart) 426.6
- arrhythmic 426.9
- atrioventricular (AV) (incomplete) (partial) 426.10
  - with
    - 2:1 atrioventricular response block 426.13
    - atrioventricular dissociation 426.0
  - first degree (incomplete) 426.11
  - second degree (Mobitz type I) 426.13
    - Mobitz (type) II 426.12
  - third degree 426.0
  - complete 426.0
    - congenital 746.86
  - congenital 746.86
  - Mobitz (incomplete)
    - type I (Wenckebach's) 426.13
    - type II 426.12
  - partial 426.13
- auriculoventricular (*see also* Block, atrioventricular) 426.10
  - complete 426.0
    - congenital 746.86
  - congenital 746.86
- bifascicular (cardiac) 426.53
- bundle branch (complete) (false) (incomplete) 426.50
  - bilateral 426.53
  - left (complete) (main stem) 426.3
    - with right bundle branch block 426.53
    - anterior fascicular 426.2
      - with
        - posterior fascicular block 426.3
        - right bundle branch block 426.52
    - hemiblock 426.2
    - incomplete 426.2
      - with right bundle branch block 426.53
    - posterior fascicular 426.2
      - with
        - anterior fascicular block 426.3
        - right bundle branch block 426.51
  - right 426.4
    - with
      - left bundle branch block (incomplete) (main stem) 426.53
      - left fascicular block 426.53
        - anterior 426.52
        - posterior 426.51
  - Wilson's type 426.4
- cardiac 426.9
- conduction 426.9
  - complete 426.0
- Eustachian tube (*see also* Obstruction, Eustachian tube) 381.60
- fascicular (left anterior) (left posterior) 426.2
- foramen Magendie (acquired) 331.3
  - congenital 742.3
    - with spina bifida (*see also* Spina bifida) 741.0 ☑
- heart 426.9
  - first degree (atrioventricular) 426.11
  - second degree (atrioventricular) 426.13
  - third degree (atrioventricular) 426.0
  - bundle branch (complete) (false) (incomplete) 426.50
    - bilateral 426.53
    - left (*see also* Block, bundle branch, left) 426.3
    - right (*see also* Block, bundle branch, right) 426.4
  - complete (atrioventricular) 426.0
  - congenital 746.86
  - incomplete 426.13
  - intra-atrial 426.6
  - intraventricular NEC 426.6
  - sinoatrial 426.6
  - specified type NEC 426.6
- hepatic vein 453.0
- intraventricular (diffuse) (myofibrillar) 426.6
  - bundle branch (complete) (false) (incomplete) 426.50
    - bilateral 426.53
    - left (*see also* Block, bundle branch, left) 426.3
    - right (*see also* Block, bundle branch, right) 426.4
- kidney (*see also* Disease, renal) 593.9
  - postcystoscopic 997.5
- myocardial (*see also* Block, heart) 426.9
- nodal 426.10
- optic nerve 377.49
- organ or site (congenital) NEC — *see* Atresia
- parietal 426.6
- peri-infarction 426.6
- portal (vein) 452
- sinoatrial 426.6
- sinoauricular 426.6
- spinal cord 336.9
- trifascicular 426.54
- tubal 628.2
- vein NEC 453.9

Blocq's disease or syndrome (astasia-abasia) 307.9

Blood
- constituents, abnormal NEC 790.6
- disease 289.9
  - specified NEC 289.89
- donor V59.01
  - other blood components V59.09
  - stem cells V59.02
  - whole blood V59.01
- dyscrasia 289.9
  - with
    - abortion — *see* Abortion, by type, with hemorrhage, delayed or excessive
    - ectopic pregnancy (*see also* categories 633.0-633.9) 639.1
    - molar pregnancy (*see also* categories 630-632) 639.1
  - fetus or newborn NEC 776.9
  - following
    - abortion 639.1
    - ectopic or molar pregnancy 639.1
  - puerperal, postpartum 666.3 ☑
- flukes NEC (*see also* Infestation, Schistosoma) 120.9
- in
  - feces (*see also* Melena) 578.1
    - occult 792.1
  - urine (*see also* Hematuria) 599.7
- mole 631
- occult 792.1
- poisoning (*see also* Septicemia) 038.9
- pressure
  - decreased, due to shock following injury 958.4
  - fluctuating 796.4
  - high (*see also* Hypertension) 401.9
    - incidental reading (isolated) (nonspecific), without diagnosis of hypertension 796.2
  - low (*see also* Hypotension) 458.9
    - incidental reading (isolated) (nonspecific), without diagnosis of hypotension 796.3
- spitting (*see also* Hemoptysis) 786.3
- staining cornea 371.12
- transfusion
  - without reported diagnosis V58.2
  - donor V59.01
    - stem cells V59.02
  - reaction or complication — *see* Complications, transfusion
- tumor — *see* Hematoma
- vessel rupture — *see* Hemorrhage

☑ Additional Digit Required — Refer to the Tabular List (Numeric Code Section) for Additional Digit Selection

▶◀ Revised Text ● New Line ▲ Revised Code

- **Blood** — *continued*
  - vomiting (*see also* Hematemesis) 578.0
- **Blood-forming organ disease** 289.9
- **Bloodgood's disease** 610.1
- **Bloodshot eye** 379.93
- **Bloom (-Machacek) (-Torre) syndrome** 757.39
- **Blotch, palpebral** 372.55
- **Blount's disease** (tibia vara) 732.4
- **Blount-Barber syndrome** (tibia vara) 732.4
- **Blue**
  - baby 746.9
  - bloater 491.20
    - with
      - acute bronchitis 491.22
      - exacerbation (acute) 491.21
  - diaper syndrome 270.0
  - disease 746.9
  - dome cyst 610.0
  - drum syndrome 381.02
  - sclera 743.47
    - with fragility of bone and deafness 756.51
  - toe syndrome 445.02
- **Blueness** (*see also* Cyanosis) 782.5
- **Blurring, visual** 368.8
- **Blushing** (abnormal) (excessive) 782.62
- **BMI** (body mass index) ●
  - adult ●
    - 25.0–25.9 V85.21 ●
    - 26.0–26.9 V85.22 ●
    - 27.0–27.9 V85.23 ●
    - 28.0–28.9 V85.24 ●
    - 29.0–29.9 V85.25 ●
    - 30.0–30.9 V85.30 ●
    - 31.0–31.9 V85.31 ●
    - 32.0–32.9 V85.32 ●
    - 33.0–33.9 V85.33 ●
    - 34.0–34.9 V85.34 ●
    - 35.0–35.9 V85.35 ●
    - 36.0–36.9 V85.36 ●
    - 37.0–37.9 V85.37 ●
    - 38.0–38.9 V85.38 ●
    - 39.0–39.9 V85.39 ●
    - 40 and over V85.4 ●
    - between 19–24 V85.1 ●
    - less than 19 V85.0 ●
- **Boarder, hospital** V65.0
  - infant V65.0
- **Bockhart's impetigo** (superficial folliculitis) 704.8
- **Bodechtel-Guttmann disease** (subacute sclerosing panencephalitis) 046.2
- **Boder-Sedgwick syndrome** (ataxia-telangiectasia) 334.8
- **Body, bodies**
  - Aschoff (*see also* Myocarditis, rheumatic) 398.0
  - asteroid, vitreous 379.22
  - choroid, colloid (degenerative) 362.57
    - hereditary 362.77
  - cytoid (retina) 362.82
  - drusen (retina) (*see also* Drusen) 362.57
    - optic disc 377.21
  - fibrin, pleura 511.0
  - foreign — *see* Foreign body
  - Hassall-Henle 371.41
  - loose
    - joint (*see also* Loose, body, joint) 718.1 ☑
      - knee 717.6
    - knee 717.6
    - sheath, tendon 727.82
  - Mallory's 034.1
  - mass index (BMI) ●
    - adult ●
      - 25.0–25.9 V85.21 ●
      - 26.0–26.9 V85.22 ●
      - 27.0–27.9 V85.23 ●
      - 28.0–28.9 V85.24 ●
      - 29.0–29.9 V85.25 ●
      - 30.0–30.9 V85.30 ●
      - 31.0–31.9 V85.31 ●
      - 32.0–32.9 V85.32 ●
      - 33.0–33.9 V85.33 ●
      - 34.0–34.9 V85.34 ●
      - 35.0–35.9 V85.35 ●
      - 36.0–36.9 V85.36 ●
      - 37.0–37.9 V85.37 ●
- **Body, bodies** — *continued*
  - mass index — *continued*
    - adult — *continued*
      - 38.0–38.9 V85.38 ●
      - 39.0–39.9 V85.39 ●
      - 40 and over V85.4 ●
      - between 19–24 V85.1 ●
      - less than 19 V85.0 ●
  - Mooser 081.0
  - Negri 071
  - rice (joint) (*see also* Loose, body, joint) 718.1 ☑
    - knee 717.6
  - rocking 307.3
- **Boeck's**
  - disease (sarcoidosis) 135
  - lupoid (miliary) 135
  - sarcoid 135
- **Boerhaave's syndrome** (spontaneous esophageal rupture) 530.4
- **Boggy**
  - cervix 622.8
  - uterus 621.8
- **Boil** (*see also* Carbuncle) 680.9
  - abdominal wall 680.2
  - Aleppo 085.1
  - ankle 680.6
  - anus 680.5
  - arm (any part, above wrist) 680.3
  - auditory canal, external 680.0
  - axilla 680.3
  - back (any part) 680.2
  - Baghdad 085.1
  - breast 680.2
  - buttock 680.5
  - chest wall 680.2
  - corpus cavernosum 607.2
  - Delhi 085.1
  - ear (any part) 680.0
  - eyelid 373.13
  - face (any part, except eye) 680.0
  - finger (any) 680.4
  - flank 680.2
  - foot (any part) 680.7
  - forearm 680.3
  - Gafsa 085.1
  - genital organ, male 608.4
  - gluteal (region) 680.5
  - groin 680.2
  - hand (any part) 680.4
  - head (any part, except face) 680.8
  - heel 680.7
  - hip 680.6
  - knee 680.6
  - labia 616.4
  - lacrimal (*see also* Dacryocystitis) 375.30
    - gland (*see also* Dacryoadenitis) 375.00
    - passages (duct) (sac) (*see also* Dacryocystitis) 375.30
  - leg, any part, except foot 680.6
  - multiple sites 680.9
  - natal 085.1
  - neck 680.1
  - nose (external) (septum) 680.0
  - orbit, orbital 376.01
  - partes posteriores 680.5
  - pectoral region 680.2
  - penis 607.2
  - perineum 680.2
  - pinna 680.0
  - scalp (any part) 680.8
  - scrotum 608.4
  - seminal vesicle 608.0
  - shoulder 680.3
  - skin NEC 680.9
  - specified site NEC 680.8
  - spermatic cord 608.4
  - temple (region) 680.0
  - testis 608.4
  - thigh 680.6
  - thumb 680.4
  - toe (any) 680.7
  - tropical 085.1
  - trunk 680.2
  - tunica vaginalis 608.4
  - umbilicus 680.2
  - upper arm 680.3
- **Boil** (*see also* Carbuncle) — *continued*
  - vas deferens 608.4
  - vulva 616.4
  - wrist 680.4
- **Bold hives** (*see also* Urticaria) 708.9
- **Bolivian hemorrhagic fever** 078.7
- **Bombé, iris** 364.74
- **Bomford-Rhoads anemia** (refractory) 238.7 ▲
- **Bone** — *see* condition
- **Bonnevie-Ullrich syndrome** 758.6
- **Bonnier's syndrome** 386.19
- **Bonvale Dam fever** 780.79
- **Bony block of joint** 718.80
  - ankle 718.87
  - elbow 718.82
  - foot 718.87
  - hand 718.84
  - hip 718.85
  - knee 718.86
  - multiple sites 718.89
  - pelvic region 718.85
  - shoulder (region) 718.81
  - specified site NEC 718.88
  - wrist 718.83
- **Borderline**
  - intellectual functioning V62.89
  - pelvis 653.1 ☑
    - with obstruction during labor 660.1 ☑
      - affecting fetus or newborn 763.1
  - psychosis (*see also* Schizophrenia) 295.5 ☑
    - of childhood (*see also* Psychosis, childhood) 299.8 ☑
  - schizophrenia (*see also* Schizophrenia) 295.5 ☑
- **Borna disease** 062.9
- **Bornholm disease** (epidemic pleurodynia) 074.1
- **Borrelia vincentii** (mouth) (pharynx) (tonsils) 101
- **Bostock's catarrh** (*see also* Fever, hay) 477.9
- **Boston exanthem** 048
- **Botalli, ductus** (patent) (persistent) 747.0
- **Bothriocephalus latus infestation** 123.4
- **Botulism** 005.1
- **Bouba** (*see also* Yaws) 102.9
- **Bouffée délirante** 298.3
- **Bouillaud's disease or syndrome** (rheumatic heart disease) 391.9
- **Bourneville's disease** (tuberous sclerosis) 759.5
- **Boutonneuse fever** 082.1
- **Boutonniere**
  - deformity (finger) 736.21
  - hand (intrinsic) 736.21
- **Bouveret (-Hoffmann) disease or syndrome** (paroxysmal tachycardia) 427.2
- **Bovine heart** — *see* Hypertrophy, cardiac
- **Bowel** — *see* condition
- **Bowen's**
  - dermatosis (precancerous) (M8081/2) — *see* Neoplasm, skin, in situ
  - disease (M8081/2) — *see* Neoplasm, skin, in situ
  - epithelioma (M8081/2) — *see* Neoplasm, skin, in situ
  - type
    - epidermoid carcinoma in situ (M8081/2) — *see* Neoplasm, skin, in situ
    - intraepidermal squamous cell carcinoma (M8081/2) — *see* Neoplasm, skin, in situ
- **Bowing**
  - femur 736.89
    - congenital 754.42
  - fibula 736.89
    - congenital 754.43
  - forearm 736.09
    - away from midline (cubitus valgus) 736.01
    - toward midline (cubitus varus) 736.02
  - leg(s), long bones, congenital 754.44
  - radius 736.09
    - away from midline (cubitus valgus) 736.01
    - toward midline (cubitus varus) 736.02
  - tibia 736.89
    - congenital 754.43

☑ Additional Digit Required — Refer to the Tabular List (Numeric Code Section) for Additional Digit Selection

▶◀ Revised Text ● New Line ▲ Revised Code

- **Bowleg(s)** 736.42
  - congenital 754.44
  - rachitic 268.1
- **Boyd's dysentery** 004.2
- **Brachial** — *see* condition
- **Brachman-de Lange syndrome** (Amsterdam dwarf, mental retardation, and brachycephaly) 759.89
- **Brachycardia** 427.89
- **Brachycephaly** 756.0
- **Brachymorphism and ectopia lentis** 759.89
- **Bradley's disease** (epidemic vomiting) 078.82
- **Bradycardia** 427.89
  - chronic (sinus) 427.81
  - newborn 779.81
  - nodal 427.89
  - postoperative 997.1
  - reflex 337.0
  - sinoatrial 427.89
    - with paroxysmal tachyarrhythmia or tachycardia 427.81
    - chronic 427.81
  - sinus 427.89
    - with paroxysmal tachyarrhythmia or tachycardia 427.81
    - chronic 427.81
    - persistent 427.81
    - severe 427.81
  - tachycardia syndrome 427.81
  - vagal 427.89
- **Bradypnea** 786.09
- **Brailsford's disease** 732.3
  - radial head 732.3
  - tarsal scaphoid 732.5
- **Brailsford-Morquio disease or syndrome** (mucopolysaccharidosis IV) 277.5
- **Brain** — *see also* condition
  - death 348.8
  - syndrome (acute) (chronic) (nonpsychotic) (organic) (with neurotic reaction) (with behavioral reaction) (*see also* Syndrome, brain) 310.9
    - with
      - presenile brain disease 290.10
      - psychosis, psychotic reaction (*see also* Psychosis, organic) 294.9
    - congenital (*see also* Retardation, mental) 319
- **Branched-chain amino-acid disease** 270.3
- **Branchial** — *see* condition
- **Brandt's syndrome** (acrodermatitis enteropathica) 686.8
- **Brash** (water) 787.1
- **Brass-founders' ague** 985.8
- **Bravais-Jacksonian epilepsy** (*see also* Epilepsy) 345.5 ☑
- **Braxton Hicks contractions** 644.1 ☑
- **Braziers' disease** 985.8
- **Brazilian**
  - blastomycosis 116.1
  - leishmaniasis 085.5
- **BRBPR** (bright red blood per rectum) 569.3
- **Break**
  - cardiorenal — *see* Hypertension, cardiorenal
  - retina (*see also* Defect, retina) 361.30
- **Breakbone fever** 061
- **Breakdown**
  - device, implant, or graft — *see* Complications, mechanical
  - nervous (*see also* Disorder, mental, nonpsychotic) 300.9
  - perineum 674.2 ☑
- **Breast** — *see* condition
- **Breast feeding difficulties** 676.8 ☑
- **Breath**
  - foul 784.9
  - holder, child 312.81
  - holding spells 786.9
  - shortness 786.05
- **Breathing**
  - asymmetrical 786.09
  - bronchial 786.09
  - exercises V57.0
  - labored 786.09
  - mouth 784.9
    - causing malocclusion 524.59 ●
  - periodic 786.09
    - high altitude 327.22 ●
  - tic 307.20
- **Breathlessness** 786.09
- **Breda's disease** (*see also* Yaws) 102.9
- **Breech**
  - delivery, affecting fetus or newborn 763.0
  - extraction, affecting fetus or newborn 763.0
  - presentation (buttocks) (complete) (frank) 652.2 ☑
    - with successful version 652.1 ☑
    - before labor, affecting fetus or newborn 761.7
    - during labor, affecting fetus or newborn 763.0
- **Breisky's disease** (kraurosis vulvae) 624.0
- **Brennemann's syndrome** (acute mesenteric lymphadenitis) 289.2
- **Brenner's**
  - tumor (benign) (M9000/0) 220
    - borderline malignancy (M9000/1) 236.2
    - malignant (M9000/3) 183.0
    - proliferating (M9000/1) 236.2
- **Bretonneau's disease** (diphtheritic malignant angina) 032.0
- **Breus' mole** 631
- **Brevicollis** 756.16
- **Bricklayers' itch** 692.89
- **Brickmakers' anemia** 126.9
- **Bridge**
  - myocardial 746.85
- **Bright red blood per rectum** (BRBPR) 569.3
- **Bright's**
  - blindness — *see* Uremia
  - disease (*see also* Nephritis) 583.9
    - arteriosclerotic (*see also* Hypertension, kidney) 403.90
- **Brill's disease** (recrudescent typhus) 081.1
  - flea-borne 081.0
  - louse-borne 081.1
- **Brill-Symmers disease** (follicular lymphoma) (M9690/3) 202.0 ☑
- **Brill-Zinsser disease** (recrudescent typhus) 081.1
- **Brinton's disease** (linitis plastica) (M8142/3) 151.9
- **Brion-Kayser disease** (*see also* Fever, paratyphoid) 002.9
- **Briquet's disorder or syndrome** 300.81
- **Brissaud's**
  - infantilism (infantile myxedema) 244.9
  - motor-verbal tic 307.23
- **Brissaud-Meige syndrome** (infantile myxedema) 244.9
- **Brittle**
  - bones (congenital) 756.51
  - nails 703.8
    - congenital 757.5
- **Broad** — *see also* condition
  - beta disease 272.2
  - ligament laceration syndrome 620.6
- **Brock's syndrome** (atelectasis due to enlarged lymph nodes) 518.0
- **Brocq's disease** 691.8
  - atopic (diffuse) neurodermatitis 691.8
  - lichen simplex chronicus 698.3
  - parakeratosis psoriasiformis 696.2
  - parapsoriasis 696.2
- **Brocq-Duhring disease** (dermatitis herpetiformis) 694.0
- **Brodie's**
  - abscess (localized) (chronic) (*see also* Osteomyelitis) 730.1 ☑
  - disease (joint) (*see also* Osteomyelitis) 730.1 ☑
- **Broken**
  - arches 734
    - congenital 755.67
  - back — *see* Fracture, vertebra, by site
  - bone — *see* Fracture, by site
  - compensation — *see* Disease, heart
  - implant or internal device — *see* listing under Complications, mechanical
  - neck — *see* Fracture, vertebra, cervical
  - nose 802.0
    - open 802.1
  - tooth, teeth 873.63
    - complicated 873.73
- **Bromhidrosis** 705.89
- **Bromidism, bromism**
  - acute 967.3
    - correct substance properly administered 349.82
    - overdose or wrong substance given or taken 967.3
  - chronic (*see also* Dependence) 304.1 ☑
- **Bromidrosiphobia** 300.23
- **Bromidrosis** 705.89
- **Bronchi, bronchial** — *see* condition
- **Bronchiectasis** (cylindrical) (diffuse) (fusiform) (localized) (moniliform) (postinfectious) (recurrent) (saccular) 494.0
  - with acute exacerbation 494.1
  - congenital 748.61
  - tuberculosis (*see also* Tuberculosis) 011.5 ☑
- **Bronchiolectasis** — *see* Bronchiectasis
- **Bronchiolitis** (acute) (infectious) (subacute) 466.19
  - with
    - bronchospasm or obstruction 466.19
    - influenza, flu, or grippe 487.1
  - catarrhal (acute) (subacute) 466.19
  - chemical 506.0
    - chronic 506.4
  - chronic (obliterative) 491.8
  - due to external agent — *see* Bronchitis, acute, due to
  - fibrosa obliterans 491.8
  - influenzal 487.1
  - obliterans 491.8
    - with organizing pneumonia (B.O.O.P.) 516.8
    - status post lung transplant 996.84
  - obliterative (chronic) (diffuse) (subacute) 491.8
    - due to fumes or vapors 506.4
  - respiratory syncytial virus 466.11
  - vesicular — *see* Pneumonia, broncho-
- **Bronchitis** (diffuse) (hypostatic) (infectious) (inflammatory) (simple) 490
  - with
    - emphysema — *see* Emphysema
    - influenza, flu, or grippe 487.1
    - obstruction airway, chronic 491.20
      - with
        - acute bronchitis 491.22
        - exacerbation (acute) 491.21
    - tracheitis 490
      - acute or subacute 466.0
        - with bronchospasm or obstruction 466.0
      - chronic 491.8
  - acute or subacute 466.0
    - with
      - bronchospasm 466.0
      - obstruction 466.0
      - tracheitis 466.0
    - chemical (due to fumes or vapors) 506.0
    - due to
      - fumes or vapors 506.0
      - radiation 508.8
  - allergic (acute) (*see also* Asthma) 493.9 ☑
  - arachidic 934.1
  - aspiration 507.0
    - due to fumes or vapors 506.0
  - asthmatic (acute) 493.90
    - with
      - acute exacerbation 493.92
      - status asthmaticus 493.91
    - chronic 493.2 ☑
  - capillary 466.19
    - with bronchospasm or obstruction 466.19

☑ Additional Digit Required — Refer to the Tabular List (Numeric Code Section) for Additional Digit Selection

▶◀ Revised Text ● New Line ▲ Revised Code

Burkitt's — *continued*
- type malignant, lymphoma, lymphoblastic, or undifferentiated (M9750/3) 200.2 ☑

Burn (acid) (cathode ray) (caustic) (chemical) (electric heating appliance) (electricity) (fire) (flame) (hot liquid or object) (irradiation) (lime) (radiation) (steam) (thermal) (x-ray) 949.0

> *Note — Use the following fifth-digit subclassification with category 948 to indicate the percent of body surface with third degree burn:*
>
> *0 Less than 10% or unspecified*
> *1 10–19%*
> *2 20–29%*
> *3 30–39%*
> *4 40–49%*
> *5 50–59%*
> *6 60–69%*
> *7 70–79%*
> *8 80–89%*
> *9 90% or more of body surface*

- with
  - blisters — *see* Burn, by site, second degree
  - erythema — *see* Burn, by site, first degree
  - skin loss (epidermal) — *see also* Burn, by site, second degree
    - full thickness — *see also* Burn, by site, third degree
      - with necrosis of underlying tissues — *see* Burn, by site, third degree, deep
- first degree — *see* Burn, by site, first degree
- second degree — *see* Burn, by site, second degree
- third degree — *see* Burn, by site, third degree
  - deep — *see* Burn, by site, third degree, deep
- abdomen, abdominal (muscle) (wall) 942.03
  - with
    - trunk — *see* Burn, trunk, multiple sites
  - first degree 942.13
  - second degree 942.23
  - third degree 942.33
    - deep 942.43
      - with loss of body part 942.53
- ankle 945.03
  - with
    - lower limb(s) — *see* Burn, leg, multiple sites
  - first degree 945.13
  - second degree 945.23
  - third degree 945.33
    - deep 945.43
      - with loss of body part 945.53
- anus — *see* Burn, trunk, specified site NEC
- arm(s) 943.00
  - first degree 943.10
  - second degree 943.20
  - third degree 943.30
    - deep 943.40
      - with loss of body part 943.50
  - lower — *see* Burn, forearm(s)
  - multiple sites, except hand(s) or wrist(s) 943.09
    - first degree 943.19
    - second degree 943.29
    - third degree 943.39
      - deep 943.49
        - with loss of body part 943.59
  - upper 943.03
    - first degree 943.13
    - second degree 943.23
    - third degree 943.33
      - deep 943.43
        - with loss of body part 943.53
- auditory canal (external) — *see* Burn, ear
- auricle (ear) — *see* Burn, ear
- axilla 943.04
  - with
    - upper limb(s), except hand(s) or wrist(s) — *see* Burn, arm(s), multiple sites
  - first degree 943.14

Burn — *continued*
- axilla — *continued*
  - second degree 943.24
  - third degree 943.34
    - deep 943.44
      - with loss of body part 943.54
- back 942.04
  - with
    - trunk — *see* Burn, trunk, multiple sites
  - first degree 942.14
  - second degree 942.24
  - third degree 942.34
    - deep 942.44
      - with loss of body part 942.54
- biceps
  - brachii — *see* Burn, arm(s), upper
  - femoris — *see* Burn, thigh
- breast(s) 942.01
  - with
    - trunk — *see* Burn, trunk, multiple sites
  - first degree 942.11
  - second degree 942.21
  - third degree 942.31
    - deep 942.41
      - with loss of body part 942.51
- brow — *see* Burn, forehead
- buttock(s) — *see* Burn, back
- canthus (eye) 940.1
  - chemical 940.0
- cervix (uteri) 947.4
- cheek (cutaneous) 941.07
  - with
    - face or head — *see* Burn, head, multiple sites
  - first degree 941.17
  - second degree 941.27
  - third degree 941.37
    - deep 941.47
      - with loss of body part 941.57
- chest wall (anterior) 942.02
  - with
    - trunk — *see* Burn, trunk, multiple sites
  - first degree 942.12
  - second degree 942.22
  - third degree 942.32
    - deep 942.42
      - with loss of body part 942.52
- chin 941.04
  - with
    - face or head — *see* Burn, head, multiple sites
  - first degree 941.14
  - second degree 941.24
  - third degree 941.34
    - deep 941.44
      - with loss of body part 941.54
- clitoris — *see* Burn, genitourinary organs, external
- colon 947.3
- conjunctiva (and cornea) 940.4
  - chemical
    - acid 940.3
    - alkaline 940.2
- cornea (and conjunctiva) 940.4
  - chemical
    - acid 940.3
    - alkaline 940.2
- costal region — *see* Burn, chest wall
- due to ingested chemical agent — *see* Burn, internal organs
- ear (auricle) (canal) (drum) (external) 941.01
  - with
    - face or head — *see* Burn, head, multiple sites
  - first degree 941.11
  - second degree 941.21
  - third degree 941.31
    - deep 941.41
      - with loss of a body part 941.51
- elbow 943.02
  - with
    - hand(s) and wrist(s) — *see* Burn, multiple specified sites
    - upper limb(s), except hand(s) or wrist(s) — *see also* Burn, arm(s), multiple sites
  - first degree 943.12

Burn — *continued*
- elbow — *continued*
  - second degree 943.22
  - third degree 943.32
    - deep 943.42
      - with loss of body part 943.52
- electricity, electric current — *see* Burn, by site
- entire body — *see* Burn, multiple, specified sites
- epididymis — *see* Burn, genitourinary organs, external
- epigastric region — *see* Burn, abdomen
- epiglottis 947.1
- esophagus 947.2
- extent (percent of body surface)
  - less than 10 percent 948.0 ☑
  - 10-19 percent 948.1 ☑
  - 20-29 percent 948.2 ☑
  - 30-39 percent 948.3 ☑
  - 40-49 percent 948.4 ☑
  - 50-59 percent 948.5 ☑
  - 60-69 percent 948.6 ☑
  - 70-79 percent 948.7 ☑
  - 80-89 percent 948.8 ☑
  - 90 percent or more 948.9 ☑
- extremity
  - lower — *see* Burn, leg
  - upper — *see* Burn, arm(s)
- eye(s) (and adnexa) (only) 940.9
  - with
    - face, head, or neck 941.02
      - first degree 941.12
      - second degree 941.22
      - third degree 941.32
        - deep 941.42
          - with loss of body part 941.52
    - other sites (classifiable to more than one category in 940-945) — *see* Burn, multiple, specified sites
    - resulting rupture and destruction of eyeball 940.5
  - specified part — *see* Burn, by site
- eyeball — *see also* Burn, eye
  - with resulting rupture and destruction of eyeball 940.5
- eyelid(s) 940.1
  - chemical 940.0
- face — *see* Burn, head
- finger (nail) (subungual) 944.01
  - with
    - hand(s) — *see* Burn, hand(s), multiple sites
    - other sites — *see* Burn, multiple, specified sites
    - thumb 944.04
      - first degree 944.14
      - second degree 944.24
      - third degree 944.34
        - deep 944.44
          - with loss of body part 944.54
  - first degree 944.11
  - second degree 944.21
  - third degree 944.31
    - deep 944.41
      - with loss of body part 944.51
  - multiple (digits) 944.03
    - with thumb — *see* Burn, finger, with thumb
    - first degree 944.13
    - second degree 944.23
    - third degree 944.33
      - deep 944.43
        - with loss of body part 944.53
- flank — *see* Burn, abdomen
- foot 945.02
  - with
    - lower limb(s) — *see* Burn, leg, multiple sites
  - first degree 945.12
  - second degree 945.22
  - third degree 945.32
    - deep 945.42
      - with loss of body part 945.52
- forearm(s) 943.01
  - with
    - upper limb(s), except hand(s) or wrist(s) — *see* Burn, arm(s), multiple sites

- **Burn** — *continued*
  - testis — *see* Burn, genitourinary organs, external
  - thigh 945.06
    - with
      - lower limb(s) — *see* Burn, leg, multiple sites
    - first degree 945.16
    - second degree 945.26
    - third degree 945.36
      - deep 945.46
        - with loss of body part 945.56
  - thorax (external) — *see* Burn, chest wall
  - throat 947.0
  - thumb(s) (nail) (subungual) 944.02
    - with
      - finger(s) — *see* Burn, finger, with other sites, thumb
      - hand(s) and wrist(s) — *see* Burn, hand(s), multiple sites
    - first degree 944.12
    - second degree 944.22
    - third degree 944.32
      - deep 944.42
        - with loss of body part 944.52
  - toe (nail) (subungual) 945.01
    - with
      - lower limb(s) — *see* Burn, leg, multiple sites
    - first degree 945.11
    - second degree 945.21
    - third degree 945.31
      - deep 945.41
        - with loss of body part 945.51
  - tongue 947.0
  - tonsil 947.0
  - trachea 947.1
  - trunk 942.00
    - first degree 942.10
    - second degree 942.20
    - third degree 942.30
      - deep 942.40
        - with loss of body part 942.50
    - multiple sites 942.09
      - first degree 942.19
      - second degree 942.29
      - third degree 942.39
        - deep 942.49
          - with loss of body part 942.59
    - specified site NEC 942.09
      - first degree 942.19
      - second degree 942.29
      - third degree 942.39
        - deep 942.49
          - with loss of body part 942.59
  - tunica vaginalis — *see* Burn, genitourinary organs, external
  - tympanic membrane — *see* Burn, ear
  - tympanum — *see* Burn, ear
  - ultraviolet 692.82
  - unspecified site (multiple) 949.0
    - with extent of body surface involved specified
      - less than 10 percent 948.0 ☑
      - 10-19 percent 948.1 ☑
      - 20-29 percent 948.2 ☑
      - 30-39 percent 948.3 ☑
      - 40-49 percent 948.4 ☑
      - 50-59 percent 948.5 ☑
      - 60-69 percent 948.6 ☑
      - 70-79 percent 948.7 ☑
      - 80-89 percent 948.8 ☑
      - 90 percent or more 948.9 ☑
    - first degree 949.1
    - second degree 949.2
    - third degree 949.3
      - deep 949.4
        - with loss of body part 949.5
  - uterus 947.4
  - uvula 947.0
  - vagina 947.4
  - vulva — *see* Burn, genitourinary organs, external
  - wrist(s) 944.07
    - with
      - hand(s) — *see* Burn, hand(s), multiple sites

- **Burn** — *continued*
  - wrist(s) — *continued*
    - first degree 944.17
    - second degree 944.27
    - third degree 944.37
      - deep 944.47
        - with loss of body part 944.57
- **Burnett's syndrome** (milk-alkali) 275.42
- **Burnier's syndrome** (hypophyseal dwarfism) 253.3
- **Burning**
  - feet syndrome 266.2
  - sensation (*see also* Disturbance, sensation) 782.0
  - tongue 529.6
- **Burns' disease** (osteochondrosis, lower ulna) 732.3
- **Bursa** — *see also* condition
  - pharynx 478.29
- **Bursitis** NEC 727.3
  - Achilles tendon 726.71
  - adhesive 726.90
    - shoulder 726.0
  - ankle 726.79
  - buttock 726.5
  - calcaneal 726.79
  - collateral ligament
    - fibular 726.63
    - tibial 726.62
  - Duplay's 726.2
  - elbow 726.33
  - finger 726.8
  - foot 726.79
  - gonococcal 098.52
  - hand 726.4
  - hip 726.5
  - infrapatellar 726.69
  - ischiogluteal 726.5
  - knee 726.60
  - occupational NEC 727.2
  - olecranon 726.33
  - pes anserinus 726.61
  - pharyngeal 478.29
  - popliteal 727.51
  - prepatellar 726.65
  - radiohumeral 727.3
  - scapulohumeral 726.19
    - adhesive 726.0
  - shoulder 726.10
    - adhesive 726.0
  - subacromial 726.19
    - adhesive 726.0
  - subcoracoid 726.19
  - subdeltoid 726.19
    - adhesive 726.0
  - subpatellar 726.69
  - syphilitic 095.7
  - Thornwaldt's, Tornwaldt's (pharyngeal) 478.29
  - toe 726.79
  - trochanteric area 726.5
  - wrist 726.4
- **Burst stitches or sutures** (complication of surgery) (external) 998.32
  - internal 998.31
- **Buruli ulcer** 031.1
- **Bury's disease** (erythema elevatum diutinum) 695.89
- **Buschke's disease or scleredema** (adultorum) 710.1
- **Busquet's disease** (osteoperiostitis) (*see also* Osteomyelitis) 730.1 ☑
- **Busse-Buschke disease** (cryptococcosis) 117.5
- **Buttock** — *see* condition
- **Button**
  - Biskra 085.1
  - Delhi 085.1
  - oriental 085.1
- **Buttonhole hand** (intrinsic) 736.21
- **Bwamba fever** (encephalitis) 066.3
- **Byssinosis** (occupational) 504
- **Bywaters' syndrome** 958.5

C

- **Cacergasia** 300.9
- **Cachexia** 799.4
  - cancerous (M8000/3) 199.1
  - cardiac — *see* Disease, heart
  - dehydration 276.51 ▲
    - with
      - hypernatremia 276.0
      - hyponatremia 276.1
  - due to malnutrition 261
  - exophthalmic 242.0 ☑
  - heart — *see* Disease, heart
  - hypophyseal 253.2
  - hypopituitary 253.2
  - lead 984.9
    - specified type of lead — *see* Table of Drugs and Chemicals
  - malaria 084.9
  - malignant (M8000/3) 199.1
  - marsh 084.9
  - nervous 300.5
  - old age 797
  - pachydermic — *see* Hypothyroidism
  - paludal 084.9
  - pituitary (postpartum) 253.2
  - renal (*see also* Disease, renal) 593.9
  - saturnine 984.9
    - specified type of lead — *see* Table of Drugs and Chemicals
  - senile 797
  - Simmonds' (pituitary cachexia) 253.2
  - splenica 289.59
  - strumipriva (*see also* Hypothyroidism) 244.9
  - tuberculous NEC (*see also* Tuberculosis) 011.9 ☑
- **Café au lait spots** 709.09
- **Caffey's disease or syndrome** (infantile cortical hyperostosis) 756.59
- **Caisson disease** 993.3
- **Caked breast** (puerperal, postpartum) 676.2 ☑
- **Cake kidney** 753.3
- **Calabar swelling** 125.2
- **Calcaneal spur** 726.73
- **Calcaneoapophysitis** 732.5
- **Calcaneonavicular bar** 755.67
- **Calcareous** — *see* condition
- **Calcicosis** (occupational) 502
- **Calciferol** (vitamin D) **deficiency** 268.9
  - with
    - osteomalacia 268.2
    - rickets (*see also* Rickets) 268.0
- **Calcification**
  - adrenal (capsule) (gland) 255.4
    - tuberculous (*see also* Tuberculosis) 017.6 ☑
  - aorta 440.0
  - artery (annular) — *see* Arteriosclerosis
  - auricle (ear) 380.89
  - bladder 596.8
    - due to S. hematobium 120.0
  - brain (cortex) — *see* Calcification, cerebral
  - bronchus 519.1
  - bursa 727.82
  - cardiac (*see also* Degeneration, myocardial) 429.1
  - cartilage (postinfectional) 733.99
  - cerebral (cortex) 348.8
    - artery 437.0
  - cervix (uteri) 622.8
  - choroid plexus 349.2
  - conjunctiva 372.54
  - corpora cavernosa (penis) 607.89
  - cortex (brain) — *see* Calcification, cerebral
  - dental pulp (nodular) 522.2
  - dentinal papilla 520.4
  - disc, intervertebral 722.90
    - cervical, cervicothoracic 722.91
    - lumbar, lumbosacral 722.93
    - thoracic, thoracolumbar 722.92
  - fallopian tube 620.8
  - falx cerebri — *see* Calcification, cerebral
  - fascia 728.89
  - gallbladder 575.8
  - general 275.40

☑ Additional Digit Required — Refer to the Tabular List (Numeric Code Section) for Additional Digit Selection

▶◀ Revised Text ● New Line ▲ Revised Code

Note — Except where otherwise indicated, the morphological varieties of carcinoma in the list below should be coded by site as for "Neoplasm, malignant."

Index Carcinoma — Carcinoma

Carcinoma — *see also* Neoplasm, by site, malignant — *continued*
sweat gland (M8400/3) — *see* Neoplasm, skin, malignant
theca cell (M8600/3) 183.0
thymic (M8580/3) 164.0
trabecular (M8190/3)
transitional (cell) (M8120/3)
papillary (M8130/3)
spindle cell type (M8122/3)
tubular (M8211/3)
undifferentiated type (M8020/3)
urothelial (M8120/3)
ventriculi 151.9
verrucous (epidermoid) (squamous cell) (M8051/3)
villous (M8262/3)
water-clear cell (M8322/3) 194.1
wolffian duct (M9110/3)
Carcinomaphobia 300.29
Carcinomatosis
peritonei (M8010/6) 197.6
specified site NEC (M8010/3) — *see* Neoplasm, by site, malignant
unspecified site (M8010/6) 199.0
Carcinosarcoma (M8980/3) — *see also* Neoplasm, by site, malignant
embryonal type (M8981/3) — *see* Neoplasm, by site, malignant
Cardia, cardial — *see* condition
Cardiac — *see also* condition
death — *see* Disease, heart
device
defibrillator, automatic implantable V45.02
in situ NEC V45.00
pacemaker
cardiac
fitting or adjustment V53.31
in situ V45.01
carotid sinus
fitting or adjustment V53.39
in situ V45.09
pacemaker — *see* Cardiac, device, pacemaker
tamponade 423.9
Cardialgia (*see also* Pain, precordial) 786.51
Cardiectasis — *see* Hypertrophy, cardiac
Cardiochalasia 530.81
Cardiomalacia (*see also* Degeneration, myocardial) 429.1
Cardiomegalia glycogenica diffusa 271.0
Cardiomegaly (*see also* Hypertrophy, cardiac) 429.3
congenital 746.89
glycogen 271.0
hypertensive (*see also* Hypertension, heart) 402.90
idiopathic 429.3
Cardiomyoliposis (*see also* Degeneration, myocardial) 429.1
Cardiomyopathy (congestive) (constrictive) (familial) (infiltrative) (obstructive) (restrictive) (sporadic) 425.4
alcoholic 425.5
amyloid 277.3 *[425.7]*
beriberi 265.0 *[425.7]*
cobalt-beer 425.5
congenital 425.3
due to
amyloidosis 277.3 *[425.7]*
beriberi 265.0 *[425.7]*
cardiac glycogenosis 271.0 *[425.7]*
Chagas' disease 086.0
Friedreich's ataxia 334.0 *[425.8]*
hypertension — *see* Hypertension, with, heart involvement
mucopolysaccharidosis 277.5 *[425.7]*
myotonia atrophica 359.2 *[425.8]*
progressive muscular dystrophy 359.1 *[425.8]*
sarcoidosis 135 *[425.8]*
glycogen storage 271.0 *[425.7]*
hypertensive — *see* Hypertension, with, heart involvement

Cardiomyopathy — *continued*
hypertrophic
nonobstructive 425.4
obstructive 425.1
congenital 746.84
idiopathic (concentric) 425.4
in
Chagas' disease 086.0
sarcoidosis 135 *[425.8]*
ischemic 414.8
metabolic NEC 277.9 *[425.7]*
amyloid 277.3 *[425.7]*
thyrotoxic (*see also* Thyrotoxicosis) 242.9 ☑ *[425.7]*
thyrotoxicosis (*see also* Thyrotoxicosis) 242.9 ☑ *[425.7]*
newborn 425.4 ●
congenital 425.3 ●
nutritional 269.9 *[425.7]*
beriberi 265.0 *[425.7]*
obscure of Africa 425.2
peripartum 674.5 ☑
postpartum 674.5 ☑
primary 425.4
secondary 425.9
takotsubo 429.89 ●
thyrotoxic (*see also* Thyrotoxicosis) 242.9 ☑ *[425.7]*
toxic NEC 425.9
tuberculous (*see also* Tuberculosis) 017.9 ☑ *[425.8]*
Cardionephritis — *see* Hypertension, cardiorenal
Cardionephropathy — *see* Hypertension, cardiorenal
Cardionephrosis — *see* Hypertension, cardiorenal
Cardioneurosis 306.2
Cardiopathia nigra 416.0
Cardiopathy (*see also* Disease, heart) 429.9
hypertensive (*see also* Hypertension, heart) 402.90
idiopathic 425.4
mucopolysaccharidosis 277.5 *[425.7]*
Cardiopericarditis (*see also* Pericarditis) 423.9
Cardiophobia 300.29
Cardioptosis 746.87
Cardiorenal — *see* condition
Cardiorrhexis (*see also* Infarct, myocardium) 410.9 ☑
Cardiosclerosis — *see* Arteriosclerosis, coronary
Cardiosis — *see* Disease, heart
Cardiospasm (esophagus) (reflex) (stomach) 530.0
congenital 750.7
Cardiostenosis — *see* Disease, heart
Cardiosymphysis 423.1
Cardiothyrotoxicosis — *see* Hyperthyroidism
Cardiovascular — *see* condition
Carditis (acute) (bacterial) (chronic) (subacute) 429.89
Coxsackie 074.20
hypertensive (*see also* Hypertension, heart) 402.90
meningococcal 036.40
rheumatic — *see* Disease, heart, rheumatic
rheumatoid 714.2
Care (of)
child (routine) V20.1
convalescent following V66.9
chemotherapy V66.2
medical NEC V66.5
psychotherapy V66.3
radiotherapy V66.1
surgery V66.0
surgical NEC V66.0
treatment (for) V66.5
combined V66.6
fracture V66.4
mental disorder NEC V66.3
specified type NEC V66.5
end-of-life V66.7
family member (handicapped) (sick)
creating problem for family V61.49
provided away from home for holiday relief V60.5

Care (of) — *continued*
family member — *continued*
unavailable, due to
absence (person rendering care) (sufferer) V60.4
inability (any reason) of person rendering care V60.4
holiday relief V60.5
hospice V66.7
lack of (at or after birth) (infant) (child) 995.52
adult 995.84
lactation of mother V24.1
palliative V66.7
postpartum
immediately after delivery V24.0
routine follow-up V24.2
prenatal V22.1
first pregnancy V22.0
high-risk pregnancy V23.9
specified problem NEC V23.89
terminal V66.7
unavailable, due to
absence of person rendering care V60.4
inability (any reason) of person rendering care V60.4
well baby V20.1
Caries (bone) (*see also* Tuberculosis, bone) 015.9 ☑ *[730.8]* ☑
arrested 521.04
cementum 521.03
cerebrospinal (tuberculous) 015.0 ☑ *[730.88]*
dental (acute) (chronic) (incipient) (infected) 521.00
with pulp exposure 521.03
extending to
dentine 521.02
pulp 521.03
other specified NEC 521.09
pit and fissure 521.06
root surface 521.08
smooth surface 521.07
dentin (acute) (chronic) 521.02
enamel (acute) (chronic) (incipient) 521.01
external meatus 380.89
hip (*see also* Tuberculosis) 015.1 ☑ *[730.85]*
initial 521.01
knee 015.2 ☑ *[730.86]*
labyrinth 386.8
limb NEC 015.7 ☑ *[730.88]*
mastoid (chronic) (process) 383.1
middle ear 385.89
nose 015.7 ☑ *[730.88]*
orbit 015.7 ☑ *[730.88]*
ossicle 385.24
petrous bone 383.20
sacrum (tuberculous) 015.0 ☑ *[730.88]*
spine, spinal (column) (tuberculous) 015.0 ☑ *[730.88]*
syphilitic 095.5
congenital 090.0 *[730.8]* ☑
teeth (internal) 521.00
initial 521.01
vertebra (column) (tuberculous) 015.0 ☑ *[730.88]*
Carini's syndrome (ichthyosis congenita) 757.1
Carious teeth 521.00
Carneous mole 631
Carnosinemia 270.5
Carotid body or sinus syndrome 337.0
Carotidynia 337.0
Carotinemia (dietary) 278.3
Carotinosis (cutis) (skin) 278.3
Carpal tunnel syndrome 354.0
Carpenter's syndrome 759.89
Carpopedal spasm (*see also* Tetany) 781.7
Carpoptosis 736.05
Carrier (suspected) **of**
amebiasis V02.2
bacterial disease (meningococcal, staphylococcal) NEC V02.59
cholera V02.0
cystic fibrosis gene V83.81
defective gene V83.89
diphtheria V02.4

- **Carrier** (suspected) **of** — *continued*
  - dysentery (bacillary) V02.3
    - amebic V02.2
  - Endamoeba histolytica V02.2
  - gastrointestinal pathogens NEC V02.3
  - genetic defect V83.89
  - gonorrhea V02.7
  - group B streptococcus V02.51
  - HAA (hepatitis Australian-antigen) V02.61
  - hemophilia A (asymptomatic) V83.01
    - symptomatic V83.02
  - hepatitis V02.60
    - Australian-antigen (HAA) V02.61
    - B V02.61
    - C V02.62
    - serum V02.61
    - specified type NEC V02.69
    - viral V02.60
  - infective organism NEC V02.9
  - malaria V02.9
  - paratyphoid V02.3
  - Salmonella V02.3
    - typhosa V02.1
  - serum hepatitis V02.61
  - Shigella V02.3
  - Staphylococcus NEC V02.59
  - Streptococcus NEC V02.52
    - group B V02.51
  - typhoid V02.1
  - venereal disease NEC V02.8
- **Carrión's disease** (Bartonellosis) 088.0
- **Car sickness** 994.6
- **Carter's**
  - relapsing fever (Asiatic) 087.0
- **Cartilage** — *see* condition
- **Caruncle** (inflamed)
  - abscess, lacrimal (*see also* Dacryocystitis) 375.30
  - conjunctiva 372.00
    - acute 372.00
  - eyelid 373.00
  - labium (majus) (minus) 616.8
  - lacrimal 375.30
  - urethra (benign) 599.3
  - vagina (wall) 616.8
- **Cascade stomach** 537.6
- **Caseation lymphatic gland** (*see also* Tuberculosis) 017.2 ☑
- **Caseous**
  - bronchitis — *see* Tuberculosis, pulmonary
  - meningitis 013.0 ☑
  - pneumonia — *see* Tuberculosis, pulmonary
- **Cassidy (-Scholte) syndrome** (malignant carcinoid) 259.2
- **Castellani's bronchitis** 104.8
- **Castleman's tumor or lymphoma** (mediastinal lymph node hyperplasia) 785.6
- **Castration, traumatic** 878.2
  - complicated 878.3
- **Casts in urine** 791.7
- **Cat's ear** 744.29
- **Catalepsy** 300.11
  - catatonic (acute) (*see also* Schizophrenia) 295.2 ☑
  - hysterical 300.11
  - schizophrenic (*see also* Schizophrenia) 295.2 ☑
- **Cataphasia** 307.0
- **Cataplexy** (idiopathic) — *see* Narcolepsy
- **Cataract** (anterior cortical) (anterior polar) (black) (capsular) (central) (cortical) (hypermature) (immature) (incipient) (mature) 366.9
  - anterior
    - and posterior axial embryonal 743.33
    - pyramidal 743.31
    - subcapsular polar
      - infantile, juvenile, or presenile 366.01
      - senile 366.13
  - associated with
    - calcinosis 275.40 *[366.42]*
    - craniofacial dysostosis 756.0 *[366.44]*
    - galactosemia 271.1 *[366.44]*
    - hypoparathyroidism 252.1 *[366.42]*
    - myotonic disorders 359.2 *[366.43]*
- **Cataract** — *continued*
  - associated with — *continued*
    - neovascularization 366.33
  - blue dot 743.39
  - cerulean 743.39
  - complicated NEC 366.30
  - congenital 743.30
    - capsular or subcapsular 743.31
    - cortical 743.32
    - nuclear 743.33
    - specified type NEC 743.39
    - total or subtotal 743.34
    - zonular 743.32
  - coronary (congenital) 743.39
    - acquired 366.12
  - cupuliform 366.14
  - diabetic 250.5 ☑ *[366.41]*
  - drug-induced 366.45
  - due to
    - chalcosis 360.24 *[366.34]*
    - chronic choroiditis (*see also* Choroiditis) 363.20 *[366.32]*
    - degenerative myopia 360.21 *[366.34]*
    - glaucoma (*see also* Glaucoma) 365.9 *[366.31]*
    - infection, intraocular NEC 366.32
    - inflammatory ocular disorder NEC 366.32
    - iridocyclitis, chronic 364.10 *[366.33]*
    - pigmentary retinal dystrophy 362.74 *[366.34]*
    - radiation 366.46
  - electric 366.46
  - glassblowers' 366.46
  - heat ray 366.46
  - heterochromic 366.33
  - in eye disease NEC 366.30
  - infantile (*see also* Cataract, juvenile) 366.00
  - intumescent 366.12
  - irradiational 366.46
  - juvenile 366.00
    - anterior subcapsular polar 366.01
    - combined forms 366.09
    - cortical 366.03
    - lamellar 366.03
    - nuclear 366.04
    - posterior subcapsular polar 366.02
    - specified NEC 366.09
    - zonular 366.03
  - lamellar 743.32
    - infantile, juvenile, or presenile 366.03
  - morgagnian 366.18
  - myotonic 359.2 *[366.43]*
  - myxedema 244.9 *[366.44]*
  - nuclear 366.16
  - posterior, polar (capsular) 743.31
    - infantile, juvenile, or presenile 366.02
    - senile 366.14
  - presenile (*see also* Cataract, juvenile) 366.00
  - punctate
    - acquired 366.12
    - congenital 743.39
  - secondary (membrane) 366.50
    - obscuring vision 366.53
    - specified type, not obscuring vision 366.52
  - senile 366.10
    - anterior subcapsular polar 366.13
    - combined forms 366.19
    - cortical 366.15
    - hypermature 366.18
    - immature 366.12
    - incipient 366.12
    - mature 366.17
    - nuclear 366.16
    - posterior subcapsular polar 366.14
    - specified NEC 366.19
    - total or subtotal 366.17
  - snowflake 250.5 ☑ *[366.41]*
  - specified NEC 366.8
  - subtotal (senile) 366.17
    - congenital 743.34
  - sunflower 360.24 *[366.34]*
  - tetanic NEC 252.1 *[366.42]*
  - total (mature) (senile) 366.17
    - congenital 743.34
    - localized 366.21
    - traumatic 366.22
  - toxic 366.45
- **Cataract** — *continued*
  - traumatic 366.20
    - partially resolved 366.23
    - total 366.22
  - zonular (perinuclear) 743.32
    - infantile, juvenile, or presenile 366.03
- **Cataracta** 366.10
  - brunescens 366.16
  - cerulea 743.39
  - complicata 366.30
  - congenita 743.30
  - coralliformis 743.39
  - coronaria (congenital) 743.39
    - acquired 366.12
  - diabetic 250.5 ☑ *[366.41]*
  - floriformis 360.24 *[366.34]*
  - membranacea
    - accreta 366.50
    - congenita 743.39
  - nigra 366.16
- **Catarrh, catarrhal** (inflammation) (*see also* condition) 460
  - acute 460
  - asthma, asthmatic (*see also* Asthma) 493.9 ☑
  - Bostock's (*see also* Fever, hay) 477.9
  - bowel — *see* Enteritis
  - bronchial 490
    - acute 466.0
    - chronic 491.0
    - subacute 466.0
  - cervix, cervical (canal) (uteri) — *see* Cervicitis
  - chest (*see also* Bronchitis) 490
  - chronic 472.0
  - congestion 472.0
  - conjunctivitis 372.03
  - due to syphilis 095.9
    - congenital 090.0
  - enteric — *see* Enteritis
  - epidemic 487.1
  - Eustachian 381.50
  - eye (acute) (vernal) 372.03
  - fauces (*see also* Pharyngitis) 462
  - febrile 460
  - fibrinous acute 466.0
  - gastroenteric — *see* Enteritis
  - gastrointestinal — *see* Enteritis
  - gingivitis 523.0
  - hay (*see also* Fever, hay) 477.9
  - infectious 460
  - intestinal — *see* Enteritis
  - larynx (*see also* Laryngitis, chronic) 476.0
  - liver 070.1
    - with hepatic coma 070.0
  - lung (*see also* Bronchitis) 490
    - acute 466.0
    - chronic 491.0
  - middle ear (chronic) — *see* Otitis media, chronic
  - mouth 528.0
  - nasal (chronic) (*see also* Rhinitis) 472.0
    - acute 460
  - nasobronchial 472.2
  - nasopharyngeal (chronic) 472.2
    - acute 460
  - nose — *see* Catarrh, nasal
  - ophthalmia 372.03
  - pneumococcal, acute 466.0
  - pulmonary (*see also* Bronchitis) 490
    - acute 466.0
    - chronic 491.0
  - spring (eye) 372.13
  - suffocating (*see also* Asthma) 493.9 ☑
  - summer (hay) (*see also* Fever, hay) 477.9
  - throat 472.1
  - tracheitis 464.10
    - with obstruction 464.11
  - tubotympanal 381.4
    - acute (*see also* Otitis media, acute, nonsuppurative) 381.00
    - chronic 381.10
  - vasomotor (*see also* Fever, hay) 477.9
  - vesical (bladder) — *see* Cystitis
- **Catarrhus aestivus** (*see also* Fever, hay) 477.9
- **Catastrophe, cerebral** (*see also* Disease, cerebrovascular, acute) 436

☑ Additional Digit Required — Refer to the Tabular List (Numeric Code Section) for Additional Digit Selection

▶◀ Revised Text ● New Line ▲ Revised Code

☑ Additional Digit Required — Refer to the Tabular List (Numeric Code Section) for Additional Digit Selection

▶◀ Revised Text ● New Line ▲ Revised Code

Cheilitis 528.5
- actinic (due to sun) 692.72
  - chronic NEC 692.74
    - due to radiation, except from sun 692.82
  - due to radiation, except from sun 692.82
- acute 528.5
- angular 528.5
- catarrhal 528.5
- chronic 528.5
- exfoliative 528.5
- gangrenous 528.5
- glandularis apostematosa 528.5
- granulomatosa 351.8
- infectional 528.5
- membranous 528.5
- Miescher's 351.8
- suppurative 528.5
- ulcerative 528.5
- vesicular 528.5

Cheilodynia 528.5

Cheilopalatoschisis (*see also* Cleft, palate, with cleft lip) 749.20

Cheilophagia 528.9

Cheiloschisis (*see also* Cleft, lip) 749.10

Cheilosis 528.5
- with pellagra 265.2
- angular 528.5
- due to
  - dietary deficiency 266.0
  - vitamin deficiency 266.0

Cheiromegaly 729.89

Cheiropompholyx 705.81

Cheloid (*see also* Keloid) 701.4

Chemical burn — *see also* Burn, by site
- from swallowing chemical — *see* Burn, internal organs

Chemodectoma (M8693/1) — *see* Paraganglioma, nonchromaffin

Chemoprophylaxis NEC V07.39

Chemosis, conjunctiva 372.73

Chemotherapy
- convalescence V66.2
- encounter (for) V58.11 ▲
- maintenance V58.11 ▲
- prophylactic NEC V07.39
  - fluoride V07.31

Cherubism 526.89

Chest — *see* condition

Cheyne-Stokes respiration (periodic) 786.04

Chiari's
- disease or syndrome (hepatic vein thrombosis) 453.0
- malformation
  - type I 348.4
  - type II (*see also* Spina bifida) 741.0 ☑
  - type III 742.0
  - type IV 742.2
- network 746.89

Chiari-Frommel syndrome 676.6 ☑

Chicago disease (North American blastomycosis) 116.0

Chickenpox (*see also* Varicella) 052.9
- exposure to V01.71
- vaccination and inoculation (prophylactic) V05.4

Chiclero ulcer 085.4

Chiggers 133.8

Chignon 111.2
- fetus or newborn (from vacuum extraction) 767.19

Chigoe disease 134.1

Chikungunya fever 066.3

Chilaiditi's syndrome (subphrenic displacement, colon) 751.4

Chilblains 991.5
- lupus 991.5

Child
- behavior causing concern V61.20

Childbed fever 670 ☑

Childbirth — *see also* Delivery
- puerperal complications — *see* Puerperal

Childhood, period of rapid growth V21.0

Chill(s) 780.99
- with fever 780.6
- congestive 780.99
  - in malarial regions 084.6
- septic — *see* Septicemia
- urethral 599.84

Chilomastigiasis 007.8

Chin — *see* condition

Chinese dysentery 004.9

Chiropractic dislocation (*see also* Lesion, nonallopathic, by site) 739.9

Chitral fever 066.0

Chlamydia, chlamydial — *see* condition

Chloasma 709.09
- cachecticorum 709.09
- eyelid 374.52
  - congenital 757.33
  - hyperthyroid 242.0 ☑
- gravidarum 646.8 ☑
- idiopathic 709.09
- skin 709.09
- symptomatic 709.09

Chloroma (M9930/3) 205.3 ☑

Chlorosis 280.9
- Egyptian (*see also* Ancylostomiasis) 126.9
- miners' (*see also* Ancylostomiasis) 126.9

Chlorotic anemia 280.9

Chocolate cyst (ovary) 617.1

Choked
- disk or disc — *see* Papilledema
- on food, phlegm, or vomitus NEC (*see also* Asphyxia, food) 933.1
- phlegm 933.1
- while vomiting NEC (*see also* Asphyxia, food) 933.1

Chokes (resulting from bends) 993.3

Choking sensation 784.9

Cholangiectasis (*see also* Disease, gallbladder) 575.8

Cholangiocarcinoma (M8160/3)
- and hepatocellular carcinoma, combined (M8180/3) 155.0
- liver 155.1
- specified site NEC — *see* Neoplasm, by site, malignant
- unspecified site 155.1

Cholangiohepatitis 575.8
- due to fluke infestation 121.1

Cholangiohepatoma (M8180/3) 155.0

Cholangiolitis (acute) (chronic) (extrahepatic) (gangrenous) 576.1
- intrahepatic 575.8
- paratyphoidal (*see also* Fever, paratyphoid) 002.9
- typhoidal 002.0

Cholangioma (M8160/0) 211.5
- malignant — *see* Cholangiocarcinoma

Cholangitis (acute) (ascending) (catarrhal) (chronic) (infective) (malignant) (primary) (recurrent) (sclerosing) (secondary) (stenosing) (suppurative) 576.1
- chronic nonsuppurative destructive 571.6
- nonsuppurative destructive (chronic) 571.6

Cholecystdocholithiasis — *see* Choledocholithiasis

Cholecystitis 575.10
- with
  - calculus, stones in
    - bile duct (common) (hepatic) — *see* Choledocholithiasis
    - gallbladder — *see* Cholelithiasis
- acute 575.0
- acute and chronic 575.12
- chronic 575.11
- emphysematous (acute) (*see also* Cholecystitis, acute) 575.0
- gangrenous (*see also* Cholecystitis, acute) 575.0
- paratyphoidal, current (*see also* Fever, paratyphoid) 002.9

Cholecystitis — *continued*
- suppurative (*see also* Cholecystitis, acute) 575.0
- typhoidal 002.0

Choledochitis (suppurative) 576.1

Choledocholith — *see* Choledocholithiasis

Choledocholithiasis 574.5 ☑

> *Note — Use the following fifth-digit subclassification with category 574:*
>
> *0 without mention of obstruction*
> *1 with obstruction*

- with
  - cholecystitis 574.4 ☑
    - acute 574.3 ☑
    - chronic 574.4 ☑
  - cholelithiasis 574.9 ☑
    - with
      - cholecystitis 574.7 ☑
        - acute 574.6 ☑
          - and chronic 574.8 ☑
        - chronic 574.7 ☑

Cholelithiasis (impacted) (multiple) 574.2 ☑

> *Note — Use the following fifth-digit subclassification with category 574:*
>
> *0 without mention of obstruction*
> *1 with obstruction*

- with
  - cholecystitis 574.1 ☑
    - acute 574.0 ☑
    - chronic 574.1 ☑
  - choledocholithiasis 574.9 ☑
    - with
      - cholecystitis 574.7 ☑
        - acute 574.6 ☑
          - and chronic 574.8 ☑
        - chronic cholecystitis 574.7 ☑

Cholemia (*see also* Jaundice) 782.4
- familial 277.4
- Gilbert's (familial nonhemolytic) 277.4

Cholemic gallstone — *see* Cholelithiasis

Choleperitoneum, choleperitonitis (*see also* Disease, gallbladder) 567.81 ▲

Cholera (algid) (Asiatic) (asphyctic) (epidemic) (gravis) (Indian) (malignant) (morbus) (pestilential) (spasmodic) 001.9
- antimonial 985.4
- carrier (suspected) of V02.0
- classical 001.0
- contact V01.0
- due to
  - Vibrio
    - cholerae (Inaba, Ogawa, Hikojima serotypes) 001.0
      - El Tor 001.1
- El Tor 001.1
- exposure to V01.0
- vaccination, prophylactic (against) V03.0

Cholerine (*see also* Cholera) 001.9

Cholestasis 576.8

Cholesteatoma (ear) 385.30
- attic (primary) 385.31
- diffuse 385.35
- external ear (canal) 380.21
- marginal (middle ear) 385.32
  - with involvement of mastoid cavity 385.33
  - secondary (with middle ear involvement) 385.33
- mastoid cavity 385.30
- middle ear (secondary) 385.32
  - with involvement of mastoid cavity 385.33
- postmastoidectomy cavity (recurrent) 383.32
- primary 385.31
- recurrent, postmastoidectomy cavity 383.32
- secondary (middle ear) 385.32
  - with involvement of mastoid cavity 385.33

Cholesteatosis (middle ear) (*see also* Cholesteatoma) 385.30
- diffuse 385.35

Cholesteremia 272.0

Cholesterin
granuloma, middle ear 385.82
in vitreous 379.22
Cholesterol
deposit
retina 362.82
vitreous 379.22
imbibition of gallbladder (*see also* Disease, gallbladder) 575.6
Cholesterolemia 272.0
essential 272.0
familial 272.0
hereditary 272.0
Cholesterosis, cholesterolosis (gallbladder) 575.6
with
cholecystitis — *see* Cholecystitis
cholelithiasis — *see* Cholelithiasis
middle ear (*see also* Cholesteatoma) 385.30
Cholocolic fistula (*see also* Fistula, gallbladder) 575.5
Choluria 791.4
Chondritis (purulent) 733.99
auricle 380.03
costal 733.6
Tietze's 733.6
patella, posttraumatic 717.7
pinna 380.03
posttraumatica patellae 717.7
tuberculous (active) (*see also* Tuberculosis) 015.9 ☑
intervertebral 015.0 ☑ *[730.88]*
Chondroangiopathia calcarea seu punctate 756.59
Chondroblastoma (M9230/0) — *see also* Neoplasm, bone, benign
malignant (M9230/3) — *see* Neoplasm, bone, malignant
Chondrocalcinosis (articular) (crystal deposition) (dihydrate) (*see also* Arthritis, due to, crystals) 275.49 *[712.3]* ☑
due to
calcium pyrophosphate 275.49 *[712.2]* ☑
dicalcium phosphate crystals 275.49 *[712.1]* ☑
pyrophosphate crystals 275.49 *[712.2]* ☑
Chondrodermatitis nodularis helicis 380.00
Chondrodysplasia 756.4
angiomatose 756.4
calcificans congenita 756.59
epiphysialis punctata 756.59
hereditary deforming 756.4
rhizomelic punctata 277.86
Chondrodystrophia (fetalis) 756.4
calcarea 756.4
calcificans congenita 756.59
fetalis hypoplastica 756.59
hypoplastica calcinosa 756.59
punctata 756.59
tarda 277.5
Chondrodystrophy (familial) (hypoplastic) 756.4
Chondroectodermal dysplasia 756.55
Chondrolysis 733.99
Chondroma (M9220/0) — *see also* Neoplasm cartilage, benign
juxtacortical (M9221/0) — *see* Neoplasm, bone, benign
periosteal (M9221/0) — *see* Neoplasm, bone, benign
Chondromalacia 733.92
epiglottis (congenital) 748.3
generalized 733.92
knee 717.7
larynx (congenital) 748.3
localized, except patella 733.92
patella, patellae 717.7
systemic 733.92
tibial plateau 733.92
trachea (congenital) 748.3
Chondromatosis (M9220/1) — *see* Neoplasm, cartilage, uncertain behavior
Chondromyxosarcoma (M9220/3) — *see* Neoplasm, cartilage, malignant
Chondro-osteodysplasia (Morquio-Brailsford type) 277.5
Chondro-osteodystrophy 277.5
Chondro-osteoma (M9210/0) — *see* Neoplasm, bone, benign
Chondropathia tuberosa 733.6
Chondrosarcoma (M9220/3) — *see also* Neoplasm, cartilage, malignant
juxtacortical (M9221/3) — *see* Neoplasm, bone, malignant
mesenchymal (M9240/3) — *see* Neoplasm, connective tissue, malignant
Chordae tendineae rupture (chronic) 429.5
Chordee (nonvenereal) 607.89
congenital 752.63
gonococcal 098.2
Chorditis (fibrinous) (nodosa) (tuberosa) 478.5
Chordoma (M9370/3) — *see* Neoplasm, by site, malignant
Chorea (gravis) (minor) (spasmodic) 333.5
with
heart involvement — *see* Chorea with rheumatic heart disease
rheumatic heart disease (chronic, inactive, or quiescent) (conditions classifiable to 393-398) — *see* rheumatic heart condition involved
active or acute (conditions classifiable to 391) 392.0
acute — *see* Chorea, Sydenham's
apoplectic (*see also* Disease, cerebrovascular, acute) 436
chronic 333.4
electric 049.8
gravidarum — *see* Eclampsia, pregnancy
habit 307.22
hereditary 333.4
Huntington's 333.4
posthemiplegic 344.89
pregnancy — *see* Eclampsia, pregnancy
progressive 333.4
chronic 333.4
hereditary 333.4
rheumatic (chronic) 392.9
with heart disease or involvement — *see* Chorea, with rheumatic heart disease
senile 333.5
Sydenham's 392.9
with heart involvement — *see* Chorea, with rheumatic heart disease
nonrheumatic 333.5
variabilis 307.23
Choreoathetosis (paroxysmal) 333.5
Chorioadenoma (destruens) (M9100/1) 236.1
Chorioamnionitis 658.4 ☑
affecting fetus or newborn 762.7
Chorioangioma (M9120/0) 219.8
Choriocarcinoma (M9100/3)
combined with
embryonal carcinoma (M9101/3) — *see* Neoplasm, by site, malignant
teratoma (M9101/3) — *see* Neoplasm, by site, malignant
specified site — *see* Neoplasm, by site, malignant
unspecified site
female 181
male 186.9
Chorioencephalitis, lymphocytic (acute) (serous) 049.0
Chorioepithelioma (M9100/3) — *see* Choriocarcinoma
Choriomeningitis (acute) (benign) (lymphocytic) (serous) 049.0
Chorionepithelioma (M9100/3) — *see* Choriocarcinoma
Chorionitis (*see also* Scleroderma) 710.1
Chorioretinitis 363.20
disseminated 363.10
generalized 363.13
in
neurosyphilis 094.83
secondary syphilis 091.51
Chorioretinitis — *continued*
disseminated — *continued*
peripheral 363.12
posterior pole 363.11
tuberculous (*see also* Tuberculosis) 017.3 ☑ *[363.13]*
due to
histoplasmosis (*see also* Histoplasmosis) 115.92
toxoplasmosis (acquired) 130.2
congenital (active) 771.2
focal 363.00
juxtapapillary 363.01
peripheral 363.04
posterior pole NEC 363.03
juxtapapillaris, juxtapapillary 363.01
progressive myopia (degeneration) 360.21
syphilitic (secondary) 091.51
congenital (early) 090.0 *[363.13]*
late 090.5 *[363.13]*
late 095.8 *[363.13]*
tuberculous (*see also* Tuberculosis) 017.3 ☑ *[363.13]*
Choristoma — *see* Neoplasm, by site, benign
Choroid — *see* condition
Choroideremia, choroidermia (initial stage) (late stage) (partial or total atrophy) 363.55
Choroiditis (*see also* Chorioretinitis) 363.20
leprous 030.9 *[363.13]*
senile guttate 363.41
sympathetic 360.11
syphilitic (secondary) 091.51
congenital (early) 090.0 *[363.13]*
late 090.5 *[363.13]*
late 095.8 *[363.13]*
Tay's 363.41
tuberculous (*see also* Tuberculosis) 017.3 ☑ *[363.13]*
Choroidopathy NEC 363.9
degenerative (*see also* Degeneration, choroid) 363.40
hereditary (*see also* Dystrophy, choroid) 363.50
specified type NEC 363.8
Choroidoretinitis — *see* Chorioretinitis
Choroidosis, central serous 362.41
Choroidretinopathy, serous 362.41
Christian's syndrome (chronic histiocytosis X) 277.89
Christian-Weber disease (nodular nonsuppurative panniculitis) 729.30
Christmas disease 286.1
Chromaffinoma (M8700/0) — *see also* Neoplasm, by site, benign
malignant (M8700/3) — *see* Neoplasm, by site, malignant
Chromatopsia 368.59
Chromhidrosis, chromidrosis 705.89
Chromoblastomycosis 117.2
Chromomycosis 117.2
Chromophytosis 111.0
Chromotrichomycosis 111.8
Chronic — *see* condition
Churg-Strauss syndrome 446.4
Chyle cyst, mesentery 457.8
Chylocele (nonfilarial) 457.8
filarial (*see also* Infestation, filarial) 125.9
tunica vaginalis (nonfilarial) 608.84
filarial (*see also* Infestation, filarial) 125.9
Chylomicronemia (fasting) (with hyperprebetalipoproteinemia) 272.3
Chylopericardium (acute) 420.90
Chylothorax (nonfilarial) 457.8
filarial (*see also* Infestation, filarial) 125.9
Chylous
ascites 457.8
cyst of peritoneum 457.8
hydrocele 603.9
hydrothorax (nonfilarial) 457.8
filarial (*see also* Infestation, filarial) 125.9
Chyluria 791.1
bilharziasis 120.0

☑ Additional Digit Required — Refer to the Tabular List (Numeric Code Section) for Additional Digit Selection
▶◀ Revised Text ● New Line ▲ Revised Code

- **Coccidioidosis** 114.9
  - lung 114.5
    - acute 114.0
    - chronic 114.4
    - primary 114.0
  - meninges 114.2
- **Coccidiosis** (colitis) (diarrhea) (dysentery) 007.2
- **Cocciuria** 791.9
- **Coccus in urine** 791.9
- **Coccydynia** 724.79
- **Coccygodynia** 724.79
- **Coccyx** — *see* condition
- **Cochin-China**
  - diarrhea 579.1
    - anguilluliasis 127.2
  - ulcer 085.1
- **Cock's peculiar tumor** 706.2
- **Cockayne's disease or syndrome** (microcephaly and dwarfism) 759.89
- **Cockayne-Weber syndrome** (epidermolysis bullosa) 757.39
- **Cocked-up toe** 735.2
- **Codman's tumor** (benign chondroblastoma) (M9230/0) — *see* Neoplasm, bone, benign
- **Coenurosis** 123.8
- **Coffee workers' lung** 495.8
- **Cogan's syndrome** 370.52
  - congenital oculomotor apraxia 379.51
  - nonsyphilitic interstitial keratitis 370.52
- **Coiling, umbilical cord** — *see* Complications, umbilical cord
- **Coitus, painful** (female) 625.0
  - male 608.89
  - psychogenic 302.76
- **Cold** 460
  - with influenza, flu, or grippe 487.1
  - abscess — *see also* Tuberculosis, abscess
    - articular — *see* Tuberculosis, joint
  - agglutinin
    - disease (chronic) or syndrome 283.0
    - hemoglobinuria 283.0
      - paroxysmal (cold) (nocturnal) 283.2
  - allergic (*see also* Fever, hay) 477.9
  - bronchus or chest — *see* Bronchitis
    - with grippe or influenza 487.1
  - common (head) 460
    - vaccination, prophylactic (against) V04.7
  - deep 464.10
  - effects of 991.9
    - specified effect NEC 991.8
  - excessive 991.9
    - specified effect NEC 991.8
  - exhaustion from 991.8
  - exposure to 991.9
    - specified effect NEC 991.8
  - grippy 487.1
  - head 460
  - injury syndrome (newborn) 778.2
  - intolerance 780.99
  - on lung — *see* Bronchitis
  - rose 477.0
  - sensitivity, autoimmune 283.0
  - virus 460
- **Coldsore** (*see also* Herpes, simplex) 054.9
- **Colibacillosis** 041.4
  - generalized 038.42
- **Colibacilluria** 791.9
- **Colic** (recurrent) 789.0 ☑
  - abdomen 789.0 ☑
    - psychogenic 307.89
  - appendicular 543.9
  - appendix 543.9
  - bile duct — *see* Choledocholithiasis
  - biliary — *see* Cholelithiasis
  - bilious — *see* Cholelithiasis
  - common duct — *see* Choledocholithiasis
  - Devonshire NEC 984.9
    - specified type of lead — *see* Table of Drugs and Chemicals
  - flatulent 787.3
  - gallbladder or gallstone — *see* Cholelithiasis
  - gastric 536.8
  - hepatic (duct) — *see* Choledocholithiasis

- **Colic** — *continued*
  - hysterical 300.11
  - infantile 789.0 ☑
  - intestinal 789.0 ☑
  - kidney 788.0
  - lead NEC 984.9
    - specified type of lead — *see* Table of Drugs and Chemicals
  - liver (duct) — *see* Choledocholithiasis
  - mucous 564.9
    - psychogenic 316 *[564.9]*
  - nephritic 788.0
  - painter's NEC 984.9
  - pancreas 577.8
  - psychogenic 306.4
  - renal 788.0
  - saturnine NEC 984.9
    - specified type of lead — *see* Table of Drugs and Chemicals
  - spasmodic 789.0 ☑
  - ureter 788.0
  - urethral 599.84
    - due to calculus 594.2
  - uterus 625.8
    - menstrual 625.3
  - vermicular 543.9
  - virus 460
  - worm NEC 128.9
- **Colicystitis** (*see also* Cystitis) 595.9
- **Colitis** (acute) (catarrhal) (croupous) (cystica superficialis) (exudative) (hemorrhagic) (noninfectious) (phlegmonous) (presumed noninfectious) 558.9
  - adaptive 564.9
  - allergic 558.3
  - amebic (*see also* Amebiasis) 006.9
    - nondysenteric 006.2
  - anthrax 022.2
  - bacillary (*see also* Infection, Shigella) 004.9
  - balantidial 007.0
  - chronic 558.9
    - ulcerative (*see also* Colitis, ulcerative) 556.9
  - coccidial 007.2
  - dietetic 558.9
  - due to radiation 558.1
  - functional 558.9
  - gangrenous 009.0
  - giardial 007.1
  - granulomatous 555.1
  - gravis (*see also* Colitis, ulcerative) 556.9
  - infectious (*see also* Enteritis, due to, specific organism) 009.0
    - presumed 009.1
  - ischemic 557.9
    - acute 557.0
    - chronic 557.1
    - due to mesenteric artery insufficiency 557.1
  - membranous 564.9
    - psychogenic 316 *[564.9]*
  - mucous 564.9
    - psychogenic 316 *[564.9]*
  - necrotic 009.0
  - polyposa (*see also* Colitis, ulcerative) 556.9
  - protozoal NEC 007.9
  - pseudomembranous 008.45
  - pseudomucinous 564.9
  - regional 555.1
  - segmental 555.1
  - septic (*see also* Enteritis, due to, specific organism) 009.0
  - spastic 564.9
    - psychogenic 316 *[564.9]*
  - Staphylococcus 008.41
    - food 005.0
  - thromboulcerative 557.0
  - toxic 558.2
  - transmural 555.1
  - trichomonal 007.3
  - tuberculous (ulcerative) 014.8 ☑
  - ulcerative (chronic) (idiopathic) (nonspecific) 556.9
    - entero- 556.0
    - fulminant 557.0
    - ileo- 556.1
    - left-sided 556.5
    - procto- 556.2

- **Colitis** — *continued*
  - ulcerative — *continued*
    - proctosigmoid 556.3
    - psychogenic 316 *[556]* ☑
    - specified NEC 556.8
    - universal 556.6
- **Collagen disease** NEC 710.9
  - nonvascular 710.9
  - vascular (allergic) (*see also* Angiitis, hypersensitivity) 446.20
- **Collagenosis** (*see also* Collagen disease) 710.9
  - cardiovascular 425.4
  - mediastinal 519.3
- **Collapse** 780.2
  - adrenal 255.8
  - cardiorenal (*see also* Hypertension, cardiorenal) 404.90
  - cardiorespiratory 785.51
    - fetus or newborn 779.89
  - cardiovascular (*see also* Disease, heart) 785.51
    - fetus or newborn 779.89
  - circulatory (peripheral) 785.59
    - with
      - abortion — *see* Abortion, by type, with shock
      - ectopic pregnancy (*see also* categories 633.0-633.9) 639.5
      - molar pregnancy (*see also* categories 630-632) 639.5
    - during or after labor and delivery 669.1 ☑
    - fetus or newborn 779.89
    - following
      - abortion 639.5
      - ectopic or molar pregnancy 639.5
  - during or after labor and delivery 669.1 ☑
    - fetus or newborn 779.89
  - external ear canal 380.50
    - secondary to
      - inflammation 380.53
      - surgery 380.52
      - trauma 380.51
  - general 780.2
  - heart — *see* Disease, heart
  - heat 992.1
  - hysterical 300.11
  - labyrinth, membranous (congenital) 744.05
  - lung (massive) (*see also* Atelectasis) 518.0
    - pressure, during labor 668.0 ☑
  - myocardial — *see* Disease, heart
  - nervous (*see also* Disorder, mental, nonpsychotic) 300.9
  - neurocirculatory 306.2
  - nose 738.0
  - postoperative (cardiovascular) 998.0
  - pulmonary (see also Atelectasis) 518.0
    - fetus or newborn 770.5
      - partial 770.5
      - primary 770.4
  - thorax 512.8
    - iatrogenic 512.1
    - postoperative 512.1
  - trachea 519.1
  - valvular — *see* Endocarditis
  - vascular (peripheral) 785.59
    - with
      - abortion — *see* Abortion, by type, with shock
      - ectopic pregnancy (*see also* categories 633.0-633.9) 639.5
      - molar pregnancy (*see also* categories 630-632) 639.5
    - cerebral (*see also* Disease, cerebrovascular, acute) 436
    - during or after labor and delivery 669.1 ☑
    - fetus or newborn 779.89
    - following
      - abortion 639.5
      - ectopic or molar pregnancy 639.5
  - vasomotor 785.59
  - vertebra 733.13
- **Collateral** — *see also* condition
  - circulation (venous) 459.89
  - dilation, veins 459.89
- **Colles' fracture** (closed) (reversed) (separation) 813.41
  - open 813.51

- **Collet's syndrome** 352.6
- **Collet-Sicard syndrome** 352.6
- **Colliculitis urethralis** (*see also* Urethritis) 597.89
- **Colliers'**
  - asthma 500
  - lung 500
  - phthisis (*see also* Tuberculosis) 011.4 ☑
- **Collodion baby** (ichthyosis congenita) 757.1
- **Colloid milium** 709.3
- **Coloboma** NEC 743.49
  - choroid 743.59
  - fundus 743.52
  - iris 743.46
  - lens 743.36
  - lids 743.62
  - optic disc (congenital) 743.57
    - acquired 377.23
  - retina 743.56
  - sclera 743.47
- **Coloenteritis** — *see* Enteritis
- **Colon** — *see* condition
- **Coloptosis** 569.89
- **Color**
  - amblyopia NEC 368.59
    - acquired 368.55
  - blindness NEC (congenital) 368.59
    - acquired 368.55
- **Colostomy**
  - attention to V55.3
  - fitting or adjustment V55.3
  - malfunctioning 569.62
  - status V44.3
- **Colpitis** (*see also* Vaginitis) 616.10
- **Colpocele** 618.6
- **Colpocystitis** (*see also* Vaginitis) 616.10
- **Colporrhexis** 665.4 ☑
- **Colpospasm** 625.1
- **Column, spinal, vertebral** — *see* condition
- **Coma** 780.01
  - apoplectic (*see also* Disease, cerebrovascular, acute) 436
  - diabetic (with ketoacidosis) 250.3 ☑
    - hyperosmolar 250.2 ☑
  - eclamptic (*see also* Eclampsia) 780.39
  - epileptic 345.3
  - hepatic 572.2
  - hyperglycemic 250.2 ☑
  - hyperosmolar (diabetic) (nonketotic) 250.2 ☑
  - hypoglycemic 251.0
    - diabetic 250.3 ☑
  - insulin 250.3 ☑
    - hyperosmolar 250.2 ☑
    - non-diabetic 251.0
    - organic hyperinsulinism 251.0
  - Kussmaul's (diabetic) 250.3 ☑
  - liver 572.2
  - newborn 779.2
  - prediabetic 250.2 ☑
  - uremic — *see* Uremia
- **Combat fatigue** (*see also* Reaction, stress, acute) 308.9
- **Combined** — *see* condition
- **Comedo** 706.1
- **Comedocarcinoma** (M8501/3) — *see also* Neoplasm, breast, malignant
  - noninfiltrating (M8501/2)
    - specified site — *see* Neoplasm, by site, in situ
    - unspecified site 233.0
- **Comedomastitis** 610.4
- **Comedones** 706.1
  - lanugo 757.4
- **Comma bacillus, carrier** (suspected) of V02.3
- **Comminuted fracture** — *see* Fracture, by site
- **Common**
  - aortopulmonary trunk 745.0
  - atrioventricular canal (defect) 745.69
  - atrium 745.69
  - cold (head) 460
    - vaccination, prophylactic (against) V04.7
  - truncus (arteriosus) 745.0
  - ventricle 745.3
- **Commotio** (current)
  - cerebri (*see also* Concussion, brain) 850.9
    - with skull fracture — *see* Fracture, skull, by site
  - retinae 921.3
  - spinalis — *see* Injury, spinal, by site
- **Commotion** (current)
  - brain (without skull fracture) (*see also* Concussion, brain) 850.9
    - with skull fracture — *see* Fracture, skull, by site
  - spinal cord — *see* Injury, spinal, by site
- **Communication**
  - abnormal — *see also* Fistula
    - between
      - base of aorta and pulmonary artery 745.0
      - left ventricle and right atrium 745.4
      - pericardial sac and pleural sac 748.8
      - pulmonary artery and pulmonary vein 747.3
    - congenital, between uterus and anterior abdominal wall 752.3
      - bladder 752.3
      - intestine 752.3
      - rectum 752.3
  - left ventricular— right atrial 745.4
  - pulmonary artery— pulmonary vein 747.3
- **Compensation**
  - broken — *see* Failure, heart
  - failure — *see* Failure, heart
  - neurosis, psychoneurosis 300.11
- **Complaint** — *see also* Disease
  - bowel, functional 564.9
    - psychogenic 306.4
  - intestine, functional 564.9
    - psychogenic 306.4
  - kidney (*see also* Disease, renal) 593.9
  - liver 573.9
  - miners' 500
- **Complete** — *see* condition
- **Complex**
  - cardiorenal (*see also* Hypertension, cardiorenal) 404.90
  - castration 300.9
  - Costen's 524.60
  - ego-dystonic homosexuality 302.0
  - Eisenmenger's (ventricular septal defect) 745.4
  - homosexual, ego-dystonic 302.0
  - hypersexual 302.89
  - inferiority 301.9
  - jumped process
    - spine — *see* Dislocation, vertebra
  - primary, tuberculosis (*see also* Tuberculosis) 010.0 ☑
  - Taussig-Bing (transposition, aorta and overriding pulmonary artery) 745.11
- **Complications**
  - abortion NEC — *see* categories 634-639
  - accidental puncture or laceration during a procedure 998.2
  - amputation stump (late) (surgical) 997.60
    - traumatic — *see* Amputation, traumatic
  - anastomosis (and bypass) — *see also* Complications, due to (presence of) any device, implant, or graft classified to 996.0-996.5 NEC
    - hemorrhage NEC 998.11
    - intestinal (internal) NEC 997.4
      - involving urinary tract 997.5
    - mechanical — *see* Complications, mechanical, graft
    - urinary tract (involving intestinal tract) 997.5
  - anesthesia, anesthetic NEC (*see also* Anesthesia, complication) 995.2
    - in labor and delivery 668.9 ☑
      - affecting fetus or newborn 763.5
      - cardiac 668.1 ☑
      - central nervous system 668.2 ☑
      - pulmonary 668.0 ☑
      - specified type NEC 668.8 ☑
  - aortocoronary (bypass) graft 996.03
    - atherosclerosis — *see* Arteriosclerosis, coronary
    - embolism 996.72

Complications — *continued*

- aortocoronary graft — *continued*
  - occlusion NEC 996.72
  - thrombus 996.72
- arthroplasty ▶(*see also* Complications, prosthetic joint)◀ 996.49 ▲
- artificial opening
  - cecostomy 569.60
  - colostomy 569.60
  - cystostomy 997.5
  - enterostomy 569.60
  - esophagostomy 530.87 ▲
    - infection 530.86
    - mechanical 530.87
  - gastrostomy 536.40
  - ileostomy 569.60
  - jejunostomy 569.60
  - nephrostomy 997.5
  - tracheostomy 519.00
  - ureterostomy 997.5
  - urethrostomy 997.5
- bariatric surgery 997.4
- bile duct implant (prosthetic) NEC 996.79
  - infection or inflammation 996.69
  - mechanical 996.59
- bleeding (intraoperative) (postoperative) 998.11
- blood vessel graft 996.1
  - aortocoronary 996.03
    - atherosclerosis — *see* Arteriosclerosis, coronary
    - embolism 996.72
    - occlusion NEC 996.72
    - thrombus 996.72
  - atherosclerosis — *see* Arteriosclerosis, extremities
  - embolism 996.74
  - occlusion NEC 996.74
  - thrombus 996.74
- bone growth stimulator NEC 996.78
  - infection or inflammation 996.67
- bone marrow transplant 996.85
- breast implant (prosthetic) NEC 996.79
  - infection or inflammation 996.69
  - mechanical 996.54
- bypass — *see also* Complications, anastomosis
  - aortocoronary 996.03
    - atherosclerosis — *see* Arteriosclerosis, coronary
    - embolism 996.72
    - occlusion NEC 996.72
    - thrombus 996.72
  - carotid artery 996.1
    - atherosclerosis — *see* Arteriosclerosis, extremities
    - embolism 996.74
    - occlusion NEC 996.74
    - thrombus 996.74
- cardiac (*see also* Disease, heart) 429.9
  - device, implant, or graft NEC 996.72
    - infection or inflammation 996.61
    - long-term effect 429.4
    - mechanical (*see also* Complications, mechanical, by type) 996.00
    - valve prosthesis 996.71
      - infection or inflammation 996.61
  - postoperative NEC 997.1
    - long-term effect 429.4
- cardiorenal (*see also* Hypertension, cardiorenal) 404.90
- carotid artery bypass graft 996.1
  - atherosclerosis — *see* Arteriosclerosis, extremities
  - embolism 996.74
  - occlusion NEC 996.74
  - thrombus 996.74
- cataract fragments in eye 998.82
- catheter device NEC — *see also* Complications, due to (presence of) any device, implant, or graft classified to 996.0-996.5 NEC
  - mechanical — *see* Complications, mechanical, catheter
- cecostomy 569.60
- cesarean section wound 674.3 ☑
- chin implant (prosthetic) NEC 996.79
  - infection or inflammation 996.69
  - mechanical 996.59
- colostomy (enterostomy) 569.60
  - specified type NEC 569.69

☑ Additional Digit Required — Refer to the Tabular List (Numeric Code Section) for Additional Digit Selection

▶◀ Revised Text ● New Line ▲ Revised Code

- **Complications** — *continued*
  - contraceptive device, intrauterine NEC 996.76
    - infection 996.65
    - inflammation 996.65
    - mechanical 996.32
  - cord (umbilical) — *see* Complications, umbilical cord
  - cornea
    - due to
      - contact lens 371.82
  - coronary (artery) bypass (graft) NEC 996.03
    - atherosclerosis — *see* Arteriosclerosis, coronary
    - embolism 996.72
    - infection or inflammation 996.61
    - mechanical 996.03
    - occlusion NEC 996.72
    - specified type NEC 996.72
    - thrombus 996.72
  - cystostomy 997.5
  - delivery 669.9 ☑
    - procedure (instrumental) (manual) (surgical) 669.4 ☑
    - specified type NEC 669.8 ☑
  - dialysis (hemodialysis) (peritoneal) (renal) NEC 999.9
    - catheter NEC — *see also* Complications, due to (presence of) any device, implant, or graft classified to 996.0-996.5 NEC
      - infection or inflammation 996.62
        - peritoneal 996.68
      - mechanical 996.1
        - peritoneal 996.56
  - due to (presence of) any device, implant, or graft classified to 996.0-996.5 NEC 996.70
    - with infection or inflammation — *see* Complications, infection or inflammation, due to (presence of) any device, implant, or graft classified to 996.0-996.5 NEC
    - arterial NEC 996.74
      - coronary NEC 996.03
        - atherosclerosis — *see* Arteriosclerosis, coronary
        - embolism 996.72
        - occlusion NEC 996.72
        - specified type NEC 996.72
        - thrombus 996.72
      - renal dialysis 996.73
    - arteriovenous fistula or shunt NEC 996.74
    - bone growth stimulator 996.78
    - breast NEC 996.79
    - cardiac NEC 996.72
      - defibrillator 996.72
      - pacemaker 996.72
      - valve prosthesis 996.71
    - catheter NEC 996.79
      - spinal 996.75
      - urinary, indwelling 996.76
      - vascular NEC 996.74
        - renal dialysis 996.73
      - ventricular shunt 996.75
    - coronary (artery) bypass (graft) NEC 996.03
      - atherosclerosis — *see* Arteriosclerosis, coronary
      - embolism 996.72
      - occlusion NEC 996.72
      - thrombus 996.72
    - electrodes
      - brain 996.75
      - heart 996.72
    - esophagostomy 530.87 ●
    - gastrointestinal NEC 996.79
    - genitourinary NEC 996.76
    - heart valve prosthesis NEC 996.71
    - infusion pump 996.74
    - insulin pump 996.57
    - internal
      - joint prosthesis 996.77
      - orthopedic NEC 996.78
      - specified type NEC 996.79
    - intrauterine contraceptive device NEC 996.76
    - joint prosthesis, internal NEC 996.77
    - mechanical — *see* Complications, mechanical
    - nervous system NEC 996.75

- **Complications** — *continued*
  - due to (presence of) any device, implant, or graft classified to 996.0-996.5 — *continued*
    - ocular lens NEC 996.79
    - orbital NEC 996.79
    - orthopedic NEC 996.78
      - joint, internal 996.77
    - renal dialysis 996.73
    - specified type NEC 996.79
    - urinary catheter, indwelling 996.76
    - vascular NEC 996.74
    - ventricular shunt 996.75
  - during dialysis NEC 999.9
  - ectopic or molar pregnancy NEC 639.9
  - electroshock therapy NEC 999.9
  - enterostomy 569.60
    - specified type NEC 569.69
  - esophagostomy 530.87 ▲
    - infection 530.86
    - mechanical 530.87
  - external (fixation) device with internal component(s) NEC 996.78
    - infection or inflammation 996.67
    - mechanical 996.49 ▲
  - extracorporeal circulation NEC 999.9
  - eye implant (prosthetic) NEC 996.79
    - infection or inflammation 996.69
    - mechanical
      - ocular lens 996.53
      - orbital globe 996.59
  - gastrointestinal, postoperative NEC (*see also* Complications, surgical procedures) 997.4
  - gastrostomy 536.40
    - specified type NEC 536.49
  - genitourinary device, implant or graft NEC 996.76
    - infection or inflammation 996.65
      - urinary catheter, indwelling 996.64
    - mechanical (*see also* Complications, mechanical, by type) 996.30
      - specified NEC 996.39
  - graft (bypass) (patch) — *see also* Complications, due to (presence of) any device, implant, or graft classified to 996.0-996.5 NEC
    - bone marrow 996.85
    - corneal NEC 996.79
      - infection or inflammation 996.69
      - rejection or reaction 996.51
    - mechanical — *see* Complications, mechanical, graft
    - organ (immune or nonimmune cause) (partial) (total) 996.80
      - bone marrow 996.85
      - heart 996.83
      - intestines 996.87
      - kidney 996.81
      - liver 996.82
      - lung 996.84
      - pancreas 996.86
      - specified NEC 996.89
    - skin NEC 996.79
      - infection or inflammation 996.69
      - rejection 996.52
        - artificial 996.55
        - decellularized allodermis 996.55
  - heart — *see also* Disease, heart transplant (immune or nonimmune cause) 996.83
  - hematoma (intraoperative) (postoperative) 998.12
  - hemorrhage (intraoperative) (postoperative) 998.11
  - hyperalimentation therapy NEC 999.9
  - immunization (procedure) — *see* Complications, vaccination
  - implant — *see also* Complications, due to (presence of) any device, implant, or graft classified to 996.0-996.5 NEC
    - mechanical — *see* Complications, mechanical, implant

- **Complications** — *continued*
  - infection and inflammation
    - due to (presence of) any device, implant or graft classified to 996.0-996.5 NEC 996.60
      - arterial NEC 996.62
        - coronary 996.61
        - renal dialysis 996.62
      - arteriovenous fistula or shunt 996.62
      - artificial heart 996.61
      - bone growth stimulator 996.67
      - breast 996.69
      - cardiac 996.61
      - catheter NEC 996.69
        - peritoneal 996.68
        - spinal 996.63
        - urinary, indwelling 996.64
        - vascular NEC 996.62
        - ventricular shunt 996.63
      - coronary artery bypass 996.61
      - electrodes
        - brain 996.63
        - heart 996.61
      - gastrointestinal NEC 996.69
      - genitourinary NEC 996.65
        - indwelling urinary catheter 996.64
      - heart assist device 996.61
      - heart valve 996.61
      - infusion pump 996.62
      - insulin pump 996.69
      - intrauterine contraceptive device 996.65
      - joint prosthesis, internal 996.66
      - ocular lens 996.69
      - orbital (implant) 996.69
      - orthopedic NEC 996.67
        - joint, internal 996.66
      - specified type NEC 996.69
      - urinary catheter, indwelling 996.64
      - ventricular shunt 996.63
  - infusion (procedure) 999.9
    - blood — *see* Complications, transfusion
    - infection NEC 999.3
    - sepsis NEC 999.3
  - inhalation therapy NEC 999.9
  - injection (procedure) 999.9
    - drug reaction (*see also* Reaction, drug) 995.2
    - infection NEC 999.3
    - sepsis NEC 999.3
    - serum (prophylactic) (therapeutic) — *see* Complications, vaccination
    - vaccine (any) — *see* Complications, vaccination
  - inoculation (any) — *see* Complications, vaccination
  - insulin pump 996.57
  - internal device (catheter) (electronic) (fixation) (prosthetic) — *see also* Complications, due to (presence of) any device, implant, or graft classified to 996.0-996.5 NEC
    - mechanical — *see* Complications, mechanical
  - intestinal transplant (immune or nonimmune cause) 996.87
  - intraoperative bleeding or hemorrhage 998.11
  - intrauterine contraceptive device (*see also* Complications, contraceptive device) 996.76
    - with fetal damage affecting management of pregnancy 655.8 ☑
    - infection or inflammation 996.65
  - jejunostomy 569.60
  - kidney transplant (immune or nonimmune cause) 996.81
  - labor 669.9 ☑
    - specified condition NEC 669.8 ☑
  - liver transplant (immune or nonimmune cause) 996.82
  - lumbar puncture 349.0
  - mechanical
    - anastomosis — *see* Complications, mechanical, graft
    - artificial heart 996.09
    - bypass — *see* Complications, mechanical, graft
    - catheter NEC 996.59
      - cardiac 996.09
      - cystostomy 996.39

☑ Additional Digit Required — Refer to the Tabular List (Numeric Code Section) for Additional Digit Selection

☑ Additional Digit Required — Refer to the Tabular List (Numeric Code Section) for Additional Digit Selection

▶◀ Revised Text ● New Line ▲ Revised Code

☑ Additional Digit Required — Refer to the Tabular List (Numeric Code Section) for Additional Digit Selection

▶◀ Revised Text ● New Line ▲ Revised Code

Note — Use the following fifth-digit subclassification with categories 851-854:

0 unspecified state of consciousness
1 with no loss of consciousness
2 with brief [less than one hour] loss of consciousness
3 with moderate [1-24 hours] loss of consciousness
4 with prolonged [more than 24 hours] loss of consciousness and return to pre-existing conscious level
5 with prolonged [more than 24 hours] loss of consciousness, without return to pre-existing conscious level
Use fifth-digit 5 to designate when a patient is unconscious and dies before regaining consciousness, regardless of the duration of the loss of consciousness
6 with loss of consciousness of unspecified duration
9 with concussion, unspecified

☑ Additional Digit Required — Refer to the Tabular List (Numeric Code Section) for Additional Digit Selection
▶◀ Revised Text ● New Line ▲ Revised Code

☑ Additional Digit Required — Refer to the Tabular List (Numeric Code Section) for Additional Digit Selection
▶◀ Revised Text ● New Line ▲ Revised Code

Counseling NEC — *continued*
  contraceptive NEC — *continued*
    management NEC V25.9
    oral contraceptive (pill) V25.01
      emergency V25.03
      postcoital V25.03
    prescription NEC V25.02
      oral contraceptive (pill) V25.01
        emergency V25.03
        postcoital V25.03
        repeat prescription V25.41
      repeat prescription V25.40
    subdermal implantable V25.43
    surveillance NEC V25.40
  dietary V65.3
  exercise V65.41
  expectant mother, pediatric pre-birth visit V65.11
  explanation of
    investigation finding NEC V65.49
    medication NEC V65.49
  family planning V25.09
  for nonattending third party V65.19
  genetic V26.33 ▲
  gonorrhea V65.45
  health (advice) (education) (instruction) NEC V65.49
  HIV V65.44
  human immunodeficiency virus V65.44
  injury prevention V65.43
  insulin pump training V65.46
  marital V61.10
  medical (for) V65.9
    boarding school resident V60.6
    condition not demonstrated V65.5
    feared complaint and no disease found V65.5
    institutional resident V60.6
    on behalf of another V65.19
    person living alone V60.3
  parent-child conflict V61.20
    specified problem NEC V61.29
  partner abuse
    perpetrator V61.12
    victim V61.11
  pediatric pre-birth visit for expectant mother V65.11
  perpetrator of
    child abuse V62.83
      parental V61.22
    partner abuse V61.12
    spouse abuse V61.12
  procreative V65.49
  sex NEC V65.49
    transmitted disease NEC V65.45
      HIV V65.44
  specified reason NEC V65.49
  spousal abuse
    perpetrator V61.12
    victim V61.11
  substance use and abuse V65.42
  syphilis V65.45
  victim (of)
    abuse NEC V62.89
    child abuse V61.21
    partner abuse V61.11
    spousal abuse V61.11
Coupled rhythm 427.89
Couvelaire uterus (complicating delivery) — *see* Placenta, separation
Cowper's gland — *see* condition
Cowperitis (*see also* Urethritis) 597.89
  gonorrheal (acute) 098.0
    chronic or duration of 2 months or over 098.2
Cowpox (abortive) 051.0
  due to vaccination 999.0
  eyelid 051.0 *[373.5]*
    postvaccination 999.0 *[373.5]*
Coxa
  plana 732.1
  valga (acquired) 736.31
    congenital 755.61
    late effect of rickets 268.1
  vara (acquired) 736.32
    congenital 755.62
    late effect of rickets 268.1
Coxae malum senilis 715.25
Coxalgia (nontuberculous) 719.45
  tuberculous (*see also* Tuberculosis) 015.1 ☑ *[730.85]*
Coxalgic pelvis 736.30
Coxitis 716.65
Coxsackie (infection) (virus) 079.2
  central nervous system NEC 048
  endocarditis 074.22
  enteritis 008.67
  meningitis (aseptic) 047.0
  myocarditis 074.23
  pericarditis 074.21
  pharyngitis 074.0
  pleurodynia 074.1
  specific disease NEC 074.8
Crabs, meaning pubic lice 132.2
Crack baby 760.75
Cracked nipple 611.2
  puerperal, postpartum 676.1 ☑
Cradle cap 690.11
Craft neurosis 300.89
Craigiasis 007.8
Cramp(s) 729.82
  abdominal 789.0 ☑
  bathing 994.1
  colic 789.0 ☑
    psychogenic 306.4
  due to immersion 994.1
  extremity (lower) (upper) NEC 729.82
  fireman 992.2
  heat 992.2
  hysterical 300.11
  immersion 994.1
  intestinal 789.0 ☑
    psychogenic 306.4
  linotypist's 300.89
    organic 333.84
  muscle (extremity) (general) 729.82
    due to immersion 994.1
    hysterical 300.11
  occupational (hand) 300.89
    organic 333.84
  psychogenic 307.89
  salt depletion 276.1
  sleep related, leg 327.52 ●
  stoker 992.2
  stomach 789.0 ☑
  telegraphers' 300.89
    organic 333.84
  typists' 300.89
    organic 333.84
  uterus 625.8
    menstrual 625.3
  writers' 333.84
    organic 333.84
    psychogenic 300.89
Cranial — *see* condition
Cranioclasis, fetal 763.89
Craniocleidodysostosis 755.59
Craniofenestria (skull) 756.0
Craniolacunia (skull) 756.0
Craniopagus 759.4
Craniopathy, metabolic 733.3
Craniopharyngeal — *see* condition
Craniopharyngioma (M9350/1) 237.0
Craniorachischisis (totalis) 740.1
Cranioschisis 756.0
Craniostenosis 756.0
Craniosynostosis 756.0
Craniotabes (cause unknown) 733.3
  rachitic 268.1
  syphilitic 090.5
Craniotomy, fetal 763.89
Cranium — *see* condition
Craw-craw 125.3
Creaking joint 719.60
  ankle 719.67
  elbow 719.62
  foot 719.67
  hand 719.64
Creaking joint — *continued*
  hip 719.65
  knee 719.66
  multiple sites 719.69
  pelvic region 719.65
  shoulder (region) 719.61
  specified site NEC 719.68
  wrist 719.63
Creeping
  eruption 126.9
  palsy 335.21
  paralysis 335.21
Crenated tongue 529.8
Creotoxism 005.9
Crepitus
  caput 756.0
  joint 719.60
    ankle 719.67
    elbow 719.62
    foot 719.67
    hand 719.64
    hip 719.65
    knee 719.66
    multiple sites 719.69
    pelvic region 719.65
    shoulder (region) 719.61
    specified site NEC 719.68
    wrist 719.63
Crescent or conus choroid, congenital 743.57
Cretin, cretinism (athyrotic) (congenital) (endemic) (metabolic) (nongoitrous) (sporadic) 243
  goitrous (sporadic) 246.1
  pelvis (dwarf type) (male type) 243
    with disproportion (fetopelvic) 653.1 ☑
      affecting fetus or newborn 763.1
      causing obstructed labor 660.1 ☑
        affecting fetus or newborn 763.1
  pituitary 253.3
Cretinoid degeneration 243
Creutzfeldt-Jakob disease (syndrome) ▶(new variant)◀ 046.1
  with dementia
    with behavioral disturbance 046.1 *[294.11]*
    without behavioral disturbance 046.1 *[294.10]*
Crib death 798.0
Cribriform hymen 752.49
Cri-du-chat syndrome 758.31
Crigler-Najjar disease or syndrome (congenital hyperbilirubinemia) 277.4
Crimean hemorrhagic fever 065.0
Criminalism 301.7
Crisis
  abdomen 789.0 ☑
  addisonian (acute adrenocortical insufficiency) 255.4
  adrenal (cortical) 255.4
  asthmatic — *see* Asthma
  brain, cerebral (*see also* Disease, cerebrovascular, acute) 436
  celiac 579.0
  Dietl's 593.4
  emotional NEC 309.29
    acute reaction to stress 308.0
    adjustment reaction 309.9
    specific to childhood or adolescence 313.9
  gastric (tabetic) 094.0
  glaucomatocyclitic 364.22
  heart (*see also* Failure, heart) 428.9
  hypertensive — *see* Hypertension
  nitritoid
    correct substance properly administered 458.29
    overdose or wrong substance given or taken 961.1
  oculogyric 378.87
    psychogenic 306.7
  Pel's 094.0
  psychosexual identity 302.6
  rectum 094.0
  renal 593.81
  sickle cell 282.62
  stomach (tabetic) 094.0

☑ Additional Digit Required — Refer to the Tabular List (Numeric Code Section) for Additional Digit Selection

▶◀ Revised Text ● New Line ▲ Revised Code

- **Cycle**
  - anovulatory 628.0
  - menstrual, irregular 626.4
- **Cyclencephaly** 759.89
- **Cyclical vomiting** 536.2
  - psychogenic 306.4
- **Cyclitic membrane** 364.74
- **Cyclitis** (*see also* Iridocyclitis) 364.3
  - acute 364.00
    - primary 364.01
    - recurrent 364.02
  - chronic 364.10
    - in
      - sarcoidosis 135 *[364.11]*
      - tuberculosis (*see also* Tuberculosis) 017.3 ☑ *[364.11]*
  - Fuchs' heterochromic 364.21
  - granulomatous 364.10
  - lens induced 364.23
  - nongranulomatous 364.00
  - posterior 363.21
  - primary 364.01
  - recurrent 364.02
  - secondary (noninfectious) 364.04
    - infectious 364.03
  - subacute 364.00
    - primary 364.01
    - recurrent 364.02
- **Cyclokeratitis** — *see* Keratitis
- **Cyclophoria** 378.44
- **Cyclopia, cyclops** 759.89
- **Cycloplegia** 367.51
- **Cyclospasm** 367.53
- **Cyclosporiasis** 007.5
- **Cyclothymia** 301.13
- **Cyclothymic personality** 301.13
- **Cyclotropia** 378.33
- **Cyesis** — *see* Pregnancy
- **Cylindroma** (M8200/3) — *see also* Neoplasm, by site, malignant
  - eccrine dermal (M8200/0) — *see* Neoplasm, skin, benign
  - skin (M8200/0) — *see* Neoplasm, skin, benign
- **Cylindruria** 791.7
- **Cyllosoma** 759.89
- **Cynanche**
  - diphtheritic 032.3
  - tonsillaris 475
- **Cynorexia** 783.6
- **Cyphosis** — *see* Kyphosis
- **Cyprus fever** (*see also* Brucellosis) 023.9
- **Cyriax's syndrome** (slipping rib) 733.99
- **Cyst** (mucus) (retention) (serous) (simple)

> *Note — In general, cysts are not neoplastic and are classified to the appropriate category for disease of the specified anatomical site. This generalization does not apply to certain types of cysts which are neoplastic in nature, for example, dermoid, nor does it apply to cysts of certain structures, for example, branchial cleft, which are classified as developmental anomalies.*
>
> *The following listing includes some of the most frequently reported sites of cysts as well as qualifiers which indicate the type of cyst. The latter qualifiers usually are not repeated under the anatomical sites. Since the code assignment for a given site may vary depending upon the type of cyst, the coder should refer to the listings under the specified type of cyst before consideration is given to the site.*

- **Cyst** (continued)
  - accessory, fallopian tube 752.11
  - adenoid (infected) 474.8
  - adrenal gland 255.8
    - congenital 759.1
  - air, lung 518.89
  - allantoic 753.7
  - alveolar process (jaw bone) 526.2
  - amnion, amniotic 658.8 ☑

Cyst — *continued*

  - anterior chamber (eye) 364.60
    - exudative 364.62
    - implantation (surgical) (traumatic) 364.61
    - parasitic 360.13
  - anterior nasopalatine 526.1
  - antrum 478.1
  - anus 569.49
  - apical (periodontal) (tooth) 522.8
  - appendix 543.9
  - arachnoid, brain 348.0
  - arytenoid 478.79
  - auricle 706.2
  - Baker's (knee) 727.51
    - tuberculous (*see also* Tuberculosis) 015.2 ☑
  - Bartholin's gland or duct 616.2
  - bile duct (*see also* Disease, biliary) 576.8
  - bladder (multiple) (trigone) 596.8
  - Blessig's 362.62
  - blood, endocardial (*see also* Endocarditis) 424.90
  - blue dome 610.0
  - bone (local) 733.20
    - aneurysmal 733.22
    - jaw 526.2
      - developmental (odontogenic) 526.0
      - fissural 526.1
      - latent 526.89
    - solitary 733.21
    - unicameral 733.21
  - brain 348.0
    - congenital 742.4
    - hydatid (*see also* Echinococcus) 122.9
    - third ventricle (colloid) 742.4
  - branchial (cleft) 744.42
  - branchiogenic 744.42
  - breast (benign) (blue dome) (pedunculated) (solitary) (traumatic) 610.0
    - involution 610.4
    - sebaceous 610.8
  - broad ligament (benign) 620.8
    - embryonic 752.11
  - bronchogenic (mediastinal) (sequestration) 518.89
    - congenital 748.4
  - buccal 528.4
  - bulbourethral gland (Cowper's) 599.89
  - bursa, bursal 727.49
    - pharyngeal 478.26
  - calcifying odontogenic (M9301/0) 213.1
    - upper jaw (bone) 213.0
  - canal of Nuck (acquired) (serous) 629.1
    - congenital 752.41
  - canthus 372.75
  - carcinomatous (M8010/3) — *see* Neoplasm, by site, malignant
  - cartilage (joint) — *see* Derangement, joint
  - cauda equina 336.8
  - cavum septi pellucidi NEC 348.0
  - celomic (pericardium) 746.89
  - cerebellopontine (angle) — *see* Cyst, brain
  - cerebellum — *see* Cyst, brain
  - cerebral — *see* Cyst, brain
  - cervical lateral 744.42
  - cervix 622.8
    - embryonal 752.41
    - nabothian (gland) 616.0
  - chamber, anterior (eye) 364.60
    - exudative 364.62
    - implantation (surgical) (traumatic) 364.61
    - parasitic 360.13
  - chiasmal, optic NEC (*see also* Lesion, chiasmal) 377.54
  - chocolate (ovary) 617.1
  - choledochal (congenital) 751.69
    - acquired 576.8
  - choledochus 751.69
  - chorion 658.8 ☑
  - choroid plexus 348.0
  - chyle, mesentery 457.8
  - ciliary body 364.60
    - exudative 364.64
    - implantation 364.61
    - primary 364.63
  - clitoris 624.8
  - coccyx (*see also* Cyst, bone) 733.20

Cyst — *continued*

  - colloid
    - third ventricle (brain) 742.4
    - thyroid gland — *see* Goiter
  - colon 569.89
  - common (bile) duct (*see also* Disease, biliary) 576.8
  - congenital NEC 759.89
    - adrenal glands 759.1
    - epiglottis 748.3
    - esophagus 750.4
    - fallopian tube 752.11
    - kidney 753.10
      - multiple 753.19
      - single 753.11
    - larynx 748.3
    - liver 751.62
    - lung 748.4
    - mediastinum 748.8
    - ovary 752.0
    - oviduct 752.11
    - pancreas 751.7
    - periurethral (tissue) 753.8
    - prepuce NEC 752.69
      - penis 752.69
    - sublingual 750.26
    - submaxillary gland 750.26
    - thymus (gland) 759.2
    - tongue 750.19
    - ureterovesical orifice 753.4
    - vulva 752.41
  - conjunctiva 372.75
  - cornea 371.23
  - corpora quadrigemina 348.0
  - corpus
    - albicans (ovary) 620.2
    - luteum (ruptured) 620.1
  - Cowper's gland (benign) (infected) 599.89
  - cranial meninges 348.0
  - craniobuccal pouch 253.8
  - craniopharyngeal pouch 253.8
  - cystic duct (*see also* Disease, gallbladder) 575.8
  - Cysticercus (any site) 123.1
  - Dandy-Walker 742.3
    - with spina bifida (*see also* Spina bifida) 741.0 ☑
  - dental 522.8
    - developmental 526.0
    - eruption 526.0
    - lateral periodontal 526.0
    - primordial (keratocyst) 526.0
    - root 522.8
  - dentigerous 526.0
    - mandible 526.0
    - maxilla 526.0
  - dermoid (M9084/0) — *see also* Neoplasm, by site, benign
    - with malignant transformation (M9084/3) 183.0
    - implantation
      - external area or site (skin) NEC 709.8
      - iris 364.61
      - skin 709.8
      - vagina 623.8
      - vulva 624.8
    - mouth 528.4
    - oral soft tissue 528.4
    - sacrococcygeal 685.1
      - with abscess 685.0
  - developmental of ovary, ovarian 752.0
  - dura (cerebral) 348.0
    - spinal 349.2
  - ear (external) 706.2
  - echinococcal (*see also* Echinococcus) 122.9
  - embryonal
    - cervix uteri 752.41
    - genitalia, female external 752.41
    - uterus 752.3
    - vagina 752.41
  - endometrial 621.8
    - ectopic 617.9
  - endometrium (uterus) 621.8
    - ectopic — *see* Endometriosis
  - enteric 751.5
  - enterogenous 751.5
  - epidermal (inclusion) (*see also* Cyst, skin) 706.2

☑ Additional Digit Required — Refer to the Tabular List (Numeric Code Section) for Additional Digit Selection
▶◀ Revised Text ● New Line ▲ Revised Code

☑ Additional Digit Required — Refer to the Tabular List (Numeric Code Section) for Additional Digit Selection

▶◀ Revised Text ● New Line ▲ Revised Code

- **Cystadenoma** (M8440/0) — *see also* Neoplasm, by site, benign — *continued*
  - pseudomucinous — *continued*
    - papillary (M8471/0)
      - borderline malignancy (M8471/1)
        - specified site — *see* Neoplasm, by site, uncertain behavior
        - unspecified site 236.2
      - specified site — *see* Neoplasm, by site, benign
      - unspecified site 220
    - specified site — *see* Neoplasm, by site, benign
    - unspecified site 220
  - serous (M8441/0)
    - borderline malignancy (M8441/1)
      - specified site — *see* Neoplasm, by site, uncertain behavior
      - unspecified site 236.2
    - papillary (M8460/0)
      - borderline malignancy (M8460/1)
        - specified site — *see* Neoplasm, by site, uncertain behavior
        - unspecified site 236.2
      - specified site — *see* Neoplasm, by site, benign
      - unspecified site 220
    - specified site — *see* Neoplasm, by site, benign
    - unspecified site 220
  - thyroid 226
- **Cystathioninemia** 270.4
- **Cystathioninuria** 270.4
- **Cystic** — *see also* condition
  - breast, chronic 610.1
  - corpora lutea 620.1
  - degeneration, congenital
    - brain 742.4
    - kidney (*see also* Cystic, disease, degeneration, kidney) 753.10
  - disease
    - breast, chronic 610.1
    - kidney, congenital 753.10
      - medullary 753.16
      - multiple 753.19
      - polycystic — *see* Polycystic, kidney
      - single 753.11
      - specified NEC 753.19
    - liver, congenital 751.62
    - lung 518.89
      - congenital 748.4
    - pancreas, congenital 751.7
    - semilunar cartilage 717.5
  - duct — *see* condition
  - eyeball, congenital 743.03
  - fibrosis (pancreas) 277.00
    - with
      - manifestations
        - gastrointestinal 277.03
        - pulmonary 277.02
        - specified NEC 277.09
      - meconium ileus 277.01
      - pulmonary exacerbation 277.02
  - hygroma (M9173/0) 228.1
  - kidney, congenital 753.10
    - medullary 753.16
    - multiple 753.19
    - polycystic — *see* Polycystic, kidney
    - single 753.11
    - specified NEC 753.19
  - liver, congenital 751.62
  - lung 518.89
    - congenital 748.4
  - mass — *see* Cyst
  - mastitis, chronic 610.1
  - ovary 620.2
  - pancreas, congenital 751.7
- **Cysticerciasis** 123.1
- **Cysticercosis** (mammary) (subretinal) 123.1
- **Cysticercus** 123.1
  - cellulosae infestation 123.1
- **Cystinosis** (malignant) 270.0
- **Cystinuria** 270.0
- **Cystitis** (bacillary) (colli) (diffuse) (exudative) (hemorrhagic) (purulent) (recurrent) (septic) (suppurative) (ulcerative) 595.9
  - with
    - abortion — *see* Abortion, by type, with urinary tract infection
    - ectopic pregnancy (*see also* categories 633.0-633.9) 639.8
    - fibrosis 595.1
    - leukoplakia 595.1
    - malakoplakia 595.1
    - metaplasia 595.1
    - molar pregnancy (*see also* categories 630-632) 639.8
  - actinomycotic 039.8 *[595.4]*
  - acute 595.0
    - of trigone 595.3
  - allergic 595.89
  - amebic 006.8 *[595.4]*
  - bilharzial 120.9 *[595.4]*
  - blennorrhagic (acute) 098.11
    - chronic or duration of 2 months or more 098.31
  - bullous 595.89
  - calculous 594.1
    - chlamydial 099.53
  - chronic 595.2
    - interstitial 595.1
    - of trigone 595.3
  - complicating pregnancy, childbirth, or puerperium 646.6 ☑
    - affecting fetus or newborn 760.1
  - cystic(a) 595.81
  - diphtheritic 032.84
  - echinococcal
    - granulosus 122.3 *[595.4]*
    - multilocularis 122.6 *[595.4]*
  - emphysematous 595.89
  - encysted 595.81
  - follicular 595.3
  - following
    - abortion 639.8
    - ectopic or molar pregnancy 639.8
  - gangrenous 595.89
  - glandularis 595.89
  - gonococcal (acute) 098.11
    - chronic or duration of 2 months or more 098.31
  - incrusted 595.89
  - interstitial 595.1
  - irradiation 595.82
  - irritation 595.89
  - malignant 595.89
  - monilial 112.2
  - of trigone 595.3
  - panmural 595.1
  - polyposa 595.89
  - prostatic 601.3
  - radiation 595.82
  - Reiter's (abacterial) 099.3
  - specified NEC 595.89
  - subacute 595.2
  - submucous 595.1
  - syphilitic 095.8
  - trichomoniasis 131.09
  - tuberculous (*see also* Tuberculosis) 016.1 ☑
  - ulcerative 595.1
- **Cystocele** (-rectocele)
  - female (without uterine prolapse) 618.01
    - with uterine prolapse 618.4
      - complete 618.3
      - incomplete 618.2
    - lateral 618.02
    - midline 618.01
    - paravaginal 618.02
  - in pregnancy or childbirth 654.4 ☑
    - affecting fetus or newborn 763.89
    - causing obstructed labor 660.2 ☑
      - affecting fetus or newborn 763.1
  - male 596.8
- **Cystoid**
  - cicatrix limbus 372.64
  - degeneration macula 362.53
- **Cystolithiasis** 594.1
- **Cystoma** (M8440/0) — *see also* Neoplasm, by site, benign
  - endometrial, ovary 617.1
  - mucinous (M8470/0)
    - specified site — *see* Neoplasm, by site, benign
    - unspecified site 220
  - serous (M8441/0)
    - specified site — *see* Neoplasm, by site, benign
    - unspecified site 220
  - simple (ovary) 620.2
- **Cystoplegia** 596.53
- **Cystoptosis** 596.8
- **Cystopyelitis** (*see also* Pyelitis) 590.80
- **Cystorrhagia** 596.8
- **Cystosarcoma phyllodes** (M9020/1) 238.3
  - benign (M9020/0) 217
  - malignant (M9020/3) — *see* Neoplasm, breast, malignant
- **Cystostomy status** V44.50
  - appendico-vesicostomy V44.52
  - cutaneous-vesicostomy V44.51
  - specified type NEC V44.59
  - with complication 997.5
- **Cystourethritis** (*see also* Urethritis) 597.89
- **Cystourethrocele** (*see also* Cystocele)
  - female (without uterine prolapse) 618.09
    - with uterine prolapse 618.4
      - complete 618.3
      - incomplete 618.2
  - male 596.8
- **Cytomegalic inclusion disease** 078.5
  - congenital 771.1
- **Cytomycosis, reticuloendothelial** (*see also* Histoplasmosis, American) 115.00
- **Cytopenia** 289.9

D

- **Daae (-Finsen) disease** (epidemic pleurodynia) 074.1
- **Dabney's grip** 074.1
- **Da Costa's syndrome** (neurocirculatory asthenia) 306.2
- **Dacryoadenitis, dacryadenitis** 375.00
  - acute 375.01
  - chronic 375.02
- **Dacryocystitis** 375.30
  - acute 375.32
  - chronic 375.42
  - neonatal 771.6
  - phlegmonous 375.33
  - syphilitic 095.8
    - congenital 090.0
  - trachomatous, active 076.1
    - late effect 139.1
  - tuberculous (*see also* Tuberculosis) 017.3 ☑
- **Dacryocystoblenorrhea** 375.42
- **Dacryocystocele** 375.43
- **Dacryolith, dacryolithiasis** 375.57
- **Dacryoma** 375.43
- **Dacryopericystitis** (acute) (subacute) 375.32
  - chronic 375.42
- **Dacryops** 375.11
- **Dacryosialadenopathy, atrophic** 710.2
- **Dacryostenosis** 375.56
  - congenital 743.65
- **Dactylitis** 686.9
  - bone (*see also* Osteomyelitis) 730.2 ☑
  - sickle-cell 282.61
  - syphilitic 095.5
  - tuberculous (*see also* Tuberculosis) 015.5 ☑
- **Dactylolysis spontanea** 136.0
- **Dactylosymphysis** (*see also* Syndactylism) 755.10
- **Damage**
  - arteriosclerotic — *see* Arteriosclerosis
  - brain 348.9
    - anoxic, hypoxic 348.1
      - during or resulting from a procedure 997.01
    - child NEC 343.9
    - due to birth injury 767.0
    - minimal (child) (*see also* Hyperkinesia) 314.9
    - newborn 767.0
  - cardiac — *see also* Disease, heart
  - cardiorenal (vascular) (*see also* Hypertension, cardiorenal) 404.90
  - central nervous system — *see* Damage, brain
  - cerebral NEC — *see* Damage, brain
  - coccyx, complicating delivery 665.6 ☑
  - coronary (*see also* Ischemia, heart) 414.9
  - eye, birth injury 767.8
  - heart — *see also* Disease, heart
    - valve — *see* Endocarditis
  - hypothalamus NEC 348.9
  - liver 571.9
    - alcoholic 571.3
  - myocardium (*see also* Degeneration, myocardial) 429.1
  - pelvic
    - joint or ligament, during delivery 665.6 ☑
    - organ NEC
      - with
        - abortion — *see* Abortion, by type, with damage to pelvic organs
        - ectopic pregnancy (*see also* categories 633.0-633.9) 639.2
        - molar pregnancy (*see also* categories 630-632) 639.2
      - during delivery 665.5 ☑
      - following
        - abortion 639.2
        - ectopic or molar pregnancy 639.2
  - renal (*see also* Disease, renal) 593.9
  - skin, solar 692.79
    - acute 692.72
    - chronic 692.74
  - subendocardium, subendocardial (*see also* Degeneration, myocardial) 429.1
  - vascular 459.9
- **Dameshek's syndrome** (erythroblastic anemia) 282.49
- **Dana-Putnam syndrome** (subacute combined sclerosis with pernicious anemia) 281.0 *[336.2]*
- **Danbolt (-Closs) syndrome** (acrodermatitis enteropathica) 686.8
- **Dandruff** 690.18
- **Dandy fever** 061
- **Dandy-Walker deformity or syndrome** (atresia, foramen of Magendie) 742.3
  - with spina bifida (*see also* Spina bifida) 741.0 ☑
- **Dangle foot** 736.79
- **Danielssen's disease** (anesthetic leprosy) 030.1
- **Danlos' syndrome** 756.83
- **Darier's disease** (congenital) (keratosis follicularis) 757.39
  - due to vitamin A deficiency 264.8
  - meaning erythema annulare centrifugum 695.0
- **Darier-Roussy sarcoid** 135
- **Darling's**
  - disease (*see also* Histoplasmosis, American) 115.00
  - histoplasmosis (*see also* Histoplasmosis, American) 115.00
- **Dartre** 054.9
- **Darwin's tubercle** 744.29
- **Davidson's anemia** (refractory) 284.9
- **Davies' disease** 425.0
- **Davies-Colley syndrome** (slipping rib) 733.99
- **Dawson's encephalitis** 046.2
- **Day blindness** (*see also* Blindness, day) 368.60
- **Dead**
  - fetus
    - retained (in utero) 656.4 ☑
      - early pregnancy (death before 22 completed weeks gestation) 632
      - late (death after 22 completed weeks gestation) 656.4 ☑
    - syndrome 641.3 ☑
  - labyrinth 386.50
  - ovum, retained 631
- **Deaf and dumb** NEC 389.7
- **Deaf mutism** (acquired) (congenital) NEC 389.7
  - endemic 243
  - hysterical 300.11
  - syphilitic, congenital 090.0
- **Deafness** (acquired) (bilateral) (both ears) (complete) (congenital) (hereditary) (middle ear) (partial) (unilateral) 389.9
  - with blue sclera and fragility of bone 756.51
  - auditory fatigue 389.9
  - aviation 993.0
    - nerve injury 951.5
  - boilermakers' 951.5
  - central 389.14
    - with conductive hearing loss 389.2
  - conductive (air) 389.00
    - with sensorineural hearing loss 389.2
    - combined types 389.08
    - external ear 389.01
    - inner ear 389.04
    - middle ear 389.03
    - multiple types 389.08
    - tympanic membrane 389.02
  - emotional (complete) 300.11
  - functional (complete) 300.11
  - high frequency 389.8
  - hysterical (complete) 300.11
  - injury 951.5
  - low frequency 389.8
  - mental 784.69
  - mixed conductive and sensorineural 389.2
  - nerve 389.12
    - with conductive hearing loss 389.2
  - neural 389.12
    - with conductive hearing loss 389.2
  - noise-induced 388.12
    - nerve injury 951.5
  - nonspeaking 389.7

Deafness — *continued*

  - perceptive 389.10
    - with conductive hearing loss 389.2
    - central 389.14
    - combined types 389.18
    - multiple types 389.18
    - neural 389.12
    - sensory 389.11
  - psychogenic (complete) 306.7
  - sensorineural (*see also* Deafness, perceptive) 389.10
  - sensory 389.11
    - with conductive hearing loss 389.2
  - specified type NEC 389.8
  - sudden NEC 388.2
  - syphilitic 094.89
  - transient ischemic 388.02
  - transmission — *see* Deafness, conductive
  - traumatic 951.5
  - word (secondary to organic lesion) 784.69
    - developmental 315.31
- **Death**
  - after delivery (cause not stated) (sudden) 674.9 ☑
  - anesthetic
    - due to
      - correct substance properly administered 995.4
      - overdose or wrong substance given 968.4
        - specified anesthetic — *see* Table of Drugs and Chemicals
    - during delivery 668.9 ☑
  - brain 348.8
  - cardiac — *see* Disease, heart
  - cause unknown 798.2
  - cot (infant) 798.0
  - crib (infant) 798.0
  - fetus, fetal (cause not stated) (intrauterine) 779.9
    - early, with retention (before 22 completed weeks gestation) 632
    - from asphyxia or anoxia (before labor) 768.0
      - during labor 768.1
    - late, affecting management of pregnancy (after 22 completed weeks gestation) 656.4 ☑
  - from pregnancy NEC 646.9 ☑
  - instantaneous 798.1
  - intrauterine (*see also* Death, fetus) 779.9
    - complicating pregnancy 656.4 ☑
  - maternal, affecting fetus or newborn 761.6
  - neonatal NEC 779.9
  - sudden (cause unknown) 798.1
    - during delivery 669.9 ☑
      - under anesthesia NEC 668.9 ☑
    - infant, syndrome (SIDS) 798.0
    - puerperal, during puerperium 674.9 ☑
  - unattended (cause unknown) 798.9
  - under anesthesia NEC
    - due to
      - correct substance properly administered 995.4
      - overdose or wrong substance given 968.4
        - specified anesthetic — *see* Table of Drugs and Chemicals
    - during delivery 668.9 ☑
  - violent 798.1
- **de Beurmann-Gougerot disease** (sporotrichosis) 117.1
- **Debility** (general) (infantile) (postinfectional) 799.3
  - with nutritional difficulty 269.9
  - congenital or neonatal NEC 779.9
  - nervous 300.5
  - old age 797
  - senile 797
- **Débove's disease** (splenomegaly) 789.2
- **Decalcification**
  - bone (*see also* Osteoporosis) 733.00
  - teeth 521.8
- **Decapitation** 874.9
  - fetal (to facilitate delivery) 763.89
- **Decapsulation, kidney** 593.89
- **Decay**
  - dental 521.00
  - senile 797
  - tooth, teeth 521.00

Deficiency, deficient — *continued*
- immunity NEC 279.3
  - cell-mediated 279.10
    - with
      - hyperimmunoglobulinemia 279.2
      - thrombocytopenia and eczema 279.12
    - specified NEC 279.19
  - combined (severe) 279.2
    - syndrome 279.2
  - common variable 279.06
  - humoral NEC 279.00
  - IgA (secretory) 279.01
  - IgG 279.03
  - IgM 279.02
- immunoglobulin, selective NEC 279.03
  - IgA 279.01
  - IgG 279.03
  - IgM 279.02
- inositol (B complex) 266.2
- interferon 279.4
- internal organ V47.0
- interstitial cell-stimulating hormone (ICSH) 253.4
- intrinsic factor (Castle's) (congenital) 281.0
- intrinsic (urethral) sphincter (ISD) 599.82
- invertase 271.3
- iodine 269.3
- iron, anemia 280.9
- labile factor (congenital) (*see also* Defect, coagulation) 286.3
  - acquired 286.7
- lacrimal fluid (acquired) 375.15
  - congenital 743.64
- lactase 271.3
- Laki-Lorand factor (*see also* Defect, coagulation) 286.3
- lecithin-cholesterol acyltranferase 272.5
- LH (luteinizing hormone) 253.4
- limb V49.0
  - lower V49.0
    - congenital (*see also* Deficiency, lower limb, congenital) 755.30
  - upper V49.0
    - congenital (*see also* Deficiency, upper limb, congenital) 755.20
- lipocaic 577.8
- lipoid (high-density) 272.5
- lipoprotein (familial) (high density) 272.5
- liver phosphorylase 271.0
- long chain 3-hydroxyacyl CoA dehydrogenase (LCHAD) 277.85
- long chain/very long chain acyl CoA dehydrogenase (LCAD, VLCAD) 277.85
- lower limb V49.0
  - congenital 755.30
    - with complete absence of distal elements 755.31
    - longitudinal (complete) (partial) (with distal deficiencies, incomplete) 755.32
      - with complete absence of distal elements 755.31
      - combined femoral, tibial, fibular (incomplete) 755.33
      - femoral 755.34
      - fibular 755.37
      - metatarsal(s) 755.38
      - phalange(s) 755.39
        - meaning all digits 755.31
      - tarsal(s) 755.38
      - tibia 755.36
      - tibiofibular 755.35
    - transverse 755.31
- luteinizing hormone (LH) 253.4
- lysosomal alpha-1, 4 glucosidase 271.0
- magnesium 275.2
- mannosidase 271.8
- medium chain acyl CoA dehydrogenase (MCAD) 277.85
- melanocyte-stimulating hormone (MSH) 253.4
- menadione (vitamin K) 269.0
  - newborn 776.0
- mental (familial) (hereditary) (*see also* Retardation, mental) 319
- mineral NEC 269.3
- molybdenum 269.3
- moral 301.7

Deficiency, deficient — *continued*
- multiple, syndrome 260
- myocardial (*see also* Insufficiency, myocardial) 428.0
- myophosphorylase 271.0
- NADH (DPNH)-methemoglobin-reductase (congenital) 289.7
- NADH-diaphorase or reductase (congenital) 289.7
- neck V48.1
- niacin (amide) (-tryptophan) 265.2
- nicotinamide 265.2
- nicotinic acid (amide) 265.2
- nose V48.8
- number of teeth (*see also* Anodontia) 520.0
- nutrition, nutritional 269.9
  - specified NEC 269.8
- ornithine transcarbamylase 270.6
- ovarian 256.39
- oxygen (*see also* Anoxia) 799.02 ▲
- pantothenic acid 266.2
- parathyroid (gland) 252.1
- phenylalanine hydroxylase 270.1
- phosphoenolpyruvate carboxykinase 271.8
- phosphofructokinase 271.2
- phosphoglucomutase 271.0
- phosphohexosisomerase 271.0
- phosphomannomutase 271.8 ●
- phosphomannose isomerase 271.8 ●
- phosphomannosyl mutase 271.8 ●
- phosphorylase kinase, liver 271.0
- pituitary (anterior) 253.2
  - posterior 253.5
- placenta — *see* Placenta, insufficiency
- plasma
  - cell 279.00
  - protein (paraproteinemia) (pyroglobulinemia) 273.8
    - gamma globulin 279.00
  - thromboplastin
    - antecedent (PTA) 286.2
    - component (PTC) 286.1
- platelet NEC 287.1
  - constitutional 286.4
- polyglandular 258.9
- potassium (K) 276.8
- proaccelerin (congenital) (*see also* Defect, congenital) 286.3
  - acquired 286.7
- proconvertin factor (congenital) (*see also* Defect, coagulation) 286.3
  - acquired 286.7
- prolactin 253.4
- protein 260
  - anemia 281.4
  - C 289.81
  - plasma — *see* Deficiency, plasma, protein
  - S 289.81
- prothrombin (congenital) (*see also* Defect, coagulation) 286.3
  - acquired 286.7
- Prower factor (*see also* Defect, coagulation) 286.3
- PRT 277.2
- pseudocholinesterase 289.89
- psychobiological 301.6
- PTA 286.2
- PTC 286.1
- purine nucleoside phosphorylase 277.2
- pyracin (alpha) (beta) 266.1
- pyridoxal 266.1
- pyridoxamine 266.1
- pyridoxine (derivatives) 266.1
- pyruvate carboxylase 271.8
- pyruvate dehydrogenase 271.8
- pyruvate kinase (PK) 282.3
- riboflavin (vitamin B_2) 266.0
- saccadic eye movements 379.57
- salivation 527.7
- salt 276.1
- secretion
  - ovary 256.39
  - salivary gland (any) 527.7
  - urine 788.5
- selenium 269.3
- serum
  - antitrypsin, familial 273.4

Deficiency, deficient — *continued*
- serum — *continued*
  - protein (congenital) 273.8
- short chain acyl CoA dehydrogenase (SCAD) 277.85
- smooth pursuit movements (eye) 379.58
- sodium (Na) 276.1
- SPCA (*see also* Defect, coagulation) 286.3
- specified NEC 269.8
- stable factor (congenital) (*see also* Defect, coagulation) 286.3
  - acquired 286.7
- Stuart (-Prower) factor (*see also* Defect, coagulation) 286.3
- sucrase 271.3
- sucrase-isomaltase 271.3
- sulfite oxidase 270.0
- syndrome, multiple 260
- thiamine, thiaminic (chloride) 265.1
- thrombokinase (*see also* Defect, coagulation) 286.3
  - newborn 776.0
- thrombopoieten 287.39 ▲
- thymolymphatic 279.2
- thyroid (gland) 244.9
- tocopherol 269.1
- toe — *see* Absence, toe
- tooth bud (*see also* Anodontia) 520.0
- trunk V48.1
- UDPG-glycogen transferase 271.0
- upper limb V49.0
  - congenital 755.20
    - with complete absence of distal elements 755.21
    - longitudinal (complete) (partial) (with distal deficiencies, incomplete) 755.22
      - carpal(s) 755.28
      - combined humeral, radial, ulnar (incomplete) 755.23
      - humeral 755.24
      - metacarpal(s) 755.28
      - phalange(s) 755.29
        - meaning all digits 755.21
      - radial 755.26
      - radioulnar 755.25
      - ulnar 755.27
    - transverse (complete) (partial) 755.21
- vascular 459.9
- vasopressin 253.5
- viosterol (*see also* Deficiency, calciferol) 268.9
- vitamin (multiple) NEC 269.2
  - A 264.9
    - with
      - Bitôt's spot 264.1
        - corneal 264.2
          - with corneal ulceration 264.3
      - keratomalacia 264.4
      - keratosis, follicular 264.8
      - night blindness 264.5
      - scar of cornea, xerophthalmic 264.6
      - specified manifestation NEC 264.8
        - ocular 264.7
      - xeroderma 264.8
      - xerophthalmia 264.7
      - xerosis
        - conjunctival 264.0
          - with Bitôt's spot 264.1
        - corneal 264.2
          - with corneal ulceration 264.3
  - B (complex) NEC 266.9
    - with
      - beriberi 265.0
      - pellagra 265.2
    - specified type NEC 266.2
  - B_1 NEC 265.1
    - beriberi 265.0
  - B_2 266.0
  - B_6 266.1
  - B_{12} 266.2
  - B_c (folic acid) 266.2
  - C (ascorbic acid) (with scurvy) 267
  - D (calciferol) (ergosterol) 268.9
    - with
      - osteomalacia 268.2
      - rickets (*see also* Rickets) 268.0
  - E 269.1

- **Deficiency, deficient** — *continued*
  - vitamin (multiple) NEC — *continued*
    - folic acid 266.2
    - G 266.0
    - H 266.2
    - K 269.0
      - of newborn 776.0
    - nicotinic acid 265.2
    - P 269.1
    - PP 265.2
    - specified NEC 269.1
  - zinc 269.3
- **Deficient** — *see also* Deficiency
  - blink reflex 374.45
  - craniofacial axis 756.0
  - number of teeth (*see also* Anodontia) 520.0
  - secretion of urine 788.5
- **Deficit**
  - neurologic NEC 781.99
    - due to
      - cerebrovascular lesion (*see also* Disease, cerebrovascular, acute) 436
        - late effect — *see* Late effect(s) (of) cerebrovascular disease
      - transient ischemic attack 435.9
  - oxygen 799.02 ▲
- **Deflection**
  - radius 736.09
  - septum (acquired) (nasal) (nose) 470
  - spine — *see* Curvature, spine
  - turbinate (nose) 470
- **Defluvium**
  - capillorum (*see also* Alopecia) 704.00
  - ciliorum 374.55
  - unguium 703.8
- **Deformity** 738.9
  - abdomen, congenital 759.9
  - abdominal wall
    - acquired 738.8
    - congenital 756.70
    - muscle deficiency syndrome 756.79
  - acquired (unspecified site) 738.9
    - specified site NEC 738.8
  - adrenal gland (congenital) 759.1
  - alimentary tract, congenital 751.9
    - lower 751.5
    - specified type NEC 751.8
    - upper (any part, except tongue) 750.9
      - specified type NEC 750.8
      - tongue 750.10
        - specified type NEC 750.19
  - ankle (joint) (acquired) 736.70
    - abduction 718.47
    - congenital 755.69
    - contraction 718.47
    - specified NEC 736.79
  - anus (congenital) 751.5
    - acquired 569.49
  - aorta (congenital) 747.20
    - acquired 447.8
    - arch 747.21
      - acquired 447.8
    - coarctation 747.10
  - aortic
    - arch 747.21
      - acquired 447.8
    - cusp or valve (congenital) 746.9
      - acquired (*see also* Endocarditis, aortic) 424.1
    - ring 747.21
  - appendix 751.5
  - arm (acquired) 736.89
    - congenital 755.50
  - arteriovenous (congenital) (peripheral) NEC 747.60
    - gastrointestinal 747.61
    - lower limb 747.64
    - renal 747.62
    - specified NEC 747.69
    - spinal 747.82
    - upper limb 747.63
  - artery (congenital) (peripheral) NEC (*see also* Deformity, vascular) 747.60
    - acquired 447.8
    - cerebral 747.81

- **Deformity** — *continued*
  - artery NEC (*see also* Deformity, vascular) — *continued*
    - coronary (congenital) 746.85
      - acquired (*see also* Ischemia, heart) 414.9
    - retinal 743.9
    - umbilical 747.5
  - atrial septal (congenital) (heart) 745.5
  - auditory canal (congenital) (external) (*see also* Deformity, ear) 744.3
    - acquired 380.50
  - auricle
    - ear (congenital) (*see also* Deformity, ear) 744.3
      - acquired 380.32
    - heart (congenital) 746.9
  - back (acquired) — *see* Deformity, spine
  - Bartholin's duct (congenital) 750.9
  - bile duct (congenital) 751.60
    - acquired 576.8
      - with calculus, choledocholithiasis, or stones — *see* Choledocholithiasis
  - biliary duct or passage (congenital) 751.60
    - acquired 576.8
      - with calculus, choledocholithiasis, or stones — *see* Choledocholithiasis
  - bladder (neck) (sphincter) (trigone) (acquired) 596.8
    - congenital 753.9
  - bone (acquired) NEC 738.9
    - congenital 756.9
    - turbinate 738.0
  - boutonniere (finger) 736.21
  - brain (congenital) 742.9
    - acquired 348.8
    - multiple 742.4
    - reduction 742.2
    - vessel (congenital) 747.81
  - breast (acquired) 611.8
    - congenital 757.9
  - bronchus (congenital) 748.3
    - acquired 519.1
  - bursa, congenital 756.9
  - canal of Nuck 752.9
  - canthus (congenital) 743.9
    - acquired 374.89
  - capillary (acquired) 448.9
    - congenital NEC (*see also* Deformity, vascular) 747.60
  - cardiac — *see* Deformity, heart
  - cardiovascular system (congenital) 746.9
  - caruncle, lacrimal (congenital) 743.9
    - acquired 375.69
  - cascade, stomach 537.6
  - cecum (congenital) 751.5
    - acquired 569.89
  - cerebral (congenital) 742.9
    - acquired 348.8
  - cervix (acquired) (uterus) 622.8
    - congenital 752.40
  - cheek (acquired) 738.19
    - congenital 744.9
  - chest (wall) (acquired) 738.3
    - congenital 754.89
    - late effect of rickets 268.1
  - chin (acquired) 738.19
    - congenital 744.9
  - choroid (congenital) 743.9
    - acquired 363.8
    - plexus (congenital) 742.9
      - acquired 349.2
  - cicatricial — *see* Cicatrix
  - cilia (congenital) 743.9
    - acquired 374.89
  - circulatory system (congenital) 747.9
  - clavicle (acquired) 738.8
    - congenital 755.51
  - clitoris (congenital) 752.40
    - acquired 624.8
  - clubfoot — *see* Clubfoot
  - coccyx (acquired) 738.6
    - congenital 756.10
  - colon (congenital) 751.5
    - acquired 569.89
  - concha (ear) (congenital) (*see also* Deformity, ear) 744.3
    - acquired 380.32

- **Deformity** — *continued*
  - congenital, organ or site not listed (*see also* Anomaly) 759.9
  - cornea (congenital) 743.9
    - acquired 371.70
  - coronary artery (congenital) 746.85
    - acquired (*see also* Ischemia, heart) 414.9
  - cranium (acquired) 738.19
    - congenital (*see also* Deformity, skull, congenital) 756.0
  - cricoid cartilage (congenital) 748.3
    - acquired 478.79
  - cystic duct (congenital) 751.60
    - acquired 575.8
  - Dandy-Walker 742.3
    - with spina bifida (*see also* Spina bifida) 741.0 ☑
  - diaphragm (congenital) 756.6
    - acquired 738.8
  - digestive organ(s) or system (congenital) NEC 751.9
    - specified type NEC 751.8
  - ductus arteriosus 747.0
  - duodenal bulb 537.89
  - duodenum (congenital) 751.5
    - acquired 537.89
  - dura (congenital) 742.9
    - brain 742.4
      - acquired 349.2
    - spinal 742.59
      - acquired 349.2
  - ear (congenital) 744.3
    - acquired 380.32
    - auricle 744.3
      - causing impairment of hearing 744.02
    - causing impairment of hearing 744.00
    - external 744.3
      - causing impairment of hearing 744.02
    - internal 744.05
    - lobule 744.3
    - middle 744.03
      - ossicles 744.04
    - ossicles 744.04
  - ectodermal (congenital) NEC 757.9
    - specified type NEC 757.8
  - ejaculatory duct (congenital) 752.9
    - acquired 608.89
  - elbow (joint) (acquired) 736.00
    - congenital 755.50
    - contraction 718.42
  - endocrine gland NEC 759.2
  - epididymis (congenital) 752.9
    - acquired 608.89
    - torsion 608.2
  - epiglottis (congenital) 748.3
    - acquired 478.79
  - esophagus (congenital) 750.9
    - acquired 530.89
  - Eustachian tube (congenital) NEC 744.3
    - specified type NEC 744.24
  - extremity (acquired) 736.9
    - congenital, except reduction deformity 755.9
      - lower 755.60
      - upper 755.50
    - reduction — *see* Deformity, reduction
  - eye (congenital) 743.9
    - acquired 379.8
    - muscle 743.9
  - eyebrow (congenital) 744.89
  - eyelid (congenital) 743.9
    - acquired 374.89
    - specified type NEC 743.62
  - face (acquired) 738.19
    - congenital (any part) 744.9
      - due to intrauterine malposition and pressure 754.0
  - fallopian tube (congenital) 752.10
    - acquired 620.8
  - femur (acquired) 736.89
    - congenital 755.60
  - fetal
    - with fetopelvic disproportion 653.7 ☑
      - affecting fetus or newborn 763.1
    - causing obstructed labor 660.1 ☑
      - affecting fetus or newborn 763.1
    - known or suspected, affecting management of pregnancy 655.9 ☑

Deformity — *continued*
- pharynx (congenital) 750.9
  - acquired 478.29
- Pierre Robin (congenital) 756.0
- pinna (acquired) 380.32
  - congenital 744.3
- pituitary (congenital) 759.2
- pleural folds (congenital) 748.8
- portal vein (congenital) 747.40
- posture — *see* Curvature, spine
- prepuce (congenital) 752.9
  - acquired 607.89
- prostate (congenital) 752.9
  - acquired 602.8
- pulmonary valve — *see* Endocarditis, pulmonary
- pupil (congenital) 743.9
  - acquired 364.75
- pylorus (congenital) 750.9
  - acquired 537.89
- rachitic (acquired), healed or old 268.1
- radius (acquired) 736.00
  - congenital 755.50
    - reduction — *see* Deformity, reduction, upper limb
- rectovaginal septum (congenital) 752.40
  - acquired 623.8
- rectum (congenital) 751.5
  - acquired 569.49
- reduction (extremity) (limb) 755.4
  - brain 742.2
  - lower limb 755.30
    - with complete absence of distal elements 755.31
    - longitudinal (complete) (partial) (with distal deficiencies, incomplete) 755.32
      - with complete absence of distal elements 755.31
      - combined femoral, tibial, fibular (incomplete) 755.33
      - femoral 755.34
      - fibular 755.37
      - metatarsal(s) 755.38
      - phalange(s) 755.39
        - meaning all digits 755.31
      - tarsal(s) 755.38
      - tibia 755.36
      - tibiofibular 755.35
    - transverse 755.31
  - upper limb 755.20
    - with complete absence of distal elements 755.21
    - longitudinal (complete) (partial) (with distal deficiencies, incomplete) 755.22
      - with complete absence of distal elements 755.21
      - carpal(s) 755.28
      - combined humeral, radial, ulnar (incomplete) 755.23
      - humeral 755.24
      - metacarpal(s) 755.28
      - phalange(s) 755.29
        - meaning all digits 755.21
      - radial 755.26
      - radioulnar 755.25
      - ulnar 755.27
    - transverse (complete) (partial) 755.21
- renal — *see* Deformity, kidney
- respiratory system (congenital) 748.9
  - specified type NEC 748.8
- rib (acquired) 738.3
  - congenital 756.3
    - cervical 756.2
- rotation (joint) (acquired) 736.9
  - congenital 755.9
  - hip or thigh 736.39
    - congenital (*see also* Subluxation, congenital, hip) 754.32
- sacroiliac joint (congenital) 755.69
  - acquired 738.5
- sacrum (acquired) 738.5
  - congenital 756.10
- saddle
  - back 737.8
  - nose 738.0
    - syphilitic 090.5

Deformity — *continued*
- salivary gland or duct (congenital) 750.9
  - acquired 527.8
- scapula (acquired) 736.89
  - congenital 755.50
- scrotum (congenital) 752.9
  - acquired 608.89
- sebaceous gland, acquired 706.8
- seminal tract or duct (congenital) 752.9
  - acquired 608.89
- septum (nasal) (acquired) 470
  - congenital 748.1
- shoulder (joint) (acquired) 736.89
  - congenital 755.50
    - specified type NEC 755.59
  - contraction 718.41
- sigmoid (flexure) (congenital) 751.5
  - acquired 569.89
- sinus of Valsalva 747.29
- skin (congenital) 757.9
  - acquired NEC 709.8
- skull (acquired) 738.19
  - congenital 756.0
    - with
      - anencephalus 740.0
      - encephalocele 742.0
      - hydrocephalus 742.3
        - with spina bifida (*see also* Spina bifida) 741.0 ☑
      - microcephalus 742.1
    - due to intrauterine malposition and pressure 754.0
- soft parts, organs or tissues (of pelvis)
  - in pregnancy or childbirth NEC 654.9 ☑
    - affecting fetus or newborn 763.89
    - causing obstructed labor 660.2 ☑
      - affecting fetus or newborn 763.1
- spermatic cord (congenital) 752.9
  - acquired 608.89
    - torsion 608.2
- spinal
  - column — *see* Deformity, spine
  - cord (congenital) 742.9
    - acquired 336.8
    - vessel (congenital) 747.82
  - nerve root (congenital) 742.9
    - acquired 724.9
- spine (acquired) NEC 738.5
  - congenital 756.10
    - due to intrauterine malposition and pressure 754.2
  - kyphoscoliotic (*see also* Kyphoscoliosis) 737.30
  - kyphotic (*see also* Kyphosis) 737.10
  - lordotic (*see also* Lordosis) 737.20
  - rachitic 268.1
  - scoliotic (*see also* Scoliosis) 737.30
- spleen
  - acquired 289.59
  - congenital 759.0
- Sprengel's (congenital) 755.52
- sternum (acquired) 738.3
  - congenital 756.3
- stomach (congenital) 750.9
  - acquired 537.89
- submaxillary gland (congenital) 750.9
  - acquired 527.8
- swan neck (acquired)
  - finger 736.22
  - hand 736.09
- talipes — *see* Talipes
- teeth, tooth NEC 520.9
- testis (congenital) 752.9
  - acquired 608.89
    - torsion 608.2
- thigh (acquired) 736.89
  - congenital 755.60
- thorax (acquired) (wall) 738.3
  - congenital 754.89
  - late effect of rickets 268.1
- thumb (acquired) 736.20
  - congenital 755.50
- thymus (tissue) (congenital) 759.2
- thyroid (gland) (congenital) 759.2
  - cartilage 748.3
    - acquired 478.79

Deformity — *continued*
- tibia (acquired) 736.89
  - congenital 755.60
  - saber 090.5
- toe (acquired) 735.9
  - congenital 755.66
  - specified NEC 735.8
- tongue (congenital) 750.10
  - acquired 529.8
- tooth, teeth NEC 520.9
- trachea (rings) (congenital) 748.3
  - acquired 519.1
- transverse aortic arch (congenital) 747.21
- tricuspid (leaflets) (valve) (congenital) 746.9
  - acquired — *see* Endocarditis, tricuspid
  - atresia or stenosis 746.1
  - specified type NEC 746.89
- trunk (acquired) 738.3
  - congenital 759.9
- ulna (acquired) 736.00
  - congenital 755.50
- upper extremity — *see* Deformity, arm
- urachus (congenital) 753.7
- ureter (opening) (congenital) 753.9
  - acquired 593.89
- urethra (valve) (congenital) 753.9
  - acquired 599.84
- urinary tract or system (congenital) 753.9
  - urachus 753.7
- uterus (congenital) 752.3
  - acquired 621.8
- uvula (congenital) 750.9
  - acquired 528.9
- vagina (congenital) 752.40
  - acquired 623.8
- valve, valvular (heart) (congenital) 746.9
  - acquired — *see* Endocarditis
  - pulmonary 746.00
  - specified type NEC 746.89
- vascular (congenital) (peripheral) NEC 747.60
  - acquired 459.9
  - gastrointestinal 747.61
  - lower limb 747.64
  - renal 747.62
  - specified site NEC 747.69
  - spinal 747.82
  - upper limb 747.63
- vas deferens (congenital) 752.9
  - acquired 608.89
- vein (congenital) NEC (*see also* Deformity, vascular) 747.60
  - brain 747.81
  - coronary 746.9
  - great 747.40
- vena cava (inferior) (superior) (congenital) 747.40
- vertebra — *see* Deformity, spine
- vesicourethral orifice (acquired) 596.8
  - congenital NEC 753.9
    - specified type NEC 753.8
- vessels of optic papilla (congenital) 743.9
- visual field (contraction) 368.45
- vitreous humor (congenital) 743.9
  - acquired 379.29
- vulva (congenital) 752.40
  - acquired 624.8
- wrist (joint) (acquired) 736.00
  - congenital 755.50
  - contraction 718.43
  - valgus 736.03
    - congenital 755.59
  - varus 736.04
    - congenital 755.59

Degeneration, degenerative
- adrenal (capsule) (gland) 255.8
  - with hypofunction 255.4
  - fatty 255.8
  - hyaline 255.8
  - infectional 255.8
  - lardaceous 277.3
- amyloid (any site) (general) 277.3
- anterior cornua, spinal cord 336.8
- aorta, aortic 440.0
  - fatty 447.8
  - valve (heart) (*see also* Endocarditis, aortic) 424.1

☑ Additional Digit Required — Refer to the Tabular List (Numeric Code Section) for Additional Digit Selection

▶◀ Revised Text ● New Line ▲ Revised Code

Note — Use the following fifth-digit subclassification with categories 640-648, 651-676:

0	*unspecified as to episode of care*
1	*delivered, with or without mention of antepartum condition*
2	*delivered, with mention of postpartum complication*
3	*antepartum condition or complication*
4	*postpartum condition or complication*

- **Delivery** — *continued*
  - complicated (by) — *continued*
    - knot (true), umbilical cord 663.2 ☑
    - labor, premature (before 37 completed weeks gestation) 644.2 ☑
    - laceration 664.9 ☑
      - anus (sphincter) 664.2 ☑
        - with mucosa 664.3 ☑
      - bladder (urinary) 665.5 ☑
      - bowel 665.5 ☑
      - central 664.4 ☑
      - cervix (uteri) 665.3 ☑
      - fourchette 664.0 ☑
      - hymen 664.0 ☑
      - labia (majora) (minora) 664.0 ☑
      - pelvic
        - floor 664.1 ☑
        - organ NEC 665.5 ☑
      - perineum, perineal 664.4 ☑
        - first degree 664.0 ☑
        - second degree 664.1 ☑
        - third degree 664.2 ☑
        - fourth degree 664.3 ☑
        - central 664.4 ☑
        - extensive NEC 664.4 ☑
        - muscles 664.1 ☑
        - skin 664.0 ☑
        - slight 664.0 ☑
      - peritoneum 665.5 ☑
      - periurethral tissue 665.5 ☑
      - rectovaginal (septum) (without perineal laceration) 665.4 ☑
        - with perineum 664.2 ☑
          - with anal or rectal mucosa 664.3 ☑
      - skin (perineum) 664.0 ☑
      - specified site or type NEC 664.8 ☑
      - sphincter ani 664.2 ☑
        - with mucosa 664.3 ☑
      - urethra 665.5 ☑
      - uterus 665.1 ☑
        - before labor 665.0 ☑
      - vagina, vaginal (deep) (high) (sulcus) (wall) (without perineal laceration) 665.4 ☑
        - with perineum 664.0 ☑
        - muscles, with perineum 664.1 ☑
      - vulva 664.0 ☑
    - lateroversion, uterus or cervix 654.4 ☑
      - causing obstructed labor 660.2 ☑
    - locked mates 660.5 ☑
    - low implantation of placenta — *see* Delivery, complicated, placenta, previa
    - mal lie 652.9 ☑
    - malposition
      - fetus NEC 652.9 ☑
        - causing obstructed labor 660.0 ☑
      - pelvic organs or tissues NEC 654.9 ☑
        - causing obstructed labor 660.2 ☑
      - placenta 641.1 ☑
        - without hemorrhage 641.0 ☑
      - uterus NEC or cervix 654.4 ☑
        - causing obstructed labor 660.2 ☑
    - malpresentation 652.9 ☑
      - causing obstructed labor 660.0 ☑
    - marginal sinus (bleeding) (rupture) 641.2 ☑
    - maternal hypotension syndrome 669.2 ☑
    - meconium in liquor 656.8 ☑
    - membranes, retained — *see* Delivery, complicated, placenta, retained
    - mentum presentation 652.4 ☑
      - causing obstructed labor 660.0 ☑
    - metrorrhagia (myopathia) — *see* Delivery, complicated, hemorrhage
    - metrorrhexis — *see* Delivery, complicated, rupture, uterus
    - multiparity (grand) 659.4 ☑
    - myelomeningocele, fetus 653.7 ☑
      - causing obstructed labor 660.1 ☑
    - Nägele's pelvis 653.0 ☑
      - causing obstructed labor 660.1 ☑
    - nonengagement, fetal head 652.5 ☑
      - causing obstructed labor 660.0 ☑
    - oblique presentation 652.3 ☑
      - causing obstructed labor 660.0 ☑
    - obstetric
      - shock 669.1 ☑
      - trauma NEC 665.9 ☑

- **Delivery** — *continued*
  - complicated (by) — *continued*
    - obstructed labor 660.9 ☑
      - due to
        - abnormality of pelvic organs or tissues (conditions classifiable to 654.0-654.9) 660.2 ☑
        - deep transverse arrest 660.3 ☑
        - impacted shoulders 660.4 ☑
        - locked twins 660.5 ☑
        - malposition and malpresentation of fetus (conditions classifiable to 652.0-652.9) 660.0 ☑
        - persistent occipitoposterior 660.3 ☑
        - shoulder dystocia 660.4 ☑
    - occult prolapse of umbilical cord 663.0 ☑
    - oversize fetus 653.5 ☑
      - causing obstructed labor 660.1 ☑
    - pathological retraction ring, uterus 661.4 ☑
    - pelvic
      - arrest (deep) (high) (of fetal head) (transverse) 660.3 ☑
      - deformity (bone) — *see also* Deformity, pelvis, with disproportion
        - soft tissue 654.9 ☑
          - causing obstructed labor 660.2 ☑
      - tumor NEC 654.9 ☑
        - causing obstructed labor 660.2 ☑
    - penetration, pregnant uterus by instrument 665.1 ☑
    - perforation — *see* Delivery, complicated, laceration
    - persistent
      - hymen 654.8 ☑
        - causing obstructed labor 660.2 ☑
      - occipitoposterior 660.3 ☑
    - placenta, placental
      - ablatio 641.2 ☑
      - abnormality 656.7 ☑
        - with hemorrhage 641.2 ☑
      - abruptio 641.2 ☑
      - accreta 667.0 ☑
        - with hemorrhage 666.0 ☑
      - adherent (without hemorrhage) 667.0 ☑
        - with hemorrhage 666.0 ☑
      - apoplexy 641.2 ☑
      - battledore placenta — *see* Placenta, abnormal
      - detachment (premature) 641.2 ☑
      - disease 656.7 ☑
      - hemorrhage NEC 641.9 ☑
      - increta (without hemorrhage) 667.0 ☑
        - with hemorrhage 666.0 ☑
      - low (implantation) 641.0 ☑
        - without hemorrhage 641.0 ☑
      - malformation 656.7 ☑
        - with hemorrhage 641.2 ☑
      - malposition 641.1 ☑
        - without hemorrhage 641.0 ☑
      - marginal sinus rupture 641.2 ☑
      - percreta 667.0 ☑
        - with hemorrhage 666.0 ☑
      - premature separation 641.2 ☑
      - previa (central) (lateral) (marginal) (partial) 641.1 ☑
        - without hemorrhage 641.0 ☑
      - retained (with hemorrhage) 666.0 ☑
        - without hemorrhage 667.0 ☑
      - rupture of marginal sinus 641.2 ☑
      - separation (premature) 641.2 ☑
      - trapped 666.0 ☑
        - without hemorrhage 667.0 ☑
      - vicious insertion 641.1 ☑
    - polyhydramnios 657.0 ☑
    - polyp, cervix 654.6 ☑
      - causing obstructed labor 660.2 ☑
    - precipitate labor 661.3 ☑
    - premature
      - labor (before 37 completed weeks gestation) 644.2 ☑
      - rupture, membranes 658.1 ☑
        - delayed delivery following 658.2 ☑
    - presenting umbilical cord 663.0 ☑
    - previous
      - cesarean delivery, section 654.2 ☑
      - surgery
        - cervix 654.6 ☑
          - causing obstructed labor 660.2 ☑

- **Delivery** — *continued*
  - complicated (by) — *continued*
    - previous — *continued*
      - surgery — *continued*
        - gynecological NEC 654.9 ☑
          - causing obstructed labor 660.2 ☑
        - perineum 654.8 ☑
        - rectum 654.8 ☑
        - uterus NEC 654.9 ☑
          - due to previous cesarean delivery, section 654.2 ☑
        - vagina 654.7 ☑
          - causing obstructed labor 660.2 ☑
        - vulva 654.8 ☑
    - primary uterine inertia 661.0 ☑
    - primipara, elderly or old 659.5 ☑
    - prolapse
      - arm or hand 652.7 ☑
        - causing obstructed labor 660.0 ☑
      - cord (umbilical) 663.0 ☑
      - fetal extremity 652.8 ☑
      - foot or leg 652.8 ☑
        - causing obstructed labor 660.0 ☑
      - umbilical cord (complete) (occult) (partial) 663.0 ☑
      - uterus 654.4 ☑
        - causing obstructed labor 660.2 ☑
    - prolonged labor 662.1 ☑
      - first stage 662.0 ☑
      - second stage 662.2 ☑
      - active phase 661.2 ☑
      - due to
        - cervical dystocia 661.0 ☑
        - contraction ring 661.4 ☑
        - tetanic uterus 661.4 ☑
        - uterine inertia 661.2 ☑
          - primary 661.0 ☑
          - secondary 661.1 ☑
      - latent phase 661.0 ☑
    - pyrexia during labor 659.2 ☑
    - rachitic pelvis 653.2 ☑
      - causing obstructed labor 660.1 ☑
    - rectocele 654.4 ☑
      - causing obstructed labor 660.2 ☑
    - retained membranes or portions of placenta 666.2 ☑
      - without hemorrhage 667.1 ☑
    - retarded (prolonged) birth 662.1 ☑
    - retention secundines (with hemorrhage) 666.2 ☑
      - without hemorrhage 667.1 ☑
    - retroversion, uterus or cervix 654.3 ☑
      - causing obstructed labor 660.2 ☑
    - rigid
      - cervix 654.6 ☑
        - causing obstructed labor 660.2 ☑
      - pelvic floor 654.4 ☑
        - causing obstructed labor 660.2 ☑
      - perineum or vulva 654.8 ☑
        - causing obstructed labor 660.2 ☑
      - vagina 654.7 ☑
        - causing obstructed labor 660.2 ☑
    - Robert's pelvis 653.0 ☑
      - causing obstructed labor 660.1 ☑
    - rupture — *see also* Delivery, complicated, laceration
      - bladder (urinary) 665.5 ☑
      - cervix 665.3 ☑
      - marginal sinus 641.2 ☑
      - membranes, premature 658.1 ☑
      - pelvic organ NEC 665.5 ☑
      - perineum (without mention of other laceration) — *see* Delivery, complicated, laceration, perineum
      - peritoneum 665.5 ☑
      - urethra 665.5 ☑
      - uterus (during labor) 665.1 ☑
        - before labor 665.0 ☑
    - sacculation, pregnant uterus 654.4 ☑
    - sacral teratomas, fetal 653.7 ☑
      - causing obstructed labor 660.1 ☑
    - scar(s)
      - cervix 654.6 ☑
        - causing obstructed labor 660.2 ☑
      - cesarean delivery, section 654.2 ☑
        - causing obstructed labor 660.2 ☑

☑ Additional Digit Required — Refer to the Tabular List (Numeric Code Section) for Additional Digit Selection

▶◀ Revised Text ● New Line ▲ Revised Code

Delivery — *continued*
  complicated (by) — *continued*
    scar(s) — *continued*
      perineum 654.8 ☑
        causing obstructed labor 660.2 ☑
      uterus NEC 654.9 ☑
        causing obstructed labor 660.2 ☑
        due to previous cesarean delivery, section 654.2 ☑
      vagina 654.7 ☑
        causing obstructed labor 660.2 ☑
      vulva 654.8 ☑
        causing obstructed labor 660.2 ☑
    scoliotic pelvis 653.0 ☑
      causing obstructed labor 660.1 ☑
    secondary uterine inertia 661.1 ☑
    secundines, retained — *see* Delivery, complicated, placenta, retained
    separation
      placenta (premature) 641.2 ☑
      pubic bone 665.6 ☑
      symphysis pubis 665.6 ☑
    septate vagina 654.7 ☑
      causing obstructed labor 660.2 ☑
    shock (birth) (obstetric) (puerperal) 669.1 ☑
    short cord syndrome 663.4 ☑
    shoulder
      girdle dystocia 660.4 ☑
      presentation 652.8 ☑
        causing obstructed labor 660.0 ☑
    Siamese twins 653.7 ☑
      causing obstructed labor 660.1 ☑
    slow slope active phase 661.2 ☑
    spasm
      cervix 661.4 ☑
      uterus 661.4 ☑
    spondylolisthesis, pelvis 653.3 ☑
      causing obstructed labor 660.1 ☑
    spondylolysis (lumbosacral) 653.3 ☑
      causing obstructed labor 660.1 ☑
    spondylosis 653.0 ☑
      causing obstructed labor 660.1 ☑
    stenosis or stricture
      cervix 654.6 ☑
        causing obstructed labor 660.2 ☑
      vagina 654.7 ☑
        causing obstructed labor 660.2 ☑
    sudden death, unknown cause 669.9 ☑
    tear (pelvic organ) (*see also* Delivery, complicated, laceration) 664.9 ☑
    teratomas, sacral, fetal 653.7 ☑
      causing obstructed labor 660.1 ☑
    tetanic uterus 661.4 ☑
    tipping pelvis 653.0 ☑
      causing obstructed labor 660.1 ☑
    transverse
      arrest (deep) 660.3 ☑
      presentation or lie 652.3 ☑
        with successful version 652.1 ☑
        causing obstructed labor 660.0 ☑
    trauma (obstetrical) NEC 665.9 ☑
    tumor
      abdominal, fetal 653.7 ☑
        causing obstructed labor 660.1 ☑
      pelvic organs or tissues NEC 654.9 ☑
        causing obstructed labor 660.2 ☑
    umbilical cord (*see also* Delivery, complicated, cord) 663.9 ☑
      around neck tightly, or with compression 663.1 ☑
      entanglement NEC 663.3 ☑
        with compression 663.2 ☑
      prolapse (complete) (occult) (partial) 663.0 ☑
    unstable lie 652.0 ☑
      causing obstructed labor 660.0 ☑
    uterine
      inertia (*see also* Delivery, complicated, inertia, uterus) 661.2 ☑
      spasm 661.4 ☑
    vasa previa 663.5 ☑
    velamentous insertion of cord 663.8 ☑
    young maternal age 659.8 ☑
  delayed NEC 662.1 ☑
    following rupture of membranes (spontaneous) 658.2 ☑
      artificial 658.3 ☑

Delivery — *continued*
  delayed NEC — *continued*
    second twin, triplet, etc. 662.3 ☑
  difficult NEC 669.9 ☑
    previous, affecting management of pregnancy or childbirth V23.49
    specified type NEC 669.8 ☑
  early onset (spontaneous) 644.2 ☑
  footling 652.8 ☑
    with successful version 652.1 ☑
  forceps NEC 669.5 ☑
    affecting fetus or newborn 763.2
  missed (at or near term) 656.4 ☑
  multiple gestation NEC 651.9 ☑
    with fetal loss and retention of one or more fetus(es) 651.6 ☑
    following (elective) fetal reduction 651.7 ☑ ●
    specified type NEC 651.8 ☑
      with fetal loss and retention of one or more fetus(es) 651.6 ☑
      following (elective) fetal reduction 651.7 ☑ ●
  nonviable infant 656.4 ☑
  normal — *see* category 650
  precipitate 661.3 ☑
    affecting fetus or newborn 763.6
  premature NEC (before 37 completed weeks gestation) 644.2 ☑
    previous, affecting management of pregnancy V23.41
  quadruplet NEC 651.2 ☑
    with fetal loss and retention of one or more fetus(es) 651.5 ☑
    following (elective) fetal reduction 651.7 ☑ ●
  quintuplet NEC 651.8 ☑
    with fetal loss and retention of one or more fetus(es) 651.6 ☑
    following (elective) fetal reduction 651.7 ☑ ●
  sextuplet NEC 651.8 ☑
    with fetal loss and retention of one or more fetus(es) 651.6 ☑
    following (elective) fetal reduction 651.7 ☑ ●
  specified complication NEC 669.8 ☑
  stillbirth (near term) NEC 656.4 ☑
    early (before 22 completed weeks gestation) 632
  term pregnancy (live birth) NEC — *see* category 650
    stillbirth NEC 656.4 ☑
  threatened premature 644.2 ☑
  triplets NEC 651.1 ☑
    with fetal loss and retention of one or more fetus(es) 651.4 ☑
    delayed delivery (one or more mates) 662.3 ☑
    following (elective) fetal reduction 651.7 ☑ ●
    locked mates 660.5 ☑
  twins NEC 651.0 ☑
    with fetal loss and retention of one fetus 651.3 ☑
    delayed delivery (one or more mates) 662.3 ☑
    following (elective) fetal reduction 651.7 ☑ ●
    locked mates 660.5 ☑
  uncomplicated — *see* category 650
  vacuum extractor NEC 669.5 ☑
    affecting fetus or newborn 763.3
  ventouse NEC 669.5 ☑
    affecting fetus or newborn 763.3

Dellen, cornea 371.41

Delusions (paranoid) 297.9
  grandiose 297.1
  parasitosis 300.29
  systematized 297.1

Dementia 294.8
  alcohol-induced persisting (*see also* Psychosis, alcoholic) 291.2
  Alzheimer's — *see* Alzheimer's, dementia
  arteriosclerotic (simple type) (uncomplicated) 290.40
    with
      acute confusional state 290.41

Dementia — *continued*
  arteriosclerotic — *continued*
    with — *continued*
      delirium 290.41
      delusions 290.42
      depressed mood 290.43
    depressed type 290.43
    paranoid type 290.42
  Binswanger's 290.12
  catatonic (acute) (*see also* Schizophrenia) 295.2 ☑
  congenital (*see also* Retardation, mental) 319
  degenerative 290.9
    presenile-onset — *see* Dementia, presenile
    senile-onset — *see* Dementia, senile
  developmental (*see also* Schizophrenia) 295.9 ☑
  dialysis 294.8
    transient 293.9
  drug-induced persisting (*see also* Psychosis, drug) 292.82
  due to or associated with condition(s) classified elsewhere
    Alzheimer's
      with behavioral disturbance 331.0 *[294.11]*
      without behavioral disturbance 331.0 *[294.10]*
    cerebral lipidoses
      with behavioral disturbance 330.1 *[294.11]*
      without behavioral disturbance 330.1 *[294.10]*
    epilepsy
      with behavioral disturbance 345.9 ☑ *[294.11]*
      without behavioral disturbance 345.9 ☑ *[294.10]*
    hepatolenticular degeneration
      with behavioral disturbance 275.1 *[294.11]*
      without behavioral disturbance 275.1 *[294.10]*
    HIV
      with behavioral disturbance 042 *[294.11]*
      without behavioral disturbance 042 *[294.10]*
    Huntington's chorea
      with behavioral disturbance 333.4 *[294.11]*
      without behavioral disturbance 333.4 *[294.10]*
    Jakob-Creutzfeldt disease ▶(new variant)◀
      with behavioral disturbance 046.1 *[294.11]*
      without behavioral disturbance 046.1 *[294.10]*
    Lewy bodies
      with behavioral disturbance 331.82 *[294.11]*
      without behavioral disturbance 331.82 *[294.10]*
    multiple sclerosis
      with behavioral disturbance 340 *[294.11]*
      without behavioral disturbance 340 *[294.10]*
    neurosyphilis
      with behavioral disturbance 094.9 *[294.11]*
      without behavioral disturbance 094.9 *[294.10]*
    Parkinsonism
      with behavioral disturbance 331.82 *[294.11]*
      without behavioral disturbance 331.82 *[294.10]*
    Pelizaeus-Merzbacher disease
      with behavioral disturbance 333.0 *[294.11]*
      without behavioral disturbance 333.0 *[294.10]*
    Pick's disease
      with behavioral disturbance 331.11 *[294.11]*
      without behavioral disturbance 331.11 *[294.10]*
    polyarteritis nodosa
      with behavioral disturbance 446.0 *[294.11]*

Dementia — *continued*
- due to or associated with condition(s) classified elsewhere — *continued*
  - polyarteritis nodosa — *continued*
    - without behavioral disturbance 446.0 *[294.10]*
  - syphilis
    - with behavioral disturbance 094.1 *[294.11]*
    - without behavioral disturbance 094.1 *[294.10]*
  - Wilson's disease
    - with behavioral disturbance 275.1 *[294.11]*
    - without behavioral disturbance 275.1 *[294.10]*
- frontal 331.19
  - with behavioral disturbance 331.19 *[294.11]*
  - without behavioral disturbance 331.19 *[294.10]*
- frontotemporal 331.19
  - with behavioral disturbance 331.19 *[294.11]*
  - without behavioral disturbance 331.19 *[294.10]*
- hebephrenic (acute) 295.1 ☑
- Heller's (infantile psychosis) (*see also* Psychosis, childhood) 299.1 ☑
- idiopathic 290.9
  - presenile-onset — *see* Dementia, presenile
  - senile-onset — *see* Dementia, senile
- in
  - arteriosclerotic brain disease 290.40
  - senility 290.0
- induced by drug 292.82
- infantile, infantilia (*see also* Psychosis, childhood) 299.0 ☑
- Lewy body 331.82
  - with behavioral disturbance 331.82 *[294.11]*
  - without behavioral disturbance 331.82 *[294.10]*
- multi-infarct (cerebrovascular) (*see also* Dementia, arteriosclerotic) 290.40
- old age 290.0
- paralytica, paralytic 094.1
  - juvenilis 090.40
  - syphilitic 094.1
    - congenital 090.40
  - tabetic form 094.1
- paranoid (*see also* Schizophrenia) 295.3 ☑
- paraphrenic (*see also* Schizophrenia) 295.3 ☑
- paretic 094.1
- praecox (*see also* Schizophrenia) 295.9 ☑
- presenile 290.10
  - with
    - acute confusional state 290.11
    - delirium 290.11
    - delusional features 290.12
    - depressive features 290.13
  - depressed type 290.13
  - paranoid type 290.12
  - simple type 290.10
  - uncomplicated 290.10
- primary (acute) (*see also* Schizophrenia) 295.0 ☑
- progressive, syphilitic 094.1
- puerperal — *see* Psychosis, puerperal
- schizophrenic (*see also* Schizophrenia) 295.9 ☑
- senile 290.0
  - with
    - acute confusional state 290.3
    - delirium 290.3
    - delusional features 290.20
    - depressive features 290.21
  - depressed type 290.21
  - exhaustion 290.0
  - paranoid type 290.20
- simple type (acute) (*see also* Schizophrenia) 295.0 ☑
- simplex (acute) (*see also* Schizophrenia) 295.0 ☑
- syphilitic 094.1
- uremic — *see* Uremia
- vascular 290.40
  - with
    - delirium 290.41
    - delusions 290.42
    - depressed mood 290.43

Demerol dependence (*see also* Dependence) 304.0 ☑

Demineralization, ankle (*see also* Osteoporosis) 733.00

Demodex folliculorum (infestation) 133.8

de Morgan's spots (senile angiomas) 448.1

Demyelinating
- polyneuritis, chronic inflammatory 357.81

Demyelination, demyelinization
- central nervous system 341.9
  - specified NEC 341.8
- corpus callosum (central) 341.8
- global 340

Dengue (fever) 061
- sandfly 061
- vaccination, prophylactic (against) V05.1
- virus hemorrhagic fever 065.4

Dens
- evaginatus 520.2
- in dente 520.2
- invaginatus 520.2

Density
- increased, bone (disseminated) (generalized) (spotted) 733.99
- lung (nodular) 518.89

Dental — *see also* condition
- examination only V72.2

Dentia praecox 520.6

Denticles (in pulp) 522.2

Dentigerous cyst 526.0

Dentin
- irregular (in pulp) 522.3
- opalescent 520.5
- secondary (in pulp) 522.3
- sensitive 521.8

Dentinogenesis imperfecta 520.5

Dentinoma (M9271/0) 213.1
- upper jaw (bone) 213.0

Dentition 520.7
- abnormal 520.6
- anomaly 520.6
- delayed 520.6
- difficult 520.7
- disorder of 520.6
- precocious 520.6
- retarded 520.6

Denture sore (mouth) 528.9

Dependence

> *Note — Use the following fifth-digit subclassification with category 304:*
>
> 0 *unspecified*
> 1 *continuous*
> 2 *episodic*
> 3 *in remission*

- with
  - withdrawal symptoms
    - alcohol 291.81
    - drug 292.0
- 14-hydroxy-dihydromorphinone 304.0 ☑
- absinthe 304.6 ☑
- acemorphan 304.0 ☑
- acetanilid(e) 304.6 ☑
- acetophenetidin 304.6 ☑
- acetorphine 304.0 ☑
- acetyldihydrocodeine 304.0 ☑
- acetyldihydrocodeinone 304.0 ☑
- Adalin 304.1 ☑
- Afghanistan black 304.3 ☑
- agrypnal 304.1 ☑
- alcohol, alcoholic (ethyl) (methyl) (wood) 303.9 ☑
  - maternal, with suspected fetal damage affecting management of pregnancy 655.4 ☑
- allobarbitone 304.1 ☑
- allonal 304.1 ☑
- allylisopropylacetylurea 304.1 ☑
- alphaprodine (hydrochloride) 304.0 ☑
- Alurate 304.1 ☑
- Alvodine 304.0 ☑
- amethocaine 304.6 ☑
- amidone 304.0 ☑
- amidopyrine 304.6 ☑

Dependence — *continued*
- aminopyrine 304.6 ☑
- amobarbital 304.1 ☑
- amphetamine(s) (type) (drugs classifiable to 969.7) 304.4 ☑
- amylene hydrate 304.6 ☑
- amylobarbitone 304.1 ☑
- amylocaine 304.6 ☑
- Amytal (sodium) 304.1 ☑
- analgesic (drug) NEC 304.6 ☑
  - synthetic with morphine-like effect 304.0 ☑
- anesthetic (agent) (drug) (gas) (general) (local) NEC 304.6 ☑
- Angel dust 304.6 ☑
- anileridine 304.0 ☑
- antipyrine 304.6 ☑
- anxiolytic 304.1 ☑
- aprobarbital 304.1 ☑
- aprobarbitone 304.1 ☑
- atropine 304.6 ☑
- Avertin (bromide) 304.6 ☑
- barbenyl 304.1 ☑
- barbital(s) 304.1 ☑
- barbitone 304.1 ☑
- barbiturate(s) (compounds) (drugs classifiable to 967.0) 304.1 ☑
- barbituric acid (and compounds) 304.1 ☑
- benzedrine 304.4 ☑
- benzylmorphine 304.0 ☑
- Beta-chlor 304.1 ☑
- bhang 304.3 ☑
- blue velvet 304.0 ☑
- Brevital 304.1 ☑
- bromal (hydrate) 304.1 ☑
- bromide(s) NEC 304.1 ☑
- bromine compounds NEC 304.1 ☑
- bromisovalum 304.1 ☑
- bromoform 304.1 ☑
- Bromo-seltzer 304.1 ☑
- bromural 304.1 ☑
- butabarbital (sodium) 304.1 ☑
- butabarpal 304.1 ☑
- butallylonal 304.1 ☑
- butethal 304.1 ☑
- buthalitone (sodium) 304.1 ☑
- Butisol 304.1 ☑
- butobarbitone 304.1 ☑
- butyl chloral (hydrate) 304.1 ☑
- caffeine 304.4 ☑
- cannabis (indica) (sativa) (resin) (derivatives) (type) 304.3 ☑
- carbamazepine 304.6 ☑
- Carbrital 304.1 ☑
- carbromal 304.1 ☑
- carisoprodol 304.6 ☑
- Catha (edulis) 304.4 ☑
- chloral (betaine) (hydrate) 304.1 ☑
- chloralamide 304.1 ☑
- chloralformamide 304.1 ☑
- chloralose 304.1 ☑
- chlordiazepoxide 304.1 ☑
- Chloretone 304.1 ☑
- chlorobutanol 304.1 ☑
- chlorodyne 304.1 ☑
- chloroform 304.6 ☑
- Cliradon 304.0 ☑
- coca (leaf) and derivatives 304.2 ☑
- cocaine 304.2 ☑
  - hydrochloride 304.2 ☑
  - salt (any) 304.2 ☑
- codeine 304.0 ☑
- combination of drugs (excluding morphine or opioid type drug) NEC 304.8 ☑
  - morphine or opioid type drug with any other drug 304.7 ☑
- croton-chloral 304.1 ☑
- cyclobarbital 304.1 ☑
- cyclobarbitone 304.1 ☑
- dagga 304.3 ☑
- Delvinal 304.1 ☑
- Demerol 304.0 ☑
- desocodeine 304.0 ☑
- desomorphine 304.0 ☑
- desoxyephedrine 304.4 ☑
- DET 304.5 ☑
- dexamphetamine 304.4 ☑
- dexedrine 304.4 ☑

- **Dermatophytosis** — *continued*
  - hand 110.2
  - nail 110.1
  - perianal (area) 110.3
  - scalp 110.0
  - scrotal 110.8
  - specified site NEC 110.8
  - toenails 110.1
  - vulva 110.8
- **Dermatopolyneuritis** 985.0
- **Dermatorrhexis** 756.83
  - acquired 701.8
- **Dermatosclerosis** (*see also* Scleroderma) 710.1
  - localized 701.0
- **Dermatosis** 709.9
  - Andrews' 686.8
  - atopic 691.8
  - Bowen's (M8081/2) — *see* Neoplasm, skin, in situ
  - bullous 694.9
    - specified type NEC 694.8
  - erythematosquamous 690.8
  - exfoliativa 695.89
  - factitial 698.4
  - gonococcal 098.89
  - herpetiformis 694.0
    - juvenile 694.2
    - senile 694.5
  - hysterical 300.11
  - Linear IgA 694.8
  - menstrual NEC 709.8
  - neutrophilic, acute febrile 695.89
  - occupational (*see also* Dermatitis) 692.9
  - papulosa nigra 709.8
  - pigmentary NEC 709.00
    - progressive 709.09
    - Schamberg's 709.09
    - Siemens-Bloch 757.33
  - progressive pigmentary 709.09
  - psychogenic 316
  - pustular subcorneal 694.1
  - Schamberg's (progressive pigmentary) 709.09
  - senile NEC 709.3
  - specified NEC 702.8
  - Unna's (seborrheic dermatitis) 690.10
- **Dermographia** 708.3
- **Dermographism** 708.3
- **Dermoid** (cyst) (M9084/0) — *see also* Neoplasm, by site, benign
  - with malignant transformation (M9084/3) 183.0
- **Dermopathy**
  - infiltrative, with thyrotoxicosis 242.0 ☑
  - senile NEC 709.3
- **Dermophytosis** — *see* Dermatophytosis
- **Descemet's membrane** — *see* condition
- **Descemetocele** 371.72
- **Descending** — *see* condition
- **Descensus uteri** (complete) (incomplete) (partial) (without vaginal wall prolapse) 618.1
  - with mention of vaginal wall prolapse — *see* Prolapse, uterovaginal
- **Desensitization to allergens** V07.1
- **Desert**
  - rheumatism 114.0
  - sore (*see also* Ulcer, skin) 707.9
- **Desertion** (child) (newborn) 995.52
  - adult 995.84
- **Desmoid** (extra-abdominal) (tumor) (M8821/1) — *see also* Neoplasm, connective tissue, uncertain behavior
  - abdominal (M8822/1) — *see* Neoplasm, connective tissue, uncertain behavior
- **Despondency** 300.4
- **Desquamative dermatitis** NEC 695.89
- **Destruction**
  - articular facet (*see also* Derangement, joint) 718.9 ☑
    - vertebra 724.9
  - bone 733.90
    - syphilitic 095.5
  - joint (*see also* Derangement, joint) 718.9 ☑
    - sacroiliac 724.6
- **Destruction** — *continued*
  - kidney 593.89
  - live fetus to facilitate birth NEC 763.89
  - ossicles (ear) 385.24
  - rectal sphincter 569.49
  - septum (nasal) 478.1
  - tuberculous NEC (*see also* Tuberculosis) 011.9 ☑
  - tympanic membrane 384.82
  - tympanum 385.89
  - vertebral disc — *see* Degeneration, intervertebral disc
- **Destructiveness** (*see also* Disturbance, conduct) 312.9
  - adjustment reaction 309.3
- **Detachment**
  - cartilage — *see also* Sprain, by site
    - knee — *see* Tear, meniscus
  - cervix, annular 622.8
    - complicating delivery 665.3 ☑
  - choroid (old) (postinfectional) (simple) (spontaneous) 363.70
    - hemorrhagic 363.72
    - serous 363.71
  - knee, medial meniscus (old) 717.3
    - current injury 836.0
  - ligament — *see* Sprain, by site
  - placenta (premature) — *see* Placenta, separation
  - retina (recent) 361.9
    - with retinal defect (rhegmatogenous) 361.00
      - giant tear 361.03
      - multiple 361.02
      - partial
        - with
          - giant tear 361.03
          - multiple defects 361.02
          - retinal dialysis (juvenile) 361.04
          - single defect 361.01
      - retinal dialysis (juvenile) 361.04
      - single 361.01
      - subtotal 361.05
      - total 361.05
    - delimited (old) (partial) 361.06
    - old
      - delimited 361.06
      - partial 361.06
      - total or subtotal 361.07
    - pigment epithelium (RPE) (serous) 362.42
      - exudative 362.42
      - hemorrhagic 362.43
    - rhegmatogenous (*see also* Detachment, retina, with retinal defect) 361.00
    - serous (without retinal defect) 361.2
    - specified type NEC 361.89
    - traction (with vitreoretinal organization) 361.81
  - vitreous humor 379.21
- **Detergent asthma** 507.8
- **Deterioration**
  - epileptic
    - with behavioral disturbance 345.9 ☑ *[294.11]*
    - without behavioral disturbance 345.9 ☑ *[294.10]*
  - heart, cardiac (*see also* Degeneration, myocardial) 429.1
  - mental (*see also* Psychosis) 298.9
  - myocardium, myocardial (*see also* Degeneration, myocardial) 429.1
  - senile (simple) 797
  - transplanted organ — *see* Complications, transplant, organ, by site
- **de Toni-Fanconi syndrome** (cystinosis) 270.0
- **Deuteranomaly** 368.52
- **Deuteranopia** (anomalous trichromat) (complete) (incomplete) 368.52
- **Deutschländer's disease** — *see* Fracture, foot
- **Development**
  - abnormal, bone 756.9
  - arrested 783.40
    - bone 733.91
    - child 783.40
    - due to malnutrition (protein-calorie) 263.2
    - fetus or newborn 764.9 ☑
    - tracheal rings (congenital) 748.3
- **Development** — *continued*
  - defective, congenital — *see also* Anomaly
    - cauda equina 742.59
    - left ventricle 746.9
      - with atresia or hypoplasia of aortic orifice or valve with hypoplasia of ascending aorta 746.7
      - in hypoplastic left heart syndrome 746.7
  - delayed (*see also* Delay, development) 783.40
    - arithmetical skills 315.1
    - language (skills) 315.31
      - expressive 315.31
      - mixed receptive-expressive 315.32
    - learning skill, specified NEC 315.2
    - mixed skills 315.5
    - motor coordination 315.4
    - reading 315.00
    - specified
      - learning skill NEC 315.2
      - type NEC, except learning 315.8
    - speech 315.39
      - associated with hyperkinesia 314.1
      - phonological 315.39
    - spelling 315.09
    - written expression 315.2
  - imperfect, congenital — *see also* Anomaly
    - heart 746.9
    - lungs 748.60
  - improper (fetus or newborn) 764.9 ☑
  - incomplete (fetus or newborn) 764.9 ☑
    - affecting management of pregnancy 656.5 ☑
    - bronchial tree 748.3
    - organ or site not listed — *see* Hypoplasia
    - respiratory system 748.9
  - sexual, precocious NEC 259.1
  - tardy, mental (*see also* Retardation, mental) 319
- **Developmental** — *see* condition
- **Devergie's disease** (pityriasis rubra pilaris) 696.4
- **Deviation**
  - conjugate (eye) 378.87
    - palsy 378.81
    - spasm, spastic 378.82
  - esophagus 530.89
  - eye, skew 378.87
  - mandible, opening and closing 524.53
  - midline (jaw) (teeth) 524.29
    - specified site NEC — *see* Malposition
  - occlusal plane 524.76
  - organ or site, congenital NEC — *see* Malposition, congenital
  - septum (acquired) (nasal) 470
    - congenital 754.0
  - sexual 302.9
    - bestiality 302.1
    - coprophilia 302.89
    - ego-dystonic
      - homosexuality 302.0
      - lesbianism 302.0
    - erotomania 302.89
      - Clérambault's 297.8
    - exhibitionism (sexual) 302.4
    - fetishism 302.81
      - transvestic 302.3
    - frotteurism 302.89
    - homosexuality, ego-dystonic 302.0
      - pedophilic 302.2
    - lesbianism, ego-dystonic 302.0
    - masochism 302.83
    - narcissism 302.89
    - necrophilia 302.89
    - nymphomania 302.89
    - pederosis 302.2
    - pedophilia 302.2
    - sadism 302.84
    - sadomasochism 302.84
    - satyriasis 302.89
    - specified type NEC 302.89
    - transvestic fetishism 302.3
    - transvestism 302.3
    - voyeurism 302.82
    - zoophilia (erotica) 302.1
  - teeth, midline 524.29
  - trachea 519.1
  - ureter (congenital) 753.4
- **Devic's disease** 341.0

☑ Additional Digit Required — Refer to the Tabular List (Numeric Code Section) for Additional Digit Selection

▶◀ Revised Text ● New Line ▲ Revised Code

☑ Additional Digit Required — Refer to the Tabular List (Numeric Code Section) for Additional Digit Selection

▶◀ Revised Text ● New Line ▲ Revised Code

Disease, diseased — *see also* Syndrome — *continued*
- cerebrovascular NEC — *continued*
  - puerperal, postpartum, childbirth 674.0 ☑
  - specified type NEC 437.8
  - thrombotic — *see* Thrombosis, brain
- ceroid storage 272.7
- cervix (uteri)
  - inflammatory 616.9
    - specified NEC 616.8
  - noninflammatory 622.9
    - specified NEC 622.8
- Chabert's 022.9
- Chagas' (*see also* Trypanosomiasis, American) 086.2
- Chandler's (osteochondritis dissecans, hip) 732.7
- Charcôt's (joint) 094.0 *[713.5]*
  - spinal cord 094.0
- Charcôt-Marie-Tooth 356.1
- Charlouis' (*see also* Yaws) 102.9
- Cheadle (-Möller) (-Barlow) (infantile scurvy) 267
- Chédiak-Steinbrinck (-Higashi) (congenital gigantism of peroxidase granules) 288.2
- cheek, inner 528.9
- chest 519.9
- Chiari's (hepatic vein thrombosis) 453.0
- Chicago (North American blastomycosis) 116.0
- chignon (white piedra) 111.2
- chigoe, chigo (jigger) 134.1
- childhood granulomatous 288.1
- Chinese liver fluke 121.1
- chlamydial NEC 078.88
- cholecystic (*see also* Disease, gallbladder) 575.9
- choroid 363.9
  - degenerative (*see also* Degeneration, choroid) 363.40
  - hereditary (*see also* Dystrophy, choroid) 363.50
  - specified type NEC 363.8
- Christian's (chronic histiocytosis X) 277.89
- Christian-Weber (nodular nonsuppurative panniculitis) 729.30
- Christmas 286.1
- ciliary body 364.9
- circulatory (system) NEC 459.9
  - chronic, maternal, affecting fetus or newborn 760.3
  - specified NEC 459.89
  - syphilitic 093.9
    - congenital 090.5
- Civatte's (poikiloderma) 709.09
- climacteric 627.2
  - male 608.89
- coagulation factor deficiency (congenital) (*see also* Defect, coagulation) 286.9
- Coats' 362.12
- coccidioidal pulmonary 114.5
  - acute 114.0
  - chronic 114.4
  - primary 114.0
  - residual 114.4
- Cockayne's (microcephaly and dwarfism) 759.89
- Cogan's 370.52
- cold
  - agglutinin 283.0
    - or hemoglobinuria 283.0
      - paroxysmal (cold) (nocturnal) 283.2
  - hemagglutinin (chronic) 283.0
- collagen NEC 710.9
  - nonvascular 710.9
  - specified NEC 710.8
  - vascular (allergic) (*see also* Angiitis, hypersensitivity) 446.20
- colon 569.9
  - functional 564.9
    - congenital 751.3
  - ischemic 557.0
- combined system (of spinal cord) 266.2 *[336.2]*
  - with anemia (pernicious) 281.0 *[336.2]*
- compressed air 993.3
- Concato's (pericardial polyserositis) 423.2
  - peritoneal 568.82
  - pleural — *see* Pleurisy
- congenital NEC 799.89

Disease, diseased — *see also* Syndrome — *continued*
- conjunctiva 372.9
  - chlamydial 077.98
    - specified NEC 077.8
  - specified type NEC 372.89
  - viral 077.99
    - specified NEC 077.8
- connective tissue, diffuse (*see also* Disease, collagen) 710.9
- Conor and Bruch's (boutonneuse fever) 082.1
- Conradi (-Hünermann) 756.59
- Cooley's (erythroblastic anemia) 282.49
- Cooper's 610.1
- Corbus' 607.1
- cork-handlers' 495.3
- cornea (*see also* Keratopathy) 371.9
- coronary (*see also* Ischemia, heart) 414.9
  - congenital 746.85
  - ostial, syphilitic 093.20
    - aortic 093.22
    - mitral 093.21
    - pulmonary 093.24
    - tricuspid 093.23
- Corrigan's — *see* Insufficiency, aortic
- Cotugno's 724.3
- Coxsackie (virus) NEC 074.8
- cranial nerve NEC 352.9
- Creutzfeldt-Jakob ▶(new variant)◀ 046.1
  - with dementia
    - with behavioral disturbance 046.1 *[294.11]*
    - without behavioral disturbance 046.1 *[294.10]*
- Crigler-Najjar (congenital hyperbilirubinemia) 277.4
- Crocq's (acrocyanosis) 443.89
- Crohn's (intestine) (*see also* Enteritis, regional) 555.9
- Crouzon's (craniofacial dysostosis) 756.0
- Cruchet's (encephalitis lethargica) 049.8
- Cruveilhier's 335.21
- Cruz-Chagas (*see also* Trypanosomiasis, American) 086.2
- crystal deposition (*see also* Arthritis, due to, crystals) 712.9 ☑
- Csillag's (lichen sclerosus et atrophicus) 701.0
- Curschmann's 359.2
- Cushing's (pituitary basophilism) 255.0
- cystic
  - breast (chronic) 610.1
  - kidney, congenital (*see also* Cystic, disease, kidney) 753.10
  - liver, congenital 751.62
  - lung 518.89
    - congenital 748.4
  - pancreas 577.2
    - congenital 751.7
  - renal, congenital (*see also* Cystic, disease, kidney) 753.10
  - semilunar cartilage 717.5
- cysticercus 123.1
- cystine storage (with renal sclerosis) 270.0
- cytomegalic inclusion (generalized) 078.5
  - with
    - pneumonia 078.5 *[484.1]*
  - congenital 771.1
- Daae (-Finsen) (epidemic pleurodynia) 074.1
- dancing 297.8
- Danielssen's (anesthetic leprosy) 030.1
- Darier's (congenital) (keratosis follicularis) 757.39
  - erythema annulare centrifugum 695.0
  - vitamin A deficiency 264.8
- Darling's (histoplasmosis) (*see also* Histoplasmosis, American) 115.00
- Davies' 425.0
- de Beurmann-Gougerot (sporotrichosis) 117.1
- Débove's (splenomegaly) 789.2
- deer fly (*see also* Tularemia) 021.9
- deficiency 269.9
- degenerative — *see also* Degeneration
  - disc — *see* Degeneration, intervertebral disc
- Degos' 447.8
- Déjérine (-Sottas) 356.0
- Déleage's 359.89

Disease, diseased — *see also* Syndrome — *continued*
- demyelinating, demyelinizating (brain stem) (central nervous system) 341.9
  - multiple sclerosis 340
  - specified NEC 341.8
- de Quervain's (tendon sheath) 727.04
  - thyroid (subacute granulomatous thyroiditis) 245.1
- Dercum's (adiposis dolorosa) 272.8
- Deutschländer's — *see* Fracture, foot
- Devergie's (pityriasis rubra pilaris) 696.4
- Devic's 341.0
- diaphorase deficiency 289.7
- diaphragm 519.4
- diarrheal, infectious 009.2
- diatomaceous earth 502
- Diaz's (osteochondrosis astragalus) 732.5
- digestive system 569.9
- Di Guglielmo's (erythemic myelosis) (M9841/3) 207.0 ☑
- Dimitri-Sturge-Weber (encephalocutaneous angiomatosis) 759.6
- disc, degenerative — *see* Degeneration, intervertebral disc
- discogenic (*see also* Disease, intervertebral disc) 722.90
- diverticular — *see* Diverticula
- Down's (mongolism) 758.0
- Dubini's (electric chorea) 049.8
- Dubois' (thymus gland) 090.5
- Duchenne's 094.0
  - locomotor ataxia 094.0
  - muscular dystrophy 359.1
  - paralysis 335.22
  - pseudohypertrophy, muscles 359.1
- Duchenne-Griesinger 359.1
- ductless glands 259.9
- Duhring's (dermatitis herpetiformis) 694.0
- Dukes (-Filatov) 057.8
- duodenum NEC 537.9
  - specified NEC 537.89
- Duplay's 726.2
- Dupré's (meningism) 781.6
- Dupuytren's (muscle contracture) 728.6
- Durand-Nicolas-Favre (climatic bubo) 099.1
- Duroziez's (congenital mitral stenosis) 746.5
- Dutton's (trypanosomiasis) 086.9
- Eales' 362.18
- ear (chronic) (inner) NEC 388.9
  - middle 385.9
    - adhesive (*see also* Adhesions, middle ear) 385.10
    - specified NEC 385.89
- Eberth's (typhoid fever) 002.0
- Ebstein's
  - heart 746.2
  - meaning diabetes 250.4 ☑ *[581.81]*
- Echinococcus (*see also* Echinococcus) 122.9
- ECHO virus NEC 078.89
- Economo's (encephalitis lethargica) 049.8
- Eddowes' (brittle bones and blue sclera) 756.51
- Edsall's 992.2
- Eichstedt's (pityriasis versicolor) 111.0
- Ellis-van Creveld (chondroectodermal dysplasia) 756.55
- endocardium — *see* Endocarditis
- endocrine glands or system NEC 259.9
  - specified NEC 259.8
- endomyocardial, idiopathic mural 425.2
- Engel-von Recklinghausen (osteitis fibrosa cystica) 252.01
- Engelmann's (diaphyseal sclerosis) 756.59
- English (rickets) 268.0
- Engman's (infectious eczematoid dermatitis) 690.8
- enteroviral, enterovirus NEC 078.89
  - central nervous system NEC 048
- epidemic NEC 136.9
- epididymis 608.9
- epigastric, functional 536.9
  - psychogenic 306.4
- Erb (-Landouzy) 359.1
- Erb-Goldflam 358.00
- Erichsen's (railway spine) 300.16
- esophagus 530.9
  - functional 530.5
  - psychogenic 306.4

☑ Additional Digit Required — Refer to the Tabular List (Numeric Code Section) for Additional Digit Selection

▶◀ Revised Text ● New Line ▲ Revised Code

Disease, diseased — *see also* Syndrome — *continued*
`  `heart — *continued*
`    `due to — *continued*
`      `cardiac glycogenosis 271.0 *[425.7]*
`      `Friedreich's ataxia 334.0 *[425.8]*
`      `gout 274.82
`      `mucopolysaccharidosis 277.5 *[425.7]*
`      `myotonia atrophica 359.2 *[425.8]*
`      `progressive muscular dystrophy 359.1 *[425.8]*
`      `sarcoidosis 135 *[425.8]*
`    `fetal 746.9
`      `inflammatory 746.89
`    `fibroid (*see also* Myocarditis) 429.0
`    `functional 427.9
`      `postoperative 997.1
`      `psychogenic 306.2
`    `glycogen storage 271.0 *[425.7]*
`    `gonococcal NEC 098.85
`    `gouty 274.82
`    `hypertensive (*see also* Hypertension, heart) 402.90
`      `benign 402.10
`      `malignant 402.00
`    `hyperthyroid (*see also* Hyperthyroidism) 242.9 ☑ *[425.7]*
`    `incompletely diagnosed — *see* Disease, heart
`    `ischemic (chronic) (*see also* Ischemia, heart) 414.9
`      `acute (*see also* Infarct, myocardium) 410.9 ☑
`        `without myocardial infarction 411.89
`          `with coronary (artery) occlusion 411.81
`      `asymptomatic 412
`      `diagnosed on ECG or other special investigation but currently presenting no symptoms 412
`    `kyphoscoliotic 416.1
`    `mitral (*see also* Endocarditis, mitral) 394.9
`    `muscular (*see also* Degeneration, myocardial) 429.1
`    `postpartum 674.8 ☑
`    `psychogenic (functional) 306.2
`    `pulmonary (chronic) 416.9
`      `acute 415.0
`      `specified NEC 416.8
`    `rheumatic (chronic) (inactive) (old) (quiescent) (with chorea) 398.90
`      `active or acute 391.9
`        `with chorea (active) (rheumatic) (Sydenham's) 392.0
`        `specified type NEC 391.8
`      `maternal, affecting fetus or newborn 760.3
`    `rheumatoid — *see* Arthritis, rheumatoid
`    `sclerotic — *see* Arteriosclerosis, coronary
`    `senile (*see also* Myocarditis) 429.0
`    `specified type NEC 429.89
`    `syphilitic 093.89
`      `aortic 093.1
`        `aneurysm 093.0
`      `asymptomatic 093.89
`      `congenital 090.5
`    `thyroid (gland) (*see also* Hyperthyroidism) 242.9 ☑ *[425.7]*
`    `thyrotoxic (*see also* Thyrotoxicosis) 242.9 ☑ *[425.7]*
`    `tuberculous (*see also* Tuberculosis) 017.9 ☑ *[425.8]*
`    `valve, valvular (obstructive) (regurgitant) — *see also* Endocarditis
`      `congenital NEC (*see also* Anomaly, heart, valve) 746.9
`        `pulmonary 746.00
`        `specified type NEC 746.89
`    `vascular — *see* Disease, cardiovascular
`  `heavy-chain (gamma G) 273.2
`  `Heberden's 715.04
`  `Hebra's
`    `dermatitis exfoliativa 695.89
`    `erythema multiforme exudativum 695.1
`    `pityriasis
`      `maculata et circinata 696.3
`      `rubra 695.89
`        `pilaris 696.4
`    `prurigo 698.2

Disease, diseased — *see also* Syndrome — *continued*
`  `Heerfordt's (uveoparotitis) 135
`  `Heidenhain's 290.10
`    `with dementia 290.10
`  `Heilmeyer-Schöner (M9842/3) 207.1 ☑
`  `Heine-Medin (*see also* Poliomyelitis) 045.9 ☑
`  `Heller's (*see also* Psychosis, childhood) 299.1 ☑
`  `Heller-Döhle (syphilitic aortitis) 093.1
`  `hematopoietic organs 289.9
`  `hemoglobin (Hb) 282.7
`    `with thalassemia 282.49
`    `abnormal (mixed) NEC 282.7
`      `with thalassemia 282.49
`    `AS genotype 282.5
`    `Bart's 282.49 ▲
`    `C (Hb-C) 282.7
`      `with other abnormal hemoglobin NEC 282.7
`      `elliptocytosis 282.7
`      `Hb-S (without crisis) 282.63
`        `with
`          `crisis 282.64
`          `vaso-occlusive pain 282.64
`      `sickle-cell (without crisis) 282.63
`        `with
`          `crisis 282.64
`          `vaso-occlusive pain 282.64
`      `thalassemia 282.49
`    `constant spring 282.7
`    `D (Hb-D) 282.7
`      `with other abnormal hemoglobin NEC 282.7
`      `Hb-S (without crisis) 282.68
`        `with crisis 282.69
`      `sickle-cell (without crisis) 282.68
`        `with crisis 282.69
`      `thalassemia 282.49
`    `E (Hb-E) 282.7
`      `with other abnormal hemoglobin NEC 282.7
`      `Hb-S (without crisis) 282.68
`        `with crisis 282.69
`      `sickle-cell (without crisis) 282.68
`        `with crisis 282.69
`      `thalassemia 282.49
`    `elliptocytosis 282.7
`    `F (Hb-F) 282.7
`    `G (Hb-G) 282.7
`    `H (Hb-H) 282.49
`    `hereditary persistence, fetal (HPFH) ("Swiss variety") 282.7
`    `high fetal gene 282.7
`    `I thalassemia 282.49
`    `M 289.7
`    `S — *see also* Disease, sickle-cell, Hb-S
`      `thalassemia (without crisis) 282.41
`        `with
`          `crisis 282.42
`          `vaso-occlusive pain 282.42
`    `spherocytosis 282.7
`    `unstable, hemolytic 282.7
`    `Zurich (Hb-Zurich) 282.7
`  `hemolytic (fetus) (newborn) 773.2
`    `autoimmune (cold type) (warm type) 283.0
`    `due to or with
`      `incompatibility
`        `ABO (blood group) 773.1
`        `blood (group) (Duffy) (Kell) (Kidd) (Lewis) (M) (S) NEC 773.2
`        `Rh (blood group) (factor) 773.0
`      `Rh negative mother 773.0
`    `unstable hemoglobin 282.7
`  `hemorrhagic 287.9
`    `newborn 776.0
`  `Henoch (-Schönlein) (purpura nervosa) 287.0
`  `hepatic — *see* Disease, liver
`  `hepatolenticular 275.1
`  `heredodegenerative NEC
`    `brain 331.89
`    `spinal cord 336.8
`  `Hers' (glycogenosis VI) 271.0
`  `Herter (-Gee) (-Heubner) (nontropical sprue) 579.0
`  `Herxheimer's (diffuse idiopathic cutaneous atrophy) 701.8
`  `Heubner's 094.89

Disease, diseased — *see also* Syndrome — *continued*
`  `Heubner-Herter (nontropical sprue) 579.0
`  `high fetal gene or hemoglobin thalassemia 282.49
`  `Hildenbrand's (typhus) 081.9
`  `hip (joint) NEC 719.95
`    `congenital 755.63
`    `suppurative 711.05
`    `tuberculous (*see also* Tuberculosis) 015.1 ☑ *[730.85]*
`  `Hippel's (retinocerebral angiomatosis) 759.6
`  `Hirschfeld's (acute diabetes mellitus) (*see also* Diabetes) 250.0 ☑
`  `Hirschsprung's (congenital megacolon) 751.3
`  `His (-Werner) (trench fever) 083.1
`  `HIV 042
`  `Hodgkin's (M9650/3) 201.9 ☑

> *Note — Use the following fifth-digit subclassification with category 201:*
>
> | | |
> |---|---|
> | *0* | *unspecified site* |
> | *1* | *lymph nodes of head, face, and neck* |
> | *2* | *intrathoracic lymph nodes* |
> | *3* | *intra-abdominal lymph nodes* |
> | *4* | *lymph nodes of axilla and upper limb* |
> | *5* | *lymph nodes of inguinal region and lower limb* |
> | *6* | *intrapelvic lymph nodes* |
> | *7* | *spleen* |
> | *8* | *lymph nodes of multiple sites* |

`    `lymphocytic
`      `depletion (M9653/3) 201.7 ☑
`        `diffuse fibrosis (M9654/3) 201.7 ☑
`        `reticular type (M9655/3) 201.7 ☑
`      `predominance (M9651/3) 201.4 ☑
`    `lymphocytic-histiocytic predominance (M9651/3) 201.4 ☑
`    `mixed cellularity (M9652/3) 201.6 ☑
`    `nodular sclerosis (M9656/3) 201.5 ☑
`      `cellular phase (M9657/3) 201.5 ☑
`  `Hodgson's 441.9
`    `ruptured 441.5
`  `Hoffa (-Kastert) (liposynovitis prepatellaris) 272.8
`  `Holla (*see also* Spherocytosis) 282.0
`  `homozygous-Hb-S 282.61
`  `hoof and mouth 078.4
`  `hookworm (*see also* Ancylostomiasis) 126.9
`  `Horton's (temporal arteritis) 446.5
`  `host-versus-graft (immune or nonimmune cause) 996.80
`    `bone marrow 996.85
`    `heart 996.83
`    `intestines 996.87
`    `kidney 996.81
`    `liver 996.82
`    `lung 996.84
`    `pancreas 996.86
`    `specified NEC 996.89
`  `HPFH (hereditary persistence of fetal hemoglobin) ("Swiss variety") 282.7
`  `Huchard's (continued arterial hypertension) 401.9
`  `Huguier's (uterine fibroma) 218.9
`  `human immunodeficiency (virus) 042
`  `hunger 251.1
`  `Hunt's
`    `dyssynergia cerebellaris myoclonica 334.2
`    `herpetic geniculate ganglionitis 053.11
`  `Huntington's 333.4
`  `Huppert's (multiple myeloma) (M9730/3) 203.0 ☑
`  `Hurler's (mucopolysaccharidosis I) 277.5
`  `Hutchinson's, meaning
`    `angioma serpiginosum 709.1
`    `cheiropompholyx 705.81
`    `prurigo estivalis 692.72
`  `Hutchinson-Boeck (sarcoidosis) 135
`  `Hutchinson-Gilford (progeria) 259.8
`  `hyaline (diffuse) (generalized) 728.9
`    `membrane (lung) (newborn) 769
`  `hydatid (*see also* Echinococcus) 122.9
`  `Hyde's (prurigo nodularis) 698.3

☑ Additional Digit Required — Refer to the Tabular List (Numeric Code Section) for Additional Digit Selection
▶◀ Revised Text ● New Line ▲ Revised Code

☑ Additional Digit Required — Refer to the Tabular List (Numeric Code Section) for Additional Digit Selection
▶◀ Revised Text ● New Line ▲ Revised Code

☑ Additional Digit Required — Refer to the Tabular List (Numeric Code Section) for Additional Digit Selection
▶◀ Revised Text　● New Line　▲ Revised Code

☑ Additional Digit Required — Refer to the Tabular List (Numeric Code Section) for Additional Digit Selection
▶◀ Revised Text ● New Line ▲ Revised Code

Note — "Closed" includes simple, complete, partial, uncomplicated, and unspecified dislocation.

"Open" includes dislocation specified as infected or compound and dislocation with foreign body.

"Chronic," "habitual," "old," or "recurrent" dislocations should be coded as indicated under the entry "Dislocation, recurrent," and "pathological" as indicated under the entry "Dislocation, pathological."

For late effect of dislocation see Late, effect, dislocation.

Dislocation — *continued*
- sternoclavicular (joint) (closed) 839.61
  - open 839.71
- sternum (closed) 839.61
  - open 839.71
- subastragalar — *see* Dislocation, foot
- subglenoid (closed) 831.01
  - open 831.11
- symphysis
  - jaw (closed) 830.0
    - open 830.1
  - mandibular (closed) 830.0
    - open 830.1
  - pubis (closed) 839.69
    - open 839.79
- tarsal (bone) (joint) 838.01
  - open 838.11
- tarsometatarsal (joint) 838.03
  - open 838.13
- temporomandibular (joint) (closed) 830.0
  - open 830.1
  - recurrent 524.69
- thigh
  - distal end (*see also* Dislocation, femur, distal end) 836.50
  - proximal end (*see also* Dislocation, hip) 835.00
- thoracic (vertebrae) (closed) 839.21
  - open 839.31
- thumb(s) (*see also* Dislocation, finger) 834.00
- thyroid cartilage (closed) 839.69
  - open 839.79
- tibia
  - distal end (closed) 837.0
    - open 837.1
  - proximal end (closed) 836.50
    - anterior 836.51
      - open 836.61
    - lateral 836.54
      - open 836.64
    - medial 836.53
      - open 836.63
    - open 836.60
    - posterior 836.52
      - open 836.62
    - rotatory 836.59
      - open 836.69
- tibiofibular
  - distal (closed) 837.0
    - open 837.1
  - superior (closed) 836.59
    - open 836.69
- toe(s) (closed) 838.09
  - open 838.19
- trachea (closed) 839.69
  - open 839.79
- ulna
  - distal end (closed) 833.09
    - open 833.19
  - proximal end — *see* Dislocation, elbow
- vertebra (articular process) (body) (closed) 839.40
  - cervical, cervicodorsal or cervicothoracic (closed) 839.00
    - first (atlas) 839.01
      - open 839.11
    - second (axis) 839.02
      - open 839.12
    - third 839.03
      - open 839.13
    - fourth 839.04
      - open 839.14
    - fifth 839.05
      - open 839.15
    - sixth 839.06
      - open 839.16
    - seventh 839.07
      - open 839.17
    - congenital 756.19
    - multiple sites 839.08
      - open 839.18
    - open 839.10
  - congenital 756.19
  - dorsal 839.21
    - open 839.31
    - recurrent 724.9

Dislocation — *continued*
- vertebra — *continued*
  - lumbar, lumbosacral 839.20
    - open 839.30
  - open NEC 839.50
  - recurrent 724.9
  - specified region NEC 839.49
    - open 839.59
  - thoracic 839.21
    - open 839.31
- wrist (carpal bone) (scaphoid) (semilunar) (closed) 833.00
  - carpometacarpal (joint) 833.04
    - open 833.14
  - metacarpal bone, proximal end 833.05
    - open 833.15
  - midcarpal (joint) 833.03
    - open 833.13
  - open 833.10
  - radiocarpal (joint) 833.02
    - open 833.12
  - radioulnar (joint) 833.01
    - open 833.11
  - recurrent 718.33
  - specified site NEC 833.09
    - open 833.19
- xiphoid cartilage (closed) 839.61
  - open 839.71

Dislodgement
- artificial skin graft 996.55
- decellularized allodermis graft 996.55

Disobedience, hostile (covert) (overt) (*see also* Disturbance, conduct) 312.0 ☑

Disorder — *see also* Disease
- academic underachievement, childhood and adolescence 313.83
- accommodation 367.51
  - drug-induced 367.89
  - toxic 367.89
- adjustment (*see also* Reaction, adjustment) 309.9
  - with
    - anxiety 309.24
    - anxiety and depressed mood 309.28
    - depressed mood 309.0
    - disturbance of conduct 309.3
    - disturbance of emotions and conduct 309.4
- adrenal (capsule) (cortex) (gland) 255.9
  - specified type NEC 255.8
- adrenogenital 255.2
- affective (*see also* Psychosis, affective) 296.90
  - atypical 296.81
- aggressive, unsocialized (*see also* Disturbance, conduct) 312.0 ☑
- alcohol, alcoholic (*see also* Alcohol) 291.9
- allergic — *see* Allergy
- amnestic (*see also* Amnestic syndrome) 294.8
  - alcohol-induced persisting 291.1
  - drug-induced persisting 292.83
  - in conditions classified elsewhere 294.0
- amino acid (metabolic) (*see also* Disturbance, metabolism, amino acid) 270.9
  - albinism 270.2
  - alkaptonuria 270.2
  - argininosuccinicaciduria 270.6
  - beta-amino-isobutyricaciduria 277.2
  - cystathioninuria 270.4
  - cystinosis 270.0
  - cystinuria 270.0
  - glycinuria 270.0
  - homocystinuria 270.4
  - imidazole 270.5
  - maple syrup (urine) disease 270.3
  - neonatal, transitory 775.8
  - oasthouse urine disease 270.2
  - ochronosis 270.2
  - phenylketonuria 270.1
  - phenylpyruvic oligophrenia 270.1
  - purine NEC 277.2
  - pyrimidine NEC 277.2
  - renal transport NEC 270.0
  - specified type NEC 270.8
  - transport NEC 270.0
    - renal 270.0
  - xanthinuria 277.2

Disorder — *see also* Disease — *continued*
- anaerobic glycolysis with anemia 282.3
- anxiety (*see also* Anxiety) 300.00
  - due to or associated with physical condition 293.84
- arteriole 447.9
  - specified type NEC 447.8
- artery 447.9
  - specified type NEC 447.8
- articulation — *see* Disorder, joint
- Asperger's 299.8 ☑
- attachment of infancy or early childhood 313.89
- attention deficit 314.00
  - with hyperactivity 314.01
  - predominantly
    - combined hyperactive/inattentive 314.01
    - hyperactive/impulsive 314.01
    - inattentive 314.00
  - residual type 314.8
- autoimmune NEC 279.4
  - hemolytic (cold type) (warm type) 283.0
  - parathyroid 252.1
  - thyroid 245.2
- autistic 299.0 ☑
- avoidant, childhood or adolescence 313.21
- balance
  - acid-base 276.9
    - mixed (with hypercapnia) 276.4
  - electrolyte 276.9
  - fluid 276.9
- behavior NEC (*see also* Disturbance, conduct) 312.9
  - disruptive 312.9
- bilirubin excretion 277.4
- bipolar (affective) (alternating) 296.80

> *Note — Use the following fifth-digit subclassification with categories 296.0-296.6:*
>
> | | |
> |---|---|
> | *0* | *unspecifed* |
> | *1* | *mild* |
> | *2* | *moderate* |
> | *3* | *severe, without mention of psychotic behavior* |
> | *4* | *severe, specified as with psychotic behavior* |
> | *5* | *in partial or unspecified remission* |
> | *6* | *in full remission* |

  - atypical 296.7
  - currently
    - depressed 296.5 ☑
    - hypomanic 296.4 ☑
    - manic 296.4 ☑
    - mixed 296.6 ☑
  - specified type NEC 296.89
  - type I 296.7
    - most recent episode (or current)
      - depressed 296.5 ☑
      - hypomanic 296.4 ☑
      - manic 296.4 ☑
      - mixed 296.6 ☑
      - unspecified 296.7
    - single manic episode 296.0
  - type II (recurrent major depressive episodes with hypomania) 296.89
- bladder 596.9
  - functional NEC 596.59
  - specified NEC 596.8
- bone NEC 733.90
  - specified NEC 733.99
- brachial plexus 353.0
- branched-chain amino-acid degradation 270.3
- breast 611.9
  - puerperal, postpartum 676.3 ☑
  - specified NEC 611.8
- Briquet's 300.81
- bursa 727.9
  - shoulder region 726.10
- carbohydrate metabolism, congenital 271.9
- cardiac, functional 427.9
  - postoperative 997.1
  - psychogenic 306.2
- cardiovascular, psychogenic 306.2

☑ Additional Digit Required — Refer to the Tabular List (Numeric Code Section) for Additional Digit Selection

▶◀ Revised Text ● New Line ▲ Revised Code

Disproportion — *continued*
- caused by — *continued*
  - contraction, pelvis — *continued*
    - midpelvic 653.8 ☑
    - midplane 653.8 ☑
    - outlet 653.3 ☑
  - fetal
    - ascites 653.7 ☑
    - hydrocephalus 653.6 ☑
    - hydrops 653.7 ☑
    - meningomyelocele 653.7 ☑
    - sacral teratoma 653.7 ☑
    - tumor 653.7 ☑
  - hydrocephalic fetus 653.6 ☑
  - pelvis, pelvic, abnormality (bony) NEC 653.0 ☑
  - unusually large fetus 653.5 ☑
- causing obstructed labor 660.1 ☑
- cephalopelvic, normally formed fetus 653.4 ☑
  - causing obstructed labor 660.1 ☑
- fetal NEC 653.5 ☑
  - causing obstructed labor 660.1 ☑
- fetopelvic, normally formed fetus 653.4 ☑
  - causing obstructed labor 660.1 ☑
- mixed maternal and fetal origin, normally formed fetus 653.4 ☑
- pelvis, pelvic (bony) NEC 653.1 ☑
  - causing obstructed labor 660.1 ☑
- specified type NEC 653.8 ☑

Disruption
- cesarean wound 674.1 ☑
- family V61.0
- gastrointestinal anastomosis 997.4
- ligament(s) — *see also* Sprain
  - knee
    - current injury — *see* Dislocation, knee
    - old 717.89
      - capsular 717.85
      - collateral (medial) 717.82
        - lateral 717.81
      - cruciate (posterior) 717.84
        - anterior 717.83
      - specified site NEC 717.85
- marital V61.10
  - involving divorce or estrangement V61.0
- operation wound (external) 998.32
  - internal 998.31
- organ transplant, anastomosis site — *see* Complications, transplant, organ, by site
- ossicles, ossicular chain 385.23
  - traumatic — *see* Fracture, skull, base
- parenchyma
  - liver (hepatic) — *see* Laceration, liver, major
  - spleen — *see* Laceration, spleen, parenchyma, massive
- phase-shift, of 24 hour sleep wake cycle, ▶unspecified◀ 780.55
  - nonorganic origin 307.45
- sleep wake cycle (24 hour), ▶unspecified◀ 780.55
  - circadian rhythm 327.33 ▲
  - nonorganic origin 307.45
- suture line (external) 998.32
  - internal 998.31
- wound
  - cesarean operation 674.1 ☑
  - episiotomy 674.2 ☑
  - operation 998.32
    - cesarean 674.1 ☑
    - internal 998.31
  - perineal (obstetric) 674.2 ☑
  - uterine 674.1 ☑

Disruptio uteri — *see also* Rupture, uterus
- complicating delivery — *see* Delivery, complicated, rupture, uterus

Dissatisfaction with
- employment V62.2
- school environment V62.3

Dissecting — *see* condition

Dissection
- aorta 441.00
  - abdominal 441.02
  - thoracic 441.01
  - thoracoabdominal 441.03
- artery, arterial
  - carotid 443.21
  - coronary 414.12
  - iliac 443.22
  - renal 443.23
  - specified NEC 443.29
  - vertebral 443.24
- vascular 459.9
- wound — *see* Wound, open, by site

Disseminated — *see* condition

Dissociated personality NEC 300.15

Dissociation
- auriculoventricular or atrioventricular (any degree) (AV) 426.89
  - with heart block 426.0
- interference 426.89
- isorhythmic 426.89
- rhythm
  - atrioventricular (AV) 426.89
  - interference 426.89

Dissociative
- identity disorder 300.14
- reaction NEC 300.15

Dissolution, vertebra (*see also* Osteoporosis) 733.00

Distention
- abdomen (gaseous) 787.3
- bladder 596.8
- cecum 569.89
- colon 569.89
- gallbladder 575.8
- gaseous (abdomen) 787.3
- intestine 569.89
- kidney 593.89
- liver 573.9
- seminal vesicle 608.89
- stomach 536.8
  - acute 536.1
  - psychogenic 306.4
- ureter 593.5
- uterus 621.8

Distichia, distichiasis (eyelid) 743.63

Distoma hepaticum infestation 121.3

Distomiasis 121.9
- bile passages 121.3
  - due to Clonorchis sinensis 121.1
- hemic 120.9
- hepatic (liver) 121.3
  - due to Clonorchis sinensis (clonorchiasis) 121.1
- intestinal 121.4
- liver 121.3
  - due to Clonorchis sinensis 121.1
- lung 121.2
- pulmonary 121.2

Distomolar (fourth molar) 520.1
- causing crowding 524.31

Disto-occlusion (division I) (division II) 524.22

Distortion (congenital)
- adrenal (gland) 759.1
- ankle (joint) 755.69
- anus 751.5
- aorta 747.29
- appendix 751.5
- arm 755.59
- artery (peripheral) NEC (*see also* Distortion, peripheral vascular system) 747.60
  - cerebral 747.81
  - coronary 746.85
  - pulmonary 747.3
  - retinal 743.58
  - umbilical 747.5
- auditory canal 744.29
  - causing impairment of hearing 744.02
- bile duct or passage 751.69
- bladder 753.8
- brain 742.4
- bronchus 748.3
- cecum 751.5
- cervix (uteri) 752.49
- chest (wall) 756.3
- clavicle 755.51
- clitoris 752.49

Distortion — *continued*
- coccyx 756.19
- colon 751.5
- common duct 751.69
- cornea 743.41
- cricoid cartilage 748.3
- cystic duct 751.69
- duodenum 751.5
- ear 744.29
  - auricle 744.29
    - causing impairment of hearing 744.02
  - causing impairment of hearing 744.09
  - external 744.29
    - causing impairment of hearing 744.02
  - inner 744.05
  - middle, except ossicles 744.03
    - ossicles 744.04
  - ossicles 744.04
- endocrine (gland) NEC 759.2
- epiglottis 748.3
- Eustachian tube 744.24
- eye 743.8
  - adnexa 743.69
- face bone(s) 756.0
- fallopian tube 752.19
- femur 755.69
- fibula 755.69
- finger(s) 755.59
- foot 755.67
- gallbladder 751.69
- genitalia, genital organ(s)
  - female 752.89
    - external 752.49
    - internal NEC 752.89
  - male 752.89
    - penis 752.69
- glottis 748.3
- gyri 742.4
- hand bone(s) 755.59
- heart (auricle) (ventricle) 746.89
  - valve (cusp) 746.89
- hepatic duct 751.69
- humerus 755.59
- hymen 752.49
- ileum 751.5
- intestine (large) (small) 751.5
  - with anomalous adhesions, fixation or malrotation 751.4
- jaw NEC 524.89
- jejunum 751.5
- kidney 753.3
- knee (joint) 755.64
- labium (majus) (minus) 752.49
- larynx 748.3
- leg 755.69
- lens 743.36
- liver 751.69
- lumbar spine 756.19
  - with disproportion (fetopelvic) 653.0 ☑
    - affecting fetus or newborn 763.1
    - causing obstructed labor 660.1 ☑
- lumbosacral (joint) (region) 756.19
- lung (fissures) (lobe) 748.69
- nerve 742.8
- nose 748.1
- organ
  - of Corti 744.05
  - of site not listed — *see* Anomaly, specified type NEC
- ossicles, ear 744.04
- ovary 752.0
- oviduct 752.19
- pancreas 751.7
- parathyroid (gland) 759.2
- patella 755.64
- peripheral vascular system NEC 747.60
  - gastrointestinal 747.61
  - lower limb 747.64
  - renal 747.62
  - spinal 747.82
  - upper limb 747.63
- pituitary (gland) 759.2
- radius 755.59
- rectum 751.5
- rib 756.3
- sacroiliac joint 755.69
- sacrum 756.19

Note — Use the following fifth-digit subclassification with categories 312.0–312.2:

0	*unspecified*
1	*mild*
2	*moderate*
3	*severe*

- **Disturbance** — *see also* Disease — *continued*
  - motor 796.1
  - nervous functional 799.2
  - neuromuscular mechanism (eye) due to syphilis 094.84
  - nutritional 269.9
    - nail 703.8
  - ocular motion 378.87
    - psychogenic 306.7
  - oculogyric 378.87
    - psychogenic 306.7
  - oculomotor NEC 378.87
    - psychogenic 306.7
  - olfactory nerve 781.1
  - optic nerve NEC 377.49
  - oral epithelium, including tongue 528.79
    - residual ridge mucosa
      - excessive 528.72
      - minimal 528.71
  - personality (pattern) (trait) (*see also* Disorder, personality) 301.9
    - following organic brain damage 310.1
  - polyglandular 258.9
  - psychomotor 307.9
  - pupillary 379.49
  - reflex 796.1
  - rhythm, heart 427.9
    - postoperative (immediate) 997.1
      - long-term effect of cardiac surgery 429.4
    - psychogenic 306.2
  - salivary secretion 527.7
  - sensation (cold) (heat) (localization) (tactile discrimination localization) (texture) (vibratory) NEC 782.0
    - hysterical 300.11
    - skin 782.0
    - smell 781.1
    - taste 781.1
  - sensory (*see also* Disturbance, sensation) 782.0
    - innervation 782.0
  - situational (transient) (*see also* Reaction, adjustment) 309.9
    - acute 308.3
  - sleep 780.50
    - with apnea — *see* Apnea, sleep
    - initiation or maintenance (*see also* Insomnia) 780.52
      - nonorganic origin 307.41
    - nonorganic origin 307.40
      - specified type NEC 307.49
    - specified NEC 780.59
      - nonorganic origin 307.49
    - wakefulness (*see also* Hypersomnia) 780.54
      - nonorganic origin 307.43
  - sociopathic 301.7
  - speech NEC 784.5
    - developmental 315.39
      - associated with hyperkinesis 314.1
    - secondary to organic lesion 784.5
  - stomach (functional) (*see also* Disturbance, gastric) 536.9
  - sympathetic (nerve) (*see also* Neuropathy, peripheral, autonomic) 337.9
  - temperature sense 782.0
    - hysterical 300.11
  - tooth
    - eruption 520.6
    - formation 520.4
      - structure, hereditary NEC 520.5
  - touch (*see also* Disturbance, sensation) 782.0
  - vascular 459.9
    - arteriosclerotic — *see* Arteriosclerosis
  - vasomotor 443.9
  - vasospastic 443.9
  - vestibular labyrinth 386.9
  - vision, visual NEC 368.9
    - psychophysical 368.16
    - specified NEC 368.8
    - subjective 368.10
  - voice 784.40
  - wakefulness (initiation or maintenance) (*see also* Hypersomnia) 780.54
    - nonorganic origin 307.43
- **Disulfiduria, beta-mercaptolactate-cysteine** 270.0
- **Disuse atrophy, bone** 733.7
- **Ditthomska syndrome** 307.81
- **Diuresis** 788.42
- **Divers'**
  - palsy or paralysis 993.3
  - squeeze 993.3
- **Diverticula, diverticulosis, diverticulum** (acute) (multiple) (perforated) (ruptured) 562.10
  - with diverticulitis 562.11
  - aorta (Kommerell's) 747.21
  - appendix (noninflammatory) 543.9
  - bladder (acquired) (sphincter) 596.3
    - congenital 753.8
  - broad ligament 620.8
  - bronchus (congenital) 748.3
    - acquired 494.0
      - with acute exacerbation 494.1
  - calyx, calyceal (kidney) 593.89
  - cardia (stomach) 537.1
  - cecum 562.10
    - with
      - diverticulitis 562.11
        - with hemorrhage 562.13
      - hemorrhage 562.12
    - congenital 751.5
  - colon (acquired) 562.10
    - with
      - diverticulitis 562.11
        - with hemorrhage 562.13
      - hemorrhage 562.12
    - congenital 751.5
  - duodenum 562.00
    - with
      - diverticulitis 562.01
        - with hemorrhage 562.03
      - hemorrhage 562.02
    - congenital 751.5
  - epiphrenic (esophagus) 530.6
  - esophagus (congenital) 750.4
    - acquired 530.6
    - epiphrenic 530.6
    - pulsion 530.6
    - traction 530.6
    - Zenker's 530.6
  - Eustachian tube 381.89
  - fallopian tube 620.8
  - gallbladder (congenital) 751.69
  - gastric 537.1
  - heart (congenital) 746.89
  - ileum 562.00
    - with
      - diverticulitis 562.01
        - with hemorrhage 562.03
      - hemorrhage 562.02
  - intestine (large) 562.10
    - with
      - diverticulitis 562.11
        - with hemorrhage 562.13
      - hemorrhage 562.12
    - congenital 751.5
    - small 562.00
      - with
        - diverticulitis 562.01
          - with hemorrhage 562.03
        - hemorrhage 562.02
      - congenital 751.5
  - jejunum 562.00
    - with
      - diverticulitis 562.01
        - with hemorrhage 562.03
      - hemorrhage 562.02
  - kidney (calyx) (pelvis) 593.89
    - with calculus 592.0
  - Kommerell's 747.21
  - laryngeal ventricle (congenital) 748.3
  - Meckel's (displaced) (hypertrophic) 751.0
  - midthoracic 530.6
  - organ or site, congenital NEC — *see* Distortion
  - pericardium (conginital) (cyst) 746.89
    - acquired (true) 423.8
  - pharyngoesophageal (pulsion) 530.6
  - pharynx (congenital) 750.27
  - pulsion (esophagus) 530.6
  - rectosigmoid 562.10
    - with
      - diverticulitis 562.11
        - with hemorrhage 562.13
- **Diverticula, diverticulosis, diverticulum** — *continued*
  - rectosigmoid — *continued*
    - with — *continued*
      - hemorrhage 562.12
    - congenital 751.5
  - rectum 562.10
    - with
      - diverticulitis 562.11
        - with hemorrhage 562.13
      - hemorrhage 562.12
  - renal (calyces) (pelvis) 593.89
    - with calculus 592.0
  - Rokitansky's 530.6
  - seminal vesicle 608.0
  - sigmoid 562.10
    - with
      - diverticulitis 562.11
        - with hemorrhage 562.13
      - hemorrhage 562.12
    - congenital 751.5
  - small intestine 562.00
    - with
      - diverticulitis 562.01
        - with hemorrhage 562.03
      - hemorrhage 562.02
  - stomach (cardia) (juxtacardia) (juxtapyloric) (acquired) 537.1
    - congenital 750.7
  - subdiaphragmatic 530.6
  - trachea (congenital) 748.3
    - acquired 519.1
  - traction (esophagus) 530.6
  - ureter (acquired) 593.89
    - congenital 753.4
  - ureterovesical orifice 593.89
  - urethra (acquired) 599.2
    - congenital 753.8
  - ventricle, left (congenital) 746.89
  - vesical (urinary) 596.3
    - congenital 753.8
  - Zenker's (esophagus) 530.6
- **Diverticulitis** (acute) (*see also* Diverticula) 562.11
  - with hemorrhage 562.13
  - bladder (urinary) 596.3
  - cecum (perforated) 562.11
    - with hemorrhage 562.13
  - colon (perforated) 562.11
    - with hemorrhage 562.13
  - duodenum 562.01
    - with hemorrhage 562.03
  - esophagus 530.6
  - ileum (perforated) 562.01
    - with hemorrhage 562.03
  - intestine (large) (perforated) 562.11
    - with hemorrhage 562.13
    - small 562.01
      - with hemorrhage 562.03
  - jejunum (perforated) 562.01
    - with hemorrhage 562.03
  - Meckel's (perforated) 751.0
  - pharyngoesophageal 530.6
  - rectosigmoid (perforated) 562.11
    - with hemorrhage 562.13
  - rectum 562.11
    - with hemorrhage 562.13
  - sigmoid (old) (perforated) 562.11
    - with hemorrhage 562.13
  - small intestine (perforated) 562.01
    - with hemorrhage 562.03
  - vesical (urinary) 596.3
- **Diverticulosis** — *see* Diverticula
- **Division**
  - cervix uteri 622.8
    - external os into two openings by frenum 752.49
  - external (cervical) into two openings by frenum 752.49
  - glans penis 752.69
  - hymen 752.49
  - labia minora (congenital) 752.49
  - ligament (partial or complete) (current) — *see also* Sprain, by site
    - with open wound — *see* Wound, open, by site

Duchenne-Aran myelopathic, muscular atrophy (nonprogressive) (progressive) 335.21

Duchenne-Griesinger disease 359.1

Ducrey's
- bacillus 099.0
- chancre 099.0
- disease (chancroid) 099.0

Duct, ductus — *see* condition

Duengero 061

Duhring's disease (dermatitis herpetiformis) 694.0

Dukes (-Filatov) disease 057.8

Dullness
- cardiac (decreased) (increased) 785.3

Dumb ague (*see also* Malaria) 084.6

Dumbness (*see also* Aphasia) 784.3

Dumdum fever 085.0

Dumping syndrome (postgastrectomy) 564.2
- nonsurgical 536.8

Duodenitis (nonspecific) (peptic) 535.60
- with hemorrhage 535.61
- due to
  - Strongyloides stercoralis 127.2

Duodenocholangitis 575.8

Duodenum, duodenal — *see* condition

Duplay's disease, periarthritis, or syndrome 726.2

Duplex — *see also* Accessory
- kidney 753.3
- placenta — *see* Placenta, abnormal
- uterus 752.2

Duplication — *see also* Accessory
- anus 751.5
- aortic arch 747.21
- appendix 751.5
- biliary duct (any) 751.69
- bladder 753.8
- cecum 751.5
  - and appendix 751.5
- clitoris 752.49
- cystic duct 751.69
- digestive organs 751.8
- duodenum 751.5
- esophagus 750.4
- fallopian tube 752.19
- frontonasal process 756.0
- gallbladder 751.69
- ileum 751.5
- intestine (large) (small) 751.5
- jejunum 751.5
- kidney 753.3
- liver 751.69
- nose 748.1
- pancreas 751.7
- penis 752.69
- respiratory organs NEC 748.9
- salivary duct 750.22
- spinal cord (incomplete) 742.51
- stomach 750.7
- ureter 753.4
- vagina 752.49
- vas deferens 752.89
- vocal cords 748.3

Dupré's disease or syndrome (meningism) 781.6

Dupuytren's
- contraction 728.6
- disease (muscle contracture) 728.6
- fracture (closed) 824.4
  - ankle (closed) 824.4
    - open 824.5
  - fibula (closed) 824.4
    - open 824.5
  - open 824.5
  - radius (closed) 813.42
    - open 813.52
- muscle contracture 728.6

Durand-Nicolas-Favre disease (climatic bubo) 099.1

Duroziez's disease (congenital mitral stenosis) 746.5

Dust
- conjunctivitis 372.05
- reticulation (occupational) 504

Dutton's
- disease (trypanosomiasis) 086.9
- relapsing fever (West African) 087.1

Dwarf, dwarfism 259.4
- with infantilism (hypophyseal) 253.3
- achondroplastic 756.4
- Amsterdam 759.89
- bird-headed 759.89
- congenital 259.4
- constitutional 259.4
- hypophyseal 253.3
- infantile 259.4
- Levi type 253.3
- Lorain-Levi (pituitary) 253.3
- Lorain type (pituitary) 253.3
- metatropic 756.4
- nephrotic-glycosuric, with hypophosphatemic rickets 270.0
- nutritional 263.2
- ovarian 758.6
- pancreatic 577.8
- pituitary 253.3
- polydystrophic 277.5
- primordial 253.3
- psychosocial 259.4
- renal 588.0
  - with hypertension — *see* Hypertension, kidney
- Russell's (uterine dwarfism and craniofacial dysostosis) 759.89

Dyke-Young anemia or syndrome (acquired macrocytic hemolytic anemia) (secondary) (symptomatic) 283.9

Dynia abnormality (*see also* Defect, coagulation) 286.9

Dysacousis 388.40

Dysadrenocortism 255.9
- hyperfunction 255.3
- hypofunction 255.4

Dysarthria 784.5

Dysautonomia (*see also* Neuropathy, peripheral, autonomic) 337.9
- familial 742.8

Dysbarism 993.3

Dysbasia 719.7
- angiosclerotica intermittens 443.9
  - due to atherosclerosis 440.21
- hysterical 300.11
- lordotica (progressiva) 333.6
- nonorganic origin 307.9
- psychogenic 307.9

Dysbetalipoproteinemia (familial) 272.2

Dyscalculia 315.1

Dyschezia (*see also* Constipation) 564.00

Dyschondroplasia (with hemangiomata) 756.4
- Voorhoeve's 756.4

Dyschondrosteosis 756.59

Dyschromia 709.00

Dyscollagenosis 710.9

Dyscoria 743.41

Dyscraniopyophalangy 759.89

Dyscrasia
- blood 289.9
  - with antepartum hemorrhage 641.3 ☑
  - fetus or newborn NEC 776.9
  - hemorrhage, subungual 287.8
  - puerperal, postpartum 666.3 ☑
- ovary 256.8
- plasma cell 273.9
- pluriglandular 258.9
- polyglandular 258.9

Dysdiadochokinesia 781.3

Dysectasia, vesical neck 596.8

Dysendocrinism 259.9

Dysentery, dysenteric (bilious) (catarrhal) (diarrhea) (epidemic) (gangrenous) (hemorrhagic) (infectious) (sporadic) (tropical) (ulcerative) 009.0
- abscess, liver (*see also* Abscess, amebic) 006.3
- amebic (*see also* Amebiasis) 006.9
  - with abscess — *see* Abscess, amebic
  - acute 006.0

Dysentery, dysenteric — *continued*
- amebic (*see also* Amebiasis) — *continued*
  - carrier (suspected) of V02.2
  - chronic 006.1
- arthritis (*see also* Arthritis, due to, dysentery) 009.0 *[711.3]* ☑
  - bacillary 004.9 *[711.3]* ☑
- asylum 004.9
- bacillary 004.9
  - arthritis 004.9 *[711.3]* ☑
  - Boyd 004.2
  - Flexner 004.1
  - Schmitz (-Stutzer) 004.0
  - Shiga 004.0
  - Shigella 004.9
    - group A 004.0
    - group B 004.1
    - group C 004.2
    - group D 004.3
    - specified type NEC 004.8
  - Sonne 004.3
  - specified type NEC 004.8
- bacterium 004.9
- balantidial 007.0
- Balantidium coli 007.0
- Boyd's 004.2
- Chilomastix 007.8
- Chinese 004.9
- choleriform 001.1
- coccidial 007.2
- Dientamoeba fragilis 007.8
- due to specified organism NEC — *see* Enteritis, due to, by organism
- Embadomonas 007.8
- Endolimax nana — *see* Dysentery, amebic
- Entamoba, entamebic — *see* Dysentery, amebic
- Flexner's 004.1
- Flexner-Boyd 004.2
- giardial 007.1
- Giardia lamblia 007.1
- Hiss-Russell 004.1
- lamblia 007.1
- leishmanial 085.0
- malarial (*see also* Malaria) 084.6
- metazoal 127.9
- Monilia 112.89
- protozoal NEC 007.9
- Russell's 004.8
- salmonella 003.0
- schistosomal 120.1
- Schmitz (-Stutzer) 004.0
- Shiga 004.0
- Shigella NEC (*see also* Dysentery, bacillary) 004.9
  - boydii 004.2
  - dysenteriae 004.0
    - Schmitz 004.0
    - Shiga 004.0
  - flexneri 004.1
  - group A 004.0
  - group B 004.1
  - group C 004.2
  - group D 004.3
  - Schmitz 004.0
  - Shiga 004.0
  - Sonnei 004.3
- Sonne 004.3
- strongyloidiasis 127.2
- trichomonal 007.3
- tuberculous (*see also* Tuberculosis) 014.8 ☑
- viral (*see also* Enteritis, viral) 008.8

Dysequilibrium 780.4

Dysesthesia 782.0
- hysterical 300.11

Dysfibrinogenemia (congenital) (*see also* Defect, coagulation) 286.3

Dysfunction
- adrenal (cortical) 255.9
  - hyperfunction 255.3
  - hypofunction 255.4
- associated with sleep stages or arousal from sleep 780.56
  - nonorganic origin 307.47
- bladder NEC 596.59
- bleeding, uterus 626.8
- brain, minimal (*see also* Hyperkinesia) 314.9

☑ Additional Digit Required — Refer to the Tabular List (Numeric Code Section) for Additional Digit Selection
▶◀ Revised Text ● New Line ▲ Revised Code

- **Dystrophy, dystrophia** — *continued*
  - muscular 359.1
    - congenital (hereditary) 359.0
      - myotonic 359.2
    - distal 359.1
    - Duchenne's 359.1
    - Erb's 359.1
    - fascioscapulohumeral 359.1
    - Gowers' 359.1
    - hereditary (progressive) 359.1
    - Landouzy-Déjérine 359.1
    - limb-girdle 359.1
    - myotonic 359.2
    - progressive (hereditary) 359.1
      - Charcôt-Marie-Tooth 356.1
    - pseudohypertrophic (infantile) 359.1
  - myocardium, myocardial (*see also* Degeneration, myocardial) 429.1
  - myotonic 359.2
  - myotonica 359.2
  - nail 703.8
    - congenital 757.5
  - neurovascular (traumatic) (*see also* Neuropathy, peripheral, autonomic) 337.9
  - nutritional 263.9
  - ocular 359.1
  - oculocerebrorenal 270.8
  - oculopharyngeal 359.1
  - ovarian 620.8
  - papillary (and pigmentary) 701.1
  - pelvicrural atrophic 359.1
  - pigmentary (*see also* Acanthosis) 701.2
  - pituitary (gland) 253.8
  - polyglandular 258.8
  - posttraumatic sympathetic — *see* Dystrophy, sympathetic
  - progressive ophthalmoplegic 359.1
  - retina, retinal (hereditary) 362.70
    - albipunctate 362.74
    - Bruch's membrane 362.77
    - cone, progressive 362.75
    - hyaline 362.77
    - in
      - Bassen-Kornzweig syndrome 272.5 *[362.72]*
      - cerebroretinal lipidosis 330.1 *[362.71]*
      - Refsum's disease 356.3 *[362.72]*
      - systemic lipidosis 272.7 *[362.71]*
    - juvenile (Stargardt's) 362.75
    - pigmentary 362.74
    - pigment epithelium 362.76
    - progressive cone (-rod) 362.75
    - pseudoinflammatory foveal 362.77
    - rod, progressive 362.75
    - sensory 362.75
    - vitelliform 362.76
  - Salzmann's nodular 371.46
  - scapuloperoneal 359.1
  - skin NEC 709.9
  - sympathetic (posttraumatic) (reflex) 337.20
    - lower limb 337.22
    - specified site NEC 337.29
    - upper limb 337.21
  - tapetoretinal NEC 362.74
  - thoracic asphyxiating 756.4
  - unguium 703.8
    - congenital 757.5
  - vitreoretinal (primary) 362.73
    - secondary 362.66
  - vulva 624.0
- **Dysuria** 788.1
  - psychogenic 306.53

E

- **Eagle-Barrett syndrome** 756.71
- **Eales' disease** (syndrome) 362.18
- **Ear** — *see also* condition
  - ache 388.70
    - otogenic 388.71
    - referred 388.72
  - lop 744.29
  - piercing V50.3
  - swimmers' acute 380.12
  - tank 380.12
  - tropical 111.8 *[380.15]*
  - wax 380.4
- **Earache** 388.70
  - otogenic 388.71
  - referred 388.72
- **Early satiety** 780.94
- **Eaton-Lambert syndrome** (*see also* Neoplasm, by site, malignant) 199.1 *[358.1]*
- **Eberth's disease** (typhoid fever) 002.0
- **Ebstein's**
  - anomaly or syndrome (downward displacement, tricuspid valve into right ventricle) 746.2
  - disease (diabetes) 250.4 ☑ *[581.81]*
- **Eccentro-osteochondrodysplasia** 277.5
- **Ecchondroma** (M9210/0) — *see* Neoplasm, bone, benign
- **Ecchondrosis** (M9210/1) 238.0
- **Ecchordosis physaliphora** 756.0
- **Ecchymosis** (multiple) 459.89
  - conjunctiva 372.72
  - eye (traumatic) 921.0
  - eyelids (traumatic) 921.1
  - newborn 772.6
  - spontaneous 782.7
  - traumatic — *see* Contusion
- **Echinococciasis** — *see* Echinococcus
- **Echinococcosis** — *see* Echinococcus
- **Echinococcus** (infection) 122.9
  - granulosus 122.4
    - liver 122.0
    - lung 122.1
    - orbit 122.3 *[376.13]*
    - specified site NEC 122.3
    - thyroid 122.2
  - liver NEC 122.8
    - granulosus 122.0
    - multilocularis 122.5
  - lung NEC 122.9
    - granulosus 122.1
    - multilocularis 122.6
  - multilocularis 122.7
    - liver 122.5
    - specified site NEC 122.6
  - orbit 122.9 *[376.13]*
    - granulosus 122.3 *[376.13]*
    - multilocularis 122.6 *[376.13]*
  - specified site NEC 122.9
    - granulosus 122.3
    - multilocularis 122.6 *[376.13]*
  - thyroid NEC 122.9
    - granulosus 122.2
    - multilocularis 122.6
- **Echinorhynchiasis** 127.7
- **Echinostomiasis** 121.8
- **Echolalia** 784.69
- **ECHO virus infection** NEC 079.1
- **Eclampsia, eclamptic** (coma) (convulsions) (delirium) 780.39
  - female, child-bearing age NEC — *see* Eclampsia, pregnancy
  - gravidarum — *see* Eclampsia, pregnancy
  - male 780.39
  - not associated with pregnancy or childbirth 780.39
  - pregnancy, childbirth, or puerperium 642.6 ☑
    - with pre-existing hypertension 642.7 ☑
    - affecting fetus or newborn 760.0
  - uremic 586
- **Eclipse blindness** (total) 363.31
- **Economic circumstance affecting care** V60.9
  - specified type NEC V60.8
- **Economo's disease** (encephalitis lethargica) 049.8
- **Ectasia, ectasis**
  - aorta (*see also* Aneurysm, aorta) 441.9
    - ruptured 441.5
  - breast 610.4
  - capillary 448.9
  - cornea (marginal) (postinfectional) 371.71
  - duct (mammary) 610.4
  - kidney 593.89
  - mammary duct (gland) 610.4
  - papillary 448.9
  - renal 593.89
  - salivary gland (duct) 527.8
  - scar, cornea 371.71
  - sclera 379.11
- **Ecthyma** 686.8
  - contagiosum 051.2
  - gangrenosum 686.09
  - infectiosum 051.2
- **Ectocardia** 746.87
- **Ectodermal dysplasia, congenital** 757.31
- **Ectodermosis erosiva pluriorificialis** 695.1
- **Ectopic, ectopia** (congenital) 759.89
  - abdominal viscera 751.8
    - due to defect in anterior abdominal wall 756.79
  - ACTH syndrome 255.0
  - adrenal gland 759.1
  - anus 751.5
  - auricular beats 427.61
  - beats 427.60
  - bladder 753.5
  - bone and cartilage in lung 748.69
  - brain 742.4
  - breast tissue 757.6
  - cardiac 746.87
  - cerebral 742.4
  - cordis 746.87
  - endometrium 617.9
  - gallbladder 751.69
  - gastric mucosa 750.7
  - gestation — *see* Pregnancy, ectopic
  - heart 746.87
  - hormone secretion NEC 259.3
  - hyperparathyroidism 259.3
  - kidney (crossed) (intrathoracic) (pelvis) 753.3
    - in pregnancy or childbirth 654.4 ☑
      - causing obstructed labor 660.2 ☑
  - lens 743.37
  - lentis 743.37
  - mole — *see* Pregnancy, ectopic
  - organ or site NEC — *see* Malposition, congenital
  - ovary 752.0
  - pancreas, pancreatic tissue 751.7
  - pregnancy — *see* Pregnancy, ectopic
  - pupil 364.75
  - renal 753.3
  - sebaceous glands of mouth 750.26
  - secretion
    - ACTH 255.0
    - adrenal hormone 259.3
    - adrenalin 259.3
    - adrenocorticotropin 255.0
    - antidiuretic hormone (ADH) 259.3
    - epinephrine 259.3
    - hormone NEC 259.3
    - norepinephrine 259.3
    - pituitary (posterior) 259.3
  - spleen 759.0
  - testis 752.51
  - thyroid 759.2
  - ureter 753.4
  - ventricular beats 427.69
  - vesicae 753.5
- **Ectrodactyly** 755.4
  - finger (*see also* Absence, finger, congenital) 755.29
  - toe (*see also* Absence, toe, congenital) 755.39
- **Ectromelia** 755.4
  - lower limb 755.30
  - upper limb 755.20
- **Ectropion** 374.10
  - anus 569.49
  - cervix 622.0
    - with mention of cervicitis 616.0
  - cicatricial 374.14
  - congenital 743.62
  - eyelid 374.10
    - cicatricial 374.14
    - congenital 743.62
    - mechanical 374.12
    - paralytic 374.12
    - senile 374.11
    - spastic 374.13
  - iris (pigment epithelium) 364.54
  - lip (congenital) 750.26
    - acquired 528.5
  - mechanical 374.12
  - paralytic 374.12

☑ Additional Digit Required — Refer to the Tabular List (Numeric Code Section) for Additional Digit Selection
▶◀ Revised Text ● New Line ▲ Revised Code

☑ Additional Digit Required — Refer to the Tabular List (Numeric Code Section) for Additional Digit Selection

- **Encephalopathy** — *continued*
  - necrotizing, subacute 330.8
  - other specified type NEC 348.39
  - pellagrous 265.2
  - portal-systemic 572.2
  - postcontusional 310.2
  - posttraumatic 310.2
  - saturnine 984.9 *[323.7]*
  - septic 348.31
  - spongioform, subacute (viral) 046.1
  - subacute
    - necrotizing 330.8
    - spongioform 046.1
    - viral, spongioform 046.1
  - subcortical progressive (Schilder) 341.1
    - chronic (Binswanger's) 290.12
  - toxic 349.82
    - metabolic 348.31
  - traumatic (postconcussional) 310.2
    - current (*see also* Concussion, brain) 850.9
      - with skull fracture — *see* Fracture, skull, by site, with intracranial injury
  - vitamin B deficiency NEC 266.9
  - Wernicke's (superior hemorrhagic polioencephalitis) 265.1
- **Encephalorrhagia** (*see also* Hemorrhage, brain) 432.9
  - healed or old V12.59
  - late effect — *see* Late effect(s) (of) cerebrovascular disease
- **Encephalosis, posttraumatic** 310.2
- **Enchondroma** (M9220/0) — *see also* Neoplasm, bone, benign
  - multiple, congenital 756.4
- **Enchondromatosis** (cartilaginous) (congenital) (multiple) 756.4
- **Enchondroses, multiple** (cartilaginous) (congenital) 756.4
- **Encopresis** (*see also* Incontinence, feces) 787.6
  - nonorganic origin 307.7
- **Encounter for** — *see also* Admission for
  - administrative purpose only V68.9
    - referral of patient without examination or treatment V68.81
    - specified purpose NEC V68.89
  - chemotherapy, ▶antineoplastic◀ V58.11 ▲
  - dialysis
    - extracorporeal (renal) V56.0
    - peritoneal V56.8
  - end-of-life care V66.7
  - hospice care V66.7
  - immunotherapy, antineoplastic V58.12 ●
  - palliative care V66.7
  - paternity testing V70.4
  - radiotherapy V58.0
  - respirator ▶[ventilator]◀ dependence
    - during ●
      - mechanical failure V46.14 ●
      - power failure V46.12 ●
    - for weaning V46.13 ●
  - screening mammogram NEC V76.12
    - for high-risk patient V76.11
  - terminal care V66.7
  - weaning from respirator [ventilator] V46.13 ●
- **Encystment** — *see* Cyst
- **End-of-life care** V66.7
- **Endamebiasis** — *see* Amebiasis
- **Endamoeba** — *see* Amebiasis
- **Endarteritis** (bacterial, subacute) (infective) (septic) 447.6
  - brain, cerebral or cerebrospinal 437.4
    - late effect — *see* Late effect(s) (of) cerebrovascular disease
  - coronary (artery) — *see* Arteriosclerosis, coronary
  - deformans — *see* Arteriosclerosis
  - embolic (*see also* Embolism) 444.9
  - obliterans — *see also* Arteriosclerosis
    - pulmonary 417.8
  - pulmonary 417.8
  - retina 362.18
  - senile — *see* Arteriosclerosis
- **Endarteritis** — *continued*
  - syphilitic 093.89
    - brain or cerebral 094.89
    - congenital 090.5
    - spinal 094.89
  - tuberculous (*see also* Tuberculosis) 017.9 ☑
- **Endemic** — *see* condition
- **Endocarditis** (chronic) (indeterminate) (interstitial) (marantis) (nonbacterial thrombotic) (residual) (sclerotic) (sclerous) (senile) (valvular) 424.90
  - with
    - rheumatic fever (conditions classifiable to 390)
      - active — *see* Endocarditis, acute, rheumatic
      - inactive or quiescent (with chorea) 397.9
  - acute or subacute 421.9
    - rheumatic (aortic) (mitral) (pulmonary) (tricuspid) 391.1
      - with chorea (acute) (rheumatic) (Sydenham's) 392.0
  - aortic (heart) (nonrheumatic) (valve) 424.1
    - with
      - mitral (valve) disease 396.9
        - active or acute 391.1
          - with chorea (acute) (rheumatic) (Sydenham's) 392.0
          - bacterial 421.0
      - rheumatic fever (conditions classifiable to 390)
        - active — *see* Endocarditis, acute, rheumatic
        - inactive or quiescent (with chorea) 395.9
          - with mitral disease 396.9
    - acute or subacute 421.9
    - arteriosclerotic 424.1
    - congenital 746.89
    - hypertensive 424.1
    - rheumatic (chronic) (inactive) 395.9
      - with mitral (valve) disease 396.9
        - active or acute 391.1
          - with chorea (acute) (rheumatic) (Sydenham's) 392.0
      - active or acute 391.1
        - with chorea (acute) (rheumatic) (Sydenham's) 392.0
    - specified cause, except rheumatic 424.1
    - syphilitic 093.22
  - arteriosclerotic or due to arteriosclerosis 424.99
  - atypical verrucous (Libman-Sacks) 710.0 *[424.91]*
  - bacterial (acute) (any valve) (chronic) (subacute) 421.0
  - blastomycotic 116.0 *[421.1]*
  - candidal 112.81
  - congenital 425.3
  - constrictive 421.0
  - Coxsackie 074.22
  - due to
    - blastomycosis 116.0 *[421.1]*
    - candidiasis 112.81
    - Coxsackie (virus) 074.22
    - disseminated lupus erythematosus 710.0 *[424.91]*
    - histoplasmosis (*see also* Histoplasmosis) 115.94
    - hypertension (benign) 424.99
    - moniliasis 112.81
    - prosthetic cardiac valve 996.61
    - Q fever 083.0 *[421.1]*
    - serratia marcescens 421.0
    - typhoid (fever) 002.0 *[421.1]*
  - fetal 425.3
  - gonococcal 098.84
  - hypertensive 424.99
  - infectious or infective (acute) (any valve) (chronic) (subacute) 421.0
  - lenta (acute) (any valve) (chronic) (subacute) 421.0
  - Libman-Sacks 710.0 *[424.91]*
  - Loeffler's (parietal fibroplastic) 421.0
  - malignant (acute) (any valve) (chronic) (subacute) 421.0
- **Endocarditis** — *continued*
  - meningococcal 036.42
  - mitral (chronic) (double) (fibroid) (heart) (inactive) (valve) (with chorea) 394.9
    - with
      - aortic (valve) disease 396.9
        - active or acute 391.1
          - with chorea (acute) (rheumatic) (Sydenham's) 392.0
      - rheumatic fever (conditions classifiable to 390)
        - active — *see* Endocarditis, acute, rheumatic
        - inactive or quiescent (with chorea) 394.9
          - with aortic valve disease 396.9
    - active or acute 391.1
      - with chorea (acute) (rheumatic) (Sydenham's) 392.0
        - bacterial 421.0
    - arteriosclerotic 424.0
    - congenital 746.89
    - hypertensive 424.0
    - nonrheumatic 424.0
      - acute or subacute 421.9
    - syphilitic 093.21
  - monilial 112.81
  - mycotic (acute) (any valve) (chronic) (subacute) 421.0
  - pneumococcic (acute) (any valve) (chronic) (subacute) 421.0
  - pulmonary (chronic) (heart) (valve) 424.3
    - with
      - rheumatic fever (conditions classifiable to 390)
        - active — *see* Endocarditis, acute, rheumatic
        - inactive or quiescent (with chorea) 397.1
    - acute or subacute 421.9
      - rheumatic 391.1
        - with chorea (acute) (rheumatic) (Sydenham's) 392.0
    - arteriosclerotic or due to arteriosclerosis 424.3
    - congenital 746.09
    - hypertensive or due to hypertension (benign) 424.3
    - rheumatic (chronic) (inactive) (with chorea) 397.1
      - active or acute 391.1
        - with chorea (acute) (rheumatic) (Sydenham's) 392.0
    - syphilitic 093.24
  - purulent (acute) (any valve) (chronic) (subacute) 421.0
  - rheumatic (chronic) (inactive) (with chorea) 397.9
    - active or acute (aortic) (mitral) (pulmonary) (tricuspid) 391.1
      - with chorea (acute) (rheumatic) (Sydenham's) 392.0
  - septic (acute) (any valve) (chronic) (subacute) 421.0
  - specified cause, except rheumatic 424.99
  - streptococcal (acute) (any valve) (chronic) (subacute) 421.0
  - subacute — *see* Endocarditis, acute
  - suppurative (any valve) (acute) (chronic) (subacute) 421.0
  - syphilitic NEC 093.20
  - toxic (*see also* Endocarditis, acute) 421.9
  - tricuspid (chronic) (heart) (inactive) (rheumatic) (valve) (with chorea) 397.0
    - with
      - rheumatic fever (conditions classifiable to 390)
        - active — *see* Endocarditis, acute, rheumatic
        - inactive or quiescent (with chorea) 397.0
    - active or acute 391.1
      - with chorea (acute) (rheumatic) (Sydenham's) 392.0
    - arteriosclerotic 424.2
    - congenital 746.89
    - hypertensive 424.2

- **Epicondylitis** (elbow) (lateral) 726.32
  - medial 726.31
- **Epicystitis** (*see also* Cystitis) 595.9
- **Epidemic** — *see* condition
- **Epidermidalization, cervix** — *see* condition
- **Epidermidization, cervix** — *see* condition
- **Epidermis, epidermal** — *see* condition
- **Epidermization, cervix** — *see* condition
- **Epidermodysplasia verruciformis** 078.19
- **Epidermoid**
  - cholesteatoma — *see* Cholesteatoma
  - inclusion (*see also* Cyst, skin) 706.2
- **Epidermolysis**
  - acuta (combustiformis) (toxica) 695.1
  - bullosa 757.39
  - necroticans combustiformis 695.1
    - due to drug
      - correct substance properly administered 695.1
      - overdose or wrong substance given or taken 977.9
        - specified drug — *see* Table of Drugs and Chemicals
- **Epidermophytid** — *see* Dermatophytosis
- **Epidermophytosis** (infected) — *see* Dermatophytosis
- **Epidermosis, ear** (middle) (*see also* Cholesteatoma) 385.30
- **Epididymis** — *see* condition
- **Epididymitis** (nonvenereal) 604.90
  - with abscess 604.0
  - acute 604.99
  - blennorrhagic (acute) 098.0
    - chronic or duration of 2 months or over 098.2
  - caseous (*see also* Tuberculosis) 016.4 ☑
  - chlamydial 099.54
  - diphtheritic 032.89 *[604.91]*
  - filarial 125.9 *[604.91]*
  - gonococcal (acute) 098.0
    - chronic or duration of 2 months or over 098.2
  - recurrent 604.99
  - residual 604.99
  - syphilitic 095.8 *[604.91]*
  - tuberculous (*see also* Tuberculosis) 016.4 ☑
- **Epididymo-orchitis** (*see also* Epididymitis) 604.90
  - with abscess 604.0
  - chlamydial 099.54
  - gonococcal (acute) 098.13
    - chronic or duration of 2 months or over 098.33
- **Epidural** — *see* condition
- **Epigastritis** (*see also* Gastritis) 535.5 ☑
- **Epigastrium, epigastric** — *see* condition
- **Epigastrocele** (*see also* Hernia, epigastric) 553.29
- **Epiglottiditis** (acute) 464.30
  - with obstruction 464.31
  - chronic 476.1
  - viral 464.30
    - with obstruction 464.31
- **Epiglottis** — *see* condition
- **Epiglottitis** (acute) 464.30
  - with obstruction 464.31
  - chronic 476.1
  - viral 464.30
    - with obstruction 464.31
- **Epignathus** 759.4
- **Epilepsia**
  - partialis continua (*see also* Epilepsy) 345.7 ☑
  - procursiva (*see also* Epilepsy) 345.8 ☑
- **Epilepsy, epileptic** (idiopathic) 345.9 ☑

> *Note — use the following fifth-digit subclassification with categories 345.0, 345.1, 345.4–345.9:*
>
> 0 *without mention of intractable epilepsy*
>
> 1 *with intractable epilepsy*

  - abdominal 345.5 ☑
  - absence (attack) 345.0 ☑

- **Epilepsy, epileptic** — *continued*
  - akinetic 345.0 ☑
    - psychomotor 345.4 ☑
  - automatism 345.4 ☑
  - autonomic diencephalic 345.5 ☑
  - brain 345.9 ☑
  - Bravais-Jacksonian 345.5 ☑
  - cerebral 345.9 ☑
  - climacteric 345.9 ☑
  - clonic 345.1 ☑
  - clouded state 345.9 ☑
  - coma 345.3
  - communicating 345.4 ☑
  - congenital 345.9 ☑
  - convulsions 345.9 ☑
  - cortical (focal) (motor) 345.5 ☑
  - cursive (running) 345.8 ☑
  - cysticercosis 123.1
  - deterioration
    - with behavioral disturbance 345.9 ☑ *[294.11]*
    - without behavioral disturbance 345.9 ☑ *[294.10]*
  - due to syphilis 094.89
  - equivalent 345.5 ☑
  - fit 345.9 ☑
  - focal (motor) 345.5 ☑
  - gelastic 345.8 ☑
  - generalized 345.9 ☑
    - convulsive 345.1 ☑
    - flexion 345.1 ☑
    - nonconvulsive 345.0 ☑
  - grand mal (idiopathic) 345.1 ☑
  - Jacksonian (motor) (sensory) 345.5 ☑
  - Kojevnikoff's, Kojevnikov's, Kojewnikoff's 345.7 ☑
  - laryngeal 786.2
  - limbic system 345.4 ☑
  - major (motor) 345.1 ☑
  - minor 345.0 ☑
  - mixed (type) 345.9 ☑
  - motor partial 345.5 ☑
  - musicogenic 345.1 ☑
  - myoclonus, myoclonic 345.1 ☑
    - progressive (familial) 333.2
  - nonconvulsive, generalized 345.0 ☑
  - parasitic NEC 123.9
  - partial (focalized) 345.5 ☑
    - with
      - impairment of consciousness 345.4 ☑
      - memory and ideational disturbances 345.4 ☑
    - abdominal type 345.5 ☑
    - motor type 345.5 ☑
    - psychomotor type 345.4 ☑
    - psychosensory type 345.4 ☑
    - secondarily generalized 345.4 ☑
    - sensory type 345.5 ☑
    - somatomotor type 345.5 ☑
    - somatosensory type 345.5 ☑
    - temporal lobe type 345.4 ☑
    - visceral type 345.5 ☑
    - visual type 345.5 ☑
  - peripheral 345.9 ☑
  - petit mal 345.0 ☑
  - photokinetic 345.8 ☑
  - progressive myoclonic (familial) 333.2
  - psychic equivalent 345.5 ☑
  - psychomotor 345.4 ☑
  - psychosensory 345.4 ☑
  - reflex 345.1 ☑
  - seizure 345.9 ☑
  - senile 345.9 ☑
  - sensory-induced 345.5 ☑
  - sleep (*see also* Narcolepsy) 347.00
  - somatomotor type 345.5 ☑
  - somatosensory 345.5 ☑
  - specified type NEC 345.8 ☑
  - status (grand mal) 345.3
    - focal motor 345.7 ☑
    - petit mal 345.2
    - psychomotor 345.7 ☑
    - temporal lobe 345.7 ☑
  - symptomatic 345.9 ☑
  - temporal lobe 345.4 ☑
  - tonic (-clonic) 345.1 ☑

- **Epilepsy, epileptic** — *continued*
  - traumatic (injury unspecified) 907.0
    - injury specified — *see* Late, effect (of) specified injury
  - twilight 293.0
  - uncinate (gyrus) 345.4 ☑
  - Unverricht (-Lundborg) (familial myoclonic) 333.2
  - visceral 345.5 ☑
  - visual 345.5 ☑
- **Epileptiform**
  - convulsions 780.39
  - seizure 780.39
- **Epiloia** 759.5
- **Epimenorrhea** 626.2
- **Epipharyngitis** (*see also* Nasopharyngitis) 460
- **Epiphora** 375.20
  - due to
    - excess lacrimation 375.21
    - insufficient drainage 375.22
- **Epiphyseal arrest** 733.91
  - femoral head 732.2
- **Epiphyseolysis, epiphysiolysis** (*see also* Osteochondrosis) 732.9
- **Epiphysitis** (*see also* Osteochondrosis) 732.9
  - juvenile 732.6
  - marginal (Scheuermann's) 732.0
  - os calcis 732.5
  - syphilitic (congenital) 090.0
  - vertebral (Scheuermann's) 732.0
- **Epiplocele** (*see also* Hernia) 553.9
- **Epiploitis** (*see also* Peritonitis) 567.9
- **Epiplosarcomphalocele** (*see also* Hernia, umbilicus) 553.1
- **Episcleritis** 379.00
  - gouty 274.89 *[379.09]*
  - nodular 379.02
  - periodica fugax 379.01
    - angioneurotic — *see* Edema, angioneurotic
  - specified NEC 379.09
  - staphylococcal 379.00
  - suppurative 379.00
  - syphilitic 095.0
  - tuberculous (*see also* Tuberculosis) 017.3 ☑ *[379.09]*
- **Episode**
  - brain (*see also* Disease, cerebrovascular, acute) 436
  - cerebral (*see also* Disease, cerebrovascular, acute) 436
  - depersonalization (in neurotic state) 300.6
  - hyporesponsive 780.09
  - psychotic (*see also* Psychosis) 298.9
    - organic, transient 293.9
  - schizophrenic (acute) NEC (*see also* Schizophrenia) 295.4 ☑
- **Epispadias**
  - female 753.8
  - male 752.62
- **Episplenitis** 289.59
- **Epistaxis** (multiple) 784.7
  - hereditary 448.0
  - vicarious menstruation 625.8
- **Epithelioma** (malignant) (M8011/3) — *see also* Neoplasm, by site, malignant
  - adenoides cysticum (M8100/0) — *see* Neoplasm, skin, benign
  - basal cell (M8090/3) — *see* Neoplasm, skin, malignant
  - benign (M8011/0) — *see* Neoplasm, by site, benign
  - Bowen's (M8081/2) — *see* Neoplasm, skin, in situ
  - calcifying (benign) (Malherbe's) (M8110/0) — *see* Neoplasm, skin, benign
  - external site — *see* Neoplasm, skin, malignant
  - intraepidermal, Jadassohn (M8096/0) — *see* Neoplasm, skin, benign
  - squamous cell (M8070/3) — *see* Neoplasm, by site, malignant
- **Epitheliopathy**
  - pigment, retina 363.15
  - posterior multifocal placoid (acute) 363.15

Erythrogenesis imperfecta 284.0
Erythroleukemia (M9840/3) 207.0 ☑
Erythromelalgia 443.82 ▲
Erythromelia 701.8
Erythropenia 285.9
Erythrophagocytosis 289.9
Erythrophobia 300.23
Erythroplakia
- oral mucosa 528.79
- tongue 528.79

Erythroplasia (Queyrat) (M8080/2)
- specified site — *see* Neoplasm, skin, in situ
- unspecified site 233.5

Erythropoiesis, idiopathic ineffective 285.0
Escaped beats, heart 427.60
- postoperative 997.1

Esoenteritis — *see* Enteritis
Esophagalgia 530.89
Esophagectasis 530.89
- due to cardiospasm 530.0

Esophagismus 530.5
Esophagitis (alkaline) (chemical) (chronic) (infectional) (necrotic) (peptic) (postoperative) (regurgitant) 530.10
- acute 530.12
- candidal 112.84
- reflux 530.11
- specified NEC 530.19
- tuberculous (*see also* Tuberculosis) 017.8 ☑
- ulcerative 530.19

Esophagocele 530.6
Esophagodynia 530.89
Esophagomalacia 530.89
Esophagoptosis 530.89
Esophagospasm 530.5
Esophagostenosis 530.3
Esophagostomiasis 127.7
Esophagostomy
- complication 530.87 ▲
  - infection 530.86
  - malfunctioning 530.87
  - mechanical 530.87

Esophagotracheal — *see* condition
Esophagus — *see* condition
Esophoria 378.41
- convergence, excess 378.84
- divergence, insufficiency 378.85

Esotropia (nonaccommodative) 378.00
- accommodative 378.35
- alternating 378.05
  - with
    - A pattern 378.06
    - specified noncomitancy NEC 378.08
    - V pattern 378.07
    - X pattern 378.08
    - Y pattern 378.08
  - intermittent 378.22
- intermittent 378.20
  - alternating 378.22
  - monocular 378.21
- monocular 378.01
  - with
    - A pattern 378.02
    - specified noncomitancy NEC 378.04
    - V pattern 378.03
    - X pattern 378.04
    - Y pattern 378.04
  - intermittent 378.21

Espundia 085.5
Essential — *see* condition
Esterapenia 289.89
Esthesioneuroblastoma (M9522/3) 160.0
Esthesioneurocytoma (M9521/3) 160.0
Esthesioneuroepithelioma (M9523/3) 160.0
Esthiomene 099.1
Estivo-autumnal
- fever 084.0
- malaria 084.0

Estrangement V61.0
Estriasis 134.0
Ethanolaminuria 270.8
Ethanolism (*see also* Alcoholism) 303.9 ☑
Ether dependence, dependency (*see also* Dependence) 304.6 ☑
Etherism (*see also* Dependence) 304.6 ☑
Ethmoid, ethmoidal — *see* condition
Ethmoiditis (chronic) (nonpurulent) (purulent) (*see also* Sinusitis, ethmoidal) 473.2
- influenzal 487.1
- Woakes' 471.1

Ethylism (*see also* Alcoholism) 303.9 ☑
Eulenburg's disease (congenital paramyotonia) 359.2
Eunuchism 257.2
Eunuchoidism 257.2
- hypogonadotropic 257.2

European blastomycosis 117.5
Eustachian — *see* condition
Euthyroid sick syndrome 790.94
Euthyroidism 244.9
Evaluation
- fetal lung maturity 659.8 ☑
- for suspected condition (*see also* Observation) V71.9
  - abuse V71.81
  - exposure
    - anthrax V71.82
    - biologic agent NEC V71.83
    - SARS V71.83
  - neglect V71.81
  - newborn — *see* Observation, suspected, condition, newborn
  - specified condition NEC V71.89
- mental health V70.2
  - requested by authority V70.1
- nursing care V63.8
- social service V63.8

▶**Evans'**◀ **syndrome** (thrombocytopenic purpura) 287.32 ▲
Eventration
- colon into chest — *see* Hernia, diaphragm
- diaphragm (congenital) 756.6

Eversion
- bladder 596.8
- cervix (uteri) 622.0
  - with mention of cervicitis 616.0
- foot NEC 736.79
  - congenital 755.67
- lacrimal punctum 375.51
- punctum lacrimale (postinfectional) (senile) 375.51
- ureter (meatus) 593.89
- urethra (meatus) 599.84
- uterus 618.1
  - complicating delivery 665.2 ☑
    - affecting fetus or newborn 763.89
  - puerperal, postpartum 674.8 ☑

Evidence
- of malignancy
  - cytologic
    - without histologic confirmation 795.04

Evisceration
- birth injury 767.8
- bowel (congenital) — *see* Hernia, ventral
- congenital (*see also* Hernia, ventral) 553.29
- operative wound 998.32
- traumatic NEC 869.1
  - eye 871.3

Evulsion — *see* Avulsion
Ewing's
- angioendothelioma (M9260/3) — *see* Neoplasm, bone, malignant
- sarcoma (M9260/3) — *see* Neoplasm, bone, malignant
- tumor (M9260/3) — *see* Neoplasm, bone, malignant

Exaggerated lumbosacral angle (with impinging spine) 756.12
Examination (general) (routine) (of) (for) V70.9
- allergy V72.7
- annual V70.0
- cardiovascular preoperative V72.81

Examination — *continued*
- cervical Papanicolaou smear V76.2
  - as a part of routine gynecological examination V72.31
  - to confirm findings of recent normal smear following initial abnormal smear V72.32
- child care (routine) V20.2
- clinical research investigation (normal control patient) (participant) V70.7
- dental V72.2
- developmental testing (child) (infant) V20.2
- donor (potential) V70.8
- ear V72.1
- eye V72.0
- following
  - accident (motor vehicle) V71.4
  - alleged rape or seduction (victim or culprit) V71.5
  - inflicted injury (victim or culprit) NEC V71.6
  - rape or seduction, alleged (victim or culprit) V71.5
  - treatment (for) V67.9
    - combined V67.6
    - fracture V67.4
    - involving high-risk medication NEC V67.51
    - mental disorder V67.3
    - specified condition NEC V67.59
- follow-up (routine) (following) V67.9
  - cancer chemotherapy V67.2
  - chemotherapy V67.2
  - disease NEC V67.59
  - high-risk medication NEC V67.51
  - injury NEC V67.59
  - population survey V70.6
  - postpartum V24.2
  - psychiatric V67.3
  - psychotherapy V67.3
  - radiotherapy V67.1
  - specified surgery NEC V67.09
  - surgery V67.00
    - vaginal pap smear V67.01
- gynecological V72.31
  - for contraceptive maintenance V25.40
    - intrauterine device V25.42
    - pill V25.41
    - specified method NEC V25.49
- health (of)
  - armed forces personnel V70.5
  - checkup V70.0
  - child, routine V20.2
  - defined subpopulation NEC V70.5
  - inhabitants of institutions V70.5
  - occupational V70.5
  - pre-employment screening V70.5
  - preschool children V70.5
    - for admission to school V70.3
  - prisoners V70.5
    - for entrance into prison V70.3
  - prostitutes V70.5
  - refugees V70.5
  - school children V70.5
  - students V70.5
- hearing V72.1
- infant V20.2
- laboratory V72.6
- lactating mother V24.1
- medical (for) (of) V70.9
  - administrative purpose NEC V70.3
  - admission to
    - old age home V70.3
    - prison V70.3
    - school V70.3
  - adoption V70.3
  - armed forces personnel V70.5
  - at health care facility V70.0
  - camp V70.3
  - child, routine V20.2
  - clinical research (control) (normal comparison) (participant) V70.7
  - defined subpopulation NEC V70.5
  - donor (potential) V70.8
  - driving license V70.3
  - general V70.9
    - routine V70.0
    - specified reason NEC V70.8

Examination — *continued*
  medical — *continued*
    immigration V70.3
    inhabitants of institutions V70.5
    insurance certification V70.3
    marriage V70.3
    medicolegal reasons V70.4
    naturalization V70.3
    occupational V70.5
    population survey V70.6
    pre-employment V70.5
    preschool children V70.5
      for admission to school V70.3
    prison V70.3
    prisoners V70.5
      for entrance into prison V70.3
    prostitutes V70.5
    refugees V70.5
    school children V70.5
    specified reason NEC V70.8
    sport competition V70.3
    students V70.5
  medicolegal reason V70.4
  pelvic (annual) (periodic) V72.31
  periodic (annual) (routine) V70.0
  postpartum
    immediately after delivery V24.0
    routine follow-up V24.2
  pregnancy (unconfirmed) (possible) V72.40
    negative result V72.41
    positive result V72.42 ●
  prenatal V22.1
    first pregnancy V22.0
    high-risk pregnancy V23.9
      specified problem NEC V23.89
  preoperative V72.84
    cardiovascular V72.81
    respiratory V72.82
    specified NEC V72.83
  preprocedural V72.84 ●
    cardiovascular V72.81 ●
    general physical V72.83 ●
    respiratory V72.82 ●
    specified NEC V72.83 ●
  psychiatric V70.2
    follow-up not needing further care V67.3
    requested by authority V70.1
  radiological NEC V72.5
  respiratory preoperative V72.82
  screening — *see* Screening
  sensitization V72.7
  skin V72.7
    hypersensitivity V72.7
  special V72.9
  specified type or reason NEC V72.85
    preoperative V72.83
      specified NEC V72.83
  teeth V72.2
  vaginal Papanicolaou smear V76.47
    following hysterectomy for malignant condition V67.01
  victim or culprit following
    alleged rape or seduction V71.5
    inflicted injury NEC V71.6
  vision V72.0
  well baby V20.2

Exanthem, exanthema (*see also* Rash) 782.1
  Boston 048
  epidemic, with meningitis 048
  lichenoid psoriasiform 696.2
  subitum 057.8
  viral, virus NEC 057.9
    specified type NEC 057.8

Excess, excessive, excessively
  alcohol level in blood 790.3
  carbohydrate tissue, localized 278.1
  carotene (dietary) 278.3
  cold 991.9
    specified effect NEC 991.8
  convergence 378.84
  crying 780.95 ▲
    of infant (baby) 780.92 ●
  development, breast 611.1
  diaphoresis (*see also* Hyperhidrosis) 780.8
  distance, interarch 524.28
  divergence 378.85

Excess, excessive, excessively — *continued*
  drinking (alcohol) NEC (*see also* Abuse, drugs, nondependent) 305.0 ☑
    continual (*see also* Alcoholism) 303.9 ☑
    habitual (*see also* Alcoholism) 303.9 ☑
  eating 783.6
  eyelid fold (congenital) 743.62
  fat 278.02 ▲
    in heart (*see also* Degeneration, myocardial) 429.1
    tissue, localized 278.1
  foreskin 605
  gas 787.3
  gastrin 251.5
  glucagon 251.4
  heat (*see also* Heat) 992.9
  horizontal overlap 524.26
  interarch distance 524.28
  interocclusal distance of teeth 524.37
  large
    colon 564.7
      congenital 751.3
    fetus or infant 766.0
      with obstructed labor 660.1 ☑
      affecting management of pregnancy 656.6 ☑
      causing disproportion 653.5 ☑
    newborn (weight of 4500 grams or more) 766.0
    organ or site, congenital NEC — *see* Anomaly, specified type NEC
  lid fold (congenital) 743.62
  long
    colon 751.5
    organ or site, congenital NEC — *see* Anomaly, specified type NEC
    umbilical cord (entangled)
      affecting fetus or newborn 762.5
      in pregnancy or childbirth 663.3 ☑
        with compression 663.2 ☑
  menstruation 626.2
  number of teeth 520.1
    causing crowding 524.31
  nutrients (dietary) NEC 783.6
  potassium (K) 276.7
  salivation (*see also* Ptyalism) 527.7
  secretion — *see also* Hypersecretion
    milk 676.6 ☑
    sputum 786.4
    sweat (*see also* Hyperhidrosis) 780.8
  short
    organ or site, congenital NEC — *see* Anomaly, specified type NEC
    umbilical cord
      affecting fetus or newborn 762.6
      in pregnancy or childbirth 663.4 ☑
  skin NEC 701.9
    eyelid 743.62
      acquired 374.30
  sodium (Na) 276.0
  spacing of teeth 524.32
  sputum 786.4
  sweating (*see also* Hyperhidrosis) 780.8
  tearing (ducts) (eye) (*see also* Epiphora) 375.20
  thirst 783.5
    due to deprivation of water 994.3
  tuberosity 524.07
  vitamin
    A (dietary) 278.2
      administered as drug (chronic) (prolonged excessive intake) 278.2
        reaction to sudden overdose 963.5
    D (dietary) 278.4
      administered as drug (chronic) (prolonged excessive intake) 278.4
        reaction to sudden overdose 963.5
  weight 278.02 ▲
    gain 783.1
      of pregnancy 646.1 ☑
    loss 783.21

Excitability, abnormal, under minor stress 309.29

Excitation
  catatonic (*see also* Schizophrenia) 295.2 ☑
  psychogenic 298.1
  reactive (from emotional stress, psychological trauma) 298.1

Excitement
  manic (*see also* Psychosis, affective) 296.0 ☑
    recurrent episode 296.1 ☑
    single episode 296.0 ☑
  mental, reactive (from emotional stress, psychological trauma) 298.1
  state, reactive (from emotional stress, psychological trauma) 298.1

Excluded pupils 364.76

Excoriation (traumatic) (*see also* Injury, superficial, by site) 919.8
  neurotic 698.4

Excyclophoria 378.44

Excyclotropia 378.33

Exencephalus, exencephaly 742.0

Exercise
  breathing V57.0
  remedial NEC V57.1
  therapeutic NEC V57.1

Exfoliation, teeth due to systemic causes 525.0

Exfoliative — *see also* condition
  dermatitis 695.89

Exhaustion, exhaustive (physical NEC) 780.79
  battle (*see also* Reaction, stress, acute) 308.9
  cardiac (*see also* Failure, heart) 428.9
  delirium (*see also* Reaction, stress, acute) 308.9
  due to
    cold 991.8
    excessive exertion 994.5
    exposure 994.4
  fetus or newborn 779.89
  heart (*see also* Failure, heart) 428.9
  heat 992.5
    due to
      salt depletion 992.4
      water depletion 992.3
  manic (*see also* Psychosis, affective) 296.0 ☑
    recurrent episode 296.1 ☑
    single episode 296.0 ☑
  maternal, complicating delivery 669.8 ☑
    affecting fetus or newborn 763.89
  mental 300.5
  myocardium, myocardial (*see also* Failure, heart) 428.9
  nervous 300.5
  old age 797
  postinfectional NEC 780.79
  psychogenic 300.5
  psychosis (*see also* Reaction, stress, acute) 308.9
  senile 797
    dementia 290.0

Exhibitionism (sexual) 302.4

Exomphalos 756.79

Exophoria 378.42
  convergence, insufficiency 378.83
  divergence, excess 378.85

Exophthalmic
  cachexia 242.0 ☑
  goiter 242.0 ☑
  ophthalmoplegia 242.0 ☑ *[376.22]*

Exophthalmos 376.30
  congenital 743.66
  constant 376.31
  endocrine NEC 259.9 *[376.22]*
  hyperthyroidism 242.0 ☑ *[376.21]*
  intermittent NEC 376.34
  malignant 242.0 ☑ *[376.21]*
  pulsating 376.35
    endocrine NEC 259.9 *[376.22]*
  thyrotoxic 242.0 ☑ *[376.21]*

Exostosis 726.91
  cartilaginous (M9210/0) — *see* Neoplasm, bone, benign
  congenital 756.4
  ear canal, external 380.81
  gonococcal 098.89
  hip 726.5
  intracranial 733.3
  jaw (bone) 526.81
  luxurians 728.11
  multiple (cancellous) (congenital) (hereditary) 756.4

☑ Additional Digit Required — Refer to the Tabular List (Numeric Code Section) for Additional Digit Selection
▶◀ Revised Text ● New Line ▲ Revised Code

F

- **Failure, failed** — *continued*
  - heart — *continued*
    - high output NEC 428.9
    - hypertensive (*see also* Hypertension, heart) 402.91
      - with renal disease (*see also* Hypertension, cardiorenal) 404.91
        - with renal failure 404.93
      - benign 402.11
      - malignant 402.01
    - left (ventricular) (*see also* Failure, ventricular, left) 428.1
      - with right-sided failure (see also Failure, heart) 428.0
    - low output (syndrome) NEC 428.9
    - organic — *see* Disease, heart
    - postoperative (immediate) 997.1
      - long term effect of cardiac surgery 429.4
    - rheumatic (chronic) (congestive) (inactive) 398.91
    - right (secondary to left heart failure, conditions classifiable to 428.1) (ventricular) (*see also* Failure, heart) 428.0
    - senile 797
    - specified during or due to a procedure 997.1
      - long-term effect of cardiac surgery 429.4
    - systolic 428.20
      - acute 428.21
      - acute on chronic 428.23
      - chronic 428.22
    - thyrotoxic (*see also* Thyrotoxicosis) 242.9 ☑ *[425.7]*
    - valvular — *see* Endocarditis
  - hepatic 572.8
    - acute 570
    - due to a procedure 997.4
  - hepatorenal 572.4
  - hypertensive heart (*see also* Hypertension, heart) 402.91
    - benign 402.11
    - malignant 402.01
  - induction (of labor) 659.1 ☑
    - abortion (legal) (*see also* Abortion, failed) 638.9
    - affecting fetus or newborn 763.89
    - by oxytocic drugs 659.1 ☑
    - instrumental 659.0 ☑
    - mechanical 659.0 ☑
    - medical 659.1 ☑
    - surgical 659.0 ☑
  - initial alveolar expansion, newborn 770.4
  - involution, thymus (gland) 254.8
  - kidney — *see* Failure, renal
  - lactation 676.4 ☑
  - Leydig's cell, adult 257.2
  - liver 572.8
    - acute 570
  - medullary 799.89
  - mitral — *see* Endocarditis, mitral
  - myocardium, myocardial (*see also* Failure, heart) 428.9
    - chronic (*see also* Failure, heart) 428.0
    - congestive (*see also* Failure, heart) 428.0
  - ovarian (primary) 256.39
    - iatrogenic 256.2
    - postablative 256.2
    - postirradiation 256.2
    - postsurgical 256.2
  - ovulation 628.0
  - prerenal 788.9
  - renal 586
    - with
      - abortion — *see* Abortion, by type, with renal failure
      - ectopic pregnancy (*see also* categories 633.0-633.9) 639.3
      - edema (*see also* Nephrosis) 581.9
      - hypertension (*see also* Hypertension, kidney) 403.91
      - hypertensive heart disease (conditions classifiable to 402) 404.92
        - with heart failure 404.93
        - benign 404.12
          - with heart failure 404.13
        - malignant 404.02
          - with heart failure 404.03

- **Failure, failed** — *continued*
  - renal — *continued*
    - with — *continued*
      - molar pregnancy (*see also* categories 630-632) 639.3
      - tubular necrosis (acute) 584.5
    - acute 584.9
      - with lesion of
        - necrosis
          - cortical (renal) 584.6
          - medullary (renal) (papillary) 584.7
          - tubular 584.5
        - specified pathology NEC 584.8
    - chronic 585.9 ▲
      - hypertensive or with hypertension (*see also* Hypertension, kidney) 403.91
    - due to a procedure 997.5
    - following
      - abortion 639.3
      - crushing 958.5
      - ectopic or molar pregnancy 639.3
      - labor and delivery (acute) 669.3 ☑
    - hypertensive (*see also* Hypertension, kidney) 403.91
    - puerperal, postpartum 669.3 ☑
  - respiration, respiratory 518.81
    - acute 518.81
    - acute and chronic 518.84
    - center 348.8
      - newborn 770.84
    - chronic 518.83
    - due to trauma, surgery or shock 518.5
    - newborn 770.84
  - rotation
    - cecum 751.4
    - colon 751.4
    - intestine 751.4
    - kidney 753.3
  - segmentation — *see also* Fusion
    - fingers (*see also* Syndactylism, fingers) 755.11
    - toes (*see also* Syndactylism, toes) 755.13
  - seminiferous tubule, adult 257.2
  - senile (general) 797
    - with psychosis 290.20
  - testis, primary (seminal) 257.2
  - to progress 661.2 ☑
  - to thrive
    - adult 783.7
    - child 783.41
  - transplant 996.80
    - bone marrow 996.85
    - organ (immune or nonimmune cause) 996.80
      - bone marrow 996.85
      - heart 996.83
      - intestines 996.87
      - kidney 996.81
      - liver 996.82
      - lung 996.84
      - pancreas 996.86
      - specified NEC 996.89
    - skin 996.52
      - artificial 996.55
      - decellularized allodermis 996.55
      - temporary allograft or pigskin graft — *omit code*
  - trial of labor NEC 660.6 ☑
    - affecting fetus or newborn 763.1
  - tubal ligation 998.89
  - urinary 586
  - vacuum extraction
    - abortion — *see* Abortion, failed
    - delivery NEC 660.7 ☑
      - affecting fetus or newborn 763.1
  - vasectomy 998.89
  - ventouse NEC 660.7 ☑
    - affecting fetus or newborn 763.1
  - ventricular (*see also* Failure, heart) 428.9
    - left 428.1
      - with rheumatic fever (conditions classifiable to 390)
        - active 391.8
          - with chorea 392.0
        - inactive or quiescent (with chorea) 398.91

- **Failure, failed** — *continued*
  - ventricular (*see also* Failure, heart) — *continued*
    - left — *continued*
      - hypertensive (*see also* Hypertension, heart) 402.91
        - benign 402.11
        - malignant 402.01
      - rheumatic (chronic) (inactive) (with chorea) 398.91
        - active or acute 391.8
          - with chorea 392.0
    - right (*see also* Failure, heart) 428.0
  - vital centers, fetus or newborn 779.89
  - weight gain in childhood 783.41
- **Fainting** (fit) (spell) 780.2
- **Falciform hymen** 752.49
- **Fall, maternal, affecting fetus or newborn** 760.5
- **Fallen arches** 734
- **Falling, any organ or part** — *see* Prolapse
- **Fallopian**
  - insufflation
    - fertility testing V26.21
    - following sterilization reversal V26.22
  - tube — *see* condition
- **Fallot's**
  - pentalogy 745.2
  - tetrad or tetralogy 745.2
  - triad or trilogy 746.09
- **Fallout, radioactive** (adverse effect) NEC 990
- **False** — *see also* condition
  - bundle branch block 426.50
  - bursa 727.89
  - croup 478.75
  - joint 733.82
  - labor (pains) 644.1 ☑
  - opening, urinary, male 752.69
  - passage, urethra (prostatic) 599.4
  - positive
    - serological test for syphilis 795.6
    - Wassermann reaction 795.6
  - pregnancy 300.11
- **Family, familial** — *see also* condition
  - disruption V61.0
  - Li-Fraumeni (syndrome) V84.01
  - planning advice V25.09
  - problem V61.9
    - specified circumstance NEC V61.8
  - retinoblastoma (syndrome) 190.5
- **Famine** 994.2
  - edema 262
- **Fanconi's anemia** (congenital pancytopenia) 284.0
- **Fanconi (-de Toni) (-Debré) syndrome** (cystinosis) 270.0
- **Farber (-Uzman) syndrome or disease** (disseminated lipogranulomatosis) 272.8
- **Farcin** 024
- **Farcy** 024
- **Farmers'**
  - lung 495.0
  - skin 692.74
- **Farsightedness** 367.0
- **Fascia** — *see* condition
- **Fasciculation** 781.0
- **Fasciculitis optica** 377.32
- **Fasciitis** 729.4
  - eosinophilic 728.89
  - necrotizing 728.86
  - nodular 728.79
  - perirenal 593.4
  - plantar 728.71
  - pseudosarcomatous 728.79
  - traumatic (old) NEC 728.79
    - current — *see* Sprain, by site
- **Fasciola hepatica infestation** 121.3
- **Fascioliasis** 121.3
- **Fasciolopsiasis** (small intestine) 121.4
- **Fasciolopsis** (small intestine) 121.4
- **Fast pulse** 785.0

- **Fever** — *continued*
  - spotted — *continued*
    - Brazilian 082.0
    - Colombian 082.0
    - meaning
      - cerebrospinal meningitis 036.0
      - typhus 082.9
  - spring 309.23
  - steroid
    - correct substance properly administered 780.6
    - overdose or wrong substance given or taken 962.0
  - streptobacillary 026.1
  - subtertian 084.0
  - Sumatran mite 081.2
  - sun 061
  - swamp 100.89
  - sweating 078.2
  - swine 003.8
  - sylvatic yellow 060.0
  - Tahyna 062.5
  - tertian — *see* Malaria, tertian
  - Thailand hemorrhagic 065.4
  - thermic 992.0
  - three day 066.0
    - with Coxsackie exanthem 074.8
  - tick
    - American mountain 066.1
    - Colorado 066.1
    - Kemerovo 066.1
    - Mediterranean 082.1
    - mountain 066.1
    - nonexanthematous 066.1
    - Quaranfil 066.1
  - tick-bite NEC 066.1
  - tick-borne NEC 066.1
    - hemorrhagic NEC 065.3
  - transitory of newborn 778.4
  - trench 083.1
  - tsutsugamushi 081.2
  - typhogastric 002.0
  - typhoid (abortive) (ambulant) (any site) (hemorrhagic) (infection) (intermittent) (malignant) (rheumatic) 002.0
  - typhomalarial (*see also* Malaria) 084.6
  - typhus — *see* Typhus
  - undulant (*see also* Brucellosis) 023.9
  - unknown origin (*see also* Pyrexia) 780.6
  - uremic — *see* Uremia
  - uveoparotid 135
  - valley (Coccidioidomycosis) 114.0
  - Venezuelan equine 066.2
  - Volhynian 083.1
  - Wesselsbron (viral) 066.3
  - West
    - African 084.8
    - Nile (viral) 066.40
      - with
        - cranial nerve disorders 066.42
        - encephalitis 066.41
        - optic neuritis 066.42
        - other complications 066.49
        - other neurologic manifestations 066.42
        - polyradiculitis 066.42
  - Whitmore's 025
  - Wolhynian 083.1
  - worm 128.9
  - Yaroslav hemorrhagic 078.6
  - yellow 060.9
    - jungle 060.0
    - sylvatic 060.0
    - urban 060.1
    - vaccination, prophylactic (against) V04.4
  - Zika (viral) 066.3
- **Fibrillation**
  - atrial (established) (paroxysmal) 427.31
  - auricular (atrial) (established) 427.31
  - cardiac (ventricular) 427.41
  - coronary (*see also* Infarct, myocardium) 410.9 ☑
  - heart (ventricular) 427.41
  - muscular 728.9
  - postoperative 997.1
  - ventricular 427.41
- **Fibrin**
  - ball or bodies, pleural (sac) 511.0
  - chamber, anterior (eye) (gelatinous exudate) 364.04
- **Fibrinogenolysis** (hemorrhagic) — *see* Fibrinolysis
- **Fibrinogenopenia** (congenital) (hereditary) (*see also* Defect, coagulation) 286.3
  - acquired 286.6
- **Fibrinolysis** (acquired) (hemorrhagic) (pathologic) 286.6
  - with
    - abortion — *see* Abortion, by type, with hemorrhage, delayed or excessive
    - ectopic pregnancy (*see also* categories 633.0-633.9) 639.1
    - molar pregnancy (*see also* categories 630-632) 639.1
  - antepartum or intrapartum 641.3 ☑
    - affecting fetus or newborn 762.1
  - following
    - abortion 639.1
    - ectopic or molar pregnancy 639.1
  - newborn, transient 776.2
  - postpartum 666.3 ☑
- **Fibrinopenia** (hereditary) (*see also* Defect, coagulation) 286.3
  - acquired 286.6
- **Fibrinopurulent** — *see* condition
- **Fibrinous** — *see* condition
- **Fibroadenoma** (M9010/0)
  - cellular intracanalicular (M9020/0) 217
  - giant (intracanalicular) (M9020/0) 217
  - intracanalicular (M9011/0)
    - cellular (M9020/0) 217
    - giant (M9020/0) 217
    - specified site — *see* Neoplasm, by site, benign
    - unspecified site 217
  - juvenile (M9030/0) 217
  - pericanicular (M9012/0)
    - specified site — *see* Neoplasm, by site, benign
    - unspecified site 217
  - phyllodes (M9020/0) 217
  - prostate 600.20
    - with urinary retention 600.21
  - specified site — *see* Neoplasm, by site, benign
  - unspecified site 217
- **Fibroadenosis, breast** (chronic) (cystic) (diffuse) (periodic) (segmental) 610.2
- **Fibroangioma** (M9160/0) — *see also* Neoplasm, by site, benign
  - juvenile (M9160/0)
    - specified site — *see* Neoplasm, by site, benign
    - unspecified site 210.7
- **Fibrocellulitis progressiva ossificans** 728.11
- **Fibrochondrosarcoma** (M9220/3) — *see* Neoplasm, cartilage, malignant
- **Fibrocystic**
  - disease 277.00
    - bone NEC 733.29
    - breast 610.1
    - jaw 526.2
    - kidney (congenital) 753.19
    - liver 751.62
    - lung 518.89
      - congenital 748.4
    - pancreas 277.00
  - kidney (congenital) 753.19
- **Fibrodysplasia ossificans multiplex** (progressiva) 728.11
- **Fibroelastosis** (cordis) (endocardial) (endomyocardial) 425.3
- **Fibroid** (tumor) (M8890/0) — *see also* Neoplasm, connective tissue, benign
  - disease, lung (chronic) (*see also* Fibrosis, lung) 515
  - heart (disease) (*see also* Myocarditis) 429.0
  - induration, lung (chronic) (*see also* Fibrosis, lung) 515
  - in pregnancy or childbirth 654.1 ☑
    - affecting fetus or newborn 763.89
    - causing obstructed labor 660.2 ☑
      - affecting fetus or newborn 763.1
- **Fibroid** (tumor) (M8890/0) — *see also* Neoplasm, connective tissue, benign — *continued*
  - liver — *see* Cirrhosis, liver
  - lung (*see also* Fibrosis, lung) 515
  - pneumonia (chronic) (*see also* Fibrosis, lung) 515
  - uterus (M8890/0) (*see also* Leiomyoma, uterus) 218.9
- **Fibrolipoma** (M8851/0) (*see also* Lipoma, by site) 214.9
- **Fibroliposarcoma** (M8850/3) — *see* Neoplasm, connective tissue, malignant
- **Fibroma** (M8810/0) — *see also* Neoplasm, connective tissue, benign
  - ameloblastic (M9330/0) 213.1
    - upper jaw (bone) 213.0
  - bone (nonossifying) 733.99
    - ossifying (M9262/0) — *see* Neoplasm, bone, benign
  - cementifying (M9274/0) — *see* Neoplasm, bone, benign
  - chondromyxoid (M9241/0) — *see* Neoplasm, bone, benign
  - desmoplastic (M8823/1) — *see* Neoplasm, connective tissue, uncertain behavior
  - facial (M8813/0) — *see* Neoplasm, connective tissue, benign
  - invasive (M8821/1) — *see* Neoplasm, connective tissue, uncertain behavior
  - molle (M8851/0) (*see also* Lipoma, by site) 214.9
  - myxoid (M8811/0) — *see* Neoplasm, connective tissue, benign
  - nasopharynx, nasopharyngeal (juvenile) (M9160/0) 210.7
  - nonosteogenic (nonossifying) — *see* Dysplasia, fibrous
  - odontogenic (M9321/0) 213.1
    - upper jaw (bone) 213.0
  - ossifying (M9262/0) — *see* Neoplasm, bone, benign
  - periosteal (M8812/0) — *see* Neoplasm, bone, benign
  - prostate 600.20
    - with urinary retention 600.21
  - soft (M8851/0) (*see also* Lipoma, by site) 214.9
- **Fibromatosis**
  - abdominal (M8822/1) — *see* Neoplasm, connective tissue, uncertain behavior
  - aggressive (M8821/1) — *see* Neoplasm, connective tissue, uncertain behavior
  - Dupuytren's 728.6
  - gingival 523.8
  - plantar fascia 728.71
  - proliferative 728.79
  - pseudosarcomatous (proliferative) (subcutaneous) 728.79
  - subcutaneous pseudosarcomatous (proliferative) 728.79
- **Fibromyalgia** 729.1
- **Fibromyoma** (M8890/0) — *see also* Neoplasm, connective tissue, benign
  - uterus (corpus) (*see also* Leiomyoma, uterus) 218.9
    - in pregnancy or childbirth 654.1 ☑
      - affecting fetus or newborn 763.89
      - causing obstructed labor 660.2 ☑
        - affecting fetus or newborn 763.1
- **Fibromyositis** (*see also* Myositis) 729.1
  - scapulohumeral 726.2
- **Fibromyxolipoma** (M8852/0) (*see also* Lipoma, by site) 214.9
- **Fibromyxoma** (M8811/0) — *see* Neoplasm, connective tissue, benign
- **Fibromyxosarcoma** (M8811/3) — *see* Neoplasm, connective tissue, malignant
- **Fibro-odontoma, ameloblastic** (M9290/0) 213.1
  - upper jaw (bone) 213.0
- **Fibro-osteoma** (M9262/0) — *see* Neoplasm, bone, benign
- **Fibroplasia, retrolental** 362.21
- **Fibropurulent** — *see* condition
- **Fibrosarcoma** (M8810/3) — *see also* Neoplasm, connective tissue, malignant
  - ameloblastic (M9330/3) 170.1
    - upper jaw (bone) 170.0

- **Fibrosarcoma** — *see also* Neoplasm, connective tissue, malignant — *continued*
  - congenital (M8814/3) — *see* Neoplasm, connective tissue, malignant
  - fascial (M8813/3) — *see* Neoplasm, connective tissue, malignant
  - infantile (M8814/3) — *see* Neoplasm, connective tissue, malignant
  - odontogenic (M9330/3) 170.1
    - upper jaw (bone) 170.0
  - periosteal (M8812/3) — *see* Neoplasm, bone, malignant
- **Fibrosclerosis**
  - breast 610.3
  - corpora cavernosa (penis) 607.89
  - familial multifocal NEC 710.8
  - multifocal (idiopathic) NEC 710.8
  - penis (corpora cavernosa) 607.89
- **Fibrosis, fibrotic**
  - adrenal (gland) 255.8
  - alveolar (diffuse) 516.3
  - amnion 658.8 ☑
  - anal papillae 569.49
  - anus 569.49
  - appendix, appendiceal, noninflammatory 543.9
  - arteriocapillary — *see* Arteriosclerosis
  - bauxite (of lung) 503
  - biliary 576.8
    - due to Clonorchis sinensis 121.1
  - bladder 596.8
    - interstitial 595.1
    - localized submucosal 595.1
    - panmural 595.1
  - bone, diffuse 756.59
  - breast 610.3
  - capillary — *see also* Arteriosclerosis
    - lung (chronic) (*see also* Fibrosis, lung) 515
  - cardiac (*see also* Myocarditis) 429.0
  - cervix 622.8
  - chorion 658.8 ☑
  - corpus cavernosum 607.89
  - cystic (of pancreas) 277.00
    - with
      - manifestations
        - gastrointestinal 277.03
        - pulmonary 277.02
        - specified NEC 277.09
      - meconium ileus 277.01
      - pulmonary exacerbation 277.02
  - due to (presence of) any device, implant, or graft — *see* Complications, due to (presence of) any device, implant, or graft classified to 996.0-996.5 NEC
  - ejaculatory duct 608.89
  - endocardium (*see also* Endocarditis) 424.90
  - endomyocardial (African) 425.0
  - epididymis 608.89
  - eye muscle 378.62
  - graphite (of lung) 503
  - heart (*see also* Myocarditis) 429.0
  - hepatic — *see also* Cirrhosis, liver
    - due to Clonorchis sinensis 121.1
  - hepatolienal — *see* Cirrhosis, liver
  - hepatosplenic — *see* Cirrhosis, liver
  - infrapatellar fat pad 729.31
  - interstitial pulmonary, newborn 770.7
  - intrascrotal 608.89
  - kidney (*see also* Sclerosis, renal) 587
  - liver — *see* Cirrhosis, liver
  - lung (atrophic) (capillary) (chronic) (confluent) (massive) (perialveolar) (peribronchial) 515
    - with
      - anthracosilicosis (occupational) 500
      - anthracosis (occupational) 500
      - asbestosis (occupational) 501
      - bagassosis (occupational) 495.1
      - bauxite 503
      - berylliosis (occupational) 503
      - byssinosis (occupational) 504
      - calcicosis (occupational) 502
      - chalicosis (occupational) 502
      - dust reticulation (occupational) 504
      - farmers' lung 495.0
      - gannister disease (occupational) 502
      - graphite 503

- **Fibrosis, fibrotic** — *continued*
  - lung — *continued*
    - with — *continued*
      - pneumonoconiosis (occupational) 505
      - pneumosiderosis (occupational) 503
      - siderosis (occupational) 503
      - silicosis (occupational) 502
      - tuberculosis (*see also* Tuberculosis) 011.4 ☑
    - diffuse (idiopathic) (interstitial) 516.3
    - due to
      - bauxite 503
      - fumes or vapors (chemical) (inhalation) 506.4
      - graphite 503
    - following radiation 508.1
    - postinflammatory 515
    - silicotic (massive) (occupational) 502
    - tuberculous (*see also* Tuberculosis) 011.4 ☑
  - lymphatic gland 289.3
  - median bar 600.90
    - with urinary retention 600.91
  - mediastinum (idiopathic) 519.3
  - meninges 349.2
  - muscle NEC 728.2
    - iatrogenic (from injection) 999.9
  - myocardium, myocardial (*see also* Myocarditis) 429.0
  - oral submucous 528.8
  - ovary 620.8
  - oviduct 620.8
  - pancreas 577.8
    - cystic 277.00
      - with
        - manifestations
          - gastrointestinal 277.03
          - pulmonary 277.02
          - specified NEC 277.09
        - meconium ileus 277.01
        - pulmonary exacerbation 277.02
  - penis 607.89
  - periappendiceal 543.9
  - periarticular (*see also* Ankylosis) 718.5 ☑
  - pericardium 423.1
  - perineum, in pregnancy or childbirth 654.8 ☑
    - affecting fetus or newborn 763.89
    - causing obstructed labor 660.2 ☑
      - affecting fetus or newborn 763.1
  - perineural NEC 355.9
    - foot 355.6
  - periureteral 593.89
  - placenta — *see* Placenta, abnormal
  - pleura 511.0
  - popliteal fat pad 729.31
  - preretinal 362.56
  - prostate (chronic) 600.90
    - with urinary retention 600.91
  - pulmonary (chronic) (*see also* Fibrosis, lung) 515
    - alveolar capillary block 516.3
    - interstitial
      - diffuse (idiopathic) 516.3
      - newborn 770.7
  - radiation — *see* Effect, adverse, radiation
  - rectal sphincter 569.49
  - retroperitoneal, idiopathic 593.4
  - sclerosing mesenteric (idiopathic) 567.82 ●
  - scrotum 608.89
  - seminal vesicle 608.89
  - senile 797
  - skin NEC 709.2
  - spermatic cord 608.89
  - spleen 289.59
    - bilharzial (*see also* Schistosomiasis) 120.9
  - subepidermal nodular (M8832/0) — *see* Neoplasm, skin, benign
  - submucous NEC 709.2
    - oral 528.8
    - tongue 528.8
  - syncytium — *see* Placenta, abnormal
  - testis 608.89
    - chronic, due to syphilis 095.8
  - thymus (gland) 254.8
  - tunica vaginalis 608.89
  - ureter 593.89
  - urethra 599.84

- **Fibrosis, fibrotic** — *continued*
  - uterus (nonneoplastic) 621.8
    - bilharzial (*see also* Schistosomiasis) 120.9
    - neoplastic (*see also* Leiomyoma, uterus) 218.9
  - vagina 623.8
  - valve, heart (*see also* Endocarditis) 424.90
  - vas deferens 608.89
  - vein 459.89
    - lower extremities 459.89
  - vesical 595.1
- **Fibrositis** (periarticular) (rheumatoid) 729.0
  - humeroscapular region 726.2
  - nodular, chronic
    - Jaccoud's 714.4
    - rheumatoid 714.4
  - ossificans 728.11
  - scapulohumeral 726.2
- **Fibrothorax** 511.0
- **Fibrotic** — *see* Fibrosis
- **Fibrous** — *see* condition
- **Fibroxanthoma** (M8831/0) — *see also* Neoplasm, connective tissue, benign
  - atypical (M8831/1) — *see* Neoplasm, connective tissue, uncertain behavior
  - malignant (M8831/3) — *see* Neoplasm, connective tissue, malignant
- **Fibroxanthosarcoma** (M8831/3) — *see* Neoplasm, connective tissue, malignant
- **Fiedler's**
  - disease (leptospiral jaundice) 100.0
  - myocarditis or syndrome (acute isolated myocarditis) 422.91
- **Fiessinger-Leroy (-Reiter) syndrome** 099.3
- **Fiessinger-Rendu syndrome** (erythema muliforme exudativum) 695.1
- **Fifth disease** (eruptive) 057.0
  - venereal 099.1
- **Filaria, filarial** — *see* Infestation, filarial
- **Filariasis** (*see also* Infestation, filarial) 125.9
  - bancroftian 125.0
  - Brug's 125.1
  - due to
    - bancrofti 125.0
    - Brugia (Wuchereria) (malayi) 125.1
    - Loa loa 125.2
    - malayi 125.1
    - organism NEC 125.6
    - Wuchereria (bancrofti) 125.0
      - malayi 125.1
  - Malayan 125.1
  - ozzardi 125.5
  - specified type NEC 125.6
- **Filatoff's, Filatov's, Filatow's disease** (infectious mononucleosis) 075
- **File-cutters' disease** 984.9
  - specified type of lead — *see* Table of Drugs and Chemicals
- **Filling defect**
  - biliary tract 793.3
  - bladder 793.5
  - duodenum 793.4
  - gallbladder 793.3
  - gastrointestinal tract 793.4
  - intestine 793.4
  - kidney 793.5
  - stomach 793.4
  - ureter 793.5
- **Filtering bleb, eye** (postglaucoma) (status) V45.69
  - with complication or rupture 997.99
  - postcataract extraction (complication) 997.99
- **Fimbrial cyst** (congenital) 752.11
- **Fimbriated hymen** 752.49
- **Financial problem affecting care** V60.2
- **Findings, abnormal, without diagnosis** (examination) (laboratory test) 796.4
  - 17-ketosteroids, elevated 791.9
  - acetonuria 791.6
  - acid phosphatase 790.5
  - albumin-globulin ratio 790.99
  - albuminuria 791.0
  - alcohol in blood 790.3
  - alkaline phosphatase 790.5

☑ Additional Digit Required — Refer to the Tabular List (Numeric Code Section) for Additional Digit Selection

▶◀ Revised Text ● New Line ▲ Revised Code

- **Findings, abnormal, without diagnosis** — *continued*
  - structure, body NEC — *continued*
    - gastrointestinal tract 793.4
    - genitourinary organs 793.5
    - head 793.0
      - echogram (ultrasound) 794.01
    - intrathoracic organs NEC 793.2
    - lung 793.1
    - musculoskeletal 793.7
    - placenta 793.9
    - retroperitoneum 793.6
    - skin 793.9
    - subcutaneous tissue NEC 793.9
  - synovial fluid 792.9
  - thermogram — *see* Findings, abnormal, structure
  - throat culture, positive 795.39
  - thyroid (function) 794.5
    - metabolism (rate) 794.5
    - scan 794.5
    - uptake 794.5
  - total proteins 790.99
  - toxicology (drugs) (heavy metals) 796.0
  - transaminase (level) 790.4
  - triglycerides 272.9
  - tuberculin skin test (without active tuberculosis) 795.5
  - ultrasound — *see also* Findings, abnormal, structure
    - cardiogram 793.2
  - uric acid, blood 790.6
  - urine, urinary constituents 791.9
    - acetone 791.6
    - albumin 791.0
    - bacteria 791.9
    - bile 791.4
    - blood 599.7
    - casts or cells 791.7
    - chyle 791.1
    - culture, positive 791.9
    - glucose 791.5
    - hemoglobin 791.2
    - ketone 791.6
    - protein 791.0
    - pus 791.9
    - sugar 791.5
  - vaginal fluid 792.9
  - vanillylmandelic acid, elevated 791.9
  - vectorcardiogram (VCG) 794.39
  - ventriculogram (cerebral) 793.0
  - VMA, elevated 791.9
  - Wassermann reaction
    - false positive 795.6
    - positive 097.1
      - follow-up of latent syphilis — *see* Syphilis, latent
      - only finding — *see* Syphilis, latent
  - white blood cell 288.9
    - count 288.9
      - elevated 288.8
      - low 288.0
    - differential 288.9
    - morphology 288.9
  - wound culture 795.39
  - xerography 793.89
  - zinc, blood 790.6
- **Finger** — *see* condition
- **Fire, St. Anthony's** (*see also* Erysipelas) 035
- **Fish**
  - hook stomach 537.89
  - meal workers' lung 495.8
- **Fisher's syndrome** 357.0
- **Fissure, fissured**
  - abdominal wall (congenital) 756.79
  - anus, anal 565.0
    - congenital 751.5
  - buccal cavity 528.9
  - clitoris (congenital) 752.49
  - ear, lobule (congenital) 744.29
  - epiglottis (congenital) 748.3
  - larynx 478.79
    - congenital 748.3
  - lip 528.5
    - congenital (*see also* Cleft, lip) 749.10
- **Fissure, fissured** — *continued*
  - nipple 611.2
    - puerperal, postpartum 676.1 ☑
  - palate (congenital) (*see also* Cleft, palate) 749.00
  - postanal 565.0
  - rectum 565.0
  - skin 709.8
    - streptococcal 686.9
  - spine (congenital) (*see also* Spina bifida) 741.9 ☑
  - sternum (congenital) 756.3
  - tongue (acquired) 529.5
    - congenital 750.13
- **Fistula** (sinus) 686.9
  - abdomen (wall) 569.81
    - bladder 596.2
    - intestine 569.81
    - ureter 593.82
    - uterus 619.2
  - abdominorectal 569.81
  - abdominosigmoidal 569.81
  - abdominothoracic 510.0
  - abdominouterine 619.2
    - congenital 752.3
  - abdominovesical 596.2
  - accessory sinuses (*see also* Sinusitis) 473.9
  - actinomycotic — *see* Actinomycosis
  - alveolar
    - antrum (*see also* Sinusitis, maxillary) 473.0
    - process 522.7
  - anorectal 565.1
  - antrobuccal (*see also* Sinusitis, maxillary) 473.0
  - antrum (*see also* Sinusitis, maxillary) 473.0
  - anus, anal (infectional) (recurrent) 565.1
    - congenital 751.5
    - tuberculous (*see also* Tuberculosis) 014.8 ☑
  - aortic sinus 747.29
  - aortoduodenal 447.2
  - appendix, appendicular 543.9
  - arteriovenous (acquired) 447.0
    - brain 437.3
      - congenital 747.81
        - ruptured (*see also* Hemorrhage, subarachnoid) 430
      - ruptured (*see also* Hemorrhage, subarachnoid) 430
    - cerebral 437.3
      - congenital 747.81
    - congenital (peripheral) 747.60
      - brain — *see* Fistula, arteriovenous, brain, congenital
      - coronary 746.85
      - gastrointestinal 747.61
      - lower limb 747.64
      - pulmonary 747.3
      - renal 747.62
      - specified site NEC 747.69
      - upper limb 747.63
    - coronary 414.19
      - congenital 746.85
    - heart 414.19
    - pulmonary (vessels) 417.0
      - congenital 747.3
    - surgically created (for dialysis) V45.1
      - complication NEC 996.73
        - atherosclerosis — *see* Arteriosclerosis, extremities
        - embolism 996.74
        - infection or inflammation 996.62
        - mechanical 996.1
        - occlusion NEC 996.74
        - thrombus 996.74
    - traumatic — *see* Injury, blood vessel, by site
  - artery 447.2
  - aural 383.81
    - congenital 744.49
  - auricle 383.81
    - congenital 744.49
  - Bartholin's gland 619.8
  - bile duct (*see also* Fistula, biliary) 576.4
  - biliary (duct) (tract) 576.4
    - congenital 751.69
  - bladder (neck) (sphincter) 596.2
    - into seminal vesicle 596.2
- **Fistula** — *continued*
  - bone 733.99
  - brain 348.8
    - arteriovenous — *see* Fistula, arteriovenous, brain
  - branchial (cleft) 744.41
  - branchiogenous 744.41
  - breast 611.0
    - puerperal, postpartum 675.1 ☑
  - bronchial 510.0
  - bronchocutaneous, bronchomediastinal, bronchopleural, bronchopleuromediastinal (infective) 510.0
    - tuberculous (*see also* Tuberculosis) 011.3 ☑
  - bronchoesophageal 530.89
    - congenital 750.3
  - buccal cavity (infective) 528.3
  - canal, ear 380.89
  - carotid-cavernous
    - congenital 747.81
      - with hemorrhage 430
    - traumatic 900.82
      - with hemorrhage (*see also* Hemorrhage, brain, traumatic) 853.0 ☑
      - late effect 908.3
  - cecosigmoidal 569.81
  - cecum 569.81
  - cerebrospinal (fluid) 349.81
  - cervical, lateral (congenital) 744.41
  - cervicoaural (congenital) 744.49
  - cervicosigmoidal 619.1
  - cervicovesical 619.0
  - cervix 619.8
  - chest (wall) 510.0
  - cholecystocolic (*see also* Fistula, gallbladder) 575.5
  - cholecystocolonic (*see also* Fistula, gallbladder) 575.5
  - cholecystoduodenal (*see also* Fistula, gallbladder) 575.5
  - cholecystoenteric (*see also* Fistula, gallbladder) 575.5
  - cholecystogastric (*see also* Fistula, gallbladder) 575.5
  - cholecystointestinal (*see also* Fistula, gallbladder) 575.5
  - choledochoduodenal 576.4
  - cholocolic (*see also* Fistula, gallbladder) 575.5
  - coccyx 685.1
    - with abscess 685.0
  - colon 569.81
  - colostomy 569.69
  - colovaginal (acquired) 619.1
  - common duct (bile duct) 576.4
  - congenital, NEC — *see* Anomaly, specified type NEC
  - cornea, causing hypotony 360.32
  - coronary, arteriovenous 414.19
    - congenital 746.85
  - costal region 510.0
  - cul-de-sac, Douglas' 619.8
  - cutaneous 686.9
  - cystic duct (*see also* Fistula, gallbladder) 575.5
    - congenital 751.69
  - dental 522.7
  - diaphragm 510.0
    - bronchovisceral 510.0
    - pleuroperitoneal 510.0
    - pulmonoperitoneal 510.0
  - duodenum 537.4
  - ear (canal) (external) 380.89
  - enterocolic 569.81
  - enterocutaneous 569.81
  - enteroenteric 569.81
  - entero-uterine 619.1
    - congenital 752.3
  - enterovaginal 619.1
    - congenital 752.49
  - enterovesical 596.1
  - epididymis 608.89
    - tuberculous (*see also* Tuberculosis) 016.4 ☑
  - esophagobronchial 530.89
    - congenital 750.3
  - esophagocutaneous 530.89
  - esophagopleurocutaneous 530.89

Fistula — *continued*
  esophagotracheal 530.84
    congenital 750.3
  esophagus 530.89
    congenital 750.4
  ethmoid (*see also* Sinusitis, ethmoidal) 473.2
  eyeball (cornea) (sclera) 360.32
  eyelid 373.11
  fallopian tube (external) 619.2
  fecal 569.81
    congenital 751.5
  from periapical lesion 522.7
  frontal sinus (*see also* Sinusitis, frontal) 473.1
  gallbladder 575.5
    with calculus, cholelithiasis, stones (*see also* Cholelithiasis) 574.2 ☑
    congenital 751.69
  gastric 537.4
  gastrocolic 537.4
    congenital 750.7
    tuberculous (*see also* Tuberculosis) 014.8 ☑
  gastroenterocolic 537.4
  gastroesophageal 537.4
  gastrojejunal 537.4
  gastrojejunocolic 537.4
  genital
    organs
      female 619.9
        specified site NEC 619.8
      male 608.89
    tract-skin (female) 619.2
  hepatopleural 510.0
  hepatopulmonary 510.0
  horseshoe 565.1
  ileorectal 569.81
  ileosigmoidal 569.81
  ileostomy 569.69
  ileovesical 596.1
  ileum 569.81
  in ano 565.1
    tuberculous (*see also* Tuberculosis) 014.8 ☑
  inner ear (*see also* Fistula, labyrinth) 386.40
  intestine 569.81
  intestinocolonic (abdominal) 569.81
  intestinoureteral 593.82
  intestinouterine 619.1
  intestinovaginal 619.1
    congenital 752.49
  intestinovesical 596.1
  involving female genital tract 619.9
    digestive-genital 619.1
    genital tract-skin 619.2
    specified site NEC 619.8
    urinary-genital 619.0
  ischiorectal (fossa) 566
  jejunostomy 569.69
  jejunum 569.81
  joint 719.80
    ankle 719.87
    elbow 719.82
    foot 719.87
    hand 719.84
    hip 719.85
    knee 719.86
    multiple sites 719.89
    pelvic region 719.85
    shoulder (region) 719.81
    specified site NEC 719.88
    tuberculous — *see* Tuberculosis, joint
    wrist 719.83
  kidney 593.89
  labium (majus) (minus) 619.8
  labyrinth, labyrinthine NEC 386.40
    combined sites 386.48
    multiple sites 386.48
    oval window 386.42
    round window 386.41
    semicircular canal 386.43
  lacrimal, lachrymal (duct) (gland) (sac) 375.61
  lacrimonasal duct 375.61
  laryngotracheal 748.3
  larynx 478.79
  lip 528.5
    congenital 750.25
  lumbar, tuberculous (*see also* Tuberculosis) 015.0 ☑ *[730.8]* ☑
  lung 510.0

Fistula — *continued*
  lymphatic (node) (vessel) 457.8
  mamillary 611.0
  mammary (gland) 611.0
    puerperal, postpartum 675.1 ☑
  mastoid (process) (region) 383.1
  maxillary (*see also* Sinusitis, maxillary) 473.0
  mediastinal 510.0
  mediastinobronchial 510.0
  mediastinocutaneous 510.0
  middle ear 385.89
  mouth 528.3
  nasal 478.1
    sinus (*see also* Sinusitis) 473.9
  nasopharynx 478.29
  nipple — *see* Fistula, breast
  nose 478.1
  oral (cutaneous) 528.3
    maxillary (*see also* Sinusitis, maxillary) 473.0
    nasal (with cleft palate) (*see also* Cleft, palate) 749.00
  orbit, orbital 376.10
  oro-antral (*see also* Sinusitis, maxillary) 473.0
  oval window (internal ear) 386.42
  oviduct (external) 619.2
  palate (hard) 526.89
    soft 528.9
  pancreatic 577.8
  pancreaticoduodenal 577.8
  parotid (gland) 527.4
    region 528.3
  pelvoabdominointestinal 569.81
  penis 607.89
  perianal 565.1
  pericardium (pleura) (sac) (*see also* Pericarditis) 423.8
  pericecal 569.81
  perineal — *see* Fistula, perineum
  perineorectal 569.81
  perineosigmoidal 569.81
  perineo-urethroscrotal 608.89
  perineum, perineal (with urethral involvement) NEC 599.1
    tuberculous (*see also* Tuberculosis) 017.9 ☑
    ureter 593.82
  perirectal 565.1
    tuberculous (*see also* Tuberculosis) 014.8 ☑
  peritoneum (*see also* Peritonitis) 567.22 ▲
  periurethral 599.1
  pharyngo-esophageal 478.29
  pharynx 478.29
    branchial cleft (congenital) 744.41
  pilonidal (infected) (rectum) 685.1
    with abscess 685.0
  pleura, pleural, pleurocutaneous, pleuroperitoneal 510.0
    stomach 510.0
    tuberculous (*see also* Tuberculosis) 012.0 ☑
  pleuropericardial 423.8
  postauricular 383.81
  postoperative, persistent 998.6
  preauricular (congenital) 744.46
  prostate 602.8
  pulmonary 510.0
    arteriovenous 417.0
      congenital 747.3
    tuberculous (*see also* Tuberculosis, pulmonary) 011.9 ☑
  pulmonoperitoneal 510.0
  rectolabial 619.1
  rectosigmoid (intercommunicating) 569.81
  rectoureteral 593.82
  rectourethral 599.1
    congenital 753.8
  rectouterine 619.1
    congenital 752.3
  rectovaginal 619.1
    congenital 752.49
    old, postpartal 619.1
    tuberculous (*see also* Tuberculosis) 014.8 ☑
  rectovesical 596.1
    congenital 753.8
  rectovesicovaginal 619.1
  rectovulvar 619.1
    congenital 752.49

Fistula — *continued*
  rectum (to skin) 565.1
    tuberculous (*see also* Tuberculosis) 014.8 ☑
  renal 593.89
  retroauricular 383.81
  round window (internal ear) 386.41
  salivary duct or gland 527.4
    congenital 750.24
  sclera 360.32
  scrotum (urinary) 608.89
    tuberculous (*see also* Tuberculosis) 016.5 ☑
  semicircular canals (internal ear) 386.43
  sigmoid 569.81
    vesicoabdominal 596.1
  sigmoidovaginal 619.1
    congenital 752.49
  skin 686.9
    ureter 593.82
    vagina 619.2
  sphenoidal sinus (*see also* Sinusitis, sphenoidal) 473.3
  splenocolic 289.59
  stercoral 569.81
  stomach 537.4
  sublingual gland 527.4
    congenital 750.24
  submaxillary
    gland 527.4
      congenital 750.24
    region 528.3
  thoracic 510.0
    duct 457.8
  thoracicoabdominal 510.0
  thoracicogastric 510.0
  thoracicointestinal 510.0
  thoracoabdominal 510.0
  thoracogastric 510.0
  thorax 510.0
  thyroglossal duct 759.2
  thyroid 246.8
  trachea (congenital) (external) (internal) 748.3
  tracheoesophageal 530.84
    congenital 750.3
    following tracheostomy 519.09
  traumatic
    arteriovenous (*see also* Injury, blood vessel, by site) 904.9
      brain — *see* Injury, intracranial
  tuberculous — *see* Tuberculosis, by site
  typhoid 002.0
  umbilical 759.89
  umbilico-urinary 753.8
  urachal, urachus 753.7
  ureter (persistent) 593.82
  ureteroabdominal 593.82
  ureterocervical 593.82
  ureterorectal 593.82
  ureterosigmoido-abdominal 593.82
  ureterovaginal 619.0
  ureterovesical 596.2
  urethra 599.1
    congenital 753.8
    tuberculous (*see also* Tuberculosis) 016.3 ☑
  urethroperineal 599.1
  urethroperineovesical 596.2
  urethrorectal 599.1
    congenital 753.8
  urethroscrotal 608.89
  urethrovaginal 619.0
  urethrovesical 596.2
  urethrovesicovaginal 619.0
  urinary (persistent) (recurrent) 599.1
  uteroabdominal (anterior wall) 619.2
    congenital 752.3
  uteroenteric 619.1
  uterofecal 619.1
  uterointestinal 619.1
    congenital 752.3
  uterorectal 619.1
    congenital 752.3
  uteroureteric 619.0
  uterovaginal 619.8
  uterovesical 619.0
    congenital 752.3
  uterus 619.8
  vagina (wall) 619.8
    postpartal, old 619.8

☑ Additional Digit Required — Refer to the Tabular List (Numeric Code Section) for Additional Digit Selection
▶◀ Revised Text ● New Line ▲ Revised Code

- **Flux** (bloody) (serosanguineous) 009.0
- **Focal** — *see* condition
- **Fochier's abscess** — *see* Abscess, by site
- **Focus, Assmann's** (*see also* Tuberculosis) 011.0 ☑
- **Fogo selvagem** 694.4
- **Foix-Alajouanine syndrome** 336.1
- **Folds, anomalous** — *see also* Anomaly, specified type NEC
  - Bowman's membrane 371.31
  - Descemet's membrane 371.32
  - epicanthic 743.63
  - heart 746.89
  - posterior segment of eye, congenital 743.54
- **Folie à deux** 297.3
- **Follicle**
  - cervix (nabothian) (ruptured) 616.0
  - graafian, ruptured, with hemorrhage 620.0
  - nabothian 616.0
- **Folliclis** (primary) (*see also* Tuberculosis) 017.0 ☑
- **Follicular** — *see also* condition
  - cyst (atretic) 620.0
- **Folliculitis** 704.8
  - abscedens et suffodiens 704.8
  - decalvans 704.09
  - gonorrheal (acute) 098.0
    - chronic or duration of 2 months or more 098.2
  - keloid, keloidalis 706.1
  - pustular 704.8
  - ulerythematosa reticulata 701.8
- **Folliculosis, conjunctival** 372.02
- **Følling's disease** (phenylketonuria) 270.1
- **Follow-up** (examination) (routine) (following) V67.9
  - cancer chemotherapy V67.2
  - chemotherapy V67.2
  - fracture V67.4
  - high-risk medication V67.51
  - injury NEC V67.59
  - postpartum
    - immediately after delivery V24.0
    - routine V24.2
  - psychiatric V67.3
  - psychotherapy V67.3
  - radiotherapy V67.1
  - specified condition NEC V67.59
  - specified surgery NEC V67.09
  - surgery V67.00
    - vaginal pap smear V67.01
  - treatment V67.9
    - combined NEC V67.6
    - fracture V67.4
    - involving high-risk medication NEC V67.51
    - mental disorder V67.3
    - specified NEC V67.59
- **Fong's syndrome** (hereditary osteoonychodysplasia) 756.89
- **Food**
  - allergy 693.1
  - anaphylactic shock — *see* Anaphylactic shock, due to, food
  - asphyxia (from aspiration or inhalation) (*see also* Asphyxia, food) 933.1
  - choked on (*see also* Asphyxia, food) 933.1
  - deprivation 994.2
    - specified kind of food NEC 269.8
  - intoxication (*see also* Poisoning, food) 005.9
  - lack of 994.2
  - poisoning (*see also* Poisoning, food) 005.9
  - refusal or rejection NEC 307.59
  - strangulation or suffocation (*see also* Asphyxia, food) 933.1
  - toxemia (*see also* Poisoning, food) 005.9
- **Foot** — *see also* condition
  - and mouth disease 078.4
  - process disease 581.3
- **Foramen ovale** (nonclosure) (patent) (persistent) 745.5
- **Forbes'** (glycogen storage) **disease** 271.0
- **Forbes-Albright syndrome** (nonpuerperal amenorrhea and lactation associated with pituitary tumor) 253.1
- **Forced birth or delivery** NEC 669.8 ☑
  - affecting fetus or newborn NEC 763.89
- **Forceps**
  - delivery NEC 669.5 ☑
    - affecting fetus or newborn 763.2
- **Fordyce's disease** (ectopic sebaceous glands) (mouth) 750.26
- **Fordyce-Fox disease** (apocrine miliaria) 705.82
- **Forearm** — *see* condition
- **Foreign body**

> *Note — For foreign body with open wound or other injury, see Wound, open, or the type of injury specified.*

  - accidentally left during a procedure 998.4
  - anterior chamber (eye) 871.6
    - magnetic 871.5
      - retained or old 360.51
    - retained or old 360.61
  - ciliary body (eye) 871.6
    - magnetic 871.5
      - retained or old 360.52
    - retained or old 360.62
  - entering through orifice (current) (old)
    - accessory sinus 932
    - air passage (upper) 933.0
      - lower 934.8
    - alimentary canal 938
    - alveolar process 935.0
    - antrum (Highmore) 932
    - anus 937
    - appendix 936
    - asphyxia due to (*see also* Asphyxia, food) 933.1
    - auditory canal 931
    - auricle 931
    - bladder 939.0
    - bronchioles 934.8
    - bronchus (main) 934.1
    - buccal cavity 935.0
    - canthus (inner) 930.1
    - cecum 936
    - cervix (canal) uterine 939.1
    - coil, ileocecal 936
    - colon 936
    - conjunctiva 930.1
    - conjunctival sac 930.1
    - cornea 930.0
    - digestive organ or tract NEC 938
    - duodenum 936
    - ear (external) 931
    - esophagus 935.1
    - eye (external) 930.9
      - combined sites 930.8
      - intraocular — *see* Foreign body, by site
      - specified site NEC 930.8
    - eyeball 930.8
      - intraocular — *see* Foreign body, intraocular
    - eyelid 930.1
      - retained or old 374.86
    - frontal sinus 932
    - gastrointestinal tract 938
    - genitourinary tract 939.9
    - globe 930.8
      - penetrating 871.6
        - magnetic 871.5
          - retained or old 360.50
        - retained or old 360.60
    - gum 935.0
    - Highmore's antrum 932
    - hypopharynx 933.0
    - ileocecal coil 936
    - ileum 936
    - inspiration (of) 933.1
    - intestine (large) (small) 936
    - lacrimal apparatus, duct, gland, or sac 930.2
    - larynx 933.1
    - lung 934.8
    - maxillary sinus 932
    - mouth 935.0
    - nasal sinus 932
    - nasopharynx 933.0
    - nose (passage) 932

Foreign body — *continued*

  - entering through orifice — *continued*
    - nostril 932
    - oral cavity 935.0
    - palate 935.0
    - penis 939.3
    - pharynx 933.0
    - pyriform sinus 933.0
    - rectosigmoid 937
      - junction 937
    - rectum 937
    - respiratory tract 934.9
      - specified part NEC 934.8
    - sclera 930.1
    - sinus 932
      - accessory 932
      - frontal 932
      - maxillary 932
      - nasal 932
      - pyriform 933.0
    - small intestine 936
    - stomach (hairball) 935.2
    - suffocation by (*see also* Asphyxia, food) 933.1
    - swallowed 938
      - tongue 933.0
    - tear ducts or glands 930.2
    - throat 933.0
    - tongue 935.0
      - swallowed 933.0
    - tonsil, tonsillar 933.0
      - fossa 933.0
    - trachea 934.0
    - ureter 939.0
    - urethra 939.0
    - uterus (any part) 939.1
    - vagina 939.2
    - vulva 939.2
    - wind pipe 934.0
  - granuloma (old) 728.82
    - bone 733.99
    - in operative wound (inadvertently left) 998.4
      - due to surgical material intentionally left — *see* Complications, due to (presence of) any device, implant, or graft classified to 996.0-996.5 NEC
    - muscle 728.82
    - skin 709.4
    - soft tissue 709.4
    - subcutaneous tissue 709.4
  - in
    - bone (residual) 733.99
    - open wound — *see* Wound, open, by site complicated
    - soft tissue (residual) 729.6
  - inadvertently left in operation wound (causing adhesions, obstruction, or perforation) 998.4
  - ingestion, ingested NEC 938
  - inhalation or inspiration (*see also* Asphyxia, food) 933.1
  - internal organ, not entering through an orifice — *see* Injury, internal, by site, with open wound
  - intraocular (nonmagnetic) 871.6
    - combined sites 871.6
      - magnetic 871.5
        - retained or old 360.59
      - retained or old 360.69
    - magnetic 871.5
      - retained or old 360.50
    - retained or old 360.60
    - specified site NEC 871.6
      - magnetic 871.5
        - retained or old 360.59
      - retained or old 360.69
  - iris (nonmagnetic) 871.6
    - magnetic 871.5
      - retained or old 360.52
    - retained or old 360.62
  - lens (nonmagnetic) 871.6
    - magnetic 871.5
      - retained or old 360.53
    - retained or old 360.63
  - lid, eye 930.1
  - ocular muscle 870.4
    - retained or old 376.6

Note — For fracture of any of the following sites with fracture of other bones — see Fracture, multiple.

"Closed" includes the following descriptions of fractures, with or without delayed healing, unless they are specified as open or compound:

comminuted	*linear*
depressed	*simple*
elevated	*slipped epiphysis*
fissured	*spiral*
greenstick	*unspecified*
impacted	

"Open" includes the following descriptions of fractures, with or without delayed healing:

compound	*puncture*
infected	*with foreign body*
missile	

For late effect of fracture, see Late, effect, fracture, by site.

- **Fracture** — *continued*
  - innominate bone (with visceral injury) (closed) 808.49
    - open 808.59
  - instep, of one foot (closed) 825.20
    - with toe(s) of same foot 827.0
      - open 827.1
    - open 825.30
  - internal
    - ear — *see* Fracture, skull, base
    - semilunar cartilage, knee — *see* Tear, meniscus, medial
  - intertrochanteric — *see* Fracture, femur, neck, intertrochanteric
  - ischium (with visceral injury) (closed) 808.42
    - open 808.52
  - jaw (bone) (lower) (closed) (*see also* Fracture, mandible) 802.20
    - angle 802.25
      - open 802.35
    - open 802.30
    - upper — *see* Fracture, maxilla
  - knee
    - cap (closed) 822.0
      - open 822.1
    - cartilage (semilunar) — *see* Tear, meniscus
  - labyrinth (osseous) — *see* Fracture, skull, base
  - larynx (closed) 807.5
    - open 807.6
  - late effect — *see* Late, effects (of), fracture
  - Le Fort's — *see* Fracture, maxilla
  - leg (closed) 827.0
    - with rib(s) or sternum 828.0
      - open 828.1
    - both (any bones) 828.0
      - open 828.1
    - lower — *see* Fracture, tibia
    - open 827.1
    - upper — *see* Fracture, femur
  - limb
    - lower (multiple) (closed) NEC 827.0
      - open 827.1
    - upper (multiple) (closed) NEC 818.0
      - open 818.1
  - long bones, due to birth trauma — *see* Birth injury, fracture
  - lumbar — *see* Fracture, vertebra, lumbar
  - lunate bone (closed) 814.02
    - open 814.12
  - malar bone (closed) 802.4
    - open 802.5
  - Malgaigne's (closed) 808.43
    - open 808.53
  - malleolus (closed) 824.8
    - bimalleolar 824.4
      - open 824.5
    - lateral 824.2
      - and medial — *see also* Fracture, malleolus, bimalleolar
        - with lip of tibia — *see* Fracture, malleolus, trimalleolar
      - open 824.3
    - medial (closed) 824.0
      - and lateral — *see also* Fracture, malleolus, bimalleolar
        - with lip of tibia — *see* Fracture, malleolus, trimalleolar
      - open 824.1
    - open 824.9
    - trimalleolar (closed) 824.6
      - open 824.7
  - malleus — *see* Fracture, skull, base
  - malunion 733.81
  - mandible (closed) 802.20
    - angle 802.25
      - open 802.35
    - body 802.28
      - alveolar border 802.27
        - open 802.37
      - open 802.38
      - symphysis 802.26
        - open 802.36
    - condylar process 802.21
      - open 802.31
    - coronoid process 802.23
      - open 802.33

- **Fracture** — *continued*
  - mandible — *continued*
    - multiple sites 802.29
      - open 802.39
    - open 802.30
    - ramus NEC 802.24
      - open 802.34
    - subcondylar 802.22
      - open 802.32
  - manubrium — *see* Fracture, sternum
  - march 733.95
    - fibula 733.93
    - metatarsals 733.94
    - tibia 733.93
  - maxilla, maxillary (superior) (upper jaw) (closed) 802.4
    - inferior — *see* Fracture, mandible
    - open 802.5
  - meniscus, knee — *see* Tear, meniscus
  - metacarpus, metacarpal (bone(s)), of one hand (closed) 815.00
    - with phalanx, phalanges, hand (finger(s)) (thumb) of same hand 817.0
      - open 817.1
    - base 815.02
      - first metacarpal 815.01
        - open 815.11
      - open 815.12
      - thumb 815.01
        - open 815.11
    - multiple sites 815.09
      - open 815.19
    - neck 815.04
      - open 815.14
    - open 815.10
    - shaft 815.03
      - open 815.13
  - metatarsus, metatarsal (bone(s)), of one foot (closed) 825.25
    - with tarsal bone(s) 825.29
      - open 825.39
    - open 825.35
  - Monteggia's (closed) 813.03
    - open 813.13
  - Moore's — *see* Fracture, radius, lower end
    - multangular bone (closed)
      - larger 814.05
        - open 814.15
      - smaller 814.06
        - open 814.16
  - multiple (closed) 829.0

> *Note — Multiple fractures of sites classifiable to the same three- or four-digit category are coded to that category, except for sites classifiable to 810-818 or 820-827 in different limbs.*
>
> *Multiple fractures of sites classifiable to different fourth-digit subdivisions within the same three-digit category should be dealt with according to coding rules.*
>
> *Multiple fractures of sites classifiable to different three-digit categories (identifiable from the listing under "Fracture"), and of sites classifiable to 810-818 or 820-827 in different limbs should be coded according to the following list, which should be referred to in the following priority order: skull or face bones, pelvis or vertebral column, legs, arms.*

-
  -
    - arm (multiple bones in same arm except in hand alone) (sites classifiable to 810-817 with sites classifiable to a different three-digit category in 810-817 in same arm) (closed) 818.0
      - open 818.1
    - arms, both or arm(s) with rib(s) or sternum (sites classifiable to 810-818 with sites classifiable to same range of categories in other limb or to 807) (closed) 819.0
      - open 819.1
    - bones of trunk NEC (closed) 809.0
      - open 809.1
    - hand, metacarpal bone(s) with phalanx or phalanges of same hand (sites classifiable to 815 with sites classifiable to 816 in same hand) (closed) 817.0
      - open 817.1

- **Fracture** — *continued*
  - multiple — *continued*
    - leg (multiple bones in same leg) (sites classifiable to 820-826 with sites classifiable to a different three-digit category in that range in same leg) (closed) 827.0
      - open 827.1
    - legs, both or leg(s) with arm(s), rib(s), or sternum (sites classifiable to 820-827 with sites classifiable to same range of categories in other leg or to 807 or 810-819) (closed) 828.0
      - open 828.1
    - open 829.1
    - pelvis with other bones except skull or face bones (sites classifiable to 808 with sites classifiable to 805-807 or 810-829) (closed) 809.0
      - open 809.1
    - skull, specified or unspecified bones, or face bone(s) with any other bone(s) (sites classifiable to 800-803 with sites classifiable to 805-829) (closed) 804.0 ☑

> *Note — Use the following fifth-digit subclassification with categories 800, 801, 803, and 804:*
>
> 0 *unspecified state of consciousness*
> 1 *with no loss of consciousness*
> 2 *with brief [less than one hour] loss of consciousness*
> 3 *with moderate [1-24 hours] loss of consciousness*
> 4 *with prolonged [more than 24 hours] loss of consciousness and return to pre-existing conscious level*
> 5 *with prolonged [more than 24 hours] loss of consciousness, without return to pre-existing conscious level*
> *Use fifth-digit 5 to designate when a patient is unconscious and dies before regaining consciousness, regardless of the duration of the loss of consciousness*
> 6 *with loss of consciousness of unspecified duration*
> 9 *with concussion, unspecified*

-
  -
    -
      - with
        - contusion, cerebral 804.1 ☑
        - epidural hemorrhage 804.2 ☑
        - extradural hemorrhage 804.2 ☑
        - hemorrhage (intracranial) NEC 804.3 ☑
        - intracranial injury NEC 804.4 ☑
        - laceration, cerebral 804.1 ☑
        - subarachnoid hemorrhage 804.2 ☑
        - subdural hemorrhage 804.2 ☑
      - open 804.5 ☑
        - with
          - contusion, cerebral 804.6 ☑
          - epidural hemorrhage 804.7 ☑
          - extradural hemorrhage 804.7 ☑
          - hemorrhage (intracranial) NEC 804.8 ☑
          - intracranial injury NEC 804.9 ☑
          - laceration, cerebral 804.6 ☑
          - subarachnoid hemorrhage 804.7 ☑
          - subdural hemorrhage 804.7 ☑
    - vertebral column with other bones, except skull or face bones (sites classifiable to 805 or 806 with sites classifiable to 807-808 or 810-829) (closed) 809.0
      - open 809.1
  - nasal (bone(s)) (closed) 802.0
    - open 802.1
    - sinus — *see* Fracture, skull, base
  - navicular
    - carpal (wrist) (closed) 814.01
      - open 814.11
    - tarsal (ankle) (closed) 825.22
      - open 825.32

- **Fracture** — *continued*
  - neck — *see* Fracture, vertebra, cervical
  - neural arch — *see* Fracture, vertebra, by site
  - nonunion 733.82
  - nose, nasal, (bone) (septum) (closed) 802.0
    - open 802.1
  - occiput — *see* Fracture, skull, base
  - odontoid process — *see* Fracture, vertebra, cervical
  - olecranon (process) (ulna) (closed) 813.01
    - open 813.11
  - open 829.1
  - orbit, orbital (bone) (region) (closed) 802.8
    - floor (blow-out) 802.6
      - open 802.7
    - open 802.9
    - roof — *see* Fracture, skull, base
    - specified part NEC 802.8
      - open 802.9
  - os
    - calcis (closed) 825.0
      - open 825.1
    - magnum (closed) 814.07
      - open 814.17
    - pubis (with visceral injury) (closed) 808.2
      - open 808.3
    - triquetrum (closed) 814.03
      - open 814.13
  - osseous
    - auditory meatus — *see* Fracture, skull, base
    - labyrinth — *see* Fracture, skull, base
  - ossicles, auditory (incus) (malleus) (stapes) — *see* Fracture, skull, base
  - osteoporotic — *see* Fracture, pathologic
  - palate (closed) 802.8
    - open 802.9
  - paratrooper — *see* Fracture, tibia, lower end
  - parietal bone — *see* Fracture, skull, vault
  - parry — *see* Fracture, Monteggia's
  - patella (closed) 822.0
    - open 822.1
  - pathologic (cause unknown) 733.10
    - ankle 733.16
    - femur (neck) 733.14
      - specified NEC 733.15
    - fibula 733.16
    - hip 733.14
    - humerus 733.11
    - radius (distal) 733.12
    - specified site NEC 733.19
    - tibia 733.16
    - ulna 733.12
    - vertebrae (collapse) 733.13
    - wrist 733.12
  - pedicle (of vertebral arch) — *see* Fracture, vertebra, by site
  - pelvis, pelvic (bone(s)) (with visceral injury) (closed) 808.8
    - multiple (with disruption of pelvic circle) 808.43
      - open 808.53
    - open 808.9
    - rim (closed) 808.49
      - open 808.59
  - peritrochanteric (closed) 820.20
    - open 820.30
  - phalanx, phalanges, of one
    - foot (closed) 826.0
      - with bone(s) of same lower limb 827.0
        - open 827.1
      - open 826.1
    - hand (closed) 816.00
      - with metacarpal bone(s) of same hand 817.0
        - open 817.1
      - distal 816.02
        - open 816.12
      - middle 816.01
        - open 816.11
      - multiple sites NEC 816.03
        - open 816.13
      - open 816.10
      - proximal 816.01
        - open 816.11
  - pisiform (closed) 814.04
    - open 814.14
  - pond — *see* Fracture, skull, vault

- **Fracture** — *continued*
  - Pott's (closed) 824.4
    - open 824.5
  - prosthetic device, internal — *see* Complications, mechanical
  - pubis (with visceral injury) (closed) 808.2
    - open 808.3
  - Quervain's (closed) 814.01
    - open 814.11
  - radius (alone) (closed) 813.81
    - with ulna NEC 813.83
      - open 813.93
    - distal end — *see* Fracture, radius, lower end
    - epiphysis
      - lower — *see* Fracture, radius, lower end
      - upper — *see* Fracture, radius, upper end
    - head — *see* Fracture, radius, upper end
    - lower end or extremity (distal end) (lower epiphysis) 813.42
      - with ulna (lower end) 813.44
        - open 813.54
      - torus 813.45
      - open 813.52
    - neck — *see* Fracture, radius, upper end
    - open NEC 813.91
    - pathologic 733.12
    - proximal end — *see* Fracture, radius, upper end
    - shaft (closed) 813.21
      - with ulna (shaft) 813.23
        - open 813.33
      - open 813.31
    - upper end 813.07
      - with ulna (upper end) 813.08
        - open 813.18
      - epiphysis 813.05
        - open 813.15
      - head 813.05
        - open 813.15
      - multiple sites 813.07
        - open 813.17
      - neck 813.06
        - open 813.16
      - open 813.17
      - specified site NEC 813.07
        - open 813.17
  - ramus
    - inferior or superior (with visceral injury) (closed) 808.2
    - open 808.3
    - ischium — *see* Fracture, ischium
    - mandible 802.24
      - open 802.34
  - rib(s) (closed) 807.0 ☑

> *Note — Use the following fifth-digit subclassification with categories 807.0-807.1:*
>
> *0 rib(s), unspecified*
> *1 one rib*
> *2 two ribs*
> *3 three ribs*
> *4 four ribs*
> *5 five ribs*
> *6 six ribs*
> *7 seven ribs*
> *8 eight or more ribs*
> *9 multiple ribs, unspecified*

-
  -
    - with flail chest (open) 807.4
    - open 807.1 ☑
  - root, tooth 873.63
    - complicated 873.73
  - sacrum — *see* Fracture, vertebra, sacrum
  - scaphoid
    - ankle (closed) 825.22
      - open 825.32
    - wrist (closed) 814.01
      - open 814.11
  - scapula (closed) 811.00
    - acromial, acromion (process) 811.01
      - open 811.11
    - body 811.09
      - open 811.19

- **Fracture** — *continued*
  - scapula — *continued*
    - coracoid process 811.02
      - open 811.12
    - glenoid (cavity) (fossa) 811.03
      - open 811.13
    - neck 811.03
      - open 811.13
    - open 811.10
  - semilunar
    - bone, wrist (closed) 814.02
      - open 814.12
    - cartilage (interior) (knee) — *see* Tear, meniscus
  - sesamoid bone — *see* Fracture, by site
  - Shepherd's (closed) 825.21
    - open 825.31
  - shoulder — *see also* Fracture, humerus, upper end
    - blade — *see* Fracture, scapula
  - silverfork — *see* Fracture, radius, lower end
  - sinus (ethmoid) (frontal) (maxillary) (nasal) (sphenoidal) — *see* Fracture, skull, base
  - Skillern's — *see* Fracture, radius, shaft
  - skull (multiple NEC) (with face bones) (closed) 803.0 ☑

> *Note — Use the following fifth-digit subclassification with categories 800, 801, 803, and 804:*
>
> *0 unspecified state of consciousness*
> *1 with no loss of consciousness*
> *2 with brief [less than one hour] loss of consciousness*
> *3 with moderate [1-24 hours] loss of consciousness*
> *4 with prolonged [more than 24 hours] loss of consciousness and return to pre-existing conscious level*
> *5 with prolonged [more than 24 hours] loss of consciousness, without return to pre-existing conscious level*
> *Use fifth-digit 5 to designate when a patient is unconscious and dies before regaining consciousness, regardless of the duration of loss of consciousness*
> *6 with loss of consciousness of unspecified duration*
> *9 with concussion, unspecified*

-
  -
    - with
      - contusion, cerebral 803.1 ☑
      - epidural hemorrhage 803.2 ☑
      - extradural hemorrhage 803.2 ☑
      - hemorrhage (intracranial) NEC 803.3 ☑
      - intracranial injury NEC 803.4 ☑
      - laceration, cerebral 803.1 ☑
      - other bones — *see* Fracture, multiple, skull
      - subarachnoid hemorrhage 803.2 ☑
      - subdural hemorrhage 803.2 ☑
    - base (antrum) (ethmoid bone) (fossa) (internal ear) (nasal sinus) (occiput) (sphenoid) (temporal bone) (closed) 801.0 ☑
      - with
        - contusion, cerebral 801.1 ☑
        - epidural hemorrhage 801.2 ☑
        - extradural hemorrhage 801.2 ☑
        - hemorrhage (intracranial) NEC 801.3 ☑
        - intracranial injury NEC 801.4 ☑
        - laceration, cerebral 801.1 ☑
        - subarachnoid hemorrhage 801.2 ☑
        - subdural hemorrhage 801.2 ☑
      - open 801.5 ☑
        - with
          - contusion, cerebral 801.6 ☑
          - epidural hemorrhage 801.7 ☑
          - extradural hemorrhage 801.7 ☑
          - hemorrhage (intracranial) NEC 801.8 ☑
          - intracranial injury NEC 801.9 ☑
          - laceration, cerebral 801.6 ☑
          - subarachnoid hemorrhage 801.7 ☑
          - subdural hemorrhage 801.7 ☑

Note — Use the following fifth-digit subclassification with categories 806.0-806.3:
C_1-C_4 or unspecified level and D_1-D_6 (T_1-T_6) or unspecified level with:
0 unspecified spinal cord injury
1 complete lesion of cord
2 anterior cord syndrome
3 central cord syndrome
4 specified injury NEC
C_5-C_7 level and D_7-D_{12} level with:
5 unspecified spinal cord injury
6 complete lesion of cord
7 anterior cord syndrome
8 central cord syndrome
9 specified injury NEC

G

- **Glomerulonephritis** (*see also* Nephritis) — *continued*
  - basement membrane NEC 583.89
    - with
      - pulmonary hemorrhage (Goodpasture's syndrome) 446.21 *[583.81]*
  - chronic 582.9
    - with
      - exudative nephritis 582.89
      - interstitial nephritis (diffuse) (focal) 582.89
      - necrotizing glomerulitis 582.4
      - specified pathology or lesion NEC 582.89
    - endothelial 582.2
    - extracapillary with epithelial crescents 582.4
    - hypocomplementemic persistent 582.2
    - lobular 582.2
    - membranoproliferative 582.2
    - membranous 582.1
      - and proliferative (mixed) 582.2
      - sclerosing 582.1
    - mesangiocapillary 582.2
    - mixed membranous and proliferative 582.2
    - proliferative (diffuse) 582.0
    - rapidly progressive 582.4
    - sclerosing 582.1
  - cirrhotic — *see* Sclerosis, renal
  - desquamative — *see* Nephrosis
  - due to or associated with
    - amyloidosis 277.3 *[583.81]*
      - with nephrotic syndrome 277.3 *[581.81]*
      - chronic 277.3 *[582.81]*
    - diabetes mellitus 250.4 ☑ *[583.81]*
      - with nephrotic syndrome 250.4 ☑ *[581.81]*
    - diphtheria 032.89 *[580.81]*
    - gonococcal infection (acute) 098.19 *[583.81]*
      - chronic or duration of 2 months or over 098.39 *[583.81]*
    - infectious hepatitis 070.9 *[580.81]*
    - malaria (with nephrotic syndrome) 084.9 *[581.81]*
    - mumps 072.79 *[580.81]*
    - polyarteritis (nodosa) (with nephrotic syndrome) 446.0 *[581.81]*
    - specified pathology NEC 583.89
      - acute 580.89
      - chronic 582.89
    - streptotrichosis 039.8 *[583.81]*
    - subacute bacterial endocarditis 421.0 *[580.81]*
    - syphilis (late) 095.4
      - congenital 090.5 *[583.81]*
      - early 091.69 *[583.81]*
    - systemic lupus erythematosus 710.0 *[583.81]*
      - with nephrotic syndrome 710.0 *[581.81]*
      - chronic 710.0 *[582.81]*
    - tuberculosis (*see also* Tuberculosis) 016.0 ☑ *[583.81]*
    - typhoid fever 002.0 *[580.81]*
  - extracapillary with epithelial crescents 583.4
    - acute 580.4
    - chronic 582.4
  - exudative 583.89
    - acute 580.89
    - chronic 582.89
  - focal (*see also* Nephritis) 583.9
    - embolic 580.4
  - granular 582.89
  - granulomatous 582.89
  - hydremic (*see also* Nephrosis) 581.9
  - hypocomplementemic persistent 583.2
    - with nephrotic syndrome 581.2
    - chronic 582.2
  - immune complex NEC 583.89
  - infective (*see also* Pyelitis) 590.80
  - interstitial (diffuse) (focal) 583.89
    - with nephrotic syndrome 581.89
    - acute 580.89
    - chronic 582.89
  - latent or quiescent 582.9
  - lobular 583.2
    - with nephrotic syndrome 581.2
    - chronic 582.2
  - membranoproliferative 583.2
    - with nephrotic syndrome 581.2
    - chronic 582.2

- **Glomerulonephritis** (*see also* Nephritis) — *continued*
  - membranous 583.1
    - with nephrotic syndrome 581.1
    - and proliferative (mixed) 583.2
      - with nephrotic syndrome 581.2
      - chronic 582.2
    - chronic 582.1
    - sclerosing 582.1
      - with nephrotic syndrome 581.1
  - mesangiocapillary 583.2
    - with nephrotic syndrome 581.2
    - chronic 582.2
  - minimal change 581.3
  - mixed membranous and proliferative 583.2
    - with nephrotic syndrome 581.2
    - chronic 582.2
  - necrotizing 583.4
    - acute 580.4
    - chronic 582.4
  - nephrotic (*see also* Nephrosis) 581.9
  - old — *see* Glomerulonephritis, chronic
  - parenchymatous 581.89
  - poststreptococcal 580.0
  - proliferative (diffuse) 583.0
    - with nephrotic syndrome 581.0
    - acute 580.0
    - chronic 582.0
  - purulent (*see also* Pyelitis) 590.80
  - quiescent — *see* Nephritis, chronic
  - rapidly progressive 583.4
    - acute 580.4
    - chronic 582.4
  - sclerosing membranous (chronic) 582.1
    - with nephrotic syndrome 581.1
  - septic (*see also* Pyelitis) 590.80
  - specified pathology or lesion NEC 583.89
    - with nephrotic syndrome 581.89
    - acute 580.89
    - chronic 582.89
  - suppurative (acute) (disseminated) (*see also* Pyelitis) 590.80
  - toxic — *see* Nephritis, acute
  - tubal, tubular — *see* Nephrosis, tubular
  - type II (Ellis) — *see* Nephrosis
  - vascular — *see* Hypertension, kidney
- **Glomerulosclerosis** (*see also* Sclerosis, renal) 587
  - focal 582.1
    - with nephrotic syndrome 581.1
  - intercapillary (nodular) (with diabetes) 250.4 ☑ *[581.81]*
- **Glossagra** 529.6
- **Glossalgia** 529.6
- **Glossitis** 529.0
  - areata exfoliativa 529.1
  - atrophic 529.4
  - benign migratory 529.1
  - gangrenous 529.0
  - Hunter's 529.4
  - median rhomboid 529.2
  - Moeller's 529.4
  - pellagrous 265.2
- **Glossocele** 529.8
- **Glossodynia** 529.6
  - exfoliativa 529.4
- **Glossoncus** 529.8
- **Glossophytia** 529.3
- **Glossoplegia** 529.8
- **Glossoptosis** 529.8
- **Glossopyrosis** 529.6
- **Glossotrichia** 529.3
- **Glossy skin** 701.9
- **Glottis** — *see* condition
- **Glottitis** — *see* Glossitis
- **Glucagonoma** (M8152/0)
  - malignant (M8152/3)
    - pancreas 157.4
    - specified site NEC — *see* Neoplasm, by site, malignant
    - unspecified site 157.4
  - pancreas 211.7
  - specified site NEC — *see* Neoplasm, by site, benign
  - unspecified site 211.7

- **Glucoglycinuria** 270.7
- **Glue ear syndrome** 381.20
- **Glue sniffing** (airplane glue) (*see also* Dependence) 304.6 ☑
- **Glycinemia** (with methylmalonic acidemia) 270.7
- **Glycinuria** (renal) (with ketosis) 270.0
- **Glycogen**
  - infiltration (*see also* Disease, glycogen storage) 271.0
  - storage disease (*see also* Disease, glycogen storage) 271.0
- **Glycogenosis** (*see also* Disease, glycogen storage) 271.0
  - cardiac 271.0 *[425.7]*
  - Cori, types I-VII 271.0
  - diabetic, secondary 250.8 ☑ *[259.8]*
  - diffuse (with hepatic cirrhosis) 271.0
  - generalized 271.0
  - glucose-6-phosphatase deficiency 271.0
  - hepatophosphorylase deficiency 271.0
  - hepatorenal 271.0
  - myophosphorylase deficiency 271.0
- **Glycopenia** 251.2
- **Glycopeptide**
  - intermediate staphylococcus aureus (GISA) V09.8
  - resistant
    - enterococcus V09.8
    - staphylococcus aureus (GRSA) V09.8
- **Glycoprolinuria** 270.8
- **Glycosuria** 791.5
  - renal 271.4
- **Gnathostoma** (spinigerum) (infection) (infestation) 128.1
  - wandering swellings from 128.1
- **Gnathostomiasis** 128.1
- **Goiter** (adolescent) (colloid) (diffuse) (dipping) (due to iodine deficiency) (endemic) (euthyroid) (heart) (hyperplastic) (internal) (intrathoracic) (juvenile) (mixed type) (nonendemic) (parenchymatous) (plunging) (sporadic) (subclavicular) (substernal) 240.9
  - with
    - hyperthyroidism (recurrent) (*see also* Goiter, toxic) 242.0 ☑
    - thyrotoxicosis (*see also* Goiter, toxic) 242.0 ☑
  - adenomatous (*see also* Goiter, nodular) 241.9
  - cancerous (M8000/3) 193
  - complicating pregnancy, childbirth, or puerperium 648.1 ☑
  - congenital 246.1
  - cystic (*see also* Goiter, nodular) 241.9
  - due to enzyme defect in synthesis of thyroid hormone (butane-insoluble iodine) (coupling) (deiodinase) (iodide trapping or organification) (iodotyrosine dehalogenase) (peroxidase) 246.1
  - dyshormonogenic 246.1
  - exophthalmic (*see also* Goiter, toxic) 242.0 ☑
  - familial (with deaf-mutism) 243
  - fibrous 245.3
  - lingual 759.2
  - lymphadenoid 245.2
  - malignant (M8000/3) 193
  - multinodular (nontoxic) 241.1
    - toxic or with hyperthyroidism (*see also* Goiter, toxic) 242.2 ☑
  - nodular (nontoxic) 241.9
    - with
      - hyperthyroidism (*see also* Goiter, toxic) 242.3 ☑
      - thyrotoxicosis (*see also* Goiter, toxic) 242.3 ☑
    - endemic 241.9
    - exophthalmic (diffuse) (*see also* Goiter, toxic) 242.0 ☑
    - multinodular (nontoxic) 241.1
    - sporadic 241.9
    - toxic (*see also* Goiter, toxic) 242.3 ☑
    - uninodular (nontoxic) 241.0
  - nontoxic (nodular) 241.9
    - multinodular 241.1
    - uninodular 241.0
  - pulsating (*see also* Goiter, toxic) 242.0 ☑

Goiter — *continued*
- simple 240.0
- toxic 242.0 ☑

> *Note — Use the following fifth-digit subclassification with category 242:*
>
> 0 *without mention of thyrotoxic crisis or storm*
>
> 1 *with mention of thyrotoxic crisis or storm*

-
  - adenomatous 242.3 ☑
    - multinodular 242.2 ☑
    - uninodular 242.1 ☑
  - multinodular 242.2 ☑
  - nodular 242.3 ☑
    - multinodular 242.2 ☑
    - uninodular 242.1 ☑
  - uninodular 242.1 ☑
- uninodular (nontoxic) 241.0
  - toxic or with hyperthyroidism (*see also* Goiter, toxic) 242.1 ☑

Goldberg (-Maxwell) (-Morris) syndrome (testicular feminization) 259.5 ▲

Goldblatt's
- hypertension 440.1
- kidney 440.1

Goldenhar's syndrome (oculoauriculovertebral dysplasia) 756.0

Goldflam-Erb disease or syndrome 358.00

Goldscheider's disease (epidermolysis bullosa) 757.39

Goldstein's disease (familial hemorrhagic telangiectasia) 448.0

Golfer's elbow 726.32

Goltz-Gorlin syndrome (dermal hypoplasia) 757.39

Gonadoblastoma (M9073/1)
- specified site — *see* Neoplasm, by site uncertain behavior
- unspecified site
  - female 236.2
  - male 236.4

Gonecystitis (*see also* Vesiculitis) 608.0

Gongylonemiasis 125.6
- mouth 125.6

Goniosynechiae 364.73

Gonococcemia 098.89

Gonococcus, gonococcal (disease) (infection) (*see also* condition) 098.0
- anus 098.7
- bursa 098.52
- chronic NEC 098.2
- complicating pregnancy, childbirth, or puerperium 647.1 ☑
  - affecting fetus or newborn 760.2
- conjunctiva, conjunctivitis (neonatorum) 098.40
- dermatosis 098.89
- endocardium 098.84
- epididymo-orchitis 098.13
  - chronic or duration of 2 months or over 098.33
- eye (newborn) 098.40
- fallopian tube (chronic) 098.37
  - acute 098.17
- genitourinary (acute) (organ) (system) (tract) (*see also* Gonorrhea) 098.0
  - lower 098.0
    - chronic 098.2
  - upper 098.10
    - chronic 098.30
- heart NEC 098.85
- joint 098.50
- keratoderma 098.81
- keratosis (blennorrhagica) 098.81
- lymphatic (gland) (node) 098.89
- meninges 098.82
- orchitis (acute) 098.13
  - chronic or duration of 2 months or over 098.33
- pelvis (acute) 098.19
  - chronic or duration of 2 months or over 098.39

Gonococcus, gonococcal (*see also* condition) — *continued*
- pericarditis 098.83
- peritonitis 098.86
- pharyngitis 098.6
- pharynx 098.6
- proctitis 098.7
- pyosalpinx (chronic) 098.37
  - acute 098.17
- rectum 098.7
- septicemia 098.89
- skin 098.89
- specified site NEC 098.89
- synovitis 098.51
- tendon sheath 098.51
- throat 098.6
- urethra (acute) 098.0
  - chronic or duration of 2 months or over 098.2
- vulva (acute) 098.0
  - chronic or duration of 2 months or over 098.2

Gonocytoma (M9073/1)
- specified site — *see* Neoplasm, by site, uncertain behavior
- unspecified site
  - female 236.2
  - male 236.4

Gonorrhea 098.0
- acute 098.0
- Bartholin's gland (acute) 098.0
  - chronic or duration of 2 months or over 098.2
- bladder (acute) 098.11
  - chronic or duration of 2 months or over 098.31
- carrier (suspected of) V02.7
- cervix (acute) 098.15
  - chronic or duration of 2 months or over 098.35
- chronic 098.2
- complicating pregnancy, childbirth, or puerperium 647.1 ☑
  - affecting fetus or newborn 760.2
- conjunctiva, conjunctivitis (neonatorum) 098.40
- contact V01.6
- Cowper's gland (acute) 098.0
  - chronic or duration of 2 months or over 098.2
- duration of two months or over 098.2
- exposure to V01.6
- fallopian tube (chronic) 098.37
  - acute 098.17
- genitourinary (acute) (organ) (system) (tract) 098.0
  - chronic 098.2
  - duration of two months or over 098.2
- kidney (acute) 098.19
  - chronic or duration of 2 months or over 098.39
- ovary (acute) 098.19
  - chronic or duration of 2 months or over 098.39
- pelvis (acute) 098.19
  - chronic or duration of 2 months or over 098.39
- penis (acute) 098.0
  - chronic or duration of 2 months or over 098.2
- prostate (acute) 098.12
  - chronic or duration of 2 months or over 098.32
- seminal vesicle (acute) 098.14
  - chronic or duration of 2 months or over 098.34
- specified site NEC — *see* Gonococcus
- spermatic cord (acute) 098.14
  - chronic or duration of 2 months or over 098.34
- urethra (acute) 098.0
  - chronic or duration of 2 months or over 098.2
- vagina (acute) 098.0
  - chronic or duration of 2 months or over 098.2

Gonorrhea — *continued*
- vas deferens (acute) 098.14
  - chronic or duration of 2 months or over 098.34
- vulva (acute) 098.0
  - chronic or duration of 2 months or over 098.2

Goodpasture's syndrome (pneumorenal) 446.21

Good's syndrome 279.06

Gopalan's syndrome (burning feet) 266.2

Gordon's disease (exudative enteropathy) 579.8

Gorlin-Chaudhry-Moss syndrome 759.89

Gougerot's syndrome (trisymptomatic) 709.1

Gougerot-Blum syndrome (pigmented purpuric lichenoid dermatitis) 709.1

Gougerot-Carteaud disease or syndrome (confluent reticulate papillomatosis) 701.8

Gougerot-Hailey-Hailey disease (benign familial chronic pemphigus) 757.39

Gougerot (-Houwer) - Sjögren syndrome (keratoconjunctivitis sicca) 710.2

Gouley's syndrome (constrictive pericarditis) 423.2

Goundou 102.6

Gout, gouty 274.9
- with specified manifestations NEC 274.89
- arthritis (acute) 274.0
- arthropathy 274.0
- degeneration, heart 274.82
- diathesis 274.9
- eczema 274.89
- episcleritis 274.89 *[379.09]*
- external ear (tophus) 274.81
- glomerulonephritis 274.10
- iritis 274.89 *[364.11]*
- joint 274.0
- kidney 274.10
- lead 984.9
  - specified type of lead — *see* Table of Drugs and Chemicals
- nephritis 274.10
- neuritis 274.89 *[357.4]*
- phlebitis 274.89 *[451.9]*
- rheumatic 714.0
- saturnine 984.9
  - specified type of lead — *see* Table of Drugs and Chemicals
- spondylitis 274.0
- synovitis 274.0
- syphilitic 095.8
- tophi 274.0
  - ear 274.81
  - heart 274.82
  - specified site NEC 274.82

Gowers'
- muscular dystrophy 359.1
- syndrome (vasovagal attack) 780.2

Gowers-Paton-Kennedy syndrome 377.04

Gradenigo's syndrome 383.02

Graft-versus-host disease (bone marrow) 996.85
- due to organ transplant NEC — *see* Complications, transplant, organ

Graham Steell's murmur (pulmonic regurgitation) (*see also* Endocarditis, pulmonary) 424.3

Grain-handlers' disease or lung 495.8

Grain mite (itch) 133.8

Grand
- mal (idiopathic) (*see also* Epilepsy) 345.1 ☑
  - hysteria of Charcôt 300.11
  - nonrecurrent or isolated 780.39
- multipara
  - affecting management of labor and delivery 659.4 ☑
  - status only (not pregnant) V61.5

Granite workers' lung 502

Granular — *see also* condition
- inflammation, pharynx 472.1
- kidney (contracting) (*see also* Sclerosis, renal) 587
- liver — *see* Cirrhosis, liver
- nephritis — *see* Nephritis

Granulation tissue, abnormal — *see also* Granuloma
- abnormal or excessive 701.5
- postmastoidectomy cavity 383.33
- postoperative 701.5
- skin 701.5

Granulocytopenia, granulocytopenic (primary) 288.0
- malignant 288.0

Granuloma NEC 686.1
- abdomen (wall) 568.89
    - skin (pyogenicum) 686.1
        - from residual foreign body 709.4
- annulare 695.89
- anus 569.49
- apical 522.6
- appendix 543.9
- aural 380.23
- beryllium (skin) 709.4
    - lung 503
- bone (*see also* Osteomyelitis) 730.1 ☑
    - eosinophilic 277.89
    - from residual foreign body 733.99
- canaliculus lacrimalis 375.81
- cerebral 348.8
- cholesterin, middle ear 385.82
- coccidioidal (progressive) 114.3
    - lung 114.4
    - meninges 114.2
    - primary (lung) 114.0
- colon 569.89
- conjunctiva 372.61
- dental 522.6
- ear, middle (cholesterin) 385.82
    - with otitis media — *see* Otitis media
- eosinophilic 277.89
    - bone 277.89
    - lung 277.89
    - oral mucosa 528.9
- exuberant 701.5
- eyelid 374.89
- facial
    - lethal midline 446.3
    - malignant 446.3
- faciale 701.8
- fissuratum (gum) 523.8
- foot NEC 686.1
- foreign body (in soft tissue) NEC 728.82
    - bone 733.99
    - in operative wound 998.4
    - muscle 728.82
    - skin 709.4
    - subcutaneous tissue 709.4
- fungoides 202.1 ☑
- gangraenescens 446.3
- giant cell (central) (jaw) (reparative) 526.3
    - gingiva 523.8
    - peripheral (gingiva) 523.8
- gland (lymph) 289.3
- Hodgkin's (M9661/3) 201.1 ☑
- ileum 569.89
- infectious NEC 136.9
- inguinale (Donovan) 099.2
    - venereal 099.2
- intestine 569.89
- iridocyclitis 364.10
- jaw (bone) 526.3
    - reparative giant cell 526.3
- kidney (*see also* Infection, kidney) 590.9
- lacrimal sac 375.81
- larynx 478.79
- lethal midline 446.3
- lipid 277.89
- lipoid 277.89
- liver 572.8
- lung (infectious) (*see also* Fibrosis, lung) 515
    - coccidioidal 114.4
    - eosinophilic 277.89
- lymph gland 289.3
- Majocchi's 110.6
- malignant, face 446.3
- mandible 526.3
- mediastinum 519.3
- midline 446.3
- monilial 112.3
- muscle 728.82
    - from residual foreign body 728.82

Granuloma — *continued*
- nasal sinus (*see also* Sinusitis) 473.9
- operation wound 998.59
    - foreign body 998.4
    - stitch (external) 998.89
        - internal organ 996.7 ☑
        - internal wound 998.89
    - talc 998.7
- oral mucosa, eosinophilic or pyogenic 528.9
- orbit, orbital 376.11
- paracoccidioidal 116.1
- penis, venereal 099.2
- periapical 522.6
- peritoneum 568.89
    - due to ova of helminths NEC (*see also* Helminthiasis) 128.9
- postmastoidectomy cavity 383.33
- postoperative — *see* Granuloma, operation wound
- prostate 601.8
- pudendi (ulcerating) 099.2
- pudendorum (ulcerative) 099.2
- pulp, internal (tooth) 521.49
- pyogenic, pyogenicum (skin) 686.1
    - maxillary alveolar ridge 522.6
    - oral mucosa 528.9
- rectum 569.49
- reticulohistiocytic 277.89
- rubrum nasi 705.89
- sarcoid 135
- Schistosoma 120.9
- septic (skin) 686.1
- silica (skin) 709.4
- sinus (accessory) (infectional) (nasal) (*see also* Sinusitis) 473.9
- skin (pyogenicum) 686.1
    - from foreign body or material 709.4
- sperm 608.89
- spine
    - syphilitic (epidural) 094.89
    - tuberculous (*see also* Tuberculosis) 015.0 ☑ *[730.88]*
- stitch (postoperative) 998.89
    - internal wound 998.89
- suppurative (skin) 686.1
- suture (postoperative) 998.89
    - internal wound 998.89
- swimming pool 031.1
- talc 728.82
    - in operation wound 998.7
- telangiectaticum (skin) 686.1
- trichophyticum 110.6
- tropicum 102.4
- umbilicus 686.1
    - newborn 771.4
- urethra 599.84
- uveitis 364.10
- vagina 099.2
- venereum 099.2
- vocal cords 478.5
- Wegener's (necrotizing respiratory granulomatosis) 446.4

Granulomatosis NEC 686.1
- disciformis chronica et progressiva 709.3
- infantiseptica 771.2
- lipoid 277.89
- lipophagic, intestinal 040.2
- miliary 027.0
- necrotizing, respiratory 446.4
- progressive, septic 288.1
- Wegener's (necrotizing respiratory) 446.4

Granulomatous tissue — *see* Granuloma

Granulosis rubra nasi 705.89

Graphite fibrosis (of lung) 503

Graphospasm 300.89
- organic 333.84

Grating scapula 733.99

Gravel (urinary) (*see also* Calculus) 592.9

Graves' disease (exophthalmic goiter) (*see also* Goiter, toxic) 242.0 ☑

Gravis — *see* condition

Grawitz's tumor (hypernephroma) (M8312/3) 189.0

Grayness, hair (premature) 704.3
- congenital 757.4

Gray or grey syndrome (chloramphenicol) (newborn) 779.4

Greenfield's disease 330.0

Green sickness 280.9

Greenstick fracture — *see* Fracture, by site

Greig's syndrome (hypertelorism) 756.0

Griesinger's disease (*see also* Ancylostomiasis) 126.9

Grinders'
- asthma 502
- lung 502
- phthisis (*see also* Tuberculosis) 011.4 ☑

Grinding, teeth 306.8

Grip
- Dabney's 074.1
- devil's 074.1

Grippe, grippal — *see also* Influenza
- Balkan 083.0
- intestinal 487.8
- summer 074.8

Grippy cold 487.1

Grisel's disease 723.5

Groin — *see* condition

Grooved
- nails (transverse) 703.8
- tongue 529.5
    - congenital 750.13

Ground itch 126.9

Growing pains, children 781.99

Growth (fungoid) (neoplastic) (new) (M8000/1) — *see also* Neoplasm, by site, unspecified nature
- adenoid (vegetative) 474.12
- benign (M8000/0) — *see* Neoplasm, by site, benign
- fetal, poor 764.9 ☑
    - affecting management of pregnancy 656.5 ☑
- malignant (M8000/3) — *see* Neoplasm, by site, malignant
- rapid, childhood V21.0
- secondary (M8000/6) — *see* Neoplasm, by site, malignant, secondary

GRSA (glycopeptide resistant staphylococcus aureus) V09.8

Gruber's hernia — *see* Hernia, Gruber's

Gruby's disease (tinea tonsurans) 110.0

G-trisomy 758.0

Guama fever 066.3

Gubler (-Millard) paralysis or syndrome 344.89

Guérin-Stern syndrome (arthrogryposis multiplex congenita) 754.89

Guertin's disease (electric chorea) 049.8

Guillain-Barré disease or syndrome 357.0

Guinea worms (infection) (infestation) 125.7

Guinon's disease (motor-verbal tic) 307.23

Gull's disease (thyroid atrophy with myxedema) 244.8

Gull and Sutton's disease — *see* Hypertension, kidney

Gum — *see* condition

Gumboil 522.7

Gumma (syphilitic) 095.9
- artery 093.89
    - cerebral or spinal 094.89
- bone 095.5
    - of yaws (late) 102.6
- brain 094.89
- cauda equina 094.89
- central nervous system NEC 094.9
- ciliary body 095.8 *[364.11]*
- congenital 090.5
    - testis 090.5
- eyelid 095.8 *[373.5]*
- heart 093.89
- intracranial 094.89
- iris 095.8 *[364.11]*
- kidney 095.4
- larynx 095.8
- leptomeninges 094.2
- liver 095.3
- meninges 094.2

☑ Additional Digit Required — Refer to the Tabular List (Numeric Code Section) for Additional Digit Selection

▶◀ Revised Text ● New Line ▲ Revised Code

H

Note — Hematomas are coded according to origin and the nature and site of the hematoma or the accompanying injury. Hematomas of unspecified origin are coded as injuries of the sites involved, except:

(a) hematomas of genital organs which are coded as diseases of the organ involved unless they complicate pregnancy or delivery

(b) hematomas of the eye which are coded as diseases of the eye.

For late effect of hematoma classifiable to 920-924 see Late, effect, contusion

Note — Use the following fifth-digit subclassification with categories 851-854:

0	*unspecified state of consciousness*
1	*with no loss of consciousness*
2	*with brief [less than one hour] loss of consciousness*
3	*with moderate [1-24 hours] loss of consciousness*
4	*with prolonged [more than 24 hours] loss of consciousness and return to pre-existing conscious level*
5	*with prolonged [more than 24 hours] loss of consciousness, without return to pre-existing conscious level*
	Use fifth-digit 5 to designate when a patient is unconscious and dies before regaining consciousness, regardless of the duration of the loss of consciousness
6	*with loss of consciousness of unspecified duration*
9	*with concussion, unspecified*

☑ Additional Digit Required — Refer to the Tabular List (Numeric Code Section) for Additional Digit Selection

▶◀ Revised Text ● New Line ▲ Revised Code

Note — Use the following fifth-digit subclassification with categories 851-854:

0	*unspecified state of consciousness*
1	*with no loss of consciousness*
2	*with brief [less than one hour] loss of consciousness*
3	*with moderate [1-24 hours] loss of consciousness*
4	*with prolonged [more than 24 hours] loss of consciousness and return to pre-existing conscious level*
5	*with prolonged [more than 24 hours] loss of consciousness, without return to pre-existing conscious level*
	Use fifth-digit 5 to designate when a patient is unconscious and dies before regaining consciousness, regardless of the duration of the loss of consciousness
6	*with loss of consciousness of unspecified duration*
9	*with concussion, unspecified*

- **Hemorrhage, hemorrhagic** — *continued*
  - postpartum (atonic) (following delivery of placenta) 666.1 ☑
    - delayed or secondary (after 24 hours) 666.2 ☑
    - retained placenta 666.0 ☑
    - third stage 666.0 ☑
  - pregnancy (concealed) 641.9 ☑
    - accidental 641.2 ☑
      - affecting fetus or newborn 762.1
    - affecting fetus or newborn 762.1
    - before 22 completed weeks gestation 640.9 ☑
      - affecting fetus or newborn 762.1
    - due to
      - abruptio placenta 641.2 ☑
        - affecting fetus or newborn 762.1
      - afibrinogenemia or other coagulation defect (conditions classifiable to 286.0-286.9) 641.3 ☑
        - affecting fetus or newborn 762.1
      - coagulation defect 641.3 ☑
        - affecting fetus or newborn 762.1
      - hyperfibrinolysis 641.3 ☑
        - affecting fetus or newborn 762.1
      - hypofibrinogenemia 641.3 ☑
        - affecting fetus or newborn 762.1
      - leiomyoma, uterus 641.8 ☑
        - affecting fetus or newborn 762.1
      - low-lying placenta 641.1 ☑
        - affecting fetus or newborn 762.1
      - marginal sinus (rupture) 641.2 ☑
        - affecting fetus or newborn 762.1
      - placenta previa 641.1 ☑
        - affecting fetus or newborn 762.0
      - premature separation of placenta (normally implanted) 641.2 ☑
        - affecting fetus or newborn 762.1
      - threatened abortion 640.0 ☑
        - affecting fetus or newborn 762.1
      - trauma 641.8 ☑
        - affecting fetus or newborn 762.1
    - early (before 22 completed weeks gestation) 640.9 ☑
      - affecting fetus or newborn 762.1
    - previous, affecting management of pregnancy or childbirth V23.49
    - unavoidable — *see* Hemorrhage, pregnancy, due to placenta previa
  - prepartum (mother) — *see* Hemorrhage, pregnancy
  - preretinal, cause unspecified 362.81
  - prostate 602.1
  - puerperal (*see also* Hemorrhage, postpartum) 666.1 ☑
  - pulmonary — *see also* Hemorrhage, lung
    - newborn (massive) 770.3
    - renal syndrome 446.21
  - purpura (primary) (*see also* Purpura, thrombocytopenic) 287.39 ▲
  - rectum (sphincter) 569.3
  - recurring, following initial hemorrhage at time of injury 958.2
  - renal 593.81
    - pulmonary syndrome 446.21
  - respiratory tract (*see also* Hemorrhage, lung) 786.3
  - retina, retinal (deep) (superficial) (vessels) 362.81
    - diabetic 250.5 ☑ *[362.01]*
    - due to birth injury 772.8
  - retrobulbar 376.89
  - retroperitoneal 459.0
  - retroplacental (*see also* Placenta, separation) 641.2 ☑
  - scalp 459.0
    - due to injury at birth 767.19
  - scrotum 608.83
  - secondary (nontraumatic) 459.0
    - following initial hemorrhage at time of injury 958.2
  - seminal vesicle 608.83
  - skin 782.7
    - newborn 772.6
  - spermatic cord 608.83
  - spinal (cord) 336.1
    - aneurysm (ruptured) 336.1
      - syphilitic 094.89
    - due to birth injury 767.4
    - fetus or newborn 767.4
  - spleen 289.59
  - spontaneous NEC 459.0
    - petechial 782.7
  - stomach 578.9
    - newborn 772.4
    - ulcer — *see* Ulcer, stomach, with hemorrhage
  - subaponeurotic, newborn 767.11
    - massive (birth injury) 767.11
  - subarachnoid (nontraumatic) 430
    - fetus or newborn (anoxic) (traumatic) 772.2
    - puerperal, postpartum, childbirth 674.0 ☑
    - traumatic — *see* Hemorrhage, brain, traumatic, subarachnoid
  - subconjunctival 372.72
    - due to birth injury 772.8
    - newborn 772.8
  - subcortical (*see also* Hemorrhage, brain) 431
  - subcutaneous 782.7
  - subdiaphragmatic 459.0
  - subdural (nontraumatic) 432.1
    - due to birth injury 767.0
    - fetus or newborn (anoxic) (hypoxic) (due to birth trauma) 767.0
    - puerperal, postpartum, childbirth 674.0 ☑
    - spinal 336.1
    - traumatic — *see* Hemorrhage, brain, traumatic, subdural
  - subgaleal 767.11
  - subhyaloid 362.81
  - subperiosteal 733.99
  - subretinal 362.81
  - subtentorial (*see also* Hemorrhage, subdural) 432.1
  - subungual 703.8
    - due to blood dyscrasia 287.8
  - suprarenal (capsule) (gland) 255.4
    - fetus or newborn 772.5
  - tentorium (traumatic) — *see also* Hemorrhage, brain, traumatic
    - fetus or newborn 767.0
    - nontraumatic — *see* Hemorrhage, subdural
  - testis 608.83
  - thigh 459.0
  - third stage 666.0 ☑
  - thorax — *see* Hemorrhage, lung
  - throat 784.8
  - thrombocythemia 238.7
  - thymus (gland) 254.8
  - thyroid (gland) 246.3
    - cyst 246.3
  - tongue 529.8
  - tonsil 474.8
    - postoperative 998.11
  - tooth socket (postextraction) 998.11
  - trachea — *see* Hemorrhage, lung
  - traumatic — *see also* nature of injury
    - brain — *see* Hemorrhage, brain, traumatic
    - recurring or secondary (following initial hemorrhage at time of injury) 958.2
  - tuberculous NEC (*see also* Tuberculosis, pulmonary) 011.9 ☑
  - tunica vaginalis 608.83
  - ulcer — *see* Ulcer, by site, with hemorrhage
  - umbilicus, umbilical cord 772.0
    - after birth, newborn 772.3
    - complicating delivery 663.8 ☑
      - affecting fetus or newborn 772.0
    - slipped ligature 772.3
    - stump 772.3
  - unavoidable (due to placenta previa) 641.1 ☑
    - affecting fetus or newborn 762.0
  - upper extremity 459.0
  - urethra (idiopathic) 599.84
  - uterus, uterine (abnormal) 626.9
    - climacteric 627.0
    - complicating delivery — *see* Hemorrhage, complicating delivery
    - due to
      - intrauterine contraceptive device 996.76
        - perforating uterus 996.32
    - functional or dysfunctional 626.8
    - in pregnancy — *see* Hemorrhage, pregnancy
    - intermenstrual 626.6
      - irregular 626.6
      - regular 626.5
    - postmenopausal 627.1
    - postpartum (*see also* Hemorrhage, postpartum) 666.1 ☑
    - prepubertal 626.8
    - pubertal 626.3
    - puerperal (immediate) 666.1 ☑
  - vagina 623.8
  - vasa previa 663.5 ☑
    - affecting fetus or newborn 772.0
  - vas deferens 608.83
  - ventricular (*see also* Hemorrhage, brain) 431
  - vesical 596.8
  - viscera 459.0
    - newborn 772.8
  - vitreous (humor) (intraocular) 379.23
  - vocal cord 478.5
  - vulva 624.8
- **Hemorrhoids** (anus) (rectum) (without complication) 455.6
  - bleeding, prolapsed, strangulated, or ulcerated NEC 455.8
    - external 455.5
    - internal 455.2
  - complicated NEC 455.8
  - complicating pregnancy and puerperium 671.8 ☑
  - external 455.3
    - with complication NEC 455.5
    - bleeding, prolapsed, strangulated, or ulcerated 455.5
    - thrombosed 455.4
  - internal 455.0
    - with complication NEC 455.2
    - bleeding, prolapsed, strangulated, or ulcerated 455.2
    - thrombosed 455.1
  - residual skin tag 455.9
  - sentinel pile 455.9
  - thrombosed NEC 455.7
    - external 455.4
    - internal 455.1
- **Hemosalpinx** 620.8
- **Hemosiderosis** 275.0
  - dietary 275.0
  - pulmonary (idiopathic) 275.0 *[516.1]*
  - transfusion NEC 999.8
    - bone marrow 996.85
- **Hemospermia** 608.82
- **Hemothorax** 511.8
  - bacterial, nontuberculous 511.1
  - newborn 772.8
  - nontuberculous 511.8
    - bacterial 511.1
  - pneumococcal 511.1
  - postoperative 998.11
  - staphylococcal 511.1
  - streptococcal 511.1
  - traumatic 860.2
    - with
      - open wound into thorax 860.3
      - pneumothorax 860.4
        - with open wound into thorax 860.5
  - tuberculous (*see also* Tuberculosis, pleura) 012.0 ☑
- **Hemotympanum** 385.89
- **Hench-Rosenberg syndrome** (palindromic arthritis) (*see also* Rheumatism, palindromic) 719.3 ☑
- **Henle's warts** 371.41
- **Henoch (-Schönlein)**
  - disease or syndrome (allergic purpura) 287.0
  - purpura (allergic) 287.0
- **Henpue, henpuye** 102.6
- **Heparitinuria** 277.5
- **Hepar lobatum** 095.3
- **Hepatalgia** 573.8
- **Hepatic** — *see also* condition
  - flexure syndrome 569.89

☑ Additional Digit Required — Refer to the Tabular List (Numeric Code Section) for Additional Digit Selection
▶◀ Revised Text ● New Line ▲ Revised Code

Hernia, hernial — *continued*
- en glissade — *see* Hernia, inguinal
- enterostomy (stoma) 569.69
- epigastric 553.29
  - with
    - gangrene (obstruction) 551.29
    - obstruction 552.29
      - and gangrene 551.29
  - recurrent 553.21
    - with
      - gangrene (obstructed) 551.21
      - obstruction 552.21
        - and gangrene 551.21
- esophageal hiatus (sliding) 553.3
  - with
    - gangrene (obstructed) 551.3
    - obstruction 552.3
      - and gangrene 551.3
  - congenital 750.6
- external (inguinal) — *see* Hernia, inguinal
- fallopian tube 620.4
- fascia 728.89
- fat 729.30
  - eyelid 374.34
  - orbital 374.34
  - pad 729.30
    - eye, eyelid 374.34
    - knee 729.31
    - orbit 374.34
    - popliteal (space) 729.31
    - specified site NEC 729.39
- femoral (unilateral) 553.00
  - with
    - gangrene (obstructed) 551.00
    - obstruction 552.00
      - with gangrene 551.00
  - bilateral 553.02
    - gangrenous (obstructed) 551.02
    - obstructed 552.02
      - with gangrene 551.02
    - recurrent 553.03
      - gangrenous (obstructed) 551.03
      - obstructed 552.03
        - with gangrene 551.03
  - recurrent (unilateral) 553.01
    - bilateral 553.03
      - gangrenous (obstructed) 551.03
      - obstructed 552.03
        - with gangrene 551.03
    - gangrenous (obstructed) 551.01
    - obstructed 552.01
      - with gangrene 551.01
- foramen
  - Bochdalek 553.3
    - with
      - gangrene (obstructed) 551.3
      - obstruction 552.3
        - and gangrene 551.3
    - congenital 756.6
  - magnum 348.4
  - Morgagni, Morgagnian 553.3
    - with
      - gangrene 551.3
      - obstruction 552.3
        - and gangrene 551.3
    - congenital 756.6
- funicular (umbilical) 553.1
  - with
    - gangrene (obstructed) 551.1
    - obstruction 552.1
      - and gangrene 551.1
  - spermatic cord — *see* Hernia, inguinal
- gangrenous — *see* Hernia, by site, with gangrene
- gastrointestinal tract 553.9
  - with
    - gangrene (obstructed) 551.9
    - obstruction 552.9
      - and gangrene 551.9
- gluteal — *see* Hernia, femoral
- Gruber's (internal mesogastric) 553.8
  - with
    - gangrene (obstructed) 551.8
    - obstruction 552.8
      - and gangrene 551.8
- Hesselbach's 553.8
  - with
    - gangrene (obstructed) 551.8

Hernia, hernial — *continued*
- Hesselbach's — *continued*
  - with — *continued*
    - obstruction 552.8
      - and gangrene 551.8
- hiatal (esophageal) (sliding) 553.3
  - with
    - gangrene (obstructed) 551.3
    - obstruction 552.3
      - and gangrene 551.3
  - congenital 750.6
- incarcerated (*see also* Hernia, by site, with obstruction) 552.9
  - gangrenous (*see also* Hernia, by site, with gangrene) 551.9
- incisional 553.21
  - with
    - gangrene (obstructed) 551.21
    - obstruction 552.21
      - and gangrene 551.21
  - lumbar — *see* Hernia, lumbar
  - recurrent 553.21
    - with
      - gangrene (obstructed) 551.21
      - obstruction 552.21
        - and gangrene 551.21
- indirect (inguinal) — *see* Hernia, inguinal
- infantile — *see* Hernia, inguinal
- infrapatellar fat pad 729.31
- inguinal (direct) (double) (encysted) (external) (funicular) (indirect) (infantile) (internal) (interstitial) (oblique) (scrotal) (sliding) 550.9 ☑

> *Note — Use the following fifth-digit subclassification with category 550:*
>
> *0 unilateral or unspecified (not specified as recurrent)*
> *1 unilateral or unspecified, recurrent*
> *2 bilateral (not specified as recurrent)*
> *3 bilateral, recurrent*

  - with
    - gangrene (obstructed) 550.0 ☑
    - obstruction 550.1 ☑
      - and gangrene 550.0 ☑
- internal 553.8
  - with
    - gangrene (obstructed) 551.8
    - obstruction 552.8
      - and gangrene 551.8
  - inguinal — *see* Hernia, inguinal
- interstitial 553.9
  - with
    - gangrene (obstructed) 551.9
    - obstruction 552.9
      - and gangrene 551.9
  - inguinal — *see* Hernia, inguinal
- intervertebral cartilage or disc — *see* Displacement, intervertebral disc
- intestine, intestinal 553.9
  - with
    - gangrene (obstructed) 551.9
    - obstruction 552.9
      - and gangrene 551.9
- intra-abdominal 553.9
  - with
    - gangrene (obstructed) 551.9
    - obstruction 552.9
      - and gangrene 551.9
- intraparietal 553.9
  - with
    - gangrene (obstructed) 551.9
    - obstruction 552.9
      - and gangrene 551.9
- iris 364.8
  - traumatic 871.1
- irreducible (*see also* Hernia, by site, with obstruction) 552.9
  - gangrenous (with obstruction) (*see also* Hernia, by site, with gangrene) 551.9
- ischiatic 553.8
  - with
    - gangrene (obstructed) 551.8
    - obstruction 552.8
      - and gangrene 551.8

Hernia, hernial — *continued*
- ischiorectal 553.8
  - with
    - gangrene (obstructed) 551.8
    - obstruction 552.8
      - and gangrene 551.8
- lens 379.32
  - traumatic 871.1
- linea
  - alba — *see* Hernia, epigastric
  - semilunaris — *see* Hernia, spigelian
- Littre's (diverticular) 553.9
  - with
    - gangrene (obstructed) 551.9
    - obstruction 552.9
      - and gangrene 551.9
- lumbar 553.8
  - with
    - gangrene (obstructed) 551.8
    - obstruction 552.8
      - and gangrene 551.8
  - intervertebral disc 722.10
- lung (subcutaneous) 518.89
  - congenital 748.69
- mediastinum 519.3
- mesenteric (internal) 553.8
  - with
    - gangrene (obstructed) 551.8
    - obstruction 552.8
      - and gangrene 551.8
- mesocolon 553.8
  - with
    - gangrene (obstructed) 551.8
    - obstruction 552.8
      - and gangrene 551.8
- muscle (sheath) 728.89
- nucleus pulposus — *see* Displacement, intervertebral disc
- oblique (inguinal) — *see* Hernia, inguinal
- obstructive (*see also* Hernia, by site, with obstruction) 552.9
  - gangrenous (with obstruction) (*see also* Hernia, by site, with gangrene) 551.9
- obturator 553.8
  - with
    - gangrene (obstructed) 551.8
    - obstruction 552.8
      - and gangrene 551.8
- omental 553.8
  - with
    - gangrene (obstructed) 551.8
    - obstruction 552.8
      - and gangrene 551.8
- orbital fat (pad) 374.34
- ovary 620.4
- oviduct 620.4
- paracolostomy (stoma) 569.69
- paraduodenal 553.8
  - with
    - gangrene (obstructed) 551.8
    - obstruction 552.8
      - and gangrene 551.8
- paraesophageal 553.3
  - with
    - gangrene (obstructed) 551.3
    - obstruction 552.3
      - and gangrene 551.3
  - congenital 750.6
- parahiatal 553.3
  - with
    - gangrene (obstructed) 551.3
    - obstruction 552.3
      - and gangrene 551.3
- paraumbilical 553.1
  - with
    - gangrene (obstructed) 551.1
    - obstruction 552.1
      - and gangrene 551.1
- parietal 553.9
  - with
    - gangrene (obstructed) 551.9
    - obstruction 552.9
      - and gangrene 551.9
- perineal 553.8
  - with
    - gangrene (obstructed) 551.8

Hiccough 786.8
- epidemic 078.89
- psychogenic 306.1

Hiccup *(see also* Hiccough) 786.8

Hicks (-Braxton) contractures 644.1 ☑

Hidden penis 752.65

Hidradenitis (axillaris) (suppurative) 705.83

Hidradenoma (nodular) (M8400/0) — *see also* Neoplasm, skin, benign
- clear cell (M8402/0) — *see* Neoplasm, skin, benign
- papillary (M8405/0) — *see* Neoplasm, skin, benign

Hidrocystoma (M8404/0) — *see* Neoplasm, skin, benign

High
- A_2 anemia 282.49
- altitude effects 993.2
  - anoxia 993.2
  - on
    - ears 993.0
    - sinuses 993.1
  - polycythemia 289.0
- arch
  - foot 755.67
  - palate 750.26
- artery (arterial) tension (*see also* Hypertension) 401.9
  - without diagnosis of hypertension 796.2
- basal metabolic rate (BMR) 794.7
- blood pressure (*see also* Hypertension) 401.9
  - incidental reading (isolated) (nonspecific), no diagnosis of hypertension 796.2
- compliance bladder 596.4
- diaphragm (congenital) 756.6
- frequency deafness (congenital) (regional) 389.8
- head at term 652.5 ☑
  - affecting fetus or newborn 763.1
- output failure (cardiac) (*see also* Failure, heart) 428.9
- oxygen-affinity hemoglobin 289.0
- palate 750.26
- risk
  - behavior — *see* Problem
  - cervical, human papillomavirus (HPV) DNA test positive 795.05
  - family situation V61.9
    - specified circumstance NEC V61.8
  - individual NEC V62.89
  - infant NEC V20.1
  - patient taking drugs (prescribed) V67.51
    - nonprescribed (*see also* Abuse, drugs, nondependent) 305.9 ☑
  - pregnancy V23.9
    - inadequate prenatal care V23.7
    - specified problem NEC V23.89
- temperature (of unknown origin) (*see also* Pyrexia) 780.6
- thoracic rib 756.3

Hildenbrand's disease (typhus) 081.9

Hilger's syndrome 337.0

Hill diarrhea 579.1

Hilliard's lupus (*see also* Tuberculosis) 017.0 ☑

Hilum — *see* condition

Hip — *see* condition

Hippel's disease (retinocerebral angiomatosis) 759.6

Hippus 379.49

Hirschfeld's disease (acute diabetes mellitus) (*see also* Diabetes) 250.0 ☑

Hirschsprung's disease or megacolon (congenital) 751.3

Hirsuties (*see also* Hypertrichosis) 704.1

Hirsutism (*see also* Hypertrichosis) 704.1

Hirudiniasis (external) (internal) 134.2

His-Werner disease (trench fever) 083.1

Hiss-Russell dysentery 004.1

Histamine cephalgia 346.2 ☑

Histidinemia 270.5

Histidinuria 270.5

Histiocytoma (M8832/0) — *see also* Neoplasm, skin, benign
- fibrous (M8830/0) — *see also* Neoplasm, skin, benign
  - atypical (M8830/1) — *see* Neoplasm, connective tissue, uncertain behavior
  - malignant (M8830/3) — *see* Neoplasm, connective tissue, malignant

Histiocytosis (acute) (chronic) (subacute) 277.89
- acute differentiated progressive (M9722/3) 202.5 ☑
- cholesterol 277.89
- essential 277.89
- lipid, lipoid (essential) 272.7
- lipochrome (familial) 288.1
- malignant (M9720/3) 202.3 ☑
- X (chronic) 277.89
  - acute (progressive) (M9722/3) 202.5 ☑

Histoplasmosis 115.90
- with
  - endocarditis 115.94
  - meningitis 115.91
  - pericarditis 115.93
  - pneumonia 115.95
  - retinitis 115.92
  - specified manifestation NEC 115.99
- African (due to Histoplasma duboisii) 115.10
  - with
    - endocarditis 115.14
    - meningitis 115.11
    - pericarditis 115.13
    - pneumonia 115.15
    - retinitis 115.12
    - specified manifestation NEC 115.19
- American (due to Histoplasma capsulatum) 115.00
  - with
    - endocarditis 115.04
    - meningitis 115.01
    - pericarditis 115.03
    - pneumonia 115.05
    - retinitis 115.02
    - specified manifestation NEC 115.09
- Darling's — *see* Histoplasmosis, American
- large form (*see also* Histoplasmosis, African) 115.10
- lung 115.05
- small form (*see also* Histoplasmosis, American) 115.00

History (personal) **of**
- abuse
  - emotional V15.42
  - neglect V15.42
  - physical V15.41
  - sexual V15.41
- affective psychosis V11.1
- alcoholism V11.3
  - specified as drinking problem (*see also* Abuse, drugs, nondependent) 305.0 ☑
- allergy to
  - analgesic agent NEC V14.6
  - anesthetic NEC V14.4
  - antibiotic agent NEC V14.1
    - penicillin V14.0
  - anti-infective agent NEC V14.3
  - diathesis V15.09
  - drug V14.9
    - specified type NEC V14.8
  - eggs V15.03
  - food additives V15.05
  - insect bite V15.06
  - latex V15.07
  - medicinal agents V14.9
    - specified type NEC V14.8
  - milk products V15.02
  - narcotic agent NEC V14.5
  - nuts V15.05
    - peanuts V15.01
  - penicillin V14.0
  - radiographic dye V15.08
  - seafood V15.04
  - serum V14.7
  - specified food NEC V15.05
  - specified nonmedicinal agents NEC V15.09
  - spider bite V15.06
  - sulfa V14.2

History (personal) **of** — *continued*
- allergy to — *continued*
  - sulfonamides V14.2
  - therapeutic agent NEC V15.09
  - vaccine V14.7
- anemia V12.3
- arthritis V13.4
- benign neoplasm of brain V12.41
- blood disease V12.3
- calculi, urinary V13.01
- cardiovascular disease V12.50
  - myocardial infarction 412
- child abuse V15.41
- cigarette smoking V15.82
- circulatory system disease V12.50
  - myocardial infarction 412
- congenital malformation V13.69
- contraception V15.7
- diathesis, allergic V15.09
- digestive system disease V12.70
  - peptic ulcer V12.71
  - polyps, colonic V12.72
  - specified NEC V12.79
- disease (of) V13.9
  - blood V12.3
  - blood-forming organs V12.3
  - cardiovascular system V12.50
  - circulatory system V12.50
  - digestive system V12.70
    - peptic ulcer V12.71
    - polyps, colonic V12.72
    - specified NEC V12.79
  - infectious V12.00
    - malaria V12.03
    - poliomyelitis V12.02
    - specified NEC V12.09
    - tuberculosis V12.01
  - parasitic V12.00
    - specified NEC V12.09
  - respiratory system V12.60 ▲
    - pneumonia V12.61 ●
    - specified NEC V12.69 ●
  - skin V13.3
  - specified site NEC V13.8
  - subcutaneous tissue V13.3
  - trophoblastic V13.1
    - affecting management of pregnancy V23.1
- disorder (of) V13.9
  - endocrine V12.2
  - genital system V13.29
  - hematological V12.3
  - immunity V12.2
  - mental V11.9
    - affective type V11.1
    - manic-depressive V11.1
    - neurosis V11.2
    - schizophrenia V11.0
    - specified type NEC V11.8
  - metabolic V12.2
  - musculoskeletal NEC V13.5
  - nervous system V12.40
    - specified type NEC V12.49
  - obstetric V13.29
    - affecting management of current pregnancy V23.49
      - pre-term labor V23.41
    - pre-term labor V13.21
  - sense organs V12.40
    - specified type NEC V12.49
  - specified site NEC V13.8
  - urinary system V13.00
    - calculi V13.01
    - infection V13.02 ●
    - nephrotic syndrome V13.03 ●
    - specified NEC V13.09
- drug use
  - nonprescribed (*see also* Abuse, drugs, nondependent) 305.9 ☑
  - patent (*see also* Abuse, drugs, nondependent) 305.9 ☑
- effect NEC of external cause V15.89
- embolism (pulmonary) V12.51
- emotional abuse V15.42
- encephalitis V12.42 ●
- endocrine disorder V12.2
- extracorporeal membrane oxygenation (ECMO) V15.87

- **History** (personal) **of** — *continued*
  - mental disorder — *continued*
    - schizophrenia V11.0
    - specified type NEC V11.8
  - metabolic disorder V12.2
  - musculoskeletal disorder NEC V13.5
  - myocardial infarction 412
  - neglect (emotional) V15.42
  - nephrotic syndrome V13.03 ●
  - nervous system disorder V12.40
    - specified type NEC V12.49
  - neurosis V11.2
  - noncompliance with medical treatment V15.81
  - nutritional deficiency V12.1
  - obstetric disorder V13.29
    - affecting management of current pregnancy V23.49
      - pre-term labor V23.41
    - pre-term labor V13.21
  - parasitic disease V12.00
    - specified NEC V12.09
  - perinatal problems V13.7
    - low birth weight (*see also* Status, low birth weight) V21.30
  - physical abuse V15.41
  - poisoning V15.6
  - poliomyelitis V12.02
  - polyps, colonic V12.72
  - poor obstetric V13.29
    - affecting management of current pregnancy V23.49
      - pre-term labor V23.41
    - pre-term labor V13.21
  - psychiatric disorder V11.9
    - affective type V11.1
    - manic-depressive V11.1
    - neurosis V11.2
    - schizophrenia V11.0
    - specified type NEC V11.8
  - psychological trauma V15.49
    - emotional abuse V15.42
    - neglect V15.42
    - physical abuse V15.41
    - rape V15.41
  - psychoneurosis V11.2
  - radiation therapy V15.3
  - rape V15.41
  - respiratory system disease V12.60 ▲
    - pneumonia V12.61 ●
    - specified NEC V12.69 ●
  - reticulosarcoma V10.71
  - schizophrenia V11.0
  - skin disease V13.3
  - smoking (tobacco) V15.82
  - subcutaneous tissue disease V13.3
  - surgery (major) to
    - great vessels V15.1
    - heart V15.1
    - major organs NEC V15.2
  - syndrome, nephrotic V13.03 ●
  - thrombophlebitis V12.52
  - thrombosis V12.51
  - tobacco use V15.82
  - trophoblastic disease V13.1
    - affecting management of pregnancy V23.1
  - tuberculosis V12.01
  - ulcer, peptic V12.71
  - urinary system disorder V13.00
    - calculi V13.01
    - infection V13.02 ●
    - nephrotic syndrome V13.03 ●
    - specified NEC V13.09
- **HIV infection** (disease) (illness) — *see* Human immunodeficiency virus (disease) (illness) (infection)
- **Hives** (bold) (*see also* Urticaria) 708.9
- **Hoarseness** 784.49
- **Hobnail liver** — *see* Cirrhosis, portal
- **Hobo, hoboism** V60.0
- **Hodgkin's**
  - disease (M9650/3) 201.9 ☑
    - lymphocytic
      - depletion (M9653/3) 201.7 ☑
        - diffuse fibrosis (M9654/3) 201.7 ☑
        - reticular type (M9655/3) 201.7 ☑
      - predominance (M9651/3) 201.4 ☑
- **Hodgkin's** — *continued*
  - disease — *continued*
    - lymphocytic-histiocytic predominance (M9651/3) 201.4 ☑
    - mixed cellularity (M9652/3) 201.6 ☑
    - nodular sclerosis (M9656/3) 201.5 ☑
      - cellular phase (M9657/3) 201.5 ☑
  - granuloma (M9661/3) 201.1 ☑
  - lymphogranulomatosis (M9650/3) 201.9 ☑
  - lymphoma (M9650/3) 201.9 ☑
  - lymphosarcoma (M9650/3) 201.9 ☑
  - paragranuloma (M9660/3) 201.0 ☑
  - sarcoma (M9662/3) 201.2 ☑
- **Hodgson's disease** (aneurysmal dilatation of aorta) 441.9
  - ruptured 441.5
- **Hodi-potsy** 111.0
- **Hoffa (-Kastert) disease or syndrome** (liposynovitis prepatellaris) 272.8
- **Hoffman's syndrome** 244.9 *[359.5]*
- **Hoffmann-Bouveret syndrome** (paroxysmal tachycardia) 427.2
- **Hole**
  - macula 362.54
  - optic disc, crater-like 377.22
  - retina (macula) 362.54
    - round 361.31
      - with detachment 361.01
- **Holla disease** (*see also* Spherocytosis) 282.0
- **Holländer-Simons syndrome** (progressive lipodystrophy) 272.6
- **Hollow foot** (congenital) 754.71
  - acquired 736.73
- **Holmes' syndrome** (visual disorientation) 368.16
- **Holoprosencephaly** 742.2
  - due to
    - trisomy 13 758.1
    - trisomy 18 758.2
- **Holthouse's hernia** — *see* Hernia, inguinal
- **Homesickness** 309.89
- **Homocystinemia** 270.4
- **Homocystinuria** 270.4
- **Homologous serum jaundice** (prophylactic) (therapeutic) — *see* Hepatitis, viral
- **Homosexuality** — *omit code*
  - ego-dystonic 302.0
  - pedophilic 302.2
  - problems with 302.0
- **Homozygous Hb-S disease** 282.61
- **Honeycomb lung** 518.89
  - congenital 748.4
- **Hong Kong ear** 117.3
- **HOOD** (hereditary osteo-onychodysplasia) 756.89
- **Hooded**
  - clitoris 752.49
  - penis 752.69
- **Hookworm** (anemia) (disease) (infestation) — *see* Ancylostomiasis
- **Hoppe-Goldflam syndrome** 358.00
- **Hordeolum** (external) (eyelid) 373.11
  - internal 373.12
- **Horn**
  - cutaneous 702.8
    - cheek 702.8
    - eyelid 702.8
    - penis 702.8
  - iliac 756.89
  - nail 703.8
    - congenital 757.5
  - papillary 700
- **Horner's**
  - syndrome (*see also* Neuropathy, peripheral, autonomic) 337.9
    - traumatic 954.0
  - teeth 520.4
- **Horseshoe kidney** (congenital) 753.3
- **Horton's**
  - disease (temporal arteritis) 446.5
  - headache or neuralgia 346.2 ☑
- **Hospice care** V66.7
- **Hospitalism** (in children) NEC 309.83
- **Hourglass contraction, contracture**
  - bladder 596.8
  - gallbladder 575.2
    - congenital 751.69
  - stomach 536.8
    - congenital 750.7
    - psychogenic 306.4
  - uterus 661.4 ☑
    - affecting fetus or newborn 763.7
- **Household circumstance affecting care** V60.9
  - specified type NEC V60.8
- **Housemaid's knee** 727.2
- **Housing circumstance affecting care** V60.9
  - specified type NEC V60.8
- **HTLV-I infection** 079.51
- **HTLV-II infection** 079.52
- **HTLV-III** (disease) (illness) (infection) — *see* Human immunodeficiency virus (disease) (illness) (infection)
- **HTLV-III/LAV** (disease) (illness) (infection) — *see* Human immunodeficiency virus (disease) (illness) (infection)
- **Huchard's disease** (continued arterial hypertension) 401.9
- **Hudson-Stähli lines** 371.11
- **Huguier's disease** (uterine fibroma) 218.9
- **Hum, venous** — *omit code*
- **Human bite** (open wound) — *see also* Wound, open, by site
  - intact skin surface — *see* Contusion
- **Human immunodeficiency virus** (disease) (illness) 042
  - infection V08
    - with symptoms, symptomatic 042
- **Human immunodeficiency virus-2 infection** 079.53
- **Human immunovirus** (disease) (illness) (infection) — *see* Human immunodeficiency virus (disease) (illness) (infection)
- **Human papillomavirus** 079.4
  - cervical
    - high risk, DNA test positive 795.05
    - low risk, DNA test positive 795.09
- **Human T-cell lymphotrophic virus-I infection** 079.51
- **Human T-cell lymphotrophic virus-II infection** 079.52
- **Human T-cell lymphotrophic virus-III** (disease) (illness) (infection) — *see* Human immunodeficiency virus (disease) (illness) (infection)
- **Humpback** (acquired) 737.9
  - congenital 756.19
- **Hunchback** (acquired) 737.9
  - congenital 756.19
- **Hunger** 994.2
  - air, psychogenic 306.1
  - disease 251.1
- **Hunner's ulcer** (*see also* Cystitis) 595.1
- **Hunt's**
  - neuralgia 053.11
  - syndrome (herpetic geniculate ganglionitis) 053.11
    - dyssynergia cerebellaris myoclonica 334.2
- **Hunter's glossitis** 529.4
- **Hunter (-Hurler) syndrome** (mucopolysaccharidosis II) 277.5
- **Hunterian chancre** 091.0
- **Huntington's**
  - chorea 333.4
  - disease 333.4
- **Huppert's disease** (multiple myeloma) (M9730/3) 203.0 ☑
- **Hurler (-Hunter) disease or syndrome** (mucopolysaccharidosis II) 277.5
- **Hürthle cell**
  - adenocarcinoma (M8290/3) 193
  - adenoma (M8290/0) 226
  - carcinoma (M8290/3) 193
  - tumor (M8290/0) 226

Index

- **Hutchinson's**
  - disease meaning
    - angioma serpiginosum 709.1
    - cheiropompholyx 705.81
    - prurigo estivalis 692.72
    - summer eruption, or summer prurigo 692.72
  - incisors 090.5
  - melanotic freckle (M8742/2) — *see also* Neoplasm, skin, in situ
    - malignant melanoma in (M8742/3) — *see* Melanoma
  - teeth or incisors (congenital syphilis) 090.5
- **Hutchinson-Boeck disease or syndrome** (sarcoidosis) 135
- **Hutchinson-Gilford disease or syndrome** (progeria) 259.8
- **Hyaline**
  - degeneration (diffuse) (generalized) 728.9
    - localized — *see* Degeneration, by site
  - membrane (disease) (lung) (newborn) 769
- **Hyalinosis cutis et mucosae** 272.8
- **Hyalin plaque, sclera, senile** 379.16
- **Hyalitis** (asteroid) 379.22
  - syphilitic 095.8
- **Hydatid**
  - cyst or tumor — *see also* Echinococcus
    - fallopian tube 752.11
  - mole — *see* Hydatidiform mole
  - Morgagni (congenital) 752.89
    - fallopian tube 752.11
- **Hydatidiform mole** (benign) (complicating pregnancy) (delivered) (undelivered) 630
  - invasive (M9100/1) 236.1
  - malignant (M9100/1) 236.1
  - previous, affecting management of pregnancy V23.1
- **Hydatidosis** — *see* Echinococcus
- **Hyde's disease** (prurigo nodularis) 698.3
- **Hydradenitis** 705.83
- **Hydradenoma** (M8400/0) — *see* Hidradenoma
- **Hydralazine lupus or syndrome**
  - correct substance properly administered 695.4
  - overdose or wrong substance given or taken 972.6
- **Hydramnios** 657.0 ☑
  - affecting fetus or newborn 761.3
- **Hydrancephaly** 742.3
  - with spina bifida (*see also* Spina bifida) 741.0 ☑
- **Hydranencephaly** 742.3
  - with spina bifida (*see also* Spina bifida) 741.0 ☑
- **Hydrargyrism** NEC 985.0
- **Hydrarthrosis** (*see also* Effusion, joint) 719.0 ☑
  - gonococcal 098.50
  - intermittent (*see also* Rheumatism, palindromic) 719.3 ☑
  - of yaws (early) (late) 102.6
  - syphilitic 095.8
    - congenital 090.5
- **Hydremia** 285.9
- **Hydrencephalocele** (congenital) 742.0
- **Hydrencephalomeningocele** (congenital) 742.0
- **Hydroa** 694.0
  - aestivale 692.72
  - gestationis 646.8 ☑
  - herpetiformis 694.0
  - pruriginosa 694.0
  - vacciniforme 692.72
- **Hydroadenitis** 705.83
- **Hydrocalycosis** (*see also* Hydronephrosis) 591
  - congenital 753.29
- **Hydrocalyx** (*see also* Hydronephrosis) 591
- **Hydrocele** (calcified) (chylous) (idiopathic) (infantile) (inguinal canal) (recurrent) (senile) (spermatic cord) (testis) (tunica vaginalis) 603.9
  - canal of Nuck (female) 629.1
    - male 603.9
  - congenital 778.6
- **Hydrocele** — *continued*
  - encysted 603.0
    - congenital 778.6
  - female NEC 629.8
  - infected 603.1
  - round ligament 629.8
  - specified type NEC 603.8
    - congenital 778.6
  - spinalis (*see also* Spina bifida) 741.9 ☑
  - vulva 624.8
- **Hydrocephalic fetus**
  - affecting management or pregnancy 655.0 ☑
  - causing disproportion 653.6 ☑
    - with obstructed labor 660.1 ☑
      - affecting fetus or newborn 763.1
- **Hydrocephalus** (acquired) (external) (internal) (malignant) (noncommunicating) (obstructive) (recurrent) 331.4
  - aqueduct of Sylvius stricture 742.3
    - with spina bifida (*see also* Spina bifida) 741.0 ☑
  - chronic 742.3
    - with spina bifida (*see also* Spina bifida) 741.0 ☑
  - communicating 331.3
  - congenital (external) (internal) 742.3
    - with spina bifida (*see also* Spina bifida) 741.0 ☑
  - due to
    - stricture of aqueduct of Sylvius 742.3
      - with spina bifida (*see also* Spina bifida) 741.0 ☑
    - toxoplasmosis (congenital) 771.2
  - fetal affecting management of pregnancy 655.0 ☑
  - foramen Magendie block (acquired) 331.3
    - congenital 742.3
      - with spina bifida (*see also* Spina bifida) 741.0 ☑
  - newborn 742.3
    - with spina bifida (*see also* Spina bifida) 741.0 ☑
  - otitic 331.4
  - syphilitic, congenital 090.49
  - tuberculous (*see also* Tuberculosis) 013.8 ☑
- **Hydrocolpos** (congenital) 623.8
- **Hydrocystoma** (M8404/0) — *see* Neoplasm, skin, benign
- **Hydroencephalocele** (congenital) 742.0
- **Hydroencephalomeningocele** (congenital) 742.0
- **Hydrohematopneumothorax** (*see also* Hemothorax) 511.8
- **Hydromeningitis** — *see* Meningitis
- **Hydromeningocele** (spinal) (*see also* Spina bifida) 741.9 ☑
  - cranial 742.0
- **Hydrometra** 621.8
- **Hydrometrocolpos** 623.8
- **Hydromicrocephaly** 742.1
- **Hydromphalus** (congenital) (since birth) 757.39
- **Hydromyelia** 742.53
- **Hydromyelocele** (*see also* Spina bifida) 741.9 ☑
- **Hydronephrosis** 591
  - atrophic 591
  - congenital 753.29
  - due to S. hematobium 120.0
  - early 591
  - functionless (infected) 591
  - infected 591
  - intermittent 591
  - primary 591
  - secondary 591
  - tuberculous (*see also* Tuberculosis) 016.0 ☑
- **Hydropericarditis** (*see also* Pericarditis) 423.9
- **Hydropericardium** (*see also* Pericarditis) 423.9
- **Hydroperitoneum** 789.5
- **Hydrophobia** 071
- **Hydrophthalmos** (*see also* Buphthalmia) 743.20
- **Hydropneumohemothorax** (*see also* Hemothorax) 511.8
- **Hydropneumopericarditis** (*see also* Pericarditis) 423.9
- **Hydropneumopericardium** (*see also* Pericarditis) 423.9
- **Hydropneumothorax** 511.8
  - nontuberculous 511.8
    - bacterial 511.1
  - pneumococcal 511.1
  - staphylococcal 511.1
  - streptococcal 511.1
  - traumatic 860.0
    - with open wound into thorax 860.1
  - tuberculous (*see also* Tuberculosis, pleura) 012.0 ☑
- **Hydrops** 782.3
  - abdominis 789.5
  - amnii (complicating pregnancy) (*see also* Hydramnios) 657.0 ☑
  - articulorum intermittens (*see also* Rheumatism, palindromic) 719.3 ☑
  - cardiac (*see also* Failure, heart) 428.0
  - congenital — *see* Hydrops, fetalis
  - endolymphatic (*see also* Disease, Ménière's) 386.00
  - fetal(is) or newborn 778.0
    - due to isoimmunization 773.3
    - not due to isoimmunization 778.0
  - gallbladder 575.3
  - idiopathic (fetus or newborn) 778.0
  - joint (see also Effusion, joint) 719.0 ☑
  - labyrinth (*see also* Disease, Ménière's) 386.00
  - meningeal NEC 331.4
  - nutritional 262
  - pericardium — *see* Pericarditis
  - pleura (*see also* Hydrothorax) 511.8
  - renal (*see also* Nephrosis) 581.9
  - spermatic cord (*see also* Hydrocele) 603.9
- **Hydropyonephrosis** (*see also* Pyelitis) 590.80
  - chronic 590.00
- **Hydrorachis** 742.53
- **Hydrorrhea** (nasal) 478.1
  - gravidarum 658.1 ☑
  - pregnancy 658.1 ☑
- **Hydrosadenitis** 705.83
- **Hydrosalpinx** (fallopian tube) (follicularis) 614.1
- **Hydrothorax** (double) (pleural) 511.8
  - chylous (nonfilarial) 457.8
    - filaria (*see also* Infestation, filarial) 125.9
  - nontuberculous 511.8
    - bacterial 511.1
  - pneumococcal 511.1
  - staphylococcal 511.1
  - streptococcal 511.1
  - traumatic 862.29
    - with open wound into thorax 862.39
  - tuberculous (*see also* Tuberculosis, pleura) 012.0 ☑
- **Hydroureter** 593.5
  - congenital 753.22
- **Hydroureteronephrosis** (*see also* Hydronephrosis) 591
- **Hydrourethra** 599.84
- **Hydroxykynureninuria** 270.2
- **Hydroxyprolinemia** 270.8
- **Hydroxyprolinuria** 270.8
- **Hygroma** (congenital) (cystic) (M9173/0) 228.1
  - prepatellar 727.3
  - subdural — *see* Hematoma, subdural
- **Hymen** — *see* condition
- **Hymenolepiasis** (diminuta) (infection) (infestation) (nana) 123.6
- **Hymenolepis** (diminuta) (infection) (infestation) (nana) 123.6
- **Hypalgesia** (*see also* Disturbance, sensation) 782.0
- **Hyperabduction syndrome** 447.8
- **Hyperacidity, gastric** 536.8
  - psychogenic 306.4
- **Hyperactive, hyperactivity**
  - basal cell, uterine cervix 622.10
  - bladder 596.51
  - bowel (syndrome) 564.9
    - sounds 787.5
  - cervix epithelial (basal) 622.10
  - child 314.01

Hutchinson's — Hyperactive, hyperactivity

☑ Additional Digit Required — Refer to the Tabular List (Numeric Code Section) for Additional Digit Selection

▶◀ Revised Text ● New Line ▲ Revised Code

☑ Additional Digit Required — Refer to the Tabular List (Numeric Code Section) for Additional Digit Selection
▶◀ Revised Text ● New Line ▲ Revised Code

Hyperplasia, hyperplastic — *continued*
- suprarenal (capsule) (gland) 255.8
- thymus (gland) (persistent) 254.0
- thyroid (*see also* Goiter) 240.9
  - primary 242.0 ☑
  - secondary 242.2 ☑
- tonsil (lymphoid tissue) 474.11
  - and adenoids 474.10
- urethrovaginal 599.89
- uterus, uterine (myometrium) 621.2
  - endometrium (*see also* Hyperplasia, endometrium) 621.30
- vitreous (humor), primary persistent 743.51
- vulva 624.3
- zygoma 738.11

Hyperpnea (*see also* Hyperventilation) 786.01

Hyperpotassemia 276.7

Hyperprebetalipoproteinemia 272.1
- with chylomicronemia 272.3
- familial 272.1

Hyperprolactinemia 253.1

Hyperprolinemia 270.8

Hyperproteinemia 273.8

Hyperprothrombinemia 289.89

Hyperpselaphesia 782.0

Hyperpyrexia 780.6
- heat (effects of) 992.0
- malarial (*see also* Malaria) 084.6
- malignant, due to anesthetic 995.86
- rheumatic — *see* Fever, rheumatic
- unknown origin (*see also* Pyrexia) 780.6

Hyperreactor, vascular 780.2

Hyperreflexia 796.1
- bladder, autonomic 596.54
  - with cauda equina 344.61
- detrusor 344.61

Hypersalivation (*see also* Ptyalism) 527.7

Hypersarcosinemia 270.8

Hypersecretion
- ACTH 255.3
- androgens (ovarian) 256.1
- calcitonin 246.0
- corticoadrenal 255.3
- cortisol 255.0
- estrogen 256.0
- gastric 536.8
  - psychogenic 306.4
- gastrin 251.5
- glucagon 251.4
- hormone
  - ACTH 255.3
  - anterior pituitary 253.1
  - growth NEC 253.0
  - ovarian androgen 256.1
  - testicular 257.0
  - thyroid stimulating 242.8 ☑
- insulin — *see* Hyperinsulinism
- lacrimal glands (*see also* Epiphora) 375.20
- medulloadrenal 255.6
- milk 676.6 ☑
- ovarian androgens 256.1
- pituitary (anterior) 253.1
- salivary gland (any) 527.7
- testicular hormones 257.0
- thyrocalcitonin 246.0
- upper respiratory 478.9

Hypersegmentation, hereditary 288.2
- eosinophils 288.2
- neutrophil nuclei 288.2

Hypersensitive, hypersensitiveness, hypersensitivity — *see also* Allergy
- angiitis 446.20
  - specified NEC 446.29
- carotid sinus 337.0
- colon 564.9
  - psychogenic 306.4
- DNA (deoxyribonucleic acid) NEC 287.2
- drug (*see also* Allergy, drug) 995.2
- esophagus 530.89

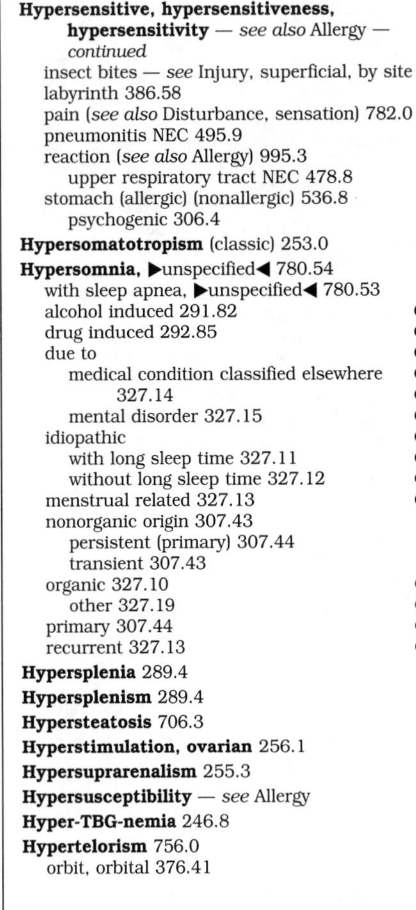

Hypersensitive, hypersensitiveness, hypersensitivity — *see also* Allergy — *continued*
- insect bites — *see* Injury, superficial, by site
- labyrinth 386.58
- pain (*see also* Disturbance, sensation) 782.0
- pneumonitis NEC 495.9
- reaction (*see also* Allergy) 995.3
  - upper respiratory tract NEC 478.8
- stomach (allergic) (nonallergic) 536.8
  - psychogenic 306.4

Hypersomatotropism (classic) 253.0

Hypersomnia, ▶unspecified◀ 780.54
- with sleep apnea, ▶unspecified◀ 780.53
- alcohol induced 291.82 ●
- drug induced 292.85 ●
- due to ●
  - medical condition classified elsewhere 327.14 ●
  - mental disorder 327.15 ●
- idiopathic ●
  - with long sleep time 327.11 ●
  - without long sleep time 327.12 ●
- menstrual related 327.13 ●
- nonorganic origin 307.43
  - persistent (primary) 307.44
  - transient 307.43
- organic 327.10 ●
  - other 327.19 ●
- primary 307.44 ●
- recurrent 327.13 ●

Hypersplenia 289.4

Hypersplenism 289.4

Hypersteatosis 706.3

Hyperstimulation, ovarian 256.1

Hypersuprarenalism 255.3

Hypersusceptibility — *see* Allergy

Hyper-TBG-nemia 246.8

Hypertelorism 756.0
- orbit, orbital 376.41

	Malignant	Benign	Unspecified
Hypertension, hypertensive (arterial) (arteriolar) (crisis) (degeneration) (disease) (essential) (fluctuating) (idiopathic) (intermittent) (labile) (low renin) (orthostatic) (paroxysmal) (primary) (systemic) (uncontrolled) (vascular)	401.0	401.1	401.9
with			
chronic kidney disease	403.01	403.11	403.91 ●
heart involvement (conditions classifiable to 429.0-429.3, 429.8, 429.9 due to hypertension) (*see also* Hypertension, heart)	402.00	402.10	402.90
with kidney involvement — *see* Hypertension, cardiorenal			
renal involvement (only conditions classifiable to 585, 586, 587) (excludes conditions classifiable to 584) (*see also* Hypertension, kidney)	403.00	403.10	403.90
with heart involvement — *see* Hypertension, cardiorenal			
failure (and sclerosis) (*see also* Hypertension, kidney)	403.01	403.11	403.91
sclerosis without failure (*see also* Hypertension, kidney)	403.00	403.10	403.90
accelerated (*see also* Hypertension, by type, malignant)	401.0	—	—
antepartum — *see* Hypertension, complicating pregnancy, childbirth, or the puerperium			
cardiorenal (disease)	404.00	404.10	404.90
with			
chronic kidney disease	403.01	403.11	403.91 ●
and heart failure	404.03	404.13	404.93 ●
heart failure	404.01	404.11	404.91
and chronic kidney disease	404.03	404.13	404.93 ●
and renal failure	404.03	404.13	404.93
renal failure	404.02	404.12	404.92
and heart failure	404.03	404.13	404.93
cardiovascular disease (arteriosclerotic) (sclerotic)	402.00	402.10	402.90
with			
heart failure	402.01	402.11	402.91
renal involvement (conditions classifiable to 403) (*see also* Hypertension, cardiorenal)	404.00	404.10	404.90
cardiovascular renal (disease) (sclerosis) (*see also* Hypertension, cardiorenal)	404.00	404.10	404.90
cerebrovascular disease NEC	437.2	437.2	437.2
complicating pregnancy, childbirth, or the puerperium	642.2 ☑	642.0 ☑	642.9 ☑
with			
albuminuria (and edema) (mild)	—	—	642.4 ☑
severe	—	—	642.5 ☑
edema (mild)	—	—	642.4 ☑
severe	—	—	642.5 ☑
heart disease	642.2 ☑	642.2 ☑	642.2 ☑
and renal disease	642.2 ☑	642.2 ☑	642.2 ☑
renal disease	642.2 ☑	642.2 ☑	642.2 ☑
and heart disease	642.2 ☑	642.2 ☑	642.2 ☑
chronic	642.2 ☑	642.0 ☑	642.0 ☑
with pre-eclampsia or eclampsia	642.7 ☑	642.7 ☑	642.7 ☑
fetus or newborn	760.0	760.0	760.0
essential	—	642.0 ☑	642.0 ☑
with pre-eclampsia or eclampsia	—	642.7 ☑	642.7 ☑
fetus or newborn	760.0	760.0	760.0
fetus or newborn	760.0	760.0	760.0
gestational	—	—	642.3 ☑
pre-existing	642.2 ☑	642.0 ☑	642.0 ☑
with pre-eclampsia or eclampsia	642.7 ☑	642.7 ☑	642.7 ☑
fetus or newborn	760.0	760.0	760.0
secondary to renal disease	642.1 ☑	642.1 ☑	642.1 ☑
with pre-eclampsia or eclampsia	642.7 ☑	642.7 ☑	642.7 ☑
fetus or newborn	760.0	760.0	760.0
transient	—	—	642.3 ☑
due to			
aldosteronism, primary	405.09	405.19	405.99
brain tumor	405.09	405.19	405.99
bulbar poliomyelitis	405.09	405.19	405.99
calculus			
kidney	405.09	405.19	405.99
ureter	405.09	405.19	405.99
coarctation, aorta	405.09	405.19	405.99
Cushing's disease	405.09	405.19	405.99
glomerulosclerosis (*see also* Hypertension, kidney)	403.00	403.10	403.90
periarteritis nodosa	405.09	405.19	405.99
pheochromocytoma	405.09	405.19	405.99
polycystic kidney(s)	405.09	405.19	405.99
polycythemia	405.09	405.19	405.99
porphyria	405.09	405.19	405.99
pyelonephritis	405.09	405.19	405.99
renal (artery)			
aneurysm	405.01	405.11	405.91
anomaly	405.01	405.11	405.91
embolism	405.01	405.11	405.91
fibromuscular hyperplasia	405.01	405.11	405.91

☑ Additional Digit Required — Refer to the Tabular List (Numeric Code Section) for Additional Digit Selection
▶◀ Revised Text ● New Line ▲ Revised Code

	Malignant	Benign	Unspecified
Hypertension, hypertensive — *continued*			
due to — *continued*			
renal — *continued*			
occlusion	405.01	405.11	405.91
stenosis	405.01	405.11	405.91
thrombosis	405.01	405.11	405.91
encephalopathy	437.2	437.2	437.2
gestational (transient) NEC	—	—	642.3 ☑
Goldblatt's	440.1	440.1	440.1
heart (disease) (conditions classifiable to 429.0-429.3, 429.8, 429.9 due to hypertension)	402.00	402.10	402.90
with heart failure	402.01	402.11	402.91
hypertensive kidney disease (conditions classifiable to 403) (*see also* Hypertension, cardiorenal)	404.00	404.10	404.90
renal sclerosis (*see also* Hypertension, cardiorenal)	404.00	404.10	404.90
intracranial, benign	—	348.2	—
intraocular	—	—	365.04
kidney	403.00	403.10	403.90
with			
chronic kidney disease	403.01	403.11	403.91 ●
heart involvement (conditions classifiable to 429.0-429.3, 429.8, 429.9 due to hypertension) (*see also* Hypertension, cardiorenal)	404.00	404.10	404.90
hypertensive heart (disease) (conditions classifiable to 402) (*see also* Hypertension, cardiorenal)	404.00	404.10	404.90
lesser circulation	—	—	416.0
necrotizing	401.0	—	—
ocular	—	—	365.04
portal (due to chronic liver disease)	—	—	572.3
postoperative	—	—	997.91
psychogenic	—	—	306.2
puerperal, postpartum — *see* Hypertension, complicating pregnancy, childbirth, or the puerperium			
pulmonary (artery)	—	—	416.8
with cor pulmonale (chronic)	—	—	416.8
acute	—	—	415.0
idiopathic	—	—	416.0
primary	—	—	416.0
of newborn	—	—	747.83
secondary	—	—	416.8
renal (disease) (*see also* Hypertension, kidney)	403.00	403.10	403.90
renovascular NEC	405.01	405.11	405.91
secondary NEC	405.09	405.19	405.99
due to			
aldosteronism, primary	405.09	405.19	405.99
brain tumor	405.09	405.19	405.99
bulbar poliomyelitis	405.09	405.19	405.99
calculus			
kidney	405.09	405.19	405.99
ureter	405.09	405.19	405.99
coarctation, aorta	405.09	405.19	405.99
Cushing's disease	405.09	405.19	405.99
glomerulosclerosis (*see also* Hypertension, kidney)	403.00	403.10	403.90
periarteritis nodosa	405.09	405.19	405.99
pheochromocytoma	405.09	405.19	405.99
polycystic kidney(s)	405.09	405.19	405.99
polycythemia	405.09	405.19	405.99
porphyria	405.09	405.19	405.99
pyelonephritis	405.09	405.19	405.99
renal (artery)			
aneurysm	405.01	405.11	405.91
anomaly	405.01	405.11	405.91
embolism	405.01	405.11	405.91
fibromuscular hyperplasia	405.01	405.11	405.91
occlusion	405.01	405.11	405.91
stenosis	405.01	405.11	405.91
thrombosis	405.01	405.11	405.91
transient	—	—	796.2
of pregnancy	—	—	642.3 ☑
venous, chronic (asymptomatic) (idiopathic)	—	—	459.30
due to			
deep vein thrombosis (*see also* Syndrome, postphlebetic)	—	—	459.10
with			
complication, NEC	—	—	459.39
inflammation	—	—	459.32
with ulcer	—	—	459.33
ulcer	—	—	459.31
with inflammation	—	—	459.33

Note — Use the following fifth-digit subclassification with category 242:

0 *without mention of thyrotoxic crisis or storm*

1 *with mention of thyrotoxic crisis or storm*

☑ Additional Digit Required — Refer to the Tabular List (Numeric Code Section) for Additional Digit Selection

▶◀ Revised Text ● New Line ▲ Revised Code

- **Hyponatremia** 276.1
- **Hypo-ovarianism** 256.39
- **Hypo-ovarism** 256.39
- **Hypoparathyroidism** (idiopathic) (surgically induced) 252.1
  - neonatal 775.4
- **Hypopharyngitis** 462
- **Hypophoria** 378.40
- **Hypophosphatasia** 275.3
- **Hypophosphatemia** (acquired) (congenital) (familial) 275.3
  - renal 275.3
- **Hypophyseal, hypophysis** — *see also* condition
  - dwarfism 253.3
  - gigantism 253.0
  - syndrome 253.8
- **Hypophyseothalamic syndrome** 253.8
- **Hypopiesis** — *see* Hypotension
- **Hypopigmentation** 709.00
  - eyelid 374.53
- **Hypopinealism** 259.8
- **Hypopituitarism** (juvenile) (syndrome) 253.2
  - due to
    - hormone therapy 253.7
    - hypophysectomy 253.7
    - radiotherapy 253.7
  - postablative 253.7
  - postpartum hemorrhage 253.2
- **Hypoplasia, hypoplasis** 759.89
  - adrenal (gland) 759.1
  - alimentary tract 751.8
    - lower 751.2
    - upper 750.8
  - anus, anal (canal) 751.2
  - aorta 747.22
  - aortic
    - arch (tubular) 747.10
    - orifice or valve with hypoplasia of ascending aorta and defective development of left ventricle (with mitral valve atresia) 746.7
  - appendix 751.2
  - areola 757.6
  - arm (*see also* Absence, arm, congenital) 755.20
  - artery (congenital) (peripheral) 747.60
    - brain 747.81
    - cerebral 747.81
    - coronary 746.85
    - gastrointestinal 747.61
    - lower limb 747.64
    - pulmonary 747.3
    - renal 747.62
    - retinal 743.58
    - specified NEC 747.69
    - spinal 747.82
    - umbilical 747.5
    - upper limb 747.63
  - auditory canal 744.29
    - causing impairment of hearing 744.02
  - biliary duct (common) or passage 751.61
  - bladder 753.8
  - bone NEC 756.9
    - face 756.0
    - malar 756.0
    - mandible 524.04
      - alveolar 524.74
    - marrow 284.9
      - acquired (secondary) 284.8
      - congenital 284.0
      - idiopathic 284.9
    - maxilla 524.03
      - alveolar 524.73
    - skull (*see also* Hypoplasia, skull) 756.0
  - brain 742.1
    - gyri 742.2
    - specified part 742.2
  - breast (areola) 757.6
  - bronchus (tree) 748.3
  - cardiac 746.89
    - valve — *see* Hypoplasia, heart, valve
    - vein 746.89
  - carpus (*see also* Absence, carpal, congenital) 755.28
  - cartilaginous 756.9
  - cecum 751.2

Hypoplasia, hypoplasis — *continued*

  - cementum 520.4
    - hereditary 520.5
  - cephalic 742.1
  - cerebellum 742.2
  - cervix (uteri) 752.49
  - chin 524.06
  - clavicle 755.51
  - coccyx 756.19
  - colon 751.2
  - corpus callosum 742.2
  - cricoid cartilage 748.3
  - dermal, focal (Goltz) 757.39
  - digestive organ(s) or tract NEC 751.8
    - lower 751.2
    - upper 750.8
  - ear 744.29
    - auricle 744.23
    - lobe 744.29
    - middle, except ossicles 744.03
      - ossicles 744.04
    - ossicles 744.04
  - enamel of teeth (neonatal) (postnatal) (prenatal) 520.4
    - hereditary 520.5
  - endocrine (gland) NEC 759.2
  - endometrium 621.8
  - epididymis 752.89
  - epiglottis 748.3
  - erythroid, congenital 284.0
  - erythropoietic, chronic acquired 284.8
  - esophagus 750.3
  - Eustachian tube 744.24
  - eye (*see also* Microphthalmos) 743.10
    - lid 743.62
  - face 744.89
    - bone(s) 756.0
  - fallopian tube 752.19
  - femur (*see also* Absence, femur, congenital) 755.34
  - fibula (*see also* Absence, fibula, congenital) 755.37
  - finger (*see also* Absence, finger, congenital) 755.29
  - focal dermal 757.39
  - foot 755.31
  - gallbladder 751.69
  - genitalia, genital organ(s)
    - female 752.89
      - external 752.49
      - internal NEC 752.89
    - in adiposogenital dystrophy 253.8
    - male 752.89
      - penis 752.69
  - glottis 748.3
  - hair 757.4
  - hand 755.21
  - heart 746.89
    - left (complex) (syndrome) 746.7
    - valve NEC 746.89
      - pulmonary 746.01
  - humerus (*see also* Absence, humerus, congenital) 755.24
  - hymen 752.49
  - intestine (small) 751.1
    - large 751.2
  - iris 743.46
  - jaw 524.09
  - kidney(s) 753.0
  - labium (majus) (minus) 752.49
  - labyrinth, membranous 744.05
  - lacrimal duct (apparatus) 743.65
  - larynx 748.3
  - leg (*see also* Absence, limb, congenital, lower) 755.30
  - limb 755.4
    - lower (*see also* Absence, limb, congenital, lower) 755.30
    - upper (*see also* Absence, limb, congenital, upper) 755.20
  - liver 751.69
  - lung (lobe) 748.5
  - mammary (areolar) 757.6
  - mandibular 524.04
    - alveolar 524.74
    - unilateral condylar 526.89

Hypoplasia, hypoplasis — *continued*

  - maxillary 524.03
    - alveolar 524.73
  - medullary 284.9
  - megakaryocytic 287.30 ▲
  - metacarpus (*see also* Absence, metacarpal, congenital) 755.28
  - metatarsus (*see also* Absence, metatarsal, congenital) 755.38
  - muscle 756.89
    - eye 743.69
  - myocardium (congenital) (Uhl's anomaly) 746.84
  - nail(s) 757.5
  - nasolacrimal duct 743.65
  - nervous system NEC 742.8
  - neural 742.8
  - nose, nasal 748.1
  - ophthalmic (*see also* Microphthalmos) 743.10
  - organ
    - of Corti 744.05
    - or site NEC — *see* Anomaly, by site
  - osseous meatus (ear) 744.03
  - ovary 752.0
  - oviduct 752.19
  - pancreas 751.7
  - parathyroid (gland) 759.2
  - parotid gland 750.26
  - patella 755.64
  - pelvis, pelvic girdle 755.69
  - penis 752.69
  - peripheral vascular system (congenital) NEC 747.60
    - gastrointestinal 747.61
    - lower limb 747.64
    - renal 747.62
    - specified NEC 747.69
    - spinal 747.82
    - upper limb 747.63
  - pituitary (gland) 759.2
  - pulmonary 748.5
    - arteriovenous 747.3
    - artery 747.3
    - valve 746.01
  - punctum lacrimale 743.65
  - radioulnar (*see also* Absence, radius, congenital, with ulna) 755.25
  - radius (*see also* Absence, radius, congenital) 755.26
  - rectum 751.2
  - respiratory system NEC 748.9
  - rib 756.3
  - sacrum 756.19
  - scapula 755.59
  - shoulder girdle 755.59
  - skin 757.39
  - skull (bone) 756.0
    - with
      - anencephalus 740.0
      - encephalocele 742.0
      - hydrocephalus 742.3
        - with spina bifida (*see also* Spina bifida) 741.0 ☑
      - microcephalus 742.1
  - spinal (cord) (ventral horn cell) 742.59
    - vessel 747.82
  - spine 756.19
  - spleen 759.0
  - sternum 756.3
  - tarsus (*see also* Absence, tarsal, congenital) 755.38
  - testis, testicle 752.89
  - thymus (gland) 279.11
  - thyroid (gland) 243
    - cartilage 748.3
  - tibiofibular (*see also* Absence, tibia, congenital, with fibula) 755.35
  - toe (*see also* Absence, toe, congenital) 755.39
  - tongue 750.16
  - trachea (cartilage) (rings) 748.3
  - Turner's (tooth) 520.4
  - ulna (*see also* Absence, ulna, congenital) 755.27
  - umbilical artery 747.5
  - ureter 753.29
  - uterus 752.3
  - vagina 752.49

Hypoplasia, hypoplasis — *continued*
vascular (peripheral) NEC (*see also* Hypoplasia, peripheral vascular system) 747.60
brain 747.81
vein(s) (peripheral) NEC (*see also* Hypoplasia, peripheral vascular system) 747.60
brain 747.81
cardiac 746.89
great 747.49
portal 747.49
pulmonary 747.49
vena cava (inferior) (superior) 747.49
vertebra 756.19
vulva 752.49
zonule (ciliary) 743.39
zygoma 738.12
Hypopotassemia 276.8
Hypoproaccelerinemia (*see also* Defect, coagulation) 286.3
Hypoproconvertinemia (congenital) (*see also* Defect, coagulation) 286.3
Hypoproteinemia (essential) (hypermetabolic) (idiopathic) 273.8
Hypoproteinosis 260
Hypoprothrombinemia (congenital) (hereditary) (idiopathic) (*see also* Defect, coagulation) 286.3
acquired 286.7
newborn 776.3
Hypopselaphesia 782.0
Hypopyon (anterior chamber) (eye) 364.05
iritis 364.05
ulcer (cornea) 370.04
Hypopyrexia 780.99
Hyporeflex 796.1
Hyporeninemia, extreme 790.99
in primary aldosteronism 255.10
Hyporesponsive episode 780.09
Hyposecretion
ACTH 253.4
ovary 256.39
postablative 256.2
salivary gland (any) 527.7
Hyposegmentation of neutrophils, hereditary 288.2
Hyposiderinemia 280.9
Hyposmolality 276.1
syndrome 276.1
Hyposomatotropism 253.3
Hyposomnia, ▶unspecified◀ (*see also* Insomnia) 780.52
with sleep apnea, unspecified 780.53 ●
Hypospadias (male) 752.61
female 753.8
Hypospermatogenesis 606.1
Hyposphagma 372.72
Hyposplenism 289.59
Hypostasis, pulmonary 514
Hypostatic — *see* condition
Hyposthenuria 593.89
Hyposuprarenalism 255.4
Hypo-TBG-nemia 246.8
Hypotension (arterial) (constitutional) 458.9
chronic 458.1
iatrogenic 458.29
maternal, syndrome (following labor and delivery) 669.2 ☑
of hemodialysis 458.21
orthostatic (chronic) 458.0
dysautonomic-dyskinetic syndrome 333.0
permanent idiopathic 458.1
postoperative 458.29
postural 458.0
specified type NEC 458.8
transient 796.3
Hypothermia (accidental) 991.6
anesthetic 995.89
newborn NEC 778.3
not associated with low environmental temperature 780.99
Hypothymergasia (*see also* Psychosis, affective) 296.2 ☑
recurrent episode 296.3 ☑
single episode 296.2 ☑
Hypothyroidism (acquired) 244.9
complicating pregnancy, childbirth, or puerperium 648.1 ☑
congenital 243
due to
ablation 244.1
radioactive iodine 244.1
surgical 244.0
iodine (administration) (ingestion) 244.2
radioactive 244.1
irradiation therapy 244.1
p-aminosalicylic acid (PAS) 244.3
phenylbutazone 244.3
resorcinol 244.3
specified cause NEC 244.8
surgery 244.0
goitrous (sporadic) 246.1
iatrogenic NEC 244.3
iodine 244.2
pituitary 244.8
postablative NEC 244.1
postsurgical 244.0
primary 244.9
secondary NEC 244.8
specified cause NEC 244.8
sporadic goitrous 246.1
Hypotonia, hypotonicity, hypotony 781.3
benign congenital 358.8
bladder 596.4
congenital 779.89
benign 358.8
eye 360.30
due to
fistula 360.32
ocular disorder NEC 360.33
following loss of aqueous or vitreous 360.33
primary 360.31
infantile muscular (benign) 359.0
muscle 728.9
uterus, uterine (contractions) — *see* Inertia, uterus
Hypotrichosis 704.09
congenital 757.4
lid (congenital) 757.4
acquired 374.55
postinfectional NEC 704.09
Hypotropia 378.32
Hypoventilation 786.09
congenital central alveolar syndrome 327.25 ●
idiopathic sleep related nonobstructive alveolar 327.24 ●
sleep related, in conditions classifiable elsewhere 327.26 ●
Hypovitaminosis (*see also* Deficiency, vitamin) 269.2
Hypovolemia 276.52 ▲
surgical shock 998.0
traumatic (shock) 958.4
Hypoxemia (*see also* Anoxia) 799.02 ▲
sleep related, in conditions classifiable elsewhere 327.26 ●
Hypoxia (*see also* Anoxia) 799.02 ▲
cerebral 348.1
during or resulting from a procedure 997.01
newborn 768.9
mild or moderate 768.6
severe 768.5
fetal, affecting newborn 768.9
intrauterine — *see* Distress, fetal
myocardial (*see also* Insufficiency, coronary) 411.89
arteriosclerotic — *see* Arteriosclerosis, coronary
newborn 768.9
sleep related 327.24 ●
Hypsarrhythmia (*see also* Epilepsy) 345.6 ☑
Hysteralgia, pregnant uterus 646.8 ☑
Hysteria, hysterical 300.10
anxiety 300.20
Charcôt's gland 300.11
Hysteria, hysterical — *continued*
conversion (any manifestation) 300.11
dissociative type NEC 300.15
psychosis, acute 298.1
Hysteroepilepsy 300.11
Hysterotomy, affecting fetus or newborn 763.89

I

Iatrogenic syndrome of excess cortisol 255.0
Iceland disease (epidemic neuromyasthenia) 049.8
Ichthyosis (congenital) 757.1
acquired 701.1
fetalis gravior 757.1
follicularis 757.1
hystrix 757.39
lamellar 757.1
lingual 528.6
palmaris and plantaris 757.39
simplex 757.1
vera 757.1
vulgaris 757.1
Ichthyotoxism 988.0
bacterial (*see also* Poisoning, food) 005.9
Icteroanemia, hemolytic (acquired) 283.9
congenital (*see also* Spherocytosis) 282.0
Icterus (*see also* Jaundice) 782.4
catarrhal — *see* Icterus, infectious
conjunctiva 782.4
newborn 774.6
epidemic — *see* Icterus, infectious
febrilis — *see* Icterus, infectious
fetus or newborn — *see* Jaundice, fetus or newborn
gravis (*see also* Necrosis, liver) 570
complicating pregnancy 646.7 ☑
affecting fetus or newborn 760.8
fetus or newborn NEC 773.0
obstetrical 646.7 ☑
affecting fetus or newborn 760.8
hematogenous (acquired) 283.9
hemolytic (acquired) 283.9
congenital (*see also* Spherocytosis) 282.0
hemorrhagic (acute) 100.0
leptospiral 100.0
newborn 776.0
spirochetal 100.0
infectious 070.1
with hepatic coma 070.0
leptospiral 100.0
spirochetal 100.0
intermittens juvenilis 277.4
malignant (*see also* Necrosis, liver) 570
neonatorum (*see also* Jaundice, fetus or newborn) 774.6
pernicious (*see also* Necrosis, liver) 570
spirochetal 100.0
Ictus solaris, solis 992.0
Ideation ●
suicidal V62.84 ●
Identity disorder 313.82
dissociative 300.14
gender role (child) 302.6
adult 302.85
psychosexual (child) 302.6
adult 302.85
Idioglossia 307.9
Idiopathic — *see* condition
Idiosyncrasy (*see also* Allergy) 995.3
drug, medicinal substance, and biological — *see* Allergy, drug
Idiot, idiocy (congenital) 318.2
amaurotic (Bielschowsky) (-Jansky) (family) (infantile (late)) (juvenile (late)) (Vogt-Spielmeyer) 330.1
microcephalic 742.1
Mongolian 758.0
oxycephalic 756.0
Id reaction (due to bacteria) 692.89
IgE asthma 493.0 ☑

☑ Additional Digit Required — Refer to the Tabular List (Numeric Code Section) for Additional Digit Selection
▶◀ Revised Text ● New Line ▲ Revised Code

- **Inadequate, inadequacy** — *continued*
  - household care, due to — *continued*
    - family member — *continued*
      - temporarily away from home V60.4
        - on vacation V60.5
    - technical defects in home V60.1
    - temporary absence from home of person rendering care V60.4
  - housing (heating) (space) V60.1
  - interarch distance 524.28
  - material resources V60.2
  - mental (*see also* Retardation, mental) 319
  - nervous system 799.2
  - personality 301.6
  - prenatal care in current pregnancy V23.7
  - pulmonary
    - function 786.09
      - newborn 770.89
    - ventilation, newborn 770.89
  - respiration 786.09
    - newborn 770.89
  - sample, Papanicolaou smear 795.08
  - social 301.6
- **Inanition** 263.9
  - with edema 262
  - due to
    - deprivation of food 994.2
    - malnutrition 263.9
  - fever 780.6
- **Inappropriate secretion**
  - ACTH 255.0
  - antidiuretic hormone (ADH) (excessive) 253.6
    - deficiency 253.5
  - ectopic hormone NEC 259.3
  - pituitary (posterior) 253.6
- **Inattention after or at birth** 995.52
- **Inborn errors of metabolism** — *see* Disorder, metabolism
- **Incarceration, incarcerated**
  - bubonocele — *see also* Hernia, inguinal, with obstruction
    - gangrenous — *see* Hernia, inguinal, with gangrene
  - colon (by hernia) — *see also* Hernia, by site with obstruction
    - gangrenous — *see* Hernia, by site, with gangrene
  - enterocele 552.9
    - gangrenous 551.9
  - epigastrocele 552.29
    - gangrenous 551.29
  - epiplocele 552.9
    - gangrenous 551.9
  - exomphalos 552.1
    - gangrenous 551.1
  - fallopian tube 620.8
  - hernia — *see also* Hernia, by site, with obstruction
    - gangrenous — *see* Hernia, by site, with gangrene
  - iris, in wound 871.1
  - lens, in wound 871.1
  - merocele (*see also* Hernia, femoral, with obstruction) 552.00
  - omentum (by hernia) — *see also* Hernia, by site, with obstruction
    - gangrenous — *see* Hernia, by site, with gangrene
  - omphalocele 756.79
  - rupture (meaning hernia) (*see also* Hernia, by site, with obstruction) 552.9
    - gangrenous (*see also* Hernia, by site, with gangrene) 551.9
  - sarcoepiplocele 552.9
    - gangrenous 551.9
  - sarcoepiplomphalocele 552.1
    - with gangrene 551.1
  - uterus 621.8
    - gravid 654.3 ☑
      - causing obstructed labor 660.2 ☑
        - affecting fetus or newborn 763.1
- **Incident, cerebrovascular** (*see also* Disease, cerebrovascular, acute) 436
- **Incineration** (entire body) (from fire, conflagration, electricity, or lightning) — *see* Burn, multiple, specified sites
- **Incised wound**
  - external — *see* Wound, open, by site
  - internal organs (abdomen, chest, or pelvis) — *see* Injury, internal, by site, with open wound
- **Incision, incisional**
  - hernia — *see* Hernia, incisional
  - surgical, complication — *see* Complications, surgical procedures
  - traumatic
    - external — *see* Wound, open, by site
    - internal organs (abdomen, chest, or pelvis) — *see* Injury, internal, by site, with open wound
- **Inclusion**
  - azurophilic leukocytic 288.2
  - blennorrhea (neonatal) (newborn) 771.6
  - cyst — *see* Cyst, skin
  - gallbladder in liver (congenital) 751.69
- **Incompatibility**
  - ABO
    - affecting management of pregnancy 656.2 ☑
    - fetus or newborn 773.1
    - infusion or transfusion reaction 999.6
  - blood (group) (Duffy) (E) (K(ell)) (Kidd) (Lewis) (M) (N) (P) (S) NEC
    - affecting management of pregnancy 656.2 ☑
    - fetus or newborn 773.2
    - infusion or transfusion reaction 999.6
  - marital V61.10
    - involving divorce or estrangement V61.0
  - Rh (blood group) (factor)
    - affecting management of pregnancy 656.1 ☑
    - fetus or newborn 773.0
    - infusion or transfusion reaction 999.7
  - Rhesus — *see* Incompatibility, Rh
- **Incompetency, incompetence, incompetent**
  - annular
    - aortic (valve) (*see also* Insufficiency, aortic) 424.1
    - mitral (valve) — (*see also* Insufficiency, mitral) 424.0
    - pulmonary valve (heart) (*see also* Endocarditis, pulmonary) 424.3
  - aortic (valve) (*see also* Insufficiency, aortic) 424.1
    - syphilitic 093.22
  - cardiac (orifice) 530.0
    - valve — *see* Endocarditis
  - cervix, cervical (os) 622.5
    - in pregnancy 654.5 ☑
      - affecting fetus or newborn 761.0
  - esophagogastric (junction) (sphincter) 530.0
  - heart valve, congenital 746.89
  - mitral (valve) — *see* Insufficiency, mitral
  - papillary muscle (heart) 429.81
  - pelvic fundus
    - pubocervical tissue 618.81
    - rectovaginal tissue 618.82
  - pulmonary valve (heart) (*see also* Endocarditis, pulmonary) 424.3
    - congenital 746.09
  - tricuspid (annular) (rheumatic) (valve) (*see also* Endocarditis, tricuspid) 397.0
  - valvular — *see* Endocarditis
  - vein, venous (saphenous) (varicose) (*see also* Varicose, vein) 454.9
  - velopharyngeal (closure)
    - acquired 528.9
    - congenital 750.29
- **Incomplete** — *see also* condition
  - bladder emptying 788.21
  - expansion lungs (newborn) 770.5
  - gestation (liveborn) — *see* Immaturity
  - rotation — *see* Malrotation
- **Incontinence** 788.30
  - without sensory awareness 788.34
  - anal sphincter 787.6
  - continuous leakage 788.37
  - feces 787.6
    - due to hysteria 300.11
    - nonorganic origin 307.7
  - hysterical 300.11
  - mixed (male) (female) (urge and stress) 788.33
  - overflow 788.38
  - paradoxical 788.39
  - rectal 787.6
- **Incontinence** — *continued*
  - specified NEC 788.39
  - stress (female) 625.6
    - male NEC 788.32
  - urethral sphincter 599.84
  - urge 788.31
    - and stress (male) (female) 788.33
  - urine 788.30
    - active 788.30
    - male 788.30
      - stress 788.32
        - and urge 788.33
    - neurogenic 788.39
    - nonorganic origin 307.6
    - stress (female) 625.6
      - male NEC 788.32
    - urge 788.31
      - and stress 788.33
- **Incontinentia pigmenti** 757.33
- **Incoordinate**
  - uterus (action) (contractions) 661.4 ☑
    - affecting fetus or newborn 763.7
- **Incoordination**
  - esophageal-pharyngeal (newborn) 787.2
  - muscular 781.3
  - papillary muscle 429.81
- **Increase, increased**
  - abnormal, in development 783.9
  - androgens (ovarian) 256.1
  - anticoagulants (antithrombin) (anti-VIIIa) (anti-IXa) (anti-Xa) (anti-XIa) 286.5
    - postpartum 666.3 ☑
  - cold sense (*see also* Disturbance, sensation) 782.0
  - estrogen 256.0
  - function
    - adrenal (cortex) 255.3
      - medulla 255.6
    - pituitary (anterior) (gland) (lobe) 253.1
      - posterior 253.6
  - heat sense (*see also* Disturbance, sensation) 782.0
  - intracranial pressure 781.99
    - injury at birth 767.8
  - light reflex of retina 362.13
  - permeability, capillary 448.9
  - pressure
    - intracranial 781.99
      - injury at birth 767.8
    - intraocular 365.00
  - pulsations 785.9
  - pulse pressure 785.9
  - sphericity, lens 743.36
  - splenic activity 289.4
  - venous pressure 459.89
    - portal 572.3
- **Incrustation, cornea, lead or zinc** 930.0
- **Incyclophoria** 378.44
- **Incyclotropia** 378.33
- **Indeterminate sex** 752.7
- **India rubber skin** 756.83
- **Indicanuria** 270.2
- **Indigestion** (bilious) (functional) 536.8
  - acid 536.8
  - catarrhal 536.8
  - due to decomposed food NEC 005.9
  - fat 579.8
  - nervous 306.4
  - psychogenic 306.4
- **Indirect** — *see* condition
- **Indolent bubo** NEC 099.8
- **Induced**
  - abortion — *see* Abortion, induced
  - birth, affecting fetus or newborn 763.89
  - delivery — *see* Delivery
  - labor — *see* Delivery
- **Induration, indurated**
  - brain 348.8
  - breast (fibrous) 611.79
    - puerperal, postpartum 676.3 ☑
  - broad ligament 620.8
  - chancre 091.0
    - anus 091.1
    - congenital 090.0
    - extragenital NEC 091.2

☑ Additional Digit Required — Refer to the Tabular List (Numeric Code Section) for Additional Digit Selection

▶◀ Revised Text ● New Line ▲ Revised Code

> *Note — Use the following fifth-digit subclassification with category 410:*
>
> *0 episode unspecified*
>
> *1 initial episode*
>
> *2 subsequent episode without recurrence*

- **Infarct, infarction** — *continued*
  - retina, retinal 362.84
    - with occlusion — *see* Occlusion, retina
  - spinal (acute) (cord) (embolic) (nonembolic) 336.1
  - spleen 289.59
    - embolic or thrombotic 444.89
  - subchorionic — *see* Infarct, placenta
  - subendocardial (*see also* Infarct, myocardium) 410.7 ☑
  - suprarenal (capsule) (gland) 255.4
  - syncytium — *see* Infarct, placenta
  - testis 608.83
  - thrombotic (*see also* Thrombosis) 453.9
    - artery, arterial — *see* Embolism
  - thyroid (gland) 246.3
  - ventricle (heart) (*see also* Infarct, myocardium) 410.9 ☑
- **Infecting** — *see* condition
- **Infection, infected, infective** (opportunistic) 136.9
  - with lymphangitis — *see* Lymphangitis
  - abortion — *see* Abortion, by type, with, sepsis
  - abscess (skin) — *see* Abscess, by site
  - Absidia 117.7
  - Acanthocheilonema (perstans) 125.4
    - streptocerca 125.6
  - accessory sinus (chronic) (*see also* Sinusitis) 473.9
  - Achorion — *see* Dermatophytosis
  - Acremonium falciforme 117.4
  - acromioclavicular (joint) 711.91
  - actinobacillus
    - lignieresii 027.8
    - mallei 024
    - muris 026.1
  - actinomadura — *see* Actinomycosis
  - Actinomyces (israelii) — *see also* Actinomycosis
    - muris-ratti 026.1
  - Actinomycetales (actinomadura) (Actinomyces) (Nocardia) (Streptomyces) — *see* Actinomycosis
  - actinomycotic NEC (*see also* Actinomycosis) 039.9
  - adenoid (chronic) 474.01
    - acute 463
    - and tonsil (chronic) 474.02
      - acute or subacute 463
  - adenovirus NEC 079.0
    - in diseases classified elsewhere — *see* category 079 ☑
    - unspecified nature or site 079.0
  - Aerobacter aerogenes NEC 041.85
    - enteritis 008.2
  - aerogenes capsulatus (*see also* Gangrene, gas) 040.0
  - aertrycke (*see also* Infection, Salmonella) 003.9
  - ajellomyces dermatitidis 116.0
  - alimentary canal NEC (*see also* Enteritis, due to, by organism) 009.0
  - Allescheria boydii 117.6
  - Alternaria 118
  - alveolus, alveolar (process) (pulpal origin) 522.4
  - ameba, amebic (histolytica) (*see also* Amebiasis) 006.9
    - acute 006.0
    - chronic 006.1
    - free-living 136.2
    - hartmanni 007.8
    - specified
      - site NEC 006.8
      - type NEC 007.8
  - amniotic fluid or cavity 658.4 ☑
    - affecting fetus or newborn 762.7
  - anaerobes (cocci) (gram-negative) (gram-positive) (mixed) NEC 041.84
  - anal canal 569.49
  - Ancylostoma braziliense 126.2
  - Angiostrongylus cantonensis 128.8
  - anisakiasis 127.1
  - Anisakis larva 127.1
  - anthrax (*see also* Anthrax) 022.9
  - antrum (chronic) (*see also* Sinusitis, maxillary) 473.0
  - anus (papillae) (sphincter) 569.49
  - arbor virus NEC 066.9
  - arbovirus NEC 066.9
- **Infection, infected, infective** — *continued*
  - argentophil-rod 027.0
  - Ascaris lumbricoides 127.0
  - ascomycetes 117.4
  - Aspergillus (flavus) (fumigatus) (terreus) 117.3
  - atypical
    - acid-fast (bacilli) (*see also* Mycobacterium, atypical) 031.9
    - mycobacteria (*see also* Mycobacterium, atypical) 031.9
  - auditory meatus (circumscribed) (diffuse) (external) (*see also* Otitis, externa) 380.10
  - auricle (ear) (*see also* Otitis, externa) 380.10
  - axillary gland 683
  - Babesiasis 088.82
  - Babesiosis 088.82
  - Bacillus NEC 041.89
    - abortus 023.1
    - anthracis (*see also* Anthrax) 022.9
    - cereus (food poisoning) 005.89
    - coli — *see* Infection, Escherichia coli
    - coliform NEC 041.85
    - Ducrey's (any location) 099.0
    - Flexner's 004.1
    - Friedländer's NEC 041.3
    - fusiformis 101
    - gas (gangrene) (*see also* Gangrene, gas) 040.0
    - mallei 024
    - melitensis 023.0
    - paratyphoid, paratyphosus 002.9
      - A 002.1
      - B 002.2
      - C 002.3
    - Schmorl's 040.3
    - Shiga 004.0
    - suipestifer (*see also* Infection, Salmonella) 003.9
    - swimming pool 031.1
    - typhosa 002.0
    - welchii (*see also* Gangrene, gas) 040.0
    - Whitmore's 025
  - bacterial NEC 041.9
    - specified NEC 041.89
      - anaerobic NEC 041.84
      - gram-negative NEC 041.85
        - anaerobic NEC 041.84
  - Bacterium
    - paratyphosum 002.9
      - A 002.1
      - B 002.2
      - C 002.3
    - typhosum 002.0
  - Bacteroides (fragilis) (melaninogenicus) (oralis) NEC 041.82
  - balantidium coli 007.0
  - Bartholin's gland 616.8
  - Basidiobolus 117.7
  - Bedsonia 079.98
    - specified NEC 079.88
  - bile duct 576.1
  - bladder (*see also* Cystitis) 595.9
  - Blastomyces, blastomycotic 116.0
    - brasiliensis 116.1
    - dermatitidis 116.0
    - European 117.5
    - loboi 116.2
    - North American 116.0
    - South American 116.1
  - blood stream — *see* Septicemia
  - bone 730.9 ☑
    - specified — *see* Osteomyelitis
  - Bordetella 033.9
    - bronchiseptica 033.8
    - parapertussis 033.1
    - pertussis 033.0
  - Borrelia
    - bergdorfi 088.81
    - vincentii (mouth) (pharynx) (tonsil) 101
  - brain (*see also* Encephalitis) 323.9
    - late effect — *see* category 326
    - membranes — (*see also* Meningitis) 322.9
    - septic 324.0
      - late effect — *see* category 326
      - meninges (*see also* Meningitis) 320.9
  - branchial cyst 744.42
- **Infection, infected, infective** — *continued*
  - breast 611.0
    - puerperal, postpartum 675.2 ☑
      - with nipple 675.9 ☑
        - specified type NEC 675.8 ☑
      - nonpurulent 675.2 ☑
      - purulent 675.1 ☑
  - bronchus (*see also* Bronchitis) 490
    - fungus NEC 117.9
  - Brucella 023.9
    - abortus 023.1
    - canis 023.3
    - melitensis 023.0
    - mixed 023.8
    - suis 023.2
  - Brugia (Wuchereria) malayi 125.1
  - bursa — *see* Bursitis
  - buttocks (skin) 686.9
  - Candida (albicans) (tropicalis) (*see also* Candidiasis) 112.9
    - congenital 771.7
  - Candiru 136.8
  - Capillaria
    - hepatica 128.8
    - philippinensis 127.5
  - cartilage 733.99
  - cat liver fluke 121.0
  - cellulitis — *see* Cellulitis, by site
  - Cephalosporum falciforme 117.4
  - Cercomonas hominis (intestinal) 007.3
  - cerebrospinal (*see also* Meningitis) 322.9
    - late effect — *see* category 326
  - cervical gland 683
  - cervix (*see also* Cervicitis) 616.0
  - cesarean section wound 674.3 ☑
  - Chilomastix (intestinal) 007.8
  - Chlamydia 079.98
    - specified NEC 079.88
  - cholera (*see also* Cholera) 001.9
  - chorionic plate 658.8 ☑
  - Cladosporium
    - bantianum 117.8
    - carrionii 117.2
    - mansoni 111.1
    - trichoides 117.8
    - wernecki 111.1
  - Clonorchis (sinensis) (liver) 121.1
  - Clostridium (haemolyticum) (novyi) NEC 041.84
    - botulinum 005.1
    - histolyticum (*see also* Gangrene, gas) 040.0
    - oedematiens (*see also* Gangrene, gas) 040.0
    - perfringens 041.83
      - due to food 005.2
    - septicum (*see also* Gangrene, gas) 040.0
    - sordellii (*see also* Gangrene, gas) 040.0
    - welchii (*see also* Gangrene, gas) 040.0
      - due to food 005.2
  - Coccidioides (immitis) (*see also* Coccidioidomycosis) 114.9
  - coccus NEC 041.89
  - colon (*see also* Enteritis, due to, by organism) 009.0
    - bacillus — *see* Infection, Escherichia coli
  - colostomy or enterostomy 569.61
  - common duct 576.1
  - complicating pregnancy, childbirth, or puerperium NEC 647.9 ☑
    - affecting fetus or newborn 760.2
  - Condiobolus 117.7
  - congenital NEC 771.89
    - Candida albicans 771.7
    - chronic 771.2
    - cytomegalovirus 771.1
    - hepatitis, viral 771.2
    - herpes simplex 771.2
    - listeriosis 771.2
    - malaria 771.2
    - poliomyelitis 771.2
    - rubella 771.0
    - toxoplasmosis 771.2
    - tuberculosis 771.2
    - urinary (tract) 771.82
    - vaccinia 771.2
  - coronavirus 079.89
    - SARS-associated 079.82
  - corpus luteum (*see also* Salpingo-oophoritis) 614.2

☑ Additional Digit Required — Refer to the Tabular List (Numeric Code Section) for Additional Digit Selection

▶◀ Revised Text ● New Line ▲ Revised Code

Infection, infected, infective — *continued*
- Corynebacterium diphtheriae — *see* Diphtheria
- Coxsackie (*see also* Coxsackie) 079.2
  - endocardium 074.22
  - heart NEC 074.20
  - in diseases classified elsewhere — *see* category 079 ☑
  - meninges 047.0
  - myocardium 074.23
  - pericardium 074.21
  - pharynx 074.0
  - specified disease NEC 074.8
  - unspecified nature or site 079.2
- Cryptococcus neoformans 117.5
- Cryptosporidia 007.4
- Cunninghamella 117.7
- cyst — *see* Cyst
- Cysticercus cellulosae 123.1
- cytomegalovirus 078.5
  - congenital 771.1
- dental (pulpal origin) 522.4
- deuteromycetes 117.4
- Dicrocoelium dendriticum 121.8
- Dipetalonema (perstans) 125.4
  - streptocerca 125.6
- diphtherial — *see* Diphtheria
- Diphyllobothrium (adult) (latum) (pacificum) 123.4
  - larval 123.5
- Diplogonoporus (grandis) 123.8
- Dipylidium (caninum) 123.8
- Dirofilaria 125.6
- dog tapeworm 123.8
- Dracunculus medinensis 125.7
- Dreschlera 118
  - hawaiiensis 117.8
- Ducrey's bacillus (any site) 099.0
- due to or resulting from
  - device, implant, or graft (any) (presence of) — *see* Complications, infection and inflammation, due to (presence of) any device, implant, or graft classified to 996.0-996.5 NEC
  - injection, inoculation, infusion, transfusion, or vaccination (prophylactic) (therapeutic) 999.3
  - injury NEC — *see* Wound, open, by site, complicated
  - surgery 998.59
- duodenum 535.6 ☑
- ear — *see also* Otitis
  - external (*see also* Otitis, externa) 380.10
  - inner (*see also* Labyrinthitis) 386.30
  - middle — *see* Otitis, media
- Eaton's agent NEC 041.81
- Eberthella typhosa 002.0
- Ebola 078.89 ▲
- echinococcosis 122.9
- Echinococcus (*see also* Echinococcus) 122.9
- Echinostoma 121.8
- ECHO virus 079.1
  - in diseases classified elsewhere — *see* category 079 ☑
  - unspecified nature or site 079.1
- Ehrlichiosis 082.40
  - chaffeensis 082.41
  - specified type NEC 082.49
- Endamoeba — *see* Infection, ameba
- endocardium (*see also* Endocarditis) 421.0
- endocervix (*see also* Cervicitis) 616.0
- Entamoeba — *see* Infection, ameba
- enteric (*see also* Enteritis, due to, by organism) 009.0
- Enterobacter aerogenes NEC 041.85
- Enterobacter sakazakii 041.85 ●
- Enterobius vermicularis 127.4
- enterococcus NEC 041.04
- enterovirus NEC 079.89
  - central nervous system NEC 048
  - enteritis 008.67
  - meningitis 047.9
- Entomophthora 117.7
- Epidermophyton — *see* Dermatophytosis
- epidermophytosis — *see* Dermatophytosis
- episiotomy 674.3 ☑
- Epstein-Barr virus 075
  - chronic 780.79 *[139.8]*

Infection, infected, infective — *continued*
- erysipeloid 027.1
- Erysipelothrix (insidiosa) (rhusiopathiae) 027.1
- erythema infectiosum 057.0
- Escherichia coli NEC 041.4
  - enteritis — *see* Enteritis, E. coli
  - generalized 038.42
  - intestinal — *see* Enteritis, E. coli
- esophagostomy 530.86
- ethmoidal (chronic) (sinus) (*see also* Sinusitis, ethmoidal) 473.2
- Eubacterium 041.84
- Eustachian tube (ear) 381.50
  - acute 381.51
  - chronic 381.52
- exanthema subitum 057.8
- external auditory canal (meatus) (*see also* Otitis, externa) 380.10
- eye NEC 360.00
- eyelid 373.9
  - specified NEC 373.8
- fallopian tube (*see also* Salpingo-oophoritis) 614.2
- fascia 728.89
- Fasciola
  - gigantica 121.3
  - hepatica 121.3
- Fasciolopsis (buski) 121.4
- fetus (intra-amniotic) — *see* Infection, congenital
- filarial — *see* Infestation, filarial
- finger (skin) 686.9
  - abscess (with lymphangitis) 681.00
    - pulp 681.01
  - cellulitis (with lymphangitis) 681.00
  - distal closed space (with lymphangitis) 681.00
  - nail 681.02
    - fungus 110.1
- fish tapeworm 123.4
  - larval 123.5
- flagellate, intestinal 007.9
- fluke — *see* Infestation, fluke
- focal
  - teeth (pulpal origin) 522.4
  - tonsils 474.00
    - and adenoids 474.02
- Fonsecaea
  - compactum 117.2
  - pedrosoi 117.2
- food (*see also* Poisoning, food) 005.9
- foot (skin) 686.9
  - fungus 110.4
- Francisella tularensis (*see also* Tularemia) 021.9
- frontal sinus (chronic) (*see also* Sinusitis, frontal) 473.1
- fungus NEC 117.9
  - beard 110.0
  - body 110.5
  - dermatiacious NEC 117.8
  - foot 110.4
  - groin 110.3
  - hand 110.2
  - nail 110.1
  - pathogenic to compromised host only 118
  - perianal (area) 110.3
  - scalp 110.0
  - scrotum 110.8
  - skin 111.9
    - foot 110.4
    - hand 110.2
  - toenails 110.1
  - trachea 117.9
- Fusarium 118
- Fusobacterium 041.84
- gallbladder (*see also* Cholecystitis, acute) 575.0
- Gardnerella vaginalis 041.89
- gas bacillus (*see also* Gas, gangrene) 040.0
- gastric (*see also* Gastritis) 535.5 ☑
- Gastrodiscoides hominis 121.8
- gastroenteric (*see also* Enteritis, due to, by organism) 009.0
- gastrointestinal (*see also* Enteritis, due to, by organism) 009.0
- gastrostomy 536.41
- generalized NEC (*see also* Septicemia) 038.9

Infection, infected, infective — *continued*
- genital organ or tract NEC
  - female 614.9
    - with
      - abortion — *see* Abortion, by type, with sepsis
      - ectopic pregnancy (*see also* categories 633.0-633.9) 639.0
      - molar pregnancy (*see also* categories 630-632) 639.0
    - complicating pregnancy 646.6 ☑
      - affecting fetus or newborn 760.8
    - following
      - abortion 639.0
      - ectopic or molar pregnancy 639.0
    - puerperal, postpartum, childbirth 670.0 ☑
      - minor or localized 646.6 ☑
        - affecting fetus or newborn 760.8
  - male 608.4
- genitourinary tract NEC 599.0
- Ghon tubercle, primary (*see also* Tuberculosis) 010.0 ☑
- Giardia lamblia 007.1
- gingival (chronic) 523.1
  - acute 523.0
  - Vincent's 101
- glanders 024
- Glenosporopsis amazonica 116.2
- Gnathostoma spinigerum 128.1
- Gongylonema 125.6
- gonococcal NEC (*see also* Gonococcus) 098.0
- gram-negative bacilli NEC 041.85
  - anaerobic 041.84
- guinea worm 125.7
- gum (*see also* Infection, gingival) 523.1
- Hantavirus 079.81
- heart 429.89
- Helicobacter pylori (H. pylori) 041.86
- helminths NEC 128.9
  - intestinal 127.9
    - mixed (types classifiable to more than one category in 120.0-127.7) 127.8
    - specified type NEC 127.7
  - specified type NEC 128.8
- Hemophilus influenzae NEC 041.5
  - generalized 038.41
- herpes (simplex) (*see also* Herpes, simplex) 054.9
  - congenital 771.2
  - zoster (*see also* Herpes, zoster) 053.9
    - eye NEC 053.29
- Heterophyes heterophyes 121.6
- Histoplasma (*see also* Histoplasmosis) 115.90
  - capsulatum (*see also* Histoplasmosis, American) 115.00
  - duboisii (*see also* Histoplasmosis, African) 115.10
- HIV V08
  - with symptoms, symptomatic 042
- hookworm (*see also* Ancylostomiasis) 126.9
- human immunodeficiency virus V08
  - with symptoms, symptomatic 042
- human papillomavirus 079.4
- hydrocele 603.1
- hydronephrosis 591
- Hymenolepis 123.6
- hypopharynx 478.29
- inguinal glands 683
  - due to soft chancre 099.0
- intestine, intestinal (*see also* Enteritis, due to, by organism) 009.0
- intrauterine (*see also* Endometritis) 615.9
  - complicating delivery 646.6 ☑
- isospora belli or hominis 007.2
- Japanese B encephalitis 062.0
- jaw (bone) (acute) (chronic) (lower) (subacute) (upper) 526.4
- joint — *see* Arthritis, infectious or infective
- kidney (cortex) (hematogenous) 590.9
  - with
    - abortion — *see* Abortion, by type, with urinary tract infection
    - calculus 592.0
    - ectopic pregnancy (*see also* categories 633.0-633.9) 639.8

Infection, infected, infective — *continued*
kidney — *continued*
with — *continued*
molar pregnancy (*see also* categories 630-632) 639.8
complicating pregnancy or puerperium 646.6 ☑
affecting fetus or newborn 760.1
following
abortion 639.8
ectopic or molar pregnancy 639.8
pelvis and ureter 590.3
Klebsiella pneumoniae NEC 041.3
knee (skin) NEC 686.9
joint — *see* Arthritis, infectious
Koch's (*see also* Tuberculosis, pulmonary) 011.9 ☑
labia (majora) (minora) (*see also* Vulvitis) 616.10
lacrimal
gland (*see also* Dacryoadenitis) 375.00
passages (duct) (sac) (*see also* Dacryocystitis) 375.30
larynx NEC 478.79
leg (skin) NEC 686.9
Leishmania (*see also* Leishmaniasis) 085.9
braziliensis 085.5
donovani 085.0
Ethiopica 085.3
furunculosa 085.1
infantum 085.0
mexicana 085.4
tropica (minor) 085.1
major 085.2
Leptosphaeria senegalensis 117.4
leptospira (*see also* Leptospirosis) 100.9
Australis 100.89
Bataviae 100.89
pyrogenes 100.89
specified type NEC 100.89
leptospirochetal NEC (*see also* Leptospirosis) 100.9
Leptothrix — *see* Actinomycosis
Listeria monocytogenes (listeriosis) 027.0
congenital 771.2
liver fluke — *see* Infestation, fluke, liver
Loa loa 125.2
eyelid 125.2 *[373.6]*
Loboa loboi 116.2
local, skin (staphylococcal) (streptococcal) NEC 686.9
abscess — *see* Abscess, by site
cellulitis — *see* Cellulitis, by site
ulcer (*see also* Ulcer, skin) 707.9
Loefflerella
mallei 024
whitmori 025
lung 518.89
atypical Mycobacterium 031.0
tuberculous (*see also* Tuberculosis, pulmonary) 011.9 ☑
basilar 518.89
chronic 518.89
fungus NEC 117.9
spirochetal 104.8
virus — *see* Pneumonia, virus
lymph gland (axillary) (cervical) (inguinal) 683
mesenteric 289.2
lymphoid tissue, base of tongue or posterior pharynx, NEC 474.00
madurella
grisea 117.4
mycetomii 117.4
major
with
abortion — *see* Abortion, by type, with sepsis
ectopic pregnancy (*see also* categories 633.0-633.9) 639.0
molar pregnancy (*see also* categories 630-632) 639.0
following
abortion 639.0
ectopic or molar pregnancy 639.0
puerperal, postpartum, childbirth 670.0 ☑
Malassezia furfur 111.0

Infection, infected, infective — *continued*
Malleomyces
mallei 024
pseudomallei 025
mammary gland 611.0
puerperal, postpartum 675.2 ☑
Mansonella (ozzardi) 125.5
mastoid (suppurative) — *see* Mastoiditis
maxilla, maxillary 526.4
sinus (chronic) (*see also* Sinusitis, maxillary) 473.0
mediastinum 519.2
medina 125.7
meibomian
cyst 373.12
gland 373.12
melioidosis 025
meninges (*see also* Meningitis) 320.9
meningococcal (*see also* condition) 036.9
brain 036.1
cerebrospinal 036.0
endocardium 036.42
generalized 036.2
meninges 036.0
meningococcemia 036.2
specified site NEC 036.89
mesenteric lymph nodes or glands NEC 289.2
Metagonimus 121.5
metatarsophalangeal 711.97
microorganism resistant to drugs — *see* Resistance (to), drugs by microorganisms
Microsporidia 136.8
microsporum, microsporic — *see* Dermatophytosis
Mima polymorpha NEC 041.85
mixed flora NEC 041.89
Monilia (*see also* Candidiasis) 112.9
neonatal 771.7
monkeypox 057.8
Monosporium apiospermum 117.6
mouth (focus) NEC 528.9
parasitic 136.9
Mucor 117.7
muscle NEC 728.89
mycelium NEC 117.9
mycetoma
actinomycotic NEC (*see also* Actinomycosis) 039.9
mycotic NEC 117.4
Mycobacterium, mycobacterial (*see also* Mycobacterium) 031.9
Mycoplasma NEC 041.81
mycotic NEC 117.9
pathogenic to compromised host only 118
skin NEC 111.9
systemic 117.9
myocardium NEC 422.90
nail (chronic) (with lymphangitis) 681.9
finger 681.02
fungus 110.1
ingrowing 703.0
toe 681.11
fungus 110.1
nasal sinus (chronic) (*see also* Sinusitis) 473.9
nasopharynx (chronic) 478.29
acute 460
navel 686.9
newborn 771.4
Neisserian — *see* Gonococcus
Neotestudina rosatii 117.4
newborn, generalized 771.89
nipple 611.0
puerperal, postpartum 675.0 ☑
with breast 675.9 ☑
specified type NEC 675.8 ☑
Nocardia — *see* Actinomycosis
nose 478.1
nostril 478.1
obstetrical surgical wound 674.3 ☑
Oesophagostomum (apiostomum) 127.7
Oestrus ovis 134.0
Oidium albicans (*see also* Candidiasis) 112.9
Onchocerca (volvulus) 125.3
eye 125.3 *[360.13]*
eyelid 125.3 *[373.6]*
operation wound 998.59

Infection, infected, infective — *continued*
Opisthorchis (felineus) (tenuicollis) (viverrini) 121.0
orbit 376.00
chronic 376.10
ovary (*see also* Salpingo-oophoritis) 614.2
Oxyuris vermicularis 127.4
pancreas 577.0
Paracoccidioides brasiliensis 116.1
Paragonimus (westermani) 121.2
parainfluenza virus 079.89
parameningococcus NEC 036.9
with meningitis 036.0
parasitic NEC 136.9
paratyphoid 002.9
type A 002.1
type B 002.2
type C 002.3
paraurethral ducts 597.89
parotid gland 527.2
Pasteurella NEC 027.2
multocida (cat-bite) (dog-bite) 027.2
pestis (*see also* Plague) 020.9
pseudotuberculosis 027.2
septica (cat-bite) (dog-bite) 027.2
tularensis (*see also* Tularemia) 021.9
pelvic, female (*see also* Disease, pelvis, inflammatory) 614.9
penis (glans) (retention) NEC 607.2
herpetic 054.13
Peptococcus 041.84
Peptostreptococcus 041.84
periapical (pulpal origin) 522.4
peridental 523.3
perineal wound (obstetrical) 674.3 ☑
periodontal 523.3
periorbital 376.00
chronic 376.10
perirectal 569.49
perirenal (*see also* Infection, kidney) 590.9
peritoneal (*see also* Peritonitis) 567.9
periureteral 593.89
periurethral 597.89
Petriellidium boydii 117.6
pharynx 478.29
Coxsackie virus 074.0
phlegmonous 462
posterior, lymphoid 474.00
Phialophora
gougerotii 117.8
jeanselmei 117.8
verrucosa 117.2
Piedraia hortai 111.3
pinna, acute 380.11
pinta 103.9
intermediate 103.1
late 103.2
mixed 103.3
primary 103.0
pinworm 127.4
pityrosporum furfur 111.0
pleuropneumonia-like organisms NEC (PPLO) 041.81
pneumococcal NEC 041.2
generalized (purulent) 038.2
Pneumococcus NEC 041.2
postoperative wound 998.59
posttraumatic NEC 958.3
postvaccinal 999.3
prepuce NEC 607.1
Proprionibacterium 041.84
prostate (capsule) (*see also* Prostatitis) 601.9
Proteus (mirabilis) (morganii) (vulgaris) NEC 041.6
enteritis 008.3
protozoal NEC 136.8
intestinal NEC 007.9
Pseudomonas NEC 041.7
mallei 024
pneumonia 482.1
pseudomallei 025
psittacosis 073.9
puerperal, postpartum (major) 670.0 ☑
minor 646.6 ☑
pulmonary — *see* Infection, lung
purulent — *see* Abscess
putrid, generalized — *see* Septicemia

☑ Additional Digit Required — Refer to the Tabular List (Numeric Code Section) for Additional Digit Selection
▶◀ Revised Text ● New Line ▲ Revised Code

☑ Additional Digit Required — Refer to the Tabular List (Numeric Code Section) for Additional Digit Selection
▶◀ Revised Text ● New Line ▲ Revised Code

☑ Additional Digit Required — Refer to the Tabular List (Numeric Code Section) for Additional Digit Selection
▶◀ Revised Text ● New Line ▲ Revised Code

☑ Additional Digit Required — Refer to the Tabular List (Numeric Code Section) for Additional Digit Selection

▶◀ Revised Text ● New Line ▲ Revised Code

- **Injury** — *continued*
  - blood vessel NEC — *continued*
    - extremity — *continued*
      - upper 903.9
        - multiple 903.8
        - specified NEC 903.8
    - femoral
      - artery (superficial) 904.1
        - above profunda origin 904.0
        - common 904.0
      - vein 904.2
    - gastric
      - artery 902.21
      - vein 902.39
    - head 900.9
      - intracranial — *see* Injury, intracranial
      - multiple 900.82
      - specified NEC 900.89
    - hemiazygos vein 901.89
    - hepatic
      - artery 902.22
      - vein 902.11
    - hypogastric 902.59
      - artery 902.51
      - vein 902.52
    - ileocolic
      - artery 902.26
      - vein 902.31
    - iliac 902.50
      - artery 902.53
      - specified branch NEC 902.59
      - vein 902.54
    - innominate
      - artery 901.1
      - vein 901.3
    - intercostal (artery) (vein) 901.81
    - jugular vein (external) 900.81
      - internal 900.1
    - leg NEC 904.8
    - mammary (artery) (vein) 901.82
    - mesenteric
      - artery 902.20
        - inferior 902.27
        - specified branch NEC 902.29
        - superior (trunk) 902.25
          - branches, primary 902.26
      - vein 902.39
        - inferior 902.32
        - superior (and primary subdivisions) 902.31
    - neck 900.9
      - multiple 900.82
      - specified NEC 900.89
    - ovarian 902.89
      - artery 902.81
      - vein 902.82
    - palmar artery 903.4
    - pelvis 902.9
      - multiple 902.87
      - specified NEC 902.89
    - plantar (deep) (artery) (vein) 904.6
    - popliteal 904.40
      - artery 904.41
      - vein 904.42
    - portal 902.33
    - pulmonary 901.40
      - artery 901.41
      - vein 901.42
    - radial (artery) (vein) 903.2
    - renal 902.40
      - artery 902.41
      - specified NEC 902.49
      - vein 902.42
    - saphenous
      - artery 904.7
      - vein (greater) (lesser) 904.3
    - splenic
      - artery 902.23
      - vein 902.34
    - subclavian
      - artery 901.1
      - vein 901.3
    - suprarenal 902.49
    - thoracic 901.9
      - multiple 901.83
      - specified NEC 901.89

- **Injury** — *continued*
  - blood vessel NEC — *continued*
    - tibial 904.50
      - artery 904.50
        - anterior 904.51
        - posterior 904.53
      - vein 904.50
        - anterior 904.52
        - posterior 904.54
    - ulnar (artery) (vein) 903.3
    - uterine 902.59
      - artery 902.55
      - vein 902.56
    - vena cava
      - inferior 902.10
        - specified branches NEC 902.19
      - superior 901.2
  - brachial plexus 953.4
    - newborn 767.6
  - brain NEC (*see also* Injury, intracranial) 854.0 ☑
  - breast 959.19
  - broad ligament — *see* Injury, internal, broad ligament
  - bronchus, bronchi — *see* Injury, internal, bronchus
  - brow 959.09
  - buttock 959.19
  - canthus, eye 921.1
  - cathode ray 990
  - cauda equina 952.4
    - with fracture, vertebra — *see* Fracture, vertebra, sacrum
  - cavernous sinus (*see also* Injury, intracranial) 854.0 ☑
  - cecum — *see* Injury, internal, cecum
  - celiac ganglion or plexus 954.1
  - cerebellum (*see also* Injury, intracranial) 854.0 ☑
  - cervix (uteri) — *see* Injury, internal, cervix
  - cheek 959.09
  - chest — *see also* Injury, internal, chest
    - wall 959.11
  - childbirth — *see also* Birth, injury
    - maternal NEC 665.9 ☑
  - chin 959.09
  - choroid (eye) 921.3
  - clitoris 959.14
  - coccyx 959.19
    - complicating delivery 665.6 ☑
  - colon — *see* Injury, internal, colon
  - common duct — *see* Injury, internal, common duct
  - conjunctiva 921.1
    - superficial 918.2
  - cord
    - spermatic — *see* Injury, internal, spermatic cord
    - spinal — *see* Injury, spinal, by site
  - cornea 921.3
    - abrasion 918.1
    - due to contact lens 371.82
    - penetrating — *see* Injury, eyeball, penetrating
    - superficial 918.1
      - due to contact lens 371.82
  - cortex (cerebral) (*see also* Injury, intracranial) 854.0 ☑
    - visual 950.3
  - costal region 959.11
  - costochondral 959.11
  - cranial
    - bones — *see* Fracture, skull, by site
    - cavity (*see also* Injury, intracranial) 854.0 ☑
    - nerve — *see* Injury, nerve, cranial
  - crushing — *see* Crush
  - cutaneous sensory nerve
    - lower limb 956.4
    - upper limb 955.5
  - delivery — *see also* Birth, injury
    - maternal NEC 665.9 ☑
  - Descemet's membrane — *see* Injury, eyeball, penetrating
  - diaphragm — *see* Injury, internal, diaphragm
  - diffuse axonal — *see* Injury, intracranial ●
  - duodenum — *see* Injury, internal, duodenum
  - ear (auricle) (canal) (drum) (external) 959.09

- **Injury** — *continued*
  - elbow (and forearm) (and wrist) 959.3
  - epididymis 959.14
  - epigastric region 959.12
  - epiglottis 959.09
  - epiphyseal, current — *see* Fracture, by site
  - esophagus — *see* Injury, internal, esophagus
  - Eustachian tube 959.09
  - extremity (lower) (upper) NEC 959.8
  - eye 921.9
    - penetrating eyeball — *see* Injury, eyeball, penetrating
    - superficial 918.9
  - eyeball 921.3
    - penetrating 871.7
      - with
        - partial loss (of intraocular tissue) 871.2
        - prolapse or exposure (of intraocular tissue) 871.1
      - without prolapse 871.0
      - foreign body (nonmagnetic) 871.6
        - magnetic 871.5
    - superficial 918.9
  - eyebrow 959.09
  - eyelid(s) 921.1
    - laceration — *see* Laceration, eyelid
    - superficial 918.0
  - face (and neck) 959.09
  - fallopian tube — *see* Injury, internal, fallopian tube
  - finger(s) (nail) 959.5
  - flank 959.19
  - foot (and ankle) (and knee) (and leg, except thigh) 959.7
  - forceps NEC 767.9
    - scalp 767.19
  - forearm (and elbow) (and wrist) 959.3
  - forehead 959.09
  - gallbladder — *see* Injury, internal, gallbladder
  - gasserian ganglion 951.2
  - gastrointestinal tract — *see* Injury, internal, gastrointestinal tract
  - genital organ(s)
    - with
      - abortion — *see* Abortion, by type, with, damage to pelvic organs
      - ectopic pregnancy (*see also* categories 633.0-633.9) 639.2
      - molar pregnancy (*see also* categories 630-632) 639.2
    - external 959.14
      - fracture of corpus cavernosum penis 959.13
    - following
      - abortion 639.2
      - ectopic or molar pregnancy 639.2
    - internal — *see* Injury, internal, genital organs
    - obstetrical trauma NEC 665.9 ☑
      - affecting fetus or newborn 763.89
  - gland
    - lacrimal 921.1
      - laceration 870.8
    - parathyroid 959.09
    - salivary 959.09
    - thyroid 959.09
  - globe (eye) (*see also* Injury, eyeball) 921.3
  - grease gun — *see* Wound, open, by site, complicated
  - groin 959.19
  - gum 959.09
  - hand(s) (except fingers) 959.4
  - head NEC 959.01
    - with
      - loss of consciousness 850.5
      - skull fracture — *see* Fracture, skull, by site
  - heart — *see* Injury, internal, heart
  - heel 959.7
  - hip (and thigh) 959.6
  - hymen 959.14
  - hyperextension (cervical) (vertebra) 847.0
  - ileum — *see* Injury, internal, ileum
  - iliac region 959.19
  - infrared rays NEC 990

- **Injury** — *continued*
  - instrumental (during surgery) 998.2
    - birth injury — *see* Birth, injury
    - nonsurgical (*see also* Injury, by site) 959.9
    - obstetrical 665.9 ☑
      - affecting fetus or newborn 763.89
      - bladder 665.5 ☑
      - cervix 665.3 ☑
      - high vaginal 665.4 ☑
      - perineal NEC 664.9 ☑
      - urethra 665.5 ☑
      - uterus 665.5 ☑
  - internal 869.0

> *Note — For injury of internal organ(s) by foreign body entering through a natural orifice (e.g., inhaled, ingested, or swallowed) — see Foreign body, entering through orifice.*
>
> *For internal injury of any of the following sites with internal injury of any other of the sites — see Injury, internal, multiple.*

-
  -
    - with
      - fracture
        - pelvis — *see* Fracture, pelvis
        - specified site, except pelvis — *see* Injury, internal, by site
      - open wound into cavity 869.1
    - abdomen, abdominal (viscera) NEC 868.00
      - with
        - fracture, pelvis — *see* Fracture, pelvis
          - open wound into cavity 868.10
        - specified site NEC 868.09
          - with open wound into cavity 868.19
    - adrenal (gland) 868.01
      - with open wound into cavity 868.11
    - aorta (thoracic) 901.0
      - abdominal 902.0
    - appendix 863.85
      - with open wound into cavity 863.95
    - bile duct 868.02
      - with open wound into cavity 868.12
    - bladder (sphincter) 867.0
      - with
        - abortion — *see* Abortion, by type, with damage to pelvic organs
        - ectopic pregnancy (*see also* categories 633.0-633.9) 639.2
        - molar pregnancy (*see also* categories 630-632) 639.2
        - open wound into cavity 867.1
      - following
        - abortion 639.2
        - ectopic or molar pregnancy 639.2
      - obstetrical trauma 665.5 ☑
        - affecting fetus or newborn 763.89
    - blood vessel — *see* Injury, blood vessel, by site
    - broad ligament 867.6
      - with open wound into cavity 867.7
    - bronchus, bronchi 862.21
      - with open wound into cavity 862.31
    - cecum 863.89
      - with open wound into cavity 863.99
    - cervix (uteri) 867.4
      - with
        - abortion — *see* Abortion, by type, with damage to pelvic organs
        - ectopic pregnancy (*see also* categories 633.0-633.9) 639.2
        - molar pregnancy (*see also* categories 630-632) 639.2
        - open wound into cavity 867.5
      - following
        - abortion 639.2
        - ectopic or molar pregnancy 639.2
      - obstetrical trauma 665.3 ☑
        - affecting fetus or newborn 763.89
    - chest (*see also* Injury, internal, intrathoracic organs) 862.8
      - with open wound into cavity 862.9
    - colon 863.40
      - with
        - open wound into cavity 863.50
        - rectum 863.46
          - with open wound into cavity 863.56
      - ascending (right) 863.41
        - with open wound into cavity 863.51

- **Injury** — *continued*
  - internal — *continued*
    - colon — *continued*
      - descending (left) 863.43
        - with open wound into cavity 863.53
      - multiple sites 863.46
        - with open wound into cavity 863.56
      - sigmoid 863.44
        - with open wound into cavity 863.54
      - specified site NEC 863.49
        - with open wound into cavity 863.59
        - transverse 863.42
          - with open wound into cavity 863.52
    - common duct 868.02
      - with open wound into cavity 868.12
    - complicating delivery 665.9 ☑
      - affecting fetus or newborn 763.89
    - diaphragm 862.0
      - with open wound into cavity 862.1
    - duodenum 863.21
      - with open wound into cavity 863.31
    - esophagus (intrathoracic) 862.22
      - with open wound into cavity 862.32
      - cervical region 874.4
        - complicated 874.5
    - fallopian tube 867.6
      - with open wound into cavity 867.7
    - gallbladder 868.02
      - with open wound into cavity 868.12
    - gastrointestinal tract NEC 863.80
      - with open wound into cavity 863.90
    - genital organ NEC 867.6
      - with open wound into cavity 867.7
    - heart 861.00
      - with open wound into thorax 861.10
    - ileum 863.29
      - with open wound into cavity 863.39
    - intestine NEC 863.89
      - with open wound into cavity 863.99
      - large NEC 863.40
        - with open wound into cavity 863.50
      - small NEC 863.20
        - with open wound into cavity 863.30
    - intra-abdominal (organ) 868.00
      - with open wound into cavity 868.10
      - multiple sites 868.09
        - with open wound into cavity 868.19
      - specified site NEC 868.09
        - with open wound into cavity 868.19
    - intrathoracic organs (multiple) 862.8
      - with open wound into cavity 862.9
      - diaphragm (only) — *see* Injury, internal, diaphragm
      - heart (only) — *see* Injury, internal, heart
      - lung (only) — *see* Injury, internal, lung
      - specified site NEC 862.29
        - with open wound into cavity 862.39
    - intrauterine (*see also* Injury, internal, uterus) 867.4
      - with open wound into cavity 867.5
    - jejunum 863.29
      - with open wound into cavity 863.39
    - kidney (subcapsular) 866.00
      - with
        - disruption of parenchyma (complete) 866.03
          - with open wound into cavity 866.13
        - hematoma (without rupture of capsule) 866.01
          - with open wound into cavity 866.11
        - laceration 866.02
          - with open wound into cavity 866.12
        - open wound into cavity 866.10
    - liver 864.00
      - with
        - contusion 864.01
          - with open wound into cavity 864.11
        - hematoma 864.01
          - with open wound into cavity 864.11
        - laceration 864.05
          - with open wound into cavity 864.15
          - major (disruption of hepatic parenchyma) 864.04
            - with open wound into cavity 864.14

- **Injury** — *continued*
  - internal — *continued*
    - liver — *continued*
      - with — *continued*
        - laceration — *continued*
          - minor (capsule only) 864.02
            - with open wound into cavity 864.12
          - moderate (involving parenchyma) 864.03
            - with open wound into cavity 864.13
            - multiple 864.04
          - stellate 864.04
            - with open wound into cavity 864.14
        - open wound into cavity 864.10
    - lung 861.20
      - with open wound into thorax 861.30
      - hemopneumothorax — *see* Hemopneumothorax, traumatic
      - hemothorax — *see* Hemothorax, traumatic
      - pneumohemothorax — *see* Pneumohemothorax, traumatic
      - pneumothorax — *see* Pneumothorax, traumatic
    - mediastinum 862.29
      - with open wound into cavity 862.39
    - mesentery 863.89
      - with open wound into cavity 863.99
    - mesosalpinx 867.6
      - with open wound into cavity 867.7
    - multiple 869.0

> *Note — Multiple internal injuries of sites classifiable to the same three- or four-digit category should be classified to that category.*
>
> *Multiple injuries classifiable to different fourth-digit subdivisions of 861 (heart and lung injuries) should be dealt with according to coding rules.*

-
  -
    -
      - internal
        - with open wound into cavity 869.1
      - intra-abdominal organ (sites classifiable to 863-868)
        - with
          - intrathoracic organ(s) (sites classifiable to 861-862) 869.0
            - with open wound into cavity 869.1
          - other intra-abdominal organ(s) (sites classifiable to 863-868, except where classifiable to the same three-digit category) 868.09
            - with open wound into cavity 868.19
      - intrathoracic organ (sites classifiable to 861-862)
        - with
          - intra-abdominal organ(s) (sites classifiable to 863-868) 869.0
            - with open wound into cavity 869.1
          - other intrathoracic organ(s) (sites classifiable to 861-862, except where classifiable to the same three-digit category) 862.8
            - with open wound into cavity 862.9
    - myocardium — *see* Injury, internal, heart
    - ovary 867.6
      - with open wound into cavity 867.7
    - pancreas (multiple sites) 863.84
      - with open wound into cavity 863.94
      - body 863.82
        - with open wound into cavity 863.92
      - head 863.81
        - with open wound into cavity 863.91
      - tail 863.83
        - with open wound into cavity 863.93
    - pelvis, pelvic (organs) (viscera) 867.8
      - with
        - fracture, pelvis — *see* Fracture, pelvis
        - open wound into cavity 867.9

Injury — *continued*
internal — *continued*
pelvis, pelvic — *continued*
specified site NEC 867.6
with open wound into cavity 867.7
peritoneum 868.03
with open wound into cavity 868.13
pleura 862.29
with open wound into cavity 862.39
prostate 867.6
with open wound into cavity 867.7
rectum 863.45
with
colon 863.46
with open wound into cavity 863.56
open wound into cavity 863.55
retroperitoneum 868.04
with open wound into cavity 868.14
round ligament 867.6
with open wound into cavity 867.7
seminal vesicle 867.6
with open wound into cavity 867.7
spermatic cord 867.6
with open wound into cavity 867.7
scrotal — *see* Wound, open, spermatic cord
spleen 865.00
with
disruption of parenchyma (massive) 865.04
with open wound into cavity 865.14
hematoma (without rupture of capsule) 865.01
with open wound into cavity 865.11
open wound into cavity 865.10
tear, capsular 865.02
with open wound into cavity 865.12
extending into parenchyma 865.03
with open wound into cavity 865.13
stomach 863.0
with open wound into cavity 863.1
suprarenal gland (multiple) 868.01
with open wound into cavity 868.11
thorax, thoracic (cavity) (organs) (multiple) (*see also* Injury, internal, intrathoracic organs) 862.8
with open wound into cavity 862.9
thymus (gland) 862.29
with open wound into cavity 862.39
trachea (intrathoracic) 862.29
with open wound into cavity 862.39
cervical region (*see also* Wound, open, trachea) 874.02
ureter 867.2
with open wound into cavity 867.3
urethra (sphincter) 867.0
with
abortion — *see* Abortion, by type, with damage to pelvic organs
ectopic pregnancy (*see also* categories 633.0-633.9) 639.2
molar pregnancy (*see also* categories 630-632) 639.2
open wound into cavity 867.1
following
abortion 639.2
ectopic or molar pregnancy 639.2
obstetrical trauma 665.5 ☑
affecting fetus or newborn 763.89
uterus 867.4
with
abortion — *see* Abortion, by type, with damage to pelvic organs
ectopic pregnancy (*see also* categories 633.0-633.9) 639.2
molar pregnancy (*see also* categories 630-632) 639.2
open wound into cavity 867.5
following
abortion 639.2
ectopic or molar pregnancy 639.2
obstetrical trauma NEC 665.5 ☑
affecting fetus or newborn 763.89
vas deferens 867.6
with open wound into cavity 867.7
vesical (sphincter) 867.0
with open wound into cavity 867.1

Injury — *continued*
internal — *continued*
viscera (abdominal) (*see also* Injury, internal, multiple) 868.00
with
fracture, pelvis — *see* Fracture, pelvis
open wound into cavity 868.10
thoracic NEC (*see also* Injury, internal, intrathoracic organs) 862.8
with open wound into cavity 862.9
interscapular region 959.19
intervertebral disc 959.19
intestine — *see* Injury, internal, intestine
intra-abdominal (organs) NEC — *see* Injury, internal, intra-abdominal
intracranial 854.0 ☑

Note — Use the following fifth-digit subclassification with categories 851-854:

0	*unspecified state of consciousness*
1	*with no loss of consciousness*
2	*with brief [less than one hour] loss of consciousness*
3	*with moderate [1-24 hours] loss of consciousness*
4	*with prolonged [more than 24 hours] loss of consciousness and return to pre-existing conscious level*
5	*with prolonged [more than 24 hours] loss of consciousness, without return to pre-existing conscious level*

Use fifth-digit 5 to designate when a patient is unconscious and dies before regaining consciousness, regardless of the duration of the loss of consciousness

6	*with loss of consciousness of unspecified duration*
9	*with concussion, unspecified*

with
open intracranial wound 854.1 ☑
skull fracture — *see* Fracture, skull, by site
contusion 851.8 ☑
with open intracranial wound 851.9 ☑
brain stem 851.4 ☑
with open intracranial wound 851.5 ☑
cerebellum 851.4 ☑
with open intracranial wound 851.5 ☑
cortex (cerebral) 851.0 ☑
with open intracranial wound 851.2 ☑
hematoma — *see* Injury, intracranial, hemorrhage
hemorrhage 853.0 ☑
with
laceration — *see* Injury, intracranial, laceration
open intracranial wound 853.1 ☑
extradural 852.4 ☑
with open intracranial wound 852.5 ☑
subarachnoid 852.0 ☑
with open intracranial wound 852.1 ☑
subdural 852.2 ☑
with open intracranial wound 852.3 ☑
laceration 851.8 ☑
with open intracranial wound 851.9 ☑
brain stem 851.6 ☑
with open intracranial wound 851.7 ☑
cerebellum 851.6 ☑
with open intracranial wound 851.7 ☑
cortex (cerebral) 851.2 ☑
with open intracranial wound 851.3 ☑
intraocular — *see* Injury, eyeball, penetrating
intrathoracic organs (multiple) — *see* Injury, internal, intrathoracic organs
intrauterine — *see* Injury, internal, intrauterine
iris 921.3
penetrating — *see* Injury, eyeball, penetrating
jaw 959.09
jejunum — *see* Injury, internal, jejunum
joint NEC 959.9
old or residual 718.80
ankle 718.87

Injury — *continued*
joint NEC — *continued*
old or residual — *continued*
elbow 718.82
foot 718.87
hand 718.84
hip 718.85
knee 718.86
multiple sites 718.89
pelvic region 718.85
shoulder (region) 718.81
specified site NEC 718.88
wrist 718.83
kidney — *see* Injury, internal, kidney
knee (and ankle) (and foot) (and leg, except thigh) 959.7
labium (majus) (minus) 959.14
labyrinth, ear 959.09
lacrimal apparatus, gland, or sac 921.1
laceration 870.8
larynx 959.09
late effect — *see* Late, effects (of), injury
leg, except thigh (and ankle) (and foot) (and knee) 959.7
upper or thigh 959.6
lens, eye 921.3
penetrating — *see* Injury, eyeball, penetrating
lid, eye — *see* Injury, eyelid
lip 959.09
liver — *see* Injury, internal, liver
lobe, parietal — *see* Injury, intracranial
lumbar (region) 959.19
plexus 953.5
lumbosacral (region) 959.19
plexus 953.5
lung — *see* Injury, internal, lung
malar region 959.09
mastoid region 959.09
maternal, during pregnancy, affecting fetus or newborn 760.5
maxilla 959.09
mediastinum — *see* Injury, internal, mediastinum
membrane
brain (*see also* Injury, intracranial) 854.0 ☑
tympanic 959.09
meningeal artery — *see* Hemorrhage, brain, traumatic, subarachnoid
meninges (cerebral) — *see* Injury, intracranial
mesenteric
artery — *see* Injury, blood vessel, mesenteric, artery
plexus, inferior 954.1
vein — *see* Injury, blood vessel, mesenteric, vein
mesentery — *see* Injury, internal, mesentery
mesosalpinx — *see* Injury, internal, mesosalpinx
middle ear 959.09
midthoracic region 959.11
mouth 959.09
multiple (sites not classifiable to the same four-digit category in 959.0-959.7) 959.8
internal 869.0
with open wound into cavity 869.1
musculocutaneous nerve 955.4
nail
finger 959.5
toe 959.7
nasal (septum) (sinus) 959.09
nasopharynx 959.09
neck (and face) 959.09
nerve 957.9
abducens 951.3
abducent 951.3
accessory 951.6
acoustic 951.5
ankle and foot 956.9
anterior crural, femoral 956.1
arm (*see also* Injury, nerve, upper limb) 955.9
auditory 951.5
axillary 955.0
brachial plexus 953.4
cervical sympathetic 954.0

Injury — *continued*
  spinal — *continued*
    nerve (root) NEC — *see* Injury, nerve, spinal, root
    plexus 953.9
      brachial 953.4
      lumbosacral 953.5
      multiple sites 953.8
    sacral 952.3
    thoracic (*see also* Injury, spinal, dorsal) 952.10
  spleen — *see* Injury, internal, spleen
  stellate ganglion 954.1
  sternal region 959.11
  stomach — *see* Injury, internal, stomach
  subconjunctival 921.1
  subcutaneous 959.9
  subdural — *see* Injury, intracranial
  submaxillary region 959.09
  submental region 959.09
  subungual
    fingers 959.5
    toes 959.7
  superficial 919 ☑

Note — Use the following fourth-digit subdivisions with categories 910-919:

0	*Abrasion or friction burn without mention of infection*
1	*Abrasion or friction burn, infected*
2	*Blister without mention of infection*
3	*Blister, infected*
4	*Insect bite, nonvenomous, without mention of infection*
5	*Insect bite, nonvenomous, infected*
6	*Superficial foreign body (splinter) without major open wound and without mention of infection*
7	*Superficial foreign body (splinter) without major open wound, infected*
8	*Other and unspecified superficial injury without mention of infection*
9	*Other and unspecified superficial injury, infected*

For late effects of superficial injury, see category 906.2.

    abdomen, abdominal (muscle) (wall) (and other part(s) of trunk) 911 ☑
    ankle (and hip, knee, leg, or thigh) 916 ☑
    anus (and other part(s) of trunk) 911 ☑
    arm 913 ☑
      upper (and shoulder) 912 ☑
    auditory canal (external) (meatus) (and other part(s) of face, neck, or scalp, except eye) 910 ☑
    axilla (and upper arm) 912 ☑
    back (and other part(s) of trunk) 911 ☑
    breast (and other part(s) of trunk) 911 ☑
    brow (and other part(s) of face, neck, or scalp, except eye) 910 ☑
    buttock (and other part(s) of trunk) 911 ☑
    canthus, eye 918.0
    cheek(s) (and other part(s) of face, neck, or scalp, except eye) 910 ☑
    chest wall (and other part(s) of trunk) 911 ☑
    chin (and other part(s) of face, neck, or scalp, except eye) 910 ☑
    clitoris (and other part(s) of trunk) 911 ☑
    conjunctiva 918.2
    cornea 918.1
      due to contact lens 371.82
    costal region (and other part(s) of trunk) 911 ☑
    ear(s) (auricle) (canal) (drum) (external) (and other part(s) of face, neck, or scalp, except eye) 910 ☑
    elbow (and forearm) (and wrist) 913 ☑
    epididymis (and other part(s) of trunk) 911 ☑
    epigastric region (and other part(s) of trunk) 911 ☑
    epiglottis (and other part(s) of face, neck, or scalp, except eye) 910 ☑
    eye(s) (and adnexa) NEC 918.9

Injury — *continued*
  superficial — *continued*
    eyelid(s) (and periocular area) 918.0
    face (any part(s), except eye) (and neck or scalp) 910 ☑
    finger(s) (nail) (any) 915 ☑
    flank (and other part(s) of trunk) 911 ☑
    foot (phalanges) (and toe(s)) 917 ☑
    forearm (and elbow) (and wrist) 913 ☑
    forehead (and other part(s) of face, neck, or scalp, except eye) 910 ☑
    globe (eye) 918.9
    groin (and other part(s) of trunk) 911 ☑
    gum(s) (and other part(s) of face, neck, or scalp, except eye) 910 ☑
    hand(s) (except fingers alone) 914 ☑
    head (and other part(s) of face, neck, or scalp, except eye) 910 ☑
    heel (and foot or toe) 917 ☑
    hip (and ankle, knee, leg, or thigh) 916 ☑
    iliac region (and other part(s) of trunk) 911 ☑
    interscapular region (and other part(s) of trunk) 911 ☑
    iris 918.9
    knee (and ankle, hip, leg, or thigh) 916 ☑
    labium (majus) (minus) (and other part(s) of trunk) 911 ☑
    lacrimal (apparatus) (gland) (sac) 918.0
    leg (lower) (upper) (and ankle, hip, knee, or thigh) 916 ☑
    lip(s) (and other part(s) of face, neck, or scalp, except eye) 910 ☑
    lower extremity (except foot) 916 ☑
    lumbar region (and other part(s) of trunk) 911 ☑
    malar region (and other part(s) of face, neck, or scalp, except eye) 910 ☑
    mastoid region (and other part(s) of face, neck, or scalp, except eye) 910 ☑
    midthoracic region (and other part(s) of trunk) 911 ☑
    mouth (and other part(s) of face, neck, or scalp, except eye) 910 ☑
    multiple sites (not classifiable to the same three-digit category) 919 ☑
    nasal (septum) (and other part(s) of face, neck, or scalp, except eye) 910 ☑
    neck (and face or scalp, any part(s), except eye) 910 ☑
    nose (septum) (and other part(s) of face, neck, or scalp, except eye) 910 ☑
    occipital region (and other part(s) of face, neck, or scalp, except eye) 910 ☑
    orbital region 918.0
    palate (soft) (and other part(s) of face, neck, or scalp, except eye) 910 ☑
    parietal region (and other part(s) of face, neck, or scalp, except eye) 910 ☑
    penis (and other part(s) of trunk) 911 ☑
    perineum (and other part(s) of trunk) 911 ☑
    periocular area 918.0
    pharynx (and other part(s) of face, neck, or scalp, except eye) 910 ☑
    popliteal space (and ankle, hip, leg, or thigh) 916 ☑
    prepuce (and other part(s) of trunk) 911 ☑
    pubic region (and other part(s) of trunk) 911 ☑
    pudenda (and other part(s) of trunk) 911 ☑
    sacral region (and other part(s) of trunk) 911 ☑
    salivary (ducts) (glands) (and other part(s) of face, neck, or scalp, except eye) 910 ☑
    scalp (and other part(s) of face or neck, except eye) 910 ☑
    scapular region (and upper arm) 912 ☑
    sclera 918.2
    scrotum (and other part(s) of trunk) 911 ☑
    shoulder (and upper arm) 912 ☑
    skin NEC 919 ☑
    specified site(s) NEC 919 ☑
    sternal region (and other part(s) of trunk) 911 ☑
    subconjunctival 918.2
    subcutaneous NEC 919 ☑

Injury — *continued*
  superficial — *continued*
    submaxillary region (and other part(s) of face, neck, or scalp, except eye) 910 ☑
    submental region (and other part(s) of face, neck, or scalp, except eye) 910 ☑
    supraclavicular fossa (and other part(s) of face, neck or scalp, except eye) 910 ☑
    supraorbital 918.0
    temple (and other part(s) of face, neck, or scalp, except eye) 910 ☑
    temporal region (and other part(s) of face, neck, or scalp, except eye) 910 ☑
    testis (and other part(s) of trunk) 911 ☑
    thigh (and ankle, hip, knee, or leg) 916 ☑
    thorax, thoracic (external) (and other part(s) of trunk) 911 ☑
    throat (and other part(s) of face, neck, or scalp, except eye) 910 ☑
    thumb(s) (nail) 915 ☑
    toe(s) (nail) (subungual) (and foot) 917 ☑
    tongue (and other part(s) of face, neck, or scalp, except eye) 910 ☑
    tooth, teeth (*see also* Abrasion, dental) 521.20
    trunk (any part(s)) 911 ☑
    tunica vaginalis 959.14
    tympanum, tympanic membrane (and other part(s) of face, neck, or scalp, except eye) 910 ☑
    upper extremity NEC 913 ☑
    uvula (and other part(s) of face, neck, or scalp, except eye) 910 ☑
    vagina (and other part(s) of trunk) 911 ☑
    vulva (and other part(s) of trunk) 911 ☑
    wrist (and elbow) (and forearm) 913 ☑
  supraclavicular fossa 959.19
  supraorbital 959.09
  surgical complication (external or internal site) 998.2
  symphysis pubis 959.19
    complicating delivery 665.6 ☑
      affecting fetus or newborn 763.89
  temple 959.09
  temporal region 959.09
  testis 959.14
  thigh (and hip) 959.6
  thorax, thoracic (external) 959.11
    cavity — *see* Injury, internal, thorax
    internal — *see* Injury, internal, intrathoracic organs
  throat 959.09
  thumb(s) (nail) 959.5
  thymus — *see* Injury, internal, thymus
  thyroid (gland) 959.09
  toe (nail) (any) 959.7
  tongue 959.09
  tonsil 959.09
  tooth NEC 873.63
    complicated 873.73
  trachea — *see* Injury, internal, trachea
  trunk 959.19
  tunica vaginalis 959.14
  tympanum, tympanic membrane 959.09
  ultraviolet rays NEC 990
  ureter — *see* Injury, internal, ureter
  urethra (sphincter) — *see* Injury, internal, urethra
  uterus — *see* Injury, internal, uterus
  uvula 959.09
  vagina 959.14
  vascular — *see* Injury, blood vessel
  vas deferens — *see* Injury, internal, vas deferens
  vein (*see also* Injury, blood vessel, by site) 904.9
  vena cava
    inferior 902.10
    superior 901.2
  vesical (sphincter) — *see* Injury, internal, vesical
  viscera (abdominal) — *see* Injury, internal, viscera
    with fracture, pelvis — *see* Fracture, pelvis
  visual 950.9
    cortex 950.3
  vitreous (humor) 871.2

☑ Additional Digit Required — Refer to the Tabular List (Numeric Code Section) for Additional Digit Selection

▶◀ Revised Text ● New Line ▲ Revised Code

☑ Additional Digit Required — Refer to the Tabular List (Numeric Code Section) for Additional Digit Selection

▶◀ Revised Text ● New Line ▲ Revised Code

Irritation — *continued*
- stomach 536.9
  - psychogenic 306.4
- sympathetic nerve NEC (*see also* Neuropathy, peripheral, autonomic) 337.9
- ulnar nerve 354.2
- vagina 623.9

Isambert's disease 012.3 ☑

Ischemia, ischemic 459.9
- basilar artery (with transient neurologic deficit) 435.0
- bone NEC 733.40
- bowel (transient) 557.9
  - acute 557.0
  - chronic 557.1
  - due to mesenteric artery insufficiency 557.1
- brain — *see also* Ischemia, cerebral
  - recurrent focal 435.9
- cardiac (*see also* Ischemia, heart) 414.9
- cardiomyopathy 414.8
- carotid artery (with transient neurologic deficit) 435.8
- cerebral (chronic) (generalized) 437.1
  - arteriosclerotic 437.0
  - intermittent (with transient neurologic deficit) 435.9
  - puerperal, postpartum, childbirth 674.0 ☑
  - recurrent focal (with transient neurologic deficit) 435.9
  - transient (with transient neurologic deficit) 435.9
- colon 557.9
  - acute 557.0
  - chronic 557.1
  - due to mesenteric artery insufficiency 557.1
- coronary (chronic) (*see also* Ischemia, heart) 414.9
- heart (chronic or with a stated duration of over 8 weeks) 414.9
  - acute or with a stated duration of 8 weeks or less (*see also* Infarct, myocardium) 410.9 ☑
    - without myocardial infarction 411.89
      - with coronary (artery) occlusion 411.81
  - subacute 411.89
- intestine (transient) 557.9
  - acute 557.0
  - chronic 557.1
  - due to mesenteric artery insufficiency 557.1
- kidney 593.81
- labyrinth 386.50
- muscles, leg 728.89

Ischemia, ischemic — *continued*
- myocardium, myocardial (chronic or with a stated duration of over 8 weeks) 414.8
  - acute (*see also* Infarct, myocardium) 410.9 ☑
    - without myocardial infarction 411.89
      - with coronary (artery) occlusion 411.81
- renal 593.81
- retina, retinal 362.84
- small bowel 557.9
  - acute 557.0
  - chronic 557.1
  - due to mesenteric artery insufficiency 557.1
- spinal cord 336.1
- subendocardial (*see also* Insufficiency, coronary) 411.89
- vertebral artery (with transient neurologic deficit) 435.1

Ischialgia (*see also* Sciatica) 724.3

Ischiopagus 759.4

Ischium, ischial — *see* condition

Ischomenia 626.8

Ischuria 788.5

Iselin's disease or osteochondrosis 732.5

Islands of
- parotid tissue in
  - lymph nodes 750.26
  - neck structures 750.26
- submaxillary glands in
  - fascia 750.26
  - lymph nodes 750.26
  - neck muscles 750.26

Islet cell tumor, pancreas (M8150/0) 211.7

Isoimmunization NEC (*see also* Incompatibility) 656.2 ☑
- fetus or newborn 773.2
  - ABO blood groups 773.1
  - Rhesus (Rh) factor 773.0

Isolation V07.0
- social V62.4

Isosporosis 007.2

Issue
- medical certificate NEC V68.0
  - cause of death V68.0
  - fitness V68.0
  - incapacity V68.0
- repeat prescription NEC V68.1
  - appliance V68.1

Issue — *continued*
- repeat prescription NEC — *continued*
  - contraceptive V25.40
    - device NEC V25.49
      - intrauterine V25.42
      - specified type NEC V25.49
    - pill V25.41
  - glasses V68.1
  - medicinal substance V68.1

Itch (*see also* Pruritus) 698.9
- bakers' 692.89
- barbers' 110.0
- bricklayers' 692.89
- cheese 133.8
- clam diggers' 120.3
- coolie 126.9
- copra 133.8
- Cuban 050.1
- dew 126.9
- dhobie 110.3
- eye 379.99
- filarial (*see also* Infestation, filarial) 125.9
- grain 133.8
- grocers' 133.8
- ground 126.9
- harvest 133.8
- jock 110.3
- Malabar 110.9
  - beard 110.0
  - foot 110.4
  - scalp 110.0
- meaning scabies 133.0
- Norwegian 133.0
- perianal 698.0
- poultrymen's 133.8
- sarcoptic 133.0
- scrub 134.1
- seven year V61.10
  - meaning scabies 133.0
- straw 133.8
- swimmers' 120.3
- washerwoman's 692.4
- water 120.3
- winter 698.8

Itsenko-Cushing syndrome (pituitary basophilism) 255.0

Ivemark's syndrome (asplenia with congenital heart disease) 759.0

Ivory bones 756.52

Ixodes 134.8

Ixodiasis 134.8

☑ Additional Digit Required — Refer to the Tabular List (Numeric Code Section) for Additional Digit Selection

▶◀ Revised Text ● New Line ▲ Revised Code

- **Kink, kinking** — *continued*
  - ileum or intestine (*see also* Obstruction, intestine) 560.9
  - Lane's (*see also* Obstruction, intestine) 560.9
  - organ or site, congenital NEC — *see* Anomaly, specified type NEC, by site
  - ureter (pelvic junction) 593.3
    - congenital 753.20
  - vein(s) 459.2
    - caval 459.2
    - peripheral 459.2
- **Kinnier Wilson's disease** (hepatolenticular degeneration) 275.1
- **Kissing**
  - osteophytes 721.5
  - spine 721.5
  - vertebra 721.5
- **Klauder's syndrome** (erythema multiforme, exudativum) 695.1
- **Klebs' disease** (*see also* Nephritis) 583.9
- **Klein-Waardenburg syndrome** (ptosisepicanthus) 270.2
- **Kleine-Levin syndrome** 327.13 ▲
- **Kleptomania** 312.32
- **Klinefelter's syndrome** 758.7
- **Klinger's disease** 446.4
- **Klippel's disease** 723.8
- **Klippel-Feil disease or syndrome** (brevicollis) 756.16
- **Klippel-Trenaunay syndrome** 759.89
- **Klumpke (-Déjérine) palsy, paralysis** (birth) (newborn) 767.6
- **Klüver-Bucy (-Terzian) syndrome** 310.0
- **Knee** — *see* condition
- **Knifegrinders' rot** (*see also* Tuberculosis) 011.4 ☑
- **Knock-knee** (acquired) 736.41
  - congenital 755.64
- **Knot**
  - intestinal, syndrome (volvulus) 560.2
  - umbilical cord (true) 663.2 ☑
    - affecting fetus or newborn 762.5
- **Knots, surfer** 919.8
  - infected 919.9
- **Knotting** (of)
  - hair 704.2
  - intestine 560.2
- **Knuckle pads** (Garrod's) 728.79
- **Köbner's disease** (epidermolysis bullosa) 757.39
- **Koch's**
  - infection (*see also* Tuberculosis, pulmonary) 011.9 ☑
  - relapsing fever 087.9
- **Koch-Weeks conjunctivitis** 372.03
- **Koenig-Wichman disease** (pemphigus) 694.4
- **Köhler's disease** (osteochondrosis) 732.5
  - first (osteochondrosis juvenilis) 732.5
  - second (Freiburg's infarction, metatarsal head) 732.5
  - patellar 732.4
  - tarsal navicular (bone) (osteoarthrosis juvenilis) 732.5
- **Köhler-Mouchet disease** (osteoarthrosis juvenilis) 732.5
- **Köhler-Pellegrini-Stieda disease or syndrome** (calcification, knee joint) 726.62
- **Koilonychia** 703.8
  - congenital 757.5
- **Kojevnikov's, Kojewnikoff's epilepsy** (*see also* Epilepsy) 345.7 ☑
- **König's**
  - disease (osteochondritis dissecans) 732.7
  - syndrome 564.89
- **Koniophthisis** (*see also* Tuberculosis) 011.4 ☑
- **Koplik's spots** 055.9
- **Kopp's asthma** 254.8
- **Korean hemorrhagic fever** 078.6
- **Korsakoff (-Wernicke) disease, psychosis, or syndrome** (nonalcoholic) 294.0
  - alcoholic 291.1
- **Korsakov's disease** — *see* Korsakoff's disease
- **Korsakow's disease** — *see* Korsakoff's disease
- **Kostmann's disease or syndrome** (infantile genetic agranulocytosis) 288.0
- **Krabbe's**
  - disease (leukodystrophy) 330.0
  - syndrome
    - congenital muscle hypoplasia 756.89
    - cutaneocerebral angioma 759.6
- **Kraepelin-Morel disease** (*see also* Schizophrenia) 295.9 ☑
- **Kraft-Weber-Dimitri disease** 759.6
- **Kraurosis**
  - ani 569.49
  - penis 607.0
  - vagina 623.8
  - vulva 624.0
- **Kreotoxism** 005.9
- **Krukenberg's**
  - spindle 371.13
  - tumor (M8490/6) 198.6
- **Kufs' disease** 330.1
- **Kugelberg-Welander disease** 335.11
- **Kuhnt-Junius degeneration or disease** 362.52
- **Kulchitsky's cell carcinoma** (carcinoid tumor of intestine) 259.2
- **Kümmell's disease or spondylitis** 721.7
- **Kundrat's disease** (lymphosarcoma) 200.1 ☑
- **Kunekune** — *see* Dermatophytosis
- **Kunkel syndrome** (lupoid hepatitis) 571.49
- **Kupffer cell sarcoma** (M9124/3) 155.0
- **Kuru** 046.0
- **Kussmaul's**
  - coma (diabetic) 250.3 ☑
  - disease (polyarteritis nodosa) 446.0
  - respiration (air hunger) 786.09
- **Kwashiorkor** (marasmus type) 260
- **Kyasanur Forest disease** 065.2
- **Kyphoscoliosis, kyphoscoliotic** (acquired) (*see also* Scoliosis) 737.30
  - congenital 756.19
  - due to radiation 737.33
  - heart (disease) 416.1
  - idiopathic 737.30
    - infantile
      - progressive 737.32
      - resolving 737.31
  - late effect of rickets 268.1 *[737.43]*
  - specified NEC 737.39
  - thoracogenic 737.34
  - tuberculous (*see also* Tuberculosis) 015.0 ☑ *[737.43]*
- **Kyphosis, kyphotic** (acquired) (postural) 737.10
  - adolescent postural 737.0
  - congenital 756.19
  - dorsalis juvenilis 732.0
  - due to or associated with
    - Charcôt-Marie-Tooth disease 356.1 *[737.41]*
    - mucopolysaccharidosis 277.5 *[737.41]*
    - neurofibromatosis 237.71 *[737.41]*
    - osteitis
      - deformans 731.0 *[737.41]*
      - fibrosa cystica 252.01 *[737.41]*
    - osteoporosis (*see also* Osteoporosis) 733.0 ☑ *[737.41]*
    - poliomyelitis (*see also* Poliomyelitis) 138 *[737.41]*
    - radiation 737.11
    - tuberculosis (*see also* Tuberculosis) 015.0 ☑ *[737.41]*
  - Kümmell's 721.7
  - late effect of rickets 268.1 *[737.41]*
  - Morquio-Brailsford type (spinal) 277.5 *[737.41]*
  - pelvis 738.6
  - postlaminectomy 737.12
  - specified cause NEC 737.19
  - syphilitic, congenital 090.5 *[737.41]*
  - tuberculous (*see also* Tuberculosis) 015.0 ☑ *[737.41]*
- **Kyrle's disease** (hyperkeratosis follicularis in cutem penetrans) 701.1

L

- **Labia, labium** — *see* condition
- **Labiated hymen** 752.49
- **Labile**
  - blood pressure 796.2
  - emotions, emotionality 301.3
  - vasomotor system 443.9
- **Labioglossal paralysis** 335.22
- **Labium leporinum** (*see also* Cleft, lip) 749.10
- **Labor** (*see also* Delivery)
  - with complications — *see* Delivery, complicated
  - abnormal NEC 661.9 ☑
    - affecting fetus or newborn 763.7
  - arrested active phase 661.1 ☑
    - affecting fetus or newborn 763.7
  - desultory 661.2 ☑
    - affecting fetus or newborn 763.7
  - dyscoordinate 661.4 ☑
    - affecting fetus or newborn 763.7
  - early onset (22-36 weeks gestation) 644.2 ☑
  - failed
    - induction 659.1 ☑
      - mechanical 659.0 ☑
      - medical 659.1 ☑
      - surgical 659.0 ☑
    - trial (vaginal delivery) 660.6 ☑
  - false 644.1 ☑
  - forced or induced, affecting fetus or newborn 763.89
  - hypertonic 661.4 ☑
    - affecting fetus or newborn 763.7
  - hypotonic 661.2 ☑
    - affecting fetus or newborn 763.7
    - primary 661.0 ☑
      - affecting fetus or newborn 763.7
    - secondary 661.1 ☑
      - affecting fetus or newborn 763.7
  - incoordinate 661.4 ☑
    - affecting fetus or newborn 763.7
  - irregular 661.2 ☑
    - affecting fetus or newborn 763.7
  - long — *see* Labor, prolonged
  - missed (at or near term) 656.4 ☑
  - obstructed NEC 660.9 ☑
    - affecting fetus or newborn 763.1
    - due to female genital mutilation 660.8 ☑ ●
    - specified cause NEC 660.8 ☑
      - affecting fetus or newborn 763.1
  - pains, spurious 644.1 ☑
  - precipitate 661.3 ☑
    - affecting fetus or newborn 763.6
  - premature 644.2 ☑
    - threatened 644.0 ☑
  - prolonged or protracted 662.1 ☑
    - affecting fetus or newborn 763.89
    - first stage 662.0 ☑
      - affecting fetus or newborn 763.89
    - second stage 662.2 ☑
      - affecting fetus or newborn 763.89
  - threatened NEC 644.1 ☑
  - undelivered 644.1 ☑
- **Labored breathing** (*see also* Hyperventilation) 786.09
- **Labyrinthitis** (inner ear) (destructive) (latent) 386.30
  - circumscribed 386.32
  - diffuse 386.31
  - focal 386.32
  - purulent 386.33
  - serous 386.31
  - suppurative 386.33
  - syphilitic 095.8
  - toxic 386.34
  - viral 386.35
- **Laceration** — *see also* Wound, open, by site
  - accidental, complicating surgery 998.2
  - Achilles tendon 845.09
    - with open wound 892.2
  - anus (sphincter) 879.6
    - with
      - abortion — *see* Abortion, by type, with damage to pelvic organs
      - ectopic pregnancy (*see also* categories 633.0-633.9) 639.2

☑ Additional Digit Required — Refer to the Tabular List (Numeric Code Section) for Additional Digit Selection

- **Laceration** — *see also* Wound, open, by site — *continued*
  - anus — *continued*
    - with — *continued*
      - molar pregnancy (*see also* categories 630-632) 639.2
    - complicated 879.7
    - complicating delivery 664.2 ☑
      - with laceration of anal or rectal mucosa 664.3 ☑
    - following
      - abortion 639.2
      - ectopic or molar pregnancy 639.2
    - nontraumatic, nonpuerperal 565.0
  - bladder (urinary)
    - with
      - abortion — *see* Abortion, by type, with damage to pelvic organs
      - ectopic pregnancy (*see also* categories 633.0-633.9) 639.2
      - molar pregnancy (*see also* categories 630-632) 639.2
    - following
      - abortion 639.2
      - ectopic or molar pregnancy 639.2
    - obstetrical trauma 665.5 ☑
  - blood vessel — *see* Injury, blood vessel, by site
  - bowel
    - with
      - abortion — *see* Abortion, by type, with damage to pelvic organs
      - ectopic pregnancy (*see also* categories 633.0-633.9) 639.2
      - molar pregnancy (*see also* categories 630-632) 639.2
    - following
      - abortion 639.2
      - ectopic or molar pregnancy 639.2
    - obstetrical trauma 665.5 ☑
  - brain (cerebral) (membrane) (with hemorrhage) 851.8 ☑

> *Note — Use the following fifth-digit subclassification with categories 851–854:*
>
> 0 *unspecified state of consciousness*
> 1 *with no loss of consciousness*
> 2 *with brief [less than one hour] loss of consciousness*
> 3 *with moderate [1-24 hours] loss of consciousness*
> 4 *with prolonged [more than 24 hours] loss of consciousness and return to pre-existing conscious level*
> 5 *with prolonged [more than 24 hours] loss of consciousness, without return to pre-existing conscious level*
>
> *Use fifth-digit 5 to designate when a patient is unconscious and dies before regaining consciousness, regardless of the duration of the loss of consciousness*
>
> 6 *with loss of consciousness of unspecified duration*
> 9 *with concussion, unspecified*

-
  -
    - with
      - open intracranial wound 851.9 ☑
      - skull fracture — *see* Fracture, skull, by site
    - cerebellum 851.6 ☑
      - with open intracranial wound 851.7 ☑
    - cortex 851.2 ☑
      - with open intracranial wound 851.3 ☑
    - during birth 767.0
    - stem 851.6 ☑
      - with open intracranial wound 851.7 ☑
  - broad ligament
    - with
      - abortion — *see* Abortion, by type, with damage to pelvic organs
      - ectopic pregnancy (*see also* categories 633.0-633.9) 639.2
      - molar pregnancy (*see also* categories 630-632) 639.2
    - following
      - abortion 639.2
      - ectopic or molar pregnancy 639.2
    - nontraumatic 620.6
    - obstetrical trauma 665.6 ☑
    - syndrome (nontraumatic) 620.6
  - capsule, joint — *see* Sprain, by site
  - cardiac — *see* Laceration, heart
  - causing eversion of cervix uteri (old) 622.0
  - central, complicating delivery 664.4 ☑
  - cerebellum — *see* Laceration, brain, cerebellum
  - cerebral — *see also* Laceration, brain
    - during birth 767.0
  - cervix (uteri)
    - with
      - abortion — *see* Abortion, by type, with damage to pelvic organs
      - ectopic pregnancy (*see also* categories 633.0-633.9) 639.2
      - molar pregnancy (*see also* categories 630-632) 639.2
    - following
      - abortion 639.2
      - ectopic or molar pregnancy 639.2
    - nonpuerperal, nontraumatic 622.3
    - obstetrical trauma (current) 665.3 ☑
    - old (postpartal) 622.3
    - traumatic — *see* Injury, internal, cervix
  - chordae heart 429.5
  - complicated 879.9
  - cornea — *see* Laceration, eyeball
    - superficial 918.1
  - cortex (cerebral) — *see* Laceration, brain, cortex
  - esophagus 530.89
  - eye(s) — *see* Laceration, ocular
  - eyeball NEC 871.4
    - with prolapse or exposure of intraocular tissue 871.1
    - penetrating — *see* Penetrating wound, eyeball
    - specified as without prolapse of intraocular tissue 871.0
  - eyelid NEC 870.8
    - full thickness 870.1
      - involving lacrimal passages 870.2
    - skin (and periocular area) 870.0
      - penetrating — *see* Penetrating wound, orbit
  - fourchette
    - with
      - abortion — *see* Abortion, by type, with damage to pelvic organs
      - ectopic pregnancy (*see also* categories 633.0-633.9) 639.2
      - molar pregnancy (*see also* categories 630-632) 639.2
    - complicating delivery 664.0 ☑
    - following
      - abortion 639.2
      - ectopic or molar pregnancy 639.2
  - heart (without penetration of heart chambers) 861.02
    - with
      - open wound into thorax 861.12
      - penetration of heart chambers 861.03
        - with open wound into thorax 861.13
  - hernial sac — *see* Hernia, by site
  - internal organ (abdomen) (chest) (pelvis) NEC — *see* Injury, internal, by site
  - kidney (parenchyma) 866.02
    - with
      - complete disruption of parenchyma (rupture) 866.03
        - with open wound into cavity 866.13
      - open wound into cavity 866.12
  - labia
    - complicating delivery 664.0 ☑
  - ligament — *see also* Sprain, by site
    - with open wound — *see* Wound, open, by site
  - liver 864.05
    - with open wound into cavity 864.15
    - major (disruption of hepatic parenchyma) 864.04
      - with open wound into cavity 864.14
    - minor (capsule only) 864.02
      - with open wound into cavity 864.12
    - moderate (involving parenchyma without major disruption) 864.03
      - with open wound into cavity 864.13
      - multiple 864.04
        - with open wound into cavity 864.14
    - stellate 864.04
      - with open wound into cavity 864.14
  - lung 861.22
    - with open wound into thorax 861.32
  - meninges — *see* Laceration, brain
  - meniscus (knee) (*see also* Tear, meniscus) 836.2
    - old 717.5
    - site other than knee — *see also* Sprain, by site
      - old NEC (*see also* Disorder, cartilage, articular) 718.0 ☑
  - muscle — *see also* Sprain, by site
    - with open wound — *see* Wound, open, by site
  - myocardium — *see* Laceration, heart
  - nerve — *see* Injury, nerve, by site
  - ocular NEC (*see also* Laceration, eyeball) 871.4
    - adnexa NEC 870.8
      - penetrating 870.3
        - with foreign body 870.4
  - orbit (eye) 870.8
    - penetrating 870.3
      - with foreign body 870.4
  - pelvic
    - floor (muscles)
      - with
        - abortion — *see* Abortion, by type, with damage to pelvic organs
        - ectopic pregnancy (*see also* categories 633.0-633.9) 639.2
        - molar pregnancy (*see also* categories 630-632) 639.2
      - complicating delivery 664.1 ☑
      - following
        - abortion 639.2
        - ectopic or molar pregnancy 639.2
      - nonpuerperal 618.7
      - old (postpartal) 618.7
    - organ NEC
      - with
        - abortion — *see* Abortion, by type, with damage to pelvic organs
        - ectopic pregnancy (*see also* categories 633.0-633.9) 639.2
        - molar pregnancy (*see also* categories 630-632) 639.2
      - complicating delivery 665.5 ☑
        - affecting fetus or newborn 763.89
      - following
        - abortion 639.2
        - ectopic or molar pregnancy 639.2
      - obstetrical trauma 665.5 ☑
  - perineum, perineal (old) (postpartal) 618.7
    - with
      - abortion — *see* Abortion, by type, with damage to pelvic floor
      - ectopic pregnancy (*see also* categories 633.0-633.9) 639.2
      - molar pregnancy (*see also* categories 630-632) 639.2
    - complicating delivery 664.4 ☑
      - first degree 664.0 ☑
      - second degree 664.1 ☑
      - third degree 664.2 ☑
      - fourth degree 664.3 ☑
      - central 664.4 ☑
      - involving
        - anal sphincter 664.2 ☑
        - fourchette 664.0 ☑
        - hymen 664.0 ☑
        - labia 664.0 ☑
        - pelvic floor 664.1 ☑
        - perineal muscles 664.1 ☑

- **Laceration** — *see also* Wound, open, by site — *continued*
  - perineum, perineal — *continued*
    - complicating delivery — *continued*
      - involving — *continued*
        - rectovaginal septum 664.2 ☑
          - with anal mucosa 664.3 ☑
        - skin 664.0 ☑
        - sphincter (anal) 664.2 ☑
          - with anal mucosa 664.3 ☑
        - vagina 664.0 ☑
        - vaginal muscles 664.1 ☑
        - vulva 664.0 ☑
      - secondary 674.2 ☑
    - following
      - abortion 639.2
      - ectopic or molar pregnancy 639.2
    - male 879.6
      - complicated 879.7
    - muscles, complicating delivery 664.1 ☑
    - nonpuerperal, current injury 879.6
      - complicated 879.7
    - secondary (postpartal) 674.2 ☑
  - peritoneum
    - with
      - abortion — *see* Abortion, by type, with damage to pelvic organs
      - ectopic pregnancy (*see also* categories 633.0-633.9) 639.2
      - molar pregnancy (*see also* categories 630-632) 639.2
    - following
      - abortion 639.2
      - ectopic or molar pregnancy 639.2
    - obstetrical trauma 665.5 ☑
  - periurethral tissue
    - with
      - abortion — *see* Abortion, by type, with damage to pelvic organs
      - ectopic pregnancy (*see also* categories 633.0-633.9) 639.2
      - molar pregnancy (*see also* categories 630-632) 639.2
    - following
      - abortion 639.2
      - ectopic or molar pregnancy 639.2
    - obstetrical trauma 665.5 ☑
  - rectovaginal (septum)
    - with
      - abortion — *see* Abortion, by type, with damage to pelvic organs
      - ectopic pregnancy (*see also* categories 633.0-633.9) 639.2
      - molar pregnancy (*see also* categories 630-632) 639.2
    - complicating delivery 665.4 ☑
      - with perineum 664.2 ☑
        - involving anal or rectal mucosa 664.3 ☑
    - following
      - abortion 639.2
      - ectopic or molar pregnancy 639.2
    - nonpuerperal 623.4
    - old (postpartal) 623.4
  - spinal cord (meninges) — *see also* Injury, spinal, by site
    - due to injury at birth 767.4
    - fetus or newborn 767.4
  - spleen 865.09
    - with
      - disruption of parenchyma (massive) 865.04
        - with open wound into cavity 865.14
      - open wound into cavity 865.19
    - capsule (without disruption of parenchyma) 865.02
      - with open wound into cavity 865.12
    - parenchyma 865.03
      - with open wound into cavity 865.13
      - massive disruption (rupture) 865.04
        - with open wound into cavity 865.14
  - tendon 848.9
    - with open wound — *see* Wound, open, by site
    - Achilles 845.09
      - with open wound 892.2

- **Laceration** — *see also* Wound, open, by site — *continued*
  - tendon — *continued*
    - lower limb NEC 844.9
      - with open wound NEC 894.2
    - upper limb NEC 840.9
      - with open wound NEC 884.2
  - tentorium cerebelli — *see* Laceration, brain, cerebellum
  - tongue 873.64
    - complicated 873.74
  - urethra
    - with
      - abortion — *see* Abortion, by type, with damage to pelvic organs
      - ectopic pregnancy (*see also* categories 633.0-633.9) 639.2
      - molar pregnancy (*see also* categories 630-632) 639.2
    - following
      - abortion 639.2
      - ectopic or molar pregnancy 639.2
    - nonpuerperal, nontraumatic 599.84
    - obstetrical trauma 665.5 ☑
  - uterus
    - with
      - abortion — *see* Abortion, by type, with damage to pelvic organs
      - ectopic pregnancy (*see also* categories 633.0-633.9) 639.2
      - molar pregnancy (*see also* categories 630-632) 639.2
    - following
      - abortion 639.2
      - ectopic or molar pregnancy 639.2
    - nonpuerperal, nontraumatic 621.8
    - obstetrical trauma NEC 665.5 ☑
    - old (postpartal) 621.8
  - vagina
    - with
      - abortion — *see* Abortion, by type, with damage to pelvic organs
      - ectopic pregnancy (*see also* categories 633.0-633.9) 639.2
      - molar pregnancy (*see also* categories 630-632) 639.2
      - perineal involvement, complicating delivery 664.0 ☑
    - complicating delivery 665.4 ☑
      - first degree 664.0 ☑
      - second degree 664.1 ☑
      - third degree 664.2 ☑
      - fourth degree 664.3 ☑
      - high 665.4 ☑
      - muscles 664.1 ☑
      - sulcus 665.4 ☑
      - wall 665.4 ☑
    - following
      - abortion 639.2
      - ectopic or molar pregnancy 639.2
    - nonpuerperal, nontraumatic 623.4
    - old (postpartal) 623.4
  - valve, heart — *see* Endocarditis
  - vulva
    - with
      - abortion — *see* Abortion, by type, with damage to pelvic organs,
      - ectopic pregnancy (*see also* categories 633.0-633.9) 639.2
      - molar pregnancy (*see also* categories 630-632) 639.2
    - complicating delivery 664.0 ☑
    - following
      - abortion 639.2
      - ectopic or molar pregnancy 639.2
    - nonpuerperal, nontraumatic 624.4
    - old (postpartal) 624.4
- **Lachrymal** — *see* condition
- **Lachrymonasal duct** — *see* condition
- **Lack of**
  - appetite (*see also* Anorexia) 783.0
  - care
    - in home V60.4
    - of adult 995.84
    - of infant (at or after birth) 995.52
  - coordination 781.3

- **Lack of** — *continued*
  - development — *see also* Hypoplasia
    - physiological in childhood 783.40
  - education V62.3
  - energy 780.79
  - financial resources V60.2
  - food 994.2
    - in environment V60.8
  - growth in childhood 783.43
  - heating V60.1
  - housing (permanent) (temporary) V60.0
    - adequate V60.1
  - material resources V60.2
  - medical attention 799.89
  - memory (*see also* Amnesia) 780.93
    - mild, following organic brain damage 310.1
  - ovulation 628.0
  - person able to render necessary care V60.4
  - physical exercise V69.0
  - physiologic development in childhood 783.40
  - posterior occlusal support 524.57
  - prenatal care in current pregnancy V23.7
  - shelter V60.0
  - sleep V69.4
  - water 994.3
- **Lacrimal** — *see* condition
- **Lacrimation, abnormal** (*see also* Epiphora) 375.20
- **Lacrimonasal duct** — *see* condition
- **Lactation, lactating** (breast) (puerperal) (postpartum)
  - defective 676.4 ☑
  - disorder 676.9 ☑
    - specified type NEC 676.8 ☑
  - excessive 676.6 ☑
  - failed 676.4 ☑
  - mastitis NEC 675.2 ☑
  - mother (care and/or examination) V24.1
  - nonpuerperal 611.6
  - suppressed 676.5 ☑
- **Lacticemia** 271.3
  - excessive 276.2
- **Lactosuria** 271.3
- **Lacunar skull** 756.0
- **Laennec's cirrhosis** (alcoholic) 571.2
  - nonalcoholic 571.5
- **Lafora's disease** 333.2
- **Lag, lid** (nervous) 374.41
- **Lagleyze-von Hippel disease** (retinocerebral angiomatosis) 759.6
- **Lagophthalmos** (eyelid) (nervous) 374.20
  - cicatricial 374.23
  - keratitis (*see also* Keratitis) 370.34
  - mechanical 374.22
  - paralytic 374.21
- **La grippe** — *see* Influenza
- **Lahore sore** 085.1
- **Lakes, venous** (cerebral) 437.8
- **Laki-Lorand factor deficiency** (*see also* Defect, coagulation) 286.3
- **Lalling** 307.9
- **Lambliasis** 007.1
- **Lame back** 724.5
- **Lancereaux's diabetes** (diabetes mellitus with marked emaciation) 250.8 ☑ *[261]*
- **Landouzy-Déjérine dystrophy** (fascioscapulohumeral atrophy) 359.1
- **Landry's disease or paralysis** 357.0
- **Landry-Guillain-Barré syndrome** 357.0
- **Lane's**
  - band 751.4
  - disease 569.89
  - kink (*see also* Obstruction, intestine) 560.9
- **Langdon Down's syndrome** (mongolism) 758.0
- **Language abolition** 784.69
- **Lanugo** (persistent) 757.4
- **Laparoscopic surgical procedure converted to open procedure** V64.41
- **Lardaceous**
  - degeneration (any site) 277.3
  - disease 277.3

Lardaceous — *continued*
- kidney 277.3 *[583.81]*
- liver 277.3

Large
- baby (regardless of gestational age) 766.1
  - exceptionally (weight of 4500 grams or more) 766.0
  - of diabetic mother 775.0
- ear 744.22
- fetus — *see also* Oversize, fetus
  - causing disproportion 653.5 ☑
    - with obstructed labor 660.1 ☑
- for dates
  - fetus or newborn (regardless of gestational age) 766.1
    - affecting management of pregnancy656.6 ☑
    - exceptionally (weight of 4500 grams or more) 766.0
- physiological cup 743.57
- stature 783.9
- waxy liver 277.3
- white kidney — *see* Nephrosis

Larsen's syndrome (flattened facies and multiple congenital dislocations) 755.8

Larsen-Johansson disease (juvenile osteopathia patellae) 732.4

Larva migrans
- cutaneous NEC 126.9
  - ancylostoma 126.9
- of Diptera in vitreous 128.0
- visceral NEC 128.0

Laryngeal — *see also* condition
- syncope 786.2

Laryngismus (acute) (infectious) (stridulous) 478.75
- congenital 748.3
- diphtheritic 032.3

Laryngitis (acute) (edematous) (fibrinous) (gangrenous) (infective) (infiltrative) (malignant) (membranous) (phlegmonous) (pneumococcal) (pseudomembranous) (septic) (subglottic) (suppurative) (ulcerative) (viral) 464.00
- with
  - influenza, flu, or grippe 487.1
  - obstruction 464.01
  - tracheitis (*see also* Laryngotracheitis) 464.20
    - with obstruction 464.21
    - acute 464.20
      - with obstruction 464.21
    - chronic 476.1
- atrophic 476.0
- Borrelia vincentii 101
- catarrhal 476.0
- chronic 476.0
  - with tracheitis (chronic) 476.1
  - due to external agent — *see* Condition, respiratory, chronic, due to
- diphtheritic (membranous) 032.3
- due to external agent — *see* Inflammation, respiratory, upper, due to
- H. influenzae 464.00
  - with obstruction 464.01
- Hemophilus influenzae 464.00
  - with obstruction 464.01
- hypertrophic 476.0
- influenzal 487.1
- pachydermic 478.79
- sicca 476.0
- spasmodic 478.75
  - acute 464.00
    - with obstruction 464.01
- streptococcal 034.0
- stridulous 478.75
- syphilitic 095.8
  - congenital 090.5
- tuberculous (*see also* Tuberculosis, larynx) 012.3 ☑
- Vincent's 101

Laryngocele (congenital) (ventricular) 748.3

Laryngofissure 478.79
- congenital 748.3

Laryngomalacia (congenital) 748.3

Laryngopharyngitis (acute) 465.0
- chronic 478.9
  - due to external agent — *see* Condition, respiratory, chronic, due to
- due to external agent — *see* Inflammation, respiratory, upper, due to
- septic 034.0

Laryngoplegia (*see also* Paralysis, vocal cord) 478.30

Laryngoptosis 478.79

Laryngospasm 478.75
- due to external agent — *see* Condition, respiratory, acute, due to

Laryngostenosis 478.74
- congenital 748.3

Laryngotracheitis (acute) (infectional) (viral) (*see also* Laryngitis) 464.20
- with obstruction 464.21
- atrophic 476.1
- Borrelia vincenti 101
- catarrhal 476.1
- chronic 476.1
  - due to external agent — *see* Condition, respiratory, chronic, due to
- diphtheritic (membranous) 032.3
- due to external agent — *see* Inflammation, respiratory, upper, due to
- H. influenzae 464.20
  - with obstruction 464.21
- hypertrophic 476.1
- influenzal 487.1
- pachydermic 478.75
- sicca 476.1
- spasmodic 478.75
  - acute 464.20
    - with obstruction 464.21
- streptococcal 034.0
- stridulous 478.75
- syphilitic 095.8
  - congenital 090.5
- tuberculous (*see also* Tuberculosis, larynx) 012.3 ☑
- Vincent's 101

Laryngotracheobronchitis (*see also* Bronchitis) 490
- acute 466.0
- chronic 491.8
- viral 466.0

Laryngotracheobronchopneumonitis — *see* Pneumonia, broncho-

Larynx, laryngeal — *see* condition

Lasègue's disease (persecution mania) 297.9

Lassa fever 078.89

Lassitude (*see also* Weakness) 780.79

Late — *see also* condition
- effect(s) (of) — *see also* condition
  - abscess
    - intracranial or intraspinal (conditions classifiable to 324) — *see* category 326
  - adverse effect of drug, medicinal or biological substance 909.5
  - allergic reaction 909.9
  - amputation
    - postoperative (late) 997.60
    - traumatic (injury classifiable to 885-887 and 895-897) 905.9
  - burn (injury classifiable to 948-949) 906.9
    - extremities NEC (injury classifiable to 943 or 945) 906.7
      - hand or wrist (injury classifiable to 944) 906.6
    - eye (injury classifiable to 940) 906.5
    - face, head, and neck (injury classifiable to 941) 906.5
    - specified site NEC (injury classifiable to 942 and 946-947) 906.8
  - cerebrovascular disease (conditions classifiable to 430-437) 438.9
    - with
      - alterations of sensations 438.6
      - aphasia 438.11
      - apraxia 438.81
      - ataxia 438.84

Late — *see also* condition — *continued*
- effect(s) (of) — *see also* condition — *continued*
  - cerebrovascular disease — *continued*
    - with — *continued*
      - cognitive deficits 438.0
      - disturbances of vision 438.7
      - dysphagia 438.82
      - dysphasia 438.12
      - facial droop 438.83
      - facial weakness 438.83
      - hemiplegia/hemiparesis
        - affecting
          - dominant side 438.21
          - nondominant side 438.22
          - unspecified side 438.20
      - monoplegia of lower limb
        - affecting
          - dominant side 438.41
          - nondominant side 438.42
          - unspecified side 438.40
      - monoplegia of upper limb
        - affecting
          - dominant side 438.31
          - nondominant side 438.32
          - unspecified side 438.30
      - paralytic syndrome NEC
        - affecting
          - bilateral 438.53
          - dominant side 438.51
          - nondominant side 438.52
          - unspecified side 438.50
      - speech and language deficit 438.10
      - specified type NEC 438.19
      - vertigo 438.85
    - specified type NEC 438.89
  - childbirth complication(s) 677
  - complication(s) of
    - childbirth 677
    - delivery 677
    - pregnancy 677
    - puerperium 677
    - surgical and medical care (conditions classifiable to 996-999) 909.3
    - trauma (conditions classifiable to 958) 908.6
  - contusion (injury classifiable to 920-924) 906.3
  - crushing (injury classifiable to 925-929) 906.4
  - delivery complication(s) 677
  - dislocation (injury classifiable to 830-839) 905.6
  - encephalitis or encephalomyelitis (conditions classifiable to 323) — *see* category 326
    - in infectious diseases 139.8
      - viral (conditions classifiable to 049.8, 049.9, 062-064) 139.0
  - external cause NEC (conditions classifiable to 995) 909.9
    - certain conditions classifiable to categories 991-994 909.4
  - foreign body in orifice (injury classifiable to 930-939) 908.5
  - fracture (multiple) (injury classifiable to 828-829) 905.5
    - extremity
      - lower (injury classifiable to 821-827) 905.4
        - neck of femur (injury classifiable to 820) 905.3
      - upper (injury classifiable to 810-819) 905.2
    - face and skull (injury classifiable to 800-804) 905.0
    - skull and face (injury classifiable to 800-804) 905.0
    - spine and trunk (injury classifiable to 805 and 807-809) 905.1
      - with spinal cord lesion (injury classifiable to 806) 907.2
  - infection
    - pyogenic, intracranial — *see* category 326
  - infectious diseases (conditions classifiable to 001-136) NEC 139.8
  - injury (injury classifiable to 959) 908.9
    - blood vessel 908.3

☑ Additional Digit Required — Refer to the Tabular List (Numeric Code Section) for Additional Digit Selection

▶◀ Revised Text ● New Line ▲ Revised Code

Lesion — *continued*
- nonallopathic — *continued*
  - in region (of) — *continued*
    - hip 739.5
    - lower extremity 739.6
    - lumbar, lumbosacral 739.3
    - occipitocervical 739.0
    - pelvic 739.5
    - pubic 739.5
    - rib cage 739.8
    - sacral, sacrococcygeal, sacroiliac 739.4
    - sternochondral 739.8
    - sternoclavicular 739.7
    - thoracic, thoracolumbar 739.2
    - upper extremity 739.7
- nose (internal) 478.1
- obstructive — *see* Obstruction
- obturator nerve 355.79
- occlusive
  - artery — *see* Embolism, artery
- organ or site NEC — *see* Disease, by site
- osteolytic 733.90
- paramacular, of retina 363.32
- peptic 537.89
- periodontal, due to traumatic occlusion 523.8
- perirectal 569.49
- peritoneum (granulomatous) 568.89
- pigmented (skin) 709.00
- pinta — *see* Pinta, lesions
- polypoid — *see* Polyp
- prechiasmal (optic) (*see also* Lesion, chiasmal) 377.54
- primary — *see also* Syphilis, primary
  - carate 103.0
  - pinta 103.0
  - yaws 102.0
- pulmonary 518.89
  - valve (*see also* Endocarditis, pulmonary) 424.3
- pylorus 537.89
- radiation NEC 990
- radium NEC 990
- rectosigmoid 569.89
- retina, retinal — *see also* Retinopathy
  - vascular 362.17
- retroperitoneal 568.89
- romanus 720.1
- sacroiliac (joint) 724.6
- salivary gland 527.8
  - benign lymphoepithelial 527.8
- saphenous nerve 355.79
- secondary — *see* Syphilis, secondary
- sigmoid 569.89
- sinus (accessory) (nasal) (*see also* Sinusitis) 473.9
- skin 709.9
  - suppurative 686.00
- SLAP (superior glenoid labrum) 840.7
- space-occupying, intracranial NEC 784.2
- spinal cord 336.9
  - congenital 742.9
  - traumatic (complete) (incomplete) (transverse) — *see* also Injury, spinal, by site
    - with
      - broken
        - back — *see* Fracture, vertebra, by site, with spinal cord injury
        - neck — *see* Fracture, vertebra, cervical, with spinal cord injury
      - fracture, vertebra — *see* Fracture, vertebra, by site, with spinal cord injury
- spleen 289.50
- stomach 537.89
- superior glenoid labrum (SLAP) 840.7
- syphilitic — *see* Syphilis
- tertiary — *see* Syphilis, tertiary
- thoracic root (nerve) 353.3
- tonsillar fossa 474.9
- tooth, teeth 525.8
  - white spot 521.01
- traumatic NEC (*see also* nature and site of injury) 959.9
- tricuspid (valve) — *see* Endocarditis, tricuspid
- trigeminal nerve 350.9
- ulcerated or ulcerative — *see* Ulcer
- uterus NEC 621.9
- vagina 623.8
- vagus nerve 352.3
- valvular — *see* Endocarditis
- vascular 459.9
  - affecting central nervous system (*see also* Lesion, cerebrovascular) 437.9
  - following trauma (*see also* Injury, blood vessel, by site) 904.9
  - retina 362.17
  - traumatic — *see* Injury, blood vessel, by site
  - umbilical cord 663.6 ☑
    - affecting fetus or newborn 762.6
- visual
  - cortex NEC (*see also* Disorder, visual, cortex) 377.73
  - pathway NEC (*see also* Disorder, visual, pathway) 377.63
- warty — *see* Verruca
- white spot, on teeth 521.01
- x-ray NEC 990

Lethargic — *see* condition

Lethargy 780.79

Letterer-Siwe disease (acute histiocytosis X) (M9722/3) 202.5 ☑

Leucinosis 270.3

Leucocoria 360.44

Leucosarcoma (M9850/3) 207.8 ☑

Leukasmus 270.2

Leukemia, leukemic (congenital) (M9800/3) 208.9 ☑

> *Note — Use the following fifth-digit subclassification for categories 203–208:*
>
> 0 *without mention of remission*
>
> 1 *with remission*

- acute NEC (M9801/3) 208.0 ☑
- aleukemic NEC (M9804/3) 208.8 ☑
  - granulocytic (M9864/3) 205.8 ☑
- basophilic (M9870/3) 205.1 ☑
- blast (cell) (M9801/3) 208.0 ☑
- blastic (M9801/3) 208.0 ☑
  - granulocytic (M9861/3) 205.0 ☑
- chronic NEC (M9803/3) 208.1 ☑
- compound (M9810/3) 207.8 ☑
- eosinophilic (M9880/3) 205.1 ☑
- giant cell (M9910/3) 207.2 ☑
- granulocytic (M9860/3) 205.9 ☑
  - acute (M9861/3) 205.0 ☑
  - aleukemic (M9864/3) 205.8 ☑
  - blastic (M9861/3) 205.0 ☑
  - chronic (M9863/3) 205.1 ☑
  - subacute (M9862/3) 205.2 ☑
  - subleukemic (M9864/3) 205.8 ☑
- hairy cell (M9940/3) 202.4 ☑
- hemoblastic (M9801/3) 208.0 ☑
- histiocytic (M9890/3) 206.9 ☑
- lymphatic (M9820/3) 204.9 ☑
  - acute (M9821/3) 204.0 ☑
  - aleukemic (M9824/3) 204.8 ☑
  - chronic (M9823/3) 204.1 ☑
  - subacute (M9822/3) 204.2 ☑
  - subleukemic (M9824/3) 204.8 ☑
- lymphoblastic (M9821/3) 204.0 ☑
- lymphocytic (M9820/3) 204.9 ☑
  - acute (M9821/3) 204.0 ☑
  - aleukemic (M9824/3) 204.8 ☑
  - chronic (M9823/3) 204.1 ☑
  - subacute (M9822/3) 204.2 ☑
  - subleukemic (M9824/3) 204.8 ☑
- lymphogenous (M9820/3) — *see* Leukemia, lymphoid
- lymphoid (M9820/3) 204.9 ☑
  - acute (M9821/3) 204.0 ☑
  - aleukemic (M9824/3) 204.8 ☑
  - blastic (M9821/3) 204.0 ☑
  - chronic (M9823/3) 204.1 ☑
  - subacute (M9822/3) 204.2 ☑
  - subleukemic (M9824/3) 204.8 ☑
- lymphosarcoma cell (M9850/3) 207.8 ☑
- mast cell (M9900/3) 207.8 ☑
- megakaryocytic (M9910/3) 207.2 ☑
- megakaryocytoid (M9910/3) 207.2 ☑
- mixed (cell) (M9810/3) 207.8 ☑
- monoblastic (M9891/3) 206.0 ☑
- monocytic (Schilling-type) (M9890/3) 206.9 ☑
  - acute (M9891/3) 206.0 ☑
  - aleukemic (M9894/3) 206.8 ☑
  - chronic (M9893/3) 206.1 ☑
  - Naegeli-type (M9863/3) 205.1 ☑
  - subacute (M9892/3) 206.2 ☑
  - subleukemic (M9894/3) 206.8 ☑
- monocytoid (M9890/3) 206.9 ☑
  - acute (M9891/3) 206.0 ☑
  - aleukemic (M9894/3) 206.8 ☑
  - chronic (M9893/3) 206.1 ☑
  - myelogenous (M9863/3) 205.1 ☑
  - subacute (M9892/3) 206.2 ☑
  - subleukemic (M9894/3) 206.8 ☑
- monomyelocytic (M9860/3) — *see* Leukemia, myelomonocytic
- myeloblastic (M9861/3) 205.0 ☑
- myelocytic (M9863/3) 205.1 ☑
  - acute (M9861/3) 205.0 ☑
- myelogenous (M9860/3) 205.9 ☑
  - acute (M9861/3) 205.0 ☑
  - aleukemic (M9864/3) 205.8 ☑
  - chronic (M9863/3) 205.1 ☑
  - monocytoid (M9863/3) 205.1 ☑
  - subacute (M9862/3) 205.2 ☑
  - subleukemic (M9864) 205.8 ☑
- myeloid (M9860/3) 205.9 ☑
  - acute (M9861/3) 205.0 ☑
  - aleukemic (M9864/3) 205.8 ☑
  - chronic (M9863/3) 205.1 ☑
  - subacute (M9862/3) 205.2 ☑
  - subleukemic (M9864/3) 205.8 ☑
- myelomonocytic (M9860/3) 205.9 ☑
  - acute (M9861/3) 205.0 ☑
  - chronic (M9863/3) 205.1 ☑
- Naegeli-type monocytic (M9863/3) 205.1 ☑
- neutrophilic (M9865/3) 205.1 ☑
- plasma cell (M9830/3) 203.1 ☑
- plasmacytic (M9830/3) 203.1 ☑
- prolymphocytic (M9825/3) — *see* Leukemia, lymphoid
- promyelocytic, acute (M9866/3) 205.0 ☑
- Schilling-type monocytic (M9890/3) — *see* Leukemia, monocytic
- stem cell (M9801/3) 208.0 ☑
- subacute NEC (M9802/3) 208.2 ☑
- subleukemic NEC (M9804/3) 208.8 ☑
- thrombocytic (M9910/3) 207.2 ☑
- undifferentiated (M9801/3) 208.0 ☑

Leukemoid reaction (lymphocytic) (monocytic) (myelocytic) 288.8

Leukoclastic vasculitis 446.29

Leukocoria 360.44

Leukocythemia — *see* Leukemia

Leukocytosis 288.8
- basophilic 288.8
- eosinophilic 288.3
- lymphocytic 288.8
- monocytic 288.8
- neutrophilic 288.8

Leukoderma 709.09
- syphilitic 091.3
  - late 095.8

Leukodermia (*see also* Leukoderma) 709.09

Leukodystrophy (cerebral) (globoid cell) (metachromatic) (progressive) (sudanophilic) 330.0

Leukoedema, mouth or tongue 528.79

Leukoencephalitis
- acute hemorrhagic (postinfectious) NEC 136.9 *[323.6]*
  - postimmunization or postvaccinal 323.5
- subacute sclerosing 046.2
  - van Bogaert's 046.2
- van Bogaert's (sclerosing) 046.2

Leukoencephalopathy (*see also* Encephalitis) 323.9
- acute necrotizing hemorrhagic (postinfectious) 136.9 *[323.6]*
  - postimmunization or postvaccinal 323.5
- metachromatic 330.0
- multifocal (progressive) 046.3
- progressive multifocal 046.3

- **Leukoerythroblastosis** 289.0
- **Leukoerythrosis** 289.0
- **Leukokeratosis** (*see also* Leukoplakia) 702.8
  - mouth 528.6
  - nicotina palati 528.79
  - tongue 528.6
- **Leukokoria** 360.44
- **Leukokraurosis vulva, vulvae** 624.0
- **Leukolymphosarcoma** (M9850/3) 207.8 ☑
- **Leukoma** (cornea) (interfering with central vision) 371.03
  - adherent 371.04
- **Leukomalacia, periventricular** 779.7
- **Leukomelanopathy, hereditary** 288.2
- **Leukonychia** (punctata) (striata) 703.8
  - congenital 757.5
- **Leukopathia**
  - unguium 703.8
    - congenital 757.5
- **Leukopenia** 288.0
  - cyclic 288.0
  - familial 288.0
  - malignant 288.0
  - periodic 288.0
  - transitory neonatal 776.7
- **Leukopenic** — *see* condition
- **Leukoplakia** 702.8
  - anus 569.49
  - bladder (postinfectional) 596.8
  - buccal 528.6
  - cervix (uteri) 622.2
  - esophagus 530.83
  - gingiva 528.6
  - kidney (pelvis) 593.89
  - larynx 478.79
  - lip 528.6
  - mouth 528.6
  - oral soft tissue (including tongue) (mucosa) 528.6
  - palate 528.6
  - pelvis (kidney) 593.89
  - penis (infectional) 607.0
  - rectum 569.49
  - syphilitic 095.8
  - tongue 528.6
  - tonsil 478.29
  - ureter (postinfectional) 593.89
  - urethra (postinfectional) 599.84
  - uterus 621.8
  - vagina 623.1
  - vesical 596.8
  - vocal cords 478.5
  - vulva 624.0
- **Leukopolioencephalopathy** 330.0
- **Leukorrhea** (vagina) 623.5
  - due to Trichomonas (vaginalis) 131.00
  - trichomonal (Trichomonas vaginalis) 131.00
- **Leukosarcoma** (M9850/3) 207.8 ☑
- **Leukosis** (M9800/3) — *see* Leukemia
- **Lev's disease or syndrome** (acquired complete heart block) 426.0
- **Levi's syndrome** (pituitary dwarfism) 253.3
- **Levocardia** (isolated) 746.87
  - with situs inversus 759.3
- **Levulosuria** 271.2
- **Lewandowski's disease** (primary) (*see also* Tuberculosis) 017.0 ☑
- **Lewandowski-Lutz disease** (epidermodysplasia verruciformis) 078.19
- **Lewy body dementia** 331.82
- **Lewy body disease** 331.82
- **Leyden's disease** (periodic vomiting) 536.2
- **Leyden-Möbius dystrophy** 359.1
- **Leydig cell**
  - carcinoma (M8650/3)
    - specified site — *see* Neoplasm, by site, malignant
    - unspecified site
      - female 183.0
      - male 186.9
- **Leydig cell** — *continued*
  - tumor (M8650/1)
    - benign (M8650/0)
      - specified site — *see* Neoplasm, by site, benign
      - unspecified site
        - female 220
        - male 222.0
    - malignant (M8650/3)
      - specified site — *see* Neoplasm, by site, malignant
      - unspecified site
        - female 183.0
        - male 186.9
    - specified site — *see* Neoplasm, by site, uncertain behavior
    - unspecified site
      - female 236.2
      - male 236.4
- **Leydig-Sertoli cell tumor** (M8631/0)
  - specified site — *see* Neoplasm, by site, benign
  - unspecified site
    - female 220
    - male 222.0
- **LGSIL** (low grade squamous intraepithelial lesion) 795.03
- **Liar, pathologic** 301.7
- **Libman-Sacks disease or syndrome** 710.0 *[424.91]*
- **Lice** (infestation) 132.9
  - body (pediculus corporis) 132.1
  - crab 132.2
  - head (pediculus capitis) 132.0
  - mixed (classifiable to more than one of the categories 132.0-132.2) 132.3
  - pubic (pediculus pubis) 132.2
- **Lichen** 697.9
  - albus 701.0
  - annularis 695.89
  - atrophicus 701.0
  - corneus obtusus 698.3
  - myxedematous 701.8
  - nitidus 697.1
  - pilaris 757.39
    - acquired 701.1
  - planopilaris 697.0
  - planus (acute) (chronicus) (hypertrophic) (verrucous) 697.0
    - morphoeicus 701.0
    - sclerosus (et atrophicus) 701.0
  - ruber 696.4
    - acuminatus 696.4
    - moniliformis 697.8
    - obtusus corneus 698.3
    - of Wilson 697.0
    - planus 697.0
  - sclerosus (et atrophicus) 701.0
  - scrofulosus (primary) (*see also* Tuberculosis) 017.0 ☑
  - simplex (Vidal's) 698.3
    - chronicus 698.3
    - circumscriptus 698.3
  - spinulosus 757.39
    - mycotic 117.9
  - striata 697.8
  - urticatus 698.2
- **Lichenification** 698.3
  - nodular 698.3
- **Lichenoides tuberculosis** (primary) (*see also* Tuberculosis) 017.0 ☑
- **Lichtheim's disease or syndrome** (subacute combined sclerosis with pernicious anemia) 281.0 *[336.2]*
- **Lien migrans** 289.59
- **Lientery** (*see also* Diarrhea) 787.91
  - infectious 009.2
- **Life circumstance problem** NEC V62.89
- **Li-Fraumeni cancer syndrome** V84.01
- **Ligament** — *see* condition
- **Light-for-dates** (infant) 764.0 ☑
  - with signs of fetal malnutrition 764.1 ☑
  - affecting management of pregnancy 656.5 ☑
- **Light-headedness** 780.4
- **Lightning** (effects) (shock) (stroke) (struck by) 994.0
  - burn — *see* Burn, by site
  - foot 266.2
- **Lightwood's disease or syndrome** (renal tubular acidosis) 588.89
- **Lignac's disease** (cystinosis) 270.0
- **Lignac (-de Toni) (-Fanconi) (-Debré) syndrome** (cystinosis) 270.0
- **Lignac (-Fanconi) syndrome** (cystinosis) 270.0
- **Ligneous thyroiditis** 245.3
- **Likoff's syndrome** (angina in menopausal women) 413.9
- **Limb** — *see* condition
- **Limitation of joint motion** (*see also* Stiffness, joint) 719.5 ☑
  - sacroiliac 724.6
- **Limit dextrinosis** 271.0
- **Limited**
  - cardiac reserve — *see* Disease, heart
  - duction, eye NEC 378.63
  - mandibular range of motion 524.52
- **Lindau's disease** (retinocerebral angiomatosis) 759.6
- **Lindau (-von Hippel) disease** (angiomatosis retinocerebellosa) 759.6
- **Linea corneae senilis** 371.41
- **Lines**
  - Beau's (transverse furrows on fingernails) 703.8
  - Harris' 733.91
  - Hudson-Stähli 371.11
  - Stähli's 371.11
- **Lingua**
  - geographical 529.1
  - nigra (villosa) 529.3
  - plicata 529.5
    - congenital 750.13
  - tylosis 528.6
- **Lingual** (tongue) — *see* also condition
  - thyroid 759.2
- **Linitis** (gastric) 535.4 ☑
  - plastica (M8142/3) 151.9
- **Lioderma essentialis** (cum melanosis et telangiectasia) 757.33
- **Lip** — *see also* condition
  - biting 528.9
- **Lipalgia** 272.8
- **Lipedema** — *see* Edema
- **Lipemia** (*see also* Hyperlipidemia) 272.4
  - retina, retinalis 272.3
- **Lipidosis** 272.7
  - cephalin 272.7
  - cerebral (infantile) (juvenile) (late) 330.1
  - cerebroretinal 330.1 *[362.71]*
  - cerebroside 272.7
  - cerebrospinal 272.7
  - chemically-induced 272.7
  - cholesterol 272.7
  - diabetic 250.8 ☑ *[272.7]*
  - dystopic (hereditary) 272.7
  - glycolipid 272.7
  - hepatosplenomegalic 272.3
  - hereditary, dystopic 272.7
  - sulfatide 330.0
- **Lipoadenoma** (M8324/0) — *see* Neoplasm, by site, benign
- **Lipoblastoma** (M8881/0) — *see* Lipoma, by site
- **Lipoblastomatosis** (M8881/0) — *see* Lipoma, by site
- **Lipochondrodystrophy** 277.5
- **Lipochrome histiocytosis** (familial) 288.1
- **Lipodystrophia progressiva** 272.6
- **Lipodystrophy** (progressive) 272.6
  - insulin 272.6
  - intestinal 040.2
  - mesenteric 567.82 ●
- **Lipofibroma** (M8851/0) — *see* Lipoma, by site
- **Lipoglycoproteinosis** 272.8
- **Lipogranuloma, sclerosing** 709.8

☑ Additional Digit Required — Refer to the Tabular List (Numeric Code Section) for Additional Digit Selection

▶◀ Revised Text ● New Line ▲ Revised Code

- **Loss** — *continued*
  - extremity or member, traumatic, current — *see* Amputation, traumatic
  - fluid (acute) 276.50 ▲
    - with
      - hypernatremia 276.0
      - hyponatremia 276.1
    - fetus or newborn 775.5
  - hair 704.00
  - hearing — *see also* Deafness
    - central 389.14
    - conductive (air) 389.00
      - with sensorineural hearing loss 389.2
      - combined types 389.08
      - external ear 389.01
      - inner ear 389.04
      - middle ear 389.03
      - multiple types 389.08
      - tympanic membrane 389.02
    - mixed type 389.2
    - nerve 389.12
    - neural 389.12
    - noise-induced 388.12
    - perceptive NEC (*see also* Loss, hearing, sensorineural) 389.10
    - sensorineural 389.10
      - with conductive hearing loss 389.2
      - central 389.14
      - combined types 389.18
      - multiple types 389.18
      - neural 389.12
      - sensory 389.11
    - sensory 389.11
    - specified type NEC 389.8
    - sudden NEC 388.2
  - height 781.91
  - labyrinthine reactivity (unilateral) 386.55
    - bilateral 386.56
  - memory (*see also* Amnesia) 780.93
    - mild, following organic brain damage 310.1
  - mind (*see also* Psychosis) 298.9
  - occlusal vertical dimension 524.37
  - organ or part — *see* Absence, by site, acquired
  - sensation 782.0
  - sense of
    - smell (*see also* Disturbance, sensation) 781.1
    - taste (*see also* Disturbance, sensation) 781.1
    - touch (*see also* Disturbance, sensation) 781.1
  - sight (acquired) (complete) (congenital) — *see* Blindness
  - spinal fluid
    - headache 349.0
  - substance of
    - bone (*see also* Osteoporosis) 733.00
    - cartilage 733.99
      - ear 380.32
    - vitreous (humor) 379.26
  - tooth, teeth
    - acquired 525.10
      - due to
        - caries 525.13
        - extraction 525.10
        - periodontal disease 525.12
        - specified NEC 525.19
        - trauma 525.11
  - vision, visual (*see also* Blindness) 369.9
    - both eyes (*see also* Blindness, both eyes) 369.3
    - complete (*see also* Blindness, both eyes) 369.00
    - one eye 369.8
    - sudden 368.11
    - transient 368.12
  - vitreous 379.26
  - voice (*see also* Aphonia) 784.41
  - weight (cause unknown) 783.21
- **Lou Gehrig's disease** 335.20
- **Louis-Bar syndrome** (ataxia-telangiectasia) 334.8
- **Louping ill** 063.1
- **Lousiness** — *see* Lice
- **Low**
  - back syndrome 724.2
  - basal metabolic rate (BMR) 794.7
  - birthweight 765.1 ☑
- **Low** — *continued*
  - birthweight — *continued*
    - extreme (less than 1000 grams) 765.0 ☑
    - for gestational age 764.0 ☑
    - status (*see also* Status, low birth weight) V21.30
  - bladder compliance 596.52
  - blood pressure (*see also* Hypotension) 458.9
    - reading (incidental) (isolated) (nonspecific) 796.3
  - cardiac reserve — *see* Disease, heart
  - compliance bladder 596.52
  - frequency deafness — *see* Disorder, hearing
  - function — *see also* Hypofunction
    - kidney (*see also* Disease, renal) 593.9
    - liver 573.9
  - hemoglobin 285.9
  - implantation, placenta — *see* Placenta, previa
  - insertion, placenta — *see* Placenta, previa
  - lying
    - kidney 593.0
    - organ or site, congenital — *see* Malposition, congenital
    - placenta — *see* Placenta, previa
  - output syndrome (cardiac) (*see also* Failure, heart) 428.9
  - platelets (blood) (*see also* Thrombocytopenia) 287.5
  - reserve, kidney (*see also* Disease, renal) 593.9
  - risk
    - cervical, human papillomavirus (HPV) DNA test positive 795.09
  - salt syndrome 593.9
  - tension glaucoma 365.12
  - vision 369.9
    - both eyes 369.20
    - one eye 369.70
- **Lowe (-Terrey-MacLachlan) syndrome** (oculocerebrorenal dystrophy) 270.8
- **Lower extremity** — *see* condition
- **Lown (-Ganong) -Levine syndrome** (short P-R interval, normal QRS complex, and paroxysmal supraventricular tachycardia) 426.81
- **LSD reaction** (*see also* Abuse, drugs, nondependent) 305.3 ☑
- **L-shaped kidney** 753.3
- **Lucas-Championnière disease** (fibrinous bronchitis) 466.0
- **Lucey-Driscoll syndrome** (jaundice due to delayed conjugation) 774.30
- **Ludwig's**
  - angina 528.3
  - disease (submaxillary cellulitis) 528.3
- **Lues** (venerea), **luetic** — *see* Syphilis
- **Luetscher's syndrome** (dehydration) 276.51 ▲
- **Lumbago** 724.2
  - due to displacement, intervertebral disc 722.10
- **Lumbalgia** 724.2
  - due to displacement, intervertebral disc 722.10
- **Lumbar** — *see* condition
- **Lumbarization, vertebra** 756.15
- **Lumbermen's itch** 133.8
- **Lump** — *see also* Mass
  - abdominal 789.3 ☑
  - breast 611.72
  - chest 786.6
  - epigastric 789.3 ☑
  - head 784.2
  - kidney 753.3
  - liver 789.1
  - lung 786.6
  - mediastinal 786.6
  - neck 784.2
  - nose or sinus 784.2
  - pelvic 789.3 ☑
  - skin 782.2
  - substernal 786.6
  - throat 784.2
  - umbilicus 789.3 ☑
- **Lunacy** (*see also* Psychosis) 298.9
- **Lunatomalacia** 732.3
- **Lung** — *see also* condition
  - donor V59.8
  - drug addict's 417.8
  - mainliners' 417.8
  - vanishing 492.0
- **Lupoid** (miliary) **of Boeck** 135
- **Lupus** 710.0
  - anticoagulant 289.81
  - Cazenave's (erythematosus) 695.4
  - discoid (local) 695.4
  - disseminated 710.0
  - erythematodes (discoid) (local) 695.4
  - erythematosus (discoid) (local) 695.4
    - disseminated 710.0
    - eyelid 373.34
    - systemic 710.0
      - with
        - encephalitis 710.0 *[323.8]*
        - lung involvement 710.0 *[517.8]*
      - inhibitor (presence of) 286.5
  - exedens 017.0 ☑
  - eyelid (*see also* Tuberculosis) 017.0 ☑ *[373.4]*
  - Hilliard's 017.0 ☑
  - hydralazine
    - correct substance properly administered 695.4
    - overdose or wrong substance given or taken 972.6
  - miliaris disseminatus faciei 017.0 ☑
  - nephritis 710.0 *[583.81]*
    - acute 710.0 *[580.81]*
    - chronic 710.0 *[582.81]*
  - nontuberculous, not disseminated 695.4
  - pernio (Besnier) 135
  - tuberculous (*see also* Tuberculosis) 017.0 ☑
    - eyelid (*see also* Tuberculosis) 017.0 ☑ *[373.4]*
  - vulgaris 017.0 ☑
- **Luschka's joint disease** 721.90
- **Luteinoma** (M8610/0) 220
- **Lutembacher's disease or syndrome** (atrial septal defect with mitral stenosis) 745.5
- **Luteoma** (M8610/0) 220
- **Lutz-Miescher disease** (elastosis perforans serpiginosa) 701.1
- **Lutz-Splendore-de Almeida disease** (Brazilian blastomycosis) 116.1
- **Luxatio**
  - bulbi due to birth injury 767.8
  - coxae congenita (*see also* Dislocation, hip, congenital) 754.30
  - erecta — *see* Dislocation, shoulder
  - imperfecta — *see* Sprain, by site
  - perinealis — *see* Dislocation, hip
- **Luxation** — *see also* Dislocation, by site
  - eyeball 360.81
    - due to birth injury 767.8
    - lateral 376.36
  - genital organs (external) NEC — *see* Wound, open, genital organs
  - globe (eye) 360.81
    - lateral 376.36
  - lacrimal gland (postinfectional) 375.16
  - lens (old) (partial) 379.32
    - congenital 743.37
      - syphilitic 090.49 *[379.32]*
    - Marfan's disease 090.49
    - spontaneous 379.32
  - penis — *see* Wound, open, penis
  - scrotum — *see* Wound, open, scrotum
  - testis — *see* Wound, open, testis
- **L-xyloketosuria** 271.8
- **Lycanthropy** (*see also* Psychosis) 298.9
- **Lyell's disease or syndrome** (toxic epidermal necrolysis) 695.1
  - due to drug
    - correct substance properly administered 695.1
    - overdose or wrong substance given or taken 977.9
      - specified drug — *see* Table of Drugs and Chemicals
- **Lyme disease** 088.81

- **Lymphoma** — *continued*
  - lymphocytic-histiocytic, mixed (diffuse) (M9613/3) 200.8 ☑
    - follicular (M9691/3) 202.0 ☑
    - nodular (M9691/3) 202.0 ☑
  - lymphoplasmacytoid type (M9611/3) 200.8 ☑
  - lymphosarcoma type (M9610/3) 200.1 ☑
  - macrofollicular (M9690/3) 202.0 ☑
  - mixed cell type (diffuse) (M9613/3) 200.8 ☑
    - follicular (M9691/3) 202.0 ☑
    - nodular (M9691/3) 202.0 ☑
  - nodular (M9690/3) 202.0 ☑
    - histiocytic (M9642/3) 200.0 ☑
    - lymphocytic (M9690/3) 202.0 ☑
      - intermediate differentiation (M9694/3) 202.0 ☑
      - poorly differentiated (M9696/3) 202.0 ☑
    - mixed (cell type) (lymphocytic-histiocytic) (small cell and large cell) (M9691/3) 202.0 ☑
  - non-Hodgkin's type NEC (M9591/3) 202.8 ☑
  - reticulum cell (type) (M9640/3) 200.0 ☑
  - small cell and large cell, mixed (diffuse) (M9613/3) 200.8 ☑
    - follicular (M9691/3) 202.0 ☑
    - nodular (9691/3) 202.0 ☑
  - stem cell (type) (M9601/3) 202.8 ☑
  - T-cell 202.1 ☑
  - undifferentiated (cell type) (non-Burkitt's) (M9600/3) 202.8 ☑
    - Burkitt's type (M9750/3) 200.2 ☑
- **Lymphomatosis** (M9590/3) — *see also* Lymphoma
  - granulomatous 099.1
- **Lymphopathia**
  - venereum 099.1
  - veneris 099.1
- **Lymphopenia** 288.8
  - familial 279.2
- **Lymphoreticulosis, benign** (of inoculation) 078.3
- **Lymphorrhea** 457.8
- **Lymphosarcoma** (M9610/3) 200.1 ☑
  - diffuse (M9610/3) 200.1 ☑
    - with plasmacytoid differentiation (M9611/3) 200.8 ☑
    - lymphoplasmacytic (M9611/3) 200.8 ☑
  - follicular (giant) (M9690/3) 202.0 ☑
    - lymphoblastic (M9696/3) 202.0 ☑
    - lymphocytic, intermediate differentiation (M9694/3) 202.0 ☑
    - mixed cell type (M9691/3) 202.0 ☑
  - giant follicular (M9690/3) 202.0 ☑
  - Hodgkin's (M9650/3) 201.9 ☑
  - immunoblastic (M9612/3) 200.8 ☑
  - lymphoblastic (diffuse) (M9630/3) 200.1 ☑
    - follicular (M9696/3) 202.0 ☑
    - nodular (M9696/3) 202.0 ☑
  - lymphocytic (diffuse) (M9620/3) 200.1 ☑
    - intermediate differentiation (diffuse) (M9621/3) 200.1 ☑
      - follicular (M9694/3) 202.0 ☑
      - nodular (M9694/3) 202.0 ☑
  - mixed cell type (diffuse) (M9613/3) 200.8 ☑
    - follicular (M9691/3) 202.0 ☑
    - nodular (M9691/3) 202.0 ☑
  - nodular (M9690/3) 202.0 ☑
    - lymphoblastic (M9696/3) 202.0 ☑
    - lymphocytic, intermediate differentiation (M9694/3) 202.0 ☑
    - mixed cell type (M9691/3) 202.0 ☑
  - prolymphocytic (M9631/3) 200.1 ☑
  - reticulum cell (M9640/3) 200.0 ☑
- **Lymphostasis** 457.8
- **Lypemania** (*see also* Melancholia) 296.2 ☑
- **Lyssa** 071

M

- **Macacus ear** 744.29
- **Maceration**
  - fetus (cause not stated) 779.9
  - wet feet, tropical (syndrome) 991.4
- **Machado-Joseph disease** 334.8
- **Machupo virus hemorrhagic fever** 078.7
- **Macleod's syndrome** (abnormal transradiancy, one lung) 492.8
- **Macrocephalia, macrocephaly** 756.0
- **Macrocheilia** (congenital) 744.81
- **Macrochilia** (congenital) 744.81
- **Macrocolon** (congenital) 751.3
- **Macrocornea** 743.41
  - associated with buphthalmos 743.22
- **Macrocytic** — *see* condition
- **Macrocytosis** 289.89
- **Macrodactylia, macrodactylism** (fingers) (thumbs) 755.57
  - toes 755.65
- **Macrodontia** 520.2
- **Macroencephaly** 742.4
- **Macrogenia** 524.05
- **Macrogenitosomia** (female) (male) (praecox) 255.2
- **Macrogingivae** 523.8
- **Macroglobulinemia** (essential) (idiopathic) (monoclonal) (primary) (syndrome) (Waldenström's) 273.3
- **Macroglossia** (congenital) 750.15
  - acquired 529.8
- **Macrognathia, macrognathism** (congenital) 524.00
  - mandibular 524.02
    - alveolar 524.72
  - maxillary 524.01
    - alveolar 524.71
- **Macrogyria** (congenital) 742.4
- **Macrohydrocephalus** (*see also* Hydrocephalus) 331.4
- **Macromastia** (*see also* Hypertrophy, breast) 611.1
- **Macropsia** 368.14
- **Macrosigmoid** 564.7
  - congenital 751.3
- **Macrospondylitis, acromegalic** 253.0
- **Macrostomia** (congenital) 744.83
- **Macrotia** (external ear) (congenital) 744.22
- **Macula**
  - cornea, corneal
    - congenital 743.43
      - interfering with vision 743.42
    - interfering with central vision 371.03
    - not interfering with central vision 371.02
  - degeneration (*see also* Degeneration, macula) 362.50
    - hereditary (*see also* Dystrophy, retina) 362.70
  - edema, cystoid 362.53
- **Maculae ceruleae** 132.1
- **Macules and papules** 709.8
- **Maculopathy, toxic** 362.55
- **Madarosis** 374.55
- **Madelung's**
  - deformity (radius) 755.54
  - disease (lipomatosis) 272.8
  - lipomatosis 272.8
- **Madness** (*see also* Psychosis) 298.9
  - myxedema (acute) 293.0
    - subacute 293.1
- **Madura**
  - disease (actinomycotic) 039.9
    - mycotic 117.4
  - foot (actinomycotic) 039.4
    - mycotic 117.4
- **Maduromycosis** (actinomycotic) 039.9
  - mycotic 117.4
- **Maffucci's syndrome** (dyschondroplasia with hemangiomas) 756.4
- **Magenblase syndrome** 306.4
- **Main en griffe** (acquired) 736.06
  - congenital 755.59
- **Maintenance**
  - chemotherapy regimen or treatment V58.11 ▲
  - dialysis regimen or treatment
    - extracorporeal (renal) V56.0
    - peritoneal V56.8
    - renal V56.0
- **Maintenance** — *continued*
  - drug therapy or regimen
    - chemotherapy, antineoplastic V58.11 ●
    - immunotherapy, antineoplastic V58.12 ●
  - external fixation NEC V54.89
  - radiotherapy V58.0
  - traction NEC V54.89
- **Majocchi's**
  - disease (purpura annularis telangiectodes) 709.1
  - granuloma 110.6
- **Major** — *see* condition
- **Mal**
  - cerebral (idiopathic) (*see also* Epilepsy) 345.9 ☑
  - comital (*see also* Epilepsy) 345.9 ☑
  - de los pintos (*see also* Pinta) 103.9
  - de Meleda 757.39
  - de mer 994.6
  - lie — *see* Presentation, fetal
  - perforant (*see also* Ulcer, lower extremity) 707.15
- **Malabar itch** 110.9
  - beard 110.0
  - foot 110.4
  - scalp 110.0
- **Malabsorption** 579.9
  - calcium 579.8
  - carbohydrate 579.8
  - disaccharide 271.3
  - drug-induced 579.8
  - due to bacterial overgrowth 579.8
  - fat 579.8
  - folate, congenital 281.2
  - galactose 271.1
  - glucose-galactose (congenital) 271.3
  - intestinal 579.9
  - isomaltose 271.3
  - lactose (hereditary) 271.3
  - methionine 270.4
  - monosaccharide 271.8
  - postgastrectomy 579.3
  - postsurgical 579.3
  - protein 579.8
  - sucrose (-isomaltose) (congenital) 271.3
  - syndrome 579.9
    - postgastrectomy 579.3
    - postsurgical 579.3
- **Malacia, bone** 268.2
  - juvenile (*see also* Rickets) 268.0
  - Kienböck's (juvenile) (lunate) (wrist) 732.3
    - adult 732.8
- **Malacoplakia**
  - bladder 596.8
  - colon 569.89
  - pelvis (kidney) 593.89
  - ureter 593.89
  - urethra 599.84
- **Malacosteon** 268.2
  - juvenile (*see also* Rickets) 268.0
- **Maladaptation** — *see* Maladjustment
- **Maladie de Roger** 745.4
- **Maladjustment**
  - conjugal V61.10
    - involving divorce or estrangement V61.0
  - educational V62.3
  - family V61.9
    - specified circumstance NEC V61.8
  - marital V61.10
    - involving divorce or estrangement V61.0
  - occupational V62.2
  - simple, adult (*see also* Reaction, adjustment) 309.9
  - situational acute (*see also* Reaction, adjustment) 309.9
  - social V62.4
- **Malaise** 780.79
- **Malakoplakia** — *see* Malacoplakia
- **Malaria, malarial** (fever) 084.6
  - algid 084.9
  - any type, with
    - algid malaria 084.9
    - blackwater fever 084.8

Malaria, malarial — *continued*
- any type, with — *continued*
  - fever
    - blackwater 084.8
    - hemoglobinuric (bilious) 084.8
  - hemoglobinuria, malarial 084.8
  - hepatitis 084.9 *[573.2]*
  - nephrosis 084.9 *[581.81]*
  - pernicious complication NEC 084.9
    - cardiac 084.9
    - cerebral 084.9
- cardiac 084.9
- carrier (suspected) of V02.9
- cerebral 084.9
- complicating pregnancy, childbirth, or puerperium 647.4 ☑
- congenital 771.2
- congestion, congestive 084.6
  - brain 084.9
- continued 084.0
- estivo-autumnal 084.0
- falciparum (malignant tertian) 084.0
- hematinuria 084.8
- hematuria 084.8
- hemoglobinuria 084.8
- hemorrhagic 084.6
- induced (therapeutically) 084.7
  - accidental — *see* Malaria, by type
- liver 084.9 *[573.2]*
- malariae (quartan) 084.2
- malignant (tertian) 084.0
- mixed infections 084.5
- monkey 084.4
- ovale 084.3
- pernicious, acute 084.0
- Plasmodium, P.
  - falciparum 084.0
  - malariae 084.2
  - ovale 084.3
  - vivax 084.1
- quartan 084.2
- quotidian 084.0
- recurrent 084.6
  - induced (therapeutically) 084.7
    - accidental — *see* Malaria, by type
- remittent 084.6
- specified types NEC 084.4
- spleen 084.6
- subtertian 084.0
- tertian (benign) 084.1
  - malignant 084.0
- tropical 084.0
- typhoid 084.6
- vivax (benign tertian) 084.1

Malassez's disease (testicular cyst) 608.89

Malassimilation 579.9

Maldescent, testis 752.51

Maldevelopment — *see also* Anomaly, by site
- brain 742.9
- colon 751.5
- hip (joint) 755.63
  - congenital dislocation (*see also* Dislocation, hip, congenital) 754.30
- mastoid process 756.0
- middle ear, except ossicles 744.03
  - ossicles 744.04
- newborn (not malformation) 764.9 ☑
- ossicles, ear 744.04
- spine 756.10
- toe 755.66

Male type pelvis 755.69
- with disproportion (fetopelvic) 653.2 ☑
  - affecting fetus or newborn 763.1
  - causing obstructed labor 660.1 ☑
    - affecting fetus or newborn 763.1

Malformation (congenital) — *see also* Anomaly
- bone 756.9
- bursa 756.9
- circulatory system NEC 747.9
  - specified type NEC 747.89
- Chiari
  - type I 348.4
  - type II (*see also* Spina bifida) 741.0 ☑
  - type III 742.0
  - type IV 742.2
- cochlea 744.05

Malformation — *see also* Anomaly — *continued*
- digestive system NEC 751.9
  - lower 751.5
  - specified type NEC 751.8
  - upper 750.9
- eye 743.9
- gum 750.9
- heart NEC 746.9
  - specified type NEC 746.89
  - valve 746.9
- internal ear 744.05
- joint NEC 755.9
  - specified type NEC 755.8
- Mondini's (congenital) (malformation, cochlea) 744.05
- muscle 756.9
- nervous system (central) 742.9
- pelvic organs or tissues
  - in pregnancy or childbirth 654.9 ☑
    - affecting fetus or newborn 763.89
    - causing obstructed labor 660.2 ☑
      - affecting fetus or newborn 763.1
- placenta (*see also* Placenta, abnormal) 656.7 ☑
- respiratory organs 748.9
  - specified type NEC 748.8
- Rieger's 743.44
- sense organs NEC 742.9
  - specified type NEC 742.8
- skin 757.9
  - specified type NEC 757.8
- spinal cord 742.9
- teeth, tooth NEC 520.9
- tendon 756.9
- throat 750.9
- umbilical cord (complicating delivery) 663.9 ☑
  - affecting fetus or newborn 762.6
- umbilicus 759.9
- urinary system NEC 753.9
  - specified type NEC 753.8

Malfunction — *see also* Dysfunction
- arterial graft 996.1
- cardiac pacemaker 996.01
- catheter device — *see* Complications, mechanical, catheter
- colostomy 569.62
- cystostomy 997.5
- device, implant, or graft NEC — *see* Complications, mechanical
- enteric stoma 569.62
- enterostomy 569.62
- esophagostomy 530.87
- gastroenteric 536.8
- gastrostomy 536.42
- nephrostomy 997.5
- pacemaker — *see* Complications, mechanical, pacemaker
- prosthetic device, internal — *see* Complications, mechanical
- tracheostomy 519.02
- vascular graft or shunt 996.1

Malgaigne's fracture (closed) 808.43
- open 808.53

Malherbe's
- calcifying epithelioma (M8110/0) — *see* Neoplasm, skin, benign
- tumor (M8110/0) — *see* Neoplasm, skin, benign

Malibu disease 919.8
- infected 919.9

Malignancy (M8000/3) — *see* Neoplasm, by site, malignant

Malignant — *see* condition

Malingerer, malingering V65.2

Mallet, finger (acquired) 736.1
- congenital 755.59
- late effect of rickets 268.1

Malleus 024

Mallory's bodies 034.1

Mallory-Weiss syndrome 530.7

Malnutrition (calorie) 263.9
- complicating pregnancy 648.9 ☑
- degree
  - first 263.1
  - second 263.0
  - third 262

Malnutrition — *continued*
- degree — *continued*
  - mild 263.1
  - moderate 263.0
  - severe 261
    - protein-calorie 262
- fetus 764.2 ☑
  - "light-for-dates" 764.1 ☑
- following gastrointestinal surgery 579.3
- intrauterine or fetal 764.2 ☑
  - fetus or infant "light-for-dates" 764.1 ☑
- lack of care, or neglect (child) (infant) 995.52
  - adult 995.84
- malignant 260
- mild 263.1
- moderate 263.0
- protein 260
- protein-calorie 263.9
  - severe 262
  - specified type NEC 263.8
- severe 261
  - protein-calorie NEC 262

Malocclusion (teeth) 524.4
- due to
  - abnormal swallowing 524.59
  - accessory teeth (causing crowding) 524.31
  - dentofacial abnormality NEC 524.89
  - impacted teeth (causing crowding) 520.6
  - missing teeth 524.30
  - mouth breathing 524.59
  - sleep postures 524.59
  - supernumerary teeth (causing crowding) 524.31
  - thumb sucking 524.59
  - tongue, lip, or finger habits 524.59
- temporomandibular (joint) 524.69

Malposition
- cardiac apex (congenital) 746.87
- cervix — *see* Malposition, uterus
- congenital
  - adrenal (gland) 759.1
  - alimentary tract 751.8
    - lower 751.5
    - upper 750.8
  - aorta 747.21
  - appendix 751.5
  - arterial trunk 747.29
  - artery (peripheral) NEC (*see also* Malposition, congenital, peripheral vascular system) 747.60
    - coronary 746.85
    - pulmonary 747.3
  - auditory canal 744.29
    - causing impairment of hearing 744.02
  - auricle (ear) 744.29
    - causing impairment of hearing 744.02
    - cervical 744.43
  - biliary duct or passage 751.69
  - bladder (mucosa) 753.8
    - exteriorized or extroverted 753.5
  - brachial plexus 742.8
  - brain tissue 742.4
  - breast 757.6
  - bronchus 748.3
  - cardiac apex 746.87
  - cecum 751.5
  - clavicle 755.51
  - colon 751.5
  - digestive organ or tract NEC 751.8
    - lower 751.5
    - upper 750.8
  - ear (auricle) (external) 744.29
    - ossicles 744.04
  - endocrine (gland) NEC 759.2
  - epiglottis 748.3
  - Eustachian tube 744.24
  - eye 743.8
  - facial features 744.89
  - fallopian tube 752.19
  - finger(s) 755.59
    - supernumerary 755.01
  - foot 755.67
  - gallbladder 751.69
  - gastrointestinal tract 751.8

- **Malposition** — *continued*
  - congenital — *continued*
    - genitalia, genital organ(s) or tract
      - female 752.89
        - external 752.49
        - internal NEC 752.89
      - male 752.89
        - penis 752.69
        - scrotal transposition 752.81
    - glottis 748.3
    - hand 755.59
    - heart 746.87
      - dextrocardia 746.87
        - with complete transposition of viscera 759.3
    - hepatic duct 751.69
    - hip (joint) (*see also* Dislocation, hip, congenital) 754.30
    - intestine (large) (small) 751.5
      - with anomalous adhesions, fixation, or malrotation 751.4
    - joint NEC 755.8
    - kidney 753.3
    - larynx 748.3
    - limb 755.8
      - lower 755.69
      - upper 755.59
    - liver 751.69
    - lung (lobe) 748.69
    - nail(s) 757.5
    - nerve 742.8
    - nervous system NEC 742.8
    - nose, nasal (septum) 748.1
    - organ or site NEC — *see* Anomaly, specified type NEC, by site
    - ovary 752.0
    - pancreas 751.7
    - parathyroid (gland) 759.2
    - patella 755.64
    - peripheral vascular system 747.60
      - gastrointestinal 747.61
      - lower limb 747.64
      - renal 747.62
      - specified NEC 747.69
      - spinal 747.82
      - upper limb 747.63
    - pituitary (gland) 759.2
    - respiratory organ or system NEC 748.9
    - rib (cage) 756.3
      - supernumerary in cervical region 756.2
    - scapula 755.59
    - shoulder 755.59
    - spinal cord 742.59
    - spine 756.19
    - spleen 759.0
    - sternum 756.3
    - stomach 750.7
    - symphysis pubis 755.69
    - testis (undescended) 752.51
    - thymus (gland) 759.2
    - thyroid (gland) (tissue) 759.2
      - cartilage 748.3
    - toe(s) 755.66
      - supernumerary 755.02
    - tongue 750.19
    - trachea 748.3
    - uterus 752.3
    - vein(s) (peripheral) NEC (*see also* Malposition, congenital, peripheral vascular system) 747.60
      - great 747.49
      - portal 747.49
      - pulmonary 747.49
    - vena cava (inferior) (superior) 747.49
  - device, implant, or graft — *see* Complications, mechanical
  - fetus NEC (*see also* Presentation, fetal) 652.9 ☑
    - with successful version 652.1 ☑
    - affecting fetus or newborn 763.1
    - before labor, affecting fetus or newborn 761.7
    - causing obstructed labor 660.0 ☑
    - in multiple gestation (one fetus or more) 652.6 ☑
      - with locking 660.5 ☑
      - causing obstructed labor 660.0 ☑

- **Malposition** — *continued*
  - gallbladder (*see also* Disease, gallbladder) 575.8
  - gastrointestinal tract 569.89
    - congenital 751.8
  - heart (*see also* Malposition, congenital, heart) 746.87
  - intestine 569.89
    - congenital 751.5
  - pelvic organs or tissues
    - in pregnancy or childbirth 654.4 ☑
      - affecting fetus or newborn 763.89
      - causing obstructed labor 660.2 ☑
        - affecting fetus or newborn 763.1
  - placenta — *see* Placenta, previa
  - stomach 537.89
    - congenital 750.7
  - tooth, teeth 524.30
    - with impaction 520.6
  - uterus or cervix (acquired) (acute) (adherent) (any degree) (asymptomatic) (postinfectional) (postpartal, old) 621.6
    - anteflexion or anteversion (*see also* Anteversion, uterus) 621.6
    - congenital 752.3
    - flexion 621.6
      - lateral (*see also* Lateroversion, uterus) 621.6
    - in pregnancy or childbirth 654.4 ☑
      - affecting fetus or newborn 763.89
      - causing obstructed labor 660.2 ☑
        - affecting fetus or newborn 763.1
    - inversion 621.6
    - lateral (flexion) (version) (*see also* Lateroversion, uterus) 621.6
    - lateroflexion (*see also* Lateroversion, uterus) 621.6
    - lateroversion (*see also* Lateroversion, uterus) 621.6
    - retroflexion or retroversion (*see also* Retroversion, uterus) 621.6
- **Malposture** 729.9
- **Malpresentation, fetus** (*see also* Presentation, fetal) 652.9 ☑
- **Malrotation**
  - cecum 751.4
  - colon 751.4
  - intestine 751.4
  - kidney 753.3
- **Malta fever** (*see also* Brucellosis) 023.9
- **Maltosuria** 271.3
- **Maltreatment** (of)
  - adult 995.80
    - emotional 995.82
    - multiple forms 995.85
    - neglect (nutritional) 995.84
    - physical 995.81
    - psychological 995.82
    - sexual 995.83
  - child 995.50
    - emotional 995.51
    - multiple forms 995.59
    - neglect (nutritional) 995.52
    - physical 995.54
      - shaken infant syndrome 995.55
    - psychological 995.51
    - sexual 995.53
  - spouse (*see also* Maltreatment, adult) 995.80
- **Malt workers' lung** 495.4
- **Malum coxae senilis** 715.25
- **Malunion, fracture** 733.81
- **Mammillitis** (*see also* Mastitis) 611.0
  - puerperal, postpartum 675.2 ☑
- **Mammitis** (*see also* Mastitis) 611.0
  - puerperal, postpartum 675.2 ☑
- **Mammographic microcalcification** 793.81
- **Mammoplasia** 611.1
- **Management**
  - contraceptive V25.9
    - specified type NEC V25.8
  - procreative V26.9
    - specified type NEC V26.8
- **Mangled** NEC (*see also* nature and site of injury) 959.9

- **Mania** (monopolar) (*see also* Psychosis, affective) 296.0 ☑
  - alcoholic (acute) (chronic) 291.9
  - Bell's — *see* Mania, chronic
  - chronic 296.0 ☑
    - recurrent episode 296.1 ☑
    - single episode 296.0 ☑
  - compulsive 300.3
  - delirious (acute) 296.0 ☑
    - recurrent episode 296.1 ☑
    - single episode 296.0 ☑
  - epileptic (*see also* Epilepsy) 345.4 ☑
  - hysterical 300.10
  - inhibited 296.89
  - puerperal (after delivery) 296.0 ☑
    - recurrent episode 296.1 ☑
    - single episode 296.0 ☑
  - recurrent episode 296.1 ☑
  - senile 290.8
  - single episode 296.0 ☑
  - stupor 296.89
  - stuporous 296.89
  - unproductive 296.89
- **Manic-depressive insanity, psychosis, reaction, or syndrome** (*see also* Psychosis, affective) 296.80
  - circular (alternating) 296.7
    - currently
      - depressed 296.5 ☑
      - episode unspecified 296.7
      - hypomanic, previously depressed 296.4 ☑
      - manic 296.4 ☑
    - mixed 296.6 ☑
  - depressed (type), depressive 296.2 ☑
    - atypical 296.82
    - recurrent episode 296.3 ☑
    - single episode 296.2 ☑
  - hypomanic 296.0 ☑
    - recurrent episode 296.1 ☑
    - single episode 296.0 ☑
  - manic 296.0 ☑
    - atypical 296.81
    - recurrent episode 296.1 ☑
    - single episode 296.0 ☑
  - mixed NEC 296.89
  - perplexed 296.89
  - stuporous 296.89
- **Manifestations, rheumatoid**
  - lungs 714.81
  - pannus — *see* Arthritis, rheumatoid
  - subcutaneous nodules — *see* Arthritis, rheumatoid
- **Mankowsky's syndrome** (familial dysplastic osteopathy) 731.2
- **Mannoheptulosuria** 271.8
- **Mannosidosis** 271.8
- **Manson's**
  - disease (schistosomiasis) 120.1
  - pyosis (pemphigus contagiosus) 684
  - schistosomiasis 120.1
- **Mansonellosis** 125.5
- **Manual** — *see* condition
- **Maple bark disease** 495.6
- **Maple bark-strippers' lung** 495.6
- **Maple syrup (urine) disease or syndrome** 270.3
- **Marable's syndrome** (celiac artery compression) 447.4
- **Marasmus** 261
  - brain 331.9
  - due to malnutrition 261
  - intestinal 569.89
  - nutritional 261
  - senile 797
  - tuberculous NEC (*see also* Tuberculosis) 011.9 ☑
- **Marble**
  - bones 756.52
  - skin 782.61
- **Marburg disease** (virus) 078.89
- **March**
  - foot 733.94
  - hemoglobinuria 283.2

Marchand multiple nodular hyperplasia (liver) 571.5

Marchesani (-Weill) syndrome (brachymorphism and ectopia lentis) 759.89

Marchiafava (-Bignami) disease or syndrome 341.8

Marchiafava-Micheli syndrome (paroxysmal nocturnal hemoglobinuria) 283.2

Marcus Gunn's syndrome (jaw-winking syndrome) 742.8

Marfan's
- congenital syphilis 090.49
- disease 090.49
- syndrome (arachnodactyly) 759.82
  - meaning congenital syphilis 090.49
    - with luxation of lens 090.49 *[379.32]*

Marginal
- implantation, placenta — *see* Placenta, previa
- placenta — *see* Placenta, previa
- sinus (hemorrhage) (rupture) 641.2 ☑
  - affecting fetus or newborn 762.1

Marie's
- cerebellar ataxia 334.2
- syndrome (acromegaly) 253.0

Marie-Bamberger disease or syndrome (hypertrophic) (pulmonary) (secondary) 731.2
- idiopathic (acropachyderma) 757.39
- primary (acropachyderma) 757.39

Marie-Charcôt-Tooth neuropathic atrophy, muscle 356.1

Marie-Strümpell arthritis or disease (ankylosing spondylitis) 720.0

Marihuana, marijuana
- abuse (*see also* Abuse, drugs, nondependent) 305.2 ☑
- dependence (*see also* Dependence) 304.3 ☑

Marion's disease (bladder neck obstruction) 596.0

Marital conflict V61.10

Mark
- port wine 757.32
- raspberry 757.32
- strawberry 757.32
- stretch 701.3
- tattoo 709.09

Maroteaux-Lamy syndrome (mucopolysaccharidosis VI) 277.5

Marriage license examination V70.3

Marrow (bone)
- arrest 284.9
- megakaryocytic 287.30 ▲
- poor function 289.9

Marseilles fever 082.1

Marsh's disease (exophthalmic goiter) 242.0 ☑

Marshall's (hidrotic) **ectodermal dysplasia** 757.31

Marsh fever (*see also* Malaria) 084.6

Martin's disease 715.27

Martin-Albright syndrome (pseudohypoparathyroidism) 275.49

Martorell-Fabre syndrome (pulseless disease) 446.7

Masculinization, female, with adrenal hyperplasia 255.2

Masculinovoblastoma (M8670/0) 220

Masochism 302.83

Masons' lung 502

Mass
- abdominal 789.3 ☑
- anus 787.99
- bone 733.90
- breast 611.72
- cheek 784.2
- chest 786.6
- cystic — *see* Cyst
- ear 388.8
- epigastric 789.3 ☑
- eye 379.92
- female genital organ 625.8
- gum 784.2

Mass — *continued*
- head 784.2
- intracranial 784.2
- joint 719.60
  - ankle 719.67
  - elbow 719.62
  - foot 719.67
  - hand 719.64
  - hip 719.65
  - knee 719.66
  - multiple sites 719.69
  - pelvic region 719.65
  - shoulder (region) 719.61
  - specified site NEC 719.68
  - wrist 719.63
- kidney (*see also* Disease, kidney) 593.9
- lung 786.6
- lymph node 785.6
- malignant (M8000/3) — *see* Neoplasm, by site, malignant
- mediastinal 786.6
- mouth 784.2
- muscle (limb) 729.89
- neck 784.2
- nose or sinus 784.2
- palate 784.2
- pelvis, pelvic 789.3 ☑
- penis 607.89
- perineum 625.8
- rectum 787.99
- scrotum 608.89
- skin 782.2
- specified organ NEC — *see* Disease of specified organ or site
- splenic 789.2
- substernal 786.6
  - thyroid (*see also* Goiter) 240.9
- superficial (localized) 782.2
- testes 608.89
- throat 784.2
- tongue 784.2
- umbilicus 789.3 ☑
- uterus 625.8
- vagina 625.8
- vulva 625.8

Massive — *see* condition

Mastalgia 611.71
- psychogenic 307.89

Mast cell
- disease 757.33
  - systemic (M9741/3) 202.6 ☑
- leukemia (M9900/3) 207.8 ☑
- sarcoma (M9742/3) 202.6 ☑
- tumor (M9740/1) 238.5
  - malignant (M9740/3) 202.6 ☑

Masters-Allen syndrome 620.6

Mastitis (acute) (adolescent) (diffuse) (interstitial) (lobular) (nonpuerperal) (nonsuppurative) (parenchymatous) (phlegmonous) (simple) (subacute) (suppurative) 611.0
- chronic (cystic) (fibrocystic) 610.1
- cystic 610.1
  - Schimmelbusch's type 610.1
- fibrocystic 610.1
- infective 611.0
- lactational 675.2 ☑
- lymphangitis 611.0
- neonatal (noninfective) 778.7
  - infective 771.5
- periductal 610.4
- plasma cell 610.4
- puerperal, postpartum, (interstitial) (nonpurulent) (parenchymatous) 675.2 ☑
  - purulent 675.1 ☑
  - stagnation 676.2 ☑
- puerperalis 675.2 ☑
- retromammary 611.0
  - puerperal, postpartum 675.1 ☑
- submammary 611.0
  - puerperal, postpartum 675.1 ☑

Mastocytoma (M9740/1) 238.5
- malignant (M9740/3) 202.6 ☑

Mastocytosis 757.33
- malignant (M9741/3) 202.6 ☑
- systemic (M9741/3) 202.6 ☑

Mastodynia 611.71
- psychogenic 307.89

Mastoid — *see* condition

Mastoidalgia (*see also* Otalgia) 388.70

Mastoiditis (coalescent) (hemorrhagic) (pneumococcal) (streptococcal) (suppurative) 383.9
- acute or subacute 383.00
  - with
    - Gradenigo's syndrome 383.02
    - petrositis 383.02
    - specified complication NEC 383.02
    - subperiosteal abscess 383.01
- chronic (necrotic) (recurrent) 383.1
- tuberculous (*see also* Tuberculosis) 015.6 ☑

Mastopathy, mastopathia 611.9
- chronica cystica 610.1
- diffuse cystic 610.1
- estrogenic 611.8
- ovarian origin 611.8

Mastoplasia 611.1

Masturbation 307.9

Maternal condition, affecting fetus or newborn
- acute yellow atrophy of liver 760.8
- albuminuria 760.1
- anesthesia or analgesia 763.5
- blood loss 762.1
- chorioamnionitis 762.7
- circulatory disease, chronic (conditions classifiable to 390-459, 745-747) 760.3
- congenital heart disease (conditions classifiable to 745-746) 760.3
- cortical necrosis of kidney 760.1
- death 761.6
- diabetes mellitus 775.0
  - manifest diabetes in the infant 775.1
- disease NEC 760.9
  - circulatory system, chronic (conditions classifiable to 390-459, 745-747) 760.3
  - genitourinary system (conditions classifiable to 580-599) 760.1
  - respiratory (conditions classifiable to 490-519, 748) 760.3
- eclampsia 760.0
- hemorrhage NEC 762.1
- hepatitis acute, malignant, or subacute 760.8
- hyperemesis (gravidarum) 761.8
- hypertension (arising during pregnancy) (conditions classifiable to 642) 760.0
- infection
  - disease classifiable to 001-136 760.2
  - genital tract NEC 760.8
  - urinary tract 760.1
- influenza 760.2
  - manifest influenza in the infant 771.2
- injury (conditions classifiable to 800-996) 760.5
- malaria 760.2
  - manifest malaria in infant or fetus 771.2
- malnutrition 760.4
- necrosis of liver 760.8
- nephritis (conditions classifiable to 580-583) 760.1
- nephrosis (conditions classifiable to 581) 760.1
- noxious substance transmitted via breast milk or placenta 760.70
  - alcohol 760.71
  - anticonvulsants 760.77 ●
  - antifungals 760.74 ●
  - anti-infective agents 760.74
  - antimetabolics 760.78 ●
  - cocaine 760.75
  - "crack" 760.75
  - diethylstilbestrol [DES] 760.76
  - hallucinogenic agents 760.73
  - medicinal agents NEC 760.79
  - narcotics 760.72
  - obstetric anesthetic or analgesic drug 760.72
  - specified agent NEC 760.79
- nutritional disorder (conditions classifiable to 260-269) 760.4
- operation unrelated to current delivery 760.6
- pre-eclampsia 760.0

Melanoblastosis
- Block-Sulzberger 757.33
- cutis linearis sive systematisata 757.33

Melanocarcinoma (M8720/3) — *see* Melanoma
Melanocytoma, eyeball (M8726/0) 224.0
Melanoderma, melanodermia 709.09
- Addison's (primary adrenal insufficiency) 255.4

Melanodontia, infantile 521.05
Melanodontoclasia 521.05
Melanoepithelioma (M8720/3) — *see* Melanoma
Melanoma (malignant) (M8720/3) 172.9

> *Note — Except where otherwise indicated, the morphological varieties of melanoma in the list below should be coded by site as for "Melanoma (malignant)". Internal sites should be coded to malignant neoplasm of those sites.*

- abdominal wall 172.5
- ala nasi 172.3
- amelanotic (M8730/3) — *see* Melanoma, by site
- ankle 172.7
- anus, anal 154.3
  - canal 154.2
- arm 172.6
- auditory canal (external) 172.2
- auricle (ear) 172.2
- auricular canal (external) 172.2
- axilla 172.5
- axillary fold 172.5
- back 172.5
- balloon cell (M8722/3) — *see* Melanoma, by site
- benign (M8720/0) — *see* Neoplasm, skin, benign
- breast (female) (male) 172.5
- brow 172.3
- buttock 172.5
- canthus (eye) 172.1
- cheek (external) 172.3
- chest wall 172.5
- chin 172.3
- choroid 190.6
- conjunctiva 190.3
- ear (external) 172.2
- epithelioid cell (M8771/3) — *see also* Melanoma, by site
  - and spindle cell, mixed (M8775/3) — *see* Melanoma, by site
- external meatus (ear) 172.2
- eye 190.9
- eyebrow 172.3
- eyelid (lower) (upper) 172.1
- face NEC 172.3
- female genital organ (external) NEC 184.4
- finger 172.6
- flank 172.5
- foot 172.7
- forearm 172.6
- forehead 172.3
- foreskin 187.1
- gluteal region 172.5
- groin 172.5
- hand 172.6
- heel 172.7
- helix 172.2
- hip 172.7
- in
  - giant pigmented nevus (M8761/3) — *see* Melanoma, by site
  - Hutchinson's melanotic freckle (M8742/3) — *see* Melanoma, by site
  - junctional nevus (M8740/3) — *see* Melanoma, by site
  - precancerous melanosis (M8741/3) — *see* Melanoma, by site
- interscapular region 172.5
- iris 190.0
- jaw 172.3
- juvenile (M8770/0) — *see* Neoplasm, skin, benign
- knee 172.7
- labium
  - majus 184.1
  - minus 184.2
- lacrimal gland 190.2
- leg 172.7
- lip (lower) (upper) 172.0
- liver 197.7
- lower limb NEC 172.7
- male genital organ (external) NEC 187.9
- meatus, acoustic (external) 172.2
- meibomian gland 172.1
- metastatic
  - of or from specified site — *see* Melanoma, by site
  - site not of skin — *see* Neoplasm, by site, malignant, secondary
  - to specified site — *see* Neoplasm, by site, malignant, secondary
  - unspecified site 172.9
- nail 172.9
  - finger 172.6
  - toe 172.7
- neck 172.4
- nodular (M8721/3) — *see* Melanoma, by site
- nose, external 172.3
- orbit 190.1
- penis 187.4
- perianal skin 172.5
- perineum 172.5
- pinna 172.2
- popliteal (fossa) (space) 172.7
- prepuce 187.1
- pubes 172.5
- pudendum 184.4
- retina 190.5
- scalp 172.4
- scrotum 187.7
- septum nasal (skin) 172.3
- shoulder 172.6
- skin NEC 172.8
- spindle cell (M8772/3) — *see also* Melanoma, by site
  - type A (M8773/3) 190.0
  - type B (M8774/3) 190.0
- submammary fold 172.5
- superficial spreading (M8743/3) — *see* Melanoma, by site
- temple 172.3
- thigh 172.7
- toe 172.7
- trunk NEC 172.5
- umbilicus 172.5
- upper limb NEC 172.6
- vagina vault 184.0
- vulva 184.4

Melanoplakia 528.9
Melanosarcoma (M8720/3) — *see also* Melanoma
- epithelioid cell (M8771/3) — *see* Melanoma

Melanosis 709.09
- addisonian (primary adrenal insufficiency) 255.4
  - tuberculous (*see also* Tuberculosis) 017.6 ☑
- adrenal 255.4
- colon 569.89
- conjunctiva 372.55
  - congenital 743.49
- corii degenerativa 757.33
- cornea (presenile) (senile) 371.12
  - congenital 743.43
    - interfering with vision 743.42
- prenatal 743.43
  - interfering with vision 743.42
- eye 372.55
  - congenital 743.49
- jute spinners' 709.09
- lenticularis progressiva 757.33
- liver 573.8
- precancerous (M8741/2) — *see also* Neoplasm, skin, in situ
  - malignant melanoma in (M8741/3) — *see* Melanoma
- Riehl's 709.09
- sclera 379.19
  - congenital 743.47
- suprarenal 255.4
- tar 709.09
- toxic 709.09

Melanuria 791.9
MELAS syndrome (mitochondrial encephalopathy, lactic acidosis and stroke-like episodes) 277.87
Melasma 709.09
- adrenal (gland) 255.4
- suprarenal (gland) 255.4

Melena 578.1
- due to
  - swallowed maternal blood 777.3
  - ulcer — *see* Ulcer, by site, with hemorrhage
- newborn 772.4
  - due to swallowed maternal blood 777.3

Meleney's
- gangrene (cutaneous) 686.09
- ulcer (chronic undermining) 686.09

Melioidosis 025
Melitensis, febris 023.0
Melitococcosis 023.0
Melkersson (-Rosenthal) syndrome 351.8
Mellitus, diabetes — *see* Diabetes
Melorheostosis (bone) (leri) 733.99
Meloschisis 744.83
Melotia 744.29
Membrana
- capsularis lentis posterior 743.39
- epipapillaris 743.57

Membranacea placenta — *see* Placenta, abnormal
Membranaceous uterus 621.8
Membrane, membranous — *see also* condition
- folds, congenital — *see* Web
- Jackson's 751.4
- over face (causing asphyxia), fetus or newborn 768.9
- premature rupture — *see* Rupture, membranes, premature
- pupillary 364.74
  - persistent 743.46
- retained (complicating delivery) (with hemorrhage) 666.2 ☑
  - without hemorrhage 667.1 ☑
- secondary (eye) 366.50
- unruptured (causing asphyxia) 768.9
- vitreous humor 379.25

Membranitis, fetal 658.4 ☑
- affecting fetus or newborn 762.7

Memory disturbance, loss or lack (*see also* Amnesia) 780.93
- mild, following organic brain damage 310.1

Menadione (vitamin K) **deficiency** 269.0
Menarche, precocious 259.1
Mendacity, pathologic 301.7
Mende's syndrome (ptosis-epicanthus) 270.2
Mendelson's syndrome (resulting from a procedure) 997.3
- obstetric 668.0 ☑

Ménétrier's disease or syndrome (hypertrophic gastritis) 535.2 ☑
Ménière's disease, syndrome, or vertigo 386.00
- cochlear 386.02
- cochleovestibular 386.01
- inactive 386.04
- in remission 386.04
- vestibular 386.03

Meninges, meningeal — *see* condition
Meningioma (M9530/0) — *see also* Neoplasm, meninges, benign
- angioblastic (M9535/0) — *see* Neoplasm, meninges, benign
- angiomatous (M9534/0) — *see* Neoplasm, meninges, benign
- endotheliomatous (M9531/0) — *see* Neoplasm, meninges, benign
- fibroblastic (M9532/0) — *see* Neoplasm, meninges, benign
- fibrous (M9532/0) — *see* Neoplasm, meninges, benign
- hemangioblastic (M9535/0) — *see* Neoplasm, meninges, benign
- hemangiopericytic (M9536/0) — *see* Neoplasm, meninges, benign

☑ Additional Digit Required — Refer to the Tabular List (Numeric Code Section) for Additional Digit Selection
▶◀ Revised Text ● New Line ▲ Revised Code

☑ Additional Digit Required — Refer to the Tabular List (Numeric Code Section) for Additional Digit Selection
▶◀ Revised Text ● New Line ▲ Revised Code

Meningoencephalitis (*see also* Encephalitis) — *continued*
- late effect — *see* category 326
- Listeria monocytogenes 027.0 *[320.7]*
- lymphocytic (serous) 049.0
- mumps 072.2
- parasitic NEC 123.9 *[323.4]*
- pneumococcal 320.1
- primary amebic 136.2
- rubella 056.01
- serous 048
  - lymphocytic 049.0
- specific 094.2
- staphylococcal 320.3
- streptococcal 320.2
- syphilitic 094.2
- toxic NEC 989.9 *[323.7]*
  - due to
    - carbon tetrachloride 987.8 *[323.7]*
    - hydroxyquinoline derivatives poisoning 961.3 *[323.7]*
    - lead 984.9 *[323.7]*
    - mercury 985.0 *[323.7]*
    - thallium 985.8 *[323.7]*
- toxoplasmosis (acquired) 130.0
- trypanosomic 086.1 *[323.2]*
- tuberculous (*see also* Tuberculosis, meninges) 013.0 ☑
- virus NEC 048

Meningoencephalocele 742.0
- syphilitic 094.89
  - congenital 090.49

Meningoencephalomyelitis (*see also* Meningoencephalitis) 323.9
- acute NEC 048
  - disseminated (postinfectious) 136.9 *[323.6]*
    - postimmunization or postvaccination 323.5
- due to
  - actinomycosis 039.8 *[320.7]*
  - torula 117.5 *[323.4]*
  - toxoplasma or toxoplasmosis (acquired) 130.0
    - congenital (active) 771.2 *[323.4]*
- late effect — *see* category 326

Meningoencephalomyelopathy (*see also* Meningoencephalomyelitis) 349.9

Meningoencephalopathy (*see also* Meningoencephalitis) 348.39

Meningoencephalopoliomyelitis (*see also* Poliomyelitis, bulbar) 045.0 ☑
- late effect 138

Meningomyelitis (*see also* Meningoencephalitis) 323.9
- blastomycotic NEC (*see also* Blastomycosis) 116.0 *[323.4]*
- due to
  - actinomycosis 039.8 *[320.7]*
  - blastomycosis (*see also* Blastomycosis) 116.0 *[323.4]*
  - Meningococcus 036.0
  - sporotrichosis 117.1 *[323.4]*
  - torula 117.5 *[323.4]*
- late effect — *see* category 326
- lethargic 049.8
- meningococcal 036.0
- syphilitic 094.2
- tuberculous (*see also* Tuberculosis, meninges) 013.0 ☑

Meningomyelocele (*see also* Spina bifida) 741.9 ☑
- syphilitic 094.89

Meningomyeloneuritis — *see* Meningoencephalitis

Meningoradiculitis — *see* Meningitis

Meningovascular — *see* condition

Meniscocytosis 282.60

Menkes' syndrome — *see* Syndrome, Menkes'

Menolipsis 626.0

Menometrorrhagia 626.2

Menopause, menopausal (symptoms) (syndrome) 627.2
- arthritis (any site) NEC 716.3 ☑
- artificial 627.4
- bleeding 627.0
- crisis 627.2
- depression (*see also* Psychosis, affective) 296.2 ☑
  - agitated 296.2 ☑
    - recurrent episode 296.3 ☑
    - single episode 296.2 ☑
  - psychotic 296.2 ☑
    - recurrent episode 296.3 ☑
    - single episode 296.2 ☑
  - recurrent episode 296.3 ☑
  - single episode 296.2 ☑
- melancholia (*see also* Psychosis, affective) 296.2 ☑
  - recurrent episode 296.3 ☑
  - single episode 296.2 ☑
- paranoid state 297.2
- paraphrenia 297.2
- postsurgical 627.4
- premature 256.31
  - postirradiation 256.2
  - postsurgical 256.2
- psychoneurosis 627.2
- psychosis NEC 298.8
- surgical 627.4
- toxic polyarthritis NEC 716.39

Menorrhagia (primary) 626.2
- climacteric 627.0
- menopausal 627.0
- postclimacteric 627.1
- postmenopausal 627.1
- preclimacteric 627.0
- premenopausal 627.0
- puberty (menses retained) 626.3

Menorrhalgia 625.3

Menoschesis 626.8

Menostaxis 626.2

Menses, retention 626.8

Menstrual — *see also* Menstruation
- cycle, irregular 626.4
- disorders NEC 626.9
- extraction V25.3
- fluid, retained 626.8
- molimen 625.4
- period, normal V65.5
- regulation V25.3

Menstruation
- absent 626.0
- anovulatory 628.0
- delayed 626.8
- difficult 625.3
- disorder 626.9
  - psychogenic 306.52
  - specified NEC 626.8
- during pregnancy 640.8 ☑
- excessive 626.2
- frequent 626.2
- infrequent 626.1
- irregular 626.4
- latent 626.8
- membranous 626.8
- painful (primary) (secondary) 625.3
  - psychogenic 306.52
- passage of clots 626.2
- precocious 626.8
- protracted 626.8
- retained 626.8
- retrograde 626.8
- scanty 626.1
- suppression 626.8
- vicarious (nasal) 625.8

Mentagra (*see also* Sycosis) 704.8

Mental — *see also* condition
- deficiency (*see also* Retardation, mental) 319
- deterioration (*see also* Psychosis) 298.9
- disorder (*see also* Disorder, mental) 300.9
- exhaustion 300.5
- insufficiency (congenital) (*see also* Retardation, mental) 319
- observation without need for further medical care NEC V71.09
- retardation (*see also* Retardation, mental) 319
- subnormality (*see also* Retardation, mental) 319
  - mild 317
  - moderate 318.0
  - profound 318.2
  - severe 318.1
- upset (*see also* Disorder, mental) 300.9

Meralgia paresthetica 355.1

Mercurial — *see* condition

Mercurialism NEC 985.0

Merergasia 300.9

Merkel cell tumor — *see* Neoplasm, by site, malignant

Merocele (*see also* Hernia, femoral) 553.00

Meromelia 755.4
- lower limb 755.30
  - intercalary 755.32
    - femur 755.34
      - tibiofibular (complete) (incomplete) 755.33
    - fibula 755.37
    - metatarsal(s) 755.38
    - tarsal(s) 755.38
    - tibia 755.36
    - tibiofibular 755.35
  - terminal (complete) (partial) (transverse) 755.31
    - longitudinal 755.32
      - metatarsal(s) 755.38
      - phalange(s) 755.39
      - tarsal(s) 755.38
  - transverse 755.31
- upper limb 755.20
  - intercalary 755.22
    - carpal(s) 755.28
    - humeral 755.24
      - radioulnar (complete) (incomplete) 755.23
    - metacarpal(s) 755.28
    - phalange(s) 755.29
    - radial 755.26
    - radioulnar 755.25
    - ulnar 755.27
  - terminal (complete) (partial) (transverse) 755.21
    - longitudinal 755.22
      - carpal(s) 755.28
      - metacarpal(s) 755.28
      - phalange(s) 755.29
  - transverse 755.21

Merosmia 781.1

MERRF syndrome (myoclonus with epilepsy and with ragged red fibers) 277.87

Merycism — *see also* Vomiting
- psychogenic 307.53

Merzbacher-Pelizaeus disease 330.0

Mesaortitis — *see* Aortitis

Mesarteritis — *see* Arteritis

Mesencephalitis (*see also* Encephalitis) 323.9
- late effect — *see* category 326

Mesenchymoma (M8990/1) — *see also* Neoplasm, connective tissue, uncertain behavior
- benign (M8990/0) — *see* Neoplasm, connective tissue, benign
- malignant (M8990/3) — *see* Neoplasm, connective tissue, malignant

Mesenteritis ●
- retractile 567.82 ●
- sclerosing 567.82 ●

Mesentery, mesenteric — *see* condition

Mesiodens, mesiodentes 520.1
- causing crowding 524.31

Mesio-occlusion 524.23

Mesocardia (with asplenia) 746.87

Mesocolon — *see* condition

Mesonephroma (malignant) (M9110/3) — *see also* Neoplasm, by site, malignant
- benign (M9110/0) — *see* Neoplasm, by site, benign

Mesophlebitis — *see* Phlebitis

Mesostromal dysgenesis 743.51

Mesothelioma (malignant) (M9050/3) — *see also* Neoplasm, by site, malignant
- benign (M9050/0) — *see* Neoplasm, by site, benign
- biphasic type (M9053/3) — *see also* Neoplasm, by site, malignant
  - benign (M9053/0) — *see* Neoplasm, by site, benign
- epithelioid (M9052/3) — *see also* Neoplasm, by site, malignant
  - benign (M9052/0) — *see* Neoplasm, by site, benign
- fibrous (M9051/3) — *see also* Neoplasm, by site, malignant
  - benign (M9051/0) — *see* Neoplasm, by site, benign

Metabolic syndrome 277.7

Metabolism disorder 277.9
- specified type NEC 277.89

Metagonimiasis 121.5

Metagonimus infestation (small intestine) 121.5

Metal
- pigmentation (skin) 709.00
- polishers' disease 502

Metalliferous miners' lung 503

Metamorphopsia 368.14

Metaplasia
- bone, in skin 709.3
- breast 611.8
- cervix — *omit code*
- endometrium (squamous) 621.8
- esophagus 530.85
- intestinal, of gastric mucosa 537.89
- kidney (pelvis) (squamous) (*see also* Disease, renal) 593.89
- myelogenous 289.89
- myeloid (agnogenic) (megakaryocytic) 289.89
- spleen 289.59
- squamous cell
  - amnion 658.8 ☑
  - bladder 596.8
  - cervix — *see* condition
  - trachea 519.1
  - tracheobronchial tree 519.1
  - uterus 621.8
    - cervix — *see* condition

Metastasis, metastatic
- abscess — *see* Abscess
- calcification 275.40
- cancer, neoplasm, or disease
  - from specified site (M8000/3) — *see* Neoplasm, by site, malignant
  - to specified site (M8000/6) — *see* Neoplasm, by site, secondary
- deposits (in) (M8000/6) — *see* Neoplasm, by site, secondary
- pneumonia 038.8 *[484.8]*
- spread (to) (M8000/6) — *see* Neoplasm, by site, secondary

Metatarsalgia 726.70
- anterior 355.6
- due to Freiberg's disease 732.5
- Morton's 355.6

Metatarsus, metatarsal — *see also* condition
- abductus valgus (congenital) 754.60
- adductus varus (congenital) 754.53
- primus varus 754.52
- valgus (adductus) (congenital) 754.60
- varus (abductus) (congenital) 754.53
  - primus 754.52

Methemoglobinemia 289.7
- acquired (with sulfhemoglobinemia) 289.7
- congenital 289.7
- enzymatic 289.7
- Hb-M disease 289.7
- hereditary 289.7
- toxic 289.7

Methemoglobinuria (*see also* Hemoglobinuria) 791.2

Methicillin-resistant staphylococcus aureus (MRSA) V09.0

Methioninemia 270.4

Metritis (catarrhal) (septic) (suppurative) (*see also* Endometritis) 615.9
- blennorrhagic 098.16
  - chronic or duration of 2 months or over 098.36
- cervical (*see also* Cervicitis) 616.0
- gonococcal 098.16
  - chronic or duration of 2 months or over 098.36
- hemorrhagic 626.8
- puerperal, postpartum, childbirth 670.0 ☑
- tuberculous (*see also* Tuberculosis) 016.7 ☑

Metropathia hemorrhagica 626.8

Metroperitonitis (*see also* Peritonitis, pelvic, female) 614.5

Metrorrhagia 626.6
- arising during pregnancy — *see* Hemorrhage, pregnancy
- postpartum NEC 666.2 ☑
- primary 626.6
- psychogenic 306.59
- puerperal 666.2 ☑

Metrorrhexis — *see* Rupture, uterus

Metrosalpingitis (*see also* Salpingo-oophoritis) 614.2

Metrostaxis 626.6

Metrovaginitis (*see also* Endometritis) 615.9
- gonococcal (acute) 098.16
  - chronic or duration of 2 months or over 098.36

Mexican fever — *see* Typhus, Mexican

Meyenburg-Altherr-Uehlinger syndrome 733.99

Meyer-Schwickerath and Weyers syndrome (dysplasia oculodentodigitalis) 759.89

Meynert's amentia (nonalcoholic) 294.0
- alcoholic 291.1

Mibelli's disease 757.39

Mice, joint (*see also* Loose, body, joint) 718.1 ☑
- knee 717.6

Micheli-Rietti syndrome (thalassemia minor) 282.49

Michotte's syndrome 721.5

Micrencephalon, micrencephaly 742.1

Microalbuminuria 791.0 ●

Microaneurysm, retina 362.14
- diabetic 250.5 ☑ *[362.01]*

Microangiopathy 443.9
- diabetic (peripheral) 250.7 ☑ *[443.81]*
  - retinal 250.5 ☑ *[362.01]*
- peripheral 443.9
  - diabetic 250.7 ☑ *[443.81]*
- retinal 362.18
  - diabetic 250.5 ☑ *[362.01]*
- thrombotic 446.6
  - Moschcowitz's (thrombotic thrombocytopenic purpura) 446.6

Microcalcification, mammographic 793.81

Microcephalus, microcephalic, microcephaly 742.1
- due to toxoplasmosis (congenital) 771.2

Microcheilia 744.82

Microcolon (congenital) 751.5

Microcornea (congenital) 743.41

Microcytic — *see* condition

Microdeletions NEC 758.33

Microdontia 520.2

Microdrepanocytosis (thalassemia-Hb-S disease) 282.49

Microembolism
- atherothrombotic — *see* Atheroembolism
- retina 362.33

Microencephalon 742.1

Microfilaria streptocerca infestation 125.3

Microgastria (congenital) 750.7

Microgenia 524.06

Microgenitalia (congenital) 752.89
- penis 752.64

Microglioma (M9710/3)
- specified site — *see* Neoplasm, by site, malignant

Microglioma — *continued*
- unspecified site 191.9

Microglossia (congenital) 750.16

Micrognathia, micrognathism (congenital) 524.00
- mandibular 524.04
  - alveolar 524.74
- maxillary 524.03
  - alveolar 524.73

Microgyria (congenital) 742.2

Microinfarct, heart (*see also* Insufficiency, coronary) 411.89

Microlithiasis, alveolar, pulmonary 516.2

Micromyelia (congenital) 742.59

Micropenis 752.64

Microphakia (congenital) 743.36

Microphthalmia (congenital) (*see also* Microphthalmos) 743.10

Microphthalmos (congenital) 743.10
- associated with eye and adnexal anomalies NEC 743.12
- due to toxoplasmosis (congenital) 771.2
- isolated 743.11
- simple 743.11
- syndrome 759.89

Micropsia 368.14

Microsporidiosis 136.8

Microsporon furfur infestation 111.0

Microsporosis (*see also* Dermatophytosis) 110.9
- nigra 111.1

Microstomia (congenital) 744.84

Microthelia 757.6

Microthromboembolism — *see* Embolism

Microtia (congenital) (external ear) 744.23

Microtropia 378.34

Micturition
- disorder NEC 788.69
  - psychogenic 306.53
- frequency 788.41
  - psychogenic 306.53
- nocturnal 788.43
- painful 788.1
  - psychogenic 306.53

Middle
- ear — *see* condition
- lobe (right) syndrome 518.0

Midplane — *see* condition

Miescher's disease 709.3
- cheilitis 351.8
- granulomatosis disciformis 709.3

Miescher-Leder syndrome or granulomatosis 709.3

Mieten's syndrome 759.89

Migraine (idiopathic) 346.9 ☑
- with aura 346.0 ☑
- abdominal (syndrome) 346.2 ☑
- allergic (histamine) 346.2 ☑
- atypical 346.1 ☑
- basilar 346.2 ☑
- classical 346.0 ☑
- common 346.1 ☑
- hemiplegic 346.8 ☑
- lower-half 346.2 ☑
- menstrual 625.4
- ophthalmic 346.8 ☑
- ophthalmoplegic 346.8 ☑
- retinal 346.2 ☑
- variant 346.2 ☑

Migrant, social V60.0

Migratory, migrating — *see also* condition
- person V60.0
- testis, congenital 752.52

Mikulicz's disease or syndrome (dryness of mouth, absent or decreased lacrimation) 527.1

Milian atrophia blanche 701.3

Miliaria (crystallina) (rubra) (tropicalis) 705.1
- apocrine 705.82

Miliary — *see* condition

Milium (*see also* Cyst, sebaceous) 706.2
- colloid 709.3

☑ Additional Digit Required — Refer to the Tabular List (Numeric Code Section) for Additional Digit Selection
▶◀ Revised Text ● New Line ▲ Revised Code

Index

Myoblastoma — Myositis

- **Myoblastoma**
  - granular cell (M9580/0) — *see also* Neoplasm, connective tissue, benign
    - malignant (M9580/3) — *see* Neoplasm, connective tissue, malignant
  - tongue (M9580/0) 210.1
- **Myocardial** — *see* condition
- **Myocardiopathy** (congestive) (constrictive) (familial) (hypertrophic nonobstructive) (idiopathic) (infiltrative) (obstructive) (primary) (restrictive) (sporadic) 425.4
  - alcoholic 425.5
  - amyloid 277.3 *[425.7]*
  - beriberi 265.0 *[425.7]*
  - cobalt-beer 425.5
  - due to
    - amyloidosis 277.3 *[425.7]*
    - beriberi 265.0 *[425.7]*
    - cardiac glycogenosis 271.0 *[425.7]*
    - Chagas' disease 086.0
    - Friedreich's ataxia 334.0 *[425.8]*
    - influenza 487.8 *[425.8]*
    - mucopolysaccharidosis 277.5 *[425.7]*
    - myotonia atrophica 359.2 *[425.8]*
    - progressive muscular dystrophy 359.1 *[425.8]*
    - sarcoidosis 135 *[425.8]*
  - glycogen storage 271.0 *[425.7]*
  - hypertrophic obstructive 425.1
  - metabolic NEC 277.9 *[425.7]*
  - nutritional 269.9 *[425.7]*
  - obscure (African) 425.2
  - peripartum 674.5 ☑
  - postpartum 674.5 ☑
  - secondary 425.9
  - thyrotoxic (*see also* Thyrotoxicosis) 242.9 ☑ *[425.7]*
  - toxic NEC 425.9
- **Myocarditis** (fibroid) (interstitial) (old) (progressive) (senile) (with arteriosclerosis) 429.0
  - with
    - rheumatic fever (conditions classifiable to 390) 398.0
      - active (*see also* Myocarditis, acute, rheumatic) 391.2
      - inactive or quiescent (with chorea) 398.0
  - active (nonrheumatic) 422.90
    - rheumatic 391.2
      - with chorea (acute) (rheumatic) (Sydenham's) 392.0
  - acute or subacute (interstitial) 422.90
    - due to Streptococcus (beta-hemolytic) 391.2
    - idiopathic 422.91
    - rheumatic 391.2
      - with chorea (acute) (rheumatic) (Sydenham's) 392.0
    - specified type NEC 422.99
  - aseptic of newborn 074.23
  - bacterial (acute) 422.92
  - chagasic 086.0
  - chronic (interstitial) 429.0
  - congenital 746.89
  - constrictive 425.4
  - Coxsackie (virus) 074.23
  - diphtheritic 032.82
  - due to or in
    - Coxsackie (virus) 074.23
    - diphtheria 032.82
    - epidemic louse-borne typhus 080 *[422.0]*
    - influenza 487.8 *[422.0]*
    - Lyme disease 088.81 *[422.0]*
    - scarlet fever 034.1 *[422.0]*
    - toxoplasmosis (acquired) 130.3
    - tuberculosis (*see also* Tuberculosis) 017.9 ☑ *[422.0]*
    - typhoid 002.0 *[422.0]*
    - typhus NEC 081.9 *[422.0]*
  - eosinophilic 422.91
  - epidemic of newborn 074.23
  - Fiedler's (acute) (isolated) (subacute) 422.91
  - giant cell (acute) (subacute) 422.91
  - gonococcal 098.85
  - granulomatous (idiopathic) (isolated) (nonspecific) 422.91

- **Myocarditis** — *continued*
  - hypertensive (*see also* Hypertension, heart) 402.90
  - idiopathic 422.91
    - granulomatous 422.91
  - infective 422.92
  - influenzal 487.8 *[422.0]*
  - isolated (diffuse) (granulomatous) 422.91
  - malignant 422.99
  - meningococcal 036.43
  - nonrheumatic, active 422.90
  - parenchymatous 422.90
  - pneumococcal (acute) (subacute) 422.92
  - rheumatic (chronic) (inactive) (with chorea) 398.0
    - active or acute 391.2
      - with chorea (acute) (rheumatic) (Sydenham's) 392.0
  - septic 422.92
  - specific (giant cell) (productive) 422.91
  - staphylococcal (acute) (subacute) 422.92
  - suppurative 422.92
  - syphilitic (chronic) 093.82
  - toxic 422.93
    - rheumatic (*see also* Myocarditis, acute rheumatic) 391.2
  - tuberculous (*see also* Tuberculosis) 017.9 ☑ *[422.0]*
  - typhoid 002.0 *[422.0]*
  - valvular — *see* Endocarditis
  - viral, except Coxsackie 422.91
    - Coxsackie 074.23
    - of newborn (Coxsackie) 074.23
- **Myocardium, myocardial** — *see* condition
- **Myocardosis** (*see also* Cardiomyopathy) 425.4
- **Myoclonia** (essential) 333.2
  - epileptica 333.2
  - Friedrich's 333.2
  - massive 333.2
- **Myoclonic**
  - epilepsy, familial (progressive) 333.2
  - jerks 333.2
- **Myoclonus** (familial essential) (multifocal) (simplex) 333.2
  - with epilepsy and with ragged red fibers (MERRF syndrome) 277.87
  - facial 351.8
  - massive (infantile) 333.2
  - pharyngeal 478.29
- **Myodiastasis** 728.84
- **Myoendocarditis** — *see also* Endocarditis
  - acute or subacute 421.9
- **Myoepithelioma** (M8982/0) — *see* Neoplasm, by site, benign
- **Myofascitis** (acute) 729.1
  - low back 724.2
- **Myofibroma** (M8890/0) — *see also* Neoplasm, connective tissue, benign
  - uterus (cervix) (corpus) (*see also* Leiomyoma) 218.9
- **Myofibrosis** 728.2
  - heart (*see also* Myocarditis) 429.0
  - humeroscapular region 726.2
  - scapulohumeral 726.2
- **Myofibrositis** (*see also* Myositis) 729.1
  - scapulohumeral 726.2
- **Myogelosis** (occupational) 728.89
- **Myoglobinuria** 791.3
- **Myoglobulinuria, primary** 791.3
- **Myokymia** — *see also* Myoclonus
  - facial 351.8
- **Myolipoma** (M8860/0)
  - specified site — *see* Neoplasm, connective tissue, benign
  - unspecified site 223.0
- **Myoma** (M8895/0) — *see also* Neoplasm, connective tissue, benign
  - cervix (stump) (uterus) (*see also* Leiomyoma) 218.9
  - malignant (M8895/3) — *see* Neoplasm, connective tissue, malignant
  - prostate 600.20
    - with urinary retention 600.21

- **Myoma** — *continued*
  - uterus (cervix) (corpus) (*see also* Leiomyoma) 218.9
    - in pregnancy or childbirth 654.1 ☑
      - affecting fetus or newborn 763.89
      - causing obstructed labor 660.2 ☑
        - affecting fetus or newborn 763.1
- **Myomalacia** 728.9
  - cordis, heart (*see also* Degeneration, myocardial) 429.1
- **Myometritis** (*see also* Endometritis) 615.9
- **Myometrium** — *see* condition
- **Myonecrosis, clostridial** 040.0
- **Myopathy** 359.9
  - alcoholic 359.4
  - amyloid 277.3 *[359.6]*
  - benign congenital 359.0
  - central core 359.0
  - centronuclear 359.0
  - congenital (benign) 359.0
  - critical illness 359.81
  - distal 359.1
  - due to drugs 359.4
  - endocrine 259.9 *[359.5]*
    - specified type NEC 259.8 *[359.5]*
  - extraocular muscles 376.82
  - facioscapulohumeral 359.1
  - in
    - Addison's disease 255.4 *[359.5]*
    - amyloidosis 277.3 *[359.6]*
    - cretinism 243 *[359.5]*
    - Cushing's syndrome 255.0 *[359.5]*
    - disseminated lupus erythematosus 710.0 *[359.6]*
    - giant cell arteritis 446.5 *[359.6]*
    - hyperadrenocorticism NEC 255.3 *[359.5]*
    - hyperparathyroidism 252.01 *[359.5]*
    - hypopituitarism 253.2 *[359.5]*
    - hypothyroidism (*see also* Hypothyroidism) 244.9 *[359.5]*
    - malignant neoplasm NEC (M8000/3) 199.1 *[359.6]*
    - myxedema (*see also* Myxedema) 244.9 *[359.5]*
    - polyarteritis nodosa 446.0 *[359.6]*
    - rheumatoid arthritis 714.0 *[359.6]*
    - sarcoidosis 135 *[359.6]*
    - scleroderma 710.1 *[359.6]*
    - Sjögren's disease 710.2 *[359.6]*
    - thyrotoxicosis (*see also* Thyrotoxicosis) 242.9 ☑ *[359.5]*
  - inflammatory 359.89
  - intensive care (ICU) 359.81
  - limb-girdle 359.1
  - myotubular 359.0
  - necrotizing, acute 359.81
  - nemaline 359.0
  - ocular 359.1
  - oculopharyngeal 359.1
  - of critical illness 359.81
  - primary 359.89
  - progressive NEC 359.89
  - quadriplegic, acute 359.81
  - rod body 359.0
  - scapulohumeral 359.1
  - specified type NEC 359.89
  - toxic 359.4
- **Myopericarditis** (*see also* Pericarditis) 423.9
- **Myopia** (axial) (congenital) (increased curvature or refraction, nucleus of lens) 367.1
  - degenerative, malignant 360.21
  - malignant 360.21
  - progressive high (degenerative) 360.21
- **Myosarcoma** (M8895/3) — *see* Neoplasm, connective tissue, malignant
- **Myosis** (persistent) 379.42
  - stromal (endolymphatic) (M8931/1) 236.0
- **Myositis** 729.1
  - clostridial 040.0
  - due to posture 729.1
  - epidemic 074.1
  - fibrosa or fibrous (chronic) 728.2
    - Volkmann's (complicating trauma) 958.6
  - infective 728.0
  - interstitial 728.81

☑ Additional Digit Required — Refer to the Tabular List (Numeric Code Section) for Additional Digit Selection

▶◀ Revised Text ● New Line ▲ Revised Code

N

Necrosis, necrotic — *continued*
- bone — *continued*
  - aseptic or avascular — *continued*
    - specified site NEC 733.49
    - talus 733.44
  - ethmoid 478.1
  - ischemic 733.40
  - jaw 526.4
  - marrow 289.89
  - Paget's (osteitis deformans) 731.0
  - tuberculous — *see* Tuberculosis, bone
- brain (softening) (*see also* Softening, brain) 437.8
- breast (aseptic) (fat) (segmental) 611.3
- bronchus, bronchi 519.1
- central nervous system NEC (*see also* Softening, brain) 437.8
- cerebellar (*see also* Softening, brain) 437.8
- cerebral (softening) (*see also* Softening, brain) 437.8
- cerebrospinal (softening) (*see also* Softening, brain) 437.8
- cornea (*see also* Keratitis) 371.40
- cortical, kidney 583.6
- cystic medial (aorta) 441.00
  - abdominal 441.02
  - thoracic 441.01
  - thoracoabdominal 441.03
- dental 521.09
  - pulp 522.1
- due to swallowing corrosive substance — *see* Burn, by site
- ear (ossicle) 385.24
- esophagus 530.89
- ethmoid (bone) 478.1
- eyelid 374.50
- fat, fatty (generalized) (*see also* Degeneration, fatty) 272.8
  - abdominal wall 567.82 ▲
  - breast (aseptic) (segmental) 611.3
  - intestine 569.89
  - localized — *see* Degeneration, by site, fatty
  - mesentery 567.82 ▲
  - omentum 567.82 ▲
  - pancreas 577.8
  - peritoneum 567.82 ▲
  - skin (subcutaneous) 709.3
    - newborn 778.1
- femur (aseptic) (avascular) 733.42
  - head 733.42
  - medial condyle 733.43
  - neck 733.42
- gallbladder (*see also* Cholecystitis, acute) 575.0
- gangrenous 785.4
- gastric 537.89
- glottis 478.79
- heart (myocardium) — *see* Infarct, myocardium
- hepatic (*see also* Necrosis, liver) 570
- hip (aseptic) (avascular) 733.42
- intestine (acute) (hemorrhagic) (massive) 557.0
- ischemic 785.4
- jaw 526.4
- kidney (bilateral) 583.9
  - acute 584.9
  - cortical 583.6
    - acute 584.6
      - with
        - abortion — *see* Abortion, by type, with renal failure
        - ectopic pregnancy (*see also* categories 633.0-633.9) 639.3
        - molar pregnancy (*see also* categories 630-632) 639.3
    - complicating pregnancy 646.2 ☑
      - affecting fetus or newborn 760.1
    - following labor and delivery 669.3 ☑
  - medullary (papillary) (*see also* Pyelitis) 590.80
    - in
      - acute renal failure 584.7
      - nephritis, nephropathy 583.7
  - papillary (*see also* Pyelitis) 590.80
    - in
      - acute renal failure 584.7
      - nephritis, nephropathy 583.7

Necrosis, necrotic — *continued*
- kidney — *continued*
  - tubular 584.5
    - with
      - abortion — *see* Abortion, by type, with renal failure
      - ectopic pregnancy (*see also* categories 633.0-633.9) 639.3
      - molar pregnancy (*see also* categories 630-632) 639.3
    - complicating
      - abortion 639.3
      - ectopic or molar pregnancy 639.3
      - pregnancy 646.2 ☑
        - affecting fetus or newborn 760.1
    - following labor and delivery 669.3 ☑
    - traumatic 958.5
- larynx 478.79
- liver (acute) (congenital) (diffuse) (massive) (subacute) 570
  - with
    - abortion — *see* Abortion, by type, with specified complication NEC
    - ectopic pregnancy (*see also* categories 633.0-633.9) 639.8
    - molar pregnancy (*see also* categories 630-632) 639.8
  - complicating pregnancy 646.7 ☑
    - affecting fetus or newborn 760.8
  - following
    - abortion 639.8
    - ectopic or molar pregnancy 639.8
  - obstetrical 646.7 ☑
  - postabortal 639.8
  - puerperal, postpartum 674.8 ☑
  - toxic 573.3
- lung 513.0
- lymphatic gland 683
- mammary gland 611.3
- mastoid (chronic) 383.1
- mesentery 557.0
  - fat 567.82 ▲
- mitral valve — *see* Insufficiency, mitral
- myocardium, myocardial — *see* Infarct, myocardium
- nose (septum) 478.1
- omentum 557.0
  - with mesenteric infarction 557.0
  - fat 567.82 ▲
- orbit, orbital 376.10
- ossicles, ear (aseptic) 385.24
- ovary (*see also* Salpingo-oophoritis) 614.2
- pancreas (aseptic) (duct) (fat) 577.8
  - acute 577.0
  - infective 577.0
- papillary, kidney (*see also* Pyelitis) 590.80
- peritoneum 557.0
  - with mesenteric infarction 557.0
  - fat 567.82 ▲
- pharynx 462
  - in granulocytopenia 288.0
- phosphorus 983.9
- pituitary (gland) (postpartum) (Sheehan) 253.2
- placenta (*see also* Placenta, abnormal) 656.7 ☑
- pneumonia 513.0
- pulmonary 513.0
- pulp (dental) 522.1
- pylorus 537.89
- radiation — *see* Necrosis, by site
- radium — *see* Necrosis, by site
- renal — *see* Necrosis, kidney
- sclera 379.19
- scrotum 608.89
- skin or subcutaneous tissue 709.8
  - due to burn — see Burn, by site
  - gangrenous 785.4
- spine, spinal (column) 730.18
  - acute 730.18
  - cord 336.1
- spleen 289.59
- stomach 537.89
- stomatitis 528.1
- subcutaneous fat 709.3
  - fetus or newborn 778.1
- subendocardial — *see* Infarct, myocardium
- suprarenal (capsule) (gland) 255.8
- teeth, tooth 521.09

Necrosis, necrotic — *continued*
- testis 608.89
- thymus (gland) 254.8
- tonsil 474.8
- trachea 519.1
- tuberculous NEC — *see* Tuberculosis
- tubular (acute) (anoxic) (toxic) 584.5
  - due to a procedure 997.5
- umbilical cord, affecting fetus or newborn 762.6
- vagina 623.8
- vertebra (lumbar) 730.18
  - acute 730.18
  - tuberculous (*see also* Tuberculosis) 015.0 ☑ *[730.8]* ☑
- vesical (aseptic) (bladder) 596.8
- x-ray — *see* Necrosis, by site

Necrospermia 606.0

Necrotizing angiitis 446.0

Negativism 301.7

Neglect (child) (newborn) NEC 995.52
- adult 995.84
- after or at birth 995.52
- hemispatial 781.8
- left-sided 781.8
- sensory 781.8
- visuospatial 781.8

Negri bodies 071

Neill-Dingwall syndrome (microcephaly and dwarfism) 759.89

Neisserian infection NEC — *see* Gonococcus

Nematodiasis NEC (*see also* Infestation, Nematode) 127.9
- ancylostoma (*see also* Ancylostomiasis) 126.9

Neoformans cryptococcus infection 117.5

Neonatal — *see also* condition
- adrenoleukodystrophy 277.86
- teeth, tooth 520.6

Neonatorum — *see* condition

☑ Additional Digit Required — Refer to the Tabular List (Numeric Code Section) for Additional Digit Selection

▶◀ Revised Text ● New Line ▲ Revised Code

	Malignant – Primary	Malignant – Secondary	Malignant – Ca in situ	Benign	Uncertain Behavior	Unspecified
Neoplasm, neoplastic	199.1	199.1	234.9	229.9	238.9	239.9

Notes — 1. The list below gives the code numbers for neoplasms by anatomical site. For each site there are six possible code numbers according to whether the neoplasm in question is malignant, benign, in situ, of uncertain behavior, or of unspecified nature. The description of the neoplasm will often indicate which of the six columns is appropriate; e.g., malignant melanoma of skin, benign fibroadenoma of breast, carcinoma in situ of cervix uteri.

Where such descriptors are not present, the remainder of the Index should be consulted where guidance is given to the appropriate column for each morphological (histological) variety listed; e.g., Mesonephroma — see Neoplasm, malignant; Embryoma — see also Neoplasm, uncertain behavior; Disease, Bowen's — see Neoplasm, skin, in situ. However, the guidance in the Index can be overridden if one of the descriptors mentioned above is present; e.g., malignant adenoma of colon is coded to 153.9 and not to 211.3 as the adjective "malignant" overrides the Index entry "Adenoma — see also Neoplasm, benign."

*2. Sites marked with the sign * (e.g., face NEC*) should be classified to malignant neoplasm of skin of these sites if the variety of neoplasm is a squamous cell carcinoma or an epidermoid carcinoma, and to benign neoplasm of skin of these sites if the variety of neoplasm is a papilloma (any type).*

Neoplasm, neoplastic	Primary	Secondary	Ca in situ	Benign	Uncertain Behavior	Unspecified
abdomen, abdominal	195.2	198.89	234.8	229.8	238.8	239.8
cavity	195.2	198.89	234.8	229.8	238.8	239.8
organ	195.2	198.89	234.8	229.8	238.8	239.8
viscera	195.2	198.89	234.8	229.8	238.8	239.8
wall	173.5	198.2	232.5	216.5	238.2	239.2
connective tissue	171.5	198.89	—	215.5	238.1	239.2
abdominopelvic	195.8	198.89	234.8	229.8	238.8	239.8
accessory sinus — *see* Neoplasm, sinus						
acoustic nerve	192.0	198.4	—	225.1	237.9	239.7
acromion (process)	170.4	198.5	—	213.4	238.0	239.2
adenoid (pharynx) (tissue)	147.1	198.89	230.0	210.7	235.1	239.0
adipose tissue (*see also* Neoplasm, connective tissue)	171.9	198.89	—	215.9	238.1	239.2
adnexa (uterine)	183.9	198.82	233.3	221.8	236.3	239.5
adrenal (cortex) (gland) (medulla)	194.0	198.7	234.8	227.0	237.2	239.7
ala nasi (external)	173.3	198.2	232.3	216.3	238.2	239.2
alimentary canal or tract NEC	159.9	197.8	230.9	211.9	235.5	239.0
alveolar	143.9	198.89	230.0	210.4	235.1	239.0
mucosa	143.9	198.89	230.0	210.4	235.1	239.0
lower	143.1	198.89	230.0	210.4	235.1	239.0
upper	143.0	198.89	230.0	210.4	235.1	239.0
ridge or process	170.1	198.5	—	213.1	238.0	239.2
carcinoma	143.9	—	—	—	—	—
lower	143.1	—	—	—	—	—
upper	143.0	—	—	—	—	—
lower	170.1	198.5	—	213.1	238.0	239.2
mucosa	143.9	198.89	230.0	210.4	235.1	239.0
lower	143.1	198.89	230.0	210.4	235.1	239.0
upper	143.0	198.89	230.0	210.4	235.1	239.0
upper	170.0	198.5	—	213.0	238.0	239.2
sulcus	145.1	198.89	230.0	210.4	235.1	239.0
alveolus	143.9	198.89	230.0	210.4	235.1	239.0
lower	143.1	198.89	230.0	210.4	235.1	239.0
upper	143.0	198.89	230.0	210.4	235.1	239.0
ampulla of Vater	156.2	197.8	230.8	211.5	235.3	239.0
ankle NEC*	195.5	198.89	232.7	229.8	238.8	239.8
anorectum, anorectal (junction)	154.8	197.5	230.7	211.4	235.2	239.0
antecubital fossa or space*	195.4	198.89	232.6	229.8	238.8	239.8
antrum (Highmore) (maxillary)	160.2	197.3	231.8	212.0	235.9	239.1
pyloric	151.2	197.8	230.2	211.1	235.2	239.0
tympanicum	160.1	197.3	231.8	212.0	235.9	239.1
anus, anal	154.3	197.5	230.6	211.4	235.5	239.0
canal	154.2	197.5	230.5	211.4	235.5	239.0
contiguous sites with rectosigmoid junction or rectum	154.8	—	—	—	—	—
margin	173.5	198.2	232.5	216.5	238.2	239.2
skin	173.5	198.2	232.5	216.5	238.2	239.2
sphincter	154.2	197.5	230.5	211.4	235.5	239.0
aorta (thoracic)	171.4	198.89	—	215.4	238.1	239.2
abdominal	171.5	198.89	—	215.5	238.1	239.2
aortic body	194.6	198.89	—	227.6	237.3	239.7
aponeurosis	171.9	198.89	—	215.9	238.1	239.2
palmar	171.2	198.89	—	215.2	238.1	239.2
plantar	171.3	198.89	—	215.3	238.1	239.2
appendix	153.5	197.5	230.3	211.3	235.2	239.0
arachnoid (cerebral)	192.1	198.4	—	225.2	237.6	239.7
spinal	192.3	198.4	—	225.4	237.6	239.7
areola (female)	174.0	198.81	233.0	217	238.3	239.3
male	175.0	198.81	233.0	217	238.3	239.3
arm NEC*	195.4	198.89	232.6	229.8	238.8	239.8
artery — *see* Neoplasm, connective tissue						
aryepiglottic fold	148.2	198.89	230.0	210.8	235.1	239.0
hypopharyngeal aspect	148.2	198.89	230.0	210.8	235.1	239.0
laryngeal aspect	161.1	197.3	231.0	212.1	235.6	239.1
marginal zone	148.2	198.89	230.0	210.8	235.1	239.0
arytenoid (cartilage)	161.3	197.3	231.0	212.1	235.6	239.1
fold — *see* Neoplasm, aryepiglottic						
atlas	170.2	198.5	—	213.2	238.0	239.2
atrium, cardiac	164.1	198.89	—	212.7	238.8	239.8
auditory						
canal (external) (skin)	173.2	198.2	232.2	216.2	238.2	239.2
internal	160.1	197.3	231.8	212.0	235.9	239.1
nerve	192.0	198.4	—	225.1	237.9	239.7
tube	160.1	197.3	231.8	212.0	235.9	239.1
opening	147.2	198.89	230.0	210.7	235.1	239.0
auricle, ear	173.2	198.2	232.2	216.2	238.2	239.2
cartilage	171.0	198.89	—	215.0	238.1	239.2
auricular canal (external)	173.2	198.2	232.2	216.2	238.2	239.2
internal	160.1	197.3	231.8	212.0	235.9	239.1
autonomic nerve or nervous system NEC	171.9	198.89	—	215.9	238.1	239.2
axilla, axillary	195.1	198.89	234.8	229.8	238.8	239.8
fold	173.5	198.2	232.5	216.5	238.2	239.2
back NEC*	195.8	198.89	232.5	229.8	238.8	239.8
Bartholin's gland	184.1	198.82	233.3	221.2	236.3	239.5
basal ganglia	191.0	198.3	—	225.0	237.5	239.6
basis pedunculi	191.7	198.3	—	225.0	237.5	239.6
bile or biliary (tract)	156.9	197.8	230.8	211.5	235.3	239.0
canaliculi (biliferi) (intrahepatic)	155.1	197.8	230.8	211.5	235.3	239.0
canals, interlobular	155.1	197.8	230.8	211.5	235.3	239.0
contiguous sites	156.8	—	—	—	—	—
duct or passage (common) (cystic) (extrahepatic)	156.1	197.8	230.8	211.5	235.3	239.0
contiguous sites with gallbladder	156.8	—	—	—	—	—
interlobular	155.1	197.8	230.8	211.5	235.3	239.0
intrahepatic	155.1	197.8	230.8	211.5	235.3	239.0
and extrahepatic	156.9	197.8	230.8	211.5	235.3	239.0
bladder (urinary)	188.9	198.1	233.7	223.3	236.7	239.4
contiguous sites	188.8	—	—	—	—	—
dome	188.1	198.1	233.7	223.3	236.7	239.4
neck	188.5	198.1	233.7	223.3	236.7	239.4
orifice	188.9	198.1	233.7	223.3	236.7	239.4
ureteric	188.6	198.1	233.7	223.3	236.7	239.4
urethral	188.5	198.1	233.7	223.3	236.7	239.4
sphincter	188.8	198.1	233.7	223.3	236.7	239.4
trigone	188.0	198.1	233.7	223.3	236.7	239.4
urachus	188.7	—	233.7	223.3	236.7	239.4
wall	188.9	198.1	233.7	223.3	236.7	239.4
anterior	188.3	198.1	233.7	223.3	236.7	239.4
lateral	188.2	198.1	233.7	223.3	236.7	239.4
posterior	188.4	198.1	233.7	223.3	236.7	239.4
blood vessel — *see* Neoplasm, connective tissue						
bone (periosteum)	170.9	198.5	—	213.9	238.0	239.2

Note — Carcinomas and adenocarcinomas, of any type other than intraosseous or odontogenic, of the sites listed under "Neoplasm, bone" should be considered as constituting metastatic spread from an unspecified primary site and coded to 198.5 for morbidity coding and to 199.1 for underlying cause of death coding.

Neoplasm, neoplastic	Primary	Secondary	Ca in situ	Benign	Uncertain Behavior	Unspecified
acetabulum	170.6	198.5	—	213.6	238.0	239.2
acromion (process)	170.4	198.5	—	213.4	238.0	239.2
ankle	170.8	198.5	—	213.8	238.0	239.2
arm NEC	170.4	198.5	—	213.4	238.0	239.2
astragalus	170.8	198.5	—	213.8	238.0	239.2

Neoplasm, neoplastic — continued	Malignant					
	Primary	Secondary	Ca in situ	Benign	Uncertain Behavior	Unspecified
bone — continued						
atlas	170.2	198.5	—	213.2	238.0	239.2
axis	170.2	198.5	—	213.2	238.0	239.2
back NEC	170.2	198.5	—	213.2	238.0	239.2
calcaneus	170.8	198.5	—	213.8	238.0	239.2
calvarium	170.0	198.5	—	213.0	238.0	239.2
carpus (any)	170.5	198.5	—	213.5	238.0	239.2
cartilage NEC	170.9	198.5	—	213.9	238.0	239.2
clavicle	170.3	198.5	—	213.3	238.0	239.2
clivus	170.0	198.5	—	213.0	238.0	239.2
coccygeal vertebra	170.6	198.5	—	213.6	238.0	239.2
coccyx	170.6	198.5	—	213.6	238.0	239.2
costal cartilage	170.3	198.5	—	213.3	238.0	239.2
costovertebral joint	170.3	198.5	—	213.3	238.0	239.2
cranial	170.0	198.5	—	213.0	238.0	239.2
cuboid	170.8	198.5	—	213.8	238.0	239.2
cuneiform	170.9	198.5	—	213.9	238.0	239.2
ankle	170.8	198.5	—	213.8	238.0	239.2
wrist	170.5	198.5	—	213.5	238.0	239.2
digital	170.9	198.5	—	213.9	238.0	239.2
finger	170.5	198.5	—	213.5	238.0	239.2
toe	170.8	198.5	—	213.8	238.0	239.2
elbow	170.4	198.5	—	213.4	238.0	239.2
ethmoid (labyrinth)	170.0	198.5	—	213.0	238.0	239.2
face	170.0	198.5	—	213.0	238.0	239.2
lower jaw	170.1	198.5	—	213.1	238.0	239.2
femur (any part)	170.7	198.5	—	213.7	238.0	239.2
fibula (any part)	170.7	198.5	—	213.7	238.0	239.2
finger (any)	170.5	198.5	—	213.5	238.0	239.2
foot	170.8	198.5	—	213.8	238.0	239.2
forearm	170.4	198.5	—	213.4	238.0	239.2
frontal	170.0	198.5	—	213.0	238.0	239.2
hand	170.5	198.5	—	213.5	238.0	239.2
heel	170.8	198.5	—	213.8	238.0	239.2
hip	170.6	198.5	—	213.6	238.0	239.2
humerus (any part)	170.4	198.5	—	213.4	238.0	239.2
hyoid	170.0	198.5	—	213.0	238.0	239.2
ilium	170.6	198.5	—	213.6	238.0	239.2
innominate	170.6	198.5	—	213.6	238.0	239.2
intervertebral cartilage or disc	170.2	198.5	—	213.2	238.0	239.2
ischium	170.6	198.5	—	213.6	238.0	239.2
jaw (lower)	170.1	198.5	—	213.1	238.0	239.2
upper	170.0	198.5	—	213.0	238.0	239.2
knee	170.7	198.5	—	213.7	238.0	239.2
leg NEC	170.7	198.5	—	213.7	238.0	239.2
limb NEC	170.9	198.5	—	213.9	238.0	239.2
lower (long bones)	170.7	198.5	—	213.7	238.0	239.2
short bones	170.8	198.5	—	213.8	238.0	239.2
upper (long bones)	170.4	198.5	—	213.4	238.0	239.2
short bones	170.5	198.5	—	213.5	238.0	239.2
long	170.9	198.5	—	213.9	238.0	239.2
lower limbs NEC	170.7	198.5	—	213.7	238.0	239.2
upper limbs NEC	170.4	198.5	—	213.4	238.0	239.2
malar	170.0	198.5	—	213.0	238.0	239.2
mandible	170.1	198.5	—	213.1	238.0	239.2
marrow NEC	202.9 ☑	198.5	—	—	—	238.7
mastoid	170.0	198.5	—	213.0	238.0	239.2
maxilla, maxillary (superior)	170.0	198.5	—	213.0	238.0	239.2
inferior	170.1	198.5	—	213.1	238.0	239.2
metacarpus (any)	170.5	198.5	—	213.5	238.0	239.2
metatarsus (any)	170.8	198.5	—	213.8	238.0	239.2
navicular (ankle)	170.8	198.5	—	213.8	238.0	239.2
hand	170.5	198.5	—	213.5	238.0	239.2
nose, nasal	170.0	198.5	—	213.0	238.0	239.2
occipital	170.0	198.5	—	213.0	238.0	239.2
orbit	170.0	198.5	—	213.0	238.0	239.2
parietal	170.0	198.5	—	213.0	238.0	239.2
patella	170.8	198.5	—	213.8	238.0	239.2
pelvic	170.6	198.5	—	213.6	238.0	239.2
phalanges	170.9	198.5	—	213.9	238.0	239.2
foot	170.8	198.5	—	213.8	238.0	239.2
hand	170.5	198.5	—	213.5	238.0	239.2
pubic	170.6	198.5	—	213.6	238.0	239.2
radius (any part)	170.4	198.5	—	213.4	238.0	239.2
rib	170.3	198.5	—	213.3	238.0	239.2
sacral vertebra	170.6	198.5	—	213.6	238.0	239.2

Neoplasm, neoplastic — continued	Malignant					
	Primary	Secondary	Ca in situ	Benign	Uncertain Behavior	Unspecified
bone — continued						
sacrum	170.6	198.5	—	213.6	238.0	239.2
scaphoid (of hand)	170.5	198.5	—	213.5	238.0	239.2
of ankle	170.8	198.5	—	213.8	238.0	239.2
scapula (any part)	170.4	198.5	—	213.4	238.0	239.2
sella turcica	170.0	198.5	—	213.0	238.0	239.2
short	170.9	198.5	—	213.9	238.0	239.2
lower limb	170.8	198.5	—	213.8	238.0	239.2
upper limb	170.5	198.5	—	213.5	238.0	239.2
shoulder	170.4	198.5	—	213.4	238.0	239.2
skeleton, skeletal NEC	170.9	198.5	—	213.9	238.0	239.2
skull	170.0	198.5	—	213.0	238.0	239.2
sphenoid	170.0	198.5	—	213.0	238.0	239.2
spine, spinal (column)	170.2	198.5	—	213.2	238.0	239.2
coccyx	170.6	198.5	—	213.6	238.0	239.2
sacrum	170.6	198.5	—	213.6	238.0	239.2
sternum	170.3	198.5	—	213.3	238.0	239.2
tarsus (any)	170.8	198.5	—	213.8	238.0	239.2
temporal	170.0	198.5	—	213.0	238.0	239.2
thumb	170.5	198.5	—	213.5	238.0	239.2
tibia (any part)	170.7	198.5	—	213.7	238.0	239.2
toe (any)	170.8	198.5	—	213.8	238.0	239.2
trapezium	170.5	198.5	—	213.5	238.0	239.2
trapezoid	170.5	198.5	—	213.5	238.0	239.2
turbinate	170.0	198.5	—	213.0	238.0	239.2
ulna (any part)	170.4	198.5	—	213.4	238.0	239.2
unciform	170.5	198.5	—	213.5	238.0	239.2
vertebra (column)	170.2	198.5	—	213.2	238.0	239.2
coccyx	170.6	198.5	—	213.6	238.0	239.2
sacrum	170.6	198.5	—	213.6	238.0	239.2
vomer	170.0	198.5	—	213.0	238.0	239.2
wrist	170.5	198.5	—	213.5	238.0	239.2
xiphoid process	170.3	198.5	—	213.3	238.0	239.2
zygomatic	170.0	198.5	—	213.0	238.0	239.2
book-leaf (mouth)	145.8	198.89	230.0	210.4	235.1	239.0
bowel — *see* Neoplasm, intestine						
brachial plexus	171.2	198.89	—	215.2	238.1	239.2
brain NEC	191.9	198.3	—	225.0	237.5	239.6
basal ganglia	191.0	198.3	—	225.0	237.5	239.6
cerebellopontine angle	191.6	198.3	—	225.0	237.5	239.6
cerebellum NOS	191.6	198.3	—	225.0	237.5	239.6
cerebrum	191.0	198.3	—	225.0	237.5	239.6
choroid plexus	191.5	198.3	—	225.0	237.5	239.6
contiguous sites	191.8	—	—	—	—	—
corpus callosum	191.8	198.3	—	225.0	237.5	239.6
corpus striatum	191.0	198.3	—	225.0	237.5	239.6
cortex (cerebral)	191.0	198.3	—	225.0	237.5	239.6
frontal lobe	191.1	198.3	—	225.0	237.5	239.6
globus pallidus	191.0	198.3	—	225.0	237.5	239.6
hippocampus	191.2	198.3	—	225.0	237.5	239.6
hypothalamus	191.0	198.3	—	225.0	237.5	239.6
internal capsule	191.0	198.3	—	225.0	237.5	239.6
medulla oblongata	191.7	198.3	—	225.0	237.5	239.6
meninges	192.1	198.4	—	225.2	237.6	239.7
midbrain	191.7	198.3	—	225.0	237.5	239.6
occipital lobe	191.4	198.3	—	225.0	237.5	239.6
parietal lobe	191.3	198.3	—	225.0	237.5	239.6
peduncle	191.7	198.3	—	225.0	237.5	239.6
pons	191.7	198.3	—	225.0	237.5	239.6
stem	191.7	198.3	—	225.0	237.5	239.6
tapetum	191.8	198.3	—	225.0	237.5	239.6
temporal lobe	191.2	198.3	—	225.0	237.5	239.6
thalamus	191.0	198.3	—	225.0	237.5	239.6
uncus	191.2	198.3	—	225.0	237.5	239.6
ventricle (floor)	191.5	198.3	—	225.0	237.5	239.6
branchial (cleft) (vestiges)	146.8	198.89	230.0	210.6	235.1	239.0
breast (connective tissue) (female) (glandular tissue) (soft parts)	174.9	198.81	233.0	217	238.3	239.3
areola	174.0	198.81	233.0	217	238.3	239.3
male	175.0	198.81	233.0	217	238.3	239.3
axillary tail	174.6	198.81	233.0	217	238.3	239.3
central portion	174.1	198.81	233.0	217	238.3	239.3
contiguous sites	174.8	—	—	—	—	—
ectopic sites	174.8	198.81	233.0	217	238.3	239.3
inner	174.8	198.81	233.0	217	238.3	239.3
lower	174.8	198.81	233.0	217	238.3	239.3

☑ Additional Digit Required — Refer to the Tabular List (Numeric Code Section) for Additional Digit Selection

▶◀ Revised Text ● New Line ▲ Revised Code

Neoplasm, neoplastic — *continued*	Malignant			Benign	Uncertain Behavior	Unspecified
	Primary	Secondary	Ca in situ			
breast — *continued*						
lower-inner quadrant	174.3	198.81	233.0	217	238.3	239.3
lower-outer quadrant	174.5	198.81	233.0	217	238.3	239.3
male	175.9	198.81	233.0	217	238.3	239.3
areola	175.0	198.81	233.0	217	238.3	239.3
ectopic tissue	175.9	198.81	233.0	217	238.3	239.3
nipple	175.0	198.81	233.0	217	238.3	239.3
mastectomy site (skin)	173.5	198.2	—	—	—	—
specified as breast tissue	174.8	198.81	—	—	—	—
midline	174.8	198.81	233.0	217	238.3	239.3
nipple	174.0	198.81	233.0	217	238.3	239.3
male	175.0	198.81	233.0	217	238.3	239.3
outer	174.8	198.81	233.0	217	238.3	239.3
skin	173.5	198.2	232.5	216.5	238.2	239.2
tail (axillary)	174.6	198.81	233.0	217	238.3	239.3
upper	174.8	198.81	233.0	217	238.3	239.3
upper-inner quadrant	174.2	198.81	233.0	217	238.3	239.3
upper-outer quadrant	174.4	198.81	233.0	217	238.3	239.3
broad ligament	183.3	198.82	233.3	221.0	236.3	239.5
bronchiogenic, bronchogenic (lung)	162.9	197.0	231.2	212.3	235.7	239.1
bronchiole	162.9	197.0	231.2	212.3	235.7	239.1
bronchus	162.9	197.0	231.2	212.3	235.7	239.1
carina	162.2	197.0	231.2	212.3	235.7	239.1
contiguous sites with lung or trachea	162.8	—	—	—	—	—
lower lobe of lung	162.5	197.0	231.2	212.3	235.7	239.1
main	162.2	197.0	231.2	212.3	235.7	239.1
middle lobe of lung	162.4	197.0	231.2	212.3	235.7	239.1
upper lobe of lung	162.3	197.0	231.2	212.3	235.7	239.1
brow	173.3	198.2	232.3	216.3	238.2	239.2
buccal (cavity)	145.9	198.89	230.0	210.4	235.1	239.0
commissure	145.0	198.89	230.0	210.4	235.1	239.0
groove (lower) (upper)	145.1	198.89	230.0	210.4	235.1	239.0
mucosa	145.0	198.89	230.0	210.4	235.1	239.0
sulcus (lower) (upper)	145.1	198.89	230.0	210.4	235.1	239.0
bulbourethral gland	189.3	198.1	233.9	223.81	236.99	239.5
bursa — *see* Neoplasm, connective tissue						
buttock NEC*	195.3	198.89	232.5	229.8	238.8	239.8
calf*	195.5	198.89	232.7	229.8	238.8	239.8
calvarium	170.0	198.5	—	213.0	238.0	239.2
calyx, renal	189.1	198.0	233.9	223.1	236.91	239.5
canal						
anal	154.2	197.5	230.5	211.4	235.5	239.0
auditory (external)	173.2	198.2	232.2	216.2	238.2	239.2
auricular (external)	173.2	198.2	232.2	216.2	238.2	239.2
canaliculi, biliary (biliferi) (intrahepatic)	155.1	197.8	230.8	211.5	235.3	239.0
canthus (eye) (inner) (outer)	173.1	198.2	232.1	216.1	238.2	239.2
capillary — *see* Neoplasm, connective tissue						
caput coli	153.4	197.5	230.3	211.3	235.2	239.0
cardia (gastric)	151.0	197.8	230.2	211.1	235.2	239.0
cardiac orifice (stomach)	151.0	197.8	230.2	211.1	235.2	239.0
cardio-esophageal junction	151.0	197.8	230.2	211.1	235.2	239.0
cardio-esophagus	151.0	197.8	230.2	211.1	235.2	239.0
carina (bronchus)	162.2	197.0	231.2	212.3	235.7	239.1
carotid (artery)	171.0	198.89	—	215.0	238.1	239.2
body	194.5	198.89	—	227.5	237.3	239.7
carpus (any bone)	170.5	198.5	—	213.5	238.0	239.2
cartilage (articular) (joint) NEC — *see also* Neoplasm, bone	170.9	198.5	—	213.9	238.0	239.2
arytenoid	161.3	197.3	231.0	212.1	235.6	239.1
auricular	171.0	198.89	—	215.0	238.1	239.2
bronchi	162.2	197.3	—	212.3	235.7	239.1
connective tissue — *see* Neoplasm, connective tissue						
costal	170.3	198.5	—	213.3	238.0	239.2
cricoid	161.3	197.3	231.0	212.1	235.6	239.1
cuneiform	161.3	197.3	231.0	212.1	235.6	239.1
ear (external)	171.0	198.89	—	215.0	238.1	239.2
ensiform	170.3	198.5	—	213.3	238.0	239.2
epiglottis	161.1	197.3	231.0	212.1	235.6	239.1
anterior surface	146.4	198.89	230.0	210.6	235.1	239.0
eyelid	171.0	198.89	—	215.0	238.1	239.2
intervertebral	170.2	198.5	—	213.2	238.0	239.2
larynx, laryngeal	161.3	197.3	231.0	212.1	235.6	239.1
nose, nasal	160.0	197.3	231.8	212.0	235.9	239.1
pinna	171.0	198.89	—	215.0	238.1	239.2

Neoplasm, neoplastic — *continued*	Malignant			Benign	Uncertain Behavior	Unspecified
	Primary	Secondary	Ca in situ			
cartilage NEC — *see also* Neoplasm, bone — *continued*						
rib	170.3	198.5	—	213.3	238.0	239.2
semilunar (knee)	170.7	198.5	—	213.7	238.0	239.2
thyroid	161.3	197.3	231.0	212.1	235.6	239.1
trachea	162.0	197.3	231.1	212.2	235.7	239.1
cauda equina	192.2	198.3	—	225.3	237.5	239.7
cavity						
buccal	145.9	198.89	230.0	210.4	235.1	239.0
nasal	160.0	197.3	231.8	212.0	235.9	239.1
oral	145.9	198.89	230.0	210.4	235.1	239.0
peritoneal	158.9	197.6	—	211.8	235.4	239.0
tympanic	160.1	197.3	231.8	212.0	235.9	239.1
cecum	153.4	197.5	230.3	211.3	235.2	239.0
central						
nervous system — *see* Neoplasm, nervous system						
white matter	191.0	198.3	—	225.0	237.5	239.6
cerebellopontine (angle)	191.6	198.3	—	225.0	237.5	239.6
cerebellum, cerebellar	191.6	198.3	—	225.0	237.5	239.6
cerebrum, cerebral (cortex) (hemisphere) (white matter)	191.0	198.3	—	225.0	237.5	239.6
meninges	192.1	198.4	—	225.2	237.6	239.7
peduncle	191.7	198.3	—	225.0	237.5	239.6
ventricle (any)	191.5	198.3	—	225.0	237.5	239.6
cervical region	195.0	198.89	234.8	229.8	238.8	239.8
cervix (cervical) (uteri) (uterus)	180.9	198.82	233.1	219.0	236.0	239.5
canal	180.0	198.82	233.1	219.0	236.0	239.5
contiguous sites	180.8	—	—	—	—	—
endocervix (canal) (gland)	180.0	198.82	233.1	219.0	236.0	239.5
exocervix	180.1	198.82	233.1	219.0	236.0	239.5
external os	180.1	198.82	233.1	219.0	236.0	239.5
internal os	180.0	198.82	233.1	219.0	236.0	239.5
nabothian gland	180.0	198.82	233.1	219.0	236.0	239.5
squamocolumnar junction	180.8	198.82	233.1	219.0	236.0	239.5
stump	180.8	198.82	233.1	219.0	236.0	239.5
cheek	195.0	198.89	234.8	229.8	238.8	239.8
external	173.3	198.2	232.3	216.3	238.2	239.2
inner aspect	145.0	198.89	230.0	210.4	235.1	239.0
internal	145.0	198.89	230.0	210.4	235.1	239.0
mucosa	145.0	198.89	230.0	210.4	235.1	239.0
chest (wall) NEC	195.1	198.89	234.8	229.8	238.8	239.8
chiasma opticum	192.0	198.4	—	225.1	237.9	239.7
chin	173.3	198.2	232.3	216.3	238.2	239.2
choana	147.3	198.89	230.0	210.7	235.1	239.0
cholangiole	155.1	197.8	230.8	211.5	235.3	239.0
choledochal duct	156.1	197.8	230.8	211.5	235.3	239.0
choroid	190.6	198.4	234.0	224.6	238.8	239.8
plexus	191.5	198.3	—	225.0	237.5	239.6
ciliary body	190.0	198.4	234.0	224.0	238.8	239.8
clavicle	170.3	198.5	—	213.3	238.0	239.2
clitoris	184.3	198.82	233.3	221.2	236.3	239.5
clivus	170.0	198.5	—	213.0	238.0	239.2
cloacogenic zone	154.8	197.5	230.7	211.4	235.5	239.0
coccygeal						
body or glomus	194.6	198.89	—	227.6	237.3	239.7
vertebra	170.6	198.5	—	213.6	238.0	239.2
coccyx	170.6	198.5	—	213.6	238.0	239.2
colon — *see also* Neoplasm, intestine, large						
and rectum	154.0	197.5	230.4	211.4	235.2	239.0
column, spinal — *see* Neoplasm, spine						
columnella	173.3	198.2	232.3	216.3	238.2	239.2
commissure						
labial, lip	140.6	198.89	230.0	210.4	235.1	239.0
laryngeal	161.0	197.3	231.0	212.1	235.6	239.1
common (bile) duct	156.1	197.8	230.8	211.5	235.3	239.0
concha	173.2	198.2	232.2	216.2	238.2	239.2
nose	160.0	197.3	231.8	212.0	235.9	239.1
conjunctiva	190.3	198.4	234.0	224.3	238.8	239.8

☑ Additional Digit Required — Refer to the Tabular List (Numeric Code Section) for Additional Digit Selection

▶◀ Revised Text ● New Line ▲ Revised Code

Neoplasm, neoplastic — *continued*	Malignant					
	Primary	Secondary	Ca in situ	Benign	Uncertain Behavior	Unspecified
connective tissue NEC	171.9	198.89	—	215.9	238.1	239.2

Note — For neoplasms of connective tissue (blood vessel, bursa, fascia, ligament, muscle, peripheral nerves, sympathetic and parasympathetic nerves and ganglia, synovia, tendon, etc.) or of morphological types that indicate connective tissue, code according to the list under "Neoplasm, connective tissue"; for sites that do not appear in this list, code to neoplasm of that site; e.g.,

liposarcoma, shoulder 171.2
leiomyosarcoma, stomach 151.9
neurofibroma, chest wall 215.4

Morphological types that indicate connective tissue appear in the proper place in the alphabetic index with the instruction "see Neoplasm, connective tissue..."

Neoplasm, neoplastic — *continued*	Primary	Secondary	Ca in situ	Benign	Uncertain Behavior	Unspecified
abdomen	171.5	198.89	—	215.5	238.1	239.2
abdominal wall	171.5	198.89	—	215.5	238.1	239.2
ankle	171.3	198.89	—	215.3	238.1	239.2
antecubital fossa or space	171.2	198.89	—	215.2	238.1	239.2
arm	171.2	198.89	—	215.2	238.1	239.2
auricle (ear)	171.0	198.89	—	215.0	238.1	239.2
axilla	171.4	198.89	—	215.4	238.1	239.2
back	171.7	198.89	—	215.7	238.1	239.2
breast (female) (*see also* Neoplasm, breast)	174.9	198.81	233.0	217	238.3	239.3
male	175.9	198.81	233.0	217	238.3	239.3
buttock	171.6	198.89	—	215.6	238.1	239.2
calf	171.3	198.89	—	215.3	238.1	239.2
cervical region	171.0	198.89	—	215.0	238.1	239.2
cheek	171.0	198.89	—	215.0	238.1	239.2
chest (wall)	171.4	198.89	—	215.4	238.1	239.2
chin	171.0	198.89	—	215.0	238.1	239.2
contiguous sites	171.8	—	—	—	—	—
diaphragm	171.4	198.89	—	215.4	238.1	239.2
ear (external)	171.0	198.89	—	215.0	238.1	239.2
elbow	171.2	198.89	—	215.2	238.1	239.2
extrarectal	171.6	198.89	—	215.6	238.1	239.2
extremity	171.8	198.89	—	215.8	238.1	239.2
lower	171.3	198.89	—	215.3	238.1	239.2
upper	171.2	198.89	—	215.2	238.1	239.2
eyelid	171.0	198.89	—	215.0	238.1	239.2
face	171.0	198.89	—	215.0	238.1	239.2
finger	171.2	198.89	—	215.2	238.1	239.2
flank	171.7	198.89	—	215.7	238.1	239.2
foot	171.3	198.89	—	215.3	238.1	239.2
forearm	171.2	198.89	—	215.2	238.1	239.2
forehead	171.0	198.89	—	215.0	238.1	239.2
gastric	171.5	198.89	—	215.5	238.1	—
gastrointestinal	171.5	198.89	—	215.5	238.1	—
gluteal region	171.6	198.89	—	215.6	238.1	239.2
great vessels NEC	171.4	198.89	—	215.4	238.1	239.2
groin	171.6	198.89	—	215.6	238.1	239.2
hand	171.2	198.89	—	215.2	238.1	239.2
head	171.0	198.89	—	215.0	238.1	239.2
heel	171.3	198.89	—	215.3	238.1	239.2
hip	171.3	198.89	—	215.3	238.1	239.2
hypochondrium	171.5	198.89	—	215.5	238.1	239.2
iliopsoas muscle	171.6	198.89	—	215.5	238.1	239.2
infraclavicular region	171.4	198.89	—	215.4	238.1	239.2
inguinal (canal) (region)	171.6	198.89	—	215.6	238.1	239.2
intrathoracic	171.4	198.89	—	215.4	238.1	239.2
intestine	171.5	198.89	—	215.5	238.1	—
ischorectal fossa	171.6	198.89	—	215.6	238.1	239.2
jaw	143.9	198.89	230.0	210.4	235.1	239.0
knee	171.3	198.89	—	215.3	238.1	239.2
leg	171.3	198.89	—	215.3	238.1	239.2
limb NEC	171.9	198.89	—	215.8	238.1	239.2
lower	171.3	198.89	—	215.3	238.1	239.2
upper	171.2	198.89	—	215.2	238.1	239.2
nates	171.6	198.89	—	215.6	238.1	239.2
neck	171.0	198.89	—	215.0	238.1	239.2
orbit	190.1	198.4	234.0	224.1	238.8	239.8
pararectal	171.6	198.89	—	215.6	238.1	239.2
para-urethral	171.6	198.89	—	215.6	238.1	239.2
paravaginal	171.6	198.89	—	215.6	238.1	239.2

Neoplasm, neoplastic — *continued*	Primary	Secondary	Ca in situ	Benign	Uncertain Behavior	Unspecified
connective tissue NEC — *continued*						
pelvis (floor)	171.6	198.89	—	215.6	238.1	239.2
pelvo-abdominal	171.8	198.89	—	215.8	238.1	239.2
perineum	171.6	198.89	—	215.6	238.1	239.2
perirectal (tissue)	171.6	198.89	—	215.6	238.1	239.2
periurethral (tissue)	171.6	198.89	—	215.6	238.1	239.2
popliteal fossa or space	171.3	198.89	—	215.3	238.1	239.2
presacral	171.6	198.89	—	215.6	238.1	239.2
psoas muscle	171.5	198.89	—	215.5	238.1	239.2
pterygoid fossa	171.0	198.89	—	215.0	238.1	239.2
rectovaginal septum or wall	171.6	198.89	—	215.6	238.1	239.2
rectovesical	171.6	198.89	—	215.6	238.1	239.2
retroperitoneum	158.0	197.6	—	211.8	235.4	239.0
sacrococcygeal region	171.6	198.89	—	215.6	238.1	239.2
scalp	171.0	198.89	—	215.0	238.1	239.2
scapular region	171.4	198.89	—	215.4	238.1	239.2
shoulder	171.2	198.89	—	215.2	238.1	239.2
skin (dermis) NEC	173.9	198.2	232.9	216.9	238.2	239.2
stomach	171.5	198.89	—	215.5	238.1	—
submental	171.0	198.89	—	215.0	238.1	239.2
supraclavicular region	171.0	198.89	—	215.0	238.1	239.2
temple	171.0	198.89	—	215.0	238.1	239.2
temporal region	171.0	198.89	—	215.0	238.1	239.2
thigh	171.3	198.89	—	215.3	238.1	239.2
thoracic (duct) (wall)	171.4	198.89	—	215.4	238.1	239.2
thorax	171.4	198.89	—	215.4	238.1	239.2
thumb	171.2	198.89	—	215.2	238.1	239.2
toe	171.3	198.89	—	215.3	238.1	239.2
trunk	171.7	198.89	—	215.7	238.1	239.2
umbilicus	171.5	198.89	—	215.5	238.1	239.2
vesicorectal	171.6	198.89	—	215.6	238.1	239.2
wrist	171.2	198.89	—	215.2	238.1	239.2
conus medullaris	192.2	198.3	—	225.3	237.5	239.7
cord (true) (vocal)	161.0	197.3	231.0	212.1	235.6	239.1
false	161.1	197.3	231.0	212.1	235.6	239.1
spermatic	187.6	198.82	233.6	222.8	236.6	239.5
spinal (cervical) (lumbar) (thoracic)	192.2	198.3	—	225.3	237.5	239.7
cornea (limbus)	190.4	198.4	234.0	224.4	238.8	239.8
corpus						
albicans	183.0	198.6	233.3	220	236.2	239.5
callosum, brain	191.8	198.3	—	225.0	237.5	239.6
cavernosum	187.3	198.82	233.5	222.1	236.6	239.5
gastric	151.4	197.8	230.2	211.1	235.2	239.0
penis	187.3	198.82	233.5	222.1	236.6	239.5
striatum, cerebrum	191.0	198.3	—	225.0	237.5	239.6
uteri	182.0	198.82	233.2	219.1	236.0	239.5
isthmus	182.1	198.82	233.2	219.1	236.0	239.5
cortex						
adrenal	194.0	198.7	234.8	227.0	237.2	239.7
cerebral	191.0	198.3	—	225.0	237.5	239.6
costal cartilage	170.3	198.5	—	213.3	238.0	239.2
costovertebral joint	170.3	198.5	—	213.3	238.0	239.2
Cowper's gland	189.3	198.1	233.9	223.81	236.99	239.5
cranial (fossa, any)	191.9	198.3	—	225.0	237.5	239.6
meninges	192.1	198.4	—	225.2	237.6	239.7
nerve (any)	192.0	198.4	—	225.1	237.9	239.7
craniobuccal pouch	194.3	198.89	234.8	227.3	237.0	239.7
craniopharyngeal (duct) (pouch)	194.3	198.89	234.8	227.3	237.0	239.7
cricoid	148.0	198.89	230.0	210.8	235.1	239.0
cartilage	161.3	197.3	231.0	212.1	235.6	239.1
cricopharynx	148.0	198.89	230.0	210.8	235.1	239.0
crypt of Morgagni	154.8	197.5	230.7	211.4	235.2	239.0
crystalline lens	190.0	198.4	234.0	224.0	238.8	239.8
cul-de-sac (Douglas')	158.8	197.6	—	211.8	235.4	239.0
cuneiform cartilage	161.3	197.3	231.0	212.1	235.6	239.1
cutaneous — *see* Neoplasm, skin						
cutis — *see* Neoplasm, skin						
cystic (bile) duct (common)	156.1	197.8	230.8	211.5	235.3	239.0
dermis — *see* Neoplasm, skin						
diaphragm	171.4	198.89	—	215.4	238.1	239.2
digestive organs, system, tube, or tract NEC	159.9	197.8	230.9	211.9	235.5	239.0
contiguous sites with peritoneum	159.8	—	—	—	—	—
disc, intervertebral	170.2	198.5	—	213.2	238.0	239.2
disease, generalized	199.0	199.0	234.9	229.9	238.9	199.0
disseminated	199.0	199.0	234.9	229.9	238.9	199.0

Neoplasm, neoplastic — *continued*	Malignant					
	Primary	Secondary	Ca in situ	Benign	Uncertain Behavior	Unspecified
Douglas' cul-de-sac or pouch	158.8	197.6	—	211.8	235.4	239.0
duodenojejunal junction	152.8	197.4	230.7	211.2	235.2	239.0
duodenum	152.0	197.4	230.7	211.2	235.2	239.0
dura (cranial) (mater)	192.1	198.4	—	225.2	237.6	239.7
cerebral	192.1	198.4	—	225.2	237.6	239.7
spinal	192.3	198.4	—	225.4	237.6	239.7
ear (external)	173.2	198.2	232.2	216.2	238.2	239.2
auricle or auris	173.2	198.2	232.2	216.2	238.2	239.2
canal, external	173.2	198.2	232.2	216.2	238.2	239.2
cartilage	171.0	198.89	—	215.0	238.1	239.2
external meatus	173.2	198.2	232.2	216.2	238.2	239.2
inner	160.1	197.3	231.8	212.0	235.9	239.8
lobule	173.2	198.2	232.2	216.2	238.2	239.2
middle	160.1	197.3	231.8	212.0	235.9	239.8
contiguous sites with accessory sinuses or nasal cavities	160.8	—	—	—	—	—
skin	173.2	198.2	232.2	216.2	238.2	239.2
earlobe	173.2	198.2	232.2	216.2	238.2	239.2
ejaculatory duct	187.8	198.82	233.6	222.8	236.6	239.5
elbow NEC*	195.4	198.89	232.6	229.8	238.8	239.8
endocardium	164.1	198.89	—	212.7	238.8	239.8
endocervix (canal) (gland)	180.0	198.82	233.1	219.0	236.0	239.5
endocrine gland NEC	194.9	198.89	—	227.9	237.4	239.7
pluriglandular NEC	194.8	198.89	234.8	227.8	237.4	239.7
endometrium (gland) (stroma)	182.0	198.82	233.2	219.1	236.0	239.5
ensiform cartilage	170.3	198.5	—	213.3	238.0	239.2
enteric — *see* Neoplasm, intestine						
ependyma (brain)	191.5	198.3	—	225.0	237.5	239.6
epicardium	164.1	198.89	—	212.7	238.8	239.8
epididymis	187.5	198.82	233.6	222.3	236.6	239.5
epidural	192.9	198.4	—	225.9	237.9	239.7
epiglottis	161.1	197.3	231.0	212.1	235.6	239.1
anterior aspect or surface	146.4	198.89	230.0	210.6	235.1	239.0
cartilage	161.3	197.3	231.0	212.1	235.6	239.1
free border (margin)	146.4	198.89	230.0	210.6	235.1	239.0
junctional region	146.5	198.89	230.0	210.6	235.1	239.0
posterior (laryngeal) surface	161.1	197.3	231.0	212.1	235.6	239.1
suprahyoid portion	161.1	197.3	231.0	212.1	235.6	239.1
esophagogastric junction	151.0	197.8	230.2	211.1	235.2	239.0
esophagus	150.9	197.8	230.1	211.0	235.5	239.0
abdominal	150.2	197.8	230.1	211.0	235.5	239.0
cervical	150.0	197.8	230.1	211.0	235.5	239.0
contiguous sites	150.8	—	—	—	—	—
distal (third)	150.5	197.8	230.1	211.0	235.5	239.0
lower (third)	150.5	197.8	230.1	211.0	235.5	239.0
middle (third)	150.4	197.8	230.1	211.0	235.5	239.0
proximal (third)	150.3	197.8	230.1	211.0	235.5	239.0
specified part NEC	150.8	197.8	230.1	211.0	235.5	239.0
thoracic	150.1	197.8	230.1	211.0	235.5	239.0
upper (third)	150.3	197.8	230.1	211.0	235.5	239.0
ethmoid (sinus)	160.3	197.3	231.8	212.0	235.9	239.1
bone or labyrinth	170.0	198.5	—	213.0	238.0	239.2
Eustachian tube	160.1	197.3	231.8	212.0	235.9	239.1
exocervix	180.1	198.82	233.1	219.0	236.0	239.5
external						
meatus (ear)	173.2	198.2	232.2	216.2	238.2	239.2
os, cervix uteri	180.1	198.82	233.1	219.0	236.0	239.5
extradural	192.9	198.4	—	225.9	237.9	239.7
extrahepatic (bile) duct	156.1	197.8	230.8	211.5	235.3	239.0
contiguous sites with gallbladder	156.8	—	—	—	—	—
extraocular muscle	190.1	198.4	234.0	224.1	238.8	239.8
extrarectal	195.3	198.89	234.8	229.8	238.8	239.8
extremity*	195.8	198.89	232.8	229.8	238.8	239.8
lower*	195.5	198.89	232.7	229.8	238.8	239.8
upper*	195.4	198.89	232.6	229.8	238.8	239.8
eye NEC	190.9	198.4	234.0	224.9	238.8	239.8
contiguous sites	190.8	—	—	—	—	—
specified sites NEC	190.8	198.4	234.0	224.8	238.8	239.8
eyeball	190.0	198.4	234.0	224.0	238.8	239.8
eyebrow	173.3	198.2	232.3	216.3	238.2	239.2
eyelid (lower) (skin) (upper)	173.1	198.2	232.1	216.1	238.2	239.2
cartilage	171.0	198.89	—	215.0	238.1	239.2
face NEC*	195.0	198.89	232.3	229.8	238.8	239.8
fallopian tube (accessory)	183.2	198.82	233.3	221.0	236.3	239.5
falx (cerebelli) (cerebri)	192.1	198.4	—	225.2	237.6	239.7
fascia — *see also* Neoplasm, connective tissue						
palmar	171.2	198.89	—	215.2	238.1	239.2
plantar	171.3	198.89	—	215.3	238.1	239.2
fatty tissue — *see* Neoplasm, connective tissue						
fauces, faucial NEC	146.9	198.89	230.0	210.6	235.1	239.0
pillars	146.2	198.89	230.0	210.6	235.1	239.0
tonsil	146.0	198.89	230.0	210.5	235.1	239.0
femur (any part)	170.7	198.5	—	213.7	238.0	239.2
fetal membrane	181	198.82	233.2	219.8	236.1	239.5
fibrous tissue — *see* Neoplasm, connective tissue						
fibula (any part)	170.7	198.5	—	213.7	238.0	239.2
filum terminale	192.2	198.3	—	225.3	237.5	239.7
finger NEC*	195.4	198.89	232.6	229.8	238.8	239.8
flank NEC*	195.8	198.89	232.5	229.8	238.8	239.8
follicle, nabothian	180.0	198.82	233.1	219.0	236.0	239.5
foot NEC*	195.5	198.89	232.7	229.8	238.8	239.8
forearm NEC*	195.4	198.89	232.6	229.8	238.8	239.8
forehead (skin)	173.3	198.2	232.3	216.3	238.2	239.2
foreskin	187.1	198.82	233.5	222.1	236.6	239.5
fornix						
pharyngeal	147.3	198.89	230.0	210.7	235.1	239.0
vagina	184.0	198.82	233.3	221.1	236.3	239.5
fossa (of)						
anterior (cranial)	191.9	198.3	—	225.0	237.5	239.6
cranial	191.9	198.3	—	225.0	237.5	239.6
ischiorectal	195.3	198.89	234.8	229.8	238.8	239.8
middle (cranial)	191.9	198.3	—	225.0	237.5	239.6
pituitary	194.3	198.89	234.8	227.3	237.0	239.7
posterior (cranial)	191.9	198.3	—	225.0	237.5	239.6
pterygoid	171.0	198.89	—	215.0	238.1	239.2
pyriform	148.1	198.89	230.0	210.8	235.1	239.0
Rosenmüller	147.2	198.89	230.0	210.7	235.1	239.0
tonsillar	146.1	198.89	230.0	210.6	235.1	239.0
fourchette	184.4	198.82	233.3	221.2	236.3	239.5
frenulum						
labii — *see* Neoplasm, lip, internal						
linguae	141.3	198.89	230.0	210.1	235.1	239.0
frontal						
bone	170.0	198.5	—	213.0	238.0	239.2
lobe, brain	191.1	198.3	—	225.0	237.5	239.6
meninges	192.1	198.4	—	225.2	237.6	239.7
pole	191.1	198.3	—	225.0	237.5	239.6
sinus	160.4	197.3	231.8	212.0	235.9	239.1
fundus						
stomach	151.3	197.8	230.2	211.1	235.2	239.0
uterus	182.0	198.82	233.2	219.1	236.0	239.5
gall duct (extrahepatic)	156.1	197.8	230.8	211.5	235.3	239.0
intrahepatic	155.1	197.8	230.8	211.5	235.3	239.0
gallbladder	156.0	197.8	230.8	211.5	235.3	239.0
contiguous sites with extrahepatic bile ducts	156.8	—	—	—	—	—
ganglia (*see also* Neoplasm, connective tissue)	171.9	198.89	—	215.9	238.1	239.2
basal	191.0	198.3	—	225.0	237.5	239.6
ganglion (*see also* Neoplasm, connective tissue)	171.9	198.89	—	215.9	238.1	239.2
cranial nerve	192.0	198.4	—	225.1	237.9	239.7
Gartner's duct	184.0	198.82	233.3	221.1	236.3	239.5
gastric — *see* Neoplasm, stomach						
gastrocolic	159.8	197.8	230.9	211.9	235.5	239.0
gastroesophageal junction	151.0	197.8	230.2	211.1	235.2	239.0
gastrointestinal (tract) NEC	159.9	197.8	230.9	211.9	235.5	239.0
generalized	199.0	199.0	234.9	229.9	238.9	199.0
genital organ or tract						
female NEC	184.9	198.82	233.3	221.9	236.3	239.5
contiguous sites	184.8	—	—	—	—	—
specified site NEC	184.8	198.82	233.3	221.8	236.3	239.5
male NEC	187.9	198.82	233.6	222.9	236.6	239.5
contiguous sites	187.8	—	—	—	—	—
specified site NEC	187.8	198.82	233.6	222.8	236.6	239.5
genitourinary tract						
female	184.9	198.82	233.3	221.9	236.3	239.5
male	187.9	198.82	233.6	222.9	236.6	239.5

Neoplasm, neoplastic — *continued*	Malignant					
	Primary	Secondary	Ca in situ	Benign	Uncertain Behavior	Unspecified
gingiva (alveolar) (marginal)	143.9	198.89	230.0	210.4	235.1	239.0
lower	143.1	198.89	230.0	210.4	235.1	239.0
mandibular	143.1	198.89	230.0	210.4	235.1	239.0
maxillary	143.0	198.89	230.0	210.4	235.1	239.0
upper	143.0	198.89	230.0	210.4	235.1	239.0
gland, glandular (lymphatic) (system) — *see also* Neoplasm, lymph gland						
endocrine NEC	194.9	198.89	—	227.9	237.4	239.7
salivary — *see* Neoplasm, salivary, gland						
glans penis	187.2	198.82	233.5	222.1	236.6	239.5
globus pallidus	191.0	198.3	—	225.0	237.5	239.6
glomus						
coccygeal	194.6	198.89	—	227.6	237.3	239.7
jugularis	194.6	198.89	—	227.6	237.3	239.7
glosso-epiglottic fold(s)	146.4	198.89	230.0	210.6	235.1	239.0
glossopalatine fold	146.2	198.89	230.0	210.6	235.1	239.0
glossopharyngeal sulcus	146.1	198.89	230.0	210.6	235.1	239.0
glottis	161.0	197.3	231.0	212.1	235.6	239.1
gluteal region*	195.3	198.89	232.5	229.8	238.8	239.8
great vessels NEC	171.4	198.89	—	215.4	238.1	239.2
groin NEC	195.3	198.89	232.5	229.8	238.8	239.8
gum	143.9	198.89	230.0	210.4	235.1	239.0
contiguous sites	143.8	—	—	—	—	—
lower	143.1	198.89	230.0	210.4	235.1	239.0
upper	143.0	198.89	230.0	210.4	235.1	239.0
hand NEC*	195.4	198.89	232.6	229.8	238.8	239.8
head NEC*	195.0	198.89	232.4	229.8	238.8	239.8
heart	164.1	198.89	—	212.7	238.8	239.8
contiguous sites with mediastinum or thymus	164.8	—	—	—	—	—
heel NEC*	195.5	198.89	232.7	229.8	238.8	239.8
helix	173.2	198.2	232.2	216.2	238.2	239.2
hematopoietic, hemopoietic tissue NEC	202.8 ☑	198.89	—	—	—	238.7
hemisphere, cerebral	191.0	198.3	—	225.0	237.5	239.6
hemorrhoidal zone	154.2	197.5	230.5	211.4	235.5	239.0
hepatic	155.2	197.7	230.8	211.5	235.3	239.0
duct (bile)	156.1	197.8	230.8	211.5	235.3	239.0
flexure (colon)	153.0	197.5	230.3	211.3	235.2	239.0
primary	155.0	—	—	—	—	—
hilus of lung	162.2	197.0	231.2	212.3	235.7	239.1
hip NEC*	195.5	198.89	232.7	229.8	238.8	239.8
hippocampus, brain	191.2	198.3	—	225.0	237.5	239.6
humerus (any part)	170.4	198.5	—	213.4	238.0	239.2
hymen	184.0	198.82	233.3	221.1	236.3	239.5
hypopharynx, hypopharyngeal NEC	148.9	198.89	230.0	210.8	235.1	239.0
contiguous sites	148.8	—	—	—	—	—
postcricoid region	148.0	198.89	230.0	210.8	235.1	239.0
posterior wall	148.3	198.89	230.0	210.8	235.1	239.0
pyriform fossa (sinus)	148.1	198.89	230.0	210.8	235.1	239.0
specified site NEC	148.8	198.89	230.0	210.8	235.1	239.0
wall	148.9	198.89	230.0	210.8	235.1	239.0
posterior	148.3	198.89	230.0	210.8	235.1	239.0
hypophysis	194.3	198.89	234.8	227.3	237.0	239.7
hypothalamus	191.0	198.3	—	225.0	237.5	239.6
ileocecum, ileocecal (coil) (junction) (valve)	153.4	197.5	230.3	211.3	235.2	239.0
ileum	152.2	197.4	230.7	211.2	235.2	239.0
ilium	170.6	198.5	—	213.6	238.0	239.2
immunoproliferative NEC	203.8 ☑	—	—	—	—	—
infraclavicular (region)*	195.1	198.89	232.5	229.8	238.8	239.8
inguinal (region)*	195.3	198.89	232.5	229.8	238.8	239.8
insula	191.0	198.3	—	225.0	237.5	239.6
insular tissue (pancreas)	157.4	197.8	230.9	211.7	235.5	239.0
brain	191.0	198.3	—	225.0	237.5	239.6
interarytenoid fold	148.2	198.89	230.0	210.8	235.1	239.0
hypopharyngeal aspect	148.2	198.89	230.0	210.8	235.1	239.0
laryngeal aspect	161.1	197.3	231.0	212.1	235.6	239.1
marginal zone	148.2	198.89	230.0	210.8	235.1	239.0
interdental papillae	143.9	198.89	230.0	210.4	235.1	239.0
lower	143.1	198.89	230.0	210.4	235.1	239.0
upper	143.0	198.89	230.0	210.4	235.1	239.0
internal						
capsule	191.0	198.3	—	225.0	237.5	239.6
os (cervix)	180.0	198.82	233.1	219.0	236.0	239.5
intervertebral cartilage or disc	170.2	198.5	—	213.2	238.0	239.2

Neoplasm, neoplastic — *continued*	Malignant					
	Primary	Secondary	Ca in situ	Benign	Uncertain Behavior	Unspecified
intestine, intestinal	159.0	197.8	230.7	211.9	235.2	239.0
large	153.9	197.5	230.3	211.3	235.2	239.0
appendix	153.5	197.5	230.3	211.3	235.2	239.0
caput coli	153.4	197.5	230.3	211.3	235.2	239.0
cecum	153.4	197.5	230.3	211.3	235.2	239.0
colon	153.9	197.5	230.3	211.3	235.2	239.0
and rectum	154.0	197.5	230.4	211.4	235.2	239.0
ascending	153.6	197.5	230.3	211.3	235.2	239.0
caput	153.4	197.5	230.3	211.3	235.2	239.0
contiguous sites	153.8	—	—	—	—	—
descending	153.2	197.5	230.3	211.3	235.2	239.0
distal	153.2	197.5	230.3	211.3	235.2	239.0
left	153.2	197.5	230.3	211.3	235.2	239.0
pelvic	153.3	197.5	230.3	211.3	235.2	239.0
right	153.6	197.5	230.3	211.3	235.2	239.0
sigmoid (flexure)	153.3	197.5	230.3	211.3	235.2	239.0
transverse	153.1	197.5	230.3	211.3	235.2	239.0
contiguous sites	153.8	—	—	—	—	—
hepatic flexure	153.0	197.5	230.3	211.3	235.2	239.0
ileocecum, ileocecal (coil) (valve)	153.4	197.5	230.3	211.3	235.2	239.0
sigmoid flexure (lower) (upper)	153.3	197.5	230.3	211.3	235.2	239.0
splenic flexure	153.7	197.5	230.3	211.3	235.2	239.0
small	152.9	197.4	230.7	211.2	235.2	239.0
contiguous sites	152.8	—	—	—	—	—
duodenum	152.0	197.4	230.7	211.2	235.2	239.0
ileum	152.2	197.4	230.7	211.2	235.2	239.0
jejunum	152.1	197.4	230.7	211.2	235.2	239.0
tract NEC	159.0	197.8	230.7	211.9	235.2	239.0
intra-abdominal	195.2	198.89	234.8	229.8	238.8	239.8
intracranial NEC	191.9	198.3	—	225.0	237.5	239.6
intrahepatic (bile) duct	155.1	197.8	230.8	211.5	235.3	239.0
intraocular	190.0	198.4	234.0	224.0	238.8	239.8
intraorbital	190.1	198.4	234.0	224.1	238.8	239.8
intrasellar	194.3	198.89	234.8	227.3	237.0	239.7
intrathoracic (cavity) (organs NEC)	195.1	198.89	234.8	229.8	238.8	239.8
contiguous sites with respiratory organs	165.8	—	—	—	—	—
iris	190.0	198.4	234.0	224.0	238.8	239.8
ischiorectal (fossa)	195.3	198.89	234.8	229.8	238.8	239.8
ischium	170.6	198.5	—	213.6	238.0	239.2
island of Reil	191.0	198.3	—	225.0	237.5	239.6
islands or islets of Langerhans	157.4	197.8	230.9	211.7	235.5	239.0
isthmus uteri	182.1	198.82	233.2	219.1	236.0	239.5
jaw	195.0	198.89	234.8	229.8	238.8	239.8
bone	170.1	198.5	—	213.1	238.0	239.2
carcinoma	143.9	—	—	—	—	—
lower	143.1	—	—	—	—	—
upper	143.0	—	—	—	—	—
lower	170.1	198.5	—	213.1	238.0	239.2
upper	170.0	198.5	—	213.0	238.0	239.2
carcinoma (any type) (lower) (upper)	195.0	—	—	—	—	—
skin	173.3	198.2	232.3	216.3	238.2	239.2
soft tissues	143.9	198.89	230.0	210.4	235.1	239.0
lower	143.1	198.89	230.0	210.4	235.1	239.0
upper	143.0	198.89	230.0	210.4	235.1	239.0
jejunum	152.1	197.4	230.7	211.2	235.2	239.0
joint NEC (*see also* Neoplasm, bone)	170.9	198.5	—	213.9	238.0	239.2
acromioclavicular	170.4	198.5	—	213.4	238.0	239.2
bursa or synovial membrane — *see* Neoplasm, connective tissue						
costovertebral	170.3	198.5	—	213.3	238.0	239.2
sternocostal	170.3	198.5	—	213.3	238.0	239.2
temporomandibular	170.1	198.5	—	213.1	238.0	239.2
junction						
anorectal	154.8	197.5	230.7	211.4	235.5	239.0
cardioesophageal	151.0	197.8	230.2	211.1	235.2	239.0
esophagogastric	151.0	197.8	230.2	211.1	235.2	239.0
gastroesophageal	151.0	197.8	230.2	211.1	235.2	239.0
hard and soft palate	145.5	198.89	230.0	210.4	235.1	239.0
ileocecal	153.4	197.5	230.3	211.3	235.2	239.0
pelvirectal	154.0	197.5	230.4	211.4	235.2	239.0
pelviureteric	189.1	198.0	233.9	223.1	236.91	239.5
rectosigmoid	154.0	197.5	230.4	211.4	235.2	239.0
squamocolumnar, of cervix	180.8	198.82	233.1	219.0	236.0	239.5
kidney (parenchyma)	189.0	198.0	233.9	223.0	236.91	239.5
calyx	189.1	198.0	233.9	223.1	236.91	239.5

☑ Additional Digit Required — Refer to the Tabular List (Numeric Code Section) for Additional Digit Selection

▶◀ Revised Text ● New Line ▲ Revised Code

Neoplasm, neoplastic — continued	Malignant					
	Primary	Secondary	Ca in situ	Benign	Uncertain Behavior	Unspecified
kidney — continued						
hilus	189.1	198.0	233.9	223.1	236.91	239.5
pelvis	189.1	198.0	233.9	223.1	236.91	239.5
knee NEC*	195.5	198.89	232.7	229.8	238.8	239.8
labia (skin)	184.4	198.82	233.3	221.2	236.3	239.5
majora	184.1	198.82	233.3	221.2	236.3	239.5
minora	184.2	198.82	233.3	221.2	236.3	239.5
labial — *see also* Neoplasm, lip						
sulcus (lower) (upper)	145.1	198.89	230.0	210.4	235.1	239.0
labium (skin)	184.4	198.82	233.3	221.2	236.3	239.5
majus	184.1	198.82	233.3	221.2	236.3	239.5
minus	184.2	198.82	233.3	221.2	236.3	239.5
lacrimal						
canaliculi	190.7	198.4	234.0	224.7	238.8	239.8
duct (nasal)	190.7	198.4	234.0	224.7	238.8	239.8
gland	190.2	198.4	234.0	224.2	238.8	239.8
punctum	190.7	198.4	234.0	224.7	238.8	239.8
sac	190.7	198.4	234.0	224.7	238.8	239.8
Langerhans, islands or islets	157.4	197.8	230.9	211.7	235.5	239.0
laryngopharynx	148.9	198.89	230.0	210.8	235.1	239.0
larynx, laryngeal NEC	161.9	197.3	231.0	212.1	235.6	239.1
aryepiglottic fold	161.1	197.3	231.0	212.1	235.6	239.1
cartilage (arytenoid) (cricoid) (cuneiform) (thyroid)	161.3	197.3	231.0	212.1	235.6	239.1
commissure (anterior) (posterior)	161.0	197.3	231.0	212.1	235.6	239.1
contiguous sites	161.8	—	—	—	—	—
extrinsic NEC	161.1	197.3	231.0	212.1	235.6	239.1
meaning hypopharynx	148.9	198.89	230.0	210.8	235.1	239.0
interarytenoid fold	161.1	197.3	231.0	212.1	235.6	239.1
intrinsic	161.0	197.3	231.0	212.1	235.6	239.1
ventricular band	161.1	197.3	231.0	212.1	235.6	239.1
leg NEC*	195.5	198.89	232.7	229.8	238.8	239.8
lens, crystalline	190.0	198.4	234.0	224.0	238.8	239.8
lid (lower) (upper)	173.1	198.2	232.1	216.1	238.2	239.2
ligament — *see also* Neoplasm, connective tissue						
broad	183.3	198.82	233.3	221.0	236.3	239.5
Mackenrodt's	183.8	198.82	233.3	221.8	236.3	239.5
non-uterine — *see* Neoplasm, connective tissue						
round	183.5	198.82	—	221.0	236.3	239.5
sacro-uterine	183.4	198.82	—	221.0	236.3	239.5
uterine	183.4	198.82	—	221.0	236.3	239.5
utero-ovarian	183.8	198.82	233.3	221.8	236.3	239.5
uterosacral	183.4	198.82	—	221.0	236.3	239.5
limb*	195.8	198.89	232.8	229.8	238.8	239.8
lower*	195.5	198.89	232.7	229.8	238.8	239.8
upper*	195.4	198.89	232.6	229.8	238.8	239.8
limbus of cornea	190.4	198.4	234.0	224.4	238.8	239.8
lingual NEC (*see also* Neoplasm, tongue)	141.9	198.89	230.0	210.1	235.1	239.0
lingula, lung	162.3	197.0	231.2	212.3	235.7	239.1
lip (external) (lipstick area) (vermillion border)	140.9	198.89	230.0	210.0	235.1	239.0
buccal aspect — *see* Neoplasm, lip, internal						
commissure	140.6	198.89	230.0	210.4	235.1	239.0
contiguous sites	140.8	—	—	—	—	—
with oral cavity or pharynx	149.8	—	—	—	—	—
frenulum — *see* Neoplasm, lip, internal						
inner aspect — *see* Neoplasm, lip, internal						
internal (buccal) (frenulum) (mucosa) (oral)	140.5	198.89	230.0	210.0	235.1	239.0
lower	140.4	198.89	230.0	210.0	235.1	239.0
upper	140.3	198.89	230.0	210.0	235.1	239.0
lower	140.1	198.89	230.0	210.0	235.1	239.0
internal (buccal) (frenulum) (mucosa) (oral)	140.4	198.89	230.0	210.0	235.1	239.0
mucosa — *see* Neoplasm, lip, internal						
oral aspect — *see* Neoplasm, lip, internal						
skin (commissure) (lower) (upper)	173.0	198.2	232.0	216.0	238.2	239.2
upper	140.0	198.89	230.0	210.0	235.1	239.0
internal (buccal) (frenulum) (mucosa) (oral)	140.3	198.89	230.0	210.0	235.1	239.0

Neoplasm, neoplastic — continued	Malignant					
	Primary	Secondary	Ca in situ	Benign	Uncertain Behavior	Unspecified
liver	155.2	197.7	230.8	211.5	235.3	239.0
primary	155.0	—	—	—	—	—
lobe						
azygos	162.3	197.0	231.2	212.3	235.7	239.1
frontal	191.1	198.3	—	225.0	237.5	239.6
lower	162.5	197.0	231.2	212.3	235.7	239.1
middle	162.4	197.0	231.2	212.3	235.7	239.1
occipital	191.4	198.3	—	225.0	237.5	239.6
parietal	191.3	198.3	—	225.0	237.5	239.6
temporal	191.2	198.3	—	225.0	237.5	239.6
upper	162.3	197.0	231.2	212.3	235.7	239.1
lumbosacral plexus	171.6	198.4	—	215.6	238.1	239.2
lung	162.9	197.0	231.2	212.3	235.7	239.1
azygos lobe	162.3	197.0	231.2	212.3	235.7	239.1
carina	162.2	197.0	231.2	212.3	235.7	239.1
contiguous sites with bronchus or trachea	162.8	—	—	—	—	—
hilus	162.2	197.0	231.2	212.3	235.7	239.1
lingula	162.3	197.0	231.2	212.3	235.7	239.1
lobe NEC	162.9	197.0	231.2	212.3	235.7	239.1
lower lobe	162.5	197.0	231.2	212.3	235.7	239.1
main bronchus	162.2	197.0	231.2	212.3	235.7	239.1
middle lobe	162.4	197.0	231.2	212.3	235.7	239.1
upper lobe	162.3	197.0	231.2	212.3	235.7	239.1
lymph, lymphatic						
channel NEC (*see also* Neoplasm, connective tissue)	171.9	198.89	—	215.9	238.1	239.2
gland (secondary)	—	196.9	—	229.0	238.8	239.8
abdominal	—	196.2	—	229.0	238.8	239.8
aortic	—	196.2	—	229.0	238.8	239.8
arm	—	196.3	—	229.0	238.8	239.8
auricular (anterior) (posterior)	—	196.0	—	229.0	238.8	239.8
axilla, axillary	—	196.3	—	229.0	238.8	239.8
brachial	—	196.3	—	229.0	238.8	239.8
bronchial	—	196.1	—	229.0	238.8	239.8
bronchopulmonary	—	196.1	—	229.0	238.8	239.8
celiac	—	196.2	—	229.0	238.8	239.8
cervical	—	196.0	—	229.0	238.8	239.8
cervicofacial	—	196.0	—	229.0	238.8	239.8
Cloquet	—	196.5	—	229.0	238.8	239.8
colic	—	196.2	—	229.0	238.8	239.8
common duct	—	196.2	—	229.0	238.8	239.8
cubital	—	196.3	—	229.0	238.8	239.8
diaphragmatic	—	196.1	—	229.0	238.8	239.8
epigastric, inferior	—	196.6	—	229.0	238.8	239.8
epitrochlear	—	196.3	—	229.0	238.8	239.8
esophageal	—	196.1	—	229.0	238.8	239.8
face	—	196.0	—	229.0	238.8	239.8
femoral	—	196.5	—	229.0	238.8	239.8
gastric	—	196.2	—	229.0	238.8	239.8
groin	—	196.5	—	229.0	238.8	239.8
head	—	196.0	—	229.0	238.8	239.8
hepatic	—	196.2	—	229.0	238.8	239.8
hilar (pulmonary)	—	196.1	—	229.0	238.8	239.8
splenic	—	196.2	—	229.0	238.8	239.8
hypogastric	—	196.6	—	229.0	238.8	239.8
ileocolic	—	196.2	—	229.0	238.8	239.8
iliac	—	196.6	—	229.0	238.8	239.8
infraclavicular	—	196.3	—	229.0	238.8	239.8
inguina, inguinal	—	196.5	—	229.0	238.8	239.8
innominate	—	196.1	—	229.0	238.8	239.8
intercostal	—	196.1	—	229.0	238.8	239.8
intestinal	—	196.2	—	229.0	238.8	239.8
intra-abdominal	—	196.2	—	229.0	238.8	239.8
intrapelvic	—	196.6	—	229.0	238.8	239.8
intrathoracic	—	196.1	—	229.0	238.8	239.9
jugular	—	196.0	—	229.0	238.8	239.8
leg	—	196.5	—	229.0	238.8	239.8
limb						
lower	—	196.5	—	229.0	238.8	239.8
upper	—	196.3	—	229.0	238.8	239.8
lower limb	—	196.5	—	229.0	238.8	238.9
lumbar	—	196.2	—	229.0	238.8	239.8
mandibular	—	196.0	—	229.0	238.8	239.8
mediastinal	—	196.1	—	229.0	238.8	239.8
mesenteric (inferior) (superior)	—	196.2	—	229.0	238.8	239.8

Neoplasm, neoplastic — *continued*	Malignant					
	Primary	Secondary	Ca in situ	Benign	Uncertain Behavior	Unspecified
lymph, lymphatic — *continued*						
gland — *continued*						
midcolic	—	196.2	—	229.0	238.8	239.8
multiple sites in categories 196.0-196.6	—	196.8	—	229.0	238.8	239.8
neck	—	196.0	—	229.0	238.8	239.8
obturator	—	196.6	—	229.0	238.8	239.8
occipital	—	196.0	—	229.0	238.8	239.8
pancreatic	—	196.2	—	229.0	238.8	239.8
para-aortic	—	196.2	—	229.0	238.8	239.8
paracervical	—	196.6	—	229.0	238.8	239.8
parametrial	—	196.6	—	229.0	238.8	239.8
parasternal	—	196.1	—	229.0	238.8	239.8
parotid	—	196.0	—	229.0	238.8	239.8
pectoral	—	196.3	—	229.0	238.8	239.8
pelvic	—	196.6	—	229.0	238.8	239.8
peri-aortic	—	196.2	—	229.0	238.8	239.8
peripancreatic	—	196.2	—	229.0	238.8	239.8
popliteal	—	196.5	—	229.0	238.8	239.8
porta hepatis	—	196.2	—	229.0	238.8	239.8
portal	—	196.2	—	229.0	238.8	239.8
preauricular	—	196.0	—	229.0	238.8	239.8
prelaryngeal	—	196.0	—	229.0	238.8	239.8
presymphysial	—	196.6	—	229.0	238.8	239.8
pretracheal	—	196.0	—	229.0	238.8	239.8
primary (any site) NEC	202.9 ☑	—	—	—	—	—
pulmonary (hiler)	—	196.1	—	229.0	238.8	239.8
pyloric	—	196.2	—	229.0	238.8	239.8
retroperitoneal	—	196.2	—	229.0	238.8	239.8
retropharyngeal	—	196.0	—	229.0	238.8	239.8
Rosenmüller's	—	196.5	—	229.0	238.8	239.8
sacral	—	196.6	—	229.0	238.8	239.8
scalene	—	196.0	—	229.0	238.8	239.8
site NEC	—	196.9	—	229.0	238.8	239.8
splenic (hilar)	—	196.2	—	229.0	238.8	239.8
subclavicular	—	196.3	—	229.0	238.8	239.8
subinguinal	—	196.5	—	229.0	238.8	239.8
sublingual	—	196.0	—	229.0	238.8	239.8
submandibular	—	196.0	—	229.0	238.8	239.8
submaxillary	—	196.0	—	229.0	238.8	239.8
submental	—	196.0	—	229.0	238.8	239.8
subscapular	—	196.3	—	229.0	238.8	239.8
supraclavicular	—	196.0	—	229.0	238.8	239.8
thoracic	—	196.1	—	229.0	238.8	239.8
tibial	—	196.5	—	229.0	238.8	239.8
tracheal	—	196.1	—	229.0	238.8	239.8
tracheobronchial	—	196.1	—	229.0	238.8	239.8
upper limb	—	196.3	—	229.0	238.8	239.8
Virchow's	—	196.0	—	229.0	238.8	239.8
node — *see also* Neoplasm, lymph gland						
primary NEC	202.9 ☑	—	—	—	—	—
vessel (*see also* Neoplasm, connective tissue)	171.9	198.89	—	215.9	238.1	239.2
Nackenrodt's ligament	183.8	198.82	233.3	221.8	236.3	239.5
malar	170.0	198.5	—	213.0	238.0	239.2
region — *see* Neoplasm, cheek						
mammary gland — *see* Neoplasm, breast						
mandible	170.1	198.5	—	213.1	238.0	239.2
alveolar						
mucose	143.1	198.89	230.0	210.4	235.1	239.0
ridge or process	170.1	198.5	—	213.1	238.0	239.2
carcinoma	143.1	—	—	—	—	—
carcinoma	143.1	—	—	—	—	—
marrow (bone) NEC	202.9 ☑	198.5	—	—	—	238.7
mastectomy site (skin)	173.5	198.2	—	—	—	—
specified as breast tissue	174.8	198.81	—	—	—	—
mastoid (air cells) (antrum) (cavity)	160.1	197.3	231.8	212.0	235.9	239.1
bone or process	170.0	198.5	—	213.0	238.0	239.2
maxilla, maxillary (superior)	170.0	198.5	—	213.0	238.0	239.2
alveolar						
mucosa	143.0	198.89	230.0	210.4	235.1	239.0
ridge or process	170.0	198.5	—	213.0	238.0	239.2
carcinoma	143.0	—	—	—	—	—
antrum	160.2	197.3	231.8	212.0	235.9	239.1
carcinoma	143.0	—	—	—	—	—
maxilla, maxillary — *continued*						
inferior — *see* Neoplasm, mandible						
sinus	160.2	197.3	231.8	212.0	235.9	239.1
meatus						
external (ear)	173.2	198.2	232.2	216.2	238.2	239.2
Meckel's diverticulum	152.3	197.4	230.7	211.2	235.2	239.0
mediastinum, mediastinal	164.9	197.1	—	212.5	235.8	239.8
anterior	164.2	197.1	—	212.5	235.8	239.8
contiguous sites with heart and thymus	164.8	—	—	—	—	—
posterior	164.3	197.1	—	212.5	235.8	239.8
medulla						
adrenal	194.0	198.7	234.8	227.0	237.2	239.7
oblongata	191.7	198.3	—	225.0	237.5	239.6
meibomian gland	173.1	198.2	232.1	216.1	238.2	239.2
melanoma — *see* Melanoma						
meninges (brain) (cerebral) (cranial) (intracranial)	192.1	198.4	—	225.2	237.6	239.7
spinal (cord)	192.3	198.4	—	225.4	237.6	239.7
meniscus, knee joint (lateral) (medial)	170.7	198.5	—	213.7	238.0	239.2
mesentery, mesenteric	158.8	197.6	—	211.8	235.4	239.0
mesoappendix	158.8	197.6	—	211.8	235.4	239.0
mesocolon	158.8	197.6	—	211.8	235.4	239.0
mesopharynx — *see* Neoplasm, oropharynx						
mesosalpinx	183.3	198.82	233.3	221.0	236.3	239.5
mesovarium	183.3	198.82	233.3	221.0	236.3	239.5
metacarpus (any bone)	170.5	198.5	—	213.5	238.0	239.2
metastatic NEC — *see also* Neoplasm, by site, secondary	—	199.1	—	—	—	—
metatarsus (any bone)	170.8	198.5	—	213.8	238.0	239.2
midbrain	191.7	198.3	—	225.0	237.5	239.6
milk duct — *see* Neoplasm, breast						
mons						
pubis	184.4	198.82	233.3	221.2	236.3	239.5
veneris	184.4	198.82	233.3	221.2	236.3	239.5
motor tract	192.9	198.4	—	225.9	237.9	239.7
brain	191.9	198.3	—	225.0	237.5	239.6
spinal	192.2	198.3	—	225.3	237.5	239.7
mouth	145.9	198.89	230.0	210.4	235.1	239.0
contiguous sites	145.8	—	—	—	—	—
floor	144.9	198.89	230.0	210.3	235.1	239.0
anterior portion	144.0	198.89	230.0	210.3	235.1	239.0
contiguous sites	144.8	—	—	—	—	—
lateral portion	144.1	198.89	230.0	210.3	235.1	239.0
roof	145.5	198.89	230.0	210.4	235.1	239.0
specified part NEC	145.8	198.89	230.0	210.4	235.1	239.0
vestibule	145.1	198.89	230.0	210.4	235.1	239.0
mucosa						
alveolar (ridge or process)	143.9	198.89	230.0	210.4	235.1	239.0
lower	143.1	198.89	230.0	210.4	235.1	239.0
upper	143.0	198.89	230.0	210.4	235.1	239.0
buccal	145.0	198.89	230.0	210.4	235.1	239.0
cheek	145.0	198.89	230.0	210.4	235.1	239.0
lip — *see* Neoplasm, lip, internal						
nasal	160.0	197.3	231.8	212.0	235.9	239.1
oral	145.0	198.89	230.0	210.4	235.1	239.0
Müllerian duct						
female	184.8	198.82	233.3	221.8	236.3	239.5
male	187.8	198.82	233.6	222.8	236.6	239.5
multiple sites NEC	199.0	199.0	234.9	229.9	238.9	199.0
muscle — *see also* Neoplasm, connective tissue						
extraocular	190.1	198.4	234.0	224.1	238.8	239.8
myocardium	164.1	198.89	—	212.7	238.8	239.8
myometrium	182.0	198.82	233.2	219.1	236.0	239.5
myopericardium	164.1	198.89	—	212.7	238.8	239.8
nabothian gland (follicle)	180.0	198.82	233.1	219.0	236.0	239.5
nail	173.9	198.2	232.9	216.9	238.2	239.2
finger	173.6	198.2	232.6	216.6	238.2	239.2
toe	173.7	198.2	232.7	216.7	238.2	239.2
nares, naris (anterior) (posterior)	160.0	197.3	231.8	212.0	235.9	239.1
nasal — *see* Neoplasm, nose						
nasolabial groove	173.3	198.2	232.3	216.3	238.2	239.2
nasolacrimal duct	190.7	198.4	234.0	224.7	238.8	239.8

Index

Neoplasm, lymph, lymphatic — Neoplasm, nasolacrimal duct

Neoplasm, neoplastic — *continued*	Malignant					
	Primary	Secondary	Ca in situ	Benign	Uncertain Behavior	Unspecified
nasopharynx, nasopharyngeal	147.9	198.89	230.0	210.7	235.1	239.0
contiguous sites	147.8	—	—	—	—	—
floor	147.3	198.89	230.0	210.7	235.1	239.0
roof	147.0	198.89	230.0	210.7	235.1	239.0
specified site NEC	147.8	198.89	230.0	210.7	235.1	239.0
wall	147.9	198.89	230.0	210.7	235.1	239.0
anterior	147.3	198.89	230.0	210.7	235.1	239.0
lateral	147.2	198.89	230.0	210.7	235.1	239.0
posterior	147.1	198.89	230.0	210.7	235.1	239.0
superior	147.0	198.89	230.0	210.7	235.1	239.0
nates	173.5	198.2	232.5	216.5	238.2	239.2
neck NEC*	195.0	198.89	234.8	229.8	238.8	239.8
nerve (autonomic) (ganglion) (parasympathetic) (peripheral) (sympathetic) — *see also* Neoplasm, connective tissue						
abducens	192.0	198.4	—	225.1	237.9	239.7
accessory (spinal)	192.0	198.4	—	225.1	237.9	239.7
acoustic	192.0	198.4	—	225.1	237.9	239.7
auditory	192.0	198.4	—	225.1	237.9	239.7
brachial	171.2	198.89	—	215.2	238.1	239.2
cranial (any)	192.0	198.4	—	225.1	237.9	239.7
facial	192.0	198.4	—	225.1	237.9	239.7
femoral	171.3	198.89	—	215.3	238.1	239.2
glossopharyngeal	192.0	198.4	—	225.1	237.9	239.7
hypoglossal	192.0	198.4	—	225.1	237.9	239.7
intercostal	171.4	198.89	—	215.4	238.1	239.2
lumbar	171.7	198.89	—	215.7	238.1	239.2
median	171.2	198.89	—	215.2	238.1	239.2
obturator	171.3	198.89	—	215.3	238.1	239.2
oculomotor	192.0	198.4	—	225.1	237.9	239.7
olfactory	192.0	198.4	—	225.1	237.9	239.7
optic	192.0	198.4	—	225.1	237.9	239.7
peripheral NEC	171.9	198.89	—	215.9	238.1	239.2
radial	171.2	198.89	—	215.2	238.1	239.2
sacral	171.6	198.89	—	215.6	238.1	239.2
sciatic	171.3	198.89	—	215.3	238.1	239.2
spinal NEC	171.9	198.89	—	215.9	238.1	239.2
trigeminal	192.0	198.4	—	225.1	237.9	239.7
trochlear	192.0	198.4	—	225.1	237.9	239.7
ulnar	171.2	198.89	—	215.2	238.1	239.2
vagus	192.0	198.4	—	225.1	237.9	239.7
nervous system (central) NEC	192.9	198.4	—	225.9	237.9	239.7
autonomic NEC	171.9	198.89	—	215.9	238.1	239.2
brain — *see also* Neoplasm, brain						
membrane or meninges	192.1	198.4	—	225.2	237.6	239.7
contiguous sites	192.8	—	—	—	—	—
parasympathetic NEC	171.9	198.89	—	215.9	238.1	239.2
sympathetic NEC	171.9	198.89	—	215.9	238.1	239.2
nipple (female)	174.0	198.81	233.0	217	238.3	239.3
male	175.0	198.81	233.0	217	238.3	239.3
nose, nasal	195.0	198.89	234.8	229.8	238.8	239.8
ala (external)	173.3	198.2	232.3	216.3	238.2	239.2
bone	170.0	198.5	—	213.0	238.0	239.2
cartilage	160.0	197.3	231.8	212.0	235.9	239.1
cavity	160.0	197.3	231.8	212.0	235.9	239.1
contiguous sites with accessory sinuses or middle ear	160.8	—	—	—	—	—
choana	147.3	198.89	230.0	210.7	235.1	239.0
external (skin)	173.3	198.2	232.3	216.3	238.2	239.2
fossa	160.0	197.3	231.8	212.0	235.9	239.1
internal	160.0	197.3	231.8	212.0	235.9	239.1
mucosa	160.0	197.3	231.8	212.0	235.9	239.1
septum	160.0	197.3	231.8	212.0	235.9	239.1
posterior margin	147.3	198.89	230.0	210.7	235.1	239.0
sinus — *see* Neoplasm, sinus						
skin	173.3	198.2	232.3	216.3	238.2	239.2
turbinate (mucosa)	160.0	197.3	231.8	212.0	235.9	239.1
bone	170.0	198.5	—	213.0	238.0	239.2
vestibule	160.0	197.3	231.8	212.0	235.9	239.1
nostril	160.0	197.3	231.8	212.0	235.9	239.1
nucleus pulposus	170.2	198.5	—	213.2	238.0	239.2
occipital						
bone	170.0	198.5	—	213.0	238.0	239.2
lobe or pole, brain	191.4	198.3	—	225.0	237.5	239.6
odontogenic — *see* Neoplasm, jaw bone						

Neoplasm, neoplastic — *continued*	Malignant					
	Primary	Secondary	Ca in situ	Benign	Uncertain Behavior	Unspecified
oesophagus — *see* Neoplasm, esophagus						
olfactory nerve or bulb	192.0	198.4	—	225.1	237.9	239.7
olive (brain)	191.7	198.3	—	225.0	237.5	239.6
omentum	158.8	197.6	—	211.8	235.4	239.0
operculum (brain)	191.0	198.3	—	225.0	237.5	239.6
optic nerve, chiasm, or tract	192.0	198.4	—	225.1	237.9	239.7
oral (cavity)	145.9	198.89	230.0	210.4	235.1	239.0
contiguous sites with lip or pharynx	149.8	—	—	—	—	—
ill-defined	149.9	198.89	230.0	210.4	235.1	239.0
mucosa	145.9	198.89	230.0	210.4	235.1	239.0
orbit	190.1	198.4	234.0	224.1	238.8	239.8
bone	170.0	198.5	—	213.0	238.0	239.2
eye	190.1	198.4	234.0	224.1	238.8	239.8
soft parts	190.1	198.4	234.0	224.1	238.8	239.8
organ of Zuckerkandl	194.6	198.89	—	227.6	237.3	239.7
oropharynx	146.9	198.89	230.0	210.6	235.1	239.0
branchial cleft (vestige)	146.8	198.89	230.0	210.6	235.1	239.0
contiguous sites	146.8	—	—	—	—	—
junctional region	146.5	198.89	230.0	210.6	235.1	239.0
lateral wall	146.6	198.89	230.0	210.6	235.1	239.0
pillars of fauces	146.2	198.89	230.0	210.6	235.1	239.0
posterior wall	146.7	198.89	230.0	210.6	235.1	239.0
specified part NEC	146.8	198.89	230.0	210.6	235.1	239.0
vallecula	146.3	198.89	230.0	210.6	235.1	239.0
os						
external	180.1	198.82	233.1	219.0	236.0	239.5
internal	180.0	198.82	233.1	219.0	236.0	239.5
ovary	183.0	198.6	233.3	220	236.2	239.5
oviduct	183.2	198.82	233.3	221.0	236.3	239.5
palate	145.5	198.89	230.0	210.4	235.1	239.0
hard	145.2	198.89	230.0	210.4	235.1	239.0
junction of hard and soft palate	145.5	198.89	230.0	210.4	235.1	239.0
soft	145.3	198.89	230.0	210.4	235.1	239.0
nasopharyngeal surface	147.3	198.89	230.0	210.7	235.1	239.0
posterior surface	147.3	198.89	230.0	210.7	235.1	239.0
superior surface	147.3	198.89	230.0	210.7	235.1	239.0
palatoglossal arch	146.2	198.89	230.0	210.6	235.1	239.0
palatopharyngeal arch	146.2	198.89	230.0	210.6	235.1	239.0
pallium	191.0	198.3	—	225.0	237.5	239.6
palpebra	173.1	198.2	232.1	216.1	238.2	239.2
pancreas	157.9	197.8	230.9	211.6	235.5	239.0
body	157.1	197.8	230.9	211.6	235.5	239.0
contiguous sites	157.8	—	—	—	—	—
duct (of Santorini) (of Wirsung)	157.3	197.8	230.9	211.6	235.5	239.0
ectopic tissue	157.8	197.8	230.9	211.6	235.5	239.0
head	157.0	197.8	230.9	211.6	235.5	239.0
islet cells	157.4	197.8	230.9	211.7	235.5	239.0
neck	157.8	197.8	230.9	211.6	235.5	239.0
tail	157.2	197.8	230.9	211.6	235.5	239.0
para-aortic body	194.6	198.89	—	227.6	237.3	239.7
paraganglion NEC	194.6	198.89	—	227.6	237.3	239.7
parametrium	183.4	198.82	—	221.0	236.3	239.5
paranephric	158.0	197.6	—	211.8	235.4	239.0
pararectal	195.3	198.89	—	229.8	238.8	239.8
parasagittal (region)	195.0	198.89	234.8	229.8	238.8	239.8
parasellar	192.9	198.4	—	225.9	237.9	239.7
parathyroid (gland)	194.1	198.89	234.8	227.1	237.4	239.7
paraurethral	195.3	198.89	—	229.8	238.8	239.8
gland	189.4	198.1	233.9	223.89	236.99	239.5
paravaginal	195.3	198.89	—	229.8	238.8	239.8
parenchyma, kidney	189.0	198.0	233.9	223.0	236.91	239.5
parietal						
bone	170.0	198.5	—	213.0	238.0	239.2
lobe, brain	191.3	198.3	—	225.0	237.5	239.6
paroophoron	183.3	198.82	233.3	221.0	236.3	239.5
parotid (duct) (gland)	142.0	198.89	230.0	210.2	235.0	239.0
parovarium	183.3	198.82	233.3	221.0	236.3	239.5
patella	170.8	198.5	—	213.8	238.0	239.2
peduncle, cerebral	191.7	198.3	—	225.0	237.5	239.6
pelvirectal junction	154.0	197.5	230.4	211.4	235.2	239.0
pelvis, pelvic	195.3	198.89	234.8	229.8	238.8	239.8
bone	170.6	198.5	—	213.6	238.0	239.2
floor	195.3	198.89	234.8	229.8	238.8	239.8
renal	189.1	198.0	233.9	223.1	236.91	239.5
viscera	195.3	198.89	234.8	229.8	238.8	239.8
wall	195.3	198.89	234.8	229.8	238.8	239.8

Neoplasm, neoplastic — *continued*	Malignant					
	Primary	Secondary	Ca in situ	Benign	Uncertain Behavior	Unspecified
pelvo-abdominal	195.8	198.89	234.8	229.8	238.8	239.8
penis	187.4	198.82	233.5	222.1	236.6	239.5
body	187.3	198.82	233.5	222.1	236.6	239.5
corpus (cavernosum)	187.3	198.82	233.5	222.1	236.6	239.5
glans	187.2	198.82	233.5	222.1	236.6	239.5
skin NEC	187.4	198.82	233.5	222.1	236.6	239.5
periadrenal (tissue)	158.0	197.6	—	211.8	235.4	239.0
perianal (skin)	173.5	198.2	232.5	216.5	238.2	239.2
pericardium	164.1	198.89	—	212.7	238.8	239.8
perinephric	158.0	197.6	—	211.8	235.4	239.0
perineum	195.3	198.89	234.8	229.8	238.8	239.8
periodontal tissue NEC	143.9	198.89	230.0	210.4	235.1	239.0
periosteum — *see* Neoplasm, bone						
peripancreatic	158.0	197.6	—	211.8	235.4	239.0
peripheral nerve NEC	171.9	198.89	—	215.9	238.1	239.2
perirectal (tissue)	195.3	198.89	—	229.8	238.8	239.8
perirenal (tissue)	158.0	197.6	—	211.8	235.4	239.0
peritoneum, peritoneal (cavity)	158.9	197.6	—	211.8	235.4	239.0
contiguous sites	158.8	—	—	—	—	—
with digestive organs	159.8	—	—	—	—	—
parietal	158.8	197.6	—	211.8	235.4	239.0
pelvic	158.8	197.6	—	211.8	235.4	239.0
specified part NEC	158.8	197.6	—	211.8	235.4	239.0
peritonsillar (tissue)	195.0	198.89	234.8	229.8	238.8	239.8
periurethral tissue	195.3	198.89	—	229.8	238.8	239.8
phalanges	170.9	198.5	—	213.9	238.0	239.2
foot	170.8	198.5	—	213.8	238.0	239.2
hand	170.5	198.5	—	213.5	238.0	239.2
pharynx, pharyngeal	149.0	198.89	230.0	210.9	235.1	239.0
bursa	147.1	198.89	230.0	210.7	235.1	239.0
fornix	147.3	198.89	230.0	210.7	235.1	239.0
recess	147.2	198.89	230.0	210.7	235.1	239.0
region	149.0	198.89	230.0	210.9	235.1	239.0
tonsil	147.1	198.89	230.0	210.7	235.1	239.0
wall (lateral) (posterior)	149.0	198.89	230.0	210.9	235.1	239.0
pia mater (cerebral) (cranial)	192.1	198.4	—	225.2	237.6	239.7
spinal	192.3	198.4	—	225.4	237.6	239.7
pillars of fauces	146.2	198.89	230.0	210.6	235.1	239.0
pineal (body) (gland)	194.4	198.89	234.8	227.4	237.1	239.7
pinna (ear) NEC	173.2	198.2	232.2	216.2	238.2	239.2
cartilage	171.0	198.89	—	215.0	238.1	239.2
piriform fossa or sinus	148.1	198.89	230.0	210.8	235.1	239.0
pituitary (body) (fossa) (gland) (lobe)	194.3	198.89	234.8	227.3	237.0	239.7
placenta	181	198.82	233.2	219.8	236.1	239.5
pleura, pleural (cavity)	163.9	197.2	—	212.4	235.8	239.1
contiguous sites	163.8	—	—	—	—	—
parietal	163.0	197.2	—	212.4	235.8	239.1
visceral	163.1	197.2	—	212.4	235.8	239.1
plexus						
brachial	171.2	198.89	—	215.2	238.1	239.2
cervical	171.0	198.89	—	215.0	238.1	239.2
choroid	191.5	198.3	—	225.0	237.5	239.6
lumbosacral	171.6	198.89	—	215.6	238.1	239.2
sacral	171.6	198.89	—	215.6	238.1	239.2
pluri-endocrine	194.8	198.89	234.8	227.8	237.4	239.7
pole						
frontal	191.1	198.3	—	225.0	237.5	239.6
occipital	191.4	198.3	—	225.0	237.5	239.6
pons (varolii)	191.7	198.3	—	225.0	237.5	239.6
popliteal fossa or space*	195.5	198.89	234.8	229.8	238.8	239.8
postcricoid (region)	148.0	198.89	230.0	210.8	235.1	239.0
posterior fossa (cranial)	191.9 ▲	198.3	—	225.0	237.5	239.6
postnasal space	147.9	198.89	230.0	210.7	235.1	239.0
prepuce	187.1	198.82	233.5	222.1	236.6	239.5
prepylorus	151.1	197.8	230.2	211.1	235.2	239.0
presacral (region)	195.3	198.89	—	229.8	238.8	239.8
prostate (gland)	185	198.82	233.4	222.2	236.5	239.5
utricle	189.3	198.1	233.9	223.81	236.99	239.5
pterygoid fossa	171.0	198.89	—	215.0	238.1	239.2
pubic bone	170.6	198.5	—	213.6	238.0	239.2
pudenda, pudendum (female)	184.4	198.82	233.3	221.2	236.3	239.5
pulmonary	162.9	197.0	231.2	212.3	235.7	239.1
putamen	191.0	198.3	—	225.0	237.5	239.6
pyloric						
antrum	151.2	197.8	230.2	211.1	235.2	239.0
canal	151.1	197.8	230.2	211.1	235.2	239.0
pylorus	151.1	197.8	230.2	211.1	235.2	239.0
pyramid (brain)	191.7	198.3	—	225.0	237.5	239.6
pyriform fossa or sinus	148.1	198.89	230.0	210.8	235.1	239.0
radius (any part)	170.4	198.5	—	213.4	238.0	239.2
Rathke's pouch	194.3	198.89	234.8	227.3	237.0	239.7
rectosigmoid (colon) (junction)	154.0	197.5	230.4	211.4	235.2	239.0
contiguous sites with anus or rectum	154.8	—	—	—	—	—
rectouterine pouch	158.8	197.6	—	211.8	235.4	239.0
rectovaginal septum or wall	195.3	198.89	234.8	229.8	238.8	239.8
rectovesical septum	195.3	198.89	234.8	229.8	238.8	239.8
rectum (ampulla)	154.1	197.5	230.4	211.4	235.2	239.0
and colon	154.0	197.5	230.4	211.4	235.2	239.0
contiguous sites with anus or rectosigmoid junction	154.8	—	—	—	—	—
renal	189.0	198.0	233.9	223.0	236.91	239.5
calyx	189.1	198.0	233.9	223.1	236.91	239.5
hilus	189.1	198.0	233.9	223.1	236.91	239.5
parenchyma	189.0	198.0	233.9	223.0	236.91	239.5
pelvis	189.1	198.0	233.9	223.1	236.91	239.5
respiratory						
organs or system NEC	165.9	197.3	231.9	212.9	235.9	239.1
contiguous sites with intrathoracic organs	165.8	—	—	—	—	—
specified sites NEC	165.8	197.3	231.8	212.8	235.9	239.1
tract NEC	165.9	197.3	231.9	212.9	235.9	239.1
upper	165.0	197.3	231.9	212.9	235.9	239.1
retina	190.5	198.4	234.0	224.5	238.8	239.8
retrobulbar	190.1	198.4	—	224.1	238.8	239.8
retrocecal	158.0	197.6	—	211.8	235.4	239.0
retromolar (area) (triangle) (trigone)	145.6	198.89	230.0	210.4	235.1	239.0
retro-orbital	195.0	198.89	234.8	229.8	238.8	239.8
retroperitoneal (space) (tissue)	158.0	197.6	—	211.8	235.4	239.0
contiguous sites	158.8	—	—	—	—	—
retroperitoneum	158.0	197.6	—	211.8	235.4	239.0
contiguous sites	158.8	—	—	—	—	—
retropharyngeal	149.0	198.89	230.0	210.9	235.1	239.0
retrovesical (septum)	195.3	198.89	234.8	229.8	238.8	239.8
rhinencephalon	191.0	198.3	—	225.0	237.5	239.6
rib	170.3	198.5	—	213.3	238.0	239.2
Rosenmüller's fossa	147.2	198.89	230.0	210.7	235.1	239.0
round ligament	183.5	198.82	—	221.0	236.3	239.5
sacrococcyx, sacrococcygeal	170.6	198.5	—	213.6	238.0	239.2
region	195.3	198.89	234.8	229.8	238.8	239.8
sacrouterine ligament	183.4	198.82	—	221.0	236.3	239.5
sacrum, sacral (vertebra)	170.6	198.5	—	213.6	238.0	239.2
salivary gland or duct (major)	142.9	198.89	230.0	210.2	235.0	239.0
contiguous sites	142.8	—	—	—	—	—
minor NEC	145.9	198.89	230.0	210.4	235.1	239.0
parotid	142.0	198.89	230.0	210.2	235.0	239.0
pluriglandular	142.8	198.89	230.0	210.2	235.0	239.0
sublingual	142.2	198.89	230.0	210.2	235.0	239.0
submandibular	142.1	198.89	230.0	210.2	235.0	239.0
submaxillary	142.1	198.89	230.0	210.2	235.0	239.0
salpinx (uterine)	183.2	198.82	233.3	221.0	236.3	239.5
Santorini's duct	157.3	197.8	230.9	211.6	235.5	239.0
scalp	173.4	198.2	232.4	216.4	238.2	239.2
scapula (any part)	170.4	198.5	—	213.4	238.0	239.2
scapular region	195.1	198.89	234.8	229.8	238.8	239.8
scar NEC (*see also* Neoplasm, skin)	173.9	198.2	232.9	216.9	238.2	239.2
sciatic nerve	171.3	198.89	—	215.3	238.1	239.2
sclera	190.0	198.4	234.0	224.0	238.8	239.8
scrotum (skin)	187.7	198.82	233.6	222.4	236.6	239.5
sebaceous gland — *see* Neoplasm, skin						
sella turcica	194.3	198.89	234.8	227.3	237.0	239.7
bone	170.0	198.5	—	213.0	238.0	239.2
semilunar cartilage (knee)	170.7	198.5	—	213.7	238.0	239.2
seminal vesicle	187.8	198.82	233.6	222.8	236.6	239.5
septum						
nasal	160.0	197.3	231.8	212.0	235.9	239.1
posterior margin	147.3	198.89	230.0	210.7	235.1	239.0
rectovaginal	195.3	198.89	234.8	229.8	238.8	239.8
rectovesical	195.3	198.89	234.8	229.8	238.8	239.8
urethrovaginal	184.9	198.82	233.3	221.9	236.3	239.5
vesicovaginal	184.9	198.82	233.3	221.9	236.3	239.5
shoulder NEC*	195.4	198.89	232.6	229.8	238.8	239.8
sigmoid flexure (lower) (upper)	153.3	197.5	230.3	211.3	235.2	239.0

Neoplasm, neoplastic — *continued*	Malignant					
	Primary	Secondary	Ca in situ	Benign	Uncertain Behavior	Unspecified
sinus (accessory)	160.9	197.3	231.8	212.0	235.9	239.1
bone (any)	170.0	198.5	—	213.0	238.0	239.2
contiguous sites with middle ear or nasal cavities	160.8	—	—	—	—	—
ethmoidal	160.3	197.3	231.8	212.0	235.9	239.1
frontal	160.4	197.3	231.8	212.0	235.9	239.1
maxillary	160.2	197.3	231.8	212.0	235.9	239.1
nasal, paranasal NEC	160.9	197.3	231.8	212.0	235.9	239.1
pyriform	148.1	198.89	230.0	210.8	235.1	239.0
sphenoidal	160.5	197.3	231.8	212.0	235.9	239.1
skeleton, skeletal NEC	170.9	198.5	—	213.9	238.0	239.2
Skene's gland	189.4	198.1	233.9	223.89	236.99	239.5
skin NEC	173.9	198.2	232.9	216.9	238.2	239.2
abdominal wall	173.5	198.2	232.5	216.5	238.2	239.2
ala nasi	173.3	198.2	232.3	216.3	238.2	239.2
ankle	173.7	198.2	232.7	216.7	238.2	239.2
antecubital space	173.6	198.2	232.6	216.6	238.2	239.2
anus	173.5	198.2	232.5	216.5	238.2	239.2
arm	173.6	198.2	232.6	216.6	238.2	239.2
auditory canal (external)	173.2	198.2	232.2	216.2	238.2	239.2
auricle (ear)	173.2	198.2	232.2	216.2	238.2	239.2
auricular canal (external)	173.2	198.2	232.2	216.2	238.2	239.2
axilla, axillary fold	173.5	198.2	232.5	216.5	238.2	239.2
back	173.5	198.2	232.5	216.5	238.2	239.2
breast	173.5	198.2	232.5	216.5	238.2	239.2
brow	173.3	198.2	232.3	216.3	238.2	239.2
buttock	173.5	198.2	232.5	216.5	238.2	239.2
calf	173.7	198.2	232.7	216.7	238.2	239.2
canthus (eye) (inner) (outer)	173.1	198.2	232.1	216.1	238.2	239.2
cervical region	173.4	198.2	232.4	216.4	238.2	239.2
cheek (external)	173.3	198.2	232.3	216.3	238.2	239.2
chest (wall)	173.5	198.2	232.5	216.5	238.2	239.2
chin	173.3	198.2	232.3	216.3	238.2	239.2
clavicular area	173.5	198.2	232.5	216.5	238.2	239.2
clitoris	184.3	198.82	233.3	221.2	236.3	239.5
columnella	173.3	198.2	232.3	216.3	238.2	239.2
concha	173.2	198.2	232.2	216.2	238.2	239.2
contiguous sites	173.8	—	—	—	—	—
ear (external)	173.2	198.2	232.2	216.2	238.2	239.2
elbow	173.6	198.2	232.6	216.6	238.2	239.2
eyebrow	173.3	198.2	232.3	216.3	238.2	239.2
eyelid	173.1	198.2	232.1	216.1	238.2	239.2
face NEC	173.3	198.2	232.3	216.3	238.2	239.2
female genital organs (external)	184.4	198.82	233.3	221.2	236.3	239.5
clitoris	184.3	198.82	233.3	221.2	236.3	239.5
labium NEC	184.4	198.82	233.3	221.2	236.3	239.5
majus	184.1	198.82	233.3	221.2	236.3	239.5
minus	184.2	198.82	233.3	221.2	236.3	239.5
pudendum	184.4	198.82	233.3	221.2	236.3	239.5
vulva	184.4	198.82	233.3	221.2	236.3	239.5
finger	173.6	198.2	232.6	216.6	238.2	239.2
flank	173.5	198.2	232.5	216.5	238.2	239.2
foot	173.7	198.2	232.7	216.7	238.2	239.2
forearm	173.6	198.2	232.6	216.6	238.2	239.2
forehead	173.3	198.2	232.3	216.3	238.2	239.2
glabella	173.3	198.2	232.3	216.3	238.2	239.2
gluteal region	173.5	198.2	232.5	216.5	238.2	239.2
groin	173.5	198.2	232.5	216.5	238.2	239.2
hand	173.6	198.2	232.6	216.6	238.2	239.2
head NEC	173.4	198.2	232.4	216.4	238.2	239.2
heel	173.7	198.2	232.7	216.7	238.2	239.2
helix	173.2	198.2	232.2	216.2	238.2	239.2
hip	173.7	198.2	232.7	216.7	238.2	239.2
infraclavicular region	173.5	198.2	232.5	216.5	238.2	239.2
inguinal region	173.5	198.2	232.5	216.5	238.2	239.2
jaw	173.3	198.2	232.3	216.3	238.2	239.2
knee	173.7	198.2	232.7	216.7	238.2	239.2
labia						
majora	184.1	198.82	233.3	221.2	236.3	239.5
minora	184.2	198.82	233.3	221.2	236.3	239.5
leg	173.7	198.2	232.7	216.7	238.2	239.2
lid (lower) (upper)	173.1	198.2	232.1	216.1	238.2	239.2
limb NEC	173.9	198.2	232.9	216.9	238.2	239.5
lower	173.7	198.2	232.7	216.7	238.2	239.2
upper	173.6	198.2	232.6	216.6	238.2	239.2
lip (lower) (upper)	173.0	198.2	232.0	216.0	238.2	239.2

Neoplasm, neoplastic — *continued*	Malignant					
	Primary	Secondary	Ca in situ	Benign	Uncertain Behavior	Unspecified
skin NEC — *continued*						
male genital organs	187.9	198.82	233.6	222.9	236.6	239.5
penis	187.4	198.82	233.5	222.1	236.6	239.5
prepuce	187.1	198.82	233.5	222.1	236.6	239.5
scrotum	187.7	198.82	233.6	222.4	236.6	239.5
mastectomy site	173.5	198.2	—	—	—	—
specified as breast tissue	174.8	198.81	—	—	—	—
meatus, acoustic (external)	173.2	198.2	232.2	216.2	238.2	239.2
nates	173.5	198.2	232.5	216.5	238.2	239.0
neck	173.4	198.2	232.4	216.4	238.2	239.2
nose (external)	173.3	198.2	232.3	216.3	238.2	239.2
palm	173.6	198.2	232.6	216.6	238.2	239.2
palpebra	173.1	198.2	232.1	216.1	238.2	239.2
penis NEC	187.4	198.82	233.5	222.1	236.6	239.5
perianal	173.5	198.2	232.5	216.5	238.2	239.2
perineum	173.5	198.2	232.5	216.5	238.2	239.2
pinna	173.2	198.2	232.2	216.2	238.2	239.2
plantar	173.7	198.2	232.7	216.7	238.2	239.2
popliteal fossa or space	173.7	198.2	232.7	216.7	238.2	239.2
prepuce	187.1	198.82	233.5	222.1	236.6	239.5
pubes	173.5	198.2	232.5	216.5	238.2	239.2
sacrococcygeal region	173.5	198.2	232.5	216.5	238.2	239.2
scalp	173.4	198.2	232.4	216.4	238.2	239.2
scapular region	173.5	198.2	232.5	216.5	238.2	239.2
scrotum	187.7	198.82	233.6	222.4	236.6	239.5
shoulder	173.6	198.2	232.6	216.6	238.2	239.2
sole (foot)	173.7	198.2	232.7	216.7	238.2	239.2
specified sites NEC	173.8	198.2	232.8	216.8	232.8	239.2
submammary fold	173.5	198.2	232.5	216.5	238.2	239.2
supraclavicular region	173.4	198.2	232.4	216.4	238.2	239.2
temple	173.3	198.2	232.3	216.3	238.2	239.2
thigh	173.7	198.2	232.7	216.7	238.2	239.2
thoracic wall	173.5	198.2	232.5	216.5	238.2	239.2
thumb	173.6	198.2	232.6	216.6	238.2	239.2
toe	173.7	198.2	232.7	216.7	238.2	239.2
tragus	173.2	198.2	232.2	216.2	238.2	239.2
trunk	173.5	198.2	232.5	216.5	238.2	239.2
umbilicus	173.5	198.2	232.5	216.5	238.2	239.2
vulva	184.4	198.82	233.3	221.2	236.3	239.5
wrist	173.6	198.2	232.6	216.6	238.2	239.2
skull	170.0	198.5	—	213.0	238.0	239.2
soft parts or tissues — *see* Neoplasm, connective tissue						
specified site NEC	195.8	198.89	234.8	229.8	238.8	239.8
spermatic cord	187.6	198.82	233.6	222.8	236.6	239.5
sphenoid	160.5	197.3	231.8	212.0	235.9	239.1
bone	170.0	198.5	—	213.0	238.0	239.2
sinus	160.5	197.3	231.8	212.0	235.9	239.1
sphincter						
anal	154.2	197.5	230.5	211.4	235.5	239.0
of Oddi	156.1	197.8	230.8	211.5	235.3	239.0
spine, spinal (column)	170.2	198.5	—	213.2	238.0	239.2
bulb	191.7	198.3	—	225.0	237.5	239.6
coccyx	170.6	198.5	—	213.6	238.0	239.2
cord (cervical) (lumbar) (sacral) (thoracic)	192.2	198.3	—	225.3	237.5	239.7
dura mater	192.3	198.4	—	225.4	237.6	239.7
lumbosacral	170.2	198.5	—	213.2	238.0	239.2
membrane	192.3	198.4	—	225.4	237.6	239.7
meninges	192.3	198.4	—	225.4	237.6	239.7
nerve (root)	171.9	198.89	—	215.9	238.1	239.2
pia mater	192.3	198.4	—	225.4	237.6	239.7
root	171.9	198.89	—	215.9	238.1	239.2
sacrum	170.6	198.5	—	213.6	238.0	239.2
spleen, splenic NEC	159.1	197.8	230.9	211.9	235.5	239.0
flexure (colon)	153.7	197.5	230.3	211.3	235.2	239.0
stem, brain	191.7	198.3	—	225.0	237.5	239.6
Stensen's duct	142.0	198.89	230.0	210.2	235.0	239.0
sternum	170.3	198.5	—	213.3	238.0	239.2
stomach	151.9	197.8	230.2	211.1	235.2	239.0
antrum (pyloric)	151.2	197.8	230.2	211.1	235.2	239.0
body	151.4	197.8	230.2	211.1	235.2	239.0
cardia	151.0	197.8	230.2	211.1	235.2	239.0
cardiac orifice	151.0	197.8	230.2	211.1	235.2	239.0
contiguous sites	151.8	—	—	—	—	—

Neoplasm, neoplastic — *continued*	Malignant					
	Primary	Secondary	Ca in situ	Benign	Uncertain Behavior	Unspecified
stomach — *continued*						
corpus	151.4	197.8	230.2	211.1	235.2	239.0
fundus	151.3	197.8	230.2	211.1	235.2	239.0
greater curvature NEC	151.6	197.8	230.2	211.1	235.2	239.0
lesser curvature NEC	151.5	197.8	230.2	211.1	235.2	239.0
prepylorus	151.1	197.8	230.2	211.1	235.2	239.0
pylorus	151.1	197.8	230.2	211.1	235.2	239.0
wall NEC	151.9	197.8	230.2	211.1	235.2	239.0
anterior NEC	151.8	197.8	230.2	211.1	235.2	239.0
posterior NEC	151.8	197.8	230.2	211.1	235.2	239.0
stroma, endometrial	182.0	198.82	233.2	219.1	236.0	239.5
stump, cervical	180.8	198.82	233.1	219.0	236.0	239.5
subcutaneous (nodule) (tissue) NEC — *see* Neoplasm, connective tissue						
subdural	192.1	198.4	—	225.2	237.6	239.7
subglottis, subglottic	161.2	197.3	231.0	212.1	235.6	239.1
sublingual	144.9	198.89	230.0	210.3	235.1	239.0
gland or duct	142.2	198.89	230.0	210.2	235.0	239.0
submandibular gland	142.1	198.89	230.0	210.2	235.0	239.0
submaxillary gland or duct	142.1	198.89	230.0	210.2	235.0	239.0
submental	195.0	198.89	234.8	229.8	238.8	239.8
subpleural	162.9	197.0	—	212.3	235.7	239.1
substernal	164.2	197.1	—	212.5	235.8	239.8
sudoriferous, sudoriparous gland, site unspecified	173.9	198.2	232.9	216.9	238.2	239.2
specified site — *see* Neoplasm, skin						
supraclavicular region	195.0	198.89	234.8	229.8	238.8	239.8
supraglottis	161.1	197.3	231.0	212.1	235.6	239.1
suprarenal (capsule) (cortex) (gland) (medulla)	194.0	198.7	234.8	227.0	237.2	239.7
suprasellar (region)	191.9	198.3	—	225.0	237.5	239.6
sweat gland (apocrine) (eccrine), site unspecified	173.9	198.2	232.9	216.9	238.2	239.2
specified site — *see* Neoplasm, skin						
sympathetic nerve or nervous system NEC	171.9	198.89	—	215.9	238.1	239.2
symphysis pubis	170.6	198.5	—	213.6	238.0	239.2
synovial membrane — *see* Neoplasm, connective tissue						
tapetum, brain	191.8	198.3	—	225.0	237.5	239.6
tarsus (any bone)	170.8	198.5	—	213.8	238.0	239.2
temple (skin)	173.3	198.2	232.3	216.3	238.2	239.2
temporal						
bone	170.0	198.5	—	213.0	238.0	239.2
lobe or pole	191.2	198.3	—	225.0	237.5	239.6
region	195.0	198.89	234.8	229.8	238.8	239.8
skin	173.3	198.2	232.3	216.3	238.2	239.2
tendon (sheath) — *see* Neoplasm, connective tissue						
tentorium (cerebelli)	192.1	198.4	—	225.2	237.6	239.7
testis, testes (descended) (scrotal)	186.9	198.82	233.6	222.0	236.4	239.5
ectopic	186.0	198.82	233.6	222.0	236.4	239.5
retained	186.0	198.82	233.6	222.0	236.4	239.5
undescended	186.0	198.82	233.6	222.0	236.4	239.5
thalamus	191.0	198.3	—	225.0	237.5	239.6
thigh NEC*	195.5	198.89	234.8	229.8	238.8	239.8
thorax, thoracic (cavity) (organs NEC)	195.1	198.89	234.8	229.8	238.8	239.8
duct	171.4	198.89	—	215.4	238.1	239.2
wall NEC	195.1	198.89	234.8	229.8	238.8	239.8
throat	149.0	198.89	230.0	210.9	235.1	239.0
thumb NEC*	195.4	198.89	232.6	229.8	238.8	239.8
thymus (gland)	164.0	198.89	—	212.6	235.8	239.8
contiguous sites with heart and mediastinum	164.8	—	—	—	—	—
thyroglossal duct	193	198.89	234.8	226	237.4	239.7
thyroid (gland)	193	198.89	234.8	226	237.4	239.7
cartilage	161.3	197.3	231.0	212.1	235.6	239.1
tibia (any part)	170.7	198.5	—	213.7	238.0	239.2
toe NEC*	195.5	198.89	232.7	229.8	238.8	239.8
tongue	141.9	198.89	230.0	210.1	235.1	239.0
anterior (two-thirds) NEC	141.4	198.89	230.0	210.1	235.1	239.0
dorsal surface	141.1	198.89	230.0	210.1	235.1	239.0
ventral surface	141.3	198.89	230.0	210.1	235.1	239.0
base (dorsal surface)	141.0	198.89	230.0	210.1	235.1	239.0
border (lateral)	141.2	198.89	230.0	210.1	235.1	239.0
contiguous sites	141.8	—	—	—	—	—

Neoplasm, neoplastic — *continued*	Malignant					
	Primary	Secondary	Ca in situ	Benign	Uncertain Behavior	Unspecified
tongue — *continued*						
dorsal surface NEC	141.1	198.89	230.0	210.1	235.1	239.0
fixed part NEC	141.0	198.89	230.0	210.1	235.1	239.0
foreamen cecum	141.1	198.89	230.0	210.1	235.1	239.0
frenulum linguae	141.3	198.89	230.0	210.1	235.1	239.0
junctional zone	141.5	198.89	230.0	210.1	235.1	239.0
margin (lateral)	141.2	198.89	230.0	210.1	235.1	239.0
midline NEC	141.1	198.89	230.0	210.1	235.1	239.0
mobile part NEC	141.4	198.89	230.0	210.1	235.1	239.0
posterior (third)	141.0	198.89	230.0	210.1	235.1	239.0
root	141.0	198.89	230.0	210.1	235.1	239.0
surface (dorsal)	141.1	198.89	230.0	210.1	235.1	239.0
base	141.0	198.89	230.0	210.1	235.1	239.0
ventral	141.3	198.89	230.0	210.1	235.1	239.0
tip	141.2	198.89	230.0	210.1	235.1	239.0
tonsil	141.6	198.89	230.0	210.1	235.1	239.0
tonsil	146.0	198.89	230.0	210.5	235.1	239.0
fauces, faucial	146.0	198.89	230.0	210.5	235.1	239.0
lingual	141.6	198.89	230.0	210.1	235.1	239.0
palatine	146.0	198.89	230.0	210.5	235.1	239.0
pharyngeal	147.1	198.89	230.0	210.7	235.1	239.0
pillar (anterior) (posterior)	146.2	198.89	230.0	210.6	235.1	239.0
tonsillar fossa	146.1	198.89	230.0	210.6	235.1	239.0
tooth socket NEC	143.9	198.89	230.0	210.4	235.1	239.0
trachea (cartilage) (mucosa)	162.0	197.3	231.1	212.2	235.7	239.1
contiguous sites with bronchus or lung	162.8	—	—	—	—	—
tracheobronchial	162.8	197.3	231.1	212.2	235.7	239.1
contiguous sites with lung	162.8	—	—	—	—	—
tragus	173.2	198.2	232.2	216.2	238.2	239.2
trunk NEC*	195.8	198.89	232.5	229.8	238.8	239.8
tubo-ovarian	183.8	198.82	233.3	221.8	236.3	239.5
tunica vaginalis	187.8	198.82	233.6	222.8	236.6	239.5
turbinate (bone)	170.0	198.5	—	213.0	238.0	239.2
nasal	160.0	197.3	231.8	212.0	235.9	239.1
tympanic cavity	160.1	197.3	231.8	212.0	235.9	239.1
ulna (any part)	170.4	198.5	—	213.4	238.0	239.2
umbilicus, umbilical	173.5	198.2	232.5	216.5	238.2	239.2
uncus, brain	191.2	198.3	—	225.0	237.5	239.6
unknown site or unspecified	199.1	199.1	234.9	229.9	238.9	239.9
urachus	188.7	198.1	233.7	223.3	236.7	239.4
ureter, ureteral	189.2	198.1	233.9	223.2	236.91	239.5
orifice (bladder)	188.6	198.1	233.7	223.3	236.7	239.4
ureter-bladder (junction)	188.6	198.1	233.7	223.3	236.7	239.4
urethra, urethral (gland)	189.3	198.1	233.9	223.81	236.99	239.5
orifice, internal	188.5	198.1	233.7	223.3	236.7	239.4
urethrovaginal (septum)	184.9	198.82	233.3	221.9	236.3	239.5
urinary organ or system NEC	189.9	198.1	233.9	223.9	236.99	239.5
bladder — *see* Neoplasm, bladder						
contiguous sites	189.8	—	—	—	—	—
specified sites NEC	189.8	198.1	233.9	223.89	236.99	239.5
utero-ovarian	183.8	198.82	233.3	221.8	236.3	239.5
ligament	183.3	198.82	—	221.0	236.3	239.5
uterosacral ligament	183.4	198.82	—	221.0	236.3	239.5
uterus, uteri, uterine	179	198.82	233.2	219.9	236.0	239.5
adnexa NEC	183.9	198.82	233.3	221.8	236.3	239.5
contiguous sites	183.8	—	—	—	—	—
body	182.0	198.82	233.2	219.1	236.0	239.5
contiguous sites	182.8	—	—	—	—	—
cervix	180.9	198.82	233.1	219.0	236.0	239.5
cornu	182.0	198.82	233.2	219.1	236.0	239.5
corpus	182.0	198.82	233.2	219.1	236.0	239.5
endocervix (canal) (gland)	180.0	198.82	233.1	219.0	236.0	239.5
endometrium	182.0	198.82	233.2	219.1	236.0	239.5
exocervix	180.1	198.82	233.1	219.0	236.0	239.5
external os	180.1	198.82	233.1	219.0	236.0	239.5
fundus	182.0	198.82	233.2	219.1	236.0	239.5
internal os	180.0	198.82	233.1	219.0	236.0	239.5
isthmus	182.1	198.82	233.2	219.1	236.0	239.5
ligament	183.4	198.82	—	221.0	236.3	239.5
broad	183.3	198.82	233.3	221.0	236.3	239.5
round	183.5	198.82	—	221.0	236.3	239.5
lower segment	182.1	198.82	233.2	219.1	236.0	239.5
myometrium	182.0	198.82	233.2	219.1	236.0	239.5
squamocolumnar junction	180.8	198.82	233.1	219.0	236.0	239.5
tube	183.2	198.82	233.3	221.0	236.3	239.5

Neoplasm, neoplastic — *continued*	Malignant Primary	Malignant Secondary	Malignant Ca in situ	Benign	Uncertain Behavior	Unspecified
utricle, prostatic	189.3	198.1	233.9	223.81	236.99	239.5
uveal tract	190.0	198.4	234.0	224.0	238.8	239.8
uvula	145.4	198.89	230.0	210.4	235.1	239.0
vagina, vaginal (fornix) (vault) (wall)	184.0	198.82	233.3	221.1	236.3	239.5
vaginovesical	184.9	198.82	233.3	221.9	236.3	239.5
septum	194.9	198.82	233.3	221.9	236.3	239.5
vallecula (epiglottis)	146.3	198.89	230.0	210.6	235.1	239.0
vascular — *see* Neoplasm, connective tissue						
vas deferens	187.6	198.82	233.6	222.8	236.6	239.5
Vater's ampulla	156.2	197.8	230.8	211.5	235.3	239.0
vein, venous — *see* Neoplasm, connective tissue						
vena cava (abdominal) (inferior)	171.5	198.89	—	215.5	238.1	239.2
superior	171.4	198.89	—	215.4	238.1	239.2
ventricle (cerebral) (floor) (fourth) (lateral) (third)	191.5	198.3	—	225.0	237.5	239.6
cardiac (left) (right)	164.1	198.89	—	212.7	238.8	239.8
ventricular band of larynx	161.1	197.3	231.0	212.1	235.6	239.1
ventriculus — see Neoplasm, stomach						
vermillion border — *see* Neoplasm, lip						
vermis, cerebellum	191.6	198.3	—	225.0	237.5	239.6
vertebra (column)	170.2	198.5	—	213.2	238.0	239.2
coccyx	170.6	198.5	—	213.6	238.0	239.2
sacrum	170.6	198.5	—	213.6	238.0	239.2
vesical — *see* Neoplasm, bladder						
vesicle, seminal	187.8	198.82	233.6	222.8	236.6	239.5
vesicocervical tissue	184.9	198.82	233.3	221.9	236.3	239.5
vesicorectal	195.3	198.89	234.8	229.8	238.8	239.8
vesicovaginal	184.9	198.82	233.3	221.9	236.3	239.5
septum	184.9	198.82	233.3	221.9	236.3	239.5
vessel (blood) — *see* Neoplasm, connective tissue						
vestibular gland, greater	184.1	198.82	233.3	221.2	236.3	239.5
vestibule						
mouth	145.1	198.89	230.0	210.4	235.1	239.0
nose	160.0	197.3	231.8	212.0	235.9	239.1
Virchow's gland	—	196.0	—	229.0	238.8	239.8
viscera NEC	195.8	198.89	234.8	229.8	238.8	239.8
vocal cords (true)	161.0	197.3	231.0	212.1	235.6	239.1
false	161.1	197.3	231.0	212.1	235.6	239.1
vomer	170.0	198.5	—	213.0	238.0	239.2
vulva	184.4	198.82	233.3	221.2	236.3	239.5
vulvovaginal gland	184.4	198.82	233.3	221.2	236.3	239.5
Waldeyer's ring	149.1	198.89	230.0	210.9	235.1	239.0
Wharton's duct	142.1	198.89	230.0	210.2	235.0	239.0
white matter (central) (cerebral)	191.0	198.3	—	225.0	237.5	239.6
windpipe	162.0	197.3	231.1	212.2	235.7	239.1
Wirsung's duct	157.3	197.8	230.9	211.6	235.5	239.0
wolffian (body) (duct)						
female	184.8	198.82	233.3	221.8	236.3	239.5
male	187.8	198.82	233.6	222.8	236.6	239.5
womb — *see* Neoplasm, uterus						
wrist NEC*	195.4	198.89	232.6	229.8	238.8	239.8
xiphoid process	170.3	198.5	—	213.3	238.0	239.2
Zuckerkandl's organ	194.6	198.89	—	227.6	237.3	239.7

Neovascularization
- choroid 362.16
- ciliary body 364.42
- cornea 370.60
  - deep 370.63
  - localized 370.61
- iris 364.42
- retina 362.16
- subretinal 362.16

Nephralgia 788.0

Nephritis, nephritic (albuminuric) (azotemic) (congenital) (degenerative) (diffuse) (disseminated) (epithelial) (familial) (focal) (granulomatous) (hemorrhagic) (infantile) (nonsuppurative, excretory) (uremic) 583.9
- with
  - edema — *see* Nephrosis
  - lesion of
    - glomerulonephritis
      - hypocomplementemic persistent 583.2
        - with nephrotic syndrome 581.2
        - chronic 582.2
      - lobular 583.2
        - with nephrotic syndrome 581.2
        - chronic 582.2
      - membranoproliferative 583.2
        - with nephrotic syndrome 581.2
        - chronic 582.2
      - membranous 583.1
        - with nephrotic syndrome 581.1
        - chronic 582.1
      - mesangiocapillary 583.2
        - with nephrotic syndrome 581.2
        - chronic 582.2
      - mixed membranous and proliferative 583.2
        - with nephrotic syndrome 581.2
        - chronic 582.2
      - proliferative (diffuse) 583.0
        - with nephrotic syndrome 581.0
        - acute 580.0
        - chronic 582.0

Nephritis, nephritic — *continued*
- with — *continued*
  - lesion of — *continued*
    - glomerulonephritis — *continued*
      - rapidly progressive 583.4
        - acute 580.4
        - chronic 582.4
    - interstitial nephritis (diffuse) (focal) 583.89
      - with nephrotic syndrome 581.89
      - acute 580.89
      - chronic 582.89
    - necrotizing glomerulitis 583.4
      - acute 580.4
      - chronic 582.4
    - renal necrosis 583.9
      - cortical 583.6
      - medullary 583.7
    - specified pathology NEC 583.89
      - with nephrotic syndrome 581.89
      - acute 580.89
      - chronic 582.89
  - necrosis, renal 583.9
    - cortical 583.6
    - medullary (papillary) 583.7
  - nephrotic syndrome (*see also* Nephrosis) 581.9
  - papillary necrosis 583.7
  - specified pathology NEC 583.89
- acute 580.9
  - extracapillary with epithelial crescents 580.4
  - hypertensive (*see also* Hypertension, kidney) 403.90
  - necrotizing 580.4
  - poststreptococcal 580.0
  - proliferative (diffuse) 580.0
  - rapidly progressive 580.4
  - specified pathology NEC 580.89
- amyloid 277.3 *[583.81]*
  - chronic 277.3 *[582.81]*
- arteriolar (*see also* Hypertension, kidney) 403.90
- arteriosclerotic (*see also* Hypertension, kidney) 403.90

Nephritis, nephritic — *continued*
- ascending (*see also* Pyelitis) 590.80
- atrophic 582.9
- basement membrane NEC 583.89
  - with
    - pulmonary hemorrhage (Goodpasture's syndrome) 446.21 *[583.81]*
- calculous, calculus 592.0
- cardiac (*see also* Hypertension, kidney) 403.90
- cardiovascular (*see also* Hypertension, kidney) 403.90
- chronic 582.9
  - arteriosclerotic (*see also* Hypertension, kidney) 403.90
  - hypertensive (*see also* Hypertension, kidney) 403.90
- cirrhotic (*see also* Sclerosis, renal) 587
- complicating pregnancy, childbirth, or puerperium 646.2 ☑
  - with hypertension 642.1 ☑
    - affecting fetus or newborn 760.0
  - affecting fetus or newborn 760.1
- croupous 580.9
- desquamative — *see* Nephrosis
- due to
  - amyloidosis 277.3 *[583.81]*
    - chronic 277.3 *[582.81]*
  - arteriosclerosis (*see also* Hypertension, kidney) 403.90
  - diabetes mellitus 250.4 ☑ *[583.81]*
    - with nephrotic syndrome 250.4 ☑ *[581.81]*
  - diphtheria 032.89 *[580.81]*
  - gonococcal infection (acute) 098.19 *[583.81]*
    - chronic or duration of 2 months or over 098.39 *[583.81]*
  - gout 274.10
  - infectious hepatitis 070.9 *[580.81]*
  - mumps 072.79 *[580.81]*
  - specified kidney pathology NEC 583.89
    - acute 580.89
    - chronic 582.89
  - streptotrichosis 039.8 *[583.81]*
  - subacute bacterial endocarditis 421.0 *[580.81]*

Nephritis, nephritic — *continued*
- due to — *continued*
  - systemic lupus erythematosus 710.0 *[583.81]*
    - chronic 710.0 *[582.81]*
  - typhoid fever 002.0 *[580.81]*
- endothelial 582.2
- end stage (chronic) (terminal) NEC 585.6 ▲
- epimembranous 581.1
- exudative 583.89
  - with nephrotic syndrome 581.89
  - acute 580.89
  - chronic 582.89
- gonococcal (acute) 098.19 *[583.81]*
  - chronic or duration of 2 months or over 098.39 *[583.81]*
- gouty 274.10
- hereditary (Alport's syndrome) 759.89
- hydremic — *see* Nephrosis
- hypertensive (*see also* Hypertension, kidney) 403.90
- hypocomplementemic persistent 583.2
  - with nephrotic syndrome 581.2
  - chronic 582.2
- immune complex NEC 583.89
- infective (*see also* Pyelitis) 590.80
- interstitial (diffuse) (focal) 583.89
  - with nephrotic syndrome 581.89
  - acute 580.89
  - chronic 582.89
- latent or quiescent — *see* Nephritis, chronic
- lead 984.9
  - specified type of lead — *see* Table of Drugs and Chemicals
- lobular 583.2
  - with nephrotic syndrome 581.2
  - chronic 582.2
- lupus 710.0 *[583.81]*
  - acute 710.0 *[580.81]*
  - chronic 710.0 *[582.81]*
- membranoproliferative 583.2
  - with nephrotic syndrome 581.2
  - chronic 582.2
- membranous 583.1
  - with nephrotic syndrome 581.1
  - chronic 582.1
- mesangiocapillary 583.2
  - with nephrotic syndrome 581.2
  - chronic 582.2
- minimal change 581.3
- mixed membranous and proliferative 583.2
  - with nephrotic syndrome 581.2
  - chronic 582.2
- necrotic, necrotizing 583.4
  - acute 580.4
  - chronic 582.4
- nephrotic — *see* Nephrosis
- old — *see* Nephritis, chronic
- parenchymatous 581.89
- polycystic 753.12
  - adult type (APKD) 753.13
  - autosomal dominant 753.13
  - autosomal recessive 753.14
  - childhood type (CPKD) 753.14
  - infantile type 753.14
- poststreptococcal 580.0
- pregnancy — *see* Nephritis, complicating pregnancy
- proliferative 583.0
  - with nephrotic syndrome 581.0
  - acute 580.0
  - chronic 582.0
- purulent (*see also* Pyelitis) 590.80
- rapidly progressive 583.4
  - acute 580.4
  - chronic 582.4
- salt-losing or salt-wasting (*see also* Disease, renal) 593.9
- saturnine 984.9
  - specified type of lead — *see* Table of Drugs and Chemicals
- septic (*see also* Pyelitis) 590.80
- specified pathology NEC 583.89
  - acute 580.89
  - chronic 582.89
- staphylococcal (*see also* Pyelitis) 590.80
- streptotrichosis 039.8 *[583.81]*
- subacute (*see also* Nephrosis) 581.9
- suppurative (*see also* Pyelitis) 590.80
- syphilitic (late) 095.4
  - congenital 090.5 *[583.81]*
  - early 091.69 *[583.81]*
- terminal (chronic) (end-stage) NEC 585.6 ▲
- toxic — *see* Nephritis, acute
- tubal, tubular — *see* Nephrosis, tubular
- tuberculous (*see also* Tuberculosis) 016.0 ☑ *[583.81]*
- type II (Ellis) — *see* Nephrosis
- vascular — *see* Hypertension, kidney
- war 580.9

Nephroblastoma (M8960/3) 189.0
- epithelial (M8961/3) 189.0
- mesenchymal (M8962/3) 189.0

Nephrocalcinosis 275.49

Nephrocystitis, pustular (*see also* Pyelitis) 590.80

Nephrolithiasis (congenital) (pelvis) (recurrent) 592.0
- uric acid 274.11

Nephroma (M8960/3) 189.0
- mesoblastic (M8960/1) 236.9 ☑

Nephronephritis (*see also* Nephrosis) 581.9

Nephronopthisis 753.16

Nephropathy (*see also* Nephritis) 583.9
- with
  - exudative nephritis 583.89
  - interstitial nephritis (diffuse) (focal) 583.89
  - medullary necrosis 583.7
  - necrosis 583.9
    - cortical 583.6
    - medullary or papillary 583.7
  - papillary necrosis 583.7
  - specified lesion or cause NEC 583.89
- analgesic 583.89
  - with medullary necrosis, acute 584.7
- arteriolar (*see also* Hypertension, kidney) 403.90
- arteriosclerotic (*see also* Hypertension, kidney) 403.90
- complicating pregnancy 646.2 ☑
- diabetic 250.4 ☑ *[583.81]*
- gouty 274.10
  - specified type NEC 274.19
- hypercalcemic 588.89
- hypertensive (*see also* Hypertension, kidney) 403.90
- hypokalemic (vacuolar) 588.89
- IgA 583.9
- obstructive 593.89
  - congenital 753.20
- phenacetin 584.7
- phosphate-losing 588.0
- potassium depletion 588.89
- proliferative (*see also* Nephritis, proliferative) 583.0
- protein-losing 588.89
- salt-losing or salt-wasting (*see also* Disease, renal) 593.9
- sickle-cell (*see also* Disease, sickle-cell) 282.60 *[583.81]*
- toxic 584.5
- vasomotor 584.5
- water-losing 588.89

Nephroptosis (*see also* Disease, renal) 593.0
- congenital (displaced) 753.3

Nephropyosis (*see also* Abscess, kidney) 590.2

Nephrorrhagia 593.81

Nephrosclerosis (arteriolar) (arteriosclerotic) (chronic) (hyaline) (*see also* Hypertension, kidney) 403.90
- gouty 274.10
- hyperplastic (arteriolar) (*see also* Hypertension, kidney) 403.90
- senile (*see also* Sclerosis, renal) 587

Nephrosis, nephrotic (Epstein's) (syndrome) 581.9
- with
  - lesion of
    - focal glomerulosclerosis 581.1
    - glomerulonephritis
      - endothelial 581.2
      - hypocomplementemic persistent 581.2
      - lobular 581.2
      - membranoproliferative 581.2
      - membranous 581.1
      - mesangiocapillary 581.2
      - minimal change 581.3
      - mixed membranous and proliferative 581.2
      - proliferative 581.0
    - segmental hyalinosis 581.1
    - specified pathology NEC 581.89
- acute — *see* Nephrosis, tubular
- anoxic — *see* Nephrosis, tubular
- arteriosclerotic (*see also* Hypertension, kidney) 403.90
- chemical — *see* Nephrosis, tubular
- cholemic 572.4
- complicating pregnancy, childbirth, or puerperium — *see* Nephritis, complicating pregnancy
- diabetic 250.4 ☑ *[581.81]*
- hemoglobinuric — *see* Nephrosis, tubular
- in
  - amyloidosis 277.3 *[581.81]*
  - diabetes mellitus 250.4 ☑ *[581.81]*
  - epidemic hemorrhagic fever 078.6
  - malaria 084.9 *[581.81]*
  - polyarteritis 446.0 *[581.81]*
  - systemic lupus erythematosus 710.0 *[581.81]*
- ischemic — *see* Nephrosis, tubular
- lipoid 581.3
- lower nephron — *see* Nephrosis, tubular
- lupoid 710.0 *[581.81]*
- lupus 710.0 *[581.81]*
- malarial 084.9 *[581.81]*
- minimal change 581.3
- necrotizing — *see* Nephrosis, tubular
- osmotic (sucrose) 588.89
- polyarteritic 446.0 *[581.81]*
- radiation 581.9
- specified lesion or cause NEC 581.89
- syphilitic 095.4
- toxic — *see* Nephrosis, tubular
- tubular (acute) 584.5
  - due to a procedure 997.5
  - radiation 581.9

Nephrosonephritis hemorrhagic (endemic) 078.6

Nephrostomy status V44.6
- with complication 997.5

Nerve — *see* condition

Nerves 799.2

Nervous (*see also* condition) 799.2
- breakdown 300.9
- heart 306.2
- stomach 306.4
- tension 799.2

Nervousness 799.2

Nesidioblastoma (M8150/0)
- pancreas 211.7
- specified site NEC — *see* Neoplasm, by site, benign
- unspecified site 211.7

Netherton's syndrome (ichthyosiform erythroderma) 757.1

Nettle rash 708.8

Nettleship's disease (urticaria pigmentosa) 757.33

Neumann's disease (pemphigus vegetans) 694.4

Neuralgia, neuralgic (acute) (*see also* Neuritis) 729.2
- accessory (nerve) 352.4
- acoustic (nerve) 388.5
- ankle 355.8
- anterior crural 355.8
- anus 787.99
- arm 723.4
- auditory (nerve) 388.5
- axilla 353.0
- bladder 788.1
- brachial 723.4
- brain — *see* Disorder, nerve, cranial
- broad ligament 625.9
- cerebral — *see* Disorder, nerve, cranial
- ciliary 346.2 ☑
- cranial nerve — *see* also Disorder, nerve, cranial

☑ Additional Digit Required — Refer to the Tabular List (Numeric Code Section) for Additional Digit Selection

▶◀ Revised Text ● New Line ▲ Revised Code

Neuralgia, neuralgic (*see also* Neuritis) — *continued*
fifth or trigeminal (*see also* Neuralgia, trigeminal) 350.1
ear 388.71
middle 352.1
facial 351.8
finger 354.9
flank 355.8
foot 355.8
forearm 354.9
Fothergill's (*see also* Neuralgia, trigeminal) 350.1
postherpetic 053.12
glossopharyngeal (nerve) 352.1
groin 355.8
hand 354.9
heel 355.8
Horton's 346.2 ☑
Hunt's 053.11
hypoglossal (nerve) 352.5
iliac region 355.8
infraorbital (*see also* Neuralgia, trigeminal) 350.1
inguinal 355.8
intercostal (nerve) 353.8
postherpetic 053.19
jaw 352.1
kidney 788.0
knee 355.8
loin 355.8
malarial (*see also* Malaria) 084.6
mastoid 385.89
maxilla 352.1
median thenar 354.1
metatarsal 355.6
middle ear 352.1
migrainous 346.2 ☑
Morton's 355.6
nerve, cranial — *see* Disorder, nerve, cranial
nose 352.0
occipital 723.8
olfactory (nerve) 352.0
ophthalmic 377.30
postherpetic 053.19
optic (nerve) 377.30
penis 607.9
perineum 355.8
pleura 511.0
postherpetic NEC 053.19
geniculate ganglion 053.11
ophthalmic 053.19
trifacial 053.12
trigeminal 053.12
pubic region 355.8
radial (nerve) 723.4
rectum 787.99
sacroiliac joint 724.3
sciatic (nerve) 724.3
scrotum 608.9
seminal vesicle 608.9
shoulder 354.9
Sluder's 337.0
specified nerve NEC — *see* Disorder, nerve
spermatic cord 608.9
sphenopalatine (ganglion) 337.0
subscapular (nerve) 723.4
suprascapular (nerve) 723.4
testis 608.89
thenar (median) 354.1
thigh 355.8
tongue 352.5
trifacial (nerve) (*see also* Neuralgia, trigeminal) 350.1
trigeminal (nerve) 350.1
postherpetic 053.12
tympanic plexus 388.71
ulnar (nerve) 723.4
vagus (nerve) 352.3
wrist 354.9
writers' 300.89
organic 333.84

Neurapraxia — *see* Injury, nerve, by site

Neurasthenia 300.5
cardiac 306.2
gastric 306.4
heart 306.2
postfebrile 780.79
postviral 780.79

Neurilemmoma (M9560/0) — *see also* Neoplasm, connective tissue, benign
acoustic (nerve) 225.1
malignant (M9560/3) — *see also* Neoplasm, connective tissue, malignant
acoustic (nerve) 192.0

Neurilemmosarcoma (M9560/3) — *see* Neoplasm, connective tissue, malignant

Neurilemoma — *see* Neurilemmoma

Neurinoma (M9560/0) — *see* Neurilemmoma

Neurinomatosis (M9560/1) — *see also* Neoplasm, connective tissue, uncertain behavior
centralis 759.5

Neuritis (*see also* Neuralgia) 729.2
abducens (nerve) 378.54
accessory (nerve) 352.4
acoustic (nerve) 388.5
syphilitic 094.86
alcoholic 357.5
with psychosis 291.1
amyloid, any site 277.3 *[357.4]*
anterior crural 355.8
arising during pregnancy 646.4 ☑
arm 723.4
ascending 355.2
auditory (nerve) 388.5
brachial (nerve) NEC 723.4
due to displacement, intervertebral disc 722.0
cervical 723.4
chest (wall) 353.8
costal region 353.8
cranial nerve — *see also* Disorder, nerve, cranial
first or olfactory 352.0
second or optic 377.30
third or oculomotor 378.52
fourth or trochlear 378.53
fifth or trigeminal (*see also* Neuralgia, trigeminal) 350.1
sixth or abducens 378.54
seventh or facial 351.8
newborn 767.5
eighth or acoustic 388.5
ninth or glossopharyngeal 352.1
tenth or vagus 352.3
eleventh or accessory 352.4
twelfth or hypoglossal 352.5
Déjérine-Sottas 356.0
diabetic 250.6 ☑ *[357.2]*
diphtheritic 032.89 *[357.4]*
due to
beriberi 265.0 *[357.4]*
displacement, prolapse, protrusion, or rupture of intervertebral disc 722.2
cervical 722.0
lumbar, lumbosacral 722.10
thoracic, thoracolumbar 722.11
herniation, nucleus pulposus 722.2
cervical 722.0
lumbar, lumbosacral 722.10
thoracic, thoracolumbar 722.11
endemic 265.0 *[357.4]*
facial (nerve) 351.8
newborn 767.5
general — *see* Polyneuropathy
geniculate ganglion 351.1
due to herpes 053.11
glossopharyngeal (nerve) 352.1
gouty 274.89 *[357.4]*
hypoglossal (nerve) 352.5
ilioinguinal (nerve) 355.8
in diseases classified elsewhere — *see* Polyneuropathy, in
infectious (multiple) 357.0
intercostal (nerve) 353.8
interstitial hypertrophic progressive NEC 356.9
leg 355.8
lumbosacral NEC 724.4
median (nerve) 354.1
thenar 354.1
multiple (acute) (infective) 356.9
endemic 265.0 *[357.4]*
multiplex endemica 265.0 *[357.4]*
nerve root (*see also* Radiculitis) 729.2
oculomotor (nerve) 378.52
olfactory (nerve) 352.0
optic (nerve) 377.30
in myelitis 341.0

Neuritis (*see also* Neuralgia) — *continued*
optic — *continued*
meningococcal 036.81
pelvic 355.8
peripheral (nerve) — *see also* Neuropathy, peripheral
complicating pregnancy or puerperium 646.4 ☑
specified nerve NEC — *see* Mononeuritis
pneumogastric (nerve) 352.3
postchickenpox 052.7
postherpetic 053.19
progressive hypertrophic interstitial NEC 356.9
puerperal, postpartum 646.4 ☑
radial (nerve) 723.4
retrobulbar 377.32
syphilitic 094.85
rheumatic (chronic) 729.2
sacral region 355.8
sciatic (nerve) 724.3
due to displacement of intervertebral disc 722.10
serum 999.5
specified nerve NEC — *see* Disorder, nerve
spinal (nerve) 355.9
root (*see also* Radiculitis) 729.2
subscapular (nerve) 723.4
suprascapular (nerve) 723.4
syphilitic 095.8
thenar (median) 354.1
thoracic NEC 724.4
toxic NEC 357.7
trochlear (nerve) 378.53
ulnar (nerve) 723.4
vagus (nerve) 352.3

Neuroangiomatosis, encephalofacial 759.6

Neuroastrocytoma (M9505/1) — *see* Neoplasm, by site, uncertain behavior

Neuro-avitaminosis 269.2

Neuroblastoma (M9500/3)
olfactory (M9522/3) 160.0
specified site — *see* Neoplasm, by site, malignant
unspecified site 194.0

Neurochorioretinitis (*see also* Chorioretinitis) 363.20

Neurocirculatory asthenia 306.2

Neurocytoma (M9506/0) — *see* Neoplasm, by site, benign

Neurodermatitis (circumscribed) (circumscripta) (local) 698.3
atopic 691.8
diffuse (Brocq) 691.8
disseminated 691.8
nodulosa 698.3

Neuroencephalomyelopathy, optic 341.0

Neuroepithelioma (M9503/3) — *see also* Neoplasm, by site, malignant
olfactory (M9521/3) 160.0

Neurofibroma (M9540/0) — *see also* Neoplasm, connective tissue, benign
melanotic (M9541/0) — *see* Neoplasm, connective tissue, benign
multiple (M9540/1) 237.70
type 1 237.71
type 2 237.72
plexiform (M9550/0) — *see* Neoplasm, connective tissue, benign

Neurofibromatosis (multiple) (M9540/1) 237.70
acoustic 237.72
malignant (M9540/3) — *see* Neoplasm, connective tissue, malignant
type 1 237.71
type 2 237.72
von Recklinghausen's 237.71

Neurofibrosarcoma (M9540/3) — *see* Neoplasm, connective tissue, malignant

Neurogenic — *see also* condition
bladder (atonic) (automatic) (autonomic) (flaccid) (hypertonic) (hypotonic) (inertia) (infranuclear) (irritable) (motor) (nonreflex) (nuclear) (paralysis) (reflex) (sensory) (spastic) (supranuclear) (uninhibited) 596.54
with cauda equina syndrome 344.61
bowel 564.81
heart 306.2

- **Neuroglioma** (M9505/1) — *see* Neoplasm, by site, uncertain behavior
- **Neurolabyrinthitis** (of Dix and Hallpike) 386.12
- **Neurolathyrism** 988.2
- **Neuroleprosy** 030.1
- **Neuroleptic malignant syndrome** 333.92
- **Neurolipomatosis** 272.8
- **Neuroma** (M9570/0) — *see also* Neoplasm, connective tissue, benign
  - acoustic (nerve) (M9560/0) 225.1
  - amputation (traumatic) — *see also* Injury, nerve, by site
    - surgical complication (late) 997.61
  - appendix 211.3
  - auditory nerve 225.1
  - digital 355.6
    - toe 355.6
  - interdigital (toe) 355.6
  - intermetatarsal 355.6
  - Morton's 355.6
  - multiple 237.70
    - type 1 237.71
    - type 2 237.72
  - nonneoplastic 355.9
    - arm NEC 354.9
    - leg NEC 355.8
    - lower extremity NEC 355.8
    - specified site NEC — *see* Mononeuritis, by site
    - upper extremity NEC 354.9
  - optic (nerve) 225.1
  - plantar 355.6
  - plexiform (M9550/0) — *see* Neoplasm, connective tissue, benign
  - surgical (nonneoplastic) 355.9
    - arm NEC 354.9
    - leg NEC 355.8
    - lower extremity NEC 355.8
    - upper extremity NEC 354.9
  - traumatic — *see also* Injury, nerve, by site
    - old — *see* Neuroma, nonneoplastic
- **Neuromyalgia** 729.1
- **Neuromyasthenia** (epidemic) 049.8
- **Neuromyelitis** 341.8
  - ascending 357.0
  - optica 341.0
- **Neuromyopathy** NEC 358.9
- **Neuromyositis** 729.1
- **Neuronevus** (M8725/0) — *see* Neoplasm, skin, benign
- **Neuronitis** 357.0
  - ascending (acute) 355.2
  - vestibular 386.12
- **Neuroparalytic** — *see* condition
- **Neuropathy, neuropathic** (*see also* Disorder, nerve) 355.9
  - acute motor 357.82
  - alcoholic 357.5
    - with psychosis 291.1
  - arm NEC 354.9
  - ataxia and retinitis pigmentosa (NARP syndrome) 277.87
  - autonomic (peripheral) — *see* Neuropathy, peripheral, autonomic
  - axillary nerve 353.0
  - brachial plexus 353.0
  - cervical plexus 353.2
  - chronic
    - progressive segmentally demyelinating 357.89
    - relapsing demyelinating 357.89
  - congenital sensory 356.2
  - Déjérine-Sottas 356.0
  - diabetic 250.6 ☑ *[357.2]*
  - entrapment 355.9
    - iliohypogastric nerve 355.79
    - ilioinguinal nerve 355.79
    - lateral cutaneous nerve of thigh 355.1
    - median nerve 354.0
    - obturator nerve 355.79
    - peroneal nerve 355.3
    - posterior tibial nerve 355.5
    - saphenous nerve 355.79
    - ulnar nerve 354.2
  - facial nerve 351.9
  - hereditary 356.9
    - peripheral 356.0
    - sensory (radicular) 356.2

- **Neuropathy, neuropathic** (*see also* Disorder, nerve) — *continued*
  - hypertrophic
    - Charcôt-Marie-Tooth 356.1
    - Déjérine-Sottas 356.0
    - interstitial 356.9
    - Refsum 356.3
  - intercostal nerve 354.8
  - ischemic — *see* Disorder, nerve
  - Jamaican (ginger) 357.7
  - leg NEC 355.8
  - lower extremity NEC 355.8
  - lumbar plexus 353.1
  - median nerve 354.1
  - motor
    - acute 357.82
  - multiple (acute) (chronic) (*see also* Polyneuropathy) 356.9
  - optic 377.39
    - ischemic 377.41
    - nutritional 377.33
    - toxic 377.34
  - peripheral (nerve) (*see also* Polyneuropathy) 356.9
    - arm NEC 354.9
    - autonomic 337.9
      - amyloid 277.3 *[337.1]*
      - idiopathic 337.0
      - in
        - amyloidosis 277.3 *[337.1]*
        - diabetes (mellitus) 250.6 ☑ *[337.1]*
        - diseases classified elsewhere 337.1
        - gout 274.89 *[337.1]*
        - hyperthyroidism 242.9 ☑ *[337.1]*
    - due to
      - antitetanus serum 357.6
      - arsenic 357.7
      - drugs 357.6
      - lead 357.7
      - organophosphate compounds 357.7
      - toxic agent NEC 357.7
    - hereditary 356.0
    - idiopathic 356.9
      - progressive 356.4
      - specified type NEC 356.8
    - in diseases classified elsewhere — *see* Polyneuropathy, in
    - leg NEC 355.8
    - lower extremity NEC 355.8
    - upper extremity NEC 354.9
  - plantar nerves 355.6
  - progressive hypertrophic interstitial 356.9
  - radicular NEC 729.2
    - brachial 723.4
    - cervical NEC 723.4
    - hereditary sensory 356.2
    - lumbar 724.4
    - lumbosacral 724.4
    - thoracic NEC 724.4
  - sacral plexus 353.1
  - sciatic 355.0
  - spinal nerve NEC 355.9
    - root (*see also* Radiculitis) 729.2
  - toxic 357.7
  - trigeminal sensory 350.8
  - ulnar nerve 354.2
  - upper extremity NEC 354.9
  - uremic 585.9 *[357.4]* ▲
  - vitamin B_{12} 266.2 *[357.4]*
    - with anemia (pernicious) 281.0 *[357.4]*
      - due to dietary deficiency 281.1 *[357.4]*
- **Neurophthisis** (*see also* Disorder, nerve)
  - diabetic 250.6 ☑ *[357.2]*
  - peripheral 356.9
- **Neuropraxia** — *see* Injury, nerve
- **Neuroretinitis** 363.05
  - syphilitic 094.85
- **Neurosarcoma** (M9540/3) — *see* Neoplasm, connective tissue, malignant
- **Neurosclerosis** — *see* Disorder, nerve
- **Neurosis, neurotic** 300.9
  - accident 300.16
  - anancastic, anankastic 300.3
  - anxiety (state) 300.00
    - generalized 300.02
    - panic type 300.01
  - asthenic 300.5
  - bladder 306.53

- **Neurosis, neurotic** — *continued*
  - cardiac (reflex) 306.2
  - cardiovascular 306.2
  - climacteric, unspecified type 627.2
  - colon 306.4
  - compensation 300.16
  - compulsive, compulsion 300.3
  - conversion 300.11
  - craft 300.89
  - cutaneous 306.3
  - depersonalization 300.6
  - depressive (reaction) (type) 300.4
  - endocrine 306.6
  - environmental 300.89
  - fatigue 300.5
  - functional (*see also* Disorder, psychosomatic) 306.9
  - gastric 306.4
  - gastrointestinal 306.4
  - genitourinary 306.50
  - heart 306.2
  - hypochondriacal 300.7
  - hysterical 300.10
    - conversion type 300.11
    - dissociative type 300.15
  - impulsive 300.3
  - incoordination 306.0
    - larynx 306.1
    - vocal cord 306.1
  - intestine 306.4
  - larynx 306.1
    - hysterical 300.11
    - sensory 306.1
  - menopause, unspecified type 627.2
  - mixed NEC 300.89
  - musculoskeletal 306.0
  - obsessional 300.3
    - phobia 300.3
  - obsessive-compulsive 300.3
  - occupational 300.89
  - ocular 306.7
  - oral 307.0
  - organ (*see also* Disorder, psychosomatic) 306.9
  - pharynx 306.1
  - phobic 300.20
  - posttraumatic (acute) (situational) 309.81
    - chronic 309.81
  - psychasthenic (type) 300.89
  - railroad 300.16
  - rectum 306.4
  - respiratory 306.1
  - rumination 306.4
  - senile 300.89
  - sexual 302.70
  - situational 300.89
  - specified type NEC 300.89
  - state 300.9
    - with depersonalization episode 300.6
  - stomach 306.4
  - vasomotor 306.2
  - visceral 306.4
  - war 300.16
- **Neurospongioblastosis diffusa** 759.5
- **Neurosyphilis** (arrested) (early) (inactive) (late) (latent) (recurrent) 094.9
  - with ataxia (cerebellar) (locomotor) (spastic) (spinal) 094.0
  - acute meningitis 094.2
  - aneurysm 094.89
  - arachnoid (adhesive) 094.2
  - arteritis (any artery) 094.89
  - asymptomatic 094.3
  - congenital 090.40
  - dura (mater) 094.89
  - general paresis 094.1
  - gumma 094.9
  - hemorrhagic 094.9
  - juvenile (asymptomatic) (meningeal) 090.40
  - leptomeninges (aseptic) 094.2
  - meningeal 094.2
  - meninges (adhesive) 094.2
  - meningovascular (diffuse) 094.2
  - optic atrophy 094.84
  - parenchymatous (degenerative) 094.1
  - paresis (*see also* Paresis, general) 094.1
  - paretic (*see also* Paresis, general) 094.1
  - relapse 094.9
  - remission in (sustained) 094.9
  - serological 094.3

☑ Additional Digit Required — Refer to the Tabular List (Numeric Code Section) for Additional Digit Selection

▶◀ Revised Text ● New Line ▲ Revised Code

- **Neurosyphilis** — *continued*
  - specified nature or site NEC 094.89
  - tabes (dorsalis) 094.0
    - juvenile 090.40
  - tabetic 094.0
    - juvenile 090.40
  - taboparesis 094.1
    - juvenile 090.40
  - thrombosis 094.89
  - vascular 094.89
- **Neurotic** (*see also* Neurosis) 300.9
  - excoriation 698.4
    - psychogenic 306.3
- **Neurotmesis** — *see* Injury, nerve, by site
- **Neurotoxemia** — *see* Toxemia
- **Neutro-occlusion** 524.21
- **Neutropenia, neutropenic** (chronic) (cyclic) (drug-induced) (genetic) (idiopathic) (immune) (infantile) (malignant) (periodic) (pernicious) (primary) (splenic) (splenomegaly) (toxic) 288.0
  - chronic hypoplastic 288.0
  - congenital (nontransient) 288.0
  - fever 288.0
  - neonatal, transitory (isoimmune) (maternal transfer) 776.7
- **Neutrophilia, hereditary giant** 288.2
- **Nevocarcinoma** (M8720/3) — *see* Melanoma
- **Nevus** (M8720/0) — *see also* Neoplasm, skin, benign

> *Note — Except where otherwise indicated, varieties of nevus in the list below that are followed by a morphology code number (M----/0) should be coded by site as for "Neoplasm, skin, benign."*

  - acanthotic 702.8
  - achromic (M8730/0)
  - amelanotic (M8730/0)
  - anemic, anemicus 709.09
  - angiomatous (M9120/0) (*see also* Hemangioma) 228.00
  - araneus 448.1
  - avasculosus 709.09
  - balloon cell (M8722/0)
  - bathing trunk (M8761/1) 238.2
  - blue (M8780/0)
    - cellular (M8790/0)
    - giant (M8790/0)
    - Jadassohn's (M8780/0)
    - malignant (M8780/3) — *see* Melanoma
  - capillary (M9131/0) (*see also* Hemangioma) 228.00
  - cavernous (M9121/0) (*see also* Hemangioma) 228.00
  - cellular (M8720/0)
    - blue (M8790/0)
  - comedonicus 757.33
  - compound (M8760/0)
  - conjunctiva (M8720/0) 224.3
  - dermal (M8750/0)
    - and epidermal (M8760/0)
  - epithelioid cell (and spindle cell) (M8770/0)
  - flammeus 757.32
    - osteohypertrophic 759.89
  - hairy (M8720/0)
  - halo (M8723/0)
  - hemangiomatous (M9120/0) (*see also* Hemangioma) 228.00
  - intradermal (M8750/0)
  - intraepidermal (M8740/0)
  - involuting (M8724/0)
  - Jadassohn's (blue) (M8780/0)
  - junction, junctional (M8740/0)
    - malignant melanoma in (M8740/3) — *see* Melanoma
  - juvenile (M8770/0)
  - lymphatic (M9170/0) 228.1
  - magnocellular (M8726/0)
    - specified site — *see* Neoplasm, by site, benign
    - unspecified site 224.0
  - malignant (M8720/3) — *see* Melanoma
  - meaning hemangioma (M9120/0) (*see also* Hemangioma) 228.00
  - melanotic (pigmented) (M8720/0)
  - multiplex 759.5
  - nonneoplastic 448.1

- **Nevus** (M8720/0) — *see also* Neoplasm, skin, benign — *continued*
  - nonpigmented (M8730/0)
  - nonvascular (M8720/0)
  - oral mucosa, white sponge 750.26
  - osteohypertrophic, flammeus 759.89
  - papillaris (M8720/0)
  - papillomatosus (M8720/0)
  - pigmented (M8720/0)
    - giant (M8761/1) — *see also* Neoplasm, skin, uncertain behavior
      - malignant melanoma in (M8761/3) — *see* Melanoma
    - systematicus 757.33
  - pilosus (M8720/0)
  - port wine 757.32
  - sanguineous 757.32
  - sebaceous (senile) 702.8
  - senile 448.1
  - spider 448.1
  - spindle cell (and epithelioid cell) (M8770/0)
  - stellar 448.1
  - strawberry 757.32
  - syringocystadenomatous papilliferous (M8406/0)
  - unius lateris 757.33
  - Unna's 757.32
  - vascular 757.32
  - verrucous 757.33
  - white sponge (oral mucosa) 750.26
- **Newborn** (infant) (liveborn)
  - affected by maternal abuse of drugs (gestational) (via placenta) (via breast milk) ▶(*see also* Noxious, substances transmitted through placenta or breast milk, affecting fetus or newborn)◀ 760.70
  - apnea 770.81 ●
    - obstructive 770.82 ●
    - specified NEC 770.82 ●
  - cardiomyopathy 425.4 ●
    - congenital 425.3 ●
  - convulsion 779.0 ●
  - electrolyte imbalance NEC (transitory) 775.5 ●
  - gestation
    - 24 completed weeks 765.22
    - 25-26 completed weeks 765.23
    - 27-28 completed weeks 765.24
    - 29-30 completed weeks 765.25
    - 31-32 completed weeks 765.26
    - 33-34 completed weeks 765.27
    - 35-36 completed weeks 765.28
    - 37 or more completed weeks 765.29
    - less than 24 completed weeks 765.21
    - unspecified completed weeks 765.20
  - infection 771.89 ●
    - candida 771.7 ●
    - mastitis 771.5 ●
    - specified NEC 771.89 ●
    - urinary tract 771.82 ●
  - mastitis 771.5 ●
  - multiple NEC
    - born in hospital (without mention of cesarean delivery or section) V37.00
      - with cesarean delivery or section V37.01
    - born outside hospital
      - hospitalized V37.1
      - not hospitalized V37.2
    - mates all liveborn
      - born in hospital (without mention of cesarean delivery or section) V34.00
        - with cesarean delivery or section V34.01
      - born outside hospital
        - hospitalized V34.1
        - not hospitalized V34.2
    - mates all stillborn
      - born in hospital (without mention of cesarean delivery or section) V35.00
        - with cesarean delivery or section V35.01
      - born outside hospital
        - hospitalized V35.1
        - not hospitalized V35.2
    - mates liveborn and stillborn
      - born in hospital (without mention of cesarean delivery or section) V36.00
        - with cesarean delivery or section V36.01

- **Newborn** (*see also* Noxious, substances transmitted through placenta or breast milk, affecting fetus or newborn) — *continued*
  - multiple — *continued*
    - mates liveborn and stillborn — *continued*
      - born outside hospital
        - hospitalized V36.1
        - not hospitalized V36.2
  - omphalitis 771.4 ●
  - seizure 779.0 ●
  - sepsis 771.81 ●
  - single
    - born in hospital (without mention of cesarean delivery or section) V30.00
      - with cesarean delivery or section V30.01
    - born outside hospital
      - hospitalized V30.1
      - not hospitalized V30.2
  - specified condition NEC 779.89 ●
  - twin NEC
    - born in hospital (without mention of cesarean delivery or section) V33.00
      - with cesarean delivery or section V33.01
    - born outside hospital
      - hospitalized V33.1
      - not hospitalized V33.2
    - mate liveborn
      - born in hospital V31.0 ☑
      - born outside hospital
        - hospitalized V31.1
        - not hospitalized V31.2
    - mate stillborn
      - born in hospital V32.0 ☑
      - born outside hospital
        - hospitalized V32.1
        - not hospitalized V32.2
  - unspecified as to single or multiple birth
    - born in hospital (without mention of cesarean delivery or section) V39.00
      - with cesarean delivery or section V39.01
    - born outside hospital
      - hospitalized V39.1
      - not hospitalized V39.2
- **Newcastle's conjunctivitis or disease** 077.8
- **Nezelof's syndrome** (pure alymphocytosis) 279.13
- **Niacin** (amide) **deficiency** 265.2
- **Nicolas-Durand-Favre disease** (climatic bubo) 099.1
- **Nicolas-Favre disease** (climatic bubo) 099.1
- **Nicotinic acid** (amide) **deficiency** 265.2
- **Niemann-Pick disease** (lipid histiocytosis) (splenomegaly) 272.7
- **Night**
  - blindness (*see also* Blindness, night) 368.60
    - congenital 368.61
    - vitamin A deficiency 264.5
  - cramps 729.82
  - sweats 780.8
  - terrors, child 307.46
- **Nightmare** 307.47
  - REM-sleep type 307.47
- **Nipple** — *see* condition
- **Nisbet's chancre** 099.0
- **Nishimoto (-Takeuchi) disease** 437.5
- **Nitritoid crisis or reaction** — *see* Crisis, nitritoid
- **Nitrogen retention, extrarenal** 788.9
- **Nitrosohemoglobinemia** 289.89
- **Njovera** 104.0
- **No**
  - diagnosis 799.9
  - disease (found) V71.9
  - room at the inn V65.0
- **Nocardiasis** — *see* Nocardiosis
- **Nocardiosis** 039.9
  - with pneumonia 039.1
  - lung 039.1
  - specified type NEC 039.8
- **Nocturia** 788.43
  - psychogenic 306.53
- **Nocturnal** — *see also* condition
  - dyspnea (paroxysmal) 786.09
  - emissions 608.89
  - enuresis 788.36
    - psychogenic 307.6
  - frequency (micturition) 788.43
    - psychogenic 306.53

☑ Additional Digit Required — Refer to the Tabular List (Numeric Code Section) for Additional Digit Selection
▶◀ Revised Text ● New Line ▲ Revised Code

O

- **Occlusion** — *continued*
  - artery NEC (*see also* Embolism, artery) — *continued*
    - carotid 433.1 ☑
      - with other precerebral artery 433.3 ☑
      - bilateral 433.3 ☑
    - cerebellar (anterior inferior) (posterior inferior) (superior) 433.8 ☑
    - cerebral (*see also* Infarct, brain) 434.9 ☑
    - choroidal (anterior) 433.8 ☑
    - communicating posterior 433.8 ☑
    - coronary (thrombotic) (*see also* Infarct, myocardium) 410.9 ☑
      - acute 410.9 ☑
        - without myocardial infarction 411.81
      - healed or old 412
    - hypophyseal 433.8 ☑
    - iliac artery 444.81
    - mesenteric (embolic) (thrombotic) (with gangrene) 557.0
    - pontine 433.8 ☑
    - precerebral NEC 433.9 ☑
      - late effect — *see* Late effect(s) (of) cerebrovascular disease
      - multiple or bilateral 433.3 ☑
      - puerperal, postpartum, childbirth 674.0 ☑
      - specified NEC 433.8 ☑
    - renal 593.81
    - retinal — *see* Occlusion, retina, artery
    - spinal 433.8 ☑
    - vertebral 433.2 ☑
      - with other precerebral artery 433.3 ☑
      - bilateral 433.3 ☑
  - basilar (artery) — *see* Occlusion, artery, basilar
  - bile duct (any) (*see also* Obstruction, biliary) 576.2
  - bowel (*see also* Obstruction, intestine) 560.9
  - brain (artery) (vascular) (*see also* Infarct, brain) 434.9 ☑
  - breast (duct) 611.8
  - carotid (artery) (common) (internal) — *see* Occlusion, artery, carotid
  - cerebellar (anterior inferior) (artery) (posterior inferior) (superior) 433.8 ☑
  - cerebral (artery) (*see also* Infarct, brain) 434.9 ☑
  - cerebrovascular (*see also* Infarct, brain) 434.9 ☑
    - diffuse 437.0
  - cervical canal (*see also* Stricture, cervix) 622.4
    - by falciparum malaria 084.0
  - cervix (uteri) (*see also* Stricture, cervix) 622.4
  - choanal 748.0
  - choroidal (artery) 433.8 ☑
  - colon (*see also* Obstruction, intestine) 560.9
  - communicating posterior artery 433.8 ☑
  - coronary (artery) (thrombotic) (*see also* Infarct, myocardium) 410.9 ☑
    - acute 410.9 ☑
      - without myocardial infarction 411.81
    - healed or old 412
    - without myocardial infarction 411.81
  - cystic duct (*see also* Obstruction, gallbladder) 575.2
    - congenital 751.69
  - disto
    - division I 524.22
    - division II 524.22
  - embolic — *see* Embolism
  - fallopian tube 628.2
    - congenital 752.19
  - gallbladder (*see also* Obstruction, gallbladder) 575.2
    - congenital 751.69
      - jaundice from 751.69 *[774.5]*
  - gingiva, traumatic 523.8
  - hymen 623.3
    - congenital 752.42
  - hypophyseal (artery) 433.8 ☑
  - iliac artery 444.81
  - intestine (*see also* Obstruction, intestine) 560.9
  - kidney 593.89
  - lacrimal apparatus — *see* Stenosis, lacrimal
  - lung 518.89
  - lymph or lymphatic channel 457.1
  - mammary duct 611.8
  - mesenteric artery (embolic) (thrombotic) (with gangrene) 557.0
  - nose 478.1
    - congenital 748.0
  - organ or site, congenital NEC — *see* Atresia
  - oviduct 628.2
    - congenital 752.19
  - periodontal, traumatic 523.8
  - peripheral arteries (lower extremity) 444.22
    - without thrombus or embolus (*see also* Arteriosclerosis, extremities) 440.20
    - due to stricture or stenosis 447.1
    - upper extremity 444.21
      - without thrombus or embolus (*see also* Arteriosclerosis, extremities 440.20
      - due to stricture or stenosis 447.1
  - pontine (artery) 433.8 ☑
  - posterior lingual, of mandibular teeth 524.29
  - precerebral artery — *see* Occlusion, artery, precerebral NEC
  - puncta lacrimalia 375.52
  - pupil 364.74
  - pylorus (*see also* Stricture, pylorus) 537.0
  - renal artery 593.81
  - retina, retinal (vascular) 362.30
    - artery, arterial 362.30
      - branch 362.32
      - central (total) 362.31
      - partial 362.33
      - transient 362.34
      - tributary 362.32
    - vein 362.30
      - branch 362.36
      - central (total) 362.35
      - incipient 362.37
      - partial 362.37
      - tributary 362.36
  - spinal artery 433.8 ☑
  - stent
    - coronary 996.72
  - teeth (mandibular) (posterior lingual) 524.29
  - thoracic duct 457.1
  - tubal 628.2
  - ureter (complete) (partial) 593.4
    - congenital 753.29
  - urethra (*see also* Stricture, urethra) 598.9
    - congenital 753.6
  - uterus 621.8
  - vagina 623.2
  - vascular NEC 459.9
  - vein — *see* Thrombosis
  - vena cava (inferior) (superior) 453.2
  - ventricle (brain) NEC 331.4
  - vertebral (artery) — *see* Occlusion, artery, vertebral
  - vessel (blood) NEC 459.9
  - vulva 624.8
- **Occlusio pupillae** 364.74
- **Occupational**
  - problems NEC V62.2
  - therapy V57.21
- **Ochlophobia** 300.29
- **Ochronosis** (alkaptonuric) (congenital) (endogenous) 270.2
  - with chloasma of eyelid 270.2
- **Ocular muscle** — *see also* condition
  - myopathy 359.1
  - torticollis 781.93
- **Oculoauriculovertebral dysplasia** 756.0
- **Oculogyric**
  - crisis or disturbance 378.87
    - psychogenic 306.7
- **Oculomotor syndrome** 378.81
- **Oddi's sphincter spasm** 576.5
- **Odelberg's disease** (juvenile osteochondrosis) 732.1
- **Odontalgia** 525.9
- **Odontoameloblastoma** (M9311/0) 213.1
  - upper jaw (bone) 213.0
- **Odontoclasia** 521.05
- **Odontoclasis** 873.63
  - complicated 873.73
- **Odontodysplasia, regional** 520.4
- **Odontogenesis imperfecta** 520.5
- **Odontoma** (M9280/0) 213.1
  - ameloblastic (M9311/0) 213.1
    - upper jaw (bone) 213.0
  - calcified (M9280/0) 213.1
    - upper jaw (bone) 213.0
  - complex (M9282/0) 213.1
    - upper jaw (bone) 213.0
  - compound (M9281/0) 213.1
    - upper jaw (bone) 213.0
  - fibroameloblastic (M9290/0) 213.1
    - upper jaw (bone) 213.0
  - follicular 526.0
  - upper jaw (bone) 213.0
- **Odontomyelitis** (closed) (open) 522.0
- **Odontonecrosis** 521.09
- **Odontorrhagia** 525.8
- **Odontosarcoma, ameloblastic** (M9290/3) 170.1
  - upper jaw (bone) 170.0
- **Odynophagia** 787.2
- **Oesophagostomiasis** 127.7
- **Oesophagostomum infestation** 127.7
- **Oestriasis** 134.0
- **Ogilvie's syndrome** (sympathicotonic colon obstruction) 560.89
- **Oguchi's disease** (retina) 368.61
- **Ohara's disease** (*see also* Tularemia) 021.9
- **Oidiomycosis** (*see also* Candidiasis) 112.9
- **Oidiomycotic meningitis** 112.83
- **Oidium albicans infection** (*see also* Candidiasis) 112.9
- **Old age** 797
  - dementia (of) 290.0
- **Olfactory** — *see* condition
- **Oligemia** 285.9
- **Oligergasia** (*see also* Retardation, mental) 319
- **Oligoamnios** 658.0 ☑
  - affecting fetus or newborn 761.2
- **Oligoastrocytoma, mixed** (M9382/3)
  - specified site — *see* Neoplasm, by site, malignant
  - unspecified site 191.9
- **Oligocythemia** 285.9
- **Oligodendroblastoma** (M9460/3)
  - specified site — *see* Neoplasm, by site, malignant
  - unspecified site 191.9
- **Oligodendroglioma** (M9450/3)
  - anaplastic type (M9451/3)
    - specified site — *see* Neoplasm, by site, malignant
    - unspecified site 191.9
  - specified site — *see* Neoplasm, by site, malignant
  - unspecified site 191.9
- **Oligodendroma** — *see* Oligodendroglioma
- **Oligodontia** (*see also* Anodontia) 520.0
- **Oligoencephalon** 742.1
- **Oligohydramnios** 658.0 ☑
  - affecting fetus or newborn 761.2
  - due to premature rupture of membranes 658.1 ☑
    - affecting fetus or newborn 761.2
- **Oligohydrosis** 705.0
- **Oligomenorrhea** 626.1
- **Oligophrenia** (*see also* Retardation, mental) 319
  - phenylpyruvic 270.1
- **Oligospermia** 606.1
- **Oligotrichia** 704.09
  - congenita 757.4
- **Oliguria** 788.5
  - with
    - abortion — *see* Abortion, by type, with renal failure
    - ectopic pregnancy (*see also* categories 633.0-633.9) 639.3
    - molar pregnancy (*see also* categories 630-632) 639.3
  - complicating
    - abortion 639.3

- **Oliguria** — *continued*
  - complicating — *continued*
    - ectopic or molar pregnancy 639.3
    - pregnancy 646.2 ☑
      - with hypertension — *see* Toxemia, of pregnancy
  - due to a procedure 997.5
  - following labor and delivery 669.3 ☑
  - heart or cardiac — *see* Failure, heart
  - puerperal, postpartum 669.3 ☑
  - specified due to a procedure 997.5
- **Ollier's disease** (chondrodysplasia) 756.4
- **Omentitis** (*see also* Peritonitis) 567.9
- **Omentocele** (*see also* Hernia, omental) 553.8
- **Omentum, omental** — *see* condition
- **Omphalitis** (congenital) (newborn) 771.4
  - not of newborn 686.9
  - tetanus 771.3
- **Omphalocele** 756.79
- **Omphalomesenteric duct, persistent** 751.0
- **Omphalorrhagia, newborn** 772.3
- **Omsk hemorrhagic fever** 065.1
- **Onanism** 307.9
- **Onchocerciasis** 125.3
  - eye 125.3 *[360.13]*
- **Onchocercosis** 125.3
- **Oncocytoma** (M8290/0) — *see* Neoplasm, by site, benign
- **Ondine's curse** 348.8
- **Oneirophrenia** (*see also* Schizophrenia) 295.4 ☑
- **Onychauxis** 703.8
  - congenital 757.5
- **Onychia** (with lymphangitis) 681.9
  - dermatophytic 110.1
  - finger 681.02
  - toe 681.11
- **Onychitis** (with lymphangitis) 681.9
  - finger 681.02
  - toe 681.11
- **Onychocryptosis** 703.0
- **Onychodystrophy** 703.8
  - congenital 757.5
- **Onychogryphosis** 703.8
- **Onychogryposis** 703.8
- **Onycholysis** 703.8
- **Onychomadesis** 703.8
- **Onychomalacia** 703.8
- **Onychomycosis** 110.1
  - finger 110.1
  - toe 110.1
- **Onycho-osteodysplasia** 756.89
- **Onychophagy** 307.9
- **Onychoptosis** 703.8
- **Onychorrhexis** 703.8
  - congenital 757.5
- **Onychoschizia** 703.8
- **Onychotrophia** (*see also* Atrophy, nail) 703.8
- **O'nyong-nyong fever** 066.3
- **Onyxis** (finger) (toe) 703.0
- **Onyxitis** (with lymphangitis) 681.9
  - finger 681.02
  - toe 681.11
- **Oocyte (egg) (ovum)** ●
  - donor V59.70 ●
    - over age 35 V59.73 ●
      - anonymous recipient V59.73 ●
      - designated recipient V59.74 ●
    - under age 35 V59.71 ●
      - anonymous recipient V59.71 ●
      - designated recipient V59.72 ●
- **Oophoritis** (cystic) (infectional) (interstitial) (*see also* Salpingo-oophoritis) 614.2
  - complicating pregnancy 646.6 ☑
  - fetal (acute) 752.0
  - gonococcal (acute) 098.19
    - chronic or duration of 2 months or over 098.39
  - tuberculous (*see also* Tuberculosis) 016.6 ☑
- **Opacity, opacities**
  - cornea 371.00
    - central 371.03
    - congenital 743.43
      - interfering with vision 743.42
    - degenerative (*see also* Degeneration, cornea) 371.40
    - hereditary (*see also* Dystrophy, cornea) 371.50
    - inflammatory (*see also* Keratitis) 370.9
    - late effect of trachoma (healed) 139.1
    - minor 371.01
    - peripheral 371.02
  - enamel (fluoride) (nonfluoride) (teeth) 520.3
  - lens (*see also* Cataract) 366.9
  - snowball 379.22
  - vitreous (humor) 379.24
    - congenital 743.51
- **Opalescent dentin** (hereditary) 520.5
- **Open, opening**
  - abnormal, organ or site, congenital — *see* Imperfect, closure
  - angle with
    - borderline intraocular pressure 365.01
    - cupping of discs 365.01
  - bite (anterior) (posterior) 524.29
  - false — *see* Imperfect, closure
  - wound — *see* Wound, open, by site
- **Operation**
  - causing mutilation of fetus 763.89
  - destructive, on live fetus, to facilitate birth 763.89
  - for delivery, fetus or newborn 763.89
  - maternal, unrelated to current delivery, affecting fetus or newborn 760.6
- **Operational fatigue** 300.89
- **Operative** — *see* condition
- **Operculitis** (chronic) 523.4
  - acute 523.3
- **Operculum, retina** 361.32
  - with detachment 361.01
- **Ophiasis** 704.01
- **Ophthalmia** (*see also* Conjunctivitis) 372.30
  - actinic rays 370.24
  - allergic (acute) 372.05
    - chronic 372.14
  - blennorrhagic (neonatorum) 098.40
  - catarrhal 372.03
  - diphtheritic 032.81
  - Egyptian 076.1
  - electric, electrica 370.24
  - gonococcal (neonatorum) 098.40
  - metastatic 360.11
  - migraine 346.8 ☑
  - neonatorum, newborn 771.6
    - gonococcal 098.40
  - nodosa 360.14
  - phlyctenular 370.31
    - with ulcer (*see also* Ulcer, cornea) 370.00
  - sympathetic 360.11
- **Ophthalmitis** — *see* Ophthalmia
- **Ophthalmocele** (congenital) 743.66
- **Ophthalmoneuromyelitis** 341.0
- **Ophthalmopathy, infiltrative with thyrotoxicosis** 242.0 ☑
- **Ophthalmoplegia** (*see also* Strabismus) 378.9
  - anterior internuclear 378.86
  - ataxia-areflexia syndrome 357.0
  - bilateral 378.9
  - diabetic 250.5 ☑ *[378.86]*
  - exophthalmic 242.0 ☑ *[376.22]*
  - external 378.55
    - progressive 378.72
    - total 378.56
  - internal (complete) (total) 367.52
  - internuclear 378.86
  - migraine 346.8 ☑
  - painful 378.55
  - Parinaud's 378.81
  - progressive external 378.72
  - supranuclear, progressive 333.0
  - total (external) 378.56
    - internal 367.52
  - unilateral 378.9
- **Opisthognathism** 524.00
- **Opisthorchiasis** (felineus) (tenuicollis) (viverrini) 121.0
- **Opisthotonos, opisthotonus** 781.0
- **Opitz's disease** (congestive splenomegaly) 289.51
- **Opiumism** (*see also* Dependence) 304.0 ☑
- **Oppenheim's disease** 358.8
- **Oppenheim-Urbach disease or syndrome** (necrobiosis lipoidica diabeticorum) 250.8 ☑ *[709.3]*
- **Opsoclonia** 379.59
- **Optic nerve** — *see* condition
- **Orbit** — *see* condition
- **Orchioblastoma** (M9071/3) 186.9
- **Orchitis** (nonspecific) (septic) 604.90
  - with abscess 604.0
  - blennorrhagic (acute) 098.13
    - chronic or duration of 2 months or over 098.33
  - diphtheritic 032.89 *[604.91]*
  - filarial 125.9 *[604.91]*
  - gangrenous 604.99
  - gonococcal (acute) 098.13
    - chronic or duration of 2 months or over 098.33
  - mumps 072.0
  - parotidea 072.0
  - suppurative 604.99
  - syphilitic 095.8 *[604.91]*
  - tuberculous (*see also* Tuberculosis) 016.5 ☑ *[608.81]*
- **Orf** 051.2
- **Organic** — *see also* condition
  - heart — *see* Disease, heart
  - insufficiency 799.89
- **Oriental**
  - bilharziasis 120.2
  - schistosomiasis 120.2
  - sore 085.1
- **Orientation**
  - ego-dystonic sexual 302.0
- **Orifice** — *see* condition
- **Origin, both great vessels from right ventricle** 745.11
- **Ormond's disease or syndrome** 593.4
- **Ornithosis** 073.9
  - with
    - complication 073.8
      - specified NEC 073.7
    - pneumonia 073.0
    - pneumonitis (lobular) 073.0
- **Orodigitofacial dysostosis** 759.89
- **Oropouche fever** 066.3
- **Orotaciduria, oroticaciduria** (congenital) (hereditary) (pyrimidine deficiency) 281.4
- **Oroya fever** 088.0
- **Orthodontics** V58.5
  - adjustment V53.4
  - aftercare V58.5
  - fitting V53.4
- **Orthopnea** 786.02
- **Orthoptic training** V57.4
- **Os, uterus** — *see* condition
- **Osgood-Schlatter**
  - disease 732.4
  - osteochondrosis 732.4
- **Osler's**
  - disease (M9950/1) (polycythemia vera) 238.4
  - nodes 421.0
- **Osler-Rendu disease** (familial hemorrhagic telangiectasia) 448.0
- **Osler-Vaquez disease** (M9950/1) (polycythemia vera) 238.4
- **Osler-Weber-Rendu syndrome** (familial hemorrhagic telangiectasia) 448.0
- **Osmidrosis** 705.89
- **Osseous** — *see* condition
- **Ossification**
  - artery — *see* Arteriosclerosis
  - auricle (ear) 380.39

☑ Additional Digit Required — Refer to the Tabular List (Numeric Code Section) for Additional Digit Selection

▶◀ Revised Text ● New Line ▲ Revised Code

Note — Use the following fifth-digit subclassification with category 715:

0	*site unspecified*
1	*shoulder region*
2	*upper arm*
3	*forearm*
4	*hand*
5	*pelvic region and thigh*
6	*lower leg*
7	*ankle and foot*
8	*other specified sites except spine*
9	*multiple sites*

> *Note — Use the following fifth-digit subclassification with category 730:*
>
> *0 site unspecified*
> *1 shoulder region*
> *2 upper arm*
> *3 forearm*
> *4 hand*
> *5 pelvic region and thigh*
> *6 lower leg*
> *7 ankle and foot*
> *8 other specified sites*
> *9 multiple sites*

☑ Additional Digit Required — Refer to the Tabular List (Numeric Code Section) for Additional Digit Selection

▶◀ Revised Text ● New Line ▲ Revised Code

P

☑ Additional Digit Required — Refer to the Tabular List (Numeric Code Section) for Additional Digit Selection

▶◀ Revised Text ● New Line ▲ Revised Code

- **Paralysis, paralytic** — *continued*
  - diaphragm (flaccid) 519.4
    - due to accidental section of phrenic nerve during procedure 998.2
  - digestive organs NEC 564.89
  - diplegic — *see* Diplegia
  - divergence (nuclear) 378.85
  - divers' 993.3
  - Duchenne's 335.22
  - due to intracranial or spinal birth injury — *see* Palsy, cerebral
  - embolic (current episode) (*see also* Embolism, brain) 434.1 ☑
    - late effect — *see* Late effect(s) (of) cerebrovascular disease
  - enteric (*see also* Ileus) 560.1
    - with hernia — *see* Hernia, by site, with obstruction
  - Erb's syphilitic spastic spinal 094.89
  - Erb (-Duchenne) (birth) (newborn) 767.6
  - esophagus 530.89
  - essential, infancy (*see also* Poliomyelitis) 045.9 ☑
  - extremity
    - lower — *see* Paralysis, leg
    - spastic (hereditary) 343.3
      - noncongenital or noninfantile 344.1
    - transient (cause unknown) 781.4
    - upper — *see* Paralysis, arm
  - eye muscle (extrinsic) 378.55
    - intrinsic 367.51
  - facial (nerve) 351.0
    - birth injury 767.5
    - congenital 767.5
    - following operation NEC 998.2
    - newborn 767.5
  - familial 359.3
    - periodic 359.3
    - spastic 334.1
  - fauces 478.29
  - finger NEC 354.9
  - foot NEC 355.8
  - gait 781.2
  - gastric nerve 352.3
  - gaze 378.81
  - general 094.1
    - ataxic 094.1
    - insane 094.1
    - juvenile 090.40
    - progressive 094.1
    - tabetic 094.1
  - glossopharyngeal (nerve) 352.2
  - glottis (*see also* Paralysis, vocal cord) 478.30
  - gluteal 353.4
  - Gubler (-Millard) 344.89
  - hand 354.9
    - hysterical 300.11
    - psychogenic 306.0
  - heart (*see also* Failure, heart) 428.9
  - hemifacial, progressive 349.89
  - hemiplegic — *see* Hemiplegia
  - hyperkalemic periodic (familial) 359.3
  - hypertensive (current episode) 437.8
  - hypoglossal (nerve) 352.5
  - hypokalemic periodic 359.3
  - Hyrtl's sphincter (rectum) 569.49
  - hysterical 300.11
  - ileus (*see also* Ileus) 560.1
  - infantile (*see also* Poliomyelitis) 045.9 ☑
    - atrophic acute 045.1 ☑
    - bulbar 045.0 ☑
    - cerebral — *see* Palsy, cerebral
    - paralytic 045.1 ☑
    - progressive acute 045.9 ☑
    - spastic — *see* Palsy, cerebral
    - spinal 045.9 ☑
  - infective (*see also* Poliomyelitis) 045.9 ☑
  - inferior nuclear 344.9
  - insane, general or progressive 094.1
  - internuclear 378.86
  - interosseous 355.9
  - intestine (*see also* Ileus) 560.1
  - intracranial (current episode) (*see also* Paralysis, brain) 437.8
    - due to birth injury 767.0
  - iris 379.49
    - due to diphtheria (toxin) 032.81 *[379.49]*

- **Paralysis, paralytic** — *continued*
  - ischemic, Volkmann's (complicating trauma) 958.6
  - isolated sleep, recurrent 327.43 ●
  - Jackson's 344.89
  - jake 357.7
  - Jamaica ginger (jake) 357.7
  - juvenile general 090.40
  - Klumpke (-Déjérine) (birth) (newborn) 767.6
  - labioglossal (laryngeal) (pharyngeal) 335.22
  - Landry's 357.0
  - laryngeal nerve (recurrent) (superior) (*see also* Paralysis, vocal cord) 478.30
  - larynx (*see also* Paralysis, vocal cord) 478.30
    - due to diphtheria (toxin) 032.3
  - late effect
    - due to
      - birth injury, brain or spinal (cord) — *see* Palsy, cerebral
      - edema, brain or cerebral — *see* Paralysis, brain
      - lesion
        - late effect — *see* Late effect(s) (of) cerebrovascular disease
        - spinal (cord) — *see* Paralysis, spinal
  - lateral 335.24
  - lead 984.9
    - specified type of lead — *see* Table of Drugs and Chemicals
  - left side — *see* Hemiplegia
  - leg 344.30
    - affecting
      - dominant side 344.31
      - nondominant side 344.32
    - both (*see also* Paraplegia) 344.1
    - crossed 344.89
    - hysterical 300.11
    - psychogenic 306.0
    - transient or transitory 781.4
      - traumatic NEC (*see also* Injury, nerve, lower limb) 956.9
  - levator palpebrae superioris 374.31
  - limb NEC 344.5
    - all four — *see* Quadriplegia
    - quadriplegia — *see* Quadriplegia
  - lip 528.5
  - Lissauer's 094.1
  - local 355.9
  - lower limb — see also Paralysis, leg
    - both (*see also* Paraplegia) 344.1
  - lung 518.89
    - newborn 770.89
  - median nerve 354.1
  - medullary (tegmental) 344.89
  - mesencephalic NEC 344.89
    - tegmental 344.89
  - middle alternating 344.89
  - Millard-Gubler-Foville 344.89
  - monoplegic — *see* Monoplegia
  - motor NEC 344.9
    - cerebral — *see* Paralysis, brain
    - spinal — *see* Paralysis, spinal
  - multiple
    - cerebral — *see* Paralysis, brain
    - spinal — *see* Paralysis, spinal
  - muscle (flaccid) 359.9
    - due to nerve lesion NEC 355.9
    - eye (extrinsic) 378.55
      - intrinsic 367.51
      - oblique 378.51
    - iris sphincter 364.8
    - ischemic (complicating trauma) (Volkmann's) 958.6
    - pseudohypertrophic 359.1
  - muscular (atrophic) 359.9
    - progressive 335.21
  - musculocutaneous nerve 354.9
  - musculospiral 354.9
  - nerve — *see also* Disorder, nerve
    - third or oculomotor (partial) 378.51
      - total 378.52
    - fourth or trochlear 378.53
    - sixth or abducens 378.54
    - seventh or facial 351.0
      - birth injury 767.5

- **Paralysis, paralytic** — *continued*
  - nerve — *see also* Disorder, nerve — *continued*
    - seventh or facial — *continued*
      - due to
        - injection NEC 999.9
        - operation NEC 997.09
      - newborn 767.5
    - accessory 352.4
    - auditory 388.5
    - birth injury 767.7
    - cranial or cerebral (*see also* Disorder, nerve, cranial) 352.9
    - facial 351.0
      - birth injury 767.5
      - newborn 767.5
    - laryngeal (*see also* Paralysis, vocal cord) 478.30
    - newborn 767.7
    - phrenic 354.8
      - newborn 767.7
    - radial 354.3
      - birth injury 767.6
      - newborn 767.6
    - syphilitic 094.89
    - traumatic NEC (*see also* Injury, nerve, by site) 957.9
    - trigeminal 350.9
    - ulnar 354.2
  - newborn NEC 767.0
  - normokalemic periodic 359.3
  - obstetrical, newborn 767.7
  - ocular 378.9
  - oculofacial, congenital 352.6
  - oculomotor (nerve) (partial) 378.51
    - alternating 344.89
    - external bilateral 378.55
    - total 378.52
  - olfactory nerve 352.0
  - palate 528.9
  - palatopharyngolaryngeal 352.6
  - paratrigeminal 350.9
  - periodic (familial) (hyperkalemic) (hypokalemic) (normokalemic) (secondary) 359.3
  - peripheral
    - autonomic nervous system — *see* Neuropathy, peripheral, autonomic
    - nerve NEC 355.9
  - peroneal (nerve) 355.3
  - pharynx 478.29
  - phrenic nerve 354.8
  - plantar nerves 355.6
  - pneumogastric nerve 352.3
  - poliomyelitis (current) (*see also* Poliomyelitis, with paralysis) 045.1 ☑
    - bulbar 045.0 ☑
  - popliteal nerve 355.3
  - pressure (*see also* Neuropathy, entrapment) 355.9
  - progressive 335.21
    - atrophic 335.21
    - bulbar 335.22
    - general 094.1
    - hemifacial 349.89
    - infantile, acute (*see also* Poliomyelitis) 045.9 ☑
    - multiple 335.20
  - pseudobulbar 335.23
  - pseudohypertrophic 359.1
    - muscle 359.1
  - psychogenic 306.0
  - pupil, pupillary 379.49
  - quadriceps 355.8
  - quadriplegic (*see also* Quadriplegia) 344.0 ☑
  - radial nerve 354.3
    - birth injury 767.6
  - rectum (sphincter) 569.49
  - rectus muscle (eye) 378.55
  - recurrent
    - isolated sleep 327.43 ●
    - laryngeal nerve (*see also* Paralysis, vocal cord) 478.30 ●
  - respiratory (muscle) (system) (tract) 786.09
    - center NEC 344.89
      - fetus or newborn 770.89
    - congenital 768.9
    - newborn 768.9
  - right side — *see* Hemiplegia

- **Paralysis, paralytic** — *continued*
  - Saturday night 354.3
  - saturnine 984.9
    - specified type of lead — *see* Table of Drugs and Chemicals
  - sciatic nerve 355.0
  - secondary — *see* Paralysis, late effect
  - seizure (cerebral) (current episode) (*see also* Disease, cerebrovascular, acute) 436
    - late effect — *see* Late effect(s) (of) cerebrovascular disease
  - senile NEC 344.9
  - serratus magnus 355.9
  - shaking (*see also* Parkinsonism) 332.0
  - shock (*see also* Disease, cerebrovascular, acute) 436
    - late effect — *see* Late effect(s) (of) cerebrovascular disease
  - shoulder 354.9
  - soft palate 528.9
  - spasmodic — *see* Paralysis, spastic
  - spastic 344.9
    - cerebral infantile — *see* Palsy, cerebral
    - congenital (cerebral) — *see* Palsy, cerebral
    - familial 334.1
    - hereditary 334.1
    - infantile 343.9
    - noncongenital or noninfantile, cerebral 344.9
    - syphilitic 094.0
      - spinal 094.89
  - sphincter, bladder (*see also* Paralysis, bladder) 596.53
  - spinal (cord) NEC 344.1
    - accessory nerve 352.4
    - acute (*see also* Poliomyelitis) 045.9 ☑
    - ascending acute 357.0
    - atrophic (acute) (*see also* Poliomyelitis, with paralysis) 045.1 ☑
      - spastic, syphilitic 094.89
    - congenital NEC 343.9
    - hemiplegic — *see* Hemiplegia
    - hereditary 336.8
    - infantile (*see also* Poliomyelitis) 045.9 ☑
    - late effect NEC 344.89
    - monoplegic — *see* Monoplegia
    - nerve 355.9
    - progressive 335.10
    - quadriplegic — *see* Quadriplegia
    - spastic NEC 343.9
    - traumatic — *see* Injury, spinal, by site
  - sternomastoid 352.4
  - stomach 536.3
    - diabetic 250.6 ☑ *[536.3]*
    - nerve ▶(nondiabetic)◀ 352.3
  - stroke (current episode) — *see* Infarct, brain
    - late effect — *see* Late effect(s) (of) cerebrovascular disease
  - subscapularis 354.8
  - superior nuclear NEC 334.9
  - supranuclear 356.8
  - sympathetic
    - cervical NEC 337.0
    - nerve NEC (*see also* Neuropathy, peripheral, autonomic) 337.9
    - nervous system — *see* Neuropathy, peripheral, autonomic
  - syndrome 344.9
    - specified NEC 344.89
  - syphilitic spastic spinal (Erb's) 094.89
  - tabetic general 094.1
  - thigh 355.8
  - throat 478.29
    - diphtheritic 032.0
    - muscle 478.29
  - thrombotic (current episode) (*see also* Thrombosis, brain) 434.0 ☑
    - late effect — *see* Late effect(s) (of) cerebrovascular disease
  - thumb NEC 354.9
  - tick (-bite) 989.5
  - Todd's (postepileptic transitory paralysis) 344.89
  - toe 355.6
  - tongue 529.8
  - transient
    - arm or leg NEC 781.4

- **Paralysis, paralytic** — *continued*
  - transient — *continued*
    - traumatic NEC (*see also* Injury, nerve, by site) 957.9
  - trapezius 352.4
  - traumatic, transient NEC (*see also* Injury, nerve, by site) 957.9
  - trembling (*see also* Parkinsonism) 332.0
  - triceps brachii 354.9
  - trigeminal nerve 350.9
  - trochlear nerve 378.53
  - ulnar nerve 354.2
  - upper limb — *see also* Paralysis, arm
    - both (*see also* Diplegia) 344.2
  - uremic — *see* Uremia
  - uveoparotitic 135
  - uvula 528.9
    - hysterical 300.11
    - postdiphtheritic 032.0
  - vagus nerve 352.3
  - vasomotor NEC 337.9
  - velum palati 528.9
  - vesical (*see also* Paralysis, bladder) 596.53
  - vestibular nerve 388.5
  - visual field, psychic 368.16
  - vocal cord 478.30
    - bilateral (partial) 478.33
      - complete 478.34
    - complete (bilateral) 478.34
    - unilateral (partial) 478.31
      - complete 478.32
  - Volkmann's (complicating trauma) 958.6
  - wasting 335.21
  - Weber's 344.89
  - wrist NEC 354.9
- **Paramedial orifice, urethrovesical** 753.8
- **Paramenia** 626.9
- **Parametritis** (chronic) (*see also* Disease, pelvis, inflammatory) 614.4
  - acute 614.3
  - puerperal, postpartum, childbirth 670.0 ☑
- **Parametrium, parametric** — *see* condition
- **Paramnesia** (*see also* Amnesia) 780.93
- **Paramolar** 520.1
  - causing crowding 524.31
- **Paramyloidosis** 277.3
- **Paramyoclonus multiplex** 333.2
- **Paramyotonia** 359.2
  - congenita 359.2
- **Paraneoplastic syndrome** — *see* condition
- **Parangi** (*see also* Yaws) 102.9
- **Paranoia** 297.1
  - alcoholic 291.5
  - querulans 297.8
  - senile 290.20
- **Paranoid**
  - dementia (*see also* Schizophrenia) 295.3 ☑
    - praecox (acute) 295.3 ☑
    - senile 290.20
  - personality 301.0
  - psychosis 297.9
    - alcoholic 291.5
    - climacteric 297.2
    - drug-induced 292.11
    - involutional 297.2
    - menopausal 297.2
    - protracted reactive 298.4
    - psychogenic 298.4
      - acute 298.3
    - senile 290.20
  - reaction (chronic) 297.9
    - acute 298.3
  - schizophrenia (acute) (*see also* Schizophrenia) 295.3 ☑
  - state 297.9
    - alcohol-induced 291.5
    - climacteric 297.2
    - drug-induced 292.11
    - due to or associated with
      - arteriosclerosis (cerebrovascular) 290.42
      - presenile brain disease 290.12
      - senile brain disease 290.20
    - involutional 297.2
    - menopausal 297.2

- **Paranoid** — *continued*
  - state — *continued*
    - senile 290.20
    - simple 297.0
    - specified type NEC 297.8
  - tendencies 301.0
  - traits 301.0
  - trends 301.0
  - type, psychopathic personality 301.0
- **Paraparesis** (*see also* Paralysis) 344.9
- **Paraphasia** 784.3
- **Paraphilia** (*see also* Deviation, sexual) 302.9
- **Paraphimosis** (congenital) 605
  - chancroidal 099.0
- **Paraphrenia, paraphrenic** (late) 297.2
  - climacteric 297.2
  - dementia (*see also* Schizophrenia) 295.3 ☑
  - involutional 297.2
  - menopausal 297.2
  - schizophrenia (acute) (*see also* Schizophrenia) 295.3 ☑
- **Paraplegia** 344.1
  - with
    - broken back — *see* Fracture, vertebra, by site, with spinal cord injury
    - fracture, vertebra — *see* Fracture, vertebra, by site, with spinal cord injury
  - ataxic — *see* Degeneration, combined, spinal cord
  - brain (current episode) (*see also* Paralysis, brain) 437.8
  - cerebral (current episode) (*see also* Paralysis, brain) 437.8
  - congenital or infantile (cerebral) (spastic) (spinal) 343.0
  - cortical — *see* Paralysis, brain
  - familial spastic 334.1
  - functional (hysterical) 300.11
  - hysterical 300.11
  - infantile 343.0
  - late effect 344.1
  - Pott's (*see also* Tuberculosis) 015.0 ☑ *[730.88]*
  - psychogenic 306.0
  - spastic
    - Erb's spinal 094.89
    - hereditary 334.1
    - not infantile or congenital 344.1
  - spinal (cord)
    - traumatic NEC — *see* Injury, spinal, by site
  - syphilitic (spastic) 094.89
  - traumatic NEC — *see* Injury, spinal, by site
- **Paraproteinemia** 273.2
  - benign (familial) 273.1
  - monoclonal 273.1
  - secondary to malignant or inflammatory disease 273.1
- **Parapsoriasis** 696.2
  - en plaques 696.2
  - guttata 696.2
  - lichenoides chronica 696.2
  - retiformis 696.2
  - varioliformis (acuta) 696.2
- **Parascarlatina** 057.8
- **Parasitic** — *see also* condition
  - disease NEC (*see also* Infestation, parasitic) 136.9
    - contact V01.89
    - exposure to V01.89
    - intestinal NEC 129
    - skin NEC 134.9
  - stomatitis 112.0
  - sycosis 110.0
    - beard 110.0
    - scalp 110.0
  - twin 759.4
- **Parasitism** NEC 136.9
  - intestinal NEC 129
  - skin NEC 134.9
  - specified — *see* Infestation
- **Parasitophobia** 300.29
- **Parasomnia** 307.47 ▲
  - alcohol induced 291.82 ●
  - drug induced 292.85 ●

Pellegrini's disease (calcification, knee joint) 726.62
Pellegrini (-Stieda) disease or syndrome (calcification, knee joint) 726.62
Pellizzi's syndrome (pineal) 259.8
Pelvic — *see also* condition
congestion-fibrosis syndrome 625.5
kidney 753.3
Pelvioectasis 591
Pelviolithiasis 592.0
Pelviperitonitis
female (*see also* Peritonitis, pelvic, female) 614.5
male (*see also* Peritonitis) 567.21 ▲
Pelvis, pelvic — *see also* condition or type
infantile 738.6
Nägele's 738.6
obliquity 738.6
Robert's 755.69
Pemphigoid 694.5
benign, mucous membrane 694.60
with ocular involvement 694.61
bullous 694.5
cicatricial 694.60
with ocular involvement 694.61
juvenile 694.2
Pemphigus 694.4
benign 694.5
chronic familial 757.39
Brazilian 694.4
circinatus 694.0
congenital, traumatic 757.39
conjunctiva 694.61
contagiosus 684
erythematodes 694.4
erythematosus 694.4
foliaceus 694.4
frambesiodes 694.4
gangrenous (*see also* Gangrene) 785.4
malignant 694.4
neonatorum, newborn 684
ocular 694.61
papillaris 694.4
seborrheic 694.4
South American 694.4
syphilitic (congenital) 090.0
vegetans 694.4
vulgaris 694.4
wildfire 694.4
Pendred's syndrome (familial goiter with deaf-mutism) 243
Pendulous
abdomen 701.9
in pregnancy or childbirth 654.4 ☑
affecting fetus or newborn 763.89
breast 611.8
Penetrating wound — *see also* Wound, open, by site
with internal injury — *see* Injury, internal, by site, with open wound
eyeball 871.7
with foreign body (nonmagnetic) 871.6
magnetic 871.5
ocular (*see also* Penetrating wound, eyeball) 871.7
adnexa 870.3
with foreign body 870.4
orbit 870.3
with foreign body 870.4
Penetration, pregnant uterus by instrument
with
abortion — *see* Abortion, by type, with damage to pelvic organs
ectopic pregnancy (*see also* categories 633.0-633.9) 639.2
molar pregnancy (*see also* categories 630-632) 639.2
complication of delivery 665.1 ☑
affecting fetus or newborn 763.89
following
abortion 639.2
ectopic or molar pregnancy 639.2
Penfield's syndrome (*see also* Epilepsy) 345.5 ☑
Penicilliosis of lung 117.3
Penis — *see* condition
Penitis 607.2
Penta X syndrome 758.81
Pentalogy (of Fallot) 745.2
Pentosuria (benign) (essential) 271.8
Peptic acid disease 536.8
Peregrinating patient V65.2
Perforated — *see* Perforation
Perforation, perforative (nontraumatic)
antrum (*see also* Sinusitis, maxillary) 473.0
appendix 540.0
with peritoneal abscess 540.1
atrial septum, multiple 745.5
attic, ear 384.22
healed 384.81
bile duct, except cystic (*see also* Disease, biliary) 576.3
cystic 575.4
bladder (urinary) 596.6
with
abortion — *see* Abortion, by type, with damage to pelvic organs
ectopic pregnancy (*see also* categories 633.0-633.9) 639.2
molar pregnancy (*see also* categories 630-632) 639.2
following
abortion 639.2
ectopic or molar pregnancy 639.2
obstetrical trauma 665.5 ☑
bowel 569.83
with
abortion — *see* Abortion, by type, with damage to pelvic organs
ectopic pregnancy (*see also* categories 633.0-633.9) 639.2
molar pregnancy (*see also* categories 630-632) 639.2
fetus or newborn 777.6
following
abortion 639.2
ectopic or molar pregnancy 639.2
obstetrical trauma 665.5 ☑
broad ligament
with
abortion — *see* Abortion, by type, with damage to pelvic organs
ectopic pregnancy (*see also* categories 633.0-633.9) 639.2
molar pregnancy (*see also* categories 630-632) 639.2
following
abortion 639.2
ectopic or molar pregnancy 639.2
obstetrical trauma 665.6 ☑
by
device, implant, or graft — *see* Complications, mechanical
foreign body left accidentally in operation wound 998.4
instrument (any) during a procedure, accidental 998.2
cecum 540.0
with peritoneal abscess 540.1
cervix (uteri) — *see also* Injury, internal, cervix
with
abortion — *see* Abortion, by type, with damage to pelvic organs
ectopic pregnancy (*see also* categories 633.0-633.9) 639.2
molar pregnancy (*see also* categories 630-632) 639.2
following
abortion 639.2
ectopic or molar pregnancy 639.2
obstetrical trauma 665.3 ☑
colon 569.83
common duct (bile) 576.3
cornea (*see also* Ulcer, cornea) 370.00
due to ulceration 370.06
cystic duct 575.4
diverticulum (*see also* Diverticula) 562.10
small intestine 562.00
duodenum, duodenal (ulcer) — *see* Ulcer, duodenum, with perforation
Perforation, perforative — *continued*
ear drum — *see* Perforation, tympanum
enteritis — *see* Enteritis
esophagus 530.4
ethmoidal sinus (*see also* Sinusitis, ethmoidal) 473.2
foreign body (external site) — *see also* Wound, open, by site, complicated
internal site, by ingested object — *see* Foreign body
frontal sinus (*see also* Sinusitis, frontal) 473.1
gallbladder or duct (*see also* Disease, gallbladder) 575.4
gastric (ulcer) — *see* Ulcer, stomach, with perforation
heart valve — *see* Endocarditis
ileum (*see also* Perforation, intestine) 569.83
instrumental
external — *see* Wound, open, by site
pregnant uterus, complicating delivery 665.9 ☑
surgical (accidental) (blood vessel) (nerve) (organ) 998.2
intestine 569.83
with
abortion — *see* Abortion, by type, with damage to pelvic organs
ectopic pregnancy (*see also* categories 633.0-633.9) 639.2
molar pregnancy (*see also* categories 630-632) 639.2
fetus or newborn 777.6
obstetrical trauma 665.5 ☑
ulcerative NEC 569.83
jejunum, jejunal 569.83
ulcer — *see* Ulcer, gastrojejunal, with perforation
mastoid (antrum) (cell) 383.89
maxillary sinus (*see also* Sinusitis, maxillary) 473.0
membrana tympani — *see* Perforation, tympanum
nasal
septum 478.1
congenital 748.1
syphilitic 095.8
sinus (*see also* Sinusitis) 473.9
congenital 748.1
palate (hard) 526.89
soft 528.9
syphilitic 095.8
syphilitic 095.8
palatine vault 526.89
syphilitic 095.8
congenital 090.5
pelvic
floor
with
abortion — *see* Abortion, by type, with damage to pelvic organs
ectopic pregnancy (*see also* categories 633.0-633.9) 639.2
molar pregnancy (*see also* categories 630-632) 639.2
obstetrical trauma 664.1 ☑
organ
with
abortion — *see* Abortion, by type, with damage to pelvic organs
ectopic pregnancy (*see also* categories 633.0-633.9) 639.2
molar pregnancy (*see also* categories 630-632) 639.2
following
abortion 639.2
ectopic or molar pregnancy 639.2
obstetrical trauma 665.5 ☑
perineum — *see* Laceration, perineum
periurethral tissue
with
abortion — *see* Abortion, by type, with damage to pelvic organs
ectopic pregnancy (*see also* categories 630-632) 639.2
molar pregnancy (*see also* categories 630-632) 639.2
pharynx 478.29

- **Perforation, perforative** — *continued*
  - pylorus, pyloric (ulcer) — *see* Ulcer, stomach, with perforation
  - rectum 569.49
  - sigmoid 569.83
  - sinus (accessory) (chronic) (nasal) (*see also* Sinusitis) 473.9
  - sphenoidal sinus (*see also* Sinusitis, sphenoidal) 473.3
  - stomach (due to ulcer) — *see* Ulcer, stomach, with perforation
  - surgical (accidental) (by instrument) (blood vessel) (nerve) (organ) 998.2
  - traumatic
    - external — *see* Wound, open, by site
    - eye (*see also* Penetrating wound, ocular) 871.7
    - internal organ — *see* Injury, internal, by site
  - tympanum (membrane) (persistent posttraumatic) (postinflammatory) 384.20
    - with
      - otitis media — *see* Otitis media
    - attic 384.22
    - central 384.21
    - healed 384.81
    - marginal NEC 384.23
    - multiple 384.24
    - pars flaccida 384.22
    - total 384.25
    - traumatic — *see* Wound, open, ear, drum
  - typhoid, gastrointestinal 002.0
  - ulcer — *see* Ulcer, by site, with perforation
  - ureter 593.89
  - urethra
    - with
      - abortion — *see* Abortion, by type, with damage to pelvic organs
      - ectopic pregnancy (*see also* categories 633.0-633.9) 639.2
      - molar pregnancy (*see also* categories 630-632) 639.2
    - following
      - abortion 639.2
      - ectopic or molar pregnancy 639.2
    - obstetrical trauma 665.5 ☑
  - uterus — *see also* Injury, internal, uterus
    - with
      - abortion — *see* Abortion, by type, with damage to pelvic organs
      - ectopic pregnancy (*see also* categories 633.0-633.9) 639.2
      - molar pregnancy (*see also* categories 630-632) 639.2
    - by intrauterine contraceptive device 996.32
    - following
      - abortion 639.2
      - ectopic or molar pregnancy 639.2
    - obstetrical trauma — *see* Injury, internal, uterus, obstetrical trauma
  - uvula 528.9
    - syphilitic 095.8
  - vagina — *see* Laceration, vagina
  - viscus NEC 799.89
    - traumatic 868.00
      - with open wound into cavity 868.10
- **Periadenitis mucosa necrotica recurrens** 528.2
- **Periangiitis** 446.0
- **Periantritis** 535.4 ☑
- **Periappendicitis** (acute) (*see also* Appendicitis) 541
- **Periarteritis** (disseminated) (infectious) (necrotizing) (nodosa) 446.0
- **Periarthritis** (joint) 726.90
  - Duplay's 726.2
  - gonococcal 098.50
  - humeroscapularis 726.2
  - scapulohumeral 726.2
  - shoulder 726.2
  - wrist 726.4
- **Periarthrosis** (angioneural) — *see* Periarthritis
- **Peribronchitis** 491.9
  - tuberculous (*see also* Tuberculosis) 011.3 ☑
- **Pericapsulitis, adhesive** (shoulder) 726.0
- **Pericarditis** (granular) (with decompensation) (with effusion) 423.9
  - with
    - rheumatic fever (conditions classifiable to 390)
      - active (*see also* Pericarditis, rheumatic) 391.0
      - inactive or quiescent 393
  - actinomycotic 039.8 *[420.0]*
  - acute (nonrheumatic) 420.90
    - with chorea (acute) (rheumatic) (Sydenham's) 392.0
    - bacterial 420.99
    - benign 420.91
    - hemorrhagic 420.90
    - idiopathic 420.91
    - infective 420.90
    - nonspecific 420.91
    - rheumatic 391.0
      - with chorea (acute) (rheumatic) (Sydenham's) 392.0
    - sicca 420.90
    - viral 420.91
  - adhesive or adherent (external) (internal) 423.1
    - acute — *see* Pericarditis, acute
    - rheumatic (external) (internal) 393
  - amebic 006.8 *[420.0]*
  - bacterial (acute) (subacute) (with serous or seropurulent effusion) 420.99
  - calcareous 423.2
  - cholesterol (chronic) 423.8
    - acute 420.90
  - chronic (nonrheumatic) 423.8
    - rheumatic 393
  - constrictive 423.2
  - Coxsackie 074.21
  - due to
    - actinomycosis 039.8 *[420.0]*
    - amebiasis 006.8 *[420.0]*
    - Coxsackie (virus) 074.21
    - histoplasmosis (*see also* Histoplasmosis) 115.93
    - nocardiosis 039.8 *[420.0]*
    - tuberculosis (*see also* Tuberculosis) 017.9 ☑ *[420.0]*
  - fibrinocaseous (*see also* Tuberculosis) 017.9 ☑ *[420.0]*
  - fibrinopurulent 420.99
  - fibrinous — *see* Pericarditis, rheumatic
  - fibropurulent 420.99
  - fibrous 423.1
  - gonococcal 098.83
  - hemorrhagic 423.0
  - idiopathic (acute) 420.91
  - infective (acute) 420.90
  - meningococcal 036.41
  - neoplastic (chronic) 423.8
    - acute 420.90
  - nonspecific 420.91
  - obliterans, obliterating 423.1
  - plastic 423.1
  - pneumococcal (acute) 420.99
  - postinfarction 411.0
  - purulent (acute) 420.99
  - rheumatic (active) (acute) (with effusion) (with pneumonia) 391.0
    - with chorea (acute) (rheumatic) (Sydenham's) 392.0
    - chronic or inactive (with chorea) 393
  - septic (acute) 420.99
  - serofibrinous — *see* Pericarditis, rheumatic
  - staphylococcal (acute) 420.99
  - streptococcal (acute) 420.99
  - suppurative (acute) 420.99
  - syphilitic 093.81
  - tuberculous (acute) (chronic) (*see also* Tuberculosis) 017.9 ☑ *[420.0]*
  - uremic 585.9 *[420.0]* ▲
  - viral (acute) 420.91
- **Pericardium, pericardial** — *see* condition
- **Pericellulitis** (*see also* Cellulitis) 682.9
- **Pericementitis** 523.4
  - acute 523.3
  - chronic (suppurative) 523.4
- **Pericholecystitis** (*see also* Cholecystitis) 575.10
- **Perichondritis**
  - auricle 380.00
    - acute 380.01
    - chronic 380.02
  - bronchus 491.9
  - ear (external) 380.00
    - acute 380.01
    - chronic 380.02
  - larynx 478.71
    - syphilitic 095.8
    - typhoid 002.0 *[478.71]*
  - nose 478.1
  - pinna 380.00
    - acute 380.01
    - chronic 380.02
  - trachea 478.9
- **Periclasia** 523.5
- **Pericolitis** 569.89
- **Pericoronitis** (chronic) 523.4
  - acute 523.3
- **Pericystitis** (*see also* Cystitis) 595.9
- **Pericytoma** (M9150/1) — *see also* Neoplasm, connective tissue, uncertain behavior
  - benign (M9150/0) — *see* Neoplasm, connective tissue, benign
  - malignant (M9150/3) — *see* Neoplasm, connective tissue, malignant
- **Peridacryocystitis, acute** 375.32
- **Peridiverticulitis** (*see also* Diverticulitis) 562.11
- **Periduodenitis** 535.6 ☑
- **Periendocarditis** (*see also* Endocarditis) 424.90
  - acute or subacute 421.9
- **Periepididymitis** (*see also* Epididymitis) 604.90
- **Perifolliculitis** (abscedens) 704.8
  - capitis, abscedens et suffodiens 704.8
  - dissecting, scalp 704.8
  - scalp 704.8
  - superficial pustular 704.8
- **Perigastritis** (acute) 535.0 ☑
- **Perigastrojejunitis** (acute) 535.0 ☑
- **Perihepatitis** (acute) 573.3
  - chlamydial 099.56
  - gonococcal 098.86
- **Peri-ileitis** (subacute) 569.89
- **Perilabyrinthitis** (acute) — *see* Labyrinthitis
- **Perimeningitis** — *see* Meningitis
- **Perimetritis** (*see also* Endometritis) 615.9
- **Perimetrosalpingitis** (*see also* Salpingo-oophoritis) 614.2
- **Perineocele** 618.05
- **Perinephric** — *see* condition
- **Perinephritic** — *see* condition
- **Perinephritis** (*see also* Infection, kidney) 590.9
  - purulent (*see also* Abscess, kidney) 590.2
- **Perineum, perineal** — *see* condition
- **Perineuritis** NEC 729.2
- **Periodic** — *see also* condition
  - disease (familial) 277.3
  - edema 995.1
    - hereditary 277.6
  - fever 277.3
  - limb movement disorder 327.51 ▲
  - paralysis (familial) 359.3
  - peritonitis 277.3
  - polyserositis 277.3
  - somnolence (*see also* Narcolepsy) 347.00
- **Periodontal**
  - cyst 522.8
  - pocket 523.8
- **Periodontitis** (chronic) (complex) (compound) (local) (simplex) 523.4
  - acute 523.3
  - apical 522.6
    - acute (pulpal origin) 522.4
- **Periodontoclasia** 523.5
- **Periodontosis** 523.5
- **Periods** — *see also* Menstruation
  - heavy 626.2
  - irregular 626.4
- **Perionychia** (with lymphangitis) 681.9
  - finger 681.02
  - toe 681.11

Perioophoritis (*see also* Salpingo-oophoritis) 614.2
Periorchitis (*see also* Orchitis) 604.90
Periosteum, periosteal — *see* condition
Periostitis (circumscribed) (diffuse) (infective) 730.3 ☑

> *Note — Use the following fifth-digit subclassification with category 730:*
>
> *0 site unspecified*
> *1 shoulder region*
> *2 upper arm*
> *3 forearm*
> *4 hand*
> *5 pelvic region and thigh*
> *6 lower leg*
> *7 ankle and foot*
> *8 other specified sites*
> *9 multiple sites*

  with osteomyelitis (*see also* Osteomyelitis) 730.2 ☑
    acute or subacute 730.0 ☑
    chronic or old 730.1 ☑
  albuminosa, albuminosus 730.3 ☑
  alveolar 526.5
  alveolodental 526.5
  dental 526.5
  gonorrheal 098.89
  hyperplastica, generalized 731.2
  jaw (lower) (upper) 526.4
  monomelic 733.99
  orbital 376.02
  syphilitic 095.5
    congenital 090.0 *[730.8]* ☑
    secondary 091.61
  tuberculous (*see also* Tuberculosis, bone) 015.9 ☑ *[730.8]* ☑
  yaws (early) (hypertrophic) (late) 102.6
Periostosis (*see also* Periostitis) 730.3 ☑
  with osteomyelitis (*see also* Osteomyelitis) 730.2 ☑
    acute or subacute 730.0 ☑
    chronic or old 730.1 ☑
  hyperplastic 756.59
Peripartum cardiomyopathy 674.5 ☑
Periphlebitis (*see also* Phlebitis) 451.9
  lower extremity 451.2
    deep (vessels) 451.19
    superficial (vessels) 451.0
  portal 572.1
  retina 362.18
  superficial (vessels) 451.0
  tuberculous (*see also* Tuberculosis) 017.9 ☑
    retina 017.3 ☑ *[362.18]*
Peripneumonia — *see* Pneumonia
Periproctitis 569.49
Periprostatitis (*see also* Prostatitis) 601.9
Perirectal — *see* condition
Perirenal — *see* condition
Perisalpingitis (*see also* Salpingo-oophoritis) 614.2
Perisigmoiditis 569.89
Perisplenitis (infectional) 289.59
Perispondylitis — *see* Spondylitis
Peristalsis reversed or visible 787.4
Peritendinitis (*see also* Tenosynovitis) 726.90
  adhesive (shoulder) 726.0
Perithelioma (M9150/1) — *see* Pericytoma
Peritoneum, peritoneal — *see also* condition
  equilibration test V56.32
Peritonitis (acute) (adhesive) (fibrinous) (hemorrhagic) (idiopathic) (localized) (perforative) (primary) (with adhesions) (with effusion) 567.9
  with or following
    abortion — *see* Abortion, by type, with sepsis
    abscess 567.21 ▲
    appendicitis 540.0
      with peritoneal abscess 540.1

Peritonitis — *continued*
  with or following — *continued*
    ectopic pregnancy (*see also* categories 633.0-633.9) 639.0
    molar pregnancy (*see also* categories 630-632) 639.0
  aseptic 998.7
  bacterial 567.29 ▲
    spontaneous 567.23 ●
  bile, biliary 567.81 ▲
  chemical 998.7
  chlamydial 099.56
  chronic proliferative 567.89 ▲
  congenital NEC 777.6
  diaphragmatic 567.22 ▲
  diffuse NEC 567.29 ▲
  diphtheritic 032.83
  disseminated NEC 567.29 ▲
  due to
    bile 567.81 ▲
    foreign
      body or object accidentally left during a procedure (instrument) (sponge) (swab) 998.4
      substance accidentally left during a procedure (chemical) (powder) (talc) 998.7
    talc 998.7
    urine 567.89 ▲
  fibrinopurulent 567.29 ▲
  fibrinous 567.29 ▲
  fibrocaseous (*see also* Tuberculosis) 014.0 ☑
  fibropurulent 567.29 ▲
  general, generalized (acute) 567.21 ▲
  gonococcal 098.86
  in infective disease NEC 136.9 *[567.0]*
  meconium (newborn) 777.6
  pancreatic 577.8
  paroxysmal, benign 277.3
  pelvic
    female (acute) 614.5
      chronic NEC 614.7
        with adhesions 614.6
      puerperal, postpartum, childbirth 670.0 ☑
    male (acute) 567.21 ▲
  periodic (familial) 277.3
  phlegmonous 567.29 ▲
  pneumococcal 567.1
  postabortal 639.0
  proliferative, chronic 567.89 ▲
  puerperal, postpartum, childbirth 670.0 ☑
  purulent 567.29 ▲
  septic 567.29 ▲
  spontaneous bacterial 567.23 ●
  staphylococcal 567.29 ▲
  streptococcal 567.29 ▲
  subdiaphragmatic 567.29 ▲
  subphrenic 567.29 ▲
  suppurative 567.29 ▲
  syphilitic 095.2
    congenital 090.0 *[567.0]*
  talc 998.7
  tuberculous (*see also* Tuberculosis) 014.0 ☑
  urine 567.89 ▲
Peritonsillar — *see* condition
Peritonsillitis 475
Perityphlitis (*see also* Appendicitis) 541
Periureteritis 593.89
Periurethral — *see* condition
Periurethritis (gangrenous) 597.89
Periuterine — *see* condition
Perivaginitis (*see also* Vaginitis) 616.10
Perivasculitis, retinal 362.18
Perivasitis (chronic) 608.4
Periventricular leukomalacia 779.7
Perivesiculitis (seminal) (*see also* Vesiculitis) 608.0
Perlèche 686.8
  due to
    moniliasis 112.0
    riboflavin deficiency 266.0
Pernicious — *see* condition
Pernio, perniosis 991.5

Persecution
  delusion 297.9
  social V62.4
Perseveration (tonic) 784.69
Persistence, persistent (congenital) 759.89
  anal membrane 751.2
  arteria stapedia 744.04
  atrioventricular canal 745.69
  bloody ejaculate 792.2
  branchial cleft 744.41
  bulbus cordis in left ventricle 745.8
  canal of Cloquet 743.51
  capsule (opaque) 743.51
  cilioretinal artery or vein 743.51
  cloaca 751.5
  communication — *see* Fistula, congenital
  convolutions
    aortic arch 747.21
    fallopian tube 752.19
    oviduct 752.19
    uterine tube 752.19
  double aortic arch 747.21
  ductus
    arteriosus 747.0
    Botalli 747.0
  fetal
    circulation 747.83
    form of cervix (uteri) 752.49
    hemoglobin (hereditary) ("Swiss variety") 282.7
    pulmonary hypertension 747.83
  foramen
    Botalli 745.5
    ovale 745.5
  Gartner's duct 752.41 ▲
  hemoglobin, fetal (hereditary) (HPFH) 282.7
  hyaloid
    artery (generally incomplete) 743.51
    system 743.51
  hymen (tag)
    in pregnancy or childbirth 654.8 ☑
      causing obstructed labor 660.2 ☑
  lanugo 757.4
  left
    posterior cardinal vein 747.49
    root with right arch of aorta 747.21
    superior vena cava 747.49
  Meckel's diverticulum 751.0
  mesonephric duct 752.89
    fallopian tube 752.11
  mucosal disease (middle ear) (with posterior or superior marginal perforation of ear drum) 382.2
  nail(s), anomalous 757.5
  occiput, anterior or posterior 660.3 ☑
    fetus or newborn 763.1
  omphalomesenteric duct 751.0
  organ or site NEC — *see* Anomaly, specified type NEC
  ostium
    atrioventriculare commune 745.69
    primum 745.61
    secundum 745.5
  ovarian rests in fallopian tube 752.19
  pancreatic tissue in intestinal tract 751.5
  primary (deciduous)
    teeth 520.6
    vitreous hyperplasia 743.51
  pulmonary hypertension 747.83
  pupillary membrane 743.46
    iris 743.46
  Rhesus (Rh) titer 999.7
  right aortic arch 747.21
  sinus
    urogenitalis 752.89
    venosus with imperfect incorporation in right auricle 747.49
  thymus (gland) 254.8
    hyperplasia 254.0
  thyroglossal duct 759.2
  thyrolingual duct 759.2
  truncus arteriosus or communis 745.0
  tunica vasculosa lentis 743.39
  umbilical sinus 753.7
  urachus 753.7
  vegetative state 780.03

- **Pick's** — *continued*
  - disease — *continued*
    - lipid histiocytosis 272.7
    - liver (pericardial pseudocirrhosis of liver) 423.2
    - pericardium (pericardial pseudocirrhosis of liver) 423.2
  - polyserositis (pericardial pseudocirrhosis of liver) 423.2
  - syndrome
    - heart (pericardial pseudocirrhosis of liver) 423.2
    - liver (pericardial pseudocirrhosis of liver) 423.2
  - tubular adenoma (M8640/0)
    - specified site — *see* Neoplasm, by site, benign
    - unspecified site
      - female 220
      - male 222.0
- **Pick-Herxheimer syndrome** (diffuse idiopathic cutaneous atrophy) 701.8
- **Pick-Niemann disease** (lipid histiocytosis) 272.7
- **Pickwickian syndrome** (cardiopulmonary obesity) 278.8
- **Piebaldism, classic** 709.09
- **Piedra** 111.2
  - beard 111.2
    - black 111.3
    - white 111.2
  - black 111.3
  - scalp 111.3
    - black 111.3
    - white 111.2
  - white 111.2
- **Pierre Marie's syndrome** (pulmonary hypertrophic osteoarthropathy) 731.2
- **Pierre Marie-Bamberger syndrome** (hypertrophic pulmonary osteoarthropathy) 731.2
- **Pierre Mauriac's syndrome** (diabetes-dwarfism-obesity) 258.1
- **Pierre Robin deformity or syndrome** (congenital) 756.0
- **Pierson's disease or osteochondrosis** 732.1
- **Pigeon**
  - breast or chest (acquired) 738.3
    - congenital 754.82
    - rachitic (*see also* Rickets) 268.0
  - breeders' disease or lung 495.2
  - fanciers' disease or lung 495.2
  - toe 735.8
- **Pigmentation** (abnormal) 709.00
  - anomaly 709.00
    - congenital 757.33
    - specified NEC 709.09
  - conjunctiva 372.55
  - cornea 371.10
    - anterior 371.11
    - posterior 371.13
    - stromal 371.12
  - lids (congenital) 757.33
    - acquired 374.52
  - limbus corneae 371.10
  - metals 709.00
  - optic papilla, congenital 743.57
  - retina (congenital) (grouped) (nevoid) 743.53
    - acquired 362.74
  - scrotum, congenital 757.33
- **Piles** — *see* Hemorrhoids
- **Pili**
  - annulati or torti (congenital) 757.4
  - incarnati 704.8
- **Pill roller hand** (intrinsic) 736.09
- **Pilomatrixoma** (M8110/0) — *see* Neoplasm, skin, benign
- **Pilonidal** — *see* condition
- **Pimple** 709.8
- **PIN I** (prostatic intraepithelial neoplasia I) 602.3
- **PIN II** (prostatic intraepithelial neoplasia II) 602.3
- **PIN III** (prostatic intraepithelial neoplasia III) 233.4
- **Pinched nerve** — *see* Neuropathy, entrapment
- **Pineal body or gland** — *see* condition
- **Pinealoblastoma** (M9362/3) 194.4
- **Pinealoma** (M9360/1) 237.1
  - malignant (M9360/3) 194.4
- **Pineoblastoma** (M9362/3) 194.4
- **Pineocytoma** (M9361/1) 237.1
- **Pinguecula** 372.51
- **Pinhole meatus** (*see also* Stricture, urethra) 598.9
- **Pink**
  - disease 985.0
  - eye 372.03
  - puffer 492.8
- **Pinkus' disease** (lichen nitidus) 697.1
- **Pinpoint**
  - meatus (*see also* Stricture, urethra) 598.9
  - os uteri (*see also* Stricture, cervix) 622.4
- **Pinselhaare** (congenital) 757.4
- **Pinta** 103.9
  - cardiovascular lesions 103.2
  - chancre (primary) 103.0
  - erythematous plaques 103.1
  - hyperchromic lesions 103.1
  - hyperkeratosis 103.1
  - lesions 103.9
    - cardiovascular 103.2
    - hyperchromic 103.1
    - intermediate 103.1
    - late 103.2
    - mixed 103.3
    - primary 103.0
    - skin (achromic) (cicatricial) (dyschromic) 103.2
      - hyperchromic 103.1
      - mixed (achromic and hyperchromic) 103.3
  - papule (primary) 103.0
  - skin lesions (achromic) (cicatricial) (dyschromic) 103.2
    - hyperchromic 103.1
    - mixed (achromic and hyperchromic) 103.3
  - vitiligo 103.2
- **Pintid** 103.0
- **Pinworms** (disease) (infection) (infestation) 127.4
- **Piry fever** 066.8
- **Pistol wound** — *see* Gunshot wound
- **Pit, lip** (mucus), **congenital** 750.25
- **Pitchers' elbow** 718.82
- **Pithecoid pelvis** 755.69
  - with disproportion (fetopelvic) 653.2 ☑
    - affecting fetus or newborn 763.1
    - causing obstructed labor 660.1 ☑
- **Pithiatism** 300.11
- **Pitted** — *see also* Pitting
  - teeth 520.4
- **Pitting** (edema) (*see also* Edema) 782.3
  - lip 782.3
  - nail 703.8
    - congenital 757.5
- **Pituitary gland** — *see* condition
- **Pituitary snuff-takers' disease** 495.8
- **Pityriasis** 696.5
  - alba 696.5
  - capitis 690.11
  - circinata (et maculata) 696.3
  - Hebra's (exfoliative dermatitis) 695.89
  - lichenoides et varioliformis 696.2
  - maculata (et circinata) 696.3
  - nigra 111.1
  - pilaris 757.39
    - acquired 701.1
    - Hebra's 696.4
  - rosea 696.3
  - rotunda 696.3
  - rubra (Hebra) 695.89
    - pilaris 696.4
  - sicca 690.18
  - simplex 690.18
  - specified type NEC 696.5
  - streptogenes 696.5
  - versicolor 111.0
    - scrotal 111.0
- **Placenta, placental**
  - ablatio 641.2 ☑
    - affecting fetus or newborn 762.1
  - abnormal, abnormality 656.7 ☑
    - with hemorrhage 641.8 ☑
      - affecting fetus or newborn 762.1
    - affecting fetus or newborn 762.2
  - abruptio 641.2 ☑
    - affecting fetus or newborn 762.1
  - accessory lobe — *see* Placenta, abnormal
  - accreta (without hemorrhage) 667.0 ☑
    - with hemorrhage 666.0 ☑
  - adherent (without hemorrhage) 667.0 ☑
    - with hemorrhage 666.0 ☑
  - apoplexy — *see* Placenta, separation
  - battledore — *see* Placenta, abnormal
  - bilobate — *see* Placenta, abnormal
  - bipartita — *see* Placenta, abnormal
  - carneous mole 631
  - centralis — *see* Placenta, previa
  - circumvallata — *see* Placenta, abnormal
  - cyst (amniotic) — *see* Placenta, abnormal
  - deficiency — *see* Placenta, insufficiency
  - degeneration — *see* Placenta, insufficiency
  - detachment (partial) (premature) (with hemorrhage) 641.2 ☑
    - affecting fetus or newborn 762.1
  - dimidiata — *see* Placenta, abnormal
  - disease 656.7 ☑
    - affecting fetus or newborn 762.2
  - duplex — *see* Placenta, abnormal
  - dysfunction — *see* Placenta, insufficiency
  - fenestrata — *see* Placenta, abnormal
  - fibrosis — *see* Placenta, abnormal
  - fleshy mole 631
  - hematoma — *see* Placenta, abnormal
  - hemorrhage NEC — *see* Placenta, separation
  - hormone disturbance or malfunction — *see* Placenta, abnormal
  - hyperplasia — *see* Placenta, abnormal
  - increta (without hemorrhage) 667.0 ☑
    - with hemorrhage 666.0 ☑
  - infarction 656.7 ☑
    - affecting fetus or newborn 762.2
  - insertion, vicious — *see* Placenta, previa
  - insufficiency
    - affecting
      - fetus or newborn 762.2
      - management of pregnancy 656.5 ☑
  - lateral — *see* Placenta, previa
  - low implantation or insertion — *see* Placenta, previa
  - low-lying — *see* Placenta, previa
  - malformation — *see* Placenta, abnormal
  - malposition — *see* Placenta, previa
  - marginalis, marginata — *see* Placenta, previa
  - marginal sinus (hemorrhage) (rupture) 641.2 ☑
    - affecting fetus or newborn 762.1
  - membranacea — *see* Placenta, abnormal
  - multilobed — *see* Placenta, abnormal
  - multipartita — *see* Placenta, abnormal
  - necrosis — *see* Placenta, abnormal
  - percreta (without hemorrhage) 667.0 ☑
    - with hemorrhage 666.0 ☑
  - polyp 674.4 ☑
  - previa (central) (centralis) (complete) (lateral) (marginal) (marginalis) (partial) (partialis) (total) (with hemorrhage) 641.1 ☑
    - affecting fetus or newborn 762.0
    - noted
      - before labor, without hemorrhage (with cesarean delivery) 641.0 ☑
      - during pregnancy (without hemorrhage) 641.0 ☑
    - without hemorrhage (before labor and delivery) (during pregnancy) 641.0 ☑
  - retention (with hemorrhage) 666.0 ☑
    - fragments, complicating puerperium (delayed hemorrhage) 666.2 ☑
      - without hemorrhage 667.1 ☑
    - postpartum, puerperal 666.2 ☑
    - without hemorrhage 667.0 ☑
  - separation (normally implanted) (partial) (premature) (with hemorrhage) 641.2 ☑
    - affecting fetus or newborn 762.1
  - septuplex — *see* Placenta, abnormal
  - small — *see* Placenta, insufficiency
  - softening (premature) — *see* Placenta, abnormal
  - spuria — *see* Placenta, abnormal

☑ Additional Digit Required — Refer to the Tabular List (Numeric Code Section) for Additional Digit Selection
▶◀ Revised Text ● New Line ▲ Revised Code

Pneumonia — *continued*
  aspiration — *continued*
    fetal 770.18 ●
      due to ●
        blood 770.16 ●
        clear amniotic fluid 770.14 ●
        meconium 770.12 ●
        postnatal stomach contents 770.86 ●
    newborn 770.18 ▲
      due to ●
        blood 770.16 ●
        clear amniotic fluid 770.14 ●
        meconium 770.12 ●
        postnatal stomach contents 770.86 ●
  asthenic 514
  atypical (disseminated) (focal) (primary) 486
    with influenza 487.0
  bacillus 482.9
    specified type NEC 482.89
  bacterial 482.9
    specified type NEC 482.89
  Bacteroides (fragilis) (oralis) (melaninogenicus) 482.81
  basal, basic, basilar — *see* Pneumonia, lobar
  broncho-, bronchial (confluent) (croupous) (diffuse) (disseminated) (hemorrhagic) (involving lobes) (lobar) (terminal) 485
    with influenza 487.0
    allergic 518.3
    aspiration (*see also* Pneumonia, aspiration) 507.0
    bacterial 482.9
      specified type NEC 482.89
    capillary 466.19
      with bronchospasm or obstruction 466.19
    chronic (*see also* Fibrosis, lung) 515
    congenital (infective) 770.0
    diplococcal 481
    Eaton's agent 483.0
    Escherichia coli (E. coli) 482.82
    Friedländer's bacillus 482.0
    Hemophilus influenzae 482.2
    hiberno-vernal 083.0 *[484.8]*
    hypostatic 514
    influenzal 487.0
    inhalation (*see also* Pneumonia, aspiration) 507.0
      due to fumes or vapors (chemical) 506.0
    Klebsiella 482.0
    lipid 507.1
      endogenous 516.8
    Mycoplasma (pneumoniae) 483.0
    ornithosis 073.0
    pleuropneumonia-like organisms (PPLO) 483.0
    pneumococcal 481
    Proteus 482.83
    Pseudomonas 482.1
    specified organism NEC 483.8
      bacterial NEC 482.89
    staphylococcal 482.40
      aureus 482.41
      specified type NEC 482.49
    streptococcal — *see* Pneumonia, streptococcal
    typhoid 002.0 *[484.8]*
    viral, virus (*see also* Pneumonia, viral) 480.9
  Butyrivibrio (fibriosolvens) 482.81
  Candida 112.4
  capillary 466.19
    with bronchospasm or obstruction 466.19
  caseous (*see also* Tuberculosis) 011.6 ☑
  catarrhal — *see* Pneumonia, broncho-
  central — *see* Pneumonia, lobar
  Chlamydia, chlamydial 483.1
    pneumoniae 483.1
    psittaci 073.0
    specified type NEC 483.1
    trachomatis 483.1
  cholesterol 516.8
  chronic (*see also* Fibrosis, lung) 515
  cirrhotic (chronic) (*see also* Fibrosis, lung) 515
  Clostridium (haemolyticum) (novyi) NEC 482.81
  confluent — *see* Pneumonia, broncho-
  congenital (infective) 770.0
    aspiration 770.18 ▲
  croupous — *see* Pneumonia, lobar

Pneumonia — *continued*
  cytomegalic inclusion 078.5 *[484.1]*
  deglutition (*see also* Pneumonia, aspiration) 507.0
  desquamative interstitial 516.8
  diffuse — *see* Pneumonia, broncho-
  diplococcal, diplococcus (broncho-) (lobar) 481
  disseminated (focal) — *see* Pneumonia, broncho-
  due to
    adenovirus 480.0
    anaerobes 482.81
    Bacterium anitratum 482.83
    Chlamydia, chlamydial 483.1
      pneumoniae 483.1
      psittaci 073.0
      specified type NEC 483.1
      trachomatis 483.1
    coccidioidomycosis 114.0
    Diplococcus (pneumoniae) 481
    Eaton's agent 483.0
    Escherichia coli (E. coli) 482.82
    Friedländer's bacillus 482.0
    fumes or vapors (chemical) (inhalation) 506.0
    fungus NEC 117.9 *[484.7]*
      coccidioidomycosis 114.0
    Hemophilus influenzae (H. influenzae) 482.2
    Herellea 482.83
    influenza 487.0
    Klebsiella pneumoniae 482.0
    Mycoplasma (pneumoniae) 483.0
    parainfluenza virus 480.2
    pleuropneumonia-like organism (PPLO) 483.0
    Pneumococcus 481
    Pneumocystis carinii 136.3
    Proteus 482.83
    Pseudomonas 482.1
    respiratory syncytial virus 480.1
    rickettsia 083.9 *[484.8]*
    SARS-associated coronavirus 480.3
    specified
      bacteria NEC 482.89
      organism NEC 483.8
      virus NEC 480.8
    Staphylococcus 482.40
      aureus 482.41
      specified type NEC 482.49
    Streptococcus — *see also* Pneumonia, streptococcal
      pneumoniae 481
    virus (*see also* Pneumonia, viral) 480.9
      SARS-associated coronavirus 480.3
  Eaton's agent 483.0
  embolic, embolism (*see* Embolism, pulmonary)
  eosinophilic 518.3
  Escherichia coli (E. coli) 482.82
  Eubacterium 482.81
  fibrinous — *see* Pneumonia, lobar
  fibroid (chronic) (*see also* Fibrosis, lung) 515
  fibrous (*see also* Fibrosis, lung) 515
  Friedländer's bacillus 482.0
  Fusobacterium (nucleatum) 482.81
  gangrenous 513.0
  giant cell (*see also* Pneumonia, viral) 480.9
  gram-negative bacteria NEC 482.83
    anaerobic 482.81
  grippal 487.0
  Hemophilus influenzae (bronchial) (lobar) 482.2
  hypostatic (broncho-) (lobar) 514
  in
    actinomycosis 039.1
    anthrax 022.1 *[484.5]*
    aspergillosis 117.3 *[484.6]*
    candidiasis 112.4
    coccidioidomycosis 114.0
    cytomegalic inclusion disease 078.5 *[484.1]*
    histoplasmosis (*see also* Histoplasmosis) 115.95
    infectious disease NEC 136.9 *[484.8]*
    measles 055.1
    mycosis, systemic NEC 117.9 *[484.7]*
    nocardiasis, nocardiosis 039.1
    ornithosis 073.0
    pneumocystosis 136.3
    psittacosis 073.0
    Q fever 083.0 *[484.8]*

Pneumonia — *continued*
  in — *continued*
    salmonellosis 003.22
    toxoplasmosis 130.4
    tularemia 021.2
    typhoid (fever) 002.0 *[484.8]*
    varicella 052.1
    whooping cough (*see also* Whooping cough) 033.9 *[484.3]*
  infective, acquired prenatally 770.0
  influenzal (broncho) (lobar) (virus) 487.0
  inhalation (*see also* Pneumonia, aspiration) 507.0
    fumes or vapors (chemical) 506.0
  interstitial 516.8
    with influenzal 487.0
    acute 136.3
    chronic (*see also* Fibrosis, lung) 515
    desquamative 516.8
    hypostatic 514
    lipoid 507.1
    lymphoid 516.8
    plasma cell 136.3
    Pseudomonas 482.1
  intrauterine (infective) 770.0
    aspiration 770.18 ▲
      blood 770.16 ●
      clear amniotic fluid 770.14 ●
      meconium 770.12 ●
      postnatal stomach contents 770.86 ●
  Klebsiella pneumoniae 482.0
  Legionnaires' 482.84
  lipid, lipoid (exogenous) (interstitial) 507.1
    endogenous 516.8
  lobar (diplococcal) (disseminated) (double) (interstitial) (pneumococcal, any type) 481
    with influenza 487.0
    bacterial 482.9
      specified type NEC 482.89
    chronic (*see also* Fibrosis, lung) 515
    Escherichia coli (E. coli) 482.82
    Friedländer's bacillus 482.0
    Hemophilus influenzae (H. influenzae) 482.2
    hypostatic 514
    influenzal 487.0
    Klebsiella 482.0
    ornithosis 073.0
    Proteus 482.83
    Pseudomonas 482.1
    psittacosis 073.0
    specified organism NEC 483.8
      bacterial NEC 482.89
    staphylococcal 482.40
      aureus 482.41
      specified type NEC 482.49
    streptococcal — *see* Pneumonia, streptococcal
    viral, virus (*see also* Pneumonia, viral) 480.9
  lobular (confluent) — *see* Pneumonia, broncho-
  Löffler's 518.3
  massive — *see* Pneumonia, lobar
  meconium ▶aspiration◀ 770.12 ▲
  metastatic NEC 038.8 *[484.8]*
  Mycoplasma (pneumoniae) 483.0
  necrotic 513.0
  nitrogen dioxide 506.9
  orthostatic 514
  parainfluenza virus 480.2
  parenchymatous (*see also* Fibrosis, lung) 515
  passive 514
  patchy — *see* Pneumonia, broncho-
  Peptococcus 482.81
  Peptostreptococcus 482.81
  plasma cell 136.3
  pleurolobar — see Pneumonia, lobar
  pleuropneumonia-like organism (PPLO) 483.0
  pneumococcal (broncho) (lobar) 481
  Pneumocystis (carinii) 136.3
  postinfectional NEC 136.9 *[484.8]*
  postmeasles 055.1
  postoperative 997.3
  primary atypical 486
  Proprionibacterium 482.81
  Proteus 482.83
  Pseudomonas 482.1
  psittacosis 073.0
  radiation 508.0

Pneumonia — *continued*
- respiratory syncytial virus 480.1
- resulting from a procedure 997.3
- rheumatic 390 *[517.1]*
- Salmonella 003.22
- SARS-associated coronavirus 480.3
- segmented, segmental — *see* Pneumonia, broncho-
- Serratia (marcescens) 482.83
- specified
  - bacteria NEC 482.89
  - organism NEC 483.8
  - virus NEC 480.8
- spirochetal 104.8 *[484.8]*
- staphylococcal (broncho) (lobar) 482.40
  - aureus 482.41
  - specified type NEC 482.49
- static, stasis 514
- streptococcal (broncho) (lobar) NEC 482.30
  - Group
    - A 482.31
    - B 482.32
    - specified NEC 482.39
  - pneumoniae 481
  - specified type NEC 482.39
- Streptococcus pneumoniae 481
- traumatic (complication) (early) (secondary) 958.8
- tuberculous (any) (*see also* Tuberculosis) 011.6 ☑
- tularemic 021.2
- TWAR agent 483.1
- varicella 052.1
- Veillonella 482.81
- viral, virus (broncho) (interstitial) (lobar) 480.9
  - with influenza, flu, or grippe 487.0
  - adenoviral 480.0
  - parainfluenza 480.2
  - respiratory syncytial 480.1
  - SARS-associated coronavirus 480.3
  - specified type NEC 480.8
- white (congenital) 090.0

Pneumonic — *see* condition

Pneumonitis (acute) (primary) (*see also* Pneumonia) 486
- allergic 495.9
  - specified type NEC 495.8
- aspiration 507.0
  - due to fumes or gases 506.0
  - fetal 770.18 ●
    - due to ●
      - blood 770.16 ●
      - clear amniotic fluid 770.14 ●
      - meconium 770.12 ●
      - postnatal stomach contents 770.86 ●
  - newborn 770.18 ▲
    - due to ●
      - blood 770.16 ●
      - clear amniotic fluid 770.14 ●
      - meconium 770.12 ●
      - postnatal stomach contents 770.86 ●
  - obstetric 668.0 ☑
- chemical 506.0
  - due to fumes or gases 506.0
- cholesterol 516.8
- chronic (*see also* Fibrosis, lung) 515
- congenital rubella 771.0
- crack 506.0
- due to
  - crack (cocaine) 506.0
  - fumes or vapors 506.0
  - inhalation
    - food (regurgitated), milk, vomitus 507.0
    - oils, essences 507.1
    - saliva 507.0
    - solids, liquids NEC 507.8
  - toxoplasmosis (acquired) 130.4
    - congenital (active) 771.2 *[484.8]*
- eosinophilic 518.3
- fetal aspiration 770.18 ▲
  - due to ●
    - blood 770.16 ●
    - clear amniotic fluid 770.14 ●
    - meconium 770.12 ●
    - postnatal stomach contents 770.86 ●

Pneumonitis (*see also* Pneumonia) — *continued*
- hypersensitivity 495.9
- interstitial (chronic) (*see also* Fibrosis, lung) 515
  - lymphoid 516.8
- lymphoid, interstitial 516.8
- meconium ▶aspiration◀ 770.12 ▲
- postanesthetic
  - correct substance properly administered 507.0
  - obstetric 668.0 ☑
  - overdose or wrong substance given 968.4
    - specified anesthetic — *see* Table of Drugs and Chemicals
- postoperative 997.3
  - obstetric 668.0 ☑
- radiation 508.0
- rubella, congenital 771.0
- "ventilation" 495.7
- wood-dust 495.8

Pneumonoconiosis — *see* Pneumoconiosis

Pneumoparotid 527.8

Pneumopathy NEC 518.89
- alveolar 516.9
  - specified NEC 516.8
- due to dust NEC 504
- parietoalveolar 516.9
  - specified condition NEC 516.8

Pneumopericarditis (*see also* Pericarditis) 423.9
- acute 420.90

Pneumopericardium — *see also* Pericarditis
- congenital 770.2
- fetus or newborn 770.2
- traumatic (post) (*see also* Pneumothorax, traumatic) 860.0
  - with open wound into thorax 860.1

Pneumoperitoneum 568.89
- fetus or newborn 770.2

Pneumophagia (psychogenic) 306.4

Pneumopleurisy, pneumopleuritis (*see also* Pneumonia) 486

Pneumopyopericardium 420.99

Pneumopyothorax (*see also* Pyopneumothorax) 510.9
- with fistula 510.0

Pneumorrhagia 786.3
- newborn 770.3
- tuberculous (*see also* Tuberculosis, pulmonary) 011.9 ☑

Pneumosiderosis (occupational) 503

Pneumothorax (acute) (chronic) 512.8
- congenital 770.2
- due to operative injury of chest wall or lung 512.1
  - accidental puncture or laceration 512.1
- fetus or newborn 770.2
- iatrogenic 512.1
- postoperative 512.1
- spontaneous 512.8
  - fetus or newborn 770.2
  - tension 512.0
- sucking 512.8
  - iatrogenic 512.1
  - postoperative 512.1
- tense valvular, infectional 512.0
- tension 512.0
  - iatrogenic 512.1
  - postoperative 512.1
  - spontaneous 512.0
- traumatic 860.0
  - with
    - hemothorax 860.4
      - with open wound into thorax 860.5
    - open wound into thorax 860.1
- tuberculous (*see also* Tuberculosis) 011.7 ☑

Pocket(s)
- endocardial (*see also* Endocarditis) 424.90
- periodontal 523.8

Podagra 274.9

Podencephalus 759.89

Poikilocytosis 790.09

Poikiloderma 709.09
- Civatte's 709.09
- congenital 757.33
- vasculare atrophicans 696.2

Poikilodermatomyositis 710.3

Pointed ear 744.29

Poise imperfect 729.9

Poisoned — *see* Poisoning

Poisoning (acute) — *see also* Table of Drugs and Chemicals
- Bacillus, B.
  - aertrycke (*see also* Infection, Salmonella) 003.9
  - botulinus 005.1
  - cholerae (suis) (*see also* Infection, Salmonella) 003.9
  - paratyphosus (*see also* Infection, Salmonella) 003.9
  - suipestifer (*see also* Infection, Salmonella) 003.9
- bacterial toxins NEC 005.9
- berries, noxious 988.2
- blood (general) — *see* Septicemia
- botulism 005.1
- bread, moldy, mouldy — *see* Poisoning, food
- damaged meat — *see* Poisoning, food
- death-cap (Amanita phalloides) (Amanita verna) 988.1
- decomposed food — *see* Poisoning, food
- diseased food — *see* Poisoning, food
- drug — *see* Table of Drugs and Chemicals
- epidemic, fish, meat, or other food — *see* Poisoning, food
- fava bean 282.2
- fish (bacterial) — *see also* Poisoning, food
  - noxious 988.0
- food (acute) (bacterial) (diseased) (infected) NEC 005.9
  - due to
    - bacillus
      - aertrycke (*see also* Poisoning, food, due to Salmonella) 003.9
      - botulinus 005.1
      - cereus 005.89
      - choleraesuis (*see also* Poisoning, food, due to Salmonella) 003.9
      - paratyphosus (*see also* Poisoning, food, due to Salmonella) 003.9
      - suipestifer (*see also* Poisoning, food, due to Salmonella) 003.9
    - Clostridium 005.3
      - botulinum 005.1
      - perfringens 005.2
      - welchii 005.2
    - Salmonella (aertrycke) (callinarum) (choleraesuis) (enteritidis) (paratyphi) (suipestifer) 003.9
      - with
        - gastroenteritis 003.0
        - localized infection(s) (*see also* Infection, Salmonella) 003.20
        - septicemia 003.1
        - specified manifestation NEC 003.8
    - specified bacterium NEC 005.89
    - Staphylococcus 005.0
    - Streptococcus 005.89
    - Vibrio parahaemolyticus 005.4
    - Vibrio vulnificus 005.81
  - noxious or naturally toxic 988.0
    - berries 988.2
    - fish 988.0
    - mushroom 988.1
    - plants NEC 988.2
- ice cream — *see* Poisoning, food
- ichthyotoxism (bacterial) 005.9
- kreotoxism, food 005.9
- malarial — *see* Malaria
- meat — *see* Poisoning, food
- mushroom (noxious) 988.1
- mussel — *see also* Poisoning, food
  - noxious 988.0
- noxious foodstuffs (*see also* Poisoning, food, noxious) 988.9
  - specified type NEC 988.8
- plants, noxious 988.2
- pork — *see also* Poisoning, food
  - specified NEC 988.8
  - Trichinosis 124
- ptomaine — *see* Poisoning, food
- putrefaction, food — *see* Poisoning, food
- radiation 508.0

☑ Additional Digit Required — Refer to the Tabular List (Numeric Code Section) for Additional Digit Selection

▶◀ Revised Text ● New Line ▲ Revised Code

Note — Use the following fifth-digit subclassification with category 045:

0	*poliovirus, unspecified type*
1	*poliovirus, type I*
2	*poliovirus, type II*
3	*poliovirus, type III*

Polyp, polypus

> *Note — Polyps of organs or sites that do not appear in the list below should be coded to the residual category for diseases of the organ or site concerned.*

- accessory sinus 471.8
- adenoid tissue 471.0
- adenomatous (M8210/0) — *see also* Neoplasm, by site, benign
  - adenocarcinoma in (M8210/3) — *see* Neoplasm, by site, malignant
  - carcinoma in (M8210/3) — *see* Neoplasm, by site, malignant
  - multiple (M8221/0) — *see* Neoplasm, by site, benign
- antrum 471.8
- anus, anal (canal) (nonadenomatous) 569.0
  - adenomatous 211.4
- Bartholin's gland 624.6
- bladder (M8120/1) 236.7
- broad ligament 620.8
- cervix (uteri) 622.7
  - adenomatous 219.0
  - in pregnancy or childbirth 654.6 ☑
    - affecting fetus or newborn 763.89
    - causing obstructed labor 660.2 ☑
  - mucous 622.7
  - nonneoplastic 622.7
- choanal 471.0
- cholesterol 575.6
- clitoris 624.6
- colon (M8210/0) (*see also* Polyp, adenomatous) 211.3
- corpus uteri 621.0
- dental 522.0
- ear (middle) 385.30
- endometrium 621.0
- ethmoidal (sinus) 471.8
- fallopian tube 620.8
- female genital organs NEC 624.8
- frontal (sinus) 471.8
- gallbladder 575.6
- gingiva 523.8
- gum 523.8
- labia 624.6
- larynx (mucous) 478.4
- malignant (M8000/3) — *see* Neoplasm, by site, malignant
- maxillary (sinus) 471.8
- middle ear 385.30
- myometrium 621.0
- nares
  - anterior 471.9
  - posterior 471.0
- nasal (mucous) 471.9
  - cavity 471.0
  - septum 471.9
- nasopharyngeal 471.0
- neoplastic (M8210/0) — *see* Neoplasm, by site, benign
- nose (mucous) 471.9
- oviduct 620.8
- paratubal 620.8
- pharynx 478.29
  - congenital 750.29
- placenta, placental 674.4 ☑
- prostate 600.20
  - with urinary retention 600.21
- pudenda 624.6
- pulp (dental) 522.0
- rectosigmoid 211.4
- rectum (nonadenomatous) 569.0
  - adenomatous 211.4
- septum (nasal) 471.9
- sinus (accessory) (ethmoidal) (frontal) (maxillary) (sphenoidal) 471.8
- sphenoidal (sinus) 471.8
- stomach (M8210/0) 211.1
- tube, fallopian 620.8
- turbinate, mucous membrane 471.8
- ureter 593.89
- urethra 599.3
- uterine
  - ligament 620.8
  - tube 620.8
- uterus (body) (corpus) (mucous) 621.0
  - in pregnancy or childbirth 654.1 ☑
    - affecting fetus or newborn 763.89
    - causing obstructed labor 660.2 ☑
- vagina 623.7
- vocal cord (mucous) 478.4
- vulva 624.6

Polyphagia 783.6

Polypoid — *see* condition

Polyposis — *see also* Polyp
- coli (adenomatous) (M8220/0) 211.3
  - adenocarcinoma in (M8220/3) 153.9
  - carcinoma in (M8220/3) 153.9
- familial (M8220/0) 211.3
- intestinal (adenomatous) (M8220/0) 211.3
- multiple (M8221/0) — *see* Neoplasm, by site, benign

Polyradiculitis (acute) 357.0

Polyradiculoneuropathy (acute) (segmentally demyelinating) 357.0

Polysarcia 278.00

Polyserositis (peritoneal) 568.82
- due to pericarditis 423.2
- paroxysmal (familial) 277.3
- pericardial 423.2
- periodic 277.3
- pleural — *see* Pleurisy
- recurrent 277.3
- tuberculous (*see also* Tuberculosis, polyserositis) 018.9 ☑

Polysialia 527.7

Polysplenia syndrome 759.0

Polythelia 757.6

Polytrichia (*see also* Hypertrichosis) 704.1

Polyunguia (congenital) 757.5
- acquired 703.8

Polyuria 788.42

Pompe's disease (glycogenosis II) 271.0

Pompholyx 705.81

Poncet's disease (tuberculous rheumatism) (*see also* Tuberculosis) 015.9 ☑

Pond fracture — *see* Fracture, skull, vault

Ponos 085.0

Pons, pontine — *see* condition

Poor
- contractions, labor 661.2 ☑
  - affecting fetus or newborn 763.7
- fetal growth NEC 764.9 ☑
  - affecting management of pregnancy 656.5 ☑
- incorporation
  - artificial skin graft 996.55
  - decellularized allodermis graft 996.55
- obstetrical history V13.29
  - affecting management of current pregnancy V23.49
    - pre-term labor V23.41
  - pre-term labor V13.21
- sucking reflex (newborn) 796.1
- vision NEC 369.9

Poradenitis, nostras 099.1

Porencephaly (congenital) (developmental) (true) 742.4
- acquired 348.0
- nondevelopmental 348.0
- traumatic (post) 310.2

Porocephaliasis 134.1

Porokeratosis 757.39
- disseminated superficial actinic (DSAP) 692.75

Poroma, eccrine (M8402/0) — *see* Neoplasm, skin, benign

Porphyria (acute) (congenital) (constitutional) (erythropoietic) (familial) (hepatica) (idiopathic) (idiosyncratic) (intermittent) (latent) (mixed hepatic) (photosensitive) (South African genetic) (Swedish) 277.1
- acquired 277.1
- cutaneatarda
  - hereditaria 277.1
  - symptomatica 277.1
- due to drugs
  - correct substance properly administered 277.1
  - overdose or wrong substance given or taken 977.9
    - specified drug — *see* Table of Drugs and Chemicals
- secondary 277.1
- toxic NEC 277.1
- variegata 277.1

Porphyrinuria (acquired) (congenital) (secondary) 277.1

Porphyruria (acquired) (congenital) 277.1

Portal — *see* condition

Port wine nevus or mark 757.32

Posadas-Wernicke disease 114.9

Position
- fetus, abnormal (*see also* Presentation, fetal) 652.9 ☑
- teeth, faulty (*see also* Anomaly, position tooth) 524.30

Positive
- culture (nonspecific) 795.39
  - AIDS virus V08
  - blood 790.7
  - HIV V08
  - human immunodeficiency virus V08
  - nose 795.39
  - skin lesion NEC 795.39
  - spinal fluid 792.0
  - sputum 795.39
  - stool 792.1
  - throat 795.39
  - urine 791.9
  - wound 795.39
- findings, anthrax 795.31
- HIV V08
- human immunodeficiency virus (HIV) V08
- PPD 795.5
- serology
  - AIDS virus V08
    - inconclusive 795.71
  - HIV V08
    - inconclusive 795.71
  - human immunodeficiency virus (HIV) V08
    - inconclusive 795.71
  - syphilis 097.1
    - with signs or symptoms — *see* Syphilis, by site and stage
    - false 795.6
- skin test 795.7 ☑
  - tuberculin (without active tuberculosis) 795.5
- VDRL 097.1
  - with signs or symptoms — *see* Syphilis, by site and stage
  - false 795.6
- Wassermann reaction 097.1
  - false 795.6

Postcardiotomy syndrome 429.4

Postcaval ureter 753.4

Postcholecystectomy syndrome 576.0

Postclimacteric bleeding 627.1

Postcommissurotomy syndrome 429.4

Postconcussional syndrome 310.2

Postcontusional syndrome 310.2

Postcricoid region — *see* condition

Post-dates (pregnancy) — *see* Pregnancy

Postencephalitic — *see also* condition
- syndrome 310.8

Posterior — *see* condition

Posterolateral sclerosis (spinal cord) — *see* Degeneration, combined

Postexanthematous — *see* condition

Postfebrile — *see* condition

Postgastrectomy dumping syndrome 564.2

Posthemiplegic chorea 344.89

Posthemorrhagic anemia (chronic) 280.0
- acute 285.1
- newborn 776.5

Posthepatitis syndrome 780.79

Postherpetic neuralgia (intercostal) (syndrome) (zoster) 053.19
geniculate ganglion 053.11
ophthalmica 053.19
trigeminal 053.12

Posthitis 607.1

Postimmunization complication or reaction — *see* Complications, vaccination

Postinfectious — *see* condition

Postinfluenzal syndrome 780.79

Postlaminectomy syndrome 722.80
cervical, cervicothoracic 722.81
kyphosis 737.12
lumbar, lumbosacral 722.83
thoracic, thoracolumbar 722.82

Postleukotomy syndrome 310.0

Postlobectomy syndrome 310.0

Postmastectomy lymphedema (syndrome) 457.0

Postmaturity, postmature (fetus or newborn) (gestation period over 42 completed weeks) 766.22
affecting management of pregnancy
post-term pregnancy 645.1 ☑
prolonged pregnancy 645.2 ☑
syndrome 766.22

Postmeasles — *see also* condition
complication 055.8
specified NEC 055.79

Postmenopausal
endometrium (atrophic) 627.8
suppurative (see also Endometritis) 615.9
hormone replacement therapy V07.4
status (age related) (natural) V49.81

Postnasal drip — *see* Sinusitis

Postnatal — *see* condition

Postoperative — *see also* condition
confusion state 293.9
psychosis 293.9
status NEC (*see also* Status (post)) V45.89

Postpancreatectomy hyperglycemia 251.3

Postpartum — *see also* condition
anemia 648.2 ☑
cardiomyopathy 674.5 ☑
observation
immediately after delivery V24.0
routine follow-up V24.2

Postperfusion syndrome NEC 999.8
bone marrow 996.85

Postpoliomyelitic — *see* condition

Postsurgery status NEC (*see also* Status (post)) V45.89

Post-term (pregnancy) 645.1 ☑
infant (gestation period over 40 completed weeks to 42 completed weeks) 766.21

Posttraumatic — *see* condition

Posttraumatic brain syndrome, nonpsychotic 310.2

Post-typhoid abscess 002.0

Postures, hysterical 300.11

Postvaccinal reaction or complication — *see* Complications, vaccination

Postvagotomy syndrome 564.2

Postvalvulotomy syndrome 429.4

Postvasectomy sperm count V25.8

Potain's disease (pulmonary edema) 514

Potain's syndrome (gastrectasis with dyspepsia) 536.1

Pott's
curvature (spinal) (*see also* Tuberculosis) 015.0 ☑ *[737.43]*
disease or paraplegia (*see also* Tuberculosis) 015.0 ☑ *[730.88]*
fracture (closed) 824.4
open 824.5
gangrene 440.24
osteomyelitis (*see also* Tuberculosis) 015.0 ☑ *[730.88]*
spinal curvature (*see also* Tuberculosis) 015.0 ☑ *[737.43]*
tumor, puffy (*see also* Osteomyelitis) 730.2 ☑

Potter's
asthma 502
disease 753.0
facies 754.0
lung 502
syndrome (with renal agenesis) 753.0

Pouch
bronchus 748.3
Douglas' — *see* condition
esophagus, esophageal (congenital) 750.4
acquired 530.6
gastric 537.1
Hartmann's (abnormal sacculation of gallbladder neck) 575.8
of intestine V44.3
attention to V55.3
pharynx, pharyngeal (congenital) 750.27

Poulet's disease 714.2

Poultrymen's itch 133.8

Poverty V60.2

Prader-Labhart-Willi-Fanconi syndrome (hypogenital dystrophy with diabetic tendency) 759.81

Prader-Willi syndrome (hypogenital dystrophy with diabetic tendency) 759.81

Preachers' voice 784.49

Pre-AIDS — *see* Human immunodeficiency virus (disease) (illness) (infection)

Preauricular appendage 744.1

Prebetalipoproteinemia (acquired) (essential) (familial) (hereditary) (primary) (secondary) 272.1
with chylomicronemia 272.3

Precipitate labor 661.3 ☑
affecting fetus or newborn 763.6

Preclimacteric bleeding 627.0
menorrhagia 627.0

Precocious
adrenarche 259.1
menarche 259.1
menstruation 626.8
pubarche 259.1
puberty NEC 259.1
sexual development NEC 259.1
thelarche 259.1

Precocity, sexual (constitutional) (cryptogenic) (female) (idiopathic) (male) NEC 259.1
with adrenal hyperplasia 255.2

Precordial pain 786.51
psychogenic 307.89

Predeciduous teeth 520.2

Prediabetes, prediabetic 790.29
complicating pregnancy, childbirth, or puerperium 648.8 ☑
fetus or newborn 775.8

Predislocation status of hip, at birth (*see also* Subluxation, congenital, hip) 754.32

Preeclampsia (mild) 642.4 ☑
with pre-existing hypertension 642.7 ☑
affecting fetus or newborn 760.0
severe 642.5 ☑
superimposed on pre-existing hypertensive disease 642.7 ☑

Preeruptive color change, teeth, tooth 520.8

Preexcitation 426.7
atrioventricular conduction 426.7
ventricular 426.7

Preglaucoma 365.00

Pregnancy (single) (uterine) (without sickness) V22.2

Note — Use the following fifth-digit subclassification with categories 640-648, 651-676:

0	*unspecified as to episode of care*
1	*delivered, with or without mention of antepartum condition*
2	*delivered, with mention of postpartum complication*
3	*antepartum condition or complication*
4	*postpartum condition or complication*

Pregnancy — *continued*
abdominal (ectopic) 633.00
with intrauterine pregnancy 633.01
affecting fetus or newborn 761.4
abnormal NEC 646.9 ☑
ampullar — *see* Pregnancy, tubal
broad ligament — *see* Pregnancy, cornual
cervical — *see* Pregnancy, cornual
combined (extrauterine and intrauterine) — *see* Pregnancy, cornual
complicated (by) 646.9 ☑
abnormal, abnormality NEC 646.9 ☑
cervix 654.6 ☑
cord (umbilical) 663.9 ☑
glucose tolerance (conditions classifiable to 790.21-790.29) 648.8 ☑
pelvic organs or tissues NEC 654.9 ☑
pelvis (bony) 653.0 ☑
perineum or vulva 654.8 ☑
placenta, placental (vessel) 656.7 ☑
position
cervix 654.4 ☑
placenta 641.1 ☑
without hemorrhage 641.0 ☑
uterus 654.4 ☑
size, fetus 653.5 ☑
uterus (congenital) 654.0 ☑
abscess or cellulitis
bladder 646.6 ☑
genitourinary tract (conditions classifiable to 590, 595, 597, 599.0, 614.0-614.5, 614.7-614.9, 615) 646.6 ☑
kidney 646.6 ☑
urinary tract NEC 646.6 ☑
adhesion, pelvic peritoneal 648.9 ☑
air embolism 673.0 ☑
albuminuria 646.2 ☑
with hypertension — *see* Toxemia, of pregnancy
amnionitis 658.4 ☑
amniotic fluid embolism 673.1 ☑
anemia (conditions classifiable to 280-285) 648.2 ☑
atrophy, yellow (acute) (liver) (subacute) 646.7 ☑
bacilluria, asymptomatic 646.5 ☑
bacteriuria, asymptomatic 646.5 ☑
bicornis or bicornuate uterus 654.0 ☑
biliary problems 646.8 ☑
bone and joint disorders (conditions classifiable to 720-724 or conditions affecting lower limbs classifiable to 711-719, 725-738) 648.7 ☑
breech presentation (buttocks) (complete) (frank) 652.2 ☑
with successful version 652.1 ☑
cardiovascular disease (conditions classifiable to 390-398, 410-429) 648.6 ☑
congenital (conditions classifiable to 745-747) 648.5 ☑
cerebrovascular disorders (conditions classifiable to 430-434, 436-437) 674.0 ☑
cervicitis (conditions classifiable to 616.0) 646.6 ☑
chloasma (gravidarum) 646.8 ☑
chorea (gravidarum) — *see* Eclampsia, pregnancy
cholelithiasis 646.8 ☑
contraction, pelvis (general) 653.1 ☑
inlet 653.2 ☑
outlet 653.3 ☑
convulsions (eclamptic) (uremic) 642.6 ☑
with pre-existing hypertension 642.7 ☑
current disease or condition (nonobstetric)
abnormal glucose tolerance 648.8 ☑
anemia 648.2 ☑
bone and joint (lower limb) 648.7 ☑
cardiovascular 648.6 ☑
congenital 648.5 ☑
cerebrovascular 674.0 ☑
diabetic 648.0 ☑
drug dependence 648.3 ☑
female genital mutilation 648.9 ☑ ●

☑ Additional Digit Required — Refer to the Tabular List (Numeric Code Section) for Additional Digit Selection
▶◀ Revised Text ● New Line ▲ Revised Code

- **Pregnancy** — *continued*
  - quintuplet NEC — *continued*
    - affecting fetus or newborn 761.5
    - following (elective) fetal reduction 651.7 ☑ ●
  - sextuplet NEC 651.8 ☑
    - with fetal loss and retention of one or more fetus(es) 651.6 ☑
    - affecting fetus or newborn 761.5
    - following (elective) fetal reduction 651.7 ☑ ●
  - spurious 300.11
  - superfecundation NEC 651.9 ☑
    - with fetal loss and retention of one or more fetus(es) 651.6 ☑
    - following (elective) fetal reduction 651.7 ☑ ●
  - superfetation NEC 651.9 ☑
    - with fetal loss and retention of one or more fetus(es) 651.6 ☑
    - following (elective) fetal reduction 651.7 ☑ ●
  - supervision (of) (for) — *see also* Pregnancy, management affected by
    - elderly
      - multigravida V23.82
      - primigravida V23.81
    - high-risk V23.9
      - insufficient prenatal care V23.7
      - specified problem NEC V23.89
    - multiparity V23.3
    - normal NEC V22.1
      - first V22.0
    - poor
      - obstetric history V23.49
        - pre-term labor V23.41
      - reproductive history V23.5
    - previous
      - abortion V23.2
      - hydatidiform mole V23.1
      - infertility V23.0
      - neonatal death V23.5
      - stillbirth V23.5
      - trophoblastic disease V23.1
      - vesicular mole V23.1
    - specified problem NEC V23.89
    - young
      - multigravida V23.84
      - primigravida V23.83
  - triplet NEC 651.1 ☑
    - with fetal loss and retention of one or more fetus(es) 651.4 ☑
    - affecting fetus or newborn 761.5
    - following (elective) fetal reduction 651.7 ☑ ●
  - tubal (with rupture) 633.10
    - with intrauterine pregnancy 633.11
    - affecting fetus or newborn 761.4
  - twin NEC 651.0 ☑
    - with fetal loss and retention of one fetus 651.3 ☑
    - affecting fetus or newborn 761.5
    - following (elective) fetal reduction 651.7 ☑ ●
  - unconfirmed V72.40
  - undelivered (no other diagnosis) V22.2
    - with false labor 644.1 ☑
    - high-risk V23.9
      - specified problem NEC V23.89
  - unwanted NEC V61.7
- **Pregnant uterus** — *see* condition
- **Preiser's disease** (osteoporosis) 733.09
- **Prekwashiorkor** 260
- **Preleukemia** 238.7
- **Preluxation of hip, congenital** (*see also* Subluxation, congenital, hip) 754.32
- **Premature** — *see also* condition
  - beats (nodal) 427.60
    - atrial 427.61
    - auricular 427.61
    - postoperative 997.1
    - specified type NEC 427.69
    - supraventricular 427.61
    - ventricular 427.69
  - birth NEC 765.1 ☑
- **Premature** — *see also* condition — *continued*
  - closure
    - cranial suture 756.0
    - fontanel 756.0
    - foramen ovale 745.8
  - contractions 427.60
    - atrial 427.61
    - auricular 427.61
    - auriculoventricular 427.61
    - heart (extrasystole) 427.60
    - junctional 427.60
    - nodal 427.60
    - postoperative 997.1
    - ventricular 427.69
  - ejaculation 302.75
  - infant NEC 765.1 ☑
    - excessive 765.0 ☑
    - light-for-dates — *see* Light-for-dates
  - labor 644.2 ☑
    - threatened 644.0 ☑
  - lungs 770.4
  - menopause 256.31
  - puberty 259.1
  - rupture of membranes or amnion 658.1 ☑
    - affecting fetus or newborn 761.1
    - delayed delivery following 658.2 ☑
  - senility (syndrome) 259.8
  - separation, placenta (partial) — *see* Placenta, separation
  - ventricular systole 427.69
- **Prematurity** NEC 765.1 ☑
  - extreme 765.0 ☑
- **Premenstrual syndrome** 625.4
- **Premenstrual tension** 625.4
- **Premolarization, cuspids** 520.2
- **Premyeloma** 273.1
- **Prenatal**
  - care, normal pregnancy V22.1
    - first V22.0
  - death, cause unknown — *see* Death, fetus
  - screening — *see* Antenatal, screening
- **Prepartum** — *see* condition
- **Preponderance, left or right ventricular** 429.3
- **Prepuce** — *see* condition
- **Presbycardia** 797
  - hypertensive (*see also* Hypertension, heart) 402.90
- **Presbycusis** 388.01
- **Presbyesophagus** 530.89
- **Presbyophrenia** 310.1
- **Presbyopia** 367.4
- **Prescription of contraceptives** NEC V25.02
  - diaphragm V25.02
  - oral (pill) V25.01
    - emergency V25.03
    - postcoital V25.03
    - repeat V25.41
  - repeat V25.40
    - oral (pill) V25.41
- **Presenile** — *see also* condition
  - aging 259.8
  - dementia (*see also* Dementia, presenile) 290.10
- **Presenility** 259.8
- **Presentation, fetal**
  - abnormal 652.9 ☑
    - with successful version 652.1 ☑
    - before labor, affecting fetus or newborn 761.7
    - causing obstructed labor 660.0 ☑
      - affecting fetus or newborn, any, except breech 763.1
    - in multiple gestation (one or more) 652.6 ☑
    - specified NEC 652.8 ☑
  - arm 652.7 ☑
    - causing obstructed labor 660.0 ☑
  - breech (buttocks) (complete) (frank) 652.2 ☑
    - with successful version 652.1 ☑
      - before labor, affecting fetus or newborn 761.7
    - before labor, affecting fetus or newborn 761.7
  - brow 652.4 ☑
    - causing obstructed labor 660.0 ☑
- **Presentation, fetal** — *continued*
  - buttocks 652.2 ☑
  - chin 652.4 ☑
  - complete 652.2 ☑
  - compound 652.8 ☑
  - cord 663.0 ☑
  - extended head 652.4 ☑
  - face 652.4 ☑
    - to pubes 652.8 ☑
  - footling 652.8 ☑
  - frank 652.2 ☑
  - hand, leg, or foot NEC 652.8 ☑
  - incomplete 652.8 ☑
  - mentum 652.4 ☑
  - multiple gestation (one fetus or more) 652.6 ☑
  - oblique 652.3 ☑
    - with successful version 652.1 ☑
  - shoulder 652.8 ☑
    - affecting fetus or newborn 763.1
  - transverse 652.3 ☑
    - with successful version 652.1 ☑
  - umbilical cord 663.0 ☑
  - unstable 652.0 ☑
- **Prespondylolisthesis** (congenital) (lumbosacral) 756.11
- **Pressure**
  - area, skin ulcer (*see also* Decubitus) 707.00
  - atrophy, spine 733.99
  - birth, fetus or newborn NEC 767.9
  - brachial plexus 353.0
  - brain 348.4
    - injury at birth 767.0
  - cerebral — *see* Pressure, brain
  - chest 786.59
  - cone, tentorial 348.4
    - injury at birth 767.0
  - funis — *see* Compression, umbilical cord
  - hyposystolic (*see also* Hypotension) 458.9
  - increased
    - intracranial 781.99
      - due to
        - benign intracranial hypertension 348.2
        - hydrocephalus — *see* hydrocephalus
        - injury at birth 767.8
    - intraocular 365.00
  - lumbosacral plexus 353.1
  - mediastinum 519.3
  - necrosis (chronic) (skin) (*see also* Decubitus) 707.00
  - nerve — *see* Compression, nerve
  - paralysis (*see also* Neuropathy, entrapment) 355.9
  - sore (chronic) (*see also* Decubitus) 707.00
  - spinal cord 336.9
  - ulcer (chronic) (*see also* Decubitus) 707.00
  - umbilical cord — *see* Compression, umbilical cord
  - venous, increased 459.89
- **Pre-syncope** 780.2
- **Preterm infant** NEC 765.1 ☑
  - extreme 765.0 ☑
- **Priapism** (penis) 607.3
- **Prickling sensation** (*see also* Disturbance, sensation) 782.0
- **Prickly heat** 705.1
- **Primary** — *see* condition
- **Primigravida, elderly**
  - affecting
    - fetus or newborn 763.89
    - management of pregnancy, labor, and delivery 659.5 ☑
- **Primipara, old**
  - affecting
    - fetus or newborn 763.89
    - management of pregnancy, labor, and delivery 659.5 ☑
- **Primula dermatitis** 692.6
- **Primus varus** (bilateral) (metatarsus) 754.52
- **P.R.I.N.D.** 436
- **Pringle's disease** (tuberous sclerosis) 759.5
- **Prinzmetal's angina** 413.1
- **Prinzmetal-Massumi syndrome** (anterior chest wall) 786.52
- **Prizefighter ear** 738.7

Problem (with) V49.9
- academic V62.3
- acculturation V62.4
- adopted child V61.29
- aged
  - in-law V61.3
  - parent V61.3
  - person NEC V61.8
- alcoholism in family V61.41
- anger reaction (*see also* Disturbance, conduct) 312.0 ☑
- behavior, child 312.9
- behavioral V40.9
  - specified NEC V40.3
- betting V69.3
- cardiorespiratory NEC V47.2
- care of sick or handicapped person in family or household V61.49
- career choice V62.2
- communication V40.1
- conscience regarding medical care V62.6
- delinquency (juvenile) 312.9
- diet, inappropriate V69.1
- digestive NEC V47.3
- ear NEC V41.3
- eating habits, inappropriate V69.1
- economic V60.2
  - affecting care V60.9
    - specified type NEC V60.8
- educational V62.3
- enuresis, child 307.6
- exercise, lack of V69.0
- eye NEC V41.1
- family V61.9
  - specified circumstance NEC V61.8
- fear reaction, child 313.0
- feeding (elderly) (infant) 783.3
  - newborn 779.3
  - nonorganic 307.59 ▲
- fetal, affecting management of pregnancy 656.9 ☑
  - specified type NEC 656.8 ☑
- financial V60.2
- foster child V61.29
  - specified NEC V41.8
- functional V41.9
  - specified type NEC V41.8
- gambling V69.3
- genital NEC V47.5
- head V48.9
  - deficiency V48.0
  - disfigurement V48.6
  - mechanical V48.2
  - motor V48.2
  - movement of V48.2
  - sensory V48.4
  - specified condition NEC V48.8
- hearing V41.2
- high-risk sexual behavior V69.2
- identity 313.82
- influencing health status NEC V49.89
- internal organ NEC V47.9
  - deficiency V47.0
  - mechanical or motor V47.1
- interpersonal NEC V62.81
- jealousy, child 313.3
- learning V40.0
- legal V62.5
- life circumstance NEC V62.89
- lifestyle V69.9
  - specified NEC V69.8
- limb V49.9
  - deficiency V49.0
  - disfigurement V49.4
  - mechanical V49.1
  - motor V49.2
  - movement, involving
    - musculoskeletal system V49.1
    - nervous system V49.2
  - sensory V49.3
  - specified condition NEC V49.5
- litigation V62.5
- living alone V60.3
- loneliness NEC V62.89
- marital V61.10
  - involving
    - divorce V61.0

Problem (with) — *continued*
- marital — *continued*
  - involving — *continued*
    - estrangement V61.0
    - psychosexual disorder 302.9
    - sexual function V41.7
  - relationship V61.10 ●
- mastication V41.6
- medical care, within family V61.49
- mental V40.9
  - specified NEC V40.2
- mental hygiene, adult V40.9
- multiparity V61.5
- nail biting, child 307.9
- neck V48.9
  - deficiency V48.1
  - disfigurement V48.7
  - mechanical V48.3
  - motor V48.3
  - movement V48.3
  - sensory V48.5
  - specified condition NEC V48.8
- neurological NEC 781.99
- none (feared complaint unfounded) V65.5
- occupational V62.2
- parent-child V61.20
  - relationship V61.20 ●
- partner V61.10
  - relationship V61.10 ●
- personal NEC V62.89
  - interpersonal conflict NEC V62.81
- personality (*see also* Disorder, personality) 301.9
- phase of life V62.89
- placenta, affecting management of pregnancy 656.9 ☑
  - specified type NEC 656.8 ☑
- poverty V60.2
- presence of sick or handicapped person in family or household V61.49
- psychiatric 300.9
- psychosocial V62.9
  - specified type NEC V62.89
- relational NEC V62.81
- relationship, childhood 313.3
- religious or spiritual belief
  - other than medical care V62.89
  - regarding medical care V62.6
- self-damaging behavior V69.8
- sexual
  - behavior, high-risk V69.2
  - function NEC V41.7
- sibling
  - relational V61.8 ●
  - relationship V61.8 ●
- sight V41.0
- sleep, lack of V69.4
- sleep disorder, child 307.40
- smell V41.5
- speech V40.1
- spite reaction, child (*see also* Disturbance, conduct) 312.0 ☑
- spoiled child reaction (*see also* Disturbance, conduct) 312.1 ☑
- swallowing V41.6
- tantrum, child (*see also* Disturbance, conduct) 312.1 ☑
- taste V41.5
- thumb sucking, child 307.9
- tic (child) 307.21
- trunk V48.9
  - deficiency V48.1
  - disfigurement V48.7
  - mechanical V48.3
  - motor V48.3
  - movement V48.3
  - sensory V48.5
  - specified condition NEC V48.8
- unemployment V62.0
- urinary NEC V47.4
- voice production V41.4

Procedure (surgical) **not done** NEC V64.3
- because of
  - contraindication V64.1
  - patient's decision V64.2
    - for reasons of conscience or religion V62.6
  - specified reason NEC V64.3

Procidentia
- anus (sphincter) 569.1
- rectum (sphincter) 569.1
- stomach 537.89
- uteri 618.1

Proctalgia 569.42
- fugax 564.6
- spasmodic 564.6
  - psychogenic 307.89

Proctitis 569.49
- amebic 006.8
- chlamydial 099.52
- gonococcal 098.7
- granulomatous 555.1
- idiopathic 556.2
  - with ulcerative sigmoiditis 556.3
- tuberculous (*see also* Tuberculosis) 014.8 ☑
- ulcerative (chronic) (nonspecific) 556.2
  - with ulcerative sigmoiditis 556.3

Proctocele
- female (without uterine prolapse) 618.04
  - with uterine prolapse 618.4
    - complete 618.3
    - incomplete 618.2
- male 569.49

Proctocolitis, idiopathic 556.2
- with ulcerative sigmoiditis 556.3

Proctoptosis 569.1

Proctosigmoiditis 569.89
- ulcerative (chronic) 556.3

Proctospasm 564.6
- psychogenic 306.4

Prodromal-AIDS — *see* Human immunodeficiency virus (disease) (illness) (infection)

Profichet's disease or syndrome 729.9

Progeria (adultorum) (syndrome) 259.8

Prognathism (mandibular) (maxillary) 524.10

Progonoma (melanotic) (M9363/0) — *see* Neoplasm, by site, benign

Progressive — *see* condition

Prolapse, prolapsed
- anus, anal (canal) (sphincter) 569.1
- arm or hand, complicating delivery 652.7 ☑
  - causing obstructed labor 660.0 ☑
    - affecting fetus or newborn 763.1
  - fetus or newborn 763.1
- bladder (acquired) (mucosa) (sphincter)
  - congenital (female) (male) 756.71
  - female (*see also* Cystocele, female) 618.01
  - male 596.8
- breast implant (prosthetic) 996.54
- cecostomy 569.69
- cecum 569.89
- cervix, cervical (stump) (hypertrophied) 618.1
  - anterior lip, obstructing labor 660.2 ☑
    - affecting fetus or newborn 763.1
  - congenital 752.49
  - postpartal (old) 618.1
- ciliary body 871.1
- colon (pedunculated) 569.89
- colostomy 569.69
- conjunctiva 372.73
- cord — *see* Prolapse, umbilical cord
- disc (intervertebral) — *see* Displacement, intervertebral disc
- duodenum 537.89
- eye implant (orbital) 996.59
  - lens (ocular) 996.53
- fallopian tube 620.4
- fetal extremity, complicating delivery 652.8 ☑
  - causing obstructed labor 660.0 ☑
  - fetus or newborn 763.1
- funis — *see* Prolapse, umbilical cord
- gastric (mucosa) 537.89
- genital, female 618.9
  - specified NEC 618.89
- globe 360.81
- ileostomy bud 569.69
- intervertebral disc — *see* Displacement, intervertebral disc
- intestine (small) 569.89
- iris 364.8
  - traumatic 871.1

☑ Additional Digit Required — Refer to the Tabular List (Numeric Code Section) for Additional Digit Selection
▶◀ Revised Text ● New Line ▲ Revised Code

Note — Use the following fifth-digit subclassification with categories 296.0-296.6:

0	*unspecified*
1	*mild*
2	*moderate*
3	*severe, without mention of psychotic behavior*
4	*severe, specified as with psychotic behavior*
5	*in partial or unspecified remission*
6	*in full remission*

☑ Additional Digit Required — Refer to the Tabular List (Numeric Code Section) for Additional Digit Selection
▶◀ Revised Text ● New Line ▲ Revised Code

☑ Additional Digit Required — Refer to the Tabular List (Numeric Code Section) for Additional Digit Selection

▶◀ Revised Text ● New Line ▲ Revised Code

Puerperal — *continued*
- thyroid dysfunction (conditions classifiable to 240-246) 648.1 ☑
- toxemia (*see also* Toxemia, of pregnancy) 642.4 ☑
  - eclamptic 642.6 ☑
    - with pre-existing hypertension 642.7 ☑
  - pre-eclamptic (mild) 642.4 ☑
    - with
      - convulsions 642.6 ☑
      - pre-existing hypertension 642.7 ☑
    - severe 642.5 ☑
- tuberculosis (conditions classifiable to 010-018) 647.3 ☑
- uremia 669.3 ☑
- vaginitis (conditions classifiable to 616.1) 646.6 ☑
- varicose veins (legs) 671.0 ☑
  - vulva or perineum 671.1 ☑
- vulvitis (conditions classifiable to 616.1) 646.6 ☑
- vulvovaginitis (conditions classifiable to 616.1) 646.6 ☑
- white leg 671.4 ☑

Pulled muscle — *see* Sprain, by site

Pulmolithiasis 518.89

Pulmonary — *see* condition

Pulmonitis (unknown etiology) 486

Pulpitis (acute) (anachoretic) (chronic) (hyperplastic) (putrescent) (suppurative) (ulcerative) 522.0

Pulpless tooth 522.9

Pulse
- alternating 427.89
  - psychogenic 306.2
- bigeminal 427.89
- fast 785.0
- feeble, rapid, due to shock following injury 958.4
- rapid 785.0
- slow 427.89
- strong 785.9
- trigeminal 427.89
- water-hammer (*see also* Insufficiency, aortic) 424.1
- weak 785.9

Pulseless disease 446.7

Pulsus
- alternans or trigeminy 427.89
  - psychogenic 306.2

Punch drunk 310.2

Puncta lacrimalia occlusion 375.52

Punctiform hymen 752.49

Puncture (traumatic) — *see also* Wound, open, by site
- accidental, complicating surgery 998.2
- bladder, nontraumatic 596.6
- by
  - device, implant, or graft — *see* Complications, mechanical
  - foreign body
    - internal organs — *see also* Injury, internal, by site
      - by ingested object — *see* Foreign body
    - left accidentally in operation wound 998.4
  - instrument (any) during a procedure, accidental 998.2
- internal organs, abdomen, chest, or pelvis — *see* Injury, internal, by site
- kidney, nontraumatic 593.89

Pupil — *see* condition

Pupillary membrane 364.74
- persistent 743.46

Pupillotonia 379.46
- pseudotabetic 379.46

Purpura 287.2
- abdominal 287.0
- allergic 287.0
- anaphylactoid 287.0
- annularis telangiectodes 709.1
- arthritic 287.0
- autoerythrocyte sensitization 287.2
- autoimmune 287.0

Purpura — *continued*
- bacterial 287.0
- Bateman's (senile) 287.2
- capillary fragility (hereditary) (idiopathic) 287.8
- cryoglobulinemic 273.2
- devil's pinches 287.2
- fibrinolytic (*see also* Fibrinolysis) 286.6
- fulminans, fulminous 286.6
- gangrenous 287.0
- hemorrhagic (*see also* Purpura, thrombocytopenic) 287.39 ▲
  - nodular 272.7
  - nonthrombocytopenic 287.0
  - thrombocytopenic 287.39 ▲
- Henoch's (purpura nervosa) 287.0
- Henoch-Schönlein (allergic) 287.0
- hypergammaglobulinemic (benign primary) (Waldenström's) 273.0
- idiopathic 287.31 ▲
  - nonthrombocytopenic 287.0
  - thrombocytopenic 287.31 ▲
- immune thrombocytopenic 287.31 ●
- infectious 287.0
- malignant 287.0
- neonatorum 772.6
- nervosa 287.0
- newborn NEC 772.6
- nonthrombocytopenic 287.2
  - hemorrhagic 287.0
  - idiopathic 287.0
- nonthrombopenic 287.2
- peliosis rheumatica 287.0
- pigmentaria, progressiva 709.09
- posttransfusion 287.4
- primary 287.0
- primitive 287.0
- red cell membrane sensitivity 287.2
- rheumatica 287.0
- Schönlein (-Henoch) (allergic) 287.0
- scorbutic 267
- senile 287.2
- simplex 287.2
- symptomatica 287.0
- telangiectasia annularis 709.1
- thrombocytopenic (*see also* Thrombocytopenia) 287.30 ▲
  - congenital 287.33 ●
  - essential 287.30 ●
  - hereditary 287.31 ●
  - idiopathic 287.31 ●
  - immune 287.31 ●
  - neonatal, transitory (*see also* Thrombocytopenia, neonatal transitory) 776.1
  - primary 287.30 ●
  - puerperal, postpartum 666.3 ☑
  - thrombotic 446.6
- thrombohemolytic (*see also* Fibrinolysis) 286.6
- thrombopenic (*see also* Thrombocytopenia) 287.30 ▲
  - congenital 287.33 ●
  - essential 287.30 ●
- thrombotic 446.6
  - thrombocytic 446.6
  - thrombocytopenic 446.6
- toxic 287.0
- variolosa 050.0
- vascular 287.0
- visceral symptoms 287.0
- Werlhof's (*see also* Purpura, thrombocytopenic) 287.39 ▲

Purpuric spots 782.7

Purulent — *see* condition

Pus
- absorption, general — *see* Septicemia
- in
  - stool 792.1
  - urine 791.9
- tube (rupture) (*see also* Salpingo-oophoritis) 614.2

Pustular rash 782.1

Pustule 686.9
- malignant 022.0
- nonmalignant 686.9

Putnam's disease (subacute combined sclerosis with pernicious anemia) 281.0 *[336.2]*

Putnam-Dana syndrome (subacute combined sclerosis with pernicious anemia) 281.0 *[336.2]*

Putrefaction, intestinal 569.89

Putrescent pulp (dental) 522.1

Pyarthritis — *see* Pyarthrosis

Pyarthrosis (*see also* Arthritis, pyogenic) 711.0 ☑
- tuberculous — *see* Tuberculosis, joint

Pycnoepilepsy, pycnolepsy (idiopathic) (*see also* Epilepsy) 345.0 ☑

Pyelectasia 593.89

Pyelectasis 593.89

Pyelitis (congenital) (uremic) 590.80
- with
  - abortion — *see* Abortion, by type, with specified complication NEC
  - contracted kidney 590.00
  - ectopic pregnancy (*see also* categories 633.0-633.9) 639.8
  - molar pregnancy (*see also* categories 630-632) 639.8
- acute 590.10
  - with renal medullary necrosis 590.11
- chronic 590.00
  - with
    - renal medullary necrosis 590.01
- complicating pregnancy, childbirth, or puerperium 646.6 ☑
  - affecting fetus or newborn 760.1
- cystica 590.3
  - following
    - abortion 639.8
    - ectopic or molar pregnancy 639.8
- gonococcal 098.19
  - chronic or duration of 2 months or over 098.39
- tuberculous (*see also* Tuberculosis) 016.0 ☑ *[590.81]*

Pyelocaliectasis 593.89

Pyelocystitis (*see also* Pyelitis) 590.80

Pyelohydronephrosis 591

Pyelonephritis (*see also* Pyelitis) 590.80
- acute 590.10
  - with renal medullary necrosis 590.11
- chronic 590.00
- syphilitic (late) 095.4
- tuberculous (*see also* Tuberculosis) 016.0 ☑ *[590.81]*

Pyelonephrosis (*see also* Pyelitis) 590.80
- chronic 590.00

Pyelophlebitis 451.89

Pyelo-ureteritis cystica 590.3

Pyemia, pyemic (purulent) (*see also* Septicemia) 038.9
- abscess — *see* Abscess
- arthritis (*see also* Arthritis, pyogenic) 711.0 ☑
- Bacillus coli 038.42
- embolism — *see* Embolism, pyemic
- fever 038.9
- infection 038.9
- joint (*see also* Arthritis, pyogenic) 711.0 ☑
- liver 572.1
- meningococcal 036.2
- newborn 771.81
- phlebitis — *see* Phlebitis
- pneumococcal 038.2
- portal 572.1
- postvaccinal 999.3
- specified organism NEC 038.8
- staphylococcal 038.10
  - aureus 038.11
  - specified organism NEC 038.19
- streptococcal 038.0
- tuberculous — *see* Tuberculosis, miliary

Pygopagus 759.4

Pykno-epilepsy, pyknolepsy (idiopathic) (*see also* Epilepsy) 345.0 ☑

Pyle (-Cohn) disease (craniometaphyseal dysplasia) 756.89

Pylephlebitis (suppurative) 572.1

Pylethrombophlebitis 572.1

Pylethrombosis 572.1

Pyloritis (*see also* Gastritis) 535.5 ☑

Pylorospasm (reflex) 537.81
- congenital or infantile 750.5

☑ Additional Digit Required — Refer to the Tabular List (Numeric Code Section) for Additional Digit Selection

▶◀ Revised Text ● New Line ▲ Revised Code

- **Pylorospasm** — *continued*
  - neurotic 306.4
  - newborn 750.5
  - psychogenic 306.4
- **Pylorus, pyloric** — *see* condition
- **Pyoarthrosis** — *see* Pyarthrosis
- **Pyocele**
  - mastoid 383.00
  - sinus (accessory) (nasal) (*see also* Sinusitis) 473.9
  - turbinate (bone) 473.9
  - urethra (*see also* Urethritis) 597.0
- **Pyococcal dermatitis** 686.00
- **Pyococcide, skin** 686.00
- **Pyocolpos** (*see also* Vaginitis) 616.10
- **Pyocyaneus dermatitis** 686.09
- **Pyocystitis** (*see also* Cystitis) 595.9
- **Pyoderma, pyodermia** 686.00
  - gangrenosum 686.01
  - specified type NEC 686.09
  - vegetans 686.8
- **Pyodermatitis** 686.00
  - vegetans 686.8
- **Pyogenic** — *see* condition
- **Pyohemia** — *see* Septicemia
- **Pyohydronephrosis** (*see also* Pyelitis) 590.80
- **Pyometra** 615.9
- **Pyometritis** (*see also* Endometritis) 615.9
- **Pyometrium** (*see also* Endometritis) 615.9
- **Pyomyositis** 728.0
  - ossificans 728.19
  - tropical (bungpagga) 040.81
- **Pyonephritis** (*see also* Pyelitis) 590.80
  - chronic 590.00
- **Pyonephrosis** (congenital) (*see also* Pyelitis) 590.80
  - acute 590.10
- **Pyo-oophoritis** (*see also* Salpingo-oophoritis) 614.2
- **Pyo-ovarium** (*see also* Salpingo-oophoritis) 614.2
- **Pyopericarditis** 420.99
- **Pyopericardium** 420.99
- **Pyophlebitis** — *see* Phlebitis
- **Pyopneumopericardium** 420.99
- **Pyopneumothorax** (infectional) 510.9
  - with fistula 510.0
  - subdiaphragmatic (*see also* Peritonitis) 567.29 ▲
  - subphrenic (*see also* Peritonitis) 567.29 ▲
  - tuberculous (*see also* Tuberculosis, pleura) 012.0 ☑
- **Pyorrhea** (alveolar) (alveolaris) 523.4
  - degenerative 523.5
- **Pyosalpingitis** (*see also* Salpingo-oophoritis) 614.2
- **Pyosalpinx** (*see also* Salpingo-oophoritis) 614.2
- **Pyosepticemia** — *see* Septicemia
- **Pyosis**
  - Corlett's (impetigo) 684
  - Manson's (pemphigus contagiosus) 684
- **Pyothorax** 510.9
  - with fistula 510.0
  - tuberculous (*see also* Tuberculosis, pleura) 012.0 ☑
- **Pyoureter** 593.89
  - tuberculous (*see also* Tuberculosis) 016.2 ☑
- **Pyramidopallidonigral syndrome** 332.0
- **Pyrexia** (of unknown origin) (P.U.O.) 780.6
  - atmospheric 992.0
  - during labor 659.2 ☑
  - environmentally-induced newborn 778.4
  - heat 992.0
  - newborn, environmentally-induced 778.4
  - puerperal 672.0 ☑
- **Pyroglobulinemia** 273.8
- **Pyromania** 312.33
- **Pyrosis** 787.1
- **Pyrroloporphyria** 277.1
- **Pyuria** (bacterial) 791.9

Q

- **Q fever** 083.0
  - with pneumonia 083.0 *[484.8]*
- **Quadricuspid aortic valve** 746.89
- **Quadrilateral fever** 083.0
- **Quadriparesis** — *see* Quadriplegia
  - meaning muscle weakness 728.87 ●
- **Quadriplegia** 344.00
  - with fracture, vertebra (process) — *see* Fracture, vertebra, cervical, with spinal cord injury
  - brain (current episode) 437.8
  - C1-C4
    - complete 344.01
    - incomplete 344.02
  - C5-C7
    - complete 344.03
    - incomplete 344.04
  - cerebral (current episode) 437.8
  - congenital or infantile (cerebral) (spastic) (spinal) 343.2
  - cortical 437.8
  - embolic (current episode) (*see also* Embolism, brain) 434.1 ☑
  - infantile (cerebral) (spastic) (spinal) 343.2
  - newborn NEC 767.0
  - specified NEC 344.09
  - thrombotic (current episode) (*see also* Thrombosis, brain) 434.0 ☑
  - traumatic — *see* Injury, spinal, cervical
- **Quadruplet**
  - affected by maternal complications of pregnancy 761.5
  - healthy liveborn — *see* Newborn, multiple
  - pregnancy (complicating delivery) NEC 651.8 ☑
    - with fetal loss and retention of one or more fetus(es) 651.5 ☑
    - following (elective) fetal reduction 651.7 ☑ ●
- **Quarrelsomeness** 301.3
- **Quartan**
  - fever 084.2
  - malaria (fever) 084.2
- **Queensland fever** 083.0
  - coastal 083.0
  - seven-day 100.89
- **Quervain's disease** 727.04
  - thyroid (subacute granulomatous thyroiditis) 245.1
- **Queyrat's erythroplasia** (M8080/2)
  - specified site — *see* Neoplasm, skin, in situ
  - unspecified site 233.5
- **Quincke's disease or edema** — *see* Edema, angioneurotic
- **Quinquaud's disease** (acne decalvans) 704.09
- **Quinsy** (gangrenous) 475
- **Quintan fever** 083.1
- **Quintuplet**
  - affected by maternal complications of pregnancy 761.5
  - healthy liveborn — *see* Newborn, multiple
  - pregnancy (complicating delivery) NEC 651.2 ☑
    - with fetal loss and retention of one or more fetus(es) 651.6 ☑
    - following (elective) fetal reduction 651.7 ☑ ●
- **Quotidian**
  - fever 084.0
  - malaria (fever) 084.0

R

- **Rabbia** 071
- **Rabbit fever** (*see also* Tularemia) 021.9
- **Rabies** 071
  - contact V01.5
  - exposure to V01.5
  - inoculation V04.5
    - reaction — *see* Complications, vaccination
  - vaccination, prophylactic (against) V04.5
- **Rachischisis** (*see also* Spina bifida) 741.9 ☑
- **Rachitic** — *see also* condition
  - deformities of spine 268.1
  - pelvis 268.1
    - with disproportion (fetopelvic) 653.2 ☑
      - affecting fetus or newborn 763.1
      - causing obstructed labor 660.1 ☑
        - affecting fetus or newborn 763.1
- **Rachitis, rachitism** — *see* also Rickets
  - acute 268.0
  - fetalis 756.4
  - renalis 588.0
  - tarda 268.0
- **Racket nail** 757.5
- **Radial nerve** — *see* condition
- **Radiation effects or sickness** — *see also* Effect, adverse, radiation
  - cataract 366.46
  - dermatitis 692.82
    - sunburn (*see also* Sunburn) 692.71
- **Radiculitis** (pressure) (vertebrogenic) 729.2
  - accessory nerve 723.4
  - anterior crural 724.4
  - arm 723.4
  - brachial 723.4
  - cervical NEC 723.4
  - due to displacement of intervertebral disc — *see* Neuritis, due to, displacement intervertebral disc
  - leg 724.4
  - lumbar NEC 724.4
  - lumbosacral 724.4
  - rheumatic 729.2
  - syphilitic 094.89
  - thoracic (with visceral pain) 724.4
- **Radiculomyelitis** 357.0
  - toxic, due to
    - Clostridium tetani 037
    - Corynebacterium diphtheriae 032.89
- **Radiculopathy** (*see also* Radiculitis) 729.2
- **Radioactive substances, adverse effect** — *see* Effect, adverse, radioactive substance
- **Radiodermal burns** (acute) (chronic) (occupational) — *see* Burn, by site
- **Radiodermatitis** 692.82
- **Radionecrosis** — *see* Effect, adverse, radiation
- **Radiotherapy session** V58.0
- **Radium, adverse effect** — *see* Effect, adverse, radioactive substance
- **Raeder-Harbitz syndrome** (pulseless disease) 446.7
- **Rage** (*see also* Disturbance, conduct) 312.0 ☑
  - meaning rabies 071
- **Rag sorters' disease** 022.1
- **Raillietiniasis** 123.8
- **Railroad neurosis** 300.16
- **Railway spine** 300.16
- **Raised** — *see* Elevation
- **Raiva** 071
- **Rake teeth, tooth** 524.39
- **Rales** 786.7
- **Ramifying renal pelvis** 753.3
- **Ramsay Hunt syndrome** (herpetic geniculate ganglionitis) 053.11
  - meaning dyssynergia cerebellaris myoclonica 334.2
- **Ranke's primary infiltration** (*see also* Tuberculosis) 010.0 ☑
- **Ranula** 527.6
  - congenital 750.26
- **Rape**
  - adult 995.83 ●
  - alleged, observation or examination V71.5
  - child 995.53 ●
- **Rapid**
  - feeble pulse, due to shock, following injury 958.4
  - heart (beat) 785.0
    - psychogenic 306.2
  - respiration 786.06
    - psychogenic 306.1

- **Rapid** — *continued*
  - second stage (delivery) 661.3 ☑
    - affecting fetus or newborn 763.6
  - time-zone change syndrome 327.35 ▲
- **Rarefaction, bone** 733.99
- **Rash** 782.1
  - canker 034.1
  - diaper 691.0
  - drug (internal use) 693.0
    - contact 692.3
  - ECHO 9 virus 078.89
  - enema 692.89
  - food (*see also* Allergy, food) 693.1
  - heat 705.1
  - napkin 691.0
  - nettle 708.8
  - pustular 782.1
  - rose 782.1
    - epidemic 056.9
      - of infants 057.8
  - scarlet 034.1
  - serum (prophylactic) (therapeutic) 999.5
  - toxic 782.1
  - wandering tongue 529.1
- **Rasmussen's aneurysm** (*see also* Tuberculosis) 011.2 ☑
- **Rat-bite fever** 026.9
  - due to Streptobacillus moniliformis 026.1 ☑
  - spirochetal (morsus muris) 026.0 ☑
- **Rathke's pouch tumor** (M9350/1) 237.0
- **Raymond (-Céstan) syndrome** 433.8 ☑
- **Raynaud's**
  - disease or syndrome (paroxysmal digital cyanosis) 443.0
  - gangrene (symmetric) 443.0 *[785.4]*
  - phenomenon (paroxysmal digital cyanosis) (secondary) 443.0
- **RDS** 769
- **Reaction**
  - acute situational maladjustment (*see also* Reaction, adjustment) 309.9
  - adaptation (*see also* Reaction, adjustment) 309.9
  - adjustment 309.9
    - with
      - anxious mood 309.24
        - with depressed mood 309.28
      - conduct disturbance 309.3
        - combined with disturbance of emotions 309.4
      - depressed mood 309.0
        - brief 309.0
          - with anxious mood 309.28
        - prolonged 309.1
      - elective mutism 309.83
      - mixed emotions and conduct 309.4
      - mutism, elective 309.83
      - physical symptoms 309.82
      - predominant disturbance (of)
        - conduct 309.3
        - emotions NEC 309.29
          - mixed 309.28
        - mixed, emotions and conduct 309.4
        - specified type NEC 309.89
      - specific academic or work inhibition 309.23
      - withdrawal 309.83
    - depressive 309.0
      - with conduct disturbance 309.4
      - brief 309.0
      - prolonged 309.1
    - specified type NEC 309.89
  - adverse food NEC 995.7
  - affective (*see also* Psychosis, affective) 296.90
    - specified type NEC 296.99
  - aggressive 301.3
    - unsocialized (*see also* Disturbance, conduct) 312.0 ☑
  - allergic (*see also* Allergy) 995.3
    - drug, medicinal substance, and biological — *see* Allergy, drug
    - food — *see* Allergy, food
    - serum 999.5
  - anaphylactic — *see* Shock, anaphylactic
  - anesthesia — *see* Anesthesia, complication

- **Reaction** — *continued*
  - anger 312.0 ☑
  - antisocial 301.7
  - antitoxin (prophylactic) (therapeutic) — *see* Complications, vaccination
  - anxiety 300.00
  - asthenic 300.5
  - compulsive 300.3
  - conversion (anesthetic) (autonomic) (hyperkinetic) (mixed paralytic) (paresthetic) 300.11
  - deoxyribonuclease (DNA) (DNase) hypersensitivity NEC 287.2
  - depressive 300.4
    - acute 309.0
    - affective (*see also* Psychosis, affective) 296.2 ☑
      - recurrent episode 296.3 ☑
      - single episode 296.2 ☑
    - brief 309.0
    - manic (*see also* Psychosis, affective) 296.80
    - neurotic 300.4
    - psychoneurotic 300.4
    - psychotic 298.0
  - dissociative 300.15
  - drug NEC (*see also* Table of Drugs and Chemicals) 995.2
    - allergic — *see* Allergy, drug
    - correct substance properly administered 995.2
    - obstetric anesthetic or analgesic NEC 668.9 ☑
      - affecting fetus or newborn 763.5
      - specified drug — *see* Table of Drugs and Chemicals
    - overdose or poisoning 977.9
      - specified drug — *see* Table of Drugs and Chemicals
    - specific to newborn 779.4
    - transmitted via placenta or breast milk — *see* Absorption, drug, through placenta
    - withdrawal NEC 292.0
      - infant of dependent mother 779.5
    - wrong substance given or taken in error 977.9
      - specified drug — *see* Table of Drugs and Chemicals
  - dyssocial 301.7
  - erysipeloid 027.1
  - fear 300.20
    - child 313.0
  - fluid loss, cerebrospinal 349.0
  - food — *see also* Allergy, food
    - adverse NEC 995.7
    - anaphylactic shock — *see* Anaphylactic shock, due to, food
  - foreign
    - body NEC 728.82
      - in operative wound (inadvertently left) 998.4
        - due to surgical material intentionally left — *see* Complications, due to (presence of) any device, implant, or graft classified to 996.0-996.5 NEC
    - substance accidentally left during a procedure (chemical) (powder) (talc) 998.7
      - body or object (instrument) (sponge) (swab) 998.4
  - graft-versus-host (GVH) 996.85
  - grief (acute) (brief) 309.0
    - prolonged 309.1
  - gross stress (*see also* Reaction, stress, acute) 308.9
  - group delinquent (*see also* Disturbance, conduct) 312.2 ☑
  - Herxheimer's 995.0
  - hyperkinetic (*see also* Hyperkinesia) 314.9
  - hypochondriacal 300.7
  - hypoglycemic, due to insulin 251.0
    - therapeutic misadventure 962.3
  - hypomanic (*see also* Psychosis, affective) 296.0 ☑
    - recurrent episode 296.1 ☑
    - single episode 296.0 ☑

- **Reaction** — *continued*
  - hysterical 300.10
    - conversion type 300.11
    - dissociative 300.15
  - id (bacterial cause) 692.89
  - immaturity NEC 301.89
    - aggressive 301.3
    - emotional instability 301.59
  - immunization — *see* Complications, vaccination
  - incompatibility
    - blood group (ABO) (infusion) (transfusion) 999.6
    - Rh (factor) (infusion) (transfusion) 999.7
  - inflammatory — *see* Infection
  - infusion — *see* Complications, infusion
  - inoculation (immune serum) — *see* Complications, vaccination
  - insulin 995.2
  - involutional
    - paranoid 297.2
    - psychotic (*see also* Psychosis, affective, depressive) 296.2 ☑
  - leukemoid (lymphocytic) (monocytic) (myelocytic) 288.8
  - LSD (*see also* Abuse, drugs, nondependent) 305.3 ☑
  - lumbar puncture 349.0
  - manic-depressive (*see also* Psychosis, affective) 296.80
    - depressed 296.2 ☑
      - recurrent episode 296.3 ☑
      - single episode 296.2 ☑
    - hypomanic 296.0 ☑
  - neurasthenic 300.5
  - neurogenic (*see* also Neurosis) 300.9
  - neurotic NEC 300.9
  - neurotic-depressive 300.4
  - nitritoid — *see* Crisis, nitritoid
  - obsessive ▶compulsive◀ 300.3
  - organic 293.9
    - acute 293.0
    - subacute 293.1
  - overanxious, child or adolescent 313.0
  - paranoid (chronic) 297.9
    - acute 298.3
    - climacteric 297.2
    - involutional 297.2
    - menopausal 297.2
    - senile 290.20
    - simple 297.0
  - passive
    - aggressive 301.84
    - dependency 301.6
  - personality (*see also* Disorder, personality) 301.9
  - phobic 300.20
  - postradiation — *see* Effect, adverse, radiation
  - psychogenic NEC 300.9
  - psychoneurotic (*see also* Neurosis) 300.9
    - anxiety 300.00
    - compulsive 300.3
    - conversion 300.11
    - depersonalization 300.6
    - depressive 300.4
    - dissociative 300.15
    - hypochondriacal 300.7
    - hysterical 300.10
      - conversion type 300.11
      - dissociative type 300.15
    - neurasthenic 300.5
    - obsessive 300.3
    - obsessive-compulsive 300.3
    - phobic 300.20
    - tension state 300.9
  - psychophysiologic NEC (*see also* Disorder, psychosomatic) 306.9
    - cardiovascular 306.2
    - digestive 306.4
    - endocrine 306.6
    - gastrointestinal 306.4
    - genitourinary 306.50
    - heart 306.2
    - hemic 306.8
    - intestinal (large) (small) 306.4
    - laryngeal 306.1
    - lymphatic 306.8

☑ Additional Digit Required — Refer to the Tabular List (Numeric Code Section) for Additional Digit Selection
▶◀ Revised Text ● New Line ▲ Revised Code

☑ Additional Digit Required — Refer to the Tabular List (Numeric Code Section) for Additional Digit Selection

▶◀ Revised Text ● New Line ▲ Revised Code

Resistance, resistant — *continued*
- drugs by microorganisms — *continued*
  - Nitrofurtimox V09.8 ☑
  - Norfloxacin V09.5 ☑
  - Nystatin V09.2
  - Ofloxacin V09.5 ☑
  - Oleandomycin V09.2
  - Oxacillin V09.0
  - Oxytetracycline V09.3
  - Para-amino salicylic acid [PAS] V09.7 ☑
  - Paromomycin V09.4
  - Penicillin (G) (V) (VK) V09.0
  - penicillins V09.0
  - Pentamidine V09.8 ☑
  - Piperacillin V09.0
  - Primaquine V09.5 ☑
  - Proguanil V09.8 ☑
  - Pyrazinamide [PZA] V09.7 ☑
  - Pyrimethamine/Sulfalene V09.8 ☑
  - Pyrimethamine/Sulfodoxine V09.8 ☑
  - Quinacrine V09.5 ☑
  - Quinidine V09.8 ☑
  - Quinine V09.8 ☑
  - quinolones V09.5 ☑
  - Rifabutin V09.7 ☑
  - Rifampin [RIF] V09.7 ☑
  - Rifamycin V09.7 ☑
  - Rolitetracycline V09.3
  - specified drugs NEC V09.8 ☑
  - Spectinomycin V09.8 ☑
  - Spiramycin V09.2
  - Streptomycin [SM] V09.4
  - Sulfacetamide V09.6
  - Sulfacytine V09.6
  - Sulfadiazine V09.6
  - Sulfadoxine V09.6
  - Sulfamethoxazole V09.6
  - Sulfapyridine V09.6
  - Sulfasalizine V09.6
  - Sulfasoxazone V09.6
  - sulfonamides V09.6
  - Sulfasoxazole V09.7 ☑
  - tetracycline V09.3
  - tetracyclines V09.3
  - Thiamphenicol V09.8 ☑
  - Ticarcillin V09.0
  - Tinidazole V09.8 ☑
  - Tobramycin V09.4
  - Triamphenicol V09.8 ☑
  - Trimethoprim V09.8 ☑
  - Vancomycin V09.8 ☑
- insulin 277.7

Resorption
- biliary 576.8
  - purulent or putrid (*see also* Cholecystitis) 576.8
- dental (roots) 521.40
  - alveoli 525.8
  - pathological
    - external 521.42
    - internal 521.41
    - specified NEC 521.49
- septic — *see* Septicemia
- teeth (roots) 521.40
  - pathological
    - external 521.42
    - internal 521.41
    - specified NEC 521.49

Respiration
- asymmetrical 786.09
- bronchial 786.09
- Cheyne-Stokes (periodic respiration) 786.04
- decreased, due to shock following injury 958.4
- disorder of 786.00
  - psychogenic 306.1
  - specified NEC 786.09
- failure 518.81
  - acute 518.81
  - acute and chronic 518.84
  - chronic 518.83
  - newborn 770.84
- insufficiency 786.09
  - acute 518.82
  - newborn NEC 770.89
- Kussmaul (air hunger) 786.09
- painful 786.52

Respiration — *continued*
- periodic 786.09
  - high altitude 327.22 ●
- poor 786.09
  - newborn NEC 770.89
- sighing 786.7
  - psychogenic 306.1
- wheezing 786.07

Respiratory — *see also* condition
- distress 786.09
  - acute 518.82
  - fetus or newborn NEC 770.89
  - syndrome (newborn) 769
    - adult (following shock, surgery, or trauma) 518.5
      - specified NEC 518.82
- failure 518.81
  - acute 518.81
  - acute and chronic 518.84
  - chronic 518.83

Respiratory syncytial virus (RSV) 079.6
- bronchiolitis 466.11
- pneumonia 480.1
- vaccination, prophylactic (against) V04.82

Response
- photoallergic 692.72
- phototoxic 692.72

Rest, rests
- mesonephric duct 752.89
  - fallopian tube 752.11
- ovarian, in fallopian tubes 752.19
- wolffian duct 752.89

Restless leg (syndrome) 333.99

Restlessness 799.2

Restoration of organ continuity from previous sterilization (tuboplasty) (vasoplasty) V26.0

Restriction of housing space V60.1

Restzustand, schizophrenic (*see also* Schizophrenia) 295.6 ☑

Retained — *see* Retention

Retardation
- development, developmental, specific (*see also* Disorder, development, specific) 315.9
  - learning, specific 315.2
    - arithmetical 315.1
    - language (skills) 315.31
      - expressive 315.31
      - mixed receptive-expressive 315.32
    - mathematics 315.1
    - reading 315.00
      - phonological 315.39
    - written expression 315.2
  - motor 315.4
- endochondral bone growth 733.91
- growth (physical) in childhood 783.43
  - due to malnutrition 263.2
  - fetal (intrauterine) 764.9 ☑
    - affecting management of pregnancy 656.5 ☑
- intrauterine growth 764.9 ☑
  - affecting management of pregnancy 656.5 ☑
- mental 319
  - borderline V62.89
  - mild, IQ 50-70 317
  - moderate, IQ 35-49 318.0
  - profound, IQ under 20 318.2
  - severe, IQ 20-34 318.1
- motor, specific 315.4
- physical 783.43
  - child 783.43
  - due to malnutrition 263.2
  - fetus (intrauterine) 764.9 ☑
    - affecting management of pregnancy 656.5 ☑
- psychomotor NEC 307.9
- reading 315.00

Retching — *see* Vomiting

Retention, retained
- bladder (*see also* Retention, urine) 788.20
  - psychogenic 306.53
- carbon dioxide 276.2
- cyst — *see* Cyst

Retention, retained — *continued*
- dead
  - fetus (after 22 completed weeks gestation) 656.4 ☑
    - early fetal death (before 22 completed weeks gestation) 632
  - ovum 631
- decidua (following delivery) (fragments) (with hemorrhage) 666.2 ☑
  - without hemorrhage 667.1 ☑
- deciduous tooth 520.6
- dental root 525.3
- fecal (*see also* Constipation) 564.00
- fluid 276.6
- foreign body — *see also* Foreign body, retained
  - bone 733.99
  - current trauma — *see* Foreign body, by site or type
  - middle ear 385.83
  - muscle 729.6
  - soft tissue NEC 729.6
- gastric 536.8
- membranes (following delivery) (with hemorrhage) 666.2 ☑
  - with abortion — *see* Abortion, by type
  - without hemorrhage 667.1 ☑
- menses 626.8
- milk (puerperal) 676.2 ☑
- nitrogen, extrarenal 788.9
- placenta (total) (with hemorrhage) 666.0 ☑
  - with abortion — *see* Abortion, by type
  - portions or fragments 666.2 ☑
    - without hemorrhage 667.1 ☑
  - without hemorrhage 667.0 ☑
- products of conception
  - early pregnancy (fetal death before 22 completed weeks gestation) 632
  - following
    - abortion — *see* Abortion, by type
    - delivery 666.2 ☑
      - with hemorrhage 666.2 ☑
      - without hemorrhage 667.1 ☑
- secundines (following delivery) (with hemorrhage) 666.2 ☑
  - with abortion — *see* Abortion, by type
  - complicating puerperium (delayed hemorrhage) 666.2 ☑
  - without hemorrhage 667.1 ☑
- smegma, clitoris 624.8
- urine NEC 788.20
  - bladder, incomplete emptying 788.21
    - due to ●
      - benign prostatic hypertrophy (BPH) — *see* category 600 ●
  - due to ●
    - benign prostatic hypertrophy (BPH) — *see* category 600 ●
  - psychogenic 306.53
  - specified NEC 788.29
- water (in tissue) (*see also* Edema) 782.3

Reticulation, dust (occupational) 504

Reticulocytosis NEC 790.99

Reticuloendotheliosis
- acute infantile (M9722/3) 202.5 ☑
- leukemic (M9940/3) 202.4 ☑
- malignant (M9720/3) 202.3 ☑
- nonlipid (M9722/3) 202.5 ☑

Reticulohistiocytoma (giant cell) 277.89

Reticulohistiocytosis, multicentric 272.8

Reticulolymphosarcoma (diffuse) (M9613/3) 200.8 ☑
- follicular (M9691/3) 202.0 ☑
- nodular (M9691/3) 202.0 ☑

Reticulosarcoma (M9640/3) 200.0 ☑
- nodular (M9642/3) 200.0 ☑
- pleomorphic cell type (M9641/3) 200.0 ☑

Reticulosis (skin)
- acute of infancy (M9722/3) 202.5 ☑
- histiocytic medullary (M9721/3) 202.3 ☑
- lipomelanotic 695.89
- malignant (M9720/3) 202.3 ☑
- Sézary's (M9701/3) 202.2 ☑

Retina, retinal — *see* condition

☑ Additional Digit Required — Refer to the Tabular List (Numeric Code Section) for Additional Digit Selection
▶◀ Revised Text ● New Line ▲ Revised Code

☑ Additional Digit Required — Refer to the Tabular List (Numeric Code Section) for Additional Digit Selection
▶◀ Revised Text ● New Line ▲ Revised Code

☑ Additional Digit Required — Refer to the Tabular List (Numeric Code Section) for Additional Digit Selection
▶◀ Revised Text ● New Line ▲ Revised Code

☑ Additional Digit Required — Refer to the Tabular List (Numeric Code Section) for Additional Digit Selection

Sensation — *continued*
- choking 784.9
- loss of (*see also* Disturbance, sensation) 782.0
- prickling (*see also* Disturbance, sensation) 782.0
- tingling (*see also* Disturbance, sensation) 782.0

Sense loss (touch) (*see also* Disturbance, sensation) 782.0
- smell 781.1
- taste 781.1

Sensibility disturbance NEC (cortical) (deep) (vibratory) (*see also* Disturbance, sensation) 782.0

Sensitive dentine 521.8

Sensitiver Beziehungswahn 297.8

Sensitivity, sensitization — *see also* Allergy
- autoerythrocyte 287.2
- carotid sinus 337.0
- child (excessive) 313.21
- cold, autoimmune 283.0
- methemoglobin 289.7
- suxamethonium 289.89
- tuberculin, without clinical or radiological symptoms 795.5

Sensory
- extinction 781.8
- neglect 781.8

Separation
- acromioclavicular — *see* Dislocation, acromioclavicular
- anxiety, abnormal 309.21
- apophysis, traumatic — *see* Fracture, by site
- choroid 363.70
  - hemorrhagic 363.72
  - serous 363.71
- costochondral (simple) (traumatic) — *see* Dislocation, costochondral
- delayed
  - umbilical cord 779.83
- epiphysis, epiphyseal
  - nontraumatic 732.9
    - upper femoral 732.2
  - traumatic — *see* Fracture, by site
- fracture — *see* Fracture, by site
- infundibulum cardiac from right ventricle by a partition 746.83
- joint (current) (traumatic) — *see* Dislocation, by site
- placenta (normally implanted) — *see* Placenta, separation
- pubic bone, obstetrical trauma 665.6 ☑
- retina, retinal (*see also* Detachment, retina) 361.9
  - layers 362.40
    - sensory (*see also* Retinoschisis) 361.10
  - pigment epithelium (exudative) 362.42
    - hemorrhagic 362.43
- sternoclavicular (traumatic) — *see* Dislocation, sternoclavicular
- symphysis pubis, obstetrical trauma 665.6 ☑
- tracheal ring, incomplete (congenital) 748.3

Sepsis (generalized) 995.91
- with
  - abortion — *see* Abortion, by type, with sepsis
  - ectopic pregnancy (*see also* categories 633.0-633.9) 639.0
  - molar pregnancy (*see also* categories 630-632) 639.0
- buccal 528.3
- complicating labor 659.3 ☑
- dental (pulpal origin) 522.4
- female genital organ NEC 614.9
- fetus (intrauterine) 771.81
- following
  - abortion 639.0
  - ectopic or molar pregnancy 639.0
  - infusion, perfusion, or transfusion 999.3
- Friedländer's 038.49
- intraocular 360.00
- localized
  - in operation wound 998.59
  - skin (*see also* Abscess) 682.9
- malleus 024

Sepsis — *continued*
- nadir 038.9
- newborn (organism unspecified) NEC 771.81
- oral 528.3
- puerperal, postpartum, childbirth (pelvic) 670.0 ☑
- resulting from infusion, injection, transfusion, or vaccination 999.3
- severe 995.92
- skin, localized (*see also* Abscess) 682.9
- umbilical (newborn) (organism unspecified) 771.89
  - tetanus 771.3
- urinary 599.0
  - meaning sepsis 995.91
  - meaning urinary tract infection 599.0

Septate — *see also* Septum

Septic — *see also* condition
- adenoids 474.01
  - and tonsils 474.02
- arm (with lymphangitis) 682.3
- embolus — *see* Embolism
- finger (with lymphangitis) 681.00
- foot (with lymphangitis) 682.7
- gallbladder (*see also* Cholecystitis) 575.8
- hand (with lymphangitis) 682.4
- joint (*see also* Arthritis, septic) 711.0 ☑
- kidney (*see also* Infection, kidney) 590.9
- leg (with lymphangitis) 682.6
- mouth 528.3
- nail 681.9
  - finger 681.02
  - toe 681.11
- shock (endotoxic) 785.52
- sore (*see also* Abscess) 682.9
  - throat 034.0
    - milk-borne 034.0
    - streptococcal 034.0
- spleen (acute) 289.59
- teeth (pulpal origin) 522.4
- throat 034.0
- thrombus — *see* Thrombosis
- toe (with lymphangitis) 681.10
- tonsils 474.00
  - and adenoids 474.02
- umbilical cord (newborn) (organism unspecified) 771.89
- uterus (*see also* Endometritis) 615.9

Septicemia, septicemic (generalized) (suppurative) 038.9
- with
  - abortion — *see* Abortion, by type, with sepsis
  - ectopic pregnancy (*see also* categories 633.0-633.9) 639.0
  - molar pregnancy (*see also* categories 630-632) 639.0
- Aerobacter aerogenes 038.49
- anaerobic 038.3
- anthrax 022.3
- Bacillus coli 038.42
- Bacteroides 038.3
- Clostridium 038.3
- complicating labor 659.3 ☑
- cryptogenic 038.9
- enteric gram-negative bacilli 038.40
- Enterobacter aerogenes 038.49
- Erysipelothrix (insidiosa) (rhusiopathiae) 027.1
- Escherichia coli 038.42
- following
  - abortion 639.0
  - ectopic or molar pregnancy 639.0
  - infusion, injection, transfusion, or vaccination 999.3
- Friedländer's (bacillus) 038.49
- gangrenous 038.9
- gonococcal 098.89
- gram-negative (organism) 038.40
  - anaerobic 038.3
- Hemophilus influenzae 038.41
- herpes (simplex) 054.5
- herpetic 054.5
- Listeria monocytogenes 027.0
- meningeal — *see* Meningitis
- meningococcal (chronic) (fulminating) 036.2
- navel, newborn (organism unspecified) 771.89

Septicemia, septicemic — *continued*
- newborn (organism unspecified) 771.81
- plague 020.2
- pneumococcal 038.2
- postabortal 639.0
- postoperative 998.59
- Proteus vulgaris 038.49
- Pseudomonas (aeruginosa) 038.43
- puerperal, postpartum 670.0 ☑
- Salmonella (aertrycke) (callinarum) (choleraesuis) (enteritidis) (suipestifer) 003.1
- Serratia 038.44
- Shigella (*see also* Dysentery, bacillary) 004.9
- specified organism NEC 038.8
- staphylococcal 038.10
  - aureus 038.11
  - specified organism NEC 038.19
- streptococcal (anaerobic) 038.0
- Streptococcus pneumoniae 038.2
- suipestifer 003.1
- umbilicus, newborn (organism unspecified) 771.89
- viral 079.99
- Yersinia enterocolitica 038.49

Septum, septate (congenital) — *see also* Anomaly, specified type NEC
- anal 751.2
- aqueduct of Sylvius 742.3
  - with spina bifida (*see also* Spina bifida) 741.0 ☑
- hymen 752.49
- uterus (*see also* Double, uterus) 752.2
- vagina 752.49
  - in pregnancy or childbirth 654.7 ☑
    - affecting fetus or newborn 763.89
    - causing obstructed labor 660.2 ☑
      - affecting fetus or newborn 763.1

Sequestration
- lung (congenital) (extralobar) (intralobar) 748.5
- orbit 376.10
- pulmonary artery (congenital) 747.3
- splenic 289.52

Sequestrum
- bone (*see also* Osteomyelitis) 730.1 ☑
  - jaw 526.4
- dental 525.8
- jaw bone 526.4
- sinus (accessory) (nasal) (*see also* Sinusitis) 473.9
  - maxillary 473.0

Sequoiosis asthma 495.8

Serology for syphilis
- doubtful
  - with signs or symptoms — *see* Syphilis, by site and stage
  - follow-up of latent syphilis — *see* Syphilis, latent
- false positive 795.6
- negative, with signs or symptoms — *see* Syphilis, by site and stage
- positive 097.1
  - with signs or symptoms — *see* Syphilis, by site and stage
  - false 795.6
  - follow-up of latent syphilis — *see* Syphilis, latent
  - only finding — *see* Syphilis, latent
- reactivated 097.1

Seroma (postoperative) (non-infected) 998.13
- infected 998.51

Seropurulent — *see* condition

Serositis, multiple 569.89
- pericardial 423.2
- peritoneal 568.82
- pleural — *see* Pleurisy

Serotonin syndrome 333.99

Serous — *see* condition

Sertoli cell
- adenoma (M8640/0)
  - specified site — *see* Neoplasm, by site, benign
  - unspecified site
    - female 220
    - male 222.0

Shock — *continued*
- thyroxin 962.7
- toxic 040.82
- transfusion — *see* Complications, transfusion
- traumatic (immediate) (delayed) 958.4

Shoemakers' chest 738.3

Short, shortening, shortness
- Achilles tendon (acquired) 727.81
- arm 736.89
  - congenital 755.20
- back 737.9
- bowel syndrome 579.3
- breath 786.05
- chain acyl CoA dehydrogenase deficiency (SCAD) 277.85
- common bile duct, congenital 751.69
- cord (umbilical) 663.4 ☑
  - affecting fetus or newborn 762.6
- cystic duct, congenital 751.69
- esophagus (congenital) 750.4
- femur (acquired) 736.81
  - congenital 755.34
- frenulum linguae 750.0
- frenum, lingual 750.0
- hamstrings 727.81
- hip (acquired) 736.39
  - congenital 755.63
- leg (acquired) 736.81
  - congenital 755.30
- metatarsus (congenital) 754.79
  - acquired 736.79
- organ or site, congenital NEC — *see* Distortion
- palate (congenital) 750.26
- P-R interval syndrome 426.81
- radius (acquired) 736.09
  - congenital 755.26
- round ligament 629.8
- sleeper 307.49
- stature, constitutional (hereditary) 783.43
- tendon 727.81
  - Achilles (acquired) 727.81
    - congenital 754.79
  - congenital 756.89
- thigh (acquired) 736.81
  - congenital 755.34
- tibialis anticus 727.81
- umbilical cord 663.4 ☑
  - affecting fetus or newborn 762.6
- urethra 599.84
- uvula (congenital) 750.26
- vagina 623.8

Shortsightedness 367.1

Shoshin (acute fulminating beriberi) 265.0

Shoulder — *see* condition

Shovel-shaped incisors 520.2

Shower, thromboembolic — *see* Embolism

Shunt (status)
- aortocoronary bypass V45.81
- arterial-venous (dialysis) V45.1
- arteriovenous, pulmonary (acquired) 417.0
  - congenital 747.3
  - traumatic (complication) 901.40
- cerebral ventricle (communicating) in situ V45.2
- coronary artery bypass V45.81
- surgical, prosthetic, with complications — *see* Complications, shunt
- vascular NEC V45.89

Shutdown
- renal 586
  - with
    - abortion — *see* Abortion, by type, with renal failure
    - ectopic pregnancy (*see also* categories 633.0-633.9) 639.3
    - molar pregnancy (*see also* categories 630-632) 639.3
  - complicating
    - abortion 639.3
    - ectopic or molar pregnancy 639.3
  - following labor and delivery 669.3 ☑

Shwachman's syndrome 288.0

Shy-Drager syndrome (orthostatic hypotension with multisystem degeneration) 333.0

Sialadenitis (any gland) (chronic) (suppurative) 527.2
- epidemic — *see* Mumps

Sialadenosis, periodic 527.2

Sialaporia 527.7

Sialectasia 527.8

Sialitis 527.2

Sialoadenitis (*see also* Sialadenitis) 527.2

Sialoangitis 527.2

Sialodochitis (fibrinosa) 527.2

Sialodocholithiasis 527.5

Sialolithiasis 527.5

Sialorrhea (*see also* Ptyalism) 527.7
- periodic 527.2

Sialosis 527.8
- rheumatic 710.2

Siamese twin 759.4

Sicard's syndrome 352.6

Sicca syndrome (keratoconjunctivitis) 710.2

Sick 799.9
- cilia syndrome 759.89
- or handicapped person in family V61.49

Sickle-cell
- anemia (see also Disease, sickle-cell) 282.60
- disease (see also Disease, sickle-cell) 282.60
- hemoglobin
  - C disease (without crisis) 282.63
    - with
      - crisis 282.64
      - vaso-occlusive pain 282.64
  - D disease (without crisis) 282.68
    - with crisis 282.69
  - E disease (without crisis) 282.68
    - with crisis 282.69
- thalassemia (without crisis) 282.41
  - with
    - crisis 282.42
    - vaso-occlusive pain 282.42
- trait 282.5

Sicklemia (*see also* Disease, sickle-cell) 282.60
- trait 282.5

Sickness
- air (travel) 994.6
- airplane 994.6
- alpine 993.2
- altitude 993.2
- Andes 993.2
- aviators' 993.2
- balloon 993.2
- car 994.6
- compressed air 993.3
- decompression 993.3
- green 280.9
- harvest 100.89
- milk 988.8
- morning 643.0 ☑
- motion 994.6
- mountain 993.2
  - acute 289.0
- protein (*see also* Complications, vaccination) 999.5
- radiation NEC 990
- roundabout (motion) 994.6
- sea 994.6
- serum NEC 999.5
- sleeping (African) 086.5
  - by Trypanosoma 086.5
    - gambiense 086.3
    - rhodesiense 086.4
  - Gambian 086.3
  - late effect 139.8
  - Rhodesian 086.4
- sweating 078.2
- swing (motion) 994.6
- train (railway) (travel) 994.6
- travel (any vehicle) 994.6

Sick sinus syndrome 427.81

Sideropenia (*see also* Anemia, iron deficiency) 280.9

Siderosis (lung) (occupational) 503
- cornea 371.15
- eye (bulbi) (vitreous) 360.23
- lens 360.23

Siegal-Cattan-Mamou disease (periodic) 277.3

Siemens' syndrome
- ectodermal dysplasia 757.31
- keratosis follicularis spinulosa (decalvans) 757.39

Sighing respiration 786.7

Sigmoid
- flexure — *see* condition
- kidney 753.3

Sigmoiditis — *see* Enteritis

Silfverskiöld's syndrome 756.50

Silicosis, silicotic (complicated) (occupational) (simple) 502
- fibrosis, lung (confluent) (massive) (occupational) 502
- non-nodular 503
- pulmonum 502

Silicotuberculosis (*see also* Tuberculosis) 011.4 ☑

Silo fillers' disease 506.9

Silver's syndrome (congenital hemihypertrophy and short stature) 759.89

Silver wire arteries, retina 362.13

Silvestroni-Bianco syndrome (thalassemia minima) 282.49

Simian crease 757.2

Simmonds' cachexia or disease (pituitary cachexia) 253.2

Simons' disease or syndrome (progressive lipodystrophy) 272.6

Simple, simplex — *see* condition

Sinding-Larsen disease (juvenile osteopathia patellae) 732.4

Singapore hemorrhagic fever 065.4

Singers' node or nodule 478.5

Single
- atrium 745.69
- coronary artery 746.85
- umbilical artery 747.5
- ventricle 745.3

Singultus 786.8
- epidemicus 078.89

Sinus — *see also* Fistula
- abdominal 569.81
- arrest 426.6
- arrhythmia 427.89
- bradycardia 427.89
  - chronic 427.81
- branchial cleft (external) (internal) 744.41
- coccygeal (infected) 685.1
  - with abscess 685.0
- dental 522.7
- dermal (congenital) 685.1
  - with abscess 685.0
- draining — *see* Fistula
- infected, skin NEC 686.9
- marginal, ruptured or bleeding 641.2 ☑
  - affecting fetus or newborn 762.1
- pause 426.6
- pericranii 742.0
- pilonidal (infected) (rectum) 685.1
  - with abscess 685.0
- preauricular 744.46
- rectovaginal 619.1
- sacrococcygeal (dermoid) (infected) 685.1
  - with abscess 685.0
- skin
  - infected NEC 686.9
  - noninfected — *see* Ulcer, skin
- tachycardia 427.89
- tarsi syndrome 726.79
- testis 608.89
- tract (postinfectional) — *see* Fistula
- urachus 753.7

Sinuses, Rokitansky-Aschoff (*see also* Disease, gallbladder) 575.8

Sinusitis (accessory) (nasal) (hyperplastic) (nonpurulent) (purulent) (chronic) 473.9
- with influenza, flu, or grippe 487.1
- acute 461.9
  - ethmoidal 461.2
  - frontal 461.1
  - maxillary 461.0
  - specified type NEC 461.8

☑ Additional Digit Required — Refer to the Tabular List (Numeric Code Section) for Additional Digit Selection

Spider
- finger 755.59
- nevus 448.1
- vascular 448.1

Spiegler-Fendt sarcoid 686.8

Spielmeyer-Stock disease 330.1

Spielmeyer-Vogt disease 330.1

Spina bifida (aperta) 741.9 ☑

> *Note — Use the following fifth-digit subclassification with category 741:*
>
> *0 unspecified region*
> *1 cervical region*
> *2 dorsal [thoracic] region*
> *3 lumbar region*

- with hydrocephalus 741.0 ☑
  - fetal (suspected), affecting management of pregnancy 655.0 ☑
- occulta 756.17

Spindle, Krukenberg's 371.13

Spine, spinal — *see* condition

Spiradenoma (eccrine) (M8403/0) — *see* Neoplasm, skin, benign

Spirillosis NEC (*see also* Fever, relapsing) 087.9

Spirillum minus 026.0

Spirillum obermeieri infection 087.0

Spirochetal — *see* condition

Spirochetosis 104.9
- arthritic, arthritica 104.9 *[711.8]* ☑
- bronchopulmonary 104.8
- icterohemorrhagica 100.0
- lung 104.8

Spitting blood (*see also* Hemoptysis) 786.3

Splanchnomegaly 569.89

Splanchnoptosis 569.89

Spleen, splenic — *see also* condition
- agenesis 759.0
- flexure syndrome 569.89
- neutropenia syndrome 288.0
- sequestration syndrome 289.52

Splenectasis (*see also* Splenomegaly) 789.2

Splenitis (interstitial) (malignant) (nonspecific) 289.59
- malarial (*see also* Malaria) 084.6
- tuberculous (*see also* Tuberculosis) 017.7 ☑

Splenocele 289.59

Splenomegalia — *see* Splenomegaly

Splenomegalic — *see* condition

Splenomegaly 789.2
- Bengal 789.2
- cirrhotic 289.51
- congenital 759.0
- congestive, chronic 289.51
- cryptogenic 789.2
- Egyptian 120.1
- Gaucher's (cerebroside lipidosis) 272.7
- idiopathic 789.2
- malarial (*see also* Malaria) 084.6
- neutropenic 288.0
- Niemann-Pick (lipid histiocytosis) 272.7
- siderotic 289.51
- syphilitic 095.8
  - congenital 090.0
- tropical (Bengal) (idiopathic) 789.2

Splenopathy 289.50

Splenopneumonia — *see* Pneumonia

Splenoptosis 289.59

Splinter — *see* Injury, superficial, by site

Split, splitting
- heart sounds 427.89
- lip, congenital (*see also* Cleft, lip) 749.10
- nails 703.8
- urinary stream 788.61

Spoiled child reaction (*see also* Disturbance, conduct) 312.1 ☑

Spondylarthritis (*see also* Spondylosis) 721.90

Spondylarthrosis (*see also* Spondylosis) 721.90

Spondylitis 720.9
- ankylopoietica 720.0
- ankylosing (chronic) 720.0
- atrophic 720.9
  - ligamentous 720.9

Spondylitis — *continued*
- chronic (traumatic) (*see also* Spondylosis) 721.90
- deformans (chronic) (*see also* Spondylosis) 721.90
- gonococcal 098.53
- gouty 274.0
- hypertrophic (*see also* Spondylosis) 721.90
- infectious NEC 720.9
- juvenile (adolescent) 720.0
- Kümmell's 721.7
- Marie-Strümpell (ankylosing) 720.0
- muscularis 720.9
- ossificans ligamentosa 721.6
- osteoarthritica (*see also* Spondylosis) 721.90
- posttraumatic 721.7
- proliferative 720.0
- rheumatoid 720.0
- rhizomelica 720.0
- sacroiliac NEC 720.2
- senescent (*see also* Spondylosis) 721.90
- senile (*see also* Spondylosis) 721.90
- static (*see also* Spondylosis) 721.90
- traumatic (chronic) (*see also* Spondylosis) 721.90
- tuberculous (*see also* Tuberculosis) 015.0 ☑ *[720.81]*
- typhosa 002.0 *[720.81]*

Spondyloarthrosis (*see also* Spondylosis) 721.90

Spondylolisthesis (congenital) (lumbosacral) 756.12
- with disproportion (fetopelvic) 653.3 ☑
  - affecting fetus or newborn 763.1
  - causing obstructed labor 660.1 ☑
    - affecting fetus or newborn 763.1
- acquired 738.4
- degenerative 738.4
- traumatic 738.4
  - acute (lumbar) — *see* Fracture, vertebra, lumbar
    - site other than lumbosacral — *see* Fracture, vertebra, by site

Spondylolysis (congenital) 756.11
- acquired 738.4
- cervical 756.19
- lumbosacral region 756.11
  - with disproportion (fetopelvic) 653.3 ☑
    - affecting fetus or newborn 763.1
    - causing obstructed labor 660.1 ☑
      - affecting fetus or newborn 763.1

Spondylopathy
- inflammatory 720.9
  - specified type NEC 720.89
- traumatic 721.7

Spondylose rhizomelique 720.0

Spondylosis 721.90
- with
  - disproportion 653.3 ☑
    - affecting fetus or newborn 763.1
    - causing obstructed labor 660.1 ☑
      - affecting fetus or newborn 763.1
  - myelopathy NEC 721.91
- cervical, cervicodorsal 721.0
  - with myelopathy 721.1
- inflammatory 720.9
- lumbar, lumbosacral 721.3
  - with myelopathy 721.42
- sacral 721.3
  - with myelopathy 721.42
- thoracic 721.2
  - with myelopathy 721.41
- traumatic 721.7

Sponge
- divers' disease 989.5
- inadvertently left in operation wound 998.4
- kidney (medullary) 753.17

Spongioblastoma (M9422/3)
- multiforme (M9440/3)
  - specified site — *see* Neoplasm, by site, malignant
  - unspecified site 191.9
- polare (M9423/3)
  - specified site — *see* Neoplasm, by site, malignant
  - unspecified site 191.9

Spongioblastoma (M9422/3) — *continued*
- primitive polar (M9443/3)
  - specified site — *see* Neoplasm, by site, malignant
  - unspecified site 191.9
- specified site — *see* Neoplasm, by site, malignant
- unspecified site 191.9

Spongiocytoma (M9400/3)
- specified site — *see* Neoplasm, by site, malignant
- unspecified site 191.9

Spongioneuroblastoma (M9504/3) — *see* Neoplasm, by site, malignant

Spontaneous — *see also* condition
- fracture — *see* Fracture, pathologic

Spoon nail 703.8
- congenital 757.5

Sporadic — *see* condition

Sporotrichosis (bones) (cutaneous) (disseminated) (epidermal) (lymphatic) (lymphocutaneous) (mucous membranes) (pulmonary) (skeletal) (visceral) 117.1

Sporotrichum schenckii infection 117.1

Spots, spotting
- atrophic (skin) 701.3
- Bitôt's (in the young child) 264.1
- café au lait 709.09
- cayenne pepper 448.1
- cotton wool (retina) 362.83
- de Morgan's (senile angiomas) 448.1
- Fúchs' black (myopic) 360.21
- intermenstrual
  - irregular 626.6
  - regular 626.5
- interpalpebral 372.53
- Koplik's 055.9
- liver 709.09
- Mongolian (pigmented) 757.33
- of pregnancy 641.9 ☑
- purpuric 782.7
- ruby 448.1

Spotted fever — *see* Fever, spotted

Sprain, strain (joint) (ligament) (muscle) (tendon) 848.9
- abdominal wall (muscle) 848.8
- Achilles tendon 845.09
- acromioclavicular 840.0
- ankle 845.00
  - and foot 845.00
- anterior longitudinal, cervical 847.0
- arm 840.9
  - upper 840.9
    - and shoulder 840.9
- astragalus 845.00
- atlanto-axial 847.0
- atlanto-occipital 847.0
- atlas 847.0
- axis 847.0
- back (*see also* Sprain, spine) 847.9
- breast bone 848.40
- broad ligament — *see* Injury, internal, broad ligament
- calcaneofibular 845.02
- carpal 842.01
- carpometacarpal 842.11
- cartilage
  - costal, without mention of injury to sternum 848.3
    - involving sternum 848.42
  - ear 848.8
  - knee 844.9
    - with current tear (*see also* Tear, meniscus) 836.2
  - semilunar (knee) 844.8
    - with current tear (*see also* Tear, meniscus) 836.2
  - septal, nose 848.0
  - thyroid region 848.2
  - xiphoid 848.49
- cervical, cervicodorsal, cervicothoracic 847.0
- chondrocostal, without mention of injury to sternum 848.3
  - involving sternum 848.42
- chondrosternal 848.42

☑ Additional Digit Required — Refer to the Tabular List (Numeric Code Section) for Additional Digit Selection

▶◀ Revised Text ● New Line ▲ Revised Code

- **Staghorn calculus** 592.0
- **Stälh's**
  - ear 744.29
  - pigment line (cornea) 371.11
- **Stälhi's pigment lines** (cornea) 371.11
- **Stain, ▶staining◀**
  - meconium 779.84 ●
  - port wine 757.32
  - tooth, teeth (hard tissues) 521.7
    - due to
      - accretions 523.6
      - deposits (betel) (black) (green) (materia alba) (orange) (tobacco) 523.6
      - metals (copper) (silver) 521.7
      - nicotine 523.6
      - pulpal bleeding 521.7
      - tobacco 523.6
- **Stammering** 307.0
- **Standstill**
  - atrial 426.6
  - auricular 426.6
  - cardiac (*see also* Arrest, cardiac) 427.5
  - sinoatrial 426.6
  - sinus 426.6
  - ventricular (*see also* Arrest, cardiac) 427.5
- **Stannosis** 503
- **Stanton's disease** (melioidosis) 025
- **Staphylitis** (acute) (catarrhal) (chronic) (gangrenous) (membranous) (suppurative) (ulcerative) 528.3
- **Staphylococcemia** 038.10
  - aureus 038.11
  - specified organism NEC 038.19
- **Staphylococcus, staphylococcal** — *see* condition
- **Staphyloderma** (skin) 686.00
- **Staphyloma** 379.11
  - anterior, localized 379.14
  - ciliary 379.11
  - cornea 371.73
  - equatorial 379.13
  - posterior 379.12
  - posticum 379.12
  - ring 379.15
  - sclera NEC 379.11
- **Starch eating** 307.52
- **Stargardt's disease** 362.75
- **Starvation** (inanition) (due to lack of food) 994.2
  - edema 262
  - voluntary NEC 307.1
- **Stasis**
  - bile (duct) (*see also* Disease, biliary) 576.8
  - bronchus (*see also* Bronchitis) 490
  - cardiac (*see also* Failure, heart) 428.0
  - cecum 564.89
  - colon 564.89
  - dermatitis (*see also* Varix, with stasis dermatitis) 454.1
  - duodenal 536.8
  - eczema (*see also* Varix, with stasis dermatitis) 454.1
  - edema (*see also* Hypertension, venous) 459.30
  - foot 991.4
  - gastric 536.3
  - ileocecal coil 564.89
  - ileum 564.89
  - intestinal 564.89
  - jejunum 564.89
  - kidney 586
  - liver 571.9
    - cirrhotic — *see* Cirrhosis, liver
  - lymphatic 457.8
  - pneumonia 514
  - portal 571.9
  - pulmonary 514
  - rectal 564.89
  - renal 586
    - tubular 584.5
  - stomach 536.3
  - ulcer
    - with varicose veins 454.0
    - without varicose veins 459.81
  - urine NEC (*see also* Retention, urine) 788.20
  - venous 459.81
- **State**
  - affective and paranoid, mixed, organic psychotic 294.8
  - agitated 307.9
    - acute reaction to stress 308.2
  - anxiety (neurotic) (*see also* Anxiety) 300.00
    - specified type NEC 300.09
  - apprehension (*see also* Anxiety) 300.00
    - specified type NEC 300.09
  - climacteric, female 627.2
    - following induced menopause 627.4
  - clouded
    - epileptic (*see also* Epilepsy) 345.9 ☑
    - paroxysmal (idiopathic) (*see also* Epilepsy) 345.9 ☑
  - compulsive (mixed) (with obsession) 300.3
  - confusional 298.9
    - acute 293.0
      - with
        - arteriosclerotic dementia 290.41
        - presenile brain disease 290.11
        - senility 290.3
      - alcoholic 291.0
      - drug-induced 292.81
    - epileptic 293.0
    - postoperative 293.9
    - reactive (emotional stress) (psychological trauma) 298.2
    - subacute 293.1
  - constitutional psychopathic 301.9
  - convulsive (*see also* Convulsions) 780.39
  - depressive NEC 311
    - induced by drug 292.84
    - neurotic 300.4
  - dissociative 300.15
  - hallucinatory 780.1
    - induced by drug 292.12
  - hypercoagulable (primary) 289.81
    - secondary 289.82
  - hyperdynamic beta-adrenergic circulatory 429.82
  - locked-in 344.81
  - menopausal 627.2
    - artificial 627.4
    - following induced menopause 627.4
  - neurotic NEC 300.9
    - with depersonalization episode 300.6
  - obsessional 300.3
  - oneiroid (*see also* Schizophrenia) 295.4 ☑
  - panic 300.01
  - paranoid 297.9
    - alcohol-induced 291.5
    - arteriosclerotic 290.42
    - climacteric 297.2
    - drug-induced 292.11
    - in
      - presenile brain disease 290.12
      - senile brain disease 290.20
    - involutional 297.2
    - menopausal 297.2
    - senile 290.20
    - simple 297.0
  - postleukotomy 310.0
  - pregnant (*see also* Pregnancy) V22.2
  - psychogenic, twilight 298.2
  - psychotic, organic (*see also* Psychosis, organic) 294.9
    - mixed paranoid and affective 294.8
    - senile or presenile NEC 290.9
    - transient NEC 293.9
      - with
        - anxiety 293.84
        - delusions 293.81
        - depression 293.83
        - hallucinations 293.82
  - residual schizophrenic (*see also* Schizophrenia) 295.6 ☑
  - tension (*see also* Anxiety) 300.9
  - transient organic psychotic 293.9
    - anxiety type 293.84
    - depressive type 293.83
    - hallucinatory type 293.83
    - paranoid type 293.81
    - specified type NEC 293.89
  - twilight
    - epileptic 293.0
    - psychogenic 298.2

State — *continued*

  - vegetative (persistent) 780.03
- **Status** (post)
  - absence
    - epileptic (*see also* Epilepsy) 345.2
    - of organ, acquired (postsurgical) — *see* Absence, by site, acquired
  - anastomosis of intestine (for bypass) V45.3
  - angioplasty, percutaneous transluminal coronary V45.82
  - anginosus 413.9
  - ankle prosthesis V43.66
  - aortocoronary bypass or shunt V45.81
  - arthrodesis V45.4
  - artificially induced condition NEC V45.89
  - artificial opening (of) V44.9
    - gastrointestinal tract NEC V44.4
    - specified site NEC V44.8
    - urinary tract NEC V44.6
    - vagina V44.7
  - aspirator V46.0
  - awaiting organ transplant V49.83
  - asthmaticus (*see also* Asthma) 493.9 ☑
  - bed confinement V49.84 ●
  - breast implant removal V45.83
  - cardiac
    - device (in situ) V45.00
      - carotid sinus V45.09
        - fitting or adjustment V53.39
      - defibrillator, automatic implantable V45.02
      - pacemaker V45.01
        - fitting or adjustment V53.31
  - carotid sinus stimulator V45.09
  - cataract extraction V45.61
  - chemotherapy V66.2
    - current V58.69
  - circumcision, female 629.20
  - clitorectomy (female genital mutilation type I) 629.21
    - with excision of labia minora (female genital mutilation type II) 629.22
  - colostomy V44.3
  - contraceptive device V45.59
    - intrauterine V45.51
    - subdermal V45.52
  - convulsivus idiopathicus (*see also* Epilepsy) 345.3
  - coronary artery bypass or shunt V45.81
  - cystostomy V44.50
    - appendico-vesicostomy V44.52
    - cutaneous-vesicostomy V44.51
    - specified type NEC V44.59
  - defibrillator, automatic implantable cardiac V45.02
  - dental crowns V45.84
  - dental fillings V45.84
  - dental restoration V45.84
  - dental sealant V49.82
  - dialysis ▶(hemo) (peritoneal)◀ V45.1
  - donor V59.9
  - drug therapy or regimen V67.59
    - high-risk medication NEC V67.51
  - elbow prosthesis V43.62
  - enterostomy V44.4
  - epileptic, epilepticus (absence) (grand mal) (*see also* Epilepsy) 345.3
    - focal motor 345.7 ☑
    - partial 345.7 ☑
    - petit mal 345.2
    - psychomotor 345.7 ☑
    - temporal lobe 345.7 ☑
  - eye (adnexa) surgery V45.69
  - female genital mutilation 629.20
    - type I 629.21
    - type II 629.22
    - type III 629.23
  - filtering bleb (eye) (postglaucoma) V45.69
    - with rupture or complication 997.99
    - postcataract extraction (complication) 997.99
  - finger joint prosthesis V43.69
  - gastrostomy V44.1
  - grand mal 345.3
  - heart valve prosthesis V43.3
  - hemodialysis V45.1 ●

Staghorn calculus — Status

Status — *continued*
hip prosthesis (joint) (partial) (total) V43.64
ileostomy V44.2
infibulation (female genital mutilation type III) 629.23
insulin pump V45.85
intestinal bypass V45.3
intrauterine contraceptive device V45.51
jejunostomy V44.4
knee joint prosthesis V43.65
lacunaris 437.8
lacunosis 437.8
low birth weight V21.30
less than 500 grams V21.31
500-999 grams V21.32
1000-1499 grams V21.33
1500-1999 grams V21.34
2000-2500 grams V21.35
lymphaticus 254.8
malignant neoplasm, ablated or excised — *see* History, malignant neoplasm
marmoratus 333.7
mutilation, female 629.20
type I 629.21
type II 629.22
type III 629.23
nephrostomy V44.6
neuropacemaker NEC V45.89
brain V45.89
carotid sinus V45.09
neurologic NEC V45.89
organ replacement
by artificial or mechanical device or prosthesis of
artery V43.4
artificial skin V43.83
bladder V43.5
blood vessel V43.4
breast V43.82
eye globe V43.0
heart
assist device V43.21
fully implantable artificial heart V43.22
valve V43.3
intestine V43.89
joint V43.60
ankle V43.66
elbow V43.62
finger V43.69
hip (partial) (total) V43.64
knee V43.65
shoulder V43.61
specified NEC V43.69
wrist V43.63
kidney V43.89
larynx V43.81
lens V43.1
limb(s) V43.7
liver V43.89
lung V43.89
organ NEC V43.89
pancreas V43.89
skin (artificial) V43.83
tissue NEC V43.89
vein V43.4
by organ transplant (heterologous) (homologous) — *see* Status, transplant
pacemaker
brain V45.89
cardiac V45.01
carotid sinus V45.09
neurologic NEC V45.89
specified site NEC V45.89
percutaneous transluminal coronary angioplasty V45.82
peritoneal dialysis V45.1 ●
petit mal 345.2
postcommotio cerebri 310.2
postmenopausal (age related) (natural) V49.81
postoperative NEC V45.89
postpartum NEC V24.2
care immediately following delivery V24.0
routine follow-up V24.2
postsurgical NEC V45.89
renal dialysis V45.1

Status — *continued*
respirator ▶[ventilator]◀ V46.11
encounter
during ●
mechanical failure V46.14 ●
power failure V46.12 ●
for weaning V46.13 ●
reversed jejunal transposition (for bypass) V45.3
shoulder prosthesis V43.61
shunt
aortocoronary bypass V45.81
arteriovenous (for dialysis) V45.1
cerebrospinal fluid V45.2
vascular NEC V45.89
aortocoronary (bypass) V45.81
ventricular (communicating) (for drainage) V45.2
sterilization
tubal ligation V26.51
vasectomy V26.52
subdermal contraceptive device V45.52
thymicolymphaticus 254.8
thymicus 254.8
thymolymphaticus 254.8
tooth extraction 525.10
tracheostomy V44.0
transplant
blood vessel V42.89
bone V42.4
marrow V42.81
cornea V42.5
heart V42.1
valve V42.2
intestine V42.84
kidney V42.0
liver V42.7
lung V42.6
organ V42.9
specified site NEC V42.89
pancreas V42.83
peripheral stem cells V42.82
skin V42.3
stem cells, peripheral V42.82
tissue V42.9
specified type NEC V42.89
vessel, blood V42.89
tubal ligation V26.51
ureterostomy V44.6
urethrostomy V44.6
vagina, artificial V44.7
vascular shunt NEC V45.89
aortocoronary (bypass) V45.81
vasectomy V26.52
ventilator ▶[respirator]◀ V46.11
encounter
during ●
mechanical failure V46.14 ●
power failure V46.12 ●
for weaning V46.13 ●
wrist prosthesis V43.63
Stave fracture — *see* Fracture, metacarpus, metacarpal bone(s)
Steal
subclavian artery 435.2
vertebral artery 435.1
Stealing, solitary, child problem (*see also* Disturbance, conduct) 312.1 ☑
Steam burn — *see* Burn, by site
Steatocystoma multiplex 706.2
Steatoma (infected) 706.2
eyelid (cystic) 374.84
infected 373.13
Steatorrhea (chronic) 579.8
with lacteal obstruction 579.2
idiopathic 579.0
adult 579.0
infantile 579.0
pancreatic 579.4
primary 579.0
secondary 579.8
specified cause NEC 579.8
tropical 579.1
Steatosis 272.8
heart (*see also* Degeneration, myocardial) 429.1
kidney 593.89
liver 571.8

Steele-Richardson (-Olszewski) Syndrome 333.0
Stein's syndrome (polycystic ovary) 256.4
Stein-Leventhal syndrome (polycystic ovary) 256.4
Steinbrocker's syndrome (*see also* Neuropathy, peripheral, autonomic) 337.9
Steinert's disease 359.2
Stenocardia (*see also* Angina) 413.9
Stenocephaly 756.0
Stenosis (cicatricial) — *see also* Stricture
ampulla of Vater 576.2
with calculus, cholelithiasis, or stones — *see* Choledocholithiasis
anus, anal (canal) (sphincter) 569.2
congenital 751.2
aorta (ascending) 747.22
arch 747.10
arteriosclerotic 440.0
calcified 440.0
aortic (valve) 424.1
with
mitral (valve)
insufficiency or incompetence 396.2
stenosis or obstruction 396.0
atypical 396.0
congenital 746.3
rheumatic 395.0
with
insufficiency, incompetency or regurgitation 395.2
with mitral (valve) disease 396.8
mitral (valve)
disease (stenosis) 396.0
insufficiency or incompetence 396.2
stenosis or obstruction 396.0
specified cause, except rheumatic 424.1
syphilitic 093.22
aqueduct of Sylvius (congenital) 742.3
with spina bifida (*see also* Spina bifida) 741.0 ☑
acquired 331.4
artery NEC 447.1
basilar — *see* Narrowing, artery, basilar
carotid (common) (internal) — *see* Narrowing, artery, carotid
celiac 447.4
cerebral 437.0
due to
embolism (*see also* Embolism, brain) 434.1 ☑
thrombus (*see also* Thrombosis, brain) 434.0 ☑
precerebral — *see* Narrowing, artery, precerebral
pulmonary (congenital) 747.3
acquired 417.8
renal 440.1
vertebral — *see* Narrowing, artery, vertebral
bile duct or biliary passage (*see also* Obstruction, biliary) 576.2
congenital 751.61
bladder neck (acquired) 596.0
congenital 753.6
brain 348.8
bronchus 519.1
syphilitic 095.8
cardia (stomach) 537.89
congenital 750.7
cardiovascular (*see also* Disease, cardiovascular) 429.2
carotid artery — *see* Narrowing, artery, carotid
cervix, cervical (canal) 622.4
congenital 752.49
in pregnancy or childbirth 654.6 ☑
affecting fetus or newborn 763.89
causing obstructed labor 660.2 ☑
affecting fetus or newborn 763.1
colon (*see also* Obstruction, intestine) 560.9
congenital 751.2
colostomy 569.62
common bile duct (*see also* Obstruction, biliary) 576.2
congenital 751.61
coronary (artery) — *see* Arteriosclerosis, coronary

☑ Additional Digit Required — Refer to the Tabular List (Numeric Code Section) for Additional Digit Selection

Stitch
- abscess 998.59
- burst (in external operation wound) 998.32
  - internal 998.31
- in back 724.5

Stojano's (subcostal) **syndrome** 098.86

Stokes' disease (exophthalmic goiter) 242.0 ☑

Stokes-Adams syndrome (syncope with heart block) 426.9

Stokvis' (-Talma) disease (enterogenous cyanosis) 289.7

Stomach — *see* condition

Stoma malfunction
- colostomy 569.62
- cystostomy 997.5
- enterostomy 569.62
- esophagostomy 530.87
- gastrostomy 536.42
- ileostomy 569.62
- nephrostomy 997.5
- tracheostomy 519.02
- ureterostomy 997.5

Stomatitis 528.0
- angular 528.5
  - due to dietary or vitamin deficiency 266.0
- aphthous 528.2
- candidal 112.0
- catarrhal 528.0
- denture 528.9
- diphtheritic (membranous) 032.0
- due to
  - dietary deficiency 266.0
  - thrush 112.0
  - vitamin deficiency 266.0
- epidemic 078.4
- epizootic 078.4
- follicular 528.0
- gangrenous 528.1
- herpetic 054.2
- herpetiformis 528.2
- malignant 528.0
- membranous acute 528.0
- monilial 112.0
- mycotic 112.0
- necrotic 528.1
  - ulcerative 101
- necrotizing ulcerative 101
- parasitic 112.0
- septic 528.0
- spirochetal 101
- suppurative (acute) 528.0
- ulcerative 528.0
  - necrotizing 101
- ulceromembranous 101
- vesicular 528.0
  - with exanthem 074.3
- Vincent's 101

Stomatocytosis 282.8

Stomatomycosis 112.0

Stomatorrhagia 528.9

Stone(s) — *see also* Calculus
- bladder 594.1
  - diverticulum 594.0
- cystine 270.0
- heart syndrome (*see also* Failure, ventricular, left) 428.1
- kidney 592.0
- prostate 602.0
- pulp (dental) 522.2
- renal 592.0
- salivary duct or gland (any) 527.5
- ureter 592.1
- urethra (impacted) 594.2
- urinary (duct) (impacted) (passage) 592.9
  - bladder 594.1
    - diverticulum 594.0
  - lower tract NEC 594.9
  - specified site 594.8
- xanthine 277.2

Stonecutters' lung 502
- tuberculous (*see also* Tuberculosis) 011.4 ☑

Stonemasons'
- asthma, disease, or lung 502
  - tuberculous (*see also* Tuberculosis) 011.4 ☑
- phthisis (*see also* Tuberculosis) 011.4 ☑

Stoppage
- bowel (*see also* Obstruction, intestine) 560.9
- heart (*see also* Arrest, cardiac) 427.5
- intestine (*see also* Obstruction, intestine) 560.9
- urine NEC (*see also* Retention, urine) 788.20

Storm, thyroid (apathetic) (*see also* Thyrotoxicosis) 242.9 ☑

Strabismus (alternating) (congenital) (nonparalytic) 378.9
- concomitant (*see also* Heterotropia) 378.30
  - convergent (*see also* Esotropia) 378.00
  - divergent (*see also* Exotropia) 378.10
- convergent (*see also* Esotropia) 378.00
- divergent (*see also* Exotropia) 378.10
- due to adhesions, scars — *see* Strabismus, mechanical
- in neuromuscular disorder NEC 378.73
  - intermittent 378.20
    - vertical 378.31
- latent 378.40
  - convergent (esophoria) 378.41
  - divergent (exophoria) 378.42
  - vertical 378.43
- mechanical 378.60
  - due to
    - Brown's tendon sheath syndrome 378.61
    - specified musculofascial disorder NEC 378.62
- paralytic 378.50
  - third or oculomotor nerve (partial) 378.51
    - total 378.52
  - fourth or trochlear nerve 378.53
  - sixth or abducens nerve 378.54
- specified type NEC 378.73
- vertical (hypertropia) 378.31

Strain — *see also* Sprain, by site
- eye NEC 368.13
- heart — *see* Disease, heart
- meaning gonorrhea — *see* Gonorrhea
- physical NEC V62.89
- postural 729.9
- psychological NEC V62.89

Strands
- conjunctiva 372.62
- vitreous humor 379.25

Strangulation, strangulated 994.7
- appendix 543.9
- asphyxiation or suffocation by 994.7
- bladder neck 596.0
- bowel — *see* Strangulation, intestine
- colon — *see* Strangulation, intestine
- cord (umbilical) — *see* Compression, umbilical cord
- due to birth injury 767.8
- food or foreign body (*see also* Asphyxia, food) 933.1
- hemorrhoids 455.8
  - external 455.5
  - internal 455.2
- hernia — *see also* Hernia, by site, with obstruction
  - gangrenous — *see* Hernia, by site, with gangrene
- intestine (large) (small) 560.2
  - with hernia — *see also* Hernia, by site, with obstruction
    - gangrenous — *see* Hernia, by site, with gangrene
  - congenital (small) 751.1
    - large 751.2
- mesentery 560.2
- mucus (*see also* Asphyxia, mucus) 933.1
  - newborn 770.18 ▲
- omentum 560.2
- organ or site, congenital NEC — *see* Atresia
- ovary 620.8
  - due to hernia 620.4
- penis 607.89
  - foreign body 939.3
- rupture (*see also* Hernia, by site, with obstruction) 552.9
  - gangrenous (*see also* Hernia, by site, with gangrene) 551.9
- stomach, due to hernia (*see also* Hernia, by site, with obstruction) 552.9
  - with gangrene (*see also* Hernia, by site, with gangrene) 551.9

Strangulation, strangulated — *continued*
- umbilical cord — *see* Compression, umbilical cord
- vesicourethral orifice 596.0

Strangury 788.1

Strawberry
- gallbladder (*see also* Disease, gallbladder) 575.6
- mark 757.32
- tongue (red) (white) 529.3

Straw itch 133.8

Streak, ovarian 752.0

Strephosymbolia 315.01
- secondary to organic lesion 784.69

Streptobacillary fever 026.1

Streptobacillus moniliformis 026.1

Streptococcemia 038.0

Streptococcicosis — *see* Infection, streptococcal

Streptococcus, streptococcal — *see* condition

Streptoderma 686.00

Streptomycosis — *see* Actinomycosis

Streptothricosis — *see* Actinomycosis

Streptothrix — *see* Actinomycosis

Streptotrichosis — *see* Actinomycosis

Stress
- fracture — *see* Fracture, stress
- polycythemia 289.0
- reaction (gross) (*see also* Reaction, stress, acute) 308.9

Stretching, nerve — *see* Injury, nerve, by site

Striae (albicantes) (atrophicae) (cutis distensae) (distensae) 701.3

Striations of nails 703.8

Stricture (*see also* Stenosis) 799.89
- ampulla of Vater 576.2
  - with calculus, cholelithiasis, or stones — *see* Choledocholithiasis
- anus (sphincter) 569.2
  - congenital 751.2
  - infantile 751.2
- aorta (ascending) 747.22
  - arch 747.10
  - arteriosclerotic 440.0
  - calcified 440.0
- aortic (valve) (*see also* Stenosis, aortic) 424.1
  - congenital 746.3
- aqueduct of Sylvius (congenital) 742.3
  - with spina bifida (*see also* Spina bifida) 741.0 ☑
  - acquired 331.4
- artery 447.1
  - basilar — *see* Narrowing, artery, basilar
  - carotid (common) (internal) — *see* Narrowing, artery, carotid
  - celiac 447.4
  - cerebral 437.0
    - congenital 747.81
    - due to
      - embolism (*see also* Embolism, brain) 434.1 ☑
      - thrombus (*see also* Thrombosis, brain) 434.0 ☑
  - congenital (peripheral) 747.60
    - cerebral 747.81
    - coronary 746.85
    - gastrointestinal 747.61
    - lower limb 747.64
    - renal 747.62
    - retinal 743.58
    - specified NEC 747.69
    - spinal 747.82
    - umbilical 747.5
    - upper limb 747.63
  - coronary — *see* Arteriosclerosis, coronary
    - congenital 746.85
  - precerebral — *see* Narrowing, artery, precerebral NEC
  - pulmonary (congenital) 747.3
    - acquired 417.8
  - renal 440.1
  - vertebral — *see* Narrowing, artery, vertebral
- auditory canal (congenital) (external) 744.02
  - acquired (*see also* Stricture, ear canal, acquired) 380.50

☑ Additional Digit Required — Refer to the Tabular List (Numeric Code Section) for Additional Digit Selection

▶◀ Revised Text ● New Line ▲ Revised Code

☑ Additional Digit Required — Refer to the Tabular List (Numeric Code Section) for Additional Digit Selection

▶◀ Revised Text ● New Line ▲ Revised Code

☑ Additional Digit Required — Refer to the Tabular List (Numeric Code Section) for Additional Digit Selection
▶◀ Revised Text ● New Line ▲ Revised Code

☑ Additional Digit Required — Refer to the Tabular List (Numeric Code Section) for Additional Digit Selection

▶◀ Revised Text ● New Line ▲ Revised Code

Index

Syndrome — Syndrome

☑ Additional Digit Required — Refer to the Tabular List (Numeric Code Section) for Additional Digit Selection
▶◀ Revised Text ● New Line ▲ Revised Code

☑ Additional Digit Required — Refer to the Tabular List (Numeric Code Section) for Additional Digit Selection
▶◀ Revised Text ● New Line ▲ Revised Code

- **Tension** — *continued*
  - headache 307.81
  - intraocular (elevated) 365.00
  - nervous 799.2
  - ocular (elevated) 365.00
  - pneumothorax 512.0
    - iatrogenic 512.1
    - postoperative 512.1
    - spontaneous 512.0
  - premenstrual 625.4
  - state 300.9
- **Tentorium** — *see* condition
- **Teratencephalus** 759.89
- **Teratism** 759.7
- **Teratoblastoma** (malignant) (M9080/3) — *see* Neoplasm, by site, malignant
- **Teratocarcinoma** (M9081/3) — *see also* Neoplasm, by site, malignant
  - liver 155.0
- **Teratoma** (solid) (M9080/1) — *see also* Neoplasm, by site, uncertain behavior
  - adult (cystic) (M9080/0) — *see* Neoplasm, by site, benign
  - and embryonal carcinoma, mixed (M9081/3) — *see* Neoplasm, by site, malignant
  - benign (M9080/0) — *see* Neoplasm, by site, benign
  - combined with choriocarcinoma (M9101/3) — *see* Neoplasm, by site, malignant
  - cystic (adult) (M9080/0) — *see* Neoplasm, by site, benign
  - differentiated type (M9080/0) — *see* Neoplasm, by site, benign
  - embryonal (M9080/3) — *see also* Neoplasm, by site, malignant
    - liver 155.0
  - fetal
    - sacral, causing fetopelvic disproportion 653.7 ☑
  - immature (M9080/3) — *see* Neoplasm, by site, malignant
  - liver (M9080/3) 155.0
    - adult, benign, cystic, differentiated type or mature (M9080/0) 211.5
  - malignant (M9080/3) — *see also* Neoplasm, by site, malignant
    - anaplastic type (M9082/3) — *see* Neoplasm, by site, malignant
    - intermediate type (M9083/3) — *see* Neoplasm, by site, malignant
    - liver (M9080/3) 155.0
    - trophoblastic (M9102/3)
      - specified site — *see* Neoplasm, by site, malignant
      - unspecified site 186.9
    - undifferentiated type (M9082/3) — *see* Neoplasm, by site, malignant
  - mature (M9080/0) — *see* Neoplasm, by site, benign
  - ovary (M9080/0) 220
    - embryonal, immature, or malignant (M9080/3) 183.0
  - suprasellar (M9080/3) — *see* Neoplasm, by site, malignant
  - testis (M9080/3) 186.9
    - adult, benign, cystic, differentiated type or mature (M9080/0) 222.0
    - undescended 186.0
- **Terminal care** V66.7
- **Termination**
  - anomalous — *see also* Malposition, congenital
    - portal vein 747.49
    - right pulmonary vein 747.42
  - pregnancy (legal) (therapeutic) (*see* Abortion, legal) 635.9 ☑
    - fetus NEC 779.6
    - illegal (*see also* Abortion, illegal) 636.9 ☑
- **Ternidens diminutus infestation** 127.7
- **Terrors, night** (child) 307.46
- **Terry's syndrome** 362.21
- **Tertiary** — *see* condition
- **Tessellated fundus, retina** (tigroid) 362.89
- **Test(s)**
  - AIDS virus V72.6
- **Test(s)** — *continued*
  - adequacy
    - hemodialysis V56.31
    - peritoneal dialysis V56.32
  - allergen V72.7
  - bacterial disease NEC (*see also* Screening, by name of disease) V74.9
  - basal metabolic rate V72.6
  - blood-alcohol V70.4
  - blood-drug V70.4
    - for therapeutic drug monitoring V58.83
  - blood typing V72.86 ●
  - developmental, infant or child V20.2
  - Dick V74.8
  - fertility V26.21
  - genetic V26.32 ▲
    - for genetic disease carrier status V26.31 ●
  - hearing V72.1
  - HIV V72.6
  - human immunodeficiency virus V72.6
  - Kveim V82.89
  - laboratory V72.6
    - for medicolegal reason V70.4
  - Mantoux (for tuberculosis) V74.1
  - mycotic organism V75.4
  - parasitic agent NEC V75.8
  - paternity V70.4
  - peritoneal equilibration V56.32
  - pregnancy
    - negative result V72.41
    - positive ▶result◀ V72.42 ▲
      - first pregnancy V72.42 ▲
    - unconfirmed V72.40
  - preoperative V72.84
    - cardiovascular V72.81
    - respiratory V72.82
    - specified NEC V72.83
  - procreative management NEC V26.29
  - sarcoidosis V82.89
  - Schick V74.3
  - Schultz-Charlton V74.8
  - skin, diagnostic
    - allergy V72.7
    - bacterial agent NEC (*see also* Screening, by name of disease) V74.9
    - Dick V74.8
    - hypersensitivity V72.7
    - Kveim V82.89
    - Mantoux V74.1
    - mycotic organism V75.4
    - parasitic agent NEC V75.8
    - sarcoidosis V82.89
    - Schick V74.3
    - Schultz-Charlton V74.8
    - tuberculin V74.1
  - specified type NEC V72.85
  - tuberculin V74.1
  - vision V72.0
  - Wassermann
    - positive (*see also* Serology for syphilis, positive) 097.1
      - false 795.6
- **Testicle, testicular, testis** — *see also* condition
  - feminization (syndrome) 259.5 ▲
- **Tetanus, tetanic** (cephalic) (convulsions) 037
  - with
    - abortion — *see* Abortion, by type, with sepsis
    - ectopic pregnancy (*see also* categories 633.0-633.9) 639.0
    - molar pregnancy (*see* categories 630-632) 639.0
  - following
    - abortion 639.0
    - ectopic or molar pregnancy 639.0
  - inoculation V03.7
    - reaction (due to serum) — *see* Complications, vaccination
  - neonatorum 771.3
  - puerperal, postpartum, childbirth 670.0 ☑
- **Tetany, tetanic** 781.7
  - alkalosis 276.3
  - associated with rickets 268.0
  - convulsions 781.7
    - hysterical 300.11
  - functional (hysterical) 300.11
- **Tetany, tetanic** — *continued*
  - hyperkinetic 781.7
    - hysterical 300.11
  - hyperpnea 786.01
    - hysterical 300.11
    - psychogenic 306.1
  - hyperventilation 786.01
    - hysterical 300.11
    - psychogenic 306.1
  - hypocalcemic, neonatal 775.4
  - hysterical 300.11
  - neonatal 775.4
  - parathyroid (gland) 252.1
  - parathyroprival 252.1
  - postoperative 252.1
  - postthyroidectomy 252.1
  - pseudotetany 781.7
    - hysterical 300.11
  - psychogenic 306.1
    - specified as conversion reaction 300.11
- **Tetralogy of Fallot** 745.2
- **Tetraplegia** — *see* Quadriplegia
- **Thailand hemorrhagic fever** 065.4
- **Thalassanemia** 282.49
- **Thalassemia** (alpha) (beta) (disease) (Hb-C) (Hb-D) (Hb-E) (Hb-H) (Hb-I) (high fetal gene) (high fetal hemoglobin) (intermedia) (major) (minima) (minor) (mixed) (trait) (with other hemoglobinopathy) 282.49
  - Hb-S (without crisis) 282.41
    - with
      - crisis 282.42
      - vaso-occlusive pain 282.42
  - sickle-cell (without crisis) 282.41
    - with
      - crisis 282.42
      - vaso-occlusive pain 282.42
- **Thalassemic variants** 282.49
- **Thaysen-Gee disease** (nontropical sprue) 579.0
- **Thecoma** (M8600/0) 220
  - malignant (M8600/3) 183.0
- **Thelarche, precocious** 259.1
- **Thelitis** 611.0
  - puerperal, postpartum 675.0 ☑
- **Therapeutic** — *see* condition
- **Therapy** V57.9
  - blood transfusion, without reported diagnosis V58.2
  - breathing V57.0
  - chemotherapy, ▶antineoplastic◀ V58.11 ▲
    - fluoride V07.31
    - prophylactic NEC V07.39
  - dialysis (intermittent) (treatment)
    - extracorporeal V56.0
    - peritoneal V56.8
    - renal V56.0
    - specified type NEC V56.8
  - exercise NEC V57.1
    - breathing V57.0
  - extracorporeal dialysis (renal) V56.0
  - fluoride prophylaxis V07.31
  - hemodialysis V56.0
  - hormone replacement (postmenopausal) V07.4
  - immunotherapy antineoplastic V58.12 ●
  - long term oxygen therapy V46.2
  - occupational V57.21
  - orthoptic V57.4
  - orthotic V57.81
  - peritoneal dialysis V56.8
  - physical NEC V57.1
  - postmenopausal hormone replacement V07.4
  - radiation V58.0
  - speech V57.3
  - vocational V57.22
- **Thermalgesia** 782.0
- **Thermalgia** 782.0
- **Thermanalgesia** 782.0
- **Thermanesthesia** 782.0
- **Thermic** — *see* condition
- **Thermography** (abnormal) 793.9
  - breast 793.89
- **Thermoplegia** 992.0

- **Thesaurismosis**
  - amyloid 277.3
  - bilirubin 277.4
  - calcium 275.40
  - cystine 270.0
  - glycogen (*see also* Disease, glycogen storage) 271.0
  - kerasin 272.7
  - lipoid 272.7
  - melanin 255.4
  - phosphatide 272.7
  - urate 274.9
- **Thiaminic deficiency** 265.1
  - with beriberi 265.0
- **Thibierge-Weissenbach syndrome** (cutaneous systemic sclerosis) 710.1
- **Thickened endometrium** 793.5
- **Thickening**
  - bone 733.99
    - extremity 733.99
  - breast 611.79
  - hymen 623.3
  - larynx 478.79
  - nail 703.8
    - congenital 757.5
  - periosteal 733.99
  - pleura (*see also* Pleurisy) 511.0
  - skin 782.8
  - subepiglottic 478.79
  - tongue 529.8
  - valve, heart — *see* Endocarditis
- **Thiele syndrome** 724.6
- **Thigh** — *see* condition
- **Thinning vertebra** (*see also* Osteoporosis) 733.00
- **Thirst, excessive** 783.5
  - due to deprivation of water 994.3
- **Thomsen's disease** 359.2
- **Thomson's disease** (congenital poikiloderma) 757.33
- **Thoracic** — *see also* condition
  - kidney 753.3
  - outlet syndrome 353.0
  - stomach — *see* Hernia, diaphragm
- **Thoracogastroschisis** (congenital) 759.89
- **Thoracopagus** 759.4
- **Thoracoschisis** 756.3
- **Thoracoscopic surgical procedure converted to open procedure** V64.42
- **Thorax** — *see* condition
- **Thorn's syndrome** (*see also* Disease, renal) 593.9
- **Thornwaldt's, Tornwaldt's**
  - bursitis (pharyngeal) 478.29
  - cyst 478.26
  - disease (pharyngeal bursitis) 478.29
- **Thorson-Biörck syndrome** (malignant carcinoid) 259.2
- **Threadworm** (infection) (infestation) 127.4
- **Threatened**
  - abortion or miscarriage 640.0 ☑
    - with subsequent abortion (*see also* Abortion, spontaneous) 634.9 ☑
    - affecting fetus 762.1
  - labor 644.1 ☑
    - affecting fetus or newborn 761.8
    - premature 644.0 ☑
  - miscarriage 640.0 ☑
    - affecting fetus 762.1
  - premature
    - delivery 644.2 ☑
      - affecting fetus or newborn 761.8
    - labor 644.0 ☑
      - before 22 completed weeks gestation 640.0 ☑
- **Three-day fever** 066.0
- **Threshers' lung** 495.0
- **Thrix annulata** (congenital) 757.4
- **Throat** — *see* condition
- **Thrombasthenia** (Glanzmann's) (hemorrhagic) (hereditary) 287.1
- **Thromboangiitis** 443.1
  - obliterans (general) 443.1
    - cerebral 437.1
    - vessels
      - brain 437.1
      - spinal cord 437.1
- **Thromboarteritis** — *see* Arteritis
- **Thromboasthenia** (Glanzmann's) (hemorrhagic) (hereditary) 287.1
- **Thrombocytasthenia** (Glanzmann's) 287.1
- **Thrombocythemia** (essential) (hemorrhagic) (primary) (M9962/1) 238.7
  - idiopathic (M9962/1) 238.7
- **Thrombocytopathy** (dystrophic) (granulopenic) 287.1
- **Thrombocytopenia, thrombocytopenic** 287.5
  - with
    - absent radii (TAR) syndrome 287.33 ●
    - giant hemangioma 287.39 ●
  - amegakaryocytic, congenital 287.33 ▲
  - congenital 287.33 ▲
  - cyclic 287.39 ▲
  - dilutional 287.4
  - due to
    - drugs 287.4
    - extracorporeal circulation of blood 287.4
    - massive blood transfusion 287.4
    - platelet alloimmunization 287.4
  - essential 287.30 ▲
  - hereditary 287.33 ▲
  - Kasabach-Merritt 287.39 ▲
  - neonatal, transitory 776.1
    - due to
      - exchange transfusion 776.1
      - idiopathic maternal thrombocytopenia 776.1
      - isoimmunization 776.1
  - primary 287.30 ▲
  - puerperal, postpartum 666.3 ☑
  - purpura (*see also* Purpura, thrombocytopenic) 287.30 ▲
    - thrombotic 446.6
  - secondary 287.4
  - sex-linked 287.39 ▲
- **Thrombocytosis, essential** 289.9
- **Thromboembolism** — *see* Embolism
- **Thrombopathy** (Bernard-Soulier) 287.1
  - constitutional 286.4
  - Willebrand-Jürgens (angiohemophilia) 286.4
- **Thrombopenia** (*see also* Thrombocytopenia) 287.5
- **Thrombophlebitis** 451.9
  - antecubital vein 451.82
  - antepartum (superficial) 671.2 ☑
    - affecting fetus or newborn 760.3
    - deep 671.3 ☑
  - arm 451.89
    - deep 451.83
    - superficial 451.82
  - breast, superficial 451.89
  - cavernous (venous) sinus — *see* Thrombophlebitis, intracranial venous sinus
  - cephalic vein 451.82
  - cerebral (sinus) (vein) 325
    - late effect — *see* category 326
    - nonpyogenic 437.6
      - in pregnancy or puerperium 671.5 ☑
      - late effect — *see* Late effect(s) (of) cerebrovascular disease
  - due to implanted device — *see* Complications, due to (presence of) any device, implant or graft classified to 996.0-996.5 NEC
  - during or resulting from a procedure NEC 997.2
  - femoral 451.11
  - femoropopliteal 451.19
  - following infusion, perfusion, or transfusion 999.2
  - hepatic (vein) 451.89
  - idiopathic, recurrent 453.1
  - iliac vein 451.81
  - iliofemoral 451.11
  - intracranial venous sinus (any) 325
    - late effect — *see* category 326
    - nonpyogenic 437.6
      - in pregnancy or puerperium 671.5 ☑
      - late effect — *see* Late effect(s) (of) cerebrovascular disease
  - jugular vein 451.89
  - lateral (venous) sinus — *see* Thrombophlebitis, intracranial venous sinus
  - leg 451.2
    - deep (vessels) 451.19
      - femoral vein 451.11
      - specified vessel NEC 451.19
    - superficial (vessels) 451.0
      - femoral vein 451.11
  - longitudinal (venous) sinus — *see* Thrombophlebitis, intracranial venous sinus
  - lower extremity 451.2
    - deep (vessels) 451.19
      - femoral vein 451.11
      - specified vessel NEC 451.19
    - superficial (vessels) 451.0
  - migrans, migrating 453.1
  - pelvic
    - with
      - abortion — *see* Abortion, by type, with sepsis
      - ectopic pregnancy (*see also* categories 633.0-633.9) 639.0
      - molar pregnancy (*see also* categories 630-632) 639.0
    - following
      - abortion 639.0
      - ectopic or molar pregnancy 639.0
    - puerperal 671.4 ☑
  - popliteal vein 451.19
  - portal (vein) 572.1
  - postoperative 997.2
  - pregnancy (superficial) 671.2 ☑
    - affecting fetus or newborn 760.3
    - deep 671.3 ☑
  - puerperal, postpartum, childbirth (extremities) (superficial) 671.2 ☑
    - deep 671.4 ☑
    - pelvic 671.4 ☑
    - specified site NEC 671.5 ☑
  - radial vein 451.83
  - saphenous (greater) (lesser) 451.0
  - sinus (intracranial) — *see* Thrombophlebitis, intracranial venous sinus
    - specified site NEC 451.89
    - tibial vein 451.19
- **Thrombosis, thrombotic** (marantic) (multiple) (progressive) (septic) (vein) (vessel) 453.9
  - with childbirth or during the puerperium — *see* Thrombosis, puerperal, postpartum
  - antepartum — *see* Thrombosis, pregnancy
  - aorta, aortic 444.1
    - abdominal 444.0
    - bifurcation 444.0
    - saddle 444.0
    - terminal 444.0
    - thoracic 444.1
    - valve — *see* Endocarditis, aortic
  - apoplexy (*see also* Thrombosis, brain) 434.0 ☑
    - late effect — *see* Late effect(s) (of) cerebrovascular disease
  - appendix, septic — *see* Appendicitis, acute
  - arteriolar-capillary platelet, disseminated 446.6
  - artery, arteries (postinfectional) 444.9
    - auditory, internal 433.8 ☑
    - basilar (*see also* Occlusion, artery, basilar) 433.0 ☑
    - carotid (common) (internal) (*see also* Occlusion, artery, carotid) 433.1 ☑
      - with other precerebral artery 433.3 ☑
    - cerebellar (anterior inferior) (posterior inferior) (superior) 433.8 ☑
    - cerebral (*see also* Thrombosis, brain) 434.0 ☑
    - choroidal (anterior) 433.8 ☑
    - communicating posterior 433.8 ☑
    - coronary (*see also* Infarct, myocardium) 410.9 ☑
      - without myocardial infarction 411.81
      - due to syphilis 093.89

Thrombophlebitis — *continued*
- artery, arteries — *continued*
  - coronary (*see also* Infarct, myocardium) — *continued*
    - healed or specified as old 412
  - extremities 444.22
    - lower 444.22
    - upper 444.21
  - femoral 444.22
  - hepatic 444.89
  - hypophyseal 433.8 ☑
  - meningeal, anterior or posterior 433.8 ☑
  - mesenteric (with gangrene) 557.0
  - ophthalmic (*see also* Occlusion, retina) 362.30
  - pontine 433.8 ☑
  - popliteal 444.22
  - precerebral — *see* Occlusion, artery, precerebral NEC
  - pulmonary 415.19
    - iatrogenic 415.11
    - postoperative 415.11
  - renal 593.81
  - retinal (*see also* Occlusion, retina) 362.30
  - specified site NEC 444.89
  - spinal, anterior or posterior 433.8 ☑
  - traumatic (complication) (early) (*see also* Injury, blood vessel, by site) 904.9
  - vertebral (*see also* Occlusion, artery, vertebral) 433.2 ☑
    - with other precerebral artery 433.3 ☑
- atrial (endocardial) 424.90
  - due to syphilis 093.89
- auricular (*see also* Infarct, myocardium) 410.9 ☑
- axillary (vein) 453.8
- basilar (artery) (*see also* Occlusion, artery, basilar) 433.0 ☑
- bland NEC 453.9
- brain (artery) (stem) 434.0 ☑
  - due to syphilis 094.89
  - iatrogenic 997.02
  - late effect — *see* Late effect(s) (of) cerebrovascular disease
  - postoperative 997.02
  - puerperal, postpartum, childbirth 674.0 ☑
  - sinus (*see also* Thrombosis, intracranial venous sinus) 325
- capillary 448.9
  - arteriolar, generalized 446.6
- cardiac (*see also* Infarct, myocardium) 410.9 ☑
  - due to syphilis 093.89
  - healed or specified as old 412
  - valve — *see* Endocarditis
- carotid (artery) (common) (internal) (*see also* Occlusion, artery, carotid) 433.1 ☑
  - with other precerebral artery 433.3 ☑
- cavernous sinus (venous) — *see* Thrombosis, intracranial venous sinus
- cerebellar artery (anterior inferior) (posterior inferior) (superior) 433.8 ☑
  - late effect — *see* Late effect(s) (of) cerebrovascular disease
- cerebral (arteries) (*see also* Thrombosis, brain) 434.0 ☑
  - late effect — *see* Late effect(s) (of) cerebrovascular disease
- coronary (artery) (*see also* Infarct, myocardium) 410.9 ☑
  - without myocardial infarction 411.81
  - due to syphilis 093.89
  - healed or specified as old 412
- corpus cavernosum 607.82
- cortical (*see also* Thrombosis, brain) 434.0 ☑
- due to (presence of) any device, implant, or graft classifiable to 996.0-996.5 — *see* Complications, due to (presence of) any device, implant, or graft classifiable to 996.0-996.5 NEC
- effort 453.8
- endocardial — *see* Infarct, myocardium
- eye (*see also* Occlusion, retina) 362.30
- femoral (vein) 453.8
  - with inflammation or phlebitis 451.11
  - artery 444.22
  - deep 453.41
- genital organ, male 608.83

Thrombosis, thrombotic — *continued*
- heart (chamber) (*see also* Infarct, myocardium) 410.9 ☑
- hepatic (vein) 453.0
  - artery 444.89
  - infectional or septic 572.1
- iliac (vein) 453.8
  - with inflammation or phlebitis 451.81
  - artery (common) (external) (internal) 444.81
- inflammation, vein — *see* Thrombophlebitis
- internal carotid artery (*see also* Occlusion, artery, carotid) 433.1 ☑
  - with other precerebral artery 433.3 ☑
- intestine (with gangrene) 557.0
- intracranial (*see also* Thrombosis, brain) 434.0 ☑
  - venous sinus (any) 325
    - nonpyogenic origin 437.6
      - in pregnancy or puerperium 671.5 ☑
- intramural (*see also* Infarct, myocardium) 410.9 ☑
  - without
    - cardiac condition 429.89
    - coronary artery disease 429.89
    - myocardial infarction 429.89
  - healed or specified as old 412
- jugular (bulb) 453.8
- kidney 593.81
  - artery 593.81
- lateral sinus (venous) — *see* Thrombosis, intracranial venous sinus
- leg 453.8
  - with inflammation or phlebitis — *see* Thrombophlebitis
  - deep (vessels) 453.40
    - lower (distal) 453.42
    - upper (proximal) 453.41
  - superficial (vessels) 453.8
- liver (venous) 453.0
  - artery 444.89
  - infectional or septic 572.1
  - portal vein 452
- longitudinal sinus (venous) — *see* Thrombosis, intracranial venous sinus
- lower extremity 453.8
  - deep vessels 453.40
    - calf 453.42
    - distal (lower leg) 453.42
    - femoral 453.41
    - iliac 453.41
    - lower leg 453.42
    - peroneal 453.42
    - popliteal 453.41
    - proximal (upper leg) 453.41
    - thigh 453.41
    - tibial 453.42
- lung 415.19
  - iatrogenic 415.11
  - postoperative 415.11
- marantic, dural sinus 437.6
- meninges (brain) (*see also* Thrombosis, brain) 434.0 ☑
- mesenteric (artery) (with gangrene) 557.0
  - vein (inferior) (superior) 557.0
- mitral — see Insufficiency, mitral
- mural (heart chamber) (*see also* Infarct, myocardium) 410.9 ☑
  - without
    - cardiac condition 429.89
    - coronary artery disease 429.89
    - myocardial infarction 429.89
  - due to syphilis 093.89
  - following myocardial infarction 429.79
  - healed or specified as old 412
- omentum (with gangrene) 557.0
- ophthalmic (artery) (*see also* Occlusion, retina) 362.30
- pampiniform plexus (male) 608.83
  - female 620.8
- parietal (*see also* Infarct, myocardium) 410.9 ☑
- penis, penile 607.82
- peripheral arteries 444.22
  - lower 444.22
  - upper 444.21
- platelet 446.6
- portal 452
  - due to syphilis 093.89

Thrombosis, thrombotic — *continued*
- portal — *continued*
  - infectional or septic 572.1
- precerebral artery — *see also* Occlusion, artery, precerebral NEC
- pregnancy 671.9 ☑
  - deep (vein) 671.3 ☑
  - superficial (vein) 671.2 ☑
- puerperal, postpartum, childbirth 671.9 ☑
  - brain (artery) 674.0 ☑
    - venous 671.5 ☑
  - cardiac 674.8 ☑
  - cerebral (artery) 674.0 ☑
    - venous 671.5 ☑
  - deep (vein) 671.4 ☑
  - intracranial sinus (nonpyogenic) (venous) 671.5 ☑
  - pelvic 671.4 ☑
  - pulmonary (artery) 673.2 ☑
  - specified site NEC 671.5 ☑
  - superficial 671.2 ☑
- pulmonary (artery) (vein) 415.19
  - iatrogenic 415.11
  - postoperative 415.11
- renal (artery) 593.81
  - vein 453.3
- resulting from presence of shunt or other internal prosthetic device — *see* Complications, due to (presence of) any device, implant, or graft classifiable to 996.0-996.5 NEC
- retina, retinal (artery) 362.30
  - arterial branch 362.32
  - central 362.31
  - partial 362.33
  - vein
    - central 362.35
    - tributary (branch) 362.36
- scrotum 608.83
- seminal vesicle 608.83
- sigmoid (venous) sinus (*see* Thrombosis, intracranial venous sinus) 325
- silent NEC 453.9
- sinus, intracranial (venous) (any) (*see also* Thrombosis, intracranial venous sinus) 325
- softening, brain (*see also* Thrombosis, brain) 434.0 ☑
- specified site NEC 453.8
- spermatic cord 608.83
- spinal cord 336.1
  - due to syphilis 094.89
  - in pregnancy or puerperium 671.5 ☑
  - pyogenic origin 324.1
    - late effect — *see* category 326
- spleen, splenic 289.59
  - artery 444.89
- testis 608.83
- traumatic (complication) (early) (*see also* Injury, blood vessel, by site) 904.9
- tricuspid — *see* Endocarditis, tricuspid
- tumor — *see* Neoplasm, by site ●
- tunica vaginalis 608.83
- umbilical cord (vessels) 663.6 ☑
  - affecting fetus or newborn 762.6
- vas deferens 608.83
- vein
  - deep 453.40 ▲
  - lower extremity — see Thrombosis, lower extremity
- vena cava (inferior) (superior) 453.2

Thrombus — *see* Thrombosis

Thrush 112.0
- newborn 771.7

Thumb — *see also* condition
- gamekeeper's 842.12
- sucking (child problem) 307.9

Thygeson's superficial punctate keratitis 370.21

Thymergasia (*see also* Psychosis, affective) 296.80

Thymitis 254.8

Thymoma (benign) (M8580/0) 212.6
- malignant (M8580/3) 164.0

Thymus, thymic (gland) — *see* condition

Tuberculosis, tubercular, tuberculous — *continued*
- scrofulous 017.2 ☑
- scrotum 016.5 ☑
- seminal tract or vesicle 016.5 ☑ *[608.81]*
- senile NEC (*see also* Tuberculosis, pulmonary) 011.9 ☑
- septic NEC (*see also* Tuberculosis, miliary) 018.9 ☑
- shoulder 015.8 ☑
  - blade 015.7 ☑ *[730.8]* ☑
- sigmoid 014.8 ☑
- sinus (accessory) (nasal) 012.8 ☑
  - bone 015.7 ☑ *[730.88]*
  - epididymis 016.4 ☑
- skeletal NEC (*see also* Osteomyelitis, due to tuberculosis) 015.9 ☑ *[730.8]* ☑
- skin (any site) (primary) 017.0 ☑
- small intestine 014.8 ☑
- soft palate 017.9 ☑
- spermatic cord 016.5 ☑
- spinal
  - column 015.0 ☑ *[730.88]*
  - cord 013.4 ☑
  - disease 015.0 ☑ *[730.88]*
  - medulla 013.4 ☑
  - membrane 013.0 ☑
  - meninges 013.0 ☑
- spine 015.0 ☑ *[730.88]*
- spleen 017.7 ☑
- splenitis 017.7 ☑
- spondylitis 015.0 ☑ *[720.81]*
- spontaneous pneumothorax — *see* Tuberculosis, pulmonary
- sternoclavicular joint 015.8 ☑
- stomach 017.9 ☑
- stonemasons' 011.4 ☑
- struma 017.2 ☑
- subcutaneous tissue (cellular) (primary) 017.0 ☑
- subcutis (primary) 017.0 ☑
- subdeltoid bursa 017.9 ☑
- submaxillary 017.9 ☑
  - region 017.9 ☑
- supraclavicular gland 017.2 ☑
- suprarenal (capsule) (gland) 017.6 ☑
- swelling, joint (*see also* Tuberculosis, joint) 015.9 ☑
- symphysis pubis 015.7 ☑ *[730.88]*
- synovitis 015.9 ☑ *[727.01]*
  - hip 015.1 ☑ *[727.01]*
  - knee 015.2 ☑ *[727.01]*
  - specified site NEC 015.8 ☑ *[727.01]*
  - spine or vertebra 015.0 ☑ *[727.01]*
- systemic — *see* Tuberculosis, miliary
- tarsitis (eyelid) 017.0 ☑ *[373.4]*
  - ankle (bone) 015.5 ☑ *[730.87]*
- tendon (sheath) — *see* Tuberculosis, tenosynovitis
- tenosynovitis 015.9 ☑ *[727.01]*
  - hip 015.1 ☑ *[727.01]*
  - knee 015.2 ☑ *[727.01]*
  - specified site NEC 015.8 ☑ *[727.01]*
  - spine or vertebra 015.0 ☑ *[727.01]*
- testis 016.5 ☑ *[608.81]*
- throat 012.8 ☑
- thymus gland 017.9 ☑
- thyroid gland 017.5 ☑
- toe 017.9 ☑
- tongue 017.9 ☑
- tonsil (lingual) 012.8 ☑
- tonsillitis 012.8 ☑
- trachea, tracheal 012.8 ☑
  - gland 012.1 ☑
    - primary, progressive 010.8 ☑
  - isolated 012.2 ☑
- tracheobronchial 011.3 ☑
  - glandular 012.1 ☑
    - primary, progressive 010.8 ☑
  - isolated 012.2 ☑
  - lymph gland or node 012.1 ☑
    - primary, progressive 010.8 ☑
- tubal 016.6 ☑
- tunica vaginalis 016.5 ☑
- typhlitis 014.8 ☑
- ulcer (primary) (skin) 017.0 ☑
  - bowel or intestine 014.8 ☑

Tuberculosis, tubercular, tuberculous — *continued*
- ulcer — *continued*
  - specified site NEC — *see* Tuberculosis, by site
- unspecified site — *see* Tuberculosis, pulmonary
- ureter 016.2 ☑
- urethra, urethral 016.3 ☑
- urinary organ or tract 016.3 ☑
  - kidney 016.0 ☑
- uterus 016.7 ☑
- uveal tract 017.3 ☑ *[363.13]*
- uvula 017.9 ☑
- vaccination, prophylactic (against) V03.2
- vagina 016.7 ☑
- vas deferens 016.5 ☑
- vein 017.9 ☑
- verruca (primary) 017.0 ☑
- verrucosa (cutis) (primary) 017.0 ☑
- vertebra (column) 015.0 ☑ *[730.88]*
- vesiculitis 016.5 ☑ *[608.81]*
- viscera NEC 014.8 ☑
- vulva 016.7 ☑ *[616.51]*
- wrist (joint) 015.8 ☑
  - bone 015.5 ☑ *[730.83]*

Tuberculum
- auriculae 744.29
- occlusal 520.2
- paramolare 520.2

Tuberous sclerosis (brain) 759.5

Tubo-ovarian — *see* condition

Tuboplasty, after previous sterilization V26.0

Tubotympanitis 381.10

Tularemia 021.9
- with
  - conjunctivitis 021.3
  - pneumonia 021.2
- bronchopneumonic 021.2
- conjunctivitis 021.3
- cryptogenic 021.1
- disseminated 021.8
- enteric 021.1
- generalized 021.8
- glandular 021.8
- intestinal 021.1
- oculoglandular 021.3
- ophthalmic 021.3
- pneumonia 021.2
- pulmonary 021.2
- specified NEC 021.8
- typhoidal 021.1
- ulceroglandular 021.0
- vaccination, prophylactic (against) V03.4

Tularensis conjunctivitis 021.3

Tumefaction — *see also* Swelling
- liver (*see also* Hypertrophy, liver) 789.1

Tumor (M8000/1) — *see also* Neoplasm, by site, unspecified nature
- Abrikossov's (M9580/0) — *see also* Neoplasm, connective tissue, benign
  - malignant (M9580/3) — *see* Neoplasm, connective tissue, malignant
- acinar cell (M8550/1) — *see* Neoplasm, by site, uncertain behavior
- acinic cell (M8550/1) — *see* Neoplasm, by site, uncertain behavior
- adenomatoid (M9054/0) — *see also* Neoplasm, by site, benign
  - odontogenic (M9300/0) 213.1
    - upper jaw (bone) 213.0
- adnexal (skin) (M8390/0) — *see* Neoplasm, skin, benign
- adrenal
  - cortical (benign) (M8370/0) 227.0
    - malignant (M8370/3) 194.0
  - rest (M8671/0) — *see* Neoplasm, by site, benign
- alpha cell (M8152/0)
  - malignant (M8152/3)
    - pancreas 157.4
    - specified site NEC — *see* Neoplasm, by site, malignant
    - unspecified site 157.4
  - pancreas 211.7

Tumor (M8000/1) — *see also* Neoplasm, by site, unspecified nature — *continued*
- alpha cell (M8152/0) — *continued*
  - specified site NEC — *see* Neoplasm, by site, benign
  - unspecified site 211.7
- aneurysmal (*see also* Aneurysm) 442.9
- aortic body (M8691/1) 237.3
  - malignant (M8691/3) 194.6
- argentaffin (M8241/1) — *see* Neoplasm, by site, uncertain behavior
- basal cell (M8090/1) — *see also* Neoplasm, skin, uncertain behavior
- benign (M8000/0) — *see* Neoplasm, by site, benign
- beta cell (M8151/0)
  - malignant (M8151/3)
    - pancreas 157.4
    - specified site — *see* Neoplasm, by site, malignant
    - unspecified site 157.4
  - pancreas 211.7
  - specified site NEC — *see* Neoplasm, by site, benign
  - unspecified site 211.7
- blood — *see* Hematoma
- Brenner (M9000/0) 220
  - borderline malignancy (M9000/1) 236.2
  - malignant (M9000/3) 183.0
  - proliferating (M9000/1) 236.2
- Brooke's (M8100/0) — *see* Neoplasm, skin, benign
- brown fat (M8880/0) — *see* Lipoma, by site
- Burkitt's (M9750/3) 200.2 ☑
- calcifying epithelial odontogenic (M9340/0) 213.1
  - upper jaw (bone) 213.0
- carcinoid (M8240/1) — *see* Carcinoid
- carotid body (M8692/1) 237.3
  - malignant (M8692/3) 194.5
- Castleman's (mediastinal lymph node hyperplasia) 785.6
- cells (M8001/1) — *see also* Neoplasm, by site, unspecified nature
  - benign (M8001/0) — *see* Neoplasm, by site, benign
  - malignant (M8001/3) — *see* Neoplasm, by site, malignant
  - uncertain whether benign or malignant (M8001/1) — *see* Neoplasm, by site, uncertain nature
- cervix
  - in pregnancy or childbirth 654.6 ☑
    - affecting fetus or newborn 763.89
    - causing obstructed labor 660.2 ☑
      - affecting fetus or newborn 763.1
- chondromatous giant cell (M9230/0) — *see* Neoplasm, bone, benign
- chromaffin (M8700/0) — *see also* Neoplasm, by site, benign
  - malignant (M8700/3) — *see* Neoplasm, by site, malignant
- Cock's peculiar 706.2
- Codman's (benign chondroblastoma) (M9230/0) — *see* Neoplasm, bone, benign
- dentigerous, mixed (M9282/0) 213.1
  - upper jaw (bone) 213.0
- dermoid (M9084/0) — *see* Neoplasm, by site, benign
  - with malignant transformation (M9084/3) 183.0
- desmoid (extra-abdominal) (M8821/1) — *see also* Neoplasm, connective tissue, uncertain behavior
  - abdominal (M8822/1) — *see* Neoplasm, connective tissue, uncertain behavior
- embryonal (mixed) (M9080/1) — *see also* Neoplasm, by site, uncertain behavior
  - liver (M9080/3) 155.0
- endodermal sinus (M9071/3)
  - specified site — *see* Neoplasm, by site, malignant
  - unspecified site
    - female 183.0
    - male 186.9

☑ Additional Digit Required — Refer to the Tabular List (Numeric Code Section) for Additional Digit Selection

▶◀ Revised Text ● New Line ▲ Revised Code

- **Tumor** (M8000/1) — *see also* Neoplasm, by site, unspecified nature — *continued*
  - stromal — *continued*
    - stomach 238.1
      - benign 215.5
      - malignant 171.5
      - uncertain behavior 238.1
  - superior sulcus (lung) (pulmonary) (syndrome) (M8010/3) 162.3
  - suprasulcus (M8010/3) 162.3
  - sweat gland (M8400/1) — *see also* Neoplasm, skin, uncertain behavior
    - benign (M8400/0) — *see* Neoplasm, skin, benign
    - malignant (M8400/3) — *see* Neoplasm, skin, malignant
  - syphilitic brain 094.89
    - congenital 090.49
  - testicular stromal (M8590/1) 236.4
  - theca cell (M8600/0) 220
  - theca cell-granulosa cell (M8621/1) 236.2
  - theca-lutein (M8610/0) 220
  - turban (M8200/0) 216.4
  - uterus
    - in pregnancy or childbirth 654.1 ☑
      - affecting fetus or newborn 763.89
      - causing obstructed labor 660.2 ☑
        - affecting fetus or newborn 763.1
  - vagina
    - in pregnancy or childbirth 654.7 ☑
      - affecting fetus or newborn 763.89
      - causing obstructed labor 660.2 ☑
        - affecting fetus or newborn 763.1
  - varicose (*see also* Varicose, vein) 454.9
  - von Recklinghausen's (M9540/1) 237.71
  - vulva
    - in pregnancy or childbirth 654.8 ☑
      - affecting fetus or newborn 763.89
      - causing obstructed labor 660.2 ☑
        - affecting fetus or newborn 763.1
  - Warthin's (salivary gland) (M8561/0) 210.2
  - white — *see also* Tuberculosis, arthritis
  - White-Darier 757.39
  - Wilms' (nephroblastoma) (M8960/3) 189.0
  - yolk sac (M9071/3)
    - specified site — *see* Neoplasm, by site, malignant
    - unspecified site
      - female 183.0
      - male 186.9
- **Tumorlet (M8040/1)** — *see* Neoplasm, by site, uncertain behavior
- **Tungiasis** 134.1
- **Tunica vasculosa lentis** 743.39
- **Tunnel vision** 368.45
- **Turban tumor** (M8200/0) 216.4
- **Türck's trachoma** (chronic catarrhal laryngitis) 476.0
- **Türk's syndrome** (ocular retraction syndrome) 378.71
- **Turner's**
  - hypoplasia (tooth) 520.4
  - syndrome 758.6
  - tooth 520.4
- **Turner-Kieser syndrome** (hereditary osteo-onychodysplasia) 756.89
- **Turner-Varny syndrome** 758.6
- **Turricephaly** 756.0
- **Tussis convulsiva** (*see also* Whooping cough) 033.9
- **Twin**
  - affected by maternal complications of pregnancy 761.5
  - conjoined 759.4
  - healthy liveborn — *see* Newborn, twin
  - pregnancy (complicating delivery) NEC 651.0 ☑
    - with fetal loss and retention of one fetus 651.3 ☑
    - following (elective) fetal reduction 651.7 ☑ ●
- **Twinning, teeth** 520.2
- **Twist, twisted**
  - bowel, colon, or intestine 560.2
  - hair (congenital) 757.4
- **Twist, twisted** — *continued*
  - mesentery 560.2
  - omentum 560.2
  - organ or site, congenital NEC — *see* Anomaly, specified type NEC
  - ovarian pedicle 620.5
    - congenital 752.0
  - umbilical cord — *see* Compression, umbilical cord
- **Twitch** 781.0
- **Tylosis** 700
  - buccalis 528.6
  - gingiva 523.8
  - linguae 528.6
  - palmaris et plantaris 757.39
- **Tympanism** 787.3
- **Tympanites** (abdominal) (intestine) 787.3
- **Tympanitis** — *see* Myringitis
- **Tympanosclerosis** 385.00
  - involving
    - combined sites NEC 385.09
      - with tympanic membrane 385.03
    - tympanic membrane 385.01
      - with ossicles 385.02
        - and middle ear 385.03
- **Tympanum** — *see* condition
- **Tympany**
  - abdomen 787.3
  - chest 786.7
- **Typhlitis** (*see also* Appendicitis) 541
- **Typhoenteritis** 002.0
- **Typhogastric fever** 002.0
- **Typhoid** (abortive) (ambulant) (any site) (fever) (hemorrhagic) (infection) (intermittent) (malignant) (rheumatic) 002.0
  - with pneumonia 002.0 *[484.8]*
  - abdominal 002.0
  - carrier (suspected) of V02.1
  - cholecystitis (current) 002.0
  - clinical (Widal and blood test negative) 002.0
  - endocarditis 002.0 *[421.1]*
  - inoculation reaction — *see* Complications, vaccination
  - meningitis 002.0 *[320.7]*
  - mesenteric lymph nodes 002.0
  - myocarditis 002.0 *[422.0]*
  - osteomyelitis (*see also* Osteomyelitis, due to, typhoid) 002.0 *[730.8]* ☑
  - perichondritis, larynx 002.0 *[478.71]*
  - pneumonia 002.0 *[484.8]*
  - spine 002.0 *[720.81]*
  - ulcer (perforating) 002.0
  - vaccination, prophylactic (against) V03.1
  - Widal negative 002.0
- **Typhomalaria** (fever) (*see also* Malaria) 084.6
- **Typhomania** 002.0
- **Typhoperitonitis** 002.0
- **Typhus** (fever) 081.9
  - abdominal, abdominalis 002.0
  - African tick 082.1
  - amarillic (*see also* Fever, Yellow) 060.9
  - brain 081.9
  - cerebral 081.9
  - classical 080
  - endemic (flea-borne) 081.0
  - epidemic (louse-borne) 080
  - exanthematic NEC 080
  - exanthematicus SAI 080
    - brillii SAI 081.1
    - Mexicanus SAI 081.0
    - pediculo vestimenti causa 080
    - typhus murinus 081.0
  - flea-borne 081.0
  - Indian tick 082.1
  - Kenya tick 082.1
  - louse-borne 080
  - Mexican 081.0
    - flea-borne 081.0
    - louse-borne 080
    - tabardillo 080
  - mite-borne 081.2
  - murine 081.0
  - North Asian tick-borne 082.2
  - petechial 081.9
- **Typhus** — *continued*
  - Queensland tick 082.3
  - rat 081.0
  - recrudescent 081.1
  - recurrent (*see also* Fever, relapsing) 087.9
  - São Paulo 082.0
  - scrub (China) (India) (Malaya) (New Guinea) 081.2
  - shop (of Malaya) 081.0
  - Siberian tick 082.2
  - tick-borne NEC 082.9
  - tropical 081.2
  - vaccination, prophylactic (against) V05.8
- **Tyrosinemia** 270.2
  - neonatal 775.8
- **Tyrosinosis** (Medes) (Sakai) 270.2
- **Tyrosinuria** 270.2
- **Tyrosyluria** 270.2

U

- **Uehlinger's syndrome** (acropachyderma) 757.39
- **Uhl's anomaly or disease** (hypoplasia of myocardium, right ventricle) 746.84
- **Ulcer, ulcerated, ulcerating, ulceration, ulcerative** 707.9
  - with gangrene 707.9 *[785.4]*
  - abdomen (wall) (*see also* Ulcer, skin) 707.8
  - ala, nose 478.1
  - alveolar process 526.5
  - amebic (intestine) 006.9
    - skin 006.6
  - anastomotic — *see* Ulcer, gastrojejunal
  - anorectal 569.41
  - antral — *see* Ulcer, stomach
  - anus (sphincter) (solitary) 569.41
    - varicose — *see* Varicose, ulcer, anus
  - aphthous (oral) (recurrent) 528.2
    - genital organ(s)
      - female 616.8
      - male 608.89
    - mouth 528.2
  - arm (*see also* Ulcer, skin) 707.8
  - arteriosclerotic plaque — *see* Arteriosclerosis, by site
  - artery NEC 447.2
    - without rupture 447.8
  - atrophic NEC — *see* Ulcer, skin
  - Barrett's (chronic peptic ulcer of esophagus) 530.85
  - bile duct 576.8
  - bladder (solitary) (sphincter) 596.8
    - bilharzial (*see also* Schistosomiasis) 120.9 *[595.4]*
    - submucosal (*see also* Cystitis) 595.1
    - tuberculous (*see also* Tuberculosis) 016.1 ☑
  - bleeding NEC — *see* Ulcer, peptic, with hemorrhage
  - bone 730.9 ☑
  - bowel (*see also* Ulcer, intestine) 569.82
  - breast 611.0
  - bronchitis 491.8
  - bronchus 519.1
  - buccal (cavity) (traumatic) 528.9
  - burn (acute) — *see* Ulcer, duodenum
  - Buruli 031.1
  - buttock (*see also* Ulcer, skin) 707.8
    - decubitus (*see also* Ulcer, decubitus) 707.00
  - cancerous (M8000/3) — *see* Neoplasm, by site, malignant
  - cardia — *see* Ulcer, stomach
  - cardio-esophageal (peptic) 530.20
    - with bleeding 530.21
  - cecum (*see also* Ulcer, intestine) 569.82
  - cervix (uteri) (trophic) 622.0
    - with mention of cervicitis 616.0
  - chancroidal 099.0
  - chest (wall) (*see also* Ulcer, skin) 707.8
  - Chiclero 085.4
  - chin (pyogenic) (*see also* Ulcer, skin) 707.8
  - chronic (cause unknown) — *see also* Ulcer, skin
    - penis 607.89
  - Cochin-China 085.1
  - colitis — *see* Colitis, ulcerative

☑ Additional Digit Required — Refer to the Tabular List (Numeric Code Section) for Additional Digit Selection
▶◀ Revised Text ● New Line ▲ Revised Code

V

- **Vaccination**
  - complication or reaction — *see* Complications, vaccination
  - not ▶carried out◀ V64.00 ▲
    - because of
      - acute illness V64.01 ●
      - allergy to vaccine or component V64.04 ●
      - caregiver refusal V64.05 ●
      - chronic illness V64.02 ●
      - immune compromised state V64.03 ●
      - patient had disease being vaccinated against V64.08 ●
      - patient refusal V64.06 ●
      - reason NEC V64.09 ●
      - religious reasons V64.07 ●
  - prophylactic (against) V05.9
    - arthropod-borne viral
      - disease NEC V05.1
      - encephalitis V05.0
    - chickenpox V05.4
    - cholera (alone) V03.0
      - with typhoid-paratyphoid (cholera + TAB) V06.0
    - common cold V04.7
    - diphtheria (alone) V03.5
      - with
        - poliomyelitis (DTP+ polio) V06.3
        - tetanus V06.5
          - pertussis combined (DTP) (DTaP) V06.1
        - typhoid-paratyphoid (DTP + TAB) V06.2
    - disease (single) NEC V05.9
      - bacterial NEC V03.9
        - specified type NEC V03.89
      - combination NEC V06.9
        - specified type NEC V06.8
      - specified type NEC V05.8
    - encephalitis, viral, arthropod-borne V05.0
    - Hemophilus influenzae, type B [Hib] V03.81
    - hepatitis, viral V05.3
    - influenza V04.81
      - with
        - Streptococcus pneumoniae [pneumococcus] V06.6
    - leishmaniasis V05.2
    - measles (alone) V04.2
      - with mumps-rubella (MMR) V06.4
    - mumps (alone) V04.6
      - with measles and rubella (MMR) V06.4
    - pertussis alone V03.6
    - plague V03.3
    - poliomyelitis V04.0
      - with diphtheria-tetanus-pertussis (DTP + polio) V06.3
    - rabies V04.5
    - respiratory syncytial virus (RSV) V04.82
    - rubella (alone) V04.3
      - with measles and mumps (MMR) V06.4
    - smallpox V04.1
    - Streptococcus pneumoniae [pneumococcus] V03.82
      - with
        - influenza V06.6
    - tetanus toxoid (alone) V03.7
      - with diphtheria [Td] [DT] V06.5
        - with
          - pertussis (DTP) (DTaP) V06.1
            - with poliomyelitis (DTP+polio) V06.3
    - tuberculosis (BCG) V03.2
    - tularemia V03.4
    - typhoid-paratyphoid (TAB) (alone) V03.1
      - with diphtheria-tetanus-pertussis (TAB + DTP) V06.2
    - varicella V05.4
    - viral
      - disease NEC V04.89
      - encephalitis, arthropod-borne V05.0
      - hepatitis V05.3
    - yellow fever V04.4
- **Vaccinia** (generalized) 999.0
  - congenital 771.2
  - conjunctiva 999.3
  - eyelids 999.0 *[373.5]*
  - localized 999.3
  - nose 999.3
  - not from vaccination 051.0
    - eyelid 051.0 *[373.5]*
  - sine vaccinatione 051.0
  - without vaccination 051.0
- **Vacuum**
  - extraction of fetus or newborn 763.3
  - in sinus (accessory) (nasal) (*see also* Sinusitis) 473.9
- **Vagabond** V60.0
- **Vagabondage** V60.0
- **Vagabonds' disease** 132.1
- **Vagina, vaginal** — *see* condition
- **Vaginalitis** (tunica) 608.4
- **Vaginismus** (reflex) 625.1
  - functional 306.51
  - hysterical 300.11
  - psychogenic 306.51
- **Vaginitis** (acute) (chronic) (circumscribed) (diffuse) (emphysematous) (Hemophilus vaginalis) (nonspecific) (nonvenereal) (ulcerative) 616.10
  - with
    - abortion — *see* Abortion, by type, with sepsis
    - ectopic pregnancy (*see also* categories 633.0-633.9) 639.0
    - molar pregnancy (*see also* categories 630-632) 639.0
  - adhesive, congenital 752.49
  - atrophic, postmenopausal 627.3
  - bacterial 616.10
  - blennorrhagic (acute) 098.0
    - chronic or duration of 2 months or over 098.2
  - candidal 112.1
  - chlamydial 099.53
  - complicating pregnancy or puerperium 646.6 ☑
    - affecting fetus or newborn 760.8
  - congenital (adhesive) 752.49
  - due to
    - C. albicans 112.1
    - Trichomonas (vaginalis) 131.01
  - following
    - abortion 639.0
    - ectopic or molar pregnancy 639.0
  - gonococcal (acute) 098.0
    - chronic or duration of 2 months or over 098.2
  - granuloma 099.2
  - Monilia 112.1
  - mycotic 112.1
  - pinworm 127.4 *[616.11]*
  - postirradiation 616.10
  - postmenopausal atrophic 627.3
  - senile (atrophic) 627.3
  - syphilitic (early) 091.0
    - late 095.8
  - trichomonal 131.01
  - tuberculous (*see also* Tuberculosis) 016.7 ☑
  - venereal NEC 099.8
- **Vaginosis** — *see* Vaginitis
- **Vagotonia** 352.3
- **Vagrancy** V60.0
- **Vallecula** — *see* condition
- **Valley fever** 114.0
- **Valsuani's disease** (progressive pernicious anemia, puerperal) 648.2 ☑
- **Valve, valvular** (formation) — *see also* condition
  - cerebral ventricle (communicating) in situ V45.2
  - cervix, internal os 752.49
  - colon 751.5
  - congenital NEC — *see* Atresia
  - formation, congenital NEC — *see* Atresia
  - heart defect — *see* Anomaly, heart, valve
  - ureter 753.29
    - pelvic junction 753.21
    - vesical orifice 753.22
  - urethra 753.6
- **Valvulitis** (chronic) (*see also* Endocarditis) 424.90
  - rheumatic (chronic) (inactive) (with chorea) 397.9
    - active or acute (aortic) (mitral) (pulmonary) (tricuspid) 391.1
  - syphilitic NEC 093.20
    - aortic 093.22
    - mitral 093.21
    - pulmonary 093.24
    - tricuspid 093.23
- **Valvulopathy** — *see* Endocarditis
- **van Bogaert's leukoencephalitis** (sclerosing) (subacute) 046.2
- **van Bogaert-Nijssen (-Peiffer) disease** 330.0
- **van Buchem's syndrome** (hyperostosis corticalis) 733.3
- **van Creveld-von Gierke disease** (glycogenosis I) 271.0
- **van den Bergh's disease** (enterogenous cyanosis) 289.7
- **van der Hoeve's syndrome** (brittle bones and blue sclera, deafness) 756.51
- **van der Hoeve-Halbertsma-Waardenburg syndrome** (ptosis-epicanthus) 270.2
- **van der Hoeve-Waardenburg-Gualdi syndrome** (ptosis epicanthus) 270.2
- **Vancomycin** (glycopeptide)
  - intermediate staphylococcus aureus (VISA/GISA) V09.8
  - resistant
    - enterococcus (VRE) V09.8
    - staphylococcus aureus (VRSA/GRSA) V09.8
- **Vanillism** 692.89
- **Vanishing lung** 492.0
- **van Neck (-Odelberg) disease or syndrome** (juvenile osteochondrosis) 732.1
- **Vanishing twin** 651.33
- **Vapor asphyxia or suffocation** NEC 987.9
  - specified agent — *see* Table of Drugs and Chemicals
- **Vaquez's disease** (M9950/1) 238.4
- **Vaquez-Osler disease** (polycythemia vera) (M9950/1) 238.4
- **Variance, lethal ball, prosthetic heart valve** 996.02
- **Variants, thalassemic** 282.49
- **Variations in hair color** 704.3
- **Varicella** 052.9
  - with
    - complication 052.8
      - specified NEC 052.7
    - pneumonia 052.1
    - vaccination and inoculation (against) (prophylactic) V05.4
  - exposure to V01.71
- **Varices** — *see* Varix
- **Varicocele** (scrotum) (thrombosed) 456.4
  - ovary 456.5
  - perineum 456.6
  - spermatic cord (ulcerated) 456.4
- **Varicose**
  - aneurysm (ruptured) (*see also* Aneurysm) 442.9
  - dermatitis (lower extremity) — *see* Varicose, vein, inflamed or infected
  - eczema — *see* Varicose, vein
  - phlebitis — *see* Varicose, vein, inflamed or infected
  - placental vessel — *see* Placenta, abnormal
  - tumor — *see* Varicose, vein
  - ulcer (lower extremity, any part) 454.0
    - anus 455.8
      - external 455.5
      - internal 455.2
    - esophagus (*see also* Varix, esophagus) 456.1
      - bleeding (*see also* Varix, esophagus, bleeding) 456.0
    - inflamed or infected 454.2
    - nasal septum 456.8
    - perineum 456.6
    - rectum — *see* Varicose, ulcer, anus
    - scrotum 456.4
    - specified site NEC 456.8

☑ Additional Digit Required — Refer to the Tabular List (Numeric Code Section) for Additional Digit Selection
▶◀ Revised Text ● New Line ▲ Revised Code

☑ Additional Digit Required — Refer to the Tabular List (Numeric Code Section) for Additional Digit Selection
▶◀ Revised Text ● New Line ▲ Revised Code

W

☑ Additional Digit Required — Refer to the Tabular List (Numeric Code Section) for Additional Digit Selection
▶◀ Revised Text ● New Line ▲ Revised Code

Note — For fracture with open wound, see Fracture.

For laceration, traumatic rupture, tear or penetrating wound of internal organs, such as heart, lung, liver, kidney, pelvic organs, etc., whether or not accompanied by open wound or fracture in the same region, see Injury, internal.

For contused wound, see Contusion. For crush injury, see Crush. For abrasion, insect bite (nonvenomous), blister, or scratch, see Injury, superficial.

Complicated includes wounds with:
  delayed healing
  delayed treatment
  foreign body
  primary infection

For late effect of open wound, see Late, effect, wound, open, by site.

☑ Additional Digit Required — Refer to the Tabular List (Numeric Code Section) for Additional Digit Selection
▶◀ Revised Text ● New Line ▲ Revised Code

Note — Multiple open wounds of sites classifiable to the same four-digit category should be classified to that category unless they are in different limbs.

Multiple open wounds of sites classifiable to different four-digit categories, or to different limbs, should be coded separately.

X

Y

Z

SECTION 2

Alphabetic Index to Poisoning and External Causes of Adverse Effects of Drugs and Other Chemical Substances

TABLE OF DRUGS AND CHEMICALS

This table contains a classification of drugs and other chemical substances to identify poisoning states and external causes of adverse effects.

Each of the listed substances in the table is assigned a code according to the poisoning classification (960-989). These codes are used when there is a statement of poisoning, overdose, wrong substance given or taken, or intoxication.

The table also contains a listing of external causes of adverse effects. An adverse effect is a pathologic manifestation due to ingestion or exposure to drugs or other chemical substances (e.g., dermatitis, hypersensitivity reaction, aspirin gastritis). The adverse effect is to be identified by the appropriate code found in Section 1, Index to Diseases and Injuries. An external cause code can then be used to identify the circumstances involved. The table headings pertaining to external causes are defined below:

Accidental poisoning (E850-E869) — accidental overdose of drug, wrong substance given or taken, drug taken inadvertently, accidents in the usage of drugs and biologicals in medical and surgical procedures, and to show external causes of poisonings classifiable to 980-989.

Therapeutic use (E930-E949) — a correct substance properly administered in therapeutic or prophylactic dosage as the external cause of adverse effects.

Suicide attempt (E950-E952) — instances in which self-inflicted injuries or poisonings are involved.

Assault (E96I-E962) — injury or poisoning inflicted by another person with the intent to injure or kill.

Undetermined (E980-E982) — to be used when the intent of the poisoning or injury cannot be determined whether it was intentional or accidental.

The American Hospital Formulary Service list numbers are included in the table to help classify new drugs not identified in the table by name. The AHFS list numbers are keyed to the continually revised American Hospital Formulary Service (AHFS).* These listings are found in the table under the main term **Drug.**

Excluded from the table are radium and other radioactive substances. The classification of adverse effects and complications pertaining to these substances will be found in Section 1, Index to Diseases and Injuries, and Section 3, Index to External Causes of Injuries.

Although certain substances are indexed with one or more subentries, the majority are listed according to one use or state. It is recognized that many substances may be used in various ways, in medicine and in industry, and may cause adverse effects whatever the state of the agent (solid, liquid, or fumes arising from a liquid). In cases in which the reported data indicates a use or state not in the table, or which is clearly different from the one listed, an attempt should be made to classify the substance in the form which most nearly expresses the reported facts.

*American Hospital Formulary Service, 2 vol. (Washington, D.C.: American Society of Hospital Pharmacists, 1959-)

		External Cause (E-Code)				
	Poisoning	Accident	Therapeutic Use	Suicide Attempt	Assault	Undetermined
1-propanol	980.3	E860.4	—	E950.9	E962.1	E980.9
2-propanol	980.2	E860.3	—	E950.9	E962.1	E980.9
2, 4-D (dichlorophenoxyacetic acid)	989.4	E863.5	—	E950.6	E962.1	E980.7
2, 4-toluene diisocyanate	983.0	E864.0	—	E950.7	E962.1	E980.6
2, 4, 5-T (trichlorophenoxyacetic acid)	989.2	E863.5	—	E950.6	E962.1	E980.7
14-hydroxydihydromorphinone	965.09	E850.2	E935.2	E950.0	E962.0	E980.0
ABOB	961.7	E857	E931.7	E950.4	E962.0	E980.4
Abrus (seed)	988.2	E865.3	—	E950.9	E962.1	E980.9
Absinthe	980.0	E860.1	—	E950.9	E962.1	E980.9
beverage	980.0	E860.0	—	E950.9	E962.1	E980.9
Acenocoumarin, acenocoumarol	964.2	E858.2	E934.2	E950.4	E962.0	E980.4
Acepromazine	969.1	E853.0	E939.1	E950.3	E962.0	E980.3
Acetal	982.8	E862.4	—	E950.9	E962.1	E980.9
Acetaldehyde (vapor)	987.8	E869.8	—	E952.8	E962.2	E982.8
liquid	989.89	E866.8	—	E950.9	E962.1	E980.9
Acetaminophen	965.4	E850.4	E935.4	E950.0	E962.0	E980.0
Acetaminosalol	965.1	E850.3	E935.3	E950.0	E962.0	E980.0
Acetanilid(e)	965.4	E850.4	E935.4	E950.0	E962.0	E980.0
Acetarsol, acetarsone	961.1	E857	E931.1	E950.4	E962.0	E980.4
Acetazolamide	974.2	E858.5	E944.2	E950.4	E962.0	E980.4
Acetic						
acid	983.1	E864.1	—	E950.7	E962.1	E980.6
with sodium acetate (ointment)	976.3	E858.7	E946.3	E950.4	E962.0	E980.4
irrigating solution	974.5	E858.5	E944.5	E950.4	E962.0	E980.4
lotion	976.2	E858.7	E946.2	E950.4	E962.0	E980.4
anhydride	983.1	E864.1	—	E950.7	E962.1	E980.6
ether (vapor)	982.8	E862.4	—	E950.9	E962.1	E980.9
Acetohexamide	962.3	E858.0	E932.3	E950.4	E962.0	E980.4
Acetomenaphthone	964.3	E858.2	E934.3	E950.4	E962.0	E980.4
Acetomorphine	965.01	E850.0	E935.0	E950.0	E962.0	E980.0
Acetone (oils) (vapor)	982.8	E862.4	—	E950.9	E962.1	E980.9
Acetophenazine (maleate)	969.1	E853.0	E939.1	E950.3	E962.0	E980.3
Acetophenetidin	965.4	E850.4	E935.4	E950.0	E962.0	E980.0
Acetophenone	982.0	E862.4	—	E950.9	E962.1	E980.9
Acetorphine	965.09	E850.2	E935.2	E950.0	E962.0	E980.0
Acetosulfone (sodium)	961.8	E857	E931.8	E950.4	E962.0	E980.4
Acetrizoate (sodium)	977.8	E858.8	E947.8	E950.4	E962.0	E980.4
Acetylcarbromal	967.3	E852.2	E937.3	E950.2	E962.0	E980.2
Acetylcholine (chloride)	971.0	E855.3	E941.0	E950.4	E962.0	E980.4
Acetylcysteine	975.5	E858.6	E945.5	E950.4	E962.0	E980.4
Acetyldigitoxin	972.1	E858.3	E942.1	E950.4	E962.0	E980.4
Acetyldihydrocodeine	965.09	E850.2	E935.2	E950.0	E962.0	E980.0
Acetyldihydrocodeinone	965.09	E850.2	E935.2	E950.0	E962.0	E980.0
Acetylene (gas) (industrial)	987.1	E868.1	—	E951.8	E962.2	E981.8
incomplete combustion of — *see* Carbon monoxide, fuel, utility						
tetrachloride (vapor)	982.3	E862.4	—	E950.9	E962.1	E980.9
Acetyliodosalicylic acid	965.1	E850.3	E935.3	E950.0	E962.0	E980.0
Acetylphenylhydrazine	965.8	E850.8	E935.8	E950.0	E962.0	E980.0
Acetylsalicylic acid	965.1	E850.3	E935.3	E950.0	E962.0	E980.0
Achromycin	960.4	E856	E930.4	E950.4	E962.0	E980.4
ophthalmic preparation	976.5	E858.7	E946.5	E950.4	E962.0	E980.4
topical NEC	976.0	E858.7	E946.0	E950.4	E962.0	E980.4
Acidifying agents	963.2	E858.1	E933.2	E950.4	E962.0	E980.4
Acids (corrosive) NEC	983.1	E864.1	—	E950.7	E962.1	E980.6
Aconite (wild)	988.2	E865.4	—	E950.9	E962.1	E980.9
Aconitine (liniment)	976.8	E858.7	E946.8	E950.4	E962.0	E980.4
Aconitum ferox	988.2	E865.4	—	E950.9	E962.1	E980.9
Acridine	983.0	E864.0	—	E950.7	E962.1	E980.6
vapor	987.8	E869.8	—	E952.8	E962.2	E982.8
Acriflavine	961.9	E857	E931.9	E950.4	E962.0	E980.4
Acrisorcin	976.0	E858.7	E946.0	E950.4	E962.0	E980.4
Acrolein (gas)	987.8	E869.8	—	E952.8	E962.2	E982.8
liquid	989.89	E866.8	—	E950.9	E962.1	E980.9
Actaea spicata	988.2	E865.4	—	E950.9	E962.1	E980.9
Acterol	961.5	E857	E931.5	E950.4	E962.0	E980.4
ACTH	962.4	E858.0	E932.4	E950.4	E962.0	E980.4
Acthar	962.4	E858.0	E932.4	E950.4	E962.0	E980.4
Actinomycin (C)(D)	960.7	E856	E930.7	E950.4	E962.0	E980.4
Adalin (acetyl)	967.3	E852.2	E937.3	E950.2	E962.0	E980.2
Adenosine (phosphate)	977.8	E858.8	E947.8	E950.4	E962.0	E980.4
Adhesives	989.89	E866.6	—	E950.9	E962.1	E980.9

☑ Additional Digit Required — Refer to the Tabular List (Numeric Code Section) for Additional Digit Selection

▶◀ Revised Text ● New Line ▲ Revised Code

	Poisoning	External Cause (E-Code)				
		Accident	Therapeutic Use	Suicide Attempt	Assault	Undetermined
ADH	962.5	E858.0	E932.5	E950.4	E962.0	E980.4
Adicillin	960.0	E856	E930.0	E950.4	E962.0	E980.4
Adiphenine	975.1	E855.6	E945.1	E950.4	E962.0	E980.4
Adjunct, pharmaceutical	977.4	E858.8	E947.4	E950.4	E962.0	E980.4
Adrenal (extract, cortex or medulla) (glucocorticoids) (hormones) (mineralocorticoids)	962.0	E858.0	E932.0	E950.4	E962.0	E980.4
ENT agent	976.6	E858.7	E946.6	E950.4	E962.0	E980.4
ophthalmic preparation	976.5	E858.7	E946.5	E950.4	E962.0	E980.4
topical NEC	976.0	E858.7	E946.0	E950.4	E962.0	E980.4
Adrenalin	971.2	E855.5	E941.2	E950.4	E962.0	E980.4
Adrenergic blocking agents	971.3	E855.6	E941.3	E950.4	E962.0	E980.4
Adrenergics	971.2	E855.5	E941.2	E950.4	E962.0	E980.4
Adrenochrome (derivatives)	972.8	E858.3	E942.8	E950.4	E962.0	E980.4
Adrenocorticotropic hormone	962.4	E858.0	E932.4	E950.4	E962.0	E980.4
Adrenocorticotropin	962.4	E858.0	E932.4	E950.4	E962.0	E980.4
Adriamycin	960.7	E856	E930.7	E950.4	E962.0	E980.4
Aerosol spray — *see* Sprays						
Aerosporin	960.8	E856	E930.8	E950.4	E962.0	E980.4
ENT agent	976.6	E858.7	E946.6	E950.4	E962.0	E980.4
ophthalmic preparation	976.5	E858.7	E946.5	E950.4	E962.0	E980.4
topical NEC	976.0	E858.7	E946.0	E950.4	E962.0	E980.4
Aethusa cynapium	988.2	E865.4	—	E950.9	E962.1	E980.9
Afghanistan black	969.6	E854.1	E939.6	E950.3	E962.0	E980.3
Aflatoxin	989.7	E865.9	—	E950.9	E962.1	E980.9
African boxwood	988.2	E865.4	—	E950.9	E962.1	E980.9
Agar (-agar)	973.3	E858.4	E943.3	E950.4	E962.0	E980.4
Agricultural agent NEC	989.89	E863.9	—	E950.6	E962.1	E980.7
Agrypnal	967.0	E851	E937.0	E950.1	E962.0	E980.1
Air contaminant(s), source or type not specified	987.9	E869.9	—	E952.9	E962.2	E982.9
specified type — *see* specific substance						
Akee	988.2	E865.4	—	E950.9	E962.1	E980.9
Akrinol	976.0	E858.7	E946.0	E950.4	E962.0	E980.4
Alantolactone	961.6	E857	E931.6	E950.4	E962.0	E980.4
Albamycin	960.8	E856	E930.8	E950.4	E962.0	E980.4
Albumin (normal human serum)	964.7	E858.2	E934.7	E950.4	E962.0	E980.4
Albuterol	975.7	E858.6	E945.7	E950.4	E962.0	E980.4
Alcohol	980.9	E860.9	—	E950.9	E962.1	E980.9
absolute	980.0	E860.1	—	E950.9	E962.1	E980.9
beverage	980.0	E860.0	E947.8	E950.9	E962.1	E980.9
amyl	980.3	E860.4	—	E950.9	E962.1	E980.9
antifreeze	980.1	E860.2	—	E950.9	E962.1	E980.9
butyl	980.3	E860.4	—	E950.9	E962.1	E980.9
dehydrated	980.0	E860.1	—	E950.9	E862.1	E980.9
beverage	980.0	E860.0	E947.8	E950.9	E962.1	E980.9
denatured	980.0	E860.1	—	E950.9	E962.1	E980.9
deterrents	977.3	E858.8	E947.3	E950.4	E962.0	E980.4
diagnostic (gastric function)	977.8	E858.8	E947.8	E950.4	E962.0	E980.4
ethyl	980.0	E860.1	—	E950.9	E962.1	E980.9
beverage	980.0	E860.0	E947.8	E950.9	E962.1	E980.9
grain	980.0	E860.1	—	E950.9	E962.1	E980.9
beverage	980.0	E860.0	E947.8	E950.9	E962.1	E980.9
industrial	980.9	E860.9	—	E950.9	E962.1	E980.9
isopropyl	980.2	E860.3	—	E950.9	E962.1	E980.9
methyl	980.1	E860.2	—	E950.9	E962.1	E980.9
preparation for consumption	980.0	E860.0	E947.8	E950.9	E962.1	E980.9
propyl	980.3	E860.4	—	E950.9	E962.1	E980.9
secondary	980.2	E860.3	—	E950.9	E962.1	E980.9
radiator	980.1	E860.2	—	E950.9	E962.1	E980.9
rubbing	980.2	E860.3	—	E950.9	E962.1	E980.9
specified type NEC	980.8	E860.8	—	E950.9	E962.1	E980.9
surgical	980.9	E860.9	—	E950.9	E962.1	E980.9
vapor (from any type of alcohol)	987.8	E869.8	—	E952.8	E962.2	E982.8
wood	980.1	E860.2	—	E950.9	E962.1	E980.9
Alcuronium chloride	975.2	E858.6	E945.2	E950.4	E962.0	E980.4
Aldactone	974.4	E858.5	E944.4	E950.4	E962.0	E980.4
Aldicarb	989.3	E863.2	—	E950.6	E962.1	E980.7
Aldomet	972.6	E858.3	E942.6	E950.4	E962.0	E980.4
Aldosterone	962.0	E858.0	E932.0	E950.4	E962.0	E980.4
Aldrin (dust)	989.2	E863.0	—	E950.6	E962.1	E980.7
Algeldrate	973.0	E858.4	E943.0	E950.4	E962.0	E980.4
Alidase	963.4	E858.1	E933.4	E950.4	E962.0	E980.4
Aliphatic thiocyanates	989.0	E866.8	—	E950.9	E962.1	E980.9
Alkaline antiseptic solution (aromatic)	976.6	E858.7	E946.6	E950.4	E962.0	E980.4
Alkalinizing agents (medicinal)	963.3	E858.1	E933.3	E950.4	E962.0	E980.4
Alkalis, caustic	983.2	E864.2	—	E950.7	E962.1	E980.6
Alkalizing agents (medicinal)	963.3	E858.1	E933.3	E950.4	E962.0	E980.4
Alka-seltzer	965.1	E850.3	E935.3	E950.0	E962.0	E980.0
Alkavervir	972.6	E858.3	E942.6	E950.4	E962.0	E980.4
Allegron	969.0	E854.0	E939.0	E950.3	E962.0	E980.3
Alleve — *see* Naproxen						
Allobarbital, allobarbitone	967.0	E851	E937.0	E950.1	E962.0	E980.1
Allopurinol	974.7	E858.5	E944.7	E950.4	E962.0	E980.4
Allylestrenol	962.2	E858.0	E932.2	E950.4	E962.0	E980.4
Allylisopropylacetylurea	967.8	E852.8	E937.8	E950.2	E962.0	E980.2
Allylisopropylmalonylurea	967.0	E851	E937.0	E950.1	E962.0	E980.1
Allyltribromide	967.3	E852.2	E937.3	E950.2	E962.0	E980.2
Aloe, aloes, aloin	973.1	E858.4	E943.1	E950.4	E962.0	E980.4
Alosetron	973.8	E858.4	E943.8	E950.4	E962.0	E980.4
Aloxidone	966.0	E855.0	E936.0	E950.4	E962.0	E980.4
Aloxiprin	965.1	E850.3	E935.3	E950.0	E962.0	E980.0
Alpha amylase	963.4	E858.1	E933.4	E950.4	E962.0	E980.4
Alphaprodine (hydrochloride)	965.09	E850.2	E935.2	E950.0	E962.0	E980.0
Alpha tocopherol	963.5	E858.1	E933.5	E950.4	E962.0	E980.4
Alseroxylon	972.6	E858.3	E942.6	E950.4	E962.0	E980.4
Alum (ammonium) (potassium)	983.2	E864.2	—	E950.7	E962.1	E980.6
medicinal (astringent) NEC	976.2	E858.7	E946.2	E950.4	E962.0	E980.4
Aluminium, aluminum (gel) (hydroxide)	973.0	E858.4	E943.0	E950.4	E962.0	E980.4
acetate solution	976.2	E858.7	E946.2	E950.4	E962.0	E980.4
aspirin	965.1	E850.3	E935.3	E950.0	E962.0	E980.0
carbonate	973.0	E858.4	E943.0	E950.4	E962.0	E980.4
glycinate	973.0	E858.4	E943.0	E950.4	E962.0	E980.4
nicotinate	972.2	E858.3	E942.2	E950.4	E962.0	E980.4
ointment (surgical) (topical)	976.3	E858.7	E946.3	E950.4	E962.0	E980.4
phosphate	973.0	E858.4	E943.0	E950.4	E962.0	E980.4
subacetate	976.2	E858.7	E946.2	E950.4	E962.0	E980.4
topical NEC	976.3	E858.7	E946.3	E950.4	E962.0	E980.4
Alurate	967.0	E851	E937.0	E950.1	E962.0	E980.1
Alverine (citrate)	975.1	E858.6	E945.1	E950.4	E962.0	E980.4
Alvodine	965.09	E850.2	E935.2	E950.0	E962.0	E980.0
Amanita phalloides	988.1	E865.5	—	E950.9	E962.1	E980.9
Amantadine (hydrochloride)	966.4	E855.0	E936.4	E950.4	E962.0	E980.4
Ambazone	961.9	E857	E931.9	E950.4	E962.0	E980.4
Ambenonium	971.0	E855.3	E941.0	E950.4	E962.0	E980.4
Ambutonium bromide	971.1	E855.4	E941.1	E950.4	E962.0	E980.4
Ametazole	977.8	E858.8	E947.8	E950.4	E962.0	E980.4
Amethocaine (infiltration) (topical)	968.5	E855.2	E938.5	E950.4	E962.0	E980.4
nerve block (peripheral) (plexus)	968.6	E855.2	E938.6	E950.4	E962.0	E980.4
spinal	968.7	E855.2	E938.7	E950.4	E962.0	E980.4
Amethopterin	963.1	E858.1	E933.1	E950.4	E962.0	E980.4
Amfepramone	977.0	E858.8	E947.0	E950.4	E962.0	E980.4
Amidon	965.02	E850.1	E935.1	E950.0	E962.0	E980.0
Amidopyrine	965.5	E850.5	E935.5	E950.0	E962.0	E980.0
Aminacrine	976.0	E858.7	E946.0	E950.4	E962.0	E980.4
Aminitrozole	961.5	E857	E931.5	E950.4	E962.0	E980.4
Aminoacetic acid	974.5	E858.5	E944.5	E950.4	E962.0	E980.4
Amino acids	974.5	E858.5	E944.5	E950.4	E962.0	E980.4
Aminocaproic acid	964.4	E858.2	E934.4	E950.4	E962.0	E980.4
Aminoethylisothiourium	963.8	E858.1	E933.8	E950.4	E962.0	E980.4
Aminoglutethimide	966.3	E855.0	E936.3	E950.4	E962.0	E980.4
Aminometradine	974.3	E858.5	E944.3	E950.4	E962.0	E980.4
Aminopentamide	971.1	E855.4	E941.1	E950.4	E962.0	E980.4
Aminophenazone	965.5	E850.5	E935.5	E950.0	E962.0	E980.0
Aminophenol	983.0	E864.0	—	E950.7	E962.1	E980.6
Aminophenylpyridone	969.5	E853.8	E939.5	E950.3	E962.0	E980.3
Aminophyllin	975.7	E858.6	E945.7	E950.4	E962.0	E980.4
Aminopterin	963.1	E858.1	E933.1	E950.4	E962.0	E980.4
Aminopyrine	965.5	E850.5	E935.5	E950.0	E962.0	E980.0
Aminosalicylic acid	961.8	E857	E931.8	E950.4	E962.0	E980.4
Amiphenazole	970.1	E854.3	E940.1	E950.4	E962.0	E980.4
Amiquinsin	972.6	E858.3	E942.6	E950.4	E962.0	E980.4
Amisometradine	974.3	E858.5	E944.3	E950.4	E962.0	E980.4
Amitriptyline	969.0	E854.0	E939.0	E950.3	E962.0	E980.3
Ammonia (fumes) (gas) (vapor)	987.8	E869.8	—	E952.8	E962.2	E982.8
liquid (household) NEC	983.2	E861.4	—	E950.7	E962.1	E980.6
spirit, aromatic	970.8	E854.3	E940.8	E950.4	E962.0	E980.4

☑ Additional Digit Required — Refer to the Tabular List (Numeric Code Section) for Additional Digit Selection

▶◀ Revised Text ● New Line ▲ Revised Code

		External Cause (E-Code)				
	Poisoning	Accident	Therapeutic Use	Suicide Attempt	Assault	Undetermined
Ammoniated mercury	976.0	E858.7	E946.0	E950.4	E962.0	E980.4
Ammonium						
carbonate	983.2	E864.2	—	E950.7	E962.1	E980.6
chloride (acidifying agent)	963.2	E858.1	E933.2	E950.4	E962.0	E980.4
expectorant	975.5	E858.6	E945.5	E950.4	E962.0	E980.4
compounds (household) NEC	983.2	E861.4	—	E950.7	E962.1	E980.6
fumes (any usage)	987.8	E869.8	—	E952.8	E962.2	E982.8
industrial	983.2	E864.2	—	E950.7	E962.1	E980.6
ichthyosulfonate	976.4	E858.7	E946.4	E950.4	E962.0	E980.4
mandelate	961.9	E857	E931.9	E950.4	E962.0	E980.4
Amobarbital	967.0	E851	E937.0	E950.1	E962.0	E980.1
Amodiaquin(e)	961.4	E857	E931.4	E950.4	E962.0	E980.4
Amopyroquin(e)	961.4	E857	E931.4	E950.4	E962.0	E980.4
Amphenidone	969.5	E853.8	E939.5	E950.3	E962.0	E980.3
Amphetamine	969.7	E854.2	E939.7	E950.3	E962.0	E980.3
Amphomycin	960.8	E856	E930.8	E950.4	E962.0	E980.4
Amphotericin B	960.1	E856	E930.1	E950.4	E962.0	E980.4
topical	976.0	E858.7	E946.0	E950.4	E962.0	E980.4
Ampicillin	960.0	E856	E930.0	E950.4	E962.0	E980.4
Amprotropine	971.1	E855.4	E941.1	E950.4	E962.0	E980.4
Amygdalin	977.8	E858.8	E947.8	E950.4	E962.0	E980.4
Amyl						
acetate (vapor)	982.8	E862.4	—	E950.9	E962.1	E980.9
alcohol	980.3	E860.4	—	E950.9	E962.1	E980.9
nitrite (medicinal)	972.4	E858.3	E942.4	E950.4	E962.0	E980.4
Amylase (alpha)	963.4	E858.1	E933.4	E950.4	E962.0	E980.4
Amylene hydrate	980.8	E860.8	—	E950.9	E962.1	E980.9
Amylobarbitone	967.0	E851	E937.0	E950.1	E962.0	E980.1
Amylocaine	968.9	E855.2	E938.9	E950.4	E962.0	E980.4
infiltration (subcutaneous)	968.5	E855.2	E938.5	E950.4	E962.0	E980.4
nerve block (peripheral) (plexus)	968.6	E855.2	E938.6	E950.4	E962.0	E980.4
spinal	968.7	E855.2	E938.7	E950.4	E962.0	E980.4
topical (surface)	968.5	E855.2	E938.5	E950.4	E962.0	E980.4
Amytal (sodium)	967.0	E851	E937.0	E950.1	E962.0	E980.1
Analeptics	970.0	E854.3	E940.0	E950.4	E962.0	E980.4
Analgesics	965.9	E850.9	E935.9	E950.0	E962.0	E980.0
aromatic NEC	965.4	E850.4	E935.4	E950.0	E962.0	E980.0
non-narcotic NEC	965.7	E850.7	E935.7	E950.0	E962.0	E980.0
specified NEC	965.8	E850.8	E935.8	E950.0	E962.0	E980.0
Anamirta cocculus	988.2	E865.3	—	E950.9	E962.1	E980.9
Ancillin	960.0	E856	E930.0	E950.4	E962.0	E980.4
Androgens (anabolic congeners)	962.1	E858.0	E932.1	E950.4	E962.0	E980.4
Androstalone	962.1	E858.0	E932.1	E950.4	E962.0	E980.4
Androsterone	962.1	E858.0	E932.1	E950.4	E962.0	E980.4
Anemone pulsatilla	988.2	E865.4	—	E950.9	E962.1	E980.9
Anesthesia, anesthetic (general) NEC	968.4	E855.1	E938.4	E950.4	E962.0	E980.4
block (nerve) (plexus)	968.6	E855.2	E938.6	E950.4	E962.0	E980.4
gaseous NEC	968.2	E855.1	E938.2	E950.4	E962.0	E980.4
halogenated hydrocarbon derivatives NEC	968.2	E855.1	E938.2	E950.4	E962.0	E980.4
infiltration (intradermal) (subcutaneous) (submucosal)	968.5	E855.2	E938.5	E950.4	E962.0	E980.4
intravenous	968.3	E855.1	E938.3	E950.4	E962.0	E980.4
local NEC	968.9	E855.2	E938.9	E950.4	E962.0	E980.4
nerve blocking (peripheral) (plexus)	968.6	E855.2	E938.6	E950.4	E962.0	E980.4
rectal NEC	968.3	E855.1	E938.3	E950.4	E962.0	E980.4
spinal	968.7	E855.2	E938.7	E950.4	E962.0	E980.4
surface	968.5	E855.2	E938.5	E950.4	E962.0	E980.4
topical	968.5	E855.2	E938.5	E950.4	E962.0	E980.4
Aneurine	963.5	E858.1	E933.5	E950.4	E962.0	E980.4
Anginine — *see* Glyceryl trinitrate						
Angio-Conray	977.8	E858.8	E947.8	E950.4	E962.0	E980.4
Angiotensin	971.2	E855.5	E941.2	E950.4	E962.0	E980.4
Anhydrohydroxyprogesterone	962.2	E858.0	E932.2	E950.4	E962.0	E980.4
Anhydron	974.3	E858.5	E944.3	E950.4	E962.0	E980.4
Anileridine	965.09	E850.2	E935.2	E950.0	E962.0	E980.0
Aniline (dye) (liquid)	983.0	E864.0	—	E950.7	E962.1	E980.6
analgesic	965.4	E850.4	E935.4	E950.0	E962.0	E980.0
derivatives, therapeutic NEC	965.4	E850.4	E935.4	E950.0	E962.0	E980.0
vapor	987.8	E869.8	—	E952.8	E962.2	E982.8
Anisindione	964.2	E858.2	E934.2	E950.4	E962.0	E980.4
Aniscoropine	971.1	E855.4	E941.1	E950.4	E962.0	E980.4
Anorexic agents	977.0	E858.8	E947.0	E950.4	E962.0	E980.4
Ant (bite) (sting)	989.5	E905.5	—	E950.9	E962.1	E980.9

		External Cause (E-Code)				
	Poisoning	Accident	Therapeutic Use	Suicide Attempt	Assault	Undetermined
Antabuse	977.3	E858.8	E947.3	E950.4	E962.0	E980.4
Antacids	973.0	E858.4	E943.0	E950.4	E962.0	E980.4
Antazoline	963.0	E858.1	E933.0	E950.4	E962.0	E980.4
Anthelmintics	961.6	E857	E931.6	E950.4	E962.0	E980.4
Anthralin	976.4	E858.7	E946.4	E950.4	E962.0	E980.4
Anthramycin	960.7	E856	E930.7	E950.4	E962.0	E980.4
Antiadrenergics	971.3	E855.6	E941.3	E950.4	E962.0	E980.4
Antiallergic agents	963.0	E858.1	E933.0	E950.4	E962.0	E980.4
Antianemic agents NEC	964.1	E858.2	E934.1	E950.4	E962.0	E980.4
Antiaris toxicaria	988.2	E865.4	—	E950.9	E962.1	E980.9
Antiarteriosclerotic agents	972.2	E858.3	E942.2	E950.4	E962.0	E980.4
Antiasthmatics	975.7	E858.6	E945.7	E950.4	E962.0	E980.4
Antibiotics	960.9	E856	E930.9	E950.4	E962.0	E980.4
antifungal	960.1	E856	E930.1	E950.4	E962.0	E980.4
antimycobacterial	960.6	E856	E930.6	E950.4	E962.0	E980.4
antineoplastic	960.7	E856	E930.7	E950.4	E962.0	E980.4
cephalosporin (group)	960.5	E856	E930.5	E950.4	E962.0	E980.4
chloramphenicol (group)	960.2	E856	E930.2	E950.4	E962.0	E980.4
macrolides	960.3	E856	E930.3	E950.4	E962.0	E980.4
specified NEC	960.8	E856	E930.8	E950.4	E962.0	E980.4
tetracycline (group)	960.4	E856	E930.4	E950.4	E962.0	E980.4
Anticancer agents NEC	963.1	E858.1	E933.1	E950.4	E962.0	E980.4
antibiotics	960.7	E856	E930.7	E950.4	E962.0	E980.4
Anticholinergics	971.1	E855.4	E941.1	E950.4	E962.0	E980.4
Anticholinesterase (organophosphorus) (reversible)	971.0	E855.3	E941.0	E950.4	E962.0	E980.4
Anticoagulants	964.2	E858.2	E934.2	E950.4	E962.0	E980.4
antagonists	964.5	E858.2	E934.5	E950.4	E962.0	E980.4
Anti-common cold agents NEC	975.6	E858.6	E945.6	E950.4	E962.0	E980.4
Anticonvulsants NEC	966.3	E855.0	E936.3	E950.4	E962.0	E980.4
Antidepressants	969.0	E854.0	E939.0	E950.3	E962.0	E980.3
Antidiabetic agents	962.3	E858.0	E932.3	E950.4	E962.0	E980.4
Antidiarrheal agents	973.5	E858.4	E943.5	E950.4	E962.0	E980.4
Antidiuretic hormone	962.5	E858.0	E932.5	E950.4	E962.0	E980.4
Antidotes NEC	977.2	E858.8	E947.2	E950.4	E962.0	E980.4
Antiemetic agents	963.0	E858.1	E933.0	E950.4	E962.0	E980.4
Antiepilepsy agent NEC	966.3	E855.0	E936.3	E950.4	E962.0	E980.4
Antifertility pills	962.2	E858.0	E932.2	E950.4	E962.0	E980.4
Antiflatulents	973.8	E858.4	E943.8	E950.4	E962.0	E980.4
Antifreeze	989.89	E866.8	—	E950.9	E962.1	E980.9
alcohol	980.1	E860.2	—	E950.9	E962.1	E980.9
ethylene glycol	982.8	E862.4	—	E950.9	E962.1	E980.9
Antifungals (nonmedicinal) (sprays)	989.4	E863.6	—	E950.6	E962.1	E980.7
medicinal NEC	961.9	E857	E931.9	E950.4	E962.0	E980.4
antibiotic	960.1	E856	E930.1	E950.4	E962.0	E980.4
topical	976.0	E858.7	E946.0	E950.4	E962.0	E980.4
Antigastric secretion agents	973.0	E858.4	E943.0	E950.4	E962.0	E980.4
Antihelmintics	961.6	E857	E931.6	E950.4	E962.0	E980.4
Antihemophilic factor (human)	964.7	E858.2	E934.7	E950.4	E962.0	E980.4
Antihistamine	963.0	E858.1	E933.0	E950.4	E962.0	E980.4
Antihypertensive agents NEC	972.6	E858.3	E942.6	E950.4	E962.0	E980.4
Anti-infectives NEC	961.9	E857	E931.9	E950.4	E962.0	E980.4
antibiotics	960.9	E856	E930.9	E950.4	E962.0	E980.4
specified NEC	960.8	E856	E930.8	E950.4	E962.0	E980.4
antihelmintic	961.6	E857	E931.6	E950.4	E962.0	E980.4
antimalarial	961.4	E857	E931.4	E950.4	E962.0	E980.4
antimycobacterial NEC	961.8	E857	E931.8	E950.4	E962.0	E980.4
antibiotics	960.6	E856	E930.6	E950.4	E962.0	E980.4
antiprotozoal NEC	961.5	E857	E931.5	E950.4	E962.0	E980.4
blood	961.4	E857	E931.4	E950.4	E962.0	E980.4
antiviral	961.7	E857	E931.7	E950.4	E962.0	E980.4
arsenical	961.1	E857	E931.1	E950.4	E962.0	E980.4
ENT agents	976.6	E858.7	E946.6	E950.4	E962.0	E980.4
heavy metals NEC	961.2	E857	E931.2	E950.4	E962.0	E980.4
local	976.0	E858.7	E946.0	E950.4	E962.0	E980.4
ophthalmic preparation	976.5	E858.7	E946.5	E950.4	E962.0	E980.4
topical NEC	976.0	E858.7	E946.0	E950.4	E962.0	E980.4
Anti-inflammatory agents (topical)	976.0	E858.7	E946.0	E950.4	E962.0	E980.4
Antiknock (tetraethyl lead)	984.1	E862.1	—	E950.9	E962.1	E980.9
Antilipemics	972.2	E858.3	E942.2	E950.4	E962.0	E980.4
Antimalarials	961.4	E857	E931.4	E950.4	E962.0	E980.4
Antimony (compounds) (vapor) NEC	985.4	E866.2	—	E950.9	E962.1	E980.9
anti-infectives	961.2	E857	E931.2	E950.4	E962.0	E980.4

☑ Additional Digit Required — Refer to the Tabular List (Numeric Code Section) for Additional Digit Selection

▶◀ Revised Text ● New Line ▲ Revised Code

	Poisoning	External Cause (E-Code)				
		Accident	Therapeutic Use	Suicide Attempt	Assault	Undetermined
Antimony — *continued*						
pesticides (vapor)	985.4	E863.4	—	E950.6	E962.2	E980.7
potassium tartrate	961.2	E857	E931.2	E950.4	E962.0	E980.4
tartrated	961.2	E857	E931.2	E950.4	E962.0	E980.4
Antimuscarinic agents	971.1	E855.4	E941.1	E950.4	E962.0	E980.4
Antimycobacterials NEC	961.8	E857	E931.8	E950.4	E962.0	E980.4
antibiotics	960.6	E856	E930.6	E950.4	E962.0	E980.4
Antineoplastic agents	963.1	E858.1	E933.1	E950.4	E962.0	E980.4
antibiotics	960.7	E856	E930.7	E950.4	E962.0	E980.4
Anti-Parkinsonism agents	966.4	E855.0	E936.4	E950.4	E962.0	E980.4
Antiphlogistics	965.69	E850.6	E935.6	E950.0	E962.0	E980.0
Antiprotozoals NEC	961.5	E857	E931.5	E950.4	E962.0	E980.4
blood	961.4	E857	E931.4	E950.4	E962.0	E980.4
Antipruritics (local)	976.1	E858.7	E946.1	E950.4	E962.0	E980.4
Antipsychotic agents NEC	969.3	E853.8	E939.3	E950.3	E962.0	E980.3
Antipyretics	965.9	E850.9	E935.9	E950.0	E962.0	E980.0
specified NEC	965.8	E850.8	E935.8	E950.0	E962.0	E980.0
Antipyrine	965.5	E850.5	E935.5	E950.0	E962.0	E980.0
Antirabies serum (equine)	979.9	E858.8	E949.9	E950.4	E962.0	E980.4
Antirheumatics	965.69	E850.6	E935.6	E950.0	E962.0	E980.0
Antiseborrheics	976.4	E858.7	E946.4	E950.4	E962.0	E980.4
Antiseptics (external) (medicinal)	976.0	E858.7	E946.0	E950.4	E962.0	E980.4
Antistine	963.0	E858.1	E933.0	E950.4	E962.0	E980.4
Antithyroid agents	962.8	E858.0	E932.8	E950.4	E962.0	E980.4
Antitoxin, any	979.9	E858.8	E949.9	E950.4	E962.0	E980.4
Antituberculars	961.8	E857	E931.8	E950.4	E962.0	E980.4
antibiotics	960.6	E856	E930.6	E950.4	E962.0	E980.4
Antitussives	975.4	E858.6	E945.4	E950.4	E962.0	E980.4
Antivaricose agents (sclerosing)	972.7	E858.3	E942.7	E950.4	E962.0	E980.4
Antivenin (crotaline) (spider-bite)	979.9	E858.8	E949.9	E950.4	E962.0	E980.4
Antivert	963.0	E858.1	E933.0	E950.4	E962.0	E980.4
Antivirals NEC	961.7	E857	E931.7	E950.4	E962.0	E980.4
Ant poisons — *see* Pesticides						
Antrol	989.4	E863.4	—	E950.6	E962.1	E980.7
fungicide	989.4	E863.6	—	E950.6	E962.1	E980.7
Apomorphine hydrochloride (emetic)	973.6	E858.4	E943.6	E950.4	E962.0	E980.4
Appetite depressants, central	977.0	E858.8	E947.0	E950.4	E962.0	E980.4
Apresoline	972.6	E858.3	E942.6	E950.4	E962.0	E980.4
Aprobarbital, aprobarbitone	967.0	E851	E937.0	E950.1	E962.0	E980.1
Apronalide	967.8	E852.8	E937.8	E950.2	E962.0	E980.2
Aqua fortis	983.1	E864.1	—	E950.7	E962.1	E980.6
Arachis oil (topical)	976.3	E858.7	E946.3	E950.4	E962.0	E980.4
cathartic	973.2	E858.4	E943.2	E950.4	E962.0	E980.4
Aralen	961.4	E857	E931.4	E950.4	E962.0	E980.4
Arginine salts	974.5	E858.5	E944.5	E950.4	E962.0	E980.4
Argyrol	976.0	E858.7	E946.0	E950.4	E962.0	E980.4
ENT agent	976.6	E858.7	E946.6	E950.4	E962.0	E980.4
ophthalmic preparation	976.5	E858.7	E946.5	E950.4	E962.0	E980.4
Aristocort	962.0	E858.0	E932.0	E950.4	E962.0	E980.4
ENT agent	976.6	E858.7	E946.6	E950.4	E962.0	E980.4
ophthalmic preparation	976.5	E858.7	E946.5	E950.4	E962.0	E980.4
topical NEC	976.0	E858.7	E946.0	E950.4	E962.0	E980.4
Aromatics, corrosive	983.0	E864.0	—	E950.7	E962.1	E980.6
disinfectants	983.0	E861.4	—	E950.7	E962.1	E980.6
Arsenate of lead (insecticide)	985.1	E863.4	—	E950.8	E962.1	E980.8
herbicide	985.1	E863.5	—	E950.8	E962.1	E980.8
Arsenic, arsenicals (compounds) (dust) (fumes) (vapor) NEC	985.1	E866.3	—	E950.8	E962.1	E980.8
anti-infectives	961.1	E857	E931.1	E950.4	E962.0	E980.4
pesticide (dust) (fumes)	985.1	E863.4	—	E950.8	E962.1	E980.8
Arsine (gas)	985.1	E866.3	—	E950.8	E962.1	E980.8
Arsphenamine (silver)	961.1	E857	E931.1	E950.4	E962.0	E980.4
Arsthinol	961.1	E857	E931.1	E950.4	E962.0	E980.4
Artane	971.1	E855.4	E941.1	E950.4	E962.0	E980.4
Arthropod (venomous) NEC	989.5	E905.5	—	E950.9	E962.1	E980.9
Asbestos	989.81	E866.8	—	E950.9	E962.1	E980.9
Ascaridole	961.6	E857	E931.6	E950.4	E962.0	E980.4
Ascorbic acid	963.5	E858.1	E933.5	E950.4	E962.0	E980.4
Asiaticoside	976.0	E858.7	E946.0	E950.4	E962.0	E980.4
Aspidium (oleoresin)	961.6	E857	E931.6	E950.4	E962.0	E980.4
Aspirin	965.1	E850.3	E935.3	E950.0	E962.0	E980.0
Astringents (local)	976.2	E858.7	E946.2	E950.4	E962.0	E980.4
Atabrine	961.3	E857	E931.3	E950.4	E962.0	E980.4
Ataractics	969.5	E853.8	E939.5	E950.3	E962.0	E980.3
Atonia drug, intestinal	973.3	E858.4	E943.3	E950.4	E962.0	E980.4

	Poisoning	External Cause (E-Code)				
		Accident	Therapeutic Use	Suicide Attempt	Assault	Undetermined
Atophan	974.7	E858.5	E944.7	E950.4	E962.0	E980.4
Atropine	971.1	E855.4	E941.1	E950.4	E962.0	E980.4
Attapulgite	973.5	E858.4	E943.5	E950.4	E962.0	E980.4
Attenuvax	979.4	E858.8	E949.4	E950.4	E962.0	E980.4
Aureomycin	960.4	E856	E930.4	E950.4	E962.0	E980.4
ophthalmic preparation	976.5	E858.7	E946.5	E950.4	E962.0	E980.4
topical NEC	976.0	E858.7	E946.0	E950.4	E962.0	E980.4
Aurothioglucose	965.69	E850.6	E935.6	E950.0	E962.0	E980.0
Aurothioglycanide	965.69	E850.6	E935.6	E950.0	E962.0	E980.0
Aurothiomalate	965.69	E850.6	E935.6	E950.0	E962.0	E980.0
Automobile fuel	981	E862.1	—	E950.9	E962.1	E980.9
Autonomic nervous system agents NEC	971.9	E855.9	E941.9	E950.4	E962.0	E980.4
Avlosulfon	961.8	E857	E931.8	E950.4	E962.0	E980.4
Avomine	967.8	E852.8	E937.8	E950.2	E962.0	E980.2
Azacyclonol	969.5	E853.8	E939.5	E950.3	E962.0	E980.3
Azapetine	971.3	E855.6	E941.3	E950.4	E962.0	E980.4
Azaribine	963.1	E858.1	E933.1	E950.4	E962.0	E980.4
Azaserine	960.7	E856	E930.7	E950.4	E962.0	E980.4
Azathioprine	963.1	E858.1	E933.1	E950.4	E962.0	E980.4
Azosulfamide	961.0	E857	E931.0	E950.4	E962.0	E980.4
Azulfidine	961.0	E857	E931.0	E950.4	E962.0	E980.4
Azuresin	977.8	E858.8	E947.8	E950.4	E962.0	E980.4
Bacimycin	976.0	E858.7	E946.0	E950.4	E962.0	E980.4
ophthalmic preparation	976.5	E858.7	E946.5	E950.4	E962.0	E980.4
Bacitracin	960.8	E856	E930.8	E950.4	E962.0	E980.4
ENT agent	976.6	E858.7	E946.6	E950.4	E962.0	E980.4
ophthalmic preparation	976.5	E858.7	E946.5	E950.4	E962.0	E980.4
topical NEC	976.0	E858.7	E946.0	E950.4	E962.0	E980.4
Baking soda	963.3	E858.1	E933.3	E950.4	E962.0	E980.4
BAL	963.8	E858.1	E933.8	E950.4	E962.0	E980.4
Bamethan (sulfate)	972.5	E858.3	E942.5	E950.4	E962.0	E980.4
Bamipine	963.0	E858.1	E933.0	E950.4	E962.0	E980.4
Baneberry	988.2	E865.4	—	E950.9	E962.1	E980.9
Banewort	988.2	E865.4	—	E950.9	E962.1	E980.9
Barbenyl	967.0	E851	E937.0	E950.1	E962.0	E980.1
Barbital, barbitone	967.0	E851	E937.0	E950.1	E962.0	E980.1
Barbiturates, barbituric acid	967.0	E851	E937.0	E950.1	E962.0	E980.1
anesthetic (intravenous)	968.3	E855.1	E938.3	E950.4	E962.0	E980.4
Barium (carbonate) (chloride) (sulfate)	985.8	E866.4	—	E950.9	E962.1	E980.9
diagnostic agent	977.8	E858.8	E947.8	E950.4	E962.0	E980.4
pesticide	985.8	E863.4	—	E950.6	E962.1	E980.7
rodenticide	985.8	E863.7	—	E950.6	E962.1	E980.7
Barrier cream	976.3	E858.7	E946.3	E950.4	E962.0	E980.4
Battery acid or fluid	983.1	E864.1	—	E950.7	E962.1	E980.6
Bay rum	980.8	E860.8	—	E950.9	E962.1	E980.9
BCG vaccine	978.0	E858.8	E948.0	E950.4	E962.0	E980.4
Bearsfoot	988.2	E865.4	—	E950.9	E962.1	E980.9
Beclamide	966.3	E855.0	E936.3	E950.4	E962.0	E980.4
Bee (sting) (venom)	989.5	E905.3	—	E950.9	E962.1	E980.9
Belladonna (alkaloids)	971.1	E855.4	E941.1	E950.4	E962.0	E980.4
Bemegride	970.0	E854.3	E940.0	E950.4	E962.0	E980.4
Benactyzine	969.8	E855.8	E939.8	E950.3	E962.0	E980.3
Benadryl	963.0	E858.1	E933.0	E950.4	E962.0	E980.4
Bendrofluazide	974.3	E858.5	E944.3	E950.4	E962.0	E980.4
Bendroflumethiazide	974.3	E858.5	E944.3	E950.4	E962.0	E980.4
Benemid	974.7	E858.5	E944.7	E950.4	E962.0	E980.4
Benethamine penicillin G	960.0	E856	E930.0	E950.4	E962.0	E980.4
Benisone	976.0	E858.7	E946.0	E950.4	E962.0	E980.4
Benoquin	976.8	E858.7	E946.8	E950.4	E962.0	E980.4
Benoxinate	968.5	E855.2	E938.5	E950.4	E962.0	E980.4
Bentonite	976.3	E858.7	E946.3	E950.4	E962.0	E980.4
Benzalkonium (chloride)	976.0	E858.7	E946.0	E950.4	E962.0	E980.4
ophthalmic preparation	976.5	E858.7	E946.5	E950.4	E962.0	E980.4
Benzamidosalicylate (calcium)	961.8	E857	E931.8	E950.4	E962.0	E980.4
Benzathine penicillin	960.0	E856	E930.0	E950.4	E962.0	E980.4
Benzcarbimine	963.1	E858.1	E933.1	E950.4	E962.0	E980.4
Benzedrex	971.2	E855.5	E941.2	E950.4	E962.0	E980.4
Benzedrine (amphetamine)	969.7	E854.2	E939.7	E950.3	E962.0	E980.3
Benzene (acetyl) (dimethyl) (methyl) (solvent) (vapor)	982.0	E862.4	—	E950.9	E962.1	E980.9
hexachloride (gamma) (insecticide) (vapor)	989.2	E863.0	—	E950.6	E962.1	E980.7
Benzethonium	976.0	E858.7	E946.0	E950.4	E962.0	E980.4
Benzhexol (chloride)	966.4	E855.0	E936.4	E950.4	E962.0	E980.4
Benzilonium	971.1	E855.4	E941.1	E950.4	E962.0	E980.4
Benzin(e) — *see* Ligroin						

☑ Additional Digit Required — Refer to the Tabular List (Numeric Code Section) for Additional Digit Selection

▶◀ Revised Text ● New Line ▲ Revised Code

	Poisoning	External Cause (E-Code)				
		Accident	Therapeutic Use	Suicide Attempt	Assault	Undetermined
Benziodarone	972.4	E858.3	E942.4	E950.4	E962.0	E980.4
Benzocaine	968.5	E855.2	E938.5	E950.4	E962.0	E980.4
Benzodiapin	969.4	E853.2	E939.4	E950.3	E962.0	E980.3
Benzodiazepines (tranquilizers) NEC	969.4	E853.2	E939.4	E950.3	E962.0	E980.3
Benzoic acid (with salicylic acid) (anti-infective)	976.0	E858.7	E946.0	E950.4	E962.0	E980.4
Benzoin	976.3	E858.7	E946.3	E950.4	E962.0	E980.4
Benzol (vapor)	982.0	E862.4	—	E950.9	E962.1	E980.9
Benzomorphan	965.09	E850.2	E935.2	E950.0	E962.0	E980.0
Benzonatate	975.4	E858.6	E945.4	E950.4	E962.0	E980.4
Benzothiadiazides	974.3	E858.5	E944.3	E950.4	E962.0	E980.4
Benzoylpas	961.8	E857	E931.8	E950.4	E962.0	E980.4
Benzperidol	969.5	E853.8	E939.5	E950.3	E962.0	E980.3
Benzphetamine	977.0	E858.8	E947.0	E950.4	E962.0	E980.4
Benzpyrinium	971.0	E855.3	E941.0	E950.4	E962.0	E980.4
Benzquinamide	963.0	E858.1	E933.0	E950.4	E962.0	E980.4
Benzthiazide	974.3	E858.5	E944.3	E950.4	E962.0	E980.4
Benztropine	971.1	E855.4	E941.1	E950.4	E962.0	E980.4
Benzyl						
acetate	982.8	E862.4	—	E950.9	E962.1	E980.9
benzoate (anti-infective)	976.0	E858.7	E946.0	E950.4	E962.0	E980.4
morphine	965.09	E850.2	E935.2	E950.0	E962.0	E980.0
penicillin	960.0	E856	E930.0	E950.4	E962.0	E980.4
Bephenium hydroxynapthoate	961.6	E857	E931.6	E950.4	E962.0	E980.4
Bergamot oil	989.89	E866.8	—	E950.9	E962.1	E980.9
Berries, poisonous	988.2	E865.3	—	E950.9	E962.1	E980.9
Beryllium (compounds) (fumes)	985.3	E866.4	—	E950.9	E962.1	E980.9
Beta-carotene	976.3	E858.7	E946.3	E950.4	E962.0	E980.4
Beta-Chlor	967.1	E852.0	E937.1	E950.2	E962.0	E980.2
Betamethasone	962.0	E858.0	E932.0	E950.4	E962.0	E980.4
topical	976.0	E858.7	E946.0	E950.4	E962.0	E980.4
Betazole	977.8	E858.8	E947.8	E950.4	E962.0	E980.4
Bethanechol	971.0	E855.3	E941.0	E950.4	E962.0	E980.4
Bethanidine	972.6	E858.3	E942.6	E950.4	E962.0	E980.4
Betula oil	976.3	E858.7	E946.3	E950.4	E962.0	E980.4
Bhang	969.6	E854.1	E939.6	E950.3	E962.0	E980.3
Bialamicol	961.5	E857	E931.5	E950.4	E962.0	E980.4
Bichloride of mercury — *see* Mercury, chloride						
Bichromates (calcium) (crystals) (potassium) (sodium)	983.9	E864.3	—	E950.7	E962.1	E980.6
fumes	987.8	E869.8	—	E952.8	E962.2	E982.8
Biguanide derivatives, oral	962.3	E858.0	E932.3	E950.4	E962.0	E980.4
Biligrafin	977.8	E858.8	E947.8	E950.4	E962.0	E980.4
Bilopaque	977.8	E858.8	E947.8	E950.4	E962.0	E980.4
Bioflavonoids	972.8	E858.3	E942.8	E950.4	E962.0	E980.4
Biological substance NEC	979.9	E858.8	E949.9	E950.4	E962.0	E980.4
Biperiden	966.4	E855.0	E936.4	E950.4	E962.0	E980.4
Bisacodyl	973.1	E858.4	E943.1	E950.4	E962.0	E980.4
Bishydroxycoumarin	964.2	E858.2	E934.2	E950.4	E962.0	E980.4
Bismarsen	961.1	E857	E931.1	E950.4	E962.0	E980.4
Bismuth (compounds) NEC	985.8	E866.4	—	E950.9	E962.1	E980.9
anti-infectives	961.2	E857	E931.2	E950.4	E962.0	E980.4
subcarbonate	973.5	E858.4	E943.5	E950.4	E962.0	E980.4
sulfarsphenamine	961.1	E857	E931.1	E950.4	E962.0	E980.4
Bithionol	961.6	E857	E931.6	E950.4	E962.0	E980.4
Bitter almond oil	989.0	E866.8	—	E950.9	E962.1	E980.9
Bittersweet	988.2	E865.4	—	E950.9	E962.1	E930.9
Black						
flag	989.4	E863.4	—	E950.6	E962.1	E980.7
henbane	988.2	E865.4	—	E950.9	E962.1	E980.9
leaf (40)	989.4	E863.4	—	E950.6	E962.1	E980.7
widow spider (bite)	989.5	E905.1	—	E950.9	E962.1	E980.9
antivenin	979.9	E858.8	E949.9	E950.4	E962.0	E980.4
Blast furnace gas (carbon monoxide from)	986	E868.8	—	E952.1	E962.2	E982.1
Bleach NEC	983.9	E864.3	—	E950.7	E962.1	E980.6
Bleaching solutions	983.9	E864.3	—	E950.7	E962.1	E980.6
Bleomycin (sulfate)	960.7	E856	E930.7	E950.4	E962.0	E980.4
Blockain	968.9	E855.2	E938.9	E950.4	E962.0	E980.4
infiltration (subcutaneous)	968.5	E855.2	E938.5	E950.4	E962.0	E980.4
nerve block (peripheral) (plexus)	968.6	E855.2	E938.6	E950.4	E962.0	E980.4
topical (surface)	968.5	E855.2	E938.5	E950.4	E962.0	E980.4
Blood (derivatives) (natural) (plasma) (whole)	964.7	E858.2	E934.7	E950.4	E962.0	E980.4
affecting agent	964.9	E858.2	E934.9	E950.4	E962.0	E980.4
specified NEC	964.8	E858.2	E934.8	E950.4	E962.0	E980.4
Blood — *continued*						
substitute (macromolecular)	964.8	E858.2	E934.8	E950.4	E962.0	E980.4
Blue velvet	965.09	E850.2	E935.2	E950.0	E962.0	E980.0
Bone meal	989.89	E866.5	—	E950.9	E962.1	E980.9
Bonine	963.0	E858.1	E933.0	E950.4	E962.0	E980.4
Boracic acid	976.0	E858.7	E946.0	E950.4	E962.0	E980.4
ENT agent	976.6	E858.7	E946.6	E950.4	E962.0	E980.4
ophthalmic preparation	976.5	E858.7	E946.5	E950.4	E962.0	E980.4
Borate (cleanser) (sodium)	989.6	E861.3	—	E950.9	E962.1	E980.9
Borax (cleanser)	989.6	E861.3	—	E950.9	E962.1	E980.9
Boric acid	976.0	E858.7	E946.0	E950.4	E962.0	E980.4
ENT agent	976.6	E858.7	E946.6	E950.4	E962.0	E980.4
ophthalmic preparation	976.5	E858.7	E946.5	E950.4	E962.0	E980.4
Boron hydride NEC	989.89	E866.8	—	E950.9	E962.1	E980.9
fumes or gas	987.8	E869.8	—	E952.8	E962.2	E982.8
Botox	975.3	E858.6	E945.3	E950.4	E962.0	E980.4
Brake fluid vapor	987.8	E869.8	—	E952.8	E962.2	E982.8
Brass (compounds) (fumes)	985.8	E866.4	—	E950.9	E962.1	E980.9
Brasso	981	E861.3	—	E950.9	E962.1	E980.9
Bretylium (tosylate)	972.6	E858.3	E942.6	E950.4	E962.0	E980.4
Brevital (sodium)	968.3	E855.1	E938.3	E950.4	E962.0	E980.4
British antilewisite	963.8	E858.1	E933.8	E950.4	E962.0	E980.4
Bromal (hydrate)	967.3	E852.2	E937.3	E950.2	E962.0	E980.2
Bromelains	963.4	E858.1	E933.4	E950.4	E962.0	E980.4
Bromides NEC	967.3	E852.2	E937.3	E950.2	E962.0	E980.2
Bromine (vapor)	987.8	E869.8	—	E952.8	E962.2	E982.8
compounds (medicinal)	967.3	E852.2	E937.3	E950.2	E962.0	E980.2
Bromisovalum	967.3	E852.2	E937.3	E950.2	E962.0	E980.2
Bromobenzyl cyanide	987.5	E869.3	—	E952.8	E962.2	E982.8
Bromodiphenhydramine	963.0	E858.1	E933.0	E950.4	E962.0	E980.4
Bromoform	967.3	E852.2	E937.3	E950.2	E962.0	E980.2
Bromophenol blue reagent	977.8	E858.8	E947.8	E950.4	E962.0	E980.4
Bromosalicylhydroxamic acid	961.8	E857	E931.8	E950.4	E962.0	E980.4
Bromo-seltzer	965.4	E850.4	E935.4	E950.0	E962.0	E980.0
Brompheniramine	963.0	E858.1	E933.0	E950.4	E962.0	E980.4
Bromural	967.3	E852.2	E937.3	E950.2	E962.0	E980.2
Brown spider (bite) (venom)	989.5	E905.1	—	E950.9	E962.1	E980.9
Brucia	988.2	E865.3	—	E950.9	E962.1	E980.9
Brucine	989.1	E863.7	—	E950.6	E962.1	E980.7
Brunswick green — *see* Copper						
Bruten — *see* Ibuprofen						
Bryonia (alba) (dioica)	988.2	E865.4	—	E950.9	E962.1	E980.9
Buclizine	969.5	E853.8	E939.5	E950.3	E962.0	E980.3
Bufferin	965.1	E850.3	E935.3	E950.0	E962.0	E980.0
Bufotenine	969.6	E854.1	E939.6	E950.3	E962.0	E980.3
Buphenine	971.2	E855.5	E941.2	E950.4	E962.0	E980.4
Bupivacaine	968.9	E855.2	E938.9	E950.4	E962.0	E980.4
infiltration (subcutaneous)	968.5	E855.2	E938.5	E950.4	E962.0	E980.4
nerve block (peripheral) (plexus)	968.6	E855.2	E938.6	E950.4	E962.0	E980.4
Busulfan	963.1	E858.1	E933.1	E950.4	E962.0	E980.4
Butabarbital (sodium)	967.0	E851	E937.0	E950.1	E962.0	E980.1
Butabarbitone	967.0	E851	E937.0	E950.1	E962.0	E980.1
Butabarpal	967.0	E851	E937.0	E950.1	E962.0	E980.1
Butacaine	968.5	E855.2	E938.5	E950.4	E962.0	E980.4
Butallylonal	967.0	E851	E937.0	E950.1	E962.0	E980.1
Butane (distributed in mobile container)	987.0	E868.0	—	E951.1	E962.2	E981.1
distributed through pipes	987.0	E867	—	E951.0	E962.2	E981.0
incomplete combustion of — *see* Carbon monoxide, butane						
Butanol	980.3	E860.4	—	E950.9	E962.1	E980.9
Butanone	982.8	E862.4	—	E950.9	E962.1	E980.9
Butaperazine	969.1	E853.0	E939.1	E950.3	E962.0	E980.3
Butazolidin	965.5	E850.5	E935.5	E950.0	E962.0	E980.0
Butethal	967.0	E851	E937.0	E950.1	E962.0	E980.1
Butethamate	971.1	E855.4	E941.1	E950.4	E962.0	E980.4
Buthalitone (sodium)	968.3	E855.1	E938.3	E950.4	E962.0	E980.4
Butisol (sodium)	967.0	E851	E937.0	E950.1	E962.0	E980.1
Butobarbital, butobarbitone	967.0	E851	E937.0	E950.1	E962.0	E980.1
Butriptyline	969.0	E854.0	E939.0	E950.3	E962.0	E980.3
Buttercups	988.2	E865.4	—	E950.9	E962.1	E980.9
Butter of antimony — *see* Antimony						
Butyl						
acetate (secondary)	982.8	E862.4	—	E950.9	E962.1	E980.9
alcohol	980.3	E860.4	—	E950.9	E962.1	E980.9
carbinol	980.8	E860.8	—	E950.9	E962.1	E980.9
carbitol	982.8	E862.4	—	E950.9	E962.1	E980.9
cellosolve	982.8	E862.4	—	E950.9	E962.1	E980.9

	Poisoning	Accident	Therapeutic Use	Suicide Attempt	Assault	Undetermined
		External Cause (E-Code)				
Butyl — *continued*						
chloral (hydrate)	967.1	E852.0	E937.1	E950.2	E962.0	E980.2
formate	982.8	E862.4	—	E950.9	E962.1	E980.9
scopolammonium bromide	971.1	E855.4	E941.1	E950.4	E962.0	E980.4
Butyn	968.5	E855.2	E938.5	E950.4	E962.0	E980.4
Butyrophenone (-based tranquilizers)	969.2	E853.1	E939.2	E950.3	E962.0	E980.3
Cacodyl, cacodylic acid — *see* Arsenic						
Cactinomycin	960.7	E856	E930.7	E950.4	E962.0	E980.4
Cade oil	976.4	E858.7	E946.4	E950.4	E962.0	E980.4
Cadmium (chloride) (compounds) (dust) (fumes) (oxide)	985.5	E866.4	—	E950.9	E962.1	E980.9
sulfide (medicinal) NEC	976.4	E858.7	E946.4	E950.4	E962.0	E980.4
Caffeine	969.7	E854.2	E939.7	E950.3	E962.0	E980.3
Calabar bean	988.2	E865.4	—	E950.9	E962.1	E980.9
Caladium seguinium	988.2	E865.4	—	E950.9	E962.1	E980.9
Calamine (liniment) (lotion)	976.3	E858.7	E946.3	E950.4	E962.0	E980.4
Calciferol	963.5	E858.1	E933.5	E950.4	E962.0	E980.4
Calcium (salts) NEC	974.5	E858.5	E944.5	E950.4	E962.0	E980.4
acetylsalicylate	965.1	E850.3	E935.3	E950.0	E962.0	E980.0
benzamidosalicylate	961.8	E857	E931.8	E950.4	E962.0	E980.4
carbaspirin	965.1	E850.3	E935.3	E950.0	E962.0	E980.0
carbimide (citrated)	977.3	E858.8	E947.3	E950.4	E962.0	E980.4
carbonate (antacid)	973.0	E858.4	E943.0	E950.4	E962.0	E980.4
cyanide (citrated)	977.3	E858.8	E947.3	E950.4	E962.0	E980.4
dioctyl sulfosuccinate	973.2	E858.4	E943.2	E950.4	E962.0	E980.4
disodium edathamil	963.8	E858.1	E933.8	E950.4	E962.0	E980.4
disodium edetate	963.8	E858.1	E933.8	E950.4	E962.0	E980.4
EDTA	963.8	E858.1	E933.8	E950.4	E962.0	E980.4
hydrate, hydroxide	983.2	E864.2	—	E950.7	E962.1	E980.6
mandelate	961.9	E857	E931.9	E950.4	E962.0	E980.4
oxide	983.2	E864.2	—	E950.7	E962.1	E980.6
Calomel — *see* Mercury, chloride						
Caloric agents NEC	974.5	E858.5	E944.5	E950.4	E962.0	E980.4
Calusterone	963.1	E858.1	E933.1	E950.4	E962.0	E980.4
Camoquin	961.4	E857	E931.4	E950.4	E962.0	E980.4
Camphor (oil)	976.1	E858.7	E946.1	E950.4	E962.0	E980.4
Candeptin	976.0	E858.7	E946.0	E950.4	E962.0	E980.4
Candicidin	976.0	E858.7	E946.0	E950.4	E962.0	E980.4
Cannabinols	969.6	E854.1	E939.6	E950.3	E962.0	E980.3
Cannabis (derivatives) (indica) (sativa)	969.6	E854.1	E939.6	E950.3	E962.0	E980.3
Canned heat	980.1	E860.2	—	E950.9	E962.1	E980.9
Cantharides, cantharidin, cantharis	976.8	E858.7	E946.8	E950.4	E962.0	E980.4
Capillary agents	972.8	E858.3	E942.8	E950.4	E962.0	E980.4
Capreomycin	960.6	E856	E930.6	E950.4	E962.0	E980.4
Captodiame, captodiamine	969.5	E853.8	E939.5	E950.3	E962.0	E980.3
Caramiphen (hydrochloride)	971.1	E855.4	E941.1	E950.4	E962.0	E980.4
Carbachol	971.0	E855.3	E941.0	E950.4	E962.0	E980.4
Carbacrylamine resins	974.5	E858.5	E944.5	E950.4	E962.0	E980.4
Carbamate (sedative)	967.8	E852.8	E937.8	E950.2	E962.0	E980.2
herbicide	989.3	E863.5	—	E950.6	E962.1	E980.7
insecticide	989.3	E863.2	—	E950.6	E962.1	E980.7
Carbamazepine	966.3	E855.0	E936.3	E950.4	E962.0	E980.4
Carbamic esters	967.8	E852.8	E937.8	E950.2	E962.0	E980.2
Carbamide	974.4	E858.5	E944.4	E950.4	E962.0	E980.4
topical	976.8	E858.7	E946.8	E950.4	E962.0	E980.4
Carbamylcholine chloride	971.0	E855.3	E941.0	E950.4	E962.0	E980.4
Carbarsone	961.1	E857	E931.1	E950.4	E962.0	E980.4
Carbaryl	989.3	E863.2	—	E950.6	E962.1	E980.7
Carbaspirin	965.1	E850.3	E935.3	E950.0	E962.0	E980.0
Carbazochrome	972.8	E858.3	E942.8	E950.4	E962.0	E980.4
Carbenicillin	960.0	E856	E930.0	E950.4	E962.0	E980.4
Carbenoxolone	973.8	E858.4	E943.8	E950.4	E962.0	E980.4
Carbetapentane	975.4	E858.6	E945.4	E950.4	E962.0	E980.4
Carbimazole	962.8	E858.0	E932.8	E950.4	E962.0	E980.4
Carbinol	980.1	E860.2	—	E950.9	E962.1	E980.9
Carbinoxamine	963.0	E858.1	E933.0	E950.4	E962.0	E980.4
Carbitol	982.8	E862.4	—	E950.9	E962.1	E980.9
Carbocaine	968.9	E855.2	E938.9	E950.4	E962.0	E980.4
infiltration (subcutaneous)	968.5	E855.2	E938.5	E950.4	E962.0	E980.4
nerve block (peripheral) (plexus)	968.6	E855.2	E938.6	E950.4	E962.0	E980.4
topical (surface)	968.5	E855.2	E938.5	E950.4	E962.0	E980.4
Carbol-fuchsin solution	976.0	E858.7	E946.0	E950.4	E962.0	E980.4
Carbolic acid (*see also* Phenol)	983.0	E864.0	—	E950.7	E962.1	E980.6
Carbomycin	960.8	E856	E930.8	E950.4	E962.0	E980.4

	Poisoning	Accident	Therapeutic Use	Suicide Attempt	Assault	Undetermined
		External Cause (E-Code)				
Carbon						
bisulfide (liquid) (vapor)	982.2	E862.4	—	E950.9	E962.1	E980.9
dioxide (gas)	987.8	E869.8	—	E952.8	E962.2	E982.8
disulfide (liquid) (vapor)	982.2	E862.4	—	E950.9	E962.1	E980.9
monoxide (from incomplete combustion of) (in) NEC	986	E868.9	—	E952.1	E962.2	E982.1
blast furnace gas	986	E868.8	—	E952.1	E962.2	E982.1
butane (distributed in mobile container)	986	E868.0	—	E951.1	E962.2	E981.1
distributed through pipes	986	E867	—	E951.0	E962.2	E981.0
charcoal fumes	986	E868.3	—	E952.1	E962.2	E982.1
coal						
gas (piped)	986	E867	—	E951.0	E962.2	E981.0
solid (in domestic stoves, fireplaces)	986	E868.3	—	E952.1	E962.2	E982.1
coke (in domestic stoves, fireplaces)	986	E868.3	—	E952.1	E962.2	E982.1
exhaust gas (motor) not in transit	986	E868.2	—	E952.0	E962.2	E982.0
combustion engine, any not in watercraft	986	E868.2	—	E952.0	E962.2	E982.0
farm tractor, not in transit	986	E868.2	—	E952.0	E962.2	E982.0
gas engine	986	E868.2	—	E952.0	E962.2	E982.0
motor pump	986	E868.2	—	E952.0	E962.2	E982.0
motor vehicle, not in transit	986	E868.2	—	E952.0	E962.2	E982.0
fuel (in domestic use)	986	E868.3	—	E952.1	E962.2	E982.1
gas (piped)	986	E867	—	E951.0	E962.2	E981.0
in mobile container	986	E868.0	—	E951.1	E962.2	E981.1
utility	986	E868.1	—	E951.8	E962.2	E981.1
in mobile container	986	E868.0	—	E951.1	E962.2	E981.1
piped (natural)	986	E867	—	E951.0	E962.2	E981.0
illuminating gas	986	E868.1	—	E951.8	E962.2	E981.8
industrial fuels or gases, any	986	E868.8	—	E952.1	E962.2	E982.1
kerosene (in domestic stoves, fireplaces)	986	E868.3	—	E952.1	E962.2	E982.1
kiln gas or vapor	986	E868.8	—	E952.1	E962.2	E982.1
motor exhaust gas, not in transit	986	E868.2	—	E952.0	E962.2	E982.0
piped gas (manufactured) (natural)	986	E867	—	E951.0	E962.2	E981.0
producer gas	986	E868.8	—	E952.1	E962.2	E982.1
propane (distributed in mobile container)	986	E868.0	—	E951.1	E962.2	E981.1
distributed through pipes	986	E867	—	E951.0	E962.2	E981.0
specified source NEC	986	E868.8	—	E952.1	E962.2	E982.1
stove gas	986	E868.1	—	E951.8	E962.2	E981.8
piped	986	E867	—	E951.0	E962.2	E981.0
utility gas	986	E868.1	—	E951.8	E962.2	E981.8
piped	986	E867	—	E951.0	E962.2	E981.0
water gas	986	E868.1	—	E951.8	E962.2	E981.8
wood (in domestic stoves, fireplaces)	986	E868.3	—	E952.1	E962.2	E982.1
tetrachloride (vapor) NEC	987.8	E869.8	—	E952.8	E962.2	E982.8
liquid (cleansing agent) NEC	982.1	E861.3	—	E950.9	E962.1	E980.9
solvent	982.1	E862.4	—	E950.9	E962.1	E980.9
Carbonic acid (gas)	987.8	E869.8	—	E952.8	E962.2	E982.8
anhydrase inhibitors	974.2	E858.5	E944.2	E950.4	E962.0	E980.4
Carbowax	976.3	E858.7	E946.3	E950.4	E962.0	E980.4
Carbrital	967.0	E851	E937.0	E950.1	E962.0	E980.1
Carbromal (derivatives)	967.3	E852.2	E937.3	E950.2	E962.0	E980.2
Cardiac						
depressants	972.0	E858.3	E942.0	E950.4	E962.0	E980.4
rhythm regulators	972.0	E858.3	E942.0	E950.4	E962.0	E980.4

	Poisoning	External Cause (E-Code) Accident	Therapeutic Use	Suicide Attempt	Assault	Undetermined
Cardiografin	977.8	E858.8	E947.8	E950.4	E962.0	E980.4
Cardio-green	977.8	E858.8	E947.8	E950.4	E962.0	E980.4
Cardiotonic glycosides	972.1	E858.3	E942.1	E950.4	E962.0	E980.4
Cardiovascular agents NEC	972.9	E858.3	E942.9	E950.4	E962.0	E980.4
Cardrase	974.2	E858.5	E944.2	E950.4	E962.0	E980.4
Carfusin	976.0	E858.7	E946.0	E950.4	E962.0	E980.4
Carisoprodol	968.0	E855.1	E938.0	E950.4	E962.0	E980.4
Carmustine	963.1	E858.1	E933.1	E950.4	E962.0	E980.4
Carotene	963.5	E858.1	E933.5	E950.4	E962.0	E980.4
Carphenazine (maleate)	969.1	E853.0	E939.1	E950.3	E962.0	E980.3
Carter's Little Pills	973.1	E858.4	E943.1	E950.4	E962.0	E980.4
Cascara (sagrada)	973.1	E858.4	E943.1	E950.4	E962.0	E980.4
Cassava	988.2	E865.4	—	E950.9	E962.1	E980.9
Castellani's paint	976.0	E858.7	E946.0	E950.4	E962.0	E980.4
Castor						
bean	988.2	E865.3	—	E950.9	E962.1	E980.9
oil	973.1	E858.4	E943.1	E950.4	E962.0	E980.4
Caterpillar (sting)	989.5	E905.5	—	E950.9	E962.1	E980.9
Catha (edulis)	970.8	E854.3	E940.8	E950.4	E962.0	E980.4
Cathartics NEC	973.3	E858.4	E943.3	E950.4	E962.0	E980.4
contact	973.1	E858.4	E943.1	E950.4	E962.0	E980.4
emollient	973.2	E858.4	E943.2	E950.4	E962.0	E980.4
intestinal irritants	973.1	E858.4	E943.1	E950.4	E962.0	E980.4
saline	973.3	E858.4	E943.3	E950.4	E962.0	E980.4
Cathomycin	960.8	E856	E930.8	E950.4	E962.0	E980.4
Caustic(s)	983.9	E864.4	—	E950.7	E962.1	E980.6
alkali	983.2	E864.2	—	E950.7	E962.1	E980.6
hydroxide	983.2	E864.2	—	E950.7	E962.1	E980.6
potash	983.2	E864.2	—	E950.7	E962.1	E980.6
soda	983.2	E864.2	—	E950.7	E962.1	E980.6
specified NEC	983.9	E864.3	—	E950.7	E962.1	E980.6
Ceepryn	976.0	E858.7	E946.0	E950.4	E962.0	E980.4
ENT agent	976.6	E858.7	E946.6	E950.4	E962.0	E980.4
lozenges	976.6	E858.7	E946.6	E950.4	E962.0	E980.4
Celestone	962.0	E858.0	E932.0	E950.4	E962.0	E980.4
topical	976.0	E858.7	E946.0	E950.4	E962.0	E980.4
Cellosolve	982.8	E862.4	—	E950.9	E962.1	E980.9
Cell stimulants and proliferants	976.8	E858.7	E946.8	E950.4	E962.0	E980.4
Cellulose derivatives, cathartic	973.3	E858.4	E943.3	E950.4	E962.0	E980.4
nitrates (topical)	976.3	E858.7	E946.3	E950.4	E962.0	E980.4
Centipede (bite)	989.5	E905.4	—	E950.9	E962.1	E980.9
Central nervous system						
depressants	968.4	E855.1	E938.4	E950.4	E962.0	E980.4
anesthetic (general) NEC	968.4	E855.1	E938.4	E950.4	E962.0	E980.4
gases NEC	968.2	E855.1	E938.2	E950.4	E962.0	E980.4
intravenous	968.3	E855.1	E938.3	E950.4	E962.0	E980.4
barbiturates	967.0	E851	E937.0	E950.1	E962.0	E980.1
bromides	967.3	E852.2	E937.3	E950.2	E962.0	E980.2
cannabis sativa	969.6	E854.1	E939.6	E950.3	E962.0	E980.3
chloral hydrate	967.1	E852.0	E937.1	E950.2	E962.0	E980.2
hallucinogenics	969.6	E854.1	E939.6	E950.3	E962.0	E980.3
hypnotics	967.9	E852.9	E937.9	E950.2	E962.0	E980.2
specified NEC	967.8	E852.8	E937.8	E950.2	E962.0	E980.2
muscle relaxants	968.0	E855.1	E938.0	E950.4	E962.0	E980.4
paraldehyde	967.2	E852.1	E937.2	E950.2	E962.0	E980.2
sedatives	967.9	E852.9	E937.9	E950.2	E962.0	E980.2
mixed NEC	967.6	E852.5	E937.6	E950.2	E962.0	E980.2
specified NEC	967.8	E852.8	E937.8	E950.2	E962.0	E980.2
muscle-tone depressants	968.0	E855.1	E938.0	E950.4	E962.0	E980.4
stimulants	970.9	E854.3	E940.9	E950.4	E962.0	E980.4
amphetamines	969.7	E854.2	E939.7	E950.3	E962.0	E980.3
analeptics	970.0	E854.3	E940.0	E950.4	E962.0	E980.4
antidepressants	969.0	E854.0	E939.0	E950.3	E962.0	E980.3
opiate antagonists	970.1	E854.3	E940.0	E950.4	E962.0	E980.4
specified NEC	970.8	E854.3	E940.8	E950.4	E962.0	E980.4
Cephalexin	960.5	E856	E930.5	E950.4	E962.0	E980.4
Cephaloglycin	960.5	E856	E930.5	E950.4	E962.0	E980.4
Cephaloridine	960.5	E856	E930.5	E950.4	E962.0	E980.4
Cephalosporins NEC	960.5	E856	E930.5	E950.4	E962.0	E980.4
N (adicillin)	960.0	E856	E930.0	E950.4	E962.0	E980.4
Cephalothin (sodium)	960.5	E856	E930.5	E950.4	E962.0	E980.4
Cerbera (odallam)	988.2	E865.4	—	E950.9	E962.1	E980.9
Cerberin	972.1	E858.3	E942.1	E950.4	E962.0	E980.4
Cerebral stimulants	970.9	E854.3	E940.9	E950.4	E962.0	E980.4
psychotherapeutic	969.7	E854.2	E939.7	E950.3	E962.0	E980.3
specified NEC	970.8	E854.3	E940.8	E950.4	E962.0	E980.4
Cetalkonium (chloride)	976.0	E858.7	E946.0	E950.4	E962.0	E980.4
Cetoxime	963.0	E858.1	E933.0	E950.4	E962.0	E980.4
Cetrimide	976.2	E858.7	E946.2	E950.4	E962.0	E980.4
Cetylpyridinium	976.0	E858.7	E946.0	E950.4	E962.0	E980.4
ENT agent	976.6	E858.7	E946.6	E950.4	E962.0	E980.4
lozenges	976.6	E858.7	E946.6	E950.4	E962.0	E980.4
Cevadilla — *see* Sabadilla						
Cevitamic acid	963.5	E858.1	E933.5	E950.4	E962.0	E980.4
Chalk, precipitated	973.0	E858.4	E943.0	E950.4	E962.0	E980.4
Charcoal						
fumes (carbon monoxide)	986	E868.3	—	E952.1	E962.2	E982.1
industrial	986	E868.8	—	E952.1	E962.2	E982.1
medicinal (activated)	973.0	E858.4	E943.0	E950.4	E962.0	E980.4
Chelating agents NEC	977.2	E858.8	E947.2	E950.4	E962.0	E980.4
Chelidonium majus	988.2	E865.4	—	E950.9	E962.1	E980.9
Chemical substance	989.9	E866.9	—	E950.9	E962.1	E980.9
specified NEC	989.89	E866.8	—	E950.9	E962.1	E980.9
Chemotherapy, antineoplastic	963.1	E858.1	E933.1	E950.4	E962.0	E980.4
Chenopodium (oil)	961.6	E857	E931.6	E950.4	E962.0	E980.4
Cherry laurel	988.2	E865.4	—	E950.9	E962.1	E980.9
Chiniofon	961.3	E857	E931.3	E950.4	E962.0	E980.4
Chlophedianol	975.4	E858.6	E945.4	E950.4	E962.0	E980.4
Chloral (betaine) (formamide) (hydrate)	967.1	E852.0	E937.1	E950.2	E962.0	E980.2
Chloralamide	967.1	E852.0	E937.1	E950.2	E962.0	E980.2
Chlorambucil	963.1	E858.1	E933.1	E950.4	E962.0	E980.4
Chloramphenicol	960.2	E856	E930.2	E950.4	E962.0	E980.4
ENT agent	976.6	E858.7	E946.6	E950.4	E962.0	E980.4
ophthalmic preparation	976.5	E858.7	E946.5	E950.4	E962.0	E980.4
topical NEC	976.0	E858.7	E946.0	E950.4	E962.0	E980.4
Chlorate(s) (potassium) (sodium) NEC	983.9	E864.3	—	E950.7	E962.1	E980.6
herbicides	989.4	E863.5	—	E950.6	E962.1	E980.7
Chlorcylizine	963.0	E858.1	E933.0	E950.4	E962.0	E980.4
Chlordan(e) (dust)	989.2	E863.0	—	E950.6	E962.1	E980.7
Chlordantoin	976.0	E858.7	E946.0	E950.4	E962.0	E980.4
Chlordiazepoxide	969.4	E853.2	E939.4	E950.3	E962.0	E980.3
Chloresium	976.8	E858.7	E946.8	E950.4	E962.0	E980.4
Chlorethiazol	967.1	E852.0	E937.1	E950.2	E962.0	E980.2
Chlorethyl — *see* Ethyl, chloride						
Chloretone	967.1	E852.0	E937.1	E950.2	E962.0	E980.2
Chlorex	982.3	E862.4	—	E950.9	E962.1	E980.9
Chlorhexadol	967.1	E852.0	E937.1	E950.2	E962.0	E980.2
Chlorhexidine (hydrochloride)	976.0	E858.7	E946.0	E950.4	E962.0	E980.4
Chlorhydroxyquinolin	976.0	E858.7	E946.0	E950.4	E962.0	E980.4
Chloride of lime (bleach)	983.9	E864.3	—	E950.7	E962.1	E980.6
Chlorinated						
camphene	989.2	E863.0	—	E950.6	E962.1	E980.7
diphenyl	989.89	E866.8	—	E950.9	E962.1	E980.9
hydrocarbons NEC	989.2	E863.0	—	E950.6	E962.1	E980.7
solvent	982.3	E862.4	—	E950.9	E962.1	E980.9
lime (bleach)	983.9	E864.3	—	E950.7	E962.1	E980.6
naphthalene — *see* Naphthalene						
pesticides NEC	989.2	E863.0	—	E950.6	E962.1	E980.7
soda — *see* Sodium, hypochlorite						
Chlorine (fumes) (gas)	987.6	E869.8	—	E952.8	E962.2	E982.8
bleach	983.9	E864.3	—	E950.7	E962.1	E980.6
compounds NEC	983.9	E864.3	—	E950.7	E962.1	E980.6
disinfectant	983.9	E861.4	—	E950.7	E962.1	E980.6
releasing agents NEC	983.9	E864.3	—	E950.7	E962.1	E980.6
Chlorisondamine	972.3	E858.3	E942.3	E950.4	E962.0	E980.4
Chlormadinone	962.2	E858.0	E932.2	E950.4	E962.0	E980.4
Chlormerodrin	974.0	E858.5	E944.0	E950.4	E962.0	E980.4
Chlormethiazole	967.1	E852.0	E937.1	E950.2	E962.0	E980.2
Chlormethylenecycline	960.4	E856	E930.4	E950.4	E962.0	E980.4
Chlormezanone	969.5	E853.8	E939.5	E950.3	E962.0	E980.3
Chloroacetophenone	987.5	E869.3	—	E952.8	E962.2	E982.8
Chloroaniline	983.0	E864.0	—	E950.7	E962.1	E980.6
Chlorobenzene, chlorobenzol	982.0	E862.4	—	E950.9	E962.1	E980.9
Chlorobutanol	967.1	E852.0	E937.1	E950.2	E962.0	E980.2
Chlorodinitrobenzene	983.0	E864.0	—	E950.7	E962.1	E980.6
dust or vapor	987.8	E869.8	—	E952.8	E962.2	E982.8
Chloroethane — *see* Ethyl, chloride						
Chloroform (fumes) (vapor)	987.8	E869.8	—	E952.8	E962.2	E982.8
anesthetic (gas)	968.2	E855.1	E938.2	E950.4	E962.0	E980.4
liquid NEC	968.4	E855.1	E938.4	E950.4	E962.0	E980.4
solvent	982.3	E862.4	—	E950.9	E962.1	E980.9
Chloroguanide	961.4	E857	E931.4	E950.4	E962.0	E980.4

		External Cause (E-Code)				
	Poisoning	Accident	Therapeutic Use	Suicide Attempt	Assault	Undetermined
Chloromycetin	960.2	E856	E930.2	E950.4	E962.0	E980.4
ENT agent	976.6	E858.7	E946.6	E950.4	E962.0	E980.4
ophthalmic preparation	976.5	E858.7	E946.5	E950.4	E962.0	E980.4
otic solution	976.6	E858.7	E946.6	E950.4	E962.0	E980.4
topical NEC	976.0	E858.7	E946.0	E950.4	E962.0	E980.4
Chloronitrobenzene	983.0	E864.0	—	E950.7	E962.1	E980.6
dust or vapor	987.8	E869.8	—	E952.8	E962.2	E982.8
Chlorophenol	983.0	E864.0	—	E950.7	E962.1	E980.6
Chlorophenothane	989.2	E863.0	—	E950.6	E962.1	E980.7
Chlorophyll (derivatives)	976.8	E858.7	E946.8	E950.4	E962.0	E980.4
Chloropicrin (fumes)	987.8	E869.8	—	E952.8	E962.2	E982.8
fumigant	989.4	E863.8	—	E950.6	E962.1	E980.7
fungicide	989.4	E863.6	—	E950.6	E962.1	E980.7
pesticide (fumes)	989.4	E863.4	—	E950.6	E962.1	E980.7
Chloroprocaine	968.9	E855.2	E938.9	E950.4	E962.0	E980.4
infiltration (subcutaneous)	968.5	E855.2	E938.5	E950.4	E962.0	E980.4
nerve block (peripheral) (plexus)	968.6	E855.2	E938.6	E950.4	E962.0	E980.4
Chloroptic	976.5	E858.7	E946.5	E950.4	E962.0	E980.4
Chloropurine	963.1	E858.1	E933.1	E950.4	E962.0	E980.4
Chloroquine (hydrochloride) (phosphate)	961.4	E857	E931.4	E950.4	E962.0	E980.4
Chlorothen	963.0	E858.1	E933.0	E950.4	E962.0	E980.4
Chlorothiazide	974.3	E858.5	E944.3	E950.4	E962.0	E980.4
Chlorotrianisene	962.2	E858.0	E932.2	E950.4	E962.0	E980.4
Chlorovinyldichloroarsine	985.1	E866.3	—	E950.8	E962.1	E980.8
Chloroxylenol	976.0	E858.7	E946.0	E950.4	E962.0	E980.4
Chlorphenesin (carbamate)	968.0	E855.1	E938.0	E950.4	E962.0	E980.4
topical (antifungal)	976.0	E858.7	E946.0	E950.4	E962.0	E980.4
Chlorpheniramine	963.0	E858.1	E933.0	E950.4	E962.0	E980.4
Chlorphenoxamine	966.4	E855.0	E936.4	E950.4	E962.0	E980.4
Chlorphentermine	977.0	E858.8	E947.0	E950.4	E962.0	E980.4
Chlorproguanil	961.4	E857	E931.4	E950.4	E962.0	E980.4
Chlorpromazine	969.1	E853.0	E939.1	E950.3	E962.0	E980.3
Chlorpropamide	962.3	E858.0	E932.3	E950.4	E962.0	E980.4
Chlorprothixene	969.3	E853.8	E939.3	E950.3	E962.0	E980.3
Chlorquinaldol	976.0	E858.7	E946.0	E950.4	E962.0	E980.4
Chlortetracycline	960.4	E856	E930.4	E950.4	E962.0	E980.4
Chlorthalidone	974.4	E858.5	E944.4	E950.4	E962.0	E980.4
Chlortrianisene	962.2	E858.0	E932.2	E950.4	E962.0	E980.4
Chlor-Trimeton	963.0	E858.1	E933.0	E950.4	E962.0	E980.4
Chlorzoxazone	968.0	E855.1	E938.0	E950.4	E962.0	E980.4
Choke damp	987.8	E869.8	—	E952.8	E962.2	E982.8
Cholebrine	977.8	E858.8	E947.8	E950.4	E962.0	E980.4
Cholera vaccine	978.2	E858.8	E948.2	E950.4	E962.0	E980.4
Cholesterol-lowering agents	972.2	E858.3	E942.2	E950.4	E962.0	E980.4
Cholestyramine (resin)	972.2	E858.3	E942.2	E950.4	E962.0	E980.4
Cholic acid	973.4	E858.4	E943.4	E950.4	E962.0	E980.4
Choline						
dihydrogen citrate	977.1	E858.8	E947.1	E950.4	E962.0	E980.4
salicylate	965.1	E850.3	E935.3	E950.0	E962.0	E980.0
theophyllinate	974.1	E858.5	E944.1	E950.4	E962.0	E980.4
Cholinergics	971.0	E855.3	E941.0	E950.4	E962.0	E980.4
Chologrāfin	977.8	E858.8	E947.8	E950.4	E962.0	E980.4
Chorionic gonadotropin	962.4	E858.0	E932.4	E950.4	E962.0	E980.4
Chromates	983.9	E864.3	—	E950.7	E962.1	E980.6
dust or mist	987.8	E869.8	—	E952.8	E962.2	E982.8
lead	984.0	E866.0	—	E950.9	E962.1	E980.9
paint	984.0	E861.5	—	E950.9	E962.1	E980.9
Chromic acid	983.9	E864.3	—	E950.7	E962.1	E980.6
dust or mist	987.8	E869.8	—	E952.8	E962.2	E982.8
Chromium	985.6	E866.4	—	E950.9	E962.1	E980.9
compounds — *see* Chromates						
Chromonar	972.4	E858.3	E942.4	E950.4	E962.0	E980.4
Chromyl chloride	983.9	E864.3	—	E950.7	E962.1	E980.6
Chrysarobin (ointment)	976.4	E858.7	E946.4	E950.4	E962.0	E980.4
Chrysazin	973.1	E858.4	E943.1	E950.4	E962.0	E980.4
Chymar	963.4	E858.1	E933.4	E950.4	E962.0	E980.4
ophthalmic preparation	976.5	E858.7	E946.5	E950.4	E962.0	E980.4
Chymotrypsin	963.4	E858.1	E933.4	E950.4	E962.0	E980.4
ophthalmic preparation	976.5	E858.7	E946.5	E950.4	E962.0	E980.4
Cicuta maculata or virosa	988.2	E865.4	—	E950.9	E962.1	E980.9
Cigarette lighter fluid	981	E862.1	—	E950.9	E962.1	E980.9
Cinchocaine (spinal)	968.7	E855.2	E938.7	E950.4	E962.0	E980.4
topical (surface)	968.5	E855.2	E938.5	E950.4	E962.0	E980.4
Cinchona	961.4	E857	E931.4	E950.4	E962.0	E980.4
Cinchonine alkaloids	961.4	E857	E931.4	E950.4	E962.0	E980.4
Cinchophen	974.7	E858.5	E944.7	E950.4	E962.0	E980.4
Cinnarizine	963.0	E858.1	E933.0	E950.4	E962.0	E980.4
Citanest	968.9	E855.2	E938.9	E950.4	E962.0	E980.4
infiltration (subcutaneous)	968.5	E855.2	E938.5	E950.4	E962.0	E980.4
nerve block (peripheral) (plexus)	968.6	E855.2	E938.6	E950.4	E962.0	E980.4
Citric acid	989.89	E866.8	—	E950.9	E962.1	E980.9
Citrovorum factor	964.1	E858.2	E934.1	E950.4	E962.0	E980.4
Claviceps purpurea	988.2	E865.4	—	E950.9	E962.1	E980.9
Cleaner, cleansing agent NEC	989.89	E861.3	—	E950.9	E962.1	E980.9
of paint or varnish	982.8	E862.9	—	E950.9	E962.1	E980.9
Clematis vitalba	988.2	E865.4	—	E950.9	E962.1	E980.9
Clemizole	963.0	E858.1	E933.0	E950.4	E962.0	E980.4
penicillin	960.0	E856	E930.0	E950.4	E962.0	E980.4
Clidinium	971.1	E855.4	E941.1	E950.4	E962.0	E980.4
Clindamycin	960.8	E856	E930.8	E950.4	E962.0	E980.4
Cliradon	965.09	E850.2	E935.2	E950.0	E962.0	E980.0
Clocortolone	962.0	E858.0	E932.0	E950.4	E962.0	E980.4
Clofedanol	975.4	E858.6	E945.4	E950.4	E962.0	E980.4
Clofibrate	972.2	E858.3	E942.2	E950.4	E962.0	E980.4
Clomethiazole	967.1	E852.0	E937.1	E950.2	E962.0	E980.2
Clomiphene	977.8	E858.8	E947.8	E950.4	E962.0	E980.4
Clonazepam	969.4	E853.2	E939.4	E950.3	E962.0	E980.3
Clonidine	972.6	E858.3	E942.6	E950.4	E962.0	E980.4
Clopamide	974.3	E858.5	E944.3	E950.4	E962.0	E980.4
Clorazepate	969.4	E853.2	E939.4	E950.3	E962.0	E980.3
Clorexolone	974.4	E858.5	E944.4	E950.4	E962.0	E980.4
Clorox (bleach)	983.9	E864.3	—	E950.7	E962.1	E980.6
Clortermine	977.0	E858.8	E947.0	E950.4	E962.0	E980.4
Clotrimazole	976.0	E858.7	E946.0	E950.4	E962.0	E980.4
Cloxacillin	960.0	E856	E930.0	E950.4	E962.0	E980.4
Coagulants NEC	964.5	E858.2	E934.5	E950.4	E962.0	E980.4
Coal (carbon monoxide from) — *see also* Carbon, monoxide, coal						
oil — *see* Kerosene						
tar NEC	983.0	E864.0	—	E950.7	E962.1	E980.6
fumes	987.8	E869.8	—	E952.8	E962.2	E982.8
medicinal (ointment)	976.4	E858.7	E946.4	E950.4	E962.0	E980.4
analgesics NEC	965.5	E850.5	E935.5	E950.0	E962.0	E980.0
naphtha (solvent)	981	E862.0	—	E950.9	E962.1	E980.9
Cobalt (fumes) (industrial)	985.8	E866.4	—	E950.9	E962.1	E980.9
Cobra (venom)	989.5	E905.0	—	E950.9	E962.1	E980.9
Coca (leaf)	970.8	E854.3	E940.8	E950.4	E962.0	E980.4
Cocaine (hydrochloride) (salt)	970.8	E854.3	E940.8	E950.4	E962.0	E980.4
topical anesthetic	968.5	E855.2	E938.5	E950.4	E962.0	E980.4
Coccidioidin	977.8	E858.8	E947.8	E950.4	E962.0	E980.4
Cocculus indicus	988.2	E865.3	—	E950.9	E962.1	E980.9
Cochineal	989.89	E866.8	—	E950.9	E962.1	E980.9
medicinal products	977.4	E858.8	E947.4	E950.4	E962.0	E980.4
Codeine	965.09	E850.2	E935.2	E950.0	E962.0	E980.0
Coffee	989.89	E866.8	—	E950.9	E962.1	E980.9
Cogentin	971.1	E855.4	E941.1	E950.4	E962.0	E980.4
Coke fumes or gas (carbon monoxide)	986	E868.3	—	E952.1	E962.2	E982.1
industrial use	986	E868.8	—	E952.1	E962.2	E982.1
Colace	973.2	E858.4	E943.2	E950.4	E962.0	E980.4
Colchicine	974.7	E858.5	E944.7	E950.4	E962.0	E980.4
Colchicum	988.2	E865.3	—	E950.9	E962.1	E980.9
Cold cream	976.3	E858.7	E946.3	E950.4	E962.0	E980.4
Colestipol	972.2	E858.3	E942.2	E950.4	E962.0	E980.4
Colistimethate	960.8	E856	E930.8	E950.4	E962.0	E980.4
Colistin	960.8	E856	E930.8	E950.4	E962.0	E980.4
Collagenase	976.8	E858.7	E946.8	E950.4	E962.0	E980.4
Collagen	977.8	E866.8	E947.8	E950.9	E962.1	E980.9
Collodion (flexible)	976.3	E858.7	E946.3	E950.4	E962.0	E980.4
Colocynth	973.1	E858.4	E943.1	E950.4	E962.0	E980.4
Coloring matter — *see* Dye(s)						
Combustion gas — *see* Carbon, monoxide						
Compazine	969.1	E853.0	E939.1	E950.3	E962.0	E980.3
Compound						
42 (warfarin)	989.4	E863.7	—	E950.6	E962.1	E980.7
269 (endrin)	989.2	E863.0	—	E950.6	E962.1	E980.7
497 (dieldrin)	989.2	E863.0	—	E950.6	E962.1	E980.7
1080 (sodium fluoroacetate)	989.4	E863.7	—	E950.6	E962.1	E980.7
3422 (parathion)	989.3	E863.1	—	E950.6	E962.1	E980.7
3911 (phorate)	989.3	E863.1	—	E950.6	E962.1	E980.7
3956 (toxaphene)	989.2	E863.0	—	E950.6	E962.1	E980.7
4049 (malathion)	989.3	E863.1	—	E950.6	E962.1	E980.7

Substance	Poisoning	External Cause (E-Code): Accident	Therapeutic Use	Suicide Attempt	Assault	Undetermined
Compound — *continued*						
4124 (dicapthon)	989.4	E863.4	—	E950.6	E962.1	E980.7
E (cortisone)	962.0	E858.0	E932.0	E950.4	E962.0	E980.4
F (hydrocortisone)	962.0	E858.0	E932.0	E950.4	E962.0	E980.4
Congo red	977.8	E858.8	E947.8	E950.4	E962.0	E980.4
Coniine, conine	965.7	E850.7	E935.7	E950.0	E962.0	E980.0
Conium (maculatum)	988.2	E865.4	—	E950.9	E962.1	E980.9
Conjugated estrogens (equine)	962.2	E858.0	E932.2	E950.4	E962.0	E980.4
Contac	975.6	E858.6	E945.6	E950.4	E962.0	E980.4
Contact lens solution	976.5	E858.7	E946.5	E950.4	E962.0	E980.4
Contraceptives (oral)	962.2	E858.0	E932.2	E950.4	E962.0	E980.4
vaginal	976.8	E858.7	E946.8	E950.4	E962.0	E980.4
Contrast media (roentgenographic)	977.8	E858.8	E947.8	E950.4	E962.0	E980.4
Convallaria majalis	988.2	E865.4	—	E950.9	E962.1	E980.9
Copper (dust) (fumes) (salts) NEC	985.8	E866.4	—	E950.9	E962.1	E980.9
arsenate, arsenite	985.1	E866.3	—	E950.8	E962.1	E980.8
insecticide	985.1	E863.4	—	E950.8	E962.1	E980.8
emetic	973.6	E858.4	E943.6	E950.4	E962.0	E980.4
fungicide	985.8	E863.6	—	E950.6	E962.1	E980.7
insecticide	985.8	E863.4	—	E950.6	E962.1	E980.7
oleate	976.0	E858.7	E946.0	E950.4	E962.0	E980.4
sulfate	983.9	E864.3	—	E950.7	E962.1	E980.6
fungicide	983.9	E863.6	—	E950.7	E962.1	E980.6
cupric	973.6	E858.4	E943.6	E950.4	E962.0	E980.4
cuprous	983.9	E864.3	—	E950.7	E962.1	E980.6
Copperhead snake (bite) (venom)	989.5	E905.0	—	E950.9	E962.1	E980.9
Coral (sting)	989.5	E905.6	—	E950.9	E962.1	E980.9
snake (bite) (venom)	989.5	E905.0	—	E950.9	E962.1	E980.9
Cordran	976.0	E858.7	E946.0	E950.4	E962.0	E980.4
Corn cures	976.4	E858.7	E946.4	E950.4	E962.0	E980.4
Cornhusker's lotion	976.3	E858.7	E946.3	E950.4	E962.0	E980.4
Corn starch	976.3	E858.7	E946.3	E950.4	E962.0	E980.4
Corrosive	983.9	E864.4	—	E950.7	E962.1	E980.6
acids NEC	983.1	E864.1	—	E950.7	E962.1	E980.6
aromatics	983.0	E864.0	—	E950.7	E962.1	E980.6
disinfectant	983.0	E861.4	—	E950.7	E962.1	E980.6
fumes NEC	987.9	E869.9	—	E952.9	E962.2	E982.9
specified NEC	983.9	E864.3	—	E950.7	E962.1	E980.6
sublimate — *see* Mercury, chloride						
Cortate	962.0	E858.0	E932.0	E950.4	E962.0	E980.4
Cort-Dome	962.0	E858.0	E932.0	E950.4	E962.0	E980.4
ENT agent	976.6	E858.7	E946.6	E950.4	E962.0	E980.4
ophthalmic preparation	976.5	E858.7	E946.5	E950.4	E962.0	E980.4
topical NEC	976.0	E858.7	E946.0	E950.4	E962.0	E980.4
Cortef	962.0	E858.0	E932.0	E950.4	E962.0	E980.4
ENT agent	976.6	E858.7	E946.6	E950.4	E962.0	E980.4
ophthalmic preparation	976.5	E858.7	E946.5	E950.4	E962.0	E980.4
topical NEC	976.0	E858.7	E946.0	E950.4	E962.0	E980.4
Corticosteroids (fluorinated)	962.0	E858.0	E932.0	E950.4	E962.0	E980.4
ENT agent	976.6	E858.7	E946.6	E950.4	E962.0	E980.4
ophthalmic preparation	976.5	E858.7	E946.5	E950.4	E962.0	E980.4
topical NEC	976.0	E858.7	E946.0	E950.4	E962.0	E980.4
Corticotropin	962.4	E858.0	E932.4	E950.4	E962.0	E980.4
Cortisol	962.0	E858.0	E932.0	E950.4	E962.0	E980.4
ENT agent	976.6	E858.7	E946.6	E950.4	E962.0	E980.4
ophthalmic preparation	976.5	E858.7	E946.5	E950.4	E962.0	E980.4
topical NEC	976.0	E858.7	E946.0	E950.4	E962.0	E980.4
Cortisone derivatives (acetate)	962.0	E858.0	E932.0	E950.4	E962.0	E980.4
ENT agent	976.6	E858.7	E946.6	E950.4	E962.0	E980.4
ophthalmic preparation	976.5	E858.7	E946.5	E950.4	E962.0	E980.4
topical NEC	976.0	E858.7	E946.0	E950.4	E962.0	E980.4
Cortogen	962.0	E858.0	E932.0	E950.4	E962.0	E980.4
ENT agent	976.6	E858.7	E946.6	E950.4	E962.0	E980.4
ophthalmic preparation	976.5	E858.7	E946.5	E950.4	E962.0	E980.4
Cortone	962.0	E858.0	E932.0	E950.4	E962.0	E980.4
ENT agent	976.6	E858.7	E946.6	E950.4	E962.0	E980.4
ophthalmic preparation	976.5	E858.7	E946.5	E950.4	E962.0	E980.4
Cortril	962.0	E858.0	E932.0	E950.4	E962.0	E980.4
ENT agent	976.6	E858.7	E946.6	E950.4	E962.0	E980.4
ophthalmic preparation	976.5	E858.7	E946.5	E950.4	E962.0	E980.4
topical NEC	976.0	E858.7	E946.0	E950.4	E962.0	E980.4
Cosmetics	989.89	E866.7	—	E950.9	E962.1	E980.9
Cosyntropin	977.8	E858.8	E947.8	E950.4	E962.0	E980.4
Cotarnine	964.5	E858.2	E934.5	E950.4	E962.0	E980.4
Cottonseed oil	976.3	E858.7	E946.3	E950.4	E962.0	E980.4
Cough mixtures (antitussives)	975.4	E858.6	E945.4	E950.4	E962.0	E980.4
containing opiates	965.09	E850.2	E935.2	E950.0	E962.0	E980.0
expectorants	975.5	E858.6	E945.5	E950.4	E962.0	E980.4
Coumadin	964.2	E858.2	E934.2	E950.4	E962.0	E980.4
rodenticide	989.4	E863.7	—	E950.6	E962.1	E980.7
Coumarin	964.2	E858.2	E934.2	E950.4	E962.0	E980.4
Coumetarol	964.2	E858.2	E934.2	E950.4	E962.0	E980.4
Cowbane	988.2	E865.4	—	E950.9	E962.1	E980.9
Cozyme	963.5	E858.1	E933.5	E950.4	E962.0	E980.4
Crack	970.8	E854.3	E940.8	E950.4	E962.0	E980.4
Creolin	983.0	E864.0	—	E950.7	E962.1	E980.6
disinfectant	983.0	E861.4	—	E950.7	E962.1	E980.6
Creosol (compound)	983.0	E864.0	—	E950.7	E962.1	E980.6
Creosote (beechwood) (coal tar)	983.0	E864.0	—	E950.7	E962.1	E980.6
medicinal (expectorant)	975.5	E858.6	E945.5	E950.4	E962.0	E980.4
syrup	975.5	E858.6	E945.5	E950.4	E962.0	E980.4
Cresol	983.0	E864.0	—	E950.7	E962.1	E980.6
disinfectant	983.0	E861.4	—	E950.7	E962.1	E980.6
Cresylic acid	983.0	E864.0	—	E950.7	E962.1	E980.6
Cropropamide	965.7	E850.7	E935.7	E950.0	E962.0	E980.0
with crotethamide	970.0	E854.3	E940.0	E950.4	E962.0	E980.4
Crotamiton	976.0	E858.7	E946.0	E950.4	E962.0	E980.4
Crotethamide	965.7	E850.7	E935.7	E950.0	E962.0	E980.0
with cropropamide	970.0	E854.3	E940.0	E950.4	E962.0	E980.4
Croton (oil)	973.1	E858.4	E943.1	E950.4	E962.0	E980.4
chloral	967.1	E852.0	E937.1	E950.2	E962.0	E980.2
Crude oil	981	E862.1	—	E950.9	E962.1	E980.9
Cryogenine	965.8	E850.8	E935.8	E950.0	E962.0	E980.0
Cryolite (pesticide)	989.4	E863.4	—	E950.6	E962.1	E980.7
Cryptenamine	972.6	E858.3	E942.6	E950.4	E962.0	E980.4
Crystal violet	976.0	E858.7	E946.0	E950.4	E962.0	E980.4
Cuckoopint	988.2	E865.4	—	E950.9	E962.1	E980.9
Cumetharol	964.2	E858.2	E934.2	E950.4	E962.0	E980.4
Cupric sulfate	973.6	E858.4	E943.6	E950.4	E962.0	E980.4
Cuprous sulfate	983.9	E864.3	—	E950.7	E962.1	E980.6
Curare, curarine	975.2	E858.6	E945.2	E950.4	E962.0	E980.4
Cyanic acid — *see* Cyanide(s)						
Cyanide(s) (compounds) (hydrogen) (potassium) (sodium) NEC	989.0	E866.8	—	E950.9	E962.1	E980.9
dust or gas (inhalation) NEC	987.7	E869.8	—	E952.8	E962.2	E982.8
fumigant	989.0	E863.8	—	E950.6	E962.1	E980.7
mercuric — *see* Mercury						
pesticide (dust) (fumes)	989.0	E863.4	—	E950.6	E962.1	E980.7
Cyanocobalamin	964.1	E858.2	E934.1	E950.4	E962.0	E980.4
Cyanogen (chloride) (gas) NEC	987.8	E869.8	—	E952.8	E962.2	E982.8
Cyclaine	968.5	E855.2	E938.5	E950.4	E962.0	E980.4
Cyclamen europaeum	988.2	E865.4	—	E950.9	E962.1	E980.9
Cyclandelate	972.5	E858.3	E942.5	E950.4	E962.0	E980.4
Cyclazocine	965.09	E850.2	E935.2	E950.0	E962.0	E980.0
Cyclizine	963.0	E858.1	E933.0	E950.4	E962.0	E980.4
Cyclobarbital, cyclobarbitone	967.0	E851	E937.0	E950.1	E962.0	E980.1
Cycloguanil	961.4	E857	E931.4	E950.4	E962.0	E980.4
Cyclohexane	982.0	E862.4	—	E950.9	E962.1	E980.9
Cyclohexanol	980.8	E860.8	—	E950.9	E962.1	E980.9
Cyclohexanone	982.8	E862.4	—	E950.9	E962.1	E980.9
Cyclomethycaine	968.5	E855.2	E938.5	E950.4	E962.0	E980.4
Cyclopentamine	971.2	E855.5	E941.2	E950.4	E962.0	E980.4
Cyclopenthiazide	974.3	E858.5	E944.3	E950.4	E962.0	E980.4
Cyclopentolate	971.1	E855.4	E941.1	E950.4	E962.0	E980.4
Cyclophosphamide	963.1	E858.1	E933.1	E950.4	E962.0	E980.4
Cyclopropane	968.2	E855.1	E938.2	E950.4	E962.0	E980.4
Cycloserine	960.6	E856	E930.6	E950.4	E962.0	E980.4
Cyclothiazide	974.3	E858.5	E944.3	E950.4	E962.0	E980.4
Cycrimine	966.4	E855.0	E936.4	E950.4	E962.0	E980.4
Cymarin	972.1	E858.3	E942.1	E950.4	E962.0	E980.4
Cyproheptadine	963.0	E858.1	E933.0	E950.4	E962.0	E980.4
Cyprolidol	969.0	E854.0	E939.0	E950.3	E962.0	E980.3
Cytarabine	963.1	E858.1	E933.1	E950.4	E962.0	E980.4
Cytisus						
laburnum	988.2	E865.4	—	E950.9	E962.1	E980.9
scoparius	988.2	E865.4	—	E950.9	E962.1	E980.9
Cytomel	962.7	E858.0	E932.7	E950.4	E962.0	E980.4
Cytosine (antineoplastic)	963.1	E858.1	E933.1	E950.4	E962.0	E980.4
Cytoxan	963.1	E858.1	E933.1	E950.4	E962.0	E980.4
Dacarbazine	963.1	E858.1	E933.1	E950.4	E962.0	E980.4

	Poisoning	External Cause (E-Code)				
		Accident	Therapeutic Use	Suicide Attempt	Assault	Undetermined
Dactinomycin	960.7	E856	E930.7	E950.4	E962.0	E980.4
DADPS	961.8	E857	E931.8	E950.4	E962.0	E980.4
Dakin's solution (external)	976.0	E858.7	E946.0	E950.4	E962.0	E980.4
Dalmane	969.4	E853.2	E939.4	E950.3	E962.0	E980.3
DAM	977.2	E858.8	E947.2	E950.4	E962.0	E980.4
Danilone	964.2	E858.2	E934.2	E950.4	E962.0	E980.4
Danthron	973.1	E858.4	E943.1	E950.4	E962.0	E980.4
Dantrolene	975.2	E858.6	E945.2	E950.4	E962.0	E980.4
Daphne (gnidium) (mezereum)	988.2	E865.4	—	E950.9	E962.1	E980.9
berry	988.2	E865.3	—	E950.9	E962.1	E980.9
Dapsone	961.8	E857	E931.8	E950.4	E962.0	E980.4
Daraprim	961.4	E857	E931.4	E950.4	E962.0	E980.4
Darnel	988.2	E865.3	—	E950.9	E962.1	E980.9
Darvon	965.8	E850.8	E935.8	E950.0	E962.0	E980.0
Daunorubicin	960.7	E856	E930.7	E950.4	E962.0	E980.4
DBI	962.3	E858.0	E932.3	E950.4	E962.0	E980.4
D-Con (rodenticide)	989.4	E863.7	—	E950.6	E962.1	E980.7
DDS	961.8	E857	E931.8	E950.4	E962.0	E980.4
DDT	989.2	E863.0	—	E950.6	E962.1	E980.7
Deadly nightshade	988.2	E865.4	—	E950.9	E962.1	E980.9
berry	988.2	E865.3	—	E950.9	E962.1	E980.9
Deanol	969.7	E854.2	E939.7	E950.3	E962.0	E980.3
Debrisoquine	972.6	E858.3	E942.6	E950.4	E962.0	E980.4
Decaborane	989.89	E866.8	—	E950.9	E962.1	E980.9
fumes	987.8	E869.8	—	E952.8	E962.2	E982.8
Decadron	962.0	E858.0	E932.0	E950.4	E962.0	E980.4
ENT agent	976.6	E858.7	E946.6	E950.4	E962.0	E980.4
ophthalmic preparation	976.5	E858.7	E946.5	E950.4	E962.0	E980.4
topical NEC	976.0	E858.7	E946.0	E950.4	E962.0	E980.4
Decahydronaphthalene	982.0	E862.4	—	E950.9	E962.1	E980.9
Decalin	982.0	E862.4	—	E950.9	E962.1	E980.9
Decamethonium	975.2	E858.6	E945.2	E950.4	E962.0	E980.4
Decholin	973.4	E858.4	E943.4	E950.4	E962.0	E980.4
sodium (diagnostic)	977.8	E858.8	E947.8	E950.4	E962.0	E980.4
Declomycin	960.4	E856	E930.4	E950.4	E962.0	E980.4
Deferoxamine	963.8	E858.1	E933.8	E950.4	E962.0	E980.4
Dehydrocholic acid	973.4	E858.4	E943.4	E950.4	E962.0	E980.4
DeKalin	982.0	E862.4	—	E950.9	E962.1	E980.9
Delalutin	962.2	E858.0	E932.2	E950.4	E962.0	E980.4
Delphinium	988.2	E865.3	—	E950.9	E962.1	E980.9
Deltasone	962.0	E858.0	E932.0	E950.4	E962.0	E980.4
Deltra	962.0	E858.0	E932.0	E950.4	E962.0	E980.4
Delvinal	967.0	E851	E937.0	E950.1	E962.0	E980.1
Demecarium (bromide)	971.0	E855.3	E941.0	E950.4	E962.0	E980.4
Demeclocycline	960.4	E856	E930.4	E950.4	E962.0	E980.4
Demecolcine	963.1	E858.1	E933.1	E950.4	E962.0	E980.4
Demelanizing agents	976.8	E858.7	E946.8	E950.4	E962.0	E980.4
Demerol	965.09	E850.2	E935.2	E950.0	E962.0	E980.0
Demethylchlortetracycline	960.4	E856	E930.4	E950.4	E962.0	E980.4
Demethyltetracycline	960.4	E856	E930.4	E950.4	E962.0	E980.4
Demeton	989.3	E863.1	—	E950.6	E962.1	E980.7
Demulcents	976.3	E858.7	E946.3	E950.4	E962.0	E980.4
Demulen	962.2	E858.0	E932.2	E950.4	E962.0	E980.4
Denatured alcohol	980.0	E860.1	—	E950.9	E962.1	E980.9
Dendrid	976.5	E858.7	E946.5	E950.4	E962.0	E980.4
Dental agents, topical	976.7	E858.7	E946.7	E950.4	E962.0	E980.4
Deodorant spray (feminine hygiene)	976.8	E858.7	E946.8	E950.4	E962.0	E980.4
Deoxyribonuclease	963.4	E858.1	E933.4	E950.4	E962.0	E980.4
Depressants						
appetite, central	977.0	E858.8	E947.0	E950.4	E962.0	E980.4
cardiac	972.0	E858.3	E942.0	E950.4	E962.0	E980.4
central nervous system (anesthetic)	968.4	E855.1	E938.4	E950.4	E962.0	E980.4
psychotherapeutic	969.5	E853.9	E939.5	E950.3	E962.0	E980.3
Dequalinium	976.0	E858.7	E946.0	E950.4	E962.0	E980.4
Dermolate	976.2	E858.7	E946.2	E950.4	E962.0	E980.4
DES	962.2	E858.0	E932.2	E950.4	E962.0	E980.4
Desenex	976.0	E858.7	E946.0	E950.4	E962.0	E980.4
Deserpidine	972.6	E858.3	E942.6	E950.4	E962.0	E980.4
Desipramine	969.0	E854.0	E939.0	E950.3	E962.0	E980.3
Deslanoside	972.1	E858.3	E942.1	E950.4	E962.0	E980.4
Desocodeine	965.09	E850.2	E935.2	E950.0	E962.0	E980.0
Desomorphine	965.09	E850.2	E935.2	E950.0	E962.0	E980.0
Desonide	976.0	E858.7	E946.0	E950.4	E962.0	E980.4
Desoxycorticosterone derivatives	962.0	E858.0	E932.0	E950.4	E962.0	E980.4
Desoxyephedrine	969.7	E854.2	E939.7	E950.3	E962.0	E980.3
DET	969.6	E854.1	E939.6	E950.3	E962.0	E980.3
Detergents (ingested) (synthetic)	989.6	E861.0	—	E950.9	E962.1	E980.9
external medication	976.2	E858.7	E946.2	E950.4	E962.0	E980.4
Deterrent, alcohol	977.3	E858.8	E947.3	E950.4	E962.0	E980.4
Detrothyronine	962.7	E858.0	E932.7	E950.4	E962.0	E980.4
Dettol (external medication)	976.0	E858.7	E946.0	E950.4	E962.0	E980.4
Dexamethasone	962.0	E858.0	E932.0	E950.4	E962.0	E980.4
ENT agent	976.6	E858.7	E946.6	E950.4	E962.0	E980.4
ophthalmic preparation	976.5	E858.7	E946.5	E950.4	E962.0	E980.4
topical NEC	976.0	E858.7	E946.0	E950.4	E962.0	E980.4
Dexamphetamine	969.7	E854.2	E939.7	E950.3	E962.0	E980.3
Dexedrine	969.7	E854.2	E939.7	E950.3	E962.0	E980.3
Dexpanthenol	963.5	E858.1	E933.5	E950.4	E962.0	E980.4
Dextran	964.8	E858.2	E934.8	E950.4	E962.0	E980.4
Dextriferron	964.0	E858.2	E934.0	E950.4	E962.0	E980.4
Dextroamphetamine	969.7	E854.2	E939.7	E950.3	E962.0	E980.3
Dextro calcium pantothenate	963.5	E858.1	E933.5	E950.4	E962.0	E980.4
Dextromethorphan	975.4	E858.6	E945.4	E950.4	E962.0	E980.4
Dextromoramide	965.09	E850.2	E935.2	E950.0	E962.0	E980.0
Dextro pantothenyl alcohol	963.5	E858.1	E933.5	E950.4	E962.0	E980.4
topical	976.8	E858.7	E946.8	E950.4	E962.0	E980.4
Dextropropoxyphene (hydrochloride)	965.8	E850.8	E935.8	E950.0	E962.0	E980.0
Dextrorphan	965.09	E850.2	E935.2	E950.0	E962.0	E980.0
Dextrose NEC	974.5	E858.5	E944.5	E950.4	E962.0	E980.4
Dextrothyroxin	962.7	E858.0	E932.7	E950.4	E962.0	E980.4
DFP	971.0	E855.3	E941.0	E950.4	E962.0	E980.4
DHE-45	972.9	E858.3	E942.9	E950.4	E962.0	E980.4
Diabinese	962.3	E858.0	E932.3	E950.4	E962.0	E980.4
Diacetyl monoxime	977.2	E858.8	E947.2	E950.4	E962.0	E980.4
Diacetylmorphine	965.01	E850.0	E935.0	E950.0	E962.0	E980.0
Diagnostic agents	977.8	E858.8	E947.8	E950.4	E962.0	E980.4
Dial (soap)	976.2	E858.7	E946.2	E950.4	E962.0	E980.4
sedative	967.0	E851	E937.0	E950.1	E962.0	E980.1
Diallylbarbituric acid	967.0	E851	E937.0	E950.1	E962.0	E980.1
Diaminodiphenylsulfone	961.8	E857	E931.8	E950.4	E962.0	E980.4
Diamorphine	965.01	E850.0	E935.0	E950.0	E962.0	E980.0
Diamox	974.2	E858.5	E944.2	E950.4	E962.0	E980.4
Diamthazole	976.0	E858.7	E946.0	E950.4	E962.0	E980.4
Diaphenylsulfone	961.8	E857	E931.8	E950.4	E962.0	E980.4
Diasone (sodium)	961.8	E857	E931.8	E950.4	E962.0	E980.4
Diazepam	969.4	E853.2	E939.4	E950.3	E962.0	E980.3
Diazinon	989.3	E863.1	—	E950.6	E962.1	E980.7
Diazomethane (gas)	987.8	E869.8	—	E952.8	E962.2	E982.8
Diazoxide	972.5	E858.3	E942.5	E950.4	E962.0	E980.4
Dibenamine	971.3	E855.6	E941.3	E950.4	E962.0	E980.4
Dibenzheptropine	963.0	E858.1	E933.0	E950.4	E962.0	E980.4
Dibenzyline	971.3	E855.6	E941.3	E950.4	E962.0	E980.4
Diborane (gas)	987.8	E869.8	—	E952.8	E962.2	E982.8
Dibromomannitol	963.1	E858.1	E933.1	E950.4	E962.0	E980.4
Dibucaine (spinal)	968.7	E855.2	E938.7	E950.4	E962.0	E980.4
topical (surface)	968.5	E855.2	E938.5	E950.4	E962.0	E980.4
Dibunate sodium	975.4	E858.6	E945.4	E950.4	E962.0	E980.4
Dibutoline	971.1	E855.4	E941.1	E950.4	E962.0	E980.4
Dicapthon	989.4	E863.4	—	E950.6	E962.1	E980.7
Dichloralphenazone	967.1	E852.0	E937.1	E950.2	E962.0	E980.2
Dichlorodifluoromethane	987.4	E869.2	—	E952.8	E962.2	E982.8
Dichloroethane	982.3	E862.4	—	E950.9	E962.1	E980.9
Dichloroethylene	982.3	E862.4	—	E950.9	E962.1	E980.9
Dichloroethyl sulfide	987.8	E869.8	—	E952.8	E962.2	E982.8
Dichlorohydrin	982.3	E862.4	—	E950.9	E962.1	E980.9
Dichloromethane (solvent) (vapor)	982.3	E862.4	—	E950.9	E962.1	E980.9
Dichlorophen(e)	961.6	E857	E931.6	E950.4	E962.0	E980.4
Dichlorphenamide	974.2	E858.5	E944.2	E950.4	E962.0	E980.4
Dichlorvos	989.3	E863.1	—	E950.6	E962.1	E980.7
Diclofenac sodium	965.69	E850.6	E935.6	E950.0	E962.0	E980.0
Dicoumarin, dicumarol	964.2	E858.2	E934.2	E950.4	E962.0	E980.4
Dicyanogen (gas)	987.8	E869.8	—	E952.8	E962.2	E982.8
Dicyclomine	971.1	E855.4	E941.1	E950.4	E962.0	E980.4
Dieldrin (vapor)	989.2	E863.0	—	E950.6	E962.1	E980.7
Dienestrol	962.2	E858.0	E932.2	E950.4	E962.0	E980.4
Dietetics	977.0	E858.8	E947.0	E950.4	E962.0	E980.4
Diethazine	966.4	E855.0	E936.4	E950.4	E962.0	E980.4
Diethyl						
barbituric acid	967.0	E851	E937.0	E950.1	E962.0	E980.1
carbamazine	961.6	E857	E931.6	E950.4	E962.0	E980.4
carbinol	980.8	E860.8	—	E950.9	E962.1	E980.9
carbonate	982.8	E862.4	—	E950.9	E962.1	E980.9
ether (vapor) — *see* Ether(s)						
propion	977.0	E858.8	E947.0	E950.4	E962.0	E980.4
stilbestrol	962.2	E858.0	E932.2	E950.4	E962.0	E980.4

Index

Diethylene — Drug

		External Cause (E-Code)				
	Poisoning	Accident	Therapeutic Use	Suicide Attempt	Assault	Undetermined
Diethylene						
dioxide	982.8	E862.4	—	E950.9	E962.1	E980.9
glycol (monoacetate) (monoethyl ether)	982.8	E862.4	—	E950.9	E962.1	E980.9
Diethylsulfone-diethylmethane	967.8	E852.8	E937.8	E950.2	E962.0	E980.2
Difencloxazine	965.09	E850.2	E935.2	E950.0	E962.0	E980.0
Diffusin	963.4	E858.1	E933.4	E950.4	E962.0	E980.4
Diflos	971.0	E855.3	E941.0	E950.4	E962.0	E980.4
Digestants	973.4	E858.4	E943.4	E950.4	E962.0	E980.4
Digitalin(e)	972.1	E858.3	E942.1	E950.4	E962.0	E980.4
Digitalis glycosides	972.1	E858.3	E942.1	E950.4	E962.0	E980.4
Digitoxin	972.1	E858.3	E942.1	E950.4	E962.0	E980.4
Digoxin	972.1	E858.3	E942.1	E950.4	E962.0	E980.4
Dihydrocodeine	965.09	E850.2	E935.2	E950.0	E962.0	E980.0
Dihydrocodeinone	965.09	E850.2	E935.2	E950.0	E962.0	E980.0
Dihydroergocristine	972.9	E858.3	E942.9	E950.4	E962.0	E980.4
Dihydroergotamine	972.9	E858.3	E942.9	E950.4	E962.0	E980.4
Dihydroergotoxine	972.9	E858.3	E942.9	E950.4	E962.0	E980.4
Dihydrohydroxycodeinone	965.09	E850.2	E935.2	E950.0	E962.0	E980.0
Dihydrohydroxymorphinone	965.09	E850.2	E935.2	E950.0	E962.0	E980.0
Dihydroisocodeine	965.09	E850.2	E935.2	E950.0	E962.0	E980.0
Dihydromorphine	965.09	E850.2	E935.2	E950.0	E962.0	E980.0
Dihydromorphinone	965.09	E850.2	E935.2	E950.0	E962.0	E980.0
Dihydrostreptomycin	960.6	E856	E930.6	E950.4	E962.0	E980.4
Dihydrotachysterol	962.6	E858.0	E932.6	E950.4	E962.0	E980.4
Dihydroxyanthraquinone	973.1	E858.4	E943.1	E950.4	E962.0	E980.4
Dihydroxycodeinone	965.09	E850.2	E935.2	E950.0	E962.0	E980.0
Diiodohydroxyquin	961.3	E857	E931.3	E950.4	E962.0	E980.4
topical	976.0	E858.7	E946.0	E950.4	E962.0	E980.4
Diiodohydroxyquinoline	961.3	E857	E931.3	E950.4	E962.0	E980.4
Dilantin	966.1	E855.0	E936.1	E950.4	E962.0	E980.4
Dilaudid	965.09	E850.2	E935.2	E950.0	E962.0	E980.0
Diloxanide	961.5	E857	E931.5	E950.4	E962.0	E980.4
Dimefline	970.0	E854.3	E940.0	E950.4	E962.0	E980.4
Dimenhydrinate	963.0	E858.1	E933.0	E950.4	E962.0	E980.4
Dimercaprol	963.8	E858.1	E933.8	E950.4	E962.0	E980.4
Dimercaptopropanol	963.8	E858.1	E933.8	E950.4	E962.0	E980.4
Dimetane	963.0	E858.1	E933.0	E950.4	E962.0	E980.4
Dimethicone	976.3	E858.7	E946.3	E950.4	E962.0	E980.4
Dimethindene	963.0	E858.1	E933.0	E950.4	E962.0	E980.4
Dimethisoquin	968.5	E855.2	E938.5	E950.4	E962.0	E980.4
Dimethisterone	962.2	E858.0	E932.2	E950.4	E962.0	E980.4
Dimethoxanate	975.4	E858.6	E945.4	E950.4	E962.0	E980.4
Dimethyl						
arsine, arsinic acid — *see* Arsenic						
carbinol	980.2	E860.3	—	E950.9	E962.1	E980.9
diguanide	962.3	E858.0	E932.3	E950.4	E962.0	E980.4
ketone	982.8	E862.4	—	E950.9	E962.1	E980.9
vapor	987.8	E869.8	—	E952.8	E962.2	E982.8
meperidine	965.09	E850.2	E935.2	E950.0	E962.0	E980.0
parathion	989.3	E863.1	—	E950.6	E962.1	E980.7
polysiloxane	973.8	E858.4	E943.8	E950.4	E962.0	E980.4
sulfate (fumes)	987.8	E869.8	—	E952.8	E962.2	E982.8
liquid	983.9	E864.3	—	E950.7	E962.1	E980.6
sulfoxide NEC	982.8	E862.4	—	E950.9	E962.1	E980.9
medicinal	976.4	E858.7	E946.4	E950.4	E962.0	E980.4
triptamine	969.6	E854.1	E939.6	E950.3	E962.0	E980.3
tubocurarine	975.2	E858.6	E945.2	E950.4	E962.0	E980.4
Dindevan	964.2	E858.2	E934.2	E950.4	E962.0	E980.4
Dinitro (-ortho-) cresol (herbicide) (spray)	989.4	E863.5	—	E950.6	E962.1	E980.7
insecticide	989.4	E863.4	—	E950.6	E962.1	E980.7
Dinitrobenzene	983.0	E864.0	—	E950.7	E962.1	E980.6
vapor	987.8	E869.8	—	E952.8	E962.2	E982.8
Dinitro-orthocresol (herbicide)	989.4	E863.5	—	E950.6	E962.1	E980.7
insecticide	989.4	E863.4	—	E950.6	E962.1	E980.7
Dinitrophenol (herbicide) (spray)	989.4	E863.5	—	E950.6	E962.1	E980.7
insecticide	989.4	E863.4	—	E950.6	E962.1	E980.7
Dinoprost	975.0	E858.6	E945.0	E950.4	E962.0	E980.4
Dioctyl sulfosuccinate (calcium) (sodium)	973.2	E858.4	E943.2	E950.4	E962.0	E980.4
Diodoquin	961.3	E857	E931.3	E950.4	E962.0	E980.4
Dione derivatives NEC	966.3	E855.0	E936.3	E950.4	E962.0	E980.4
Dionin	965.09	E850.2	E935.2	E950.0	E962.0	E980.0
Dioxane	982.8	E862.4	—	E950.9	E962.1	E980.9
Dioxin — *see* Herbicide						
Dioxyline	972.5	E858.3	E942.5	E950.4	E962.0	E980.4
Dipentene	982.8	E862.4	—	E950.9	E962.1	E980.9
Diphemanil	971.1	E855.4	E941.1	E950.4	E962.0	E980.4
Diphenadione	964.2	E858.2	E934.2	E950.4	E962.0	E980.4
Diphenhydramine	963.0	E858.1	E933.0	E950.4	E962.0	E980.4
Diphenidol	963.0	E858.1	E933.0	E950.4	E962.0	E980.4
Diphenoxylate	973.5	E858.4	E943.5	E950.4	E962.0	E980.4
Diphenylchloroarsine	985.1	E866.3	—	E950.8	E962.1	E980.8
Diphenylhydantoin (sodium)	966.1	E855.0	E936.1	E950.4	E962.0	E980.4
Diphenylpyraline	963.0	E858.1	E933.0	E950.4	E962.0	E980.4
Diphtheria						
antitoxin	979.9	E858.8	E949.9	E950.4	E962.0	E980.4
toxoid	978.5	E858.8	E948.5	E950.4	E962.0	E980.4
with tetanus toxoid	978.9	E858.8	E948.9	E950.4	E962.0	E980.4
with pertussis component	978.6	E858.8	E948.6	E950.4	E962.0	E980.4
vaccine	978.5	E858.8	E948.5	E950.4	E962.0	E980.4
Dipipanone	965.09	E850.2	E935.2	E950.0	E962.0	E980.0
Diplovax	979.5	E858.8	E949.5	E950.4	E962.0	E980.4
Diprophylline	975.1	E858.6	E945.1	E950.4	E962.0	E980.4
Dipyridamole	972.4	E858.3	E942.4	E950.4	E962.0	E980.4
Dipyrone	965.5	E850.5	E935.5	E950.0	E962.0	E980.0
Diquat	989.4	E863.5	—	E950.6	E962.1	E980.7
Disinfectant NEC	983.9	E861.4	—	E950.7	E962.1	E980.6
alkaline	983.2	E861.4	—	E950.7	E962.1	E980.6
aromatic	983.0	E861.4	—	E950.7	E962.1	E980.6
Disipal	966.4	E855.0	E936.4	E950.4	E962.0	E980.4
Disodium edetate	963.8	E858.1	E933.8	E950.4	E962.0	E980.4
Disulfamide	974.4	E858.5	E944.4	E950.4	E962.0	E980.4
Disulfanilamide	961.0	E857	E931.0	E950.4	E962.0	E980.4
Disulfiram	977.3	E858.8	E947.3	E950.4	E962.0	E980.4
Dithiazanine	961.6	E857	E931.6	E950.4	E962.0	E980.4
Dithioglycerol	963.8	E858.1	E933.8	E950.4	E962.0	E980.4
Dithranol	976.4	E858.7	E946.4	E950.4	E962.0	E980.4
Diucardin	974.3	E858.5	E944.3	E950.4	E962.0	E980.4
Diupres	974.3	E858.5	E944.3	E950.4	E962.0	E980.4
Diuretics NEC	974.4	E858.5	E944.4	E950.4	E962.0	E980.4
carbonic acid anhydrase inhibitors	974.2	E858.5	E944.2	E950.4	E962.0	E980.4
mercurial	974.0	E858.5	E944.0	E950.4	E962.0	E980.4
osmotic	974.4	E858.5	E944.4	E950.4	E962.0	E980.4
purine derivatives	974.1	E858.5	E944.1	E950.4	E962.0	E980.4
saluretic	974.3	E858.5	E944.3	E950.4	E962.0	E980.4
Diuril	974.3	E858.5	E944.3	E950.4	E962.0	E980.4
Divinyl ether	968.2	E855.1	E938.2	E950.4	E962.0	E980.4
D-lysergic acid diethylamide	969.6	E854.1	E939.6	E950.3	E962.0	E980.3
DMCT	960.4	E856	E930.4	E950.4	E962.0	E980.4
DMSO	982.8	E862.4	—	E950.9	E962.1	E980.9
DMT	969.6	E854.1	E939.6	E950.3	E962.0	E980.3
DNOC	989.4	E863.5	—	E950.6	E962.1	E980.7
DOCA	962.0	E858.0	E932.0	E950.4	E962.0	E980.4
Dolophine	965.02	E850.1	E935.1	E950.0	E962.0	E980.0
Doloxene	965.8	E850.8	E935.8	E950.0	E962.0	E980.0
DOM	969.6	E854.1	E939.6	E950.3	E962.0	E980.3
Domestic gas — *see* Gas, utility						
Domiphen (bromide) (lozenges)	976.6	E858.7	E946.6	E950.4	E962.0	E980.4
Dopa (levo)	966.4	E855.0	E936.4	E950.4	E962.0	E980.4
Dopamine	971.2	E855.5	E941.2	E950.4	E962.0	E980.4
Doriden	967.5	E852.4	E937.5	E950.2	E962.0	E980.2
Dormiral	967.0	E851	E937.0	E950.1	E962.0	E980.1
Dormison	967.8	E852.8	E937.8	E950.2	E962.0	E980.2
Dornase	963.4	E858.1	E933.4	E950.4	E962.0	E980.4
Dorsacaine	968.5	E855.2	E938.5	E950.4	E962.0	E980.4
Dothiepin hydrochloride	969.0	E854.0	E939.0	E950.3	E962.0	E980.3
Doxapram	970.0	E854.3	E940.0	E950.4	E962.0	E980.4
Doxepin	969.0	E854.0	E939.0	E950.3	E962.0	E980.3
Doxorubicin	960.7	E856	E930.7	E950.4	E962.0	E980.4
Doxycycline	960.4	E856	E930.4	E950.4	E962.0	E980.4
Doxylamine	963.0	E858.1	E933.0	E950.4	E962.0	E980.4
Dramamine	963.0	E858.1	E933.0	E950.4	E962.0	E980.4
Drano (drain cleaner)	983.2	E864.2	—	E950.7	E962.1	E980.6
Dromoran	965.09	E850.2	E935.2	E950.0	E962.0	E980.0
Dromostanolone	962.1	E858.0	E932.1	E950.4	E962.0	E980.4
Droperidol	969.2	E853.1	E939.2	E950.3	E962.0	E980.3
Drotrecogin alfa	964.2	E858.2	E934.2	E950.4	E962.0	E980.4
Drug	977.9	E858.9	E947.9	E950.5	E962.0	E980.5
specified NEC	977.8	E858.8	E947.8	E950.4	E962.0	E980.4

☑ Additional Digit Required — Refer to the Tabular List (Numeric Code Section) for Additional Digit Selection

▶◀ Revised Text ● New Line ▲ Revised Code

		External Cause (E-Code)				
	Poisoning	Accident	Therapeutic Use	Suicide Attempt	Assault	Undetermined
Drug — *continued*						
AHFS List						
4:00 antihistamine drugs	963.0	E858.1	E933.0	E950.4	E962.0	E980.4
8:04 amebacides	961.5	E857	E931.5	E950.4	E962.0	E980.4
arsenical anti-infectives	961.1	E857	E931.1	E950.4	E962.0	E980.4
quinoline derivatives	961.3	E857	E931.3	E950.4	E962.0	E980.4
8:08 anthelmintics	961.6	E857	E931.6	E950.4	E962.0	E980.4
quinoline derivatives	961.3	E857	E931.3	E950.4	E962.0	E980.4
8:12.04 antifungal antibiotics	960.1	E856	E930.1	E950.4	E962.0	E980.4
8:12.06 cephalosporins	960.5	E856	E930.5	E950.4	E962.0	E980.4
8:12.08 chloramphenicol	960.2	E856	E930.2	E950.4	E962.0	E980.4
8:12.12 erythromycins	960.3	E856	E930.3	E950.4	E962.0	E980.4
8:12.16 penicillins	960.0	E856	E930.0	E950.4	E962.0	E980.4
8:12.20 streptomycins	960.6	E856	E930.6	E950.4	E962.0	E980.4
8:12.24 tetracyclines	960.4	E856	E930.4	E950.4	E962.0	E980.4
8:12.28 other antibiotics	960.8	E856	E930.8	E950.4	E962.0	E980.4
antimycobacterial	960.6	E856	E930.6	E950.4	E962.0	E980.4
macrolides	960.3	E856	E930.3	E950.4	E962.0	E980.4
8:16 antituberculars	961.8	E857	E931.8	E950.4	E962.0	E980.4
antibiotics	960.6	E856	E930.6	E950.4	E962.0	E980.4
8:18 antivirals	961.7	E857	E931.7	E950.4	E962.0	E980.4
8:20 plasmodicides (antimalarials)	961.4	E857	E931.4	E950.4	E962.0	E980.4
8:24 sulfonamides	961.0	E857	E931.0	E950.4	E962.0	E980.4
8:26 sulfones	961.8	E857	E931.8	E950.4	E962.0	E980.4
8:28 treponemicides	961.2	E857	E931.2	E950.4	E962.0	E980.4
8:32 trichomonacides	961.5	E857	E931.5	E950.4	E962.0	E980.4
quinoline derivatives	961.3	E857	E931.3	E950.4	E962.0	E980.4
nitrofuran derivatives	961.9	E857	E931.9	E950.4	E962.0	E980.4
8:36 urinary germicides	961.9	E857	E931.9	E950.4	E962.0	E980.4
quinoline derivatives	961.3	E857	E931.3	E950.4	E962.0	E980.4
8:40 other anti-infectives	961.9	E857	E931.9	E950.4	E962.0	E980.4
10:00 antineoplastic agents	963.1	E858.1	E933.1	E950.4	E962.0	E980.4
antibiotics	960.7	E856	E930.7	E950.4	E962.0	E980.4
progestogens	962.2	E858.0	E932.2	E950.4	E962.0	E980.4
12:04 parasympathomimetic (cholinergic) agents	971.0	E855.3	E941.0	E950.4	E962.0	E980.4
12:08 parasympatholytic (cholinergic-blocking) agents	971.1	E855.4	E941.1	E950.4	E962.0	E980.4
12:12 Sympathomimetic (adrenergic) agents	971.2	E855.5	E941.2	E950.4	E962.0	E980.4
12:16 sympatholytic (adrenergic-blocking) agents	971.3	E855.6	E941.3	E950.4	E962.0	E980.4
12:20 skeletal muscle relaxants						
central nervous system muscle-tone depressants	968.0	E855.1	E938.0	E950.4	E962.0	E980.4
myoneural blocking agents	975.2	E858.6	E945.2	E950.4	E962.0	E980.4
16:00 blood derivatives	964.7	E858.2	E934.7	E950.4	E962.0	E980.4
20:04 antianemia drugs	964.1	E858.2	E934.1	E950.4	E962.0	E980.4
20:04.04 iron preparations	964.0	E858.2	E934.0	E950.4	E962.0	E980.4
20:04.08 liver and stomach preparations	964.1	E858.2	E934.1	E950.4	E962.0	E980.4
20:12.04 anticoagulants	964.2	E858.2	E934.2	E950.4	E962.0	E980.4
20:12.08 antiheparin agents	964.5	E858.2	E934.5	E950.4	E962.0	E980.4
20:12.12 coagulants	964.5	E858.2	E934.5	E950.4	E962.0	E980.4
20:12.16 hemostatics NEC	964.5	E858.2	E934.5	E950.4	E962.0	E980.4
capillary active drugs	972.8	E858.3	E942.8	E950.4	E962.0	E980.4
24:04 cardiac drugs	972.9	E858.3	E942.9	E950.4	E962.0	E980.4
cardiotonic agents	972.1	E858.3	E942.1	E950.4	E962.0	E980.4
rhythm regulators	972.0	E858.3	E942.0	E950.4	E962.0	E980.4
24:06 antilipemic agents	972.2	E858.3	E942.2	E950.4	E962.0	E980.4
thyroid derivatives	962.7	E858.0	E932.7	E950.4	E962.0	E980.4
24:08 hypotensive agents	972.6	E858.3	E942.6	E950.4	E962.0	E980.4
adrenergic blocking agents	971.3	E855.6	E941.3	E950.4	E962.0	E980.4
ganglion blocking agents	972.3	E858.3	E942.3	E950.4	E962.0	E980.4
vasodilators	972.5	E858.3	E942.5	E950.4	E962.0	E980.4
24:12 vasodilating agents NEC	972.5	E858.3	E942.5	E950.4	E962.0	E980.4
coronary	972.4	E858.3	E942.4	E950.4	E962.0	E980.4
nicotinic acid derivatives	972.2	E858.3	E942.2	E950.4	E962.0	E980.4

		External Cause (E-Code)				
	Poisoning	Accident	Therapeutic Use	Suicide Attempt	Assault	Undetermined
Drug — *continued*						
24:16 sclerosing agents	972.7	E858.3	E942.7	E950.4	E962.0	E980.4
28:04 general anesthetics	968.4	E855.1	E938.4	E950.4	E962.0	E980.4
gaseous anesthetics	968.2	E855.1	E938.2	E950.4	E962.0	E980.4
halothane	968.1	E855.1	E938.1	E950.4	E962.0	E980.4
intravenous anesthetics	968.3	E855.1	E938.3	E950.4	E962.0	E980.4
28:08 analgesics and antipyretics	965.9	E850.9	E935.9	E950.0	E962.0	E980.0
antirheumatics	965.69	E850.6	E935.6	E950.0	E962.0	E980.0
aromatic analgesics	965.4	E850.4	E935.4	E950.0	E962.0	E980.0
non-narcotic NEC	965.7	E850.7	E935.7	E950.0	E962.0	E980.0
opium alkaloids	965.00	E850.2	E935.2	E950.0	E962.0	E980.0
heroin	965.01	E850.0	E935.0	E950.0	E962.0	E980.0
methadone	965.02	E850.1	E935.1	E950.0	E962.0	E980.0
specified type NEC	965.09	E850.2	E935.2	E950.0	E962.0	E980.0
pyrazole derivatives	965.5	E850.5	E935.5	E950.0	E962.0	E980.0
salicylates	965.1	E850.3	E935.3	E950.0	E962.0	E980.0
specified NEC	965.8	E850.8	E935.8	E950.0	E962.0	E980.0
28:10 narcotic antagonists	970.1	E854.3	E940.1	E950.4	E962.0	E980.4
28:12 anticonvulsants	966.3	E855.0	E936.3	E950.4	E962.0	E980.4
barbiturates	967.0	E851	E937.0	E950.1	E962.0	E980.1
benzodiazepine-based tranquilizers	969.4	E853.2	E939.4	E950.3	E962.0	E980.3
bromides	967.3	E852.2	E937.3	E950.2	E962.0	E980.2
hydantoin derivatives	966.1	E855.0	E936.1	E950.4	E962.0	E980.4
oxazolidine (derivatives)	966.0	E855.0	E936.0	E950.4	E962.0	E980.4
succinimides	966.2	E855.0	E936.2	E950.4	E962.0	E980.4
28:16.04 antidepressants	969.0	E854.0	E939.0	E950.3	E962.0	E980.3
28:16.08 tranquilizers	969.5	E853.9	E939.5	E950.3	E962.0	E980.3
benzodiazepine-based	969.4	E853.2	E939.4	E950.3	E962.0	E980.3
butyrophenone-based	969.2	E853.1	E939.2	E950.3	E962.0	E980.3
major NEC	969.3	E853.8	E939.3	E950.3	E962.0	E980.3
phenothiazine-based	969.1	E853.0	E939.1	E950.3	E962.0	E980.3
28:16.12 other psychotherapeutic agents	969.8	E855.8	E939.8	E950.3	E962.0	E980.3
28:20 respiratory and cerebral stimulants	970.9	E854.3	E940.9	E950.4	E962.0	E980.4
analeptics	970.0	E854.3	E940.0	E950.4	E962.0	E980.4
anorexigenic agents	977.0	E858.8	E947.0	E950.4	E962.0	E980.4
psychostimulants	969.7	E854.2	E939.7	E950.3	E962.0	E980.3
specified NEC	970.8	E854.3	E940.8	E950.4	E962.0	E980.4
28:24 sedatives and hypnotics	967.9	E852.9	E937.9	E950.2	E962.0	E980.2
barbiturates	967.0	E851	E937.0	E950.1	E962.0	E980.1
benzodiazepine-based tranquilizers	969.4	E853.2	E939.4	E950.3	E962.0	E980.3
chloral hydrate (group)	967.1	E852.0	E937.1	E950.2	E962.0	E980.2
glutethamide group	967.5	E852.4	E937.5	E950.2	E962.0	E980.2
intravenous anesthetics	968.3	E855.1	E938.3	E950.4	E962.0	E980.4
methaqualone (compounds)	967.4	E852.3	E937.4	E950.2	E962.0	E980.2
paraldehyde	967.2	E852.1	E937.2	E950.2	E962.0	E980.2
phenothiazine-based tranquilizers	969.1	E853.0	E939.1	E950.3	E962.0	E980.3
specified NEC	967.8	E852.8	E937.8	E950.2	E962.0	E980.2
thiobarbiturates	968.3	E855.1	E938.3	E950.4	E962.0	E980.4
tranquilizer NEC	969.5	E853.9	E939.5	E950.3	E962.0	E980.3
36:04 to 36:88 diagnostic agents	977.8	E858.8	E947.8	E950.4	E962.0	E980.4
40:00 electrolyte, caloric, and water balance agents NEC	974.5	E858.5	E944.5	E950.4	E962.0	E980.4
40:04 acidifying agents	963.2	E858.1	E933.2	E950.4	E962.0	E980.4
40:08 alkalinizing agents	963.3	E858.1	E933.3	E950.4	E962.0	E980.4
40:10 ammonia detoxicants	974.5	E858.5	E944.5	E950.4	E962.0	E980.4
40:12 replacement solutions	974.5	E858.5	E944.5	E950.4	E962.0	E980.4
plasma expanders	964.8	E858.2	E934.8	E950.4	E962.0	E980.4
40:16 sodium-removing resins	974.5	E858.5	E944.5	E950.4	E962.0	E980.4
40:18 potassium-removing resins	974.5	E858.5	E944.5	E950.4	E962.0	E980.4
40:20 caloric agents	974.5	E858.5	E944.5	E950.4	E962.0	E980.4
40:24 salt and sugar substitutes	974.5	E858.5	E944.5	E950.4	E962.0	E980.4

		External Cause (E-Code)				
	Poisoning	Accident	Therapeutic Use	Suicide Attempt	Assault	Undetermined
Drug — *continued*						
40:28 diuretics NEC	974.4	E858.5	E944.4	E950.4	E962.0	E980.4
carbonic acid anhydrase inhibitors	974.2	E858.5	E944.2	E950.4	E962.0	E980.4
mercurials	974.0	E858.5	E944.0	E950.4	E962.0	E980.4
purine derivatives	974.1	E858.5	E944.1	E950.4	E962.0	E980.4
saluretics	974.3	E858.5	E944.3	E950.4	E962.0	E980.4
thiazides	974.3	E858.5	E944.3	E950.4	E962.0	E980.4
40:36 irrigating solutions	974.5	E858.5	E944.5	E950.4	E962.0	E980.4
40:40 uricosuric agents	974.7	E858.5	E944.7	E950.4	E962.0	E980.4
44:00 enzymes	963.4	E858.1	E933.4	E950.4	E962.0	E980.4
fibrinolysis-affecting agents	964.4	E858.2	E934.4	E950.4	E962.0	E980.4
gastric agents	973.4	E858.4	E943.4	E950.4	E962.0	E980.4
48:00 expectorants and cough preparations						
antihistamine agents	963.0	E858.1	E933.0	E950.4	E962.0	E980.4
antitussives	975.4	E858.6	E945.4	E950.4	E962.0	E980.4
codeine derivatives	965.09	E850.2	E935.2	E950.0	E962.0	E980.0
expectorants	975.5	E858.6	E945.5	E950.4	E962.0	E980.4
narcotic agents NEC	965.09	E850.2	E935.2	E950.0	E962.0	E980.0
52:04 anti-infectives (EENT)						
ENT agent	976.6	E858.7	E946.6	E950.4	E962.0	E980.4
ophthalmic preparation	976.5	E858.7	E946.5	E950.4	E962.0	E980.4
52:04.04 antibiotics (EENT)						
ENT agent	976.6	E858.7	E946.6	E950.4	E962.0	E980.4
ophthalmic preparation	976.5	E858.7	E946.5	E950.4	E962.0	E980.4
52:04.06 antivirals (EENT)						
ENT agent	976.6	E858.7	E946.6	E950.4	E962.0	E980.4
ophthalmic preparation	976.5	E858.7	E946.5	E950.4	E962.0	E980.4
52:04.08 sulfonamides (EENT)						
ENT agent	976.6	E858.7	E946.6	E950.4	E962.0	E980.4
ophthalmic preparation	976.5	E858.7	E946.5	E950.4	E962.0	E980.4
52:04.12 miscellaneous anti-infectives (EENT)						
ENT agent	976.6	E858.7	E946.6	E950.4	E962.0	E980.4
ophthalmic preparation	976.5	E858.7	E946.5	E950.4	E962.0	E980.4
52:08 anti-inflammatory agents (EENT)						
ENT agent	976.6	E858.7	E946.6	E950.4	E962.0	E980.4
ophthalmic preparation	976.5	E858.7	E946.5	E950.4	E962.0	E980.4
52:10 carbonic anhydrase inhibitors	974.2	E858.5	E944.2	E950.4	E962.0	E980.4
52:12 contact lens solutions	976.5	E858.7	E946.5	E950.4	E962.0	E980.4
52:16 local anesthetics (EENT)	968.5	E855.2	E938.5	E950.4	E962.0	E980.4
52:20 miotics	971.0	E855.3	E941.0	E950.4	E962.0	E980.4
52:24 mydriatics						
adrenergics	971.2	E855.5	E941.2	E950.4	E962.0	E980.4
anticholinergics	971.1	E855.4	E941.1	E950.4	E962.0	E980.4
antimuscarinics	971.1	E855.4	E941.1	E950.4	E962.0	E980.4
parasympatholytics	971.1	E855.4	E941.1	E950.4	E962.0	E980.4
spasmolytics	971.1	E855.4	E941.1	E950.4	E962.0	E980.4
sympathomimetics	971.2	E855.5	E941.2	E950.4	E962.0	E980.4
52:28 mouth washes and gargles	976.6	E858.7	E946.6	E950.4	E962.0	E980.4
52:32 vasoconstrictors (EENT)	971.2	E855.5	E941.2	E950.4	E962.0	E980.4
52:36 unclassified agents (EENT)						
ENT agent	976.6	E858.7	E946.6	E950.4	E962.0	E980.4
ophthalmic preparation	976.5	E858.7	E946.5	E950.4	E962.0	E980.4
56:04 antacids and adsorbents	973.0	E858.4	E943.0	E950.4	E962.0	E980.4
56:08 antidiarrhea agents	973.5	E858.4	E943.5	E950.4	E962.0	E980.4
56:10 antiflatulents	973.8	E858.4	E943.8	E950.4	E962.0	E980.4
56:12 cathartics NEC	973.3	E858.4	E943.3	E950.4	E962.0	E980.4
emollients	973.2	E858.4	E943.2	E950.4	E962.0	E980.4
irritants	973.1	E858.4	E943.1	E950.4	E962.0	E980.4
56:16 digestants	973.4	E858.4	E943.4	E950.4	E962.0	E980.4
56:20 emetics and antiemetics						
antiemetics	963.0	E858.1	E933.0	E950.4	E962.0	E980.4
emetics	973.6	E858.4	E943.6	E950.4	E962.0	E980.4
56:24 lipotropic agents	977.1	E858.8	E947.1	E950.4	E962.0	E980.4
56:40 miscellaneous G.I. drugs	973.8	E858.4	E943.8	E950.4	E962.0	E980.4
60:00 gold compounds	965.69	E850.6	E935.6	E950.0	E962.0	E980.0
64:00 heavy metal antagonists	963.8	E858.1	E933.8	E950.4	E962.0	E980.4
Drug — *continued*						
68:04 adrenals	962.0	E858.0	E932.0	E950.4	E962.0	E980.4
68:08 androgens	962.1	E858.0	E932.1	E950.4	E962.0	E980.4
68:12 contraceptives, oral	962.2	E858.0	E932.2	E950.4	E962.0	E980.4
68:16 estrogens	962.2	E858.0	E932.2	E950.4	E962.0	E980.4
68:18 gonadotropins	962.4	E858.0	E932.4	E950.4	E962.0	E980.4
68:20 insulins and antidiabetic agents	962.3	E858.0	E932.3	E950.4	E962.0	E980.4
68:20.08 insulins	962.3	E858.0	E932.3	E950.4	E962.0	E980.4
68:24 parathyroid	962.6	E858.0	E932.6	E950.4	E962.0	E980.4
68:28 pituitary (posterior)	962.5	E858.0	E932.5	E950.4	E962.0	E980.4
anterior	962.4	E858.0	E932.4	E950.4	E962.0	E980.4
68:32 progestogens	962.2	E858.0	E932.2	E950.4	E962.0	E980.4
68:34 other corpus luteum hormones NEC	962.2	E858.0	E932.2	E950.4	E962.0	E980.4
68:36 thyroid and antithyroid						
antithyroid	962.8	E858.0	E932.8	E950.4	E962.0	E980.4
thyroid (derivatives)	962.7	E858.0	E932.7	E950.4	E962.0	E980.4
72:00 local anesthetics NEC	968.9	E855.2	E938.9	E950.4	E962.0	E980.4
topical (surface)	968.5	E855.2	E938.5	E950.4	E962.0	E980.4
infiltration (intradermal) (subcutaneous) (submucosal)	968.5	E855.2	E938.5	E950.4	E962.0	E980.4
nerve blocking (peripheral) (plexus) (regional)	968.6	E855.2	E938.6	E950.4	E962.0	E980.4
spinal	968.7	E855.2	E938.7	E950.4	E962.0	E980.4
76:00 oxytocics	975.0	E858.6	E945.0	E950.4	E962.0	E980.4
78:00 radioactive agents	990	—	—	—	—	—
80:04 serums NEC	979.9	E858.8	E949.9	E950.4	E962.0	E980.4
immune gamma globulin (human)	964.6	E858.2	E934.6	E950.4	E962.0	E980.4
80:08 toxoids NEC	978.8	E858.8	E948.8	E950.4	E962.0	E980.4
diphtheria	978.5	E858.8	E948.5	E950.4	E962.0	E980.4
and tetanus	978.9	E858.8	E948.9	E950.4	E962.0	E980.4
w/pertussis component	978.6	E858.8	E948.6	E950.4	E962.0	E980.4
tetanus	978.4	E858.8	E948.4	E950.4	E962.0	E980.4
and diphtheria	978.9	E858.8	E948.9	E950.4	E962.0	E980.4
with pertussis component	978.6	E858.8	E948.6	E950.4	E962.0	E980.4
80:12 vaccines	979.9	E858.8	E949.9	E950.4	E962.0	E980.4
bacterial NEC	978.8	E858.8	E948.8	E950.4	E962.0	E980.4
with						
other bacterial components	978.9	E858.8	E948.9	E950.4	E962.0	E980.4
pertussis component	978.6	E858.8	E948.6	E950.4	E962.0	E980.4
viral and rickettsial components	979.7	E858.8	E949.7	E950.4	E962.0	E980.4
rickettsial NEC	979.6	E858.8	E949.6	E950.4	E962.0	E980.4
with						
bacterial component	979.7	E858.8	E949.7	E950.4	E962.0	E980.4
pertussis component	978.6	E858.8	E948.6	E950.4	E962.0	E980.4
viral component	979.7	E858.8	E949.7	E950.4	E962.0	E980.4
viral NEC	979.6	E858.8	E949.6	E950.4	E962.0	E980.4
with						
bacterial component	979.7	E858.8	E949.7	E950.4	E962.0	E980.4
pertussis component	978.6	E858.8	E948.6	E950.4	E962.0	E980.4
rickettsial component	979.7	E858.8	E949.7	E950.4	E962.0	E980.4
84:04.04 antibiotics (skin and mucous membrane)	976.0	E858.7	E946.0	E950.4	E962.0	E980.4
84:04.08 fungicides (skin and mucous membrane)	976.0	E858.7	E946.0	E950.4	E962.0	E980.4
84:04.12 scabicides and pediculicides (skin and mucous membrane)	976.0	E858.7	E946.0	E950.4	E962.0	E980.4
84:04.16 miscellaneous local anti-infectives (skin and mucous membrane)	976.0	E858.7	E946.0	E950.4	E962.0	E980.4

		External Cause (E-Code)				
	Poisoning	Accident	Therapeutic Use	Suicide Attempt	Assault	Undetermined
Drug — *continued*						
84:06 anti-inflammatory agents (skin and mucous membrane)	976.0	E858.7	E946.0	E950.4	E962.0	E980.4
84:08 antipruritics and local anesthetics						
antipruritics	976.1	E858.7	E946.1	E950.4	E962.0	E980.4
local anesthetics	968.5	E855.2	E938.5	E950.4	E962.0	E980.4
84:12 astringents	976.2	E858.7	E946.2	E950.4	E962.0	E980.4
84:16 cell stimulants and proliferants	976.8	E858.7	E946.8	E950.4	E962.0	E980.4
84:20 detergents	976.2	E858.7	E946.2	E950.4	E962.0	E980.4
84:24 emollients, demulcents, and protectants	976.3	E858.7	E946.3	E950.4	E962.0	E980.4
84:28 keratolytic agents	976.4	E858.7	E946.4	E950.4	E962.0	E980.4
84:32 keratoplastic agents	976.4	E858.7	E946.4	E950.4	E962.0	E980.4
84:36 miscellaneous agents (skin and mucous membrane)	976.8	E858.7	E946.8	E950.4	E962.0	E980.4
86:00 spasmolytic agents	975.1	E858.6	E945.1	E950.4	E962.0	E980.4
antiasthmatics	975.7	E858.6	E945.7	E950.4	E962.0	E980.4
papaverine	972.5	E858.3	E942.5	E950.4	E962.0	E980.4
theophylline	974.1	E858.5	E944.1	E950.4	E962.0	E980.4
88:04 vitamin A	963.5	E858.1	E933.5	E950.4	E962.0	E980.4
88:08 vitamin B complex	963.5	E858.1	E933.5	E950.4	E962.0	E980.4
hematopoietic vitamin	964.1	E858.2	E934.1	E950.4	E962.0	E980.4
nicotinic acid derivatives	972.2	E858.3	E942.2	E950.4	E962.0	E980.4
88:12 vitamin C	963.5	E858.1	E933.5	E950.4	E962.0	E980.4
88:16 vitamin D	963.5	E858.1	E933.5	E950.4	E962.0	E980.4
88:20 vitamin E	963.5	E858.1	E933.5	E950.4	E962.0	E980.4
88:24 vitamin K activity	964.3	E858.2	E934.3	E950.4	E962.0	E980.4
88:28 multivitamin preparations	963.5	E858.1	E933.5	E950.4	E962.0	E980.4
92:00 unclassified therapeutic agents	977.8	E858.8	E947.8	E950.4	E962.0	E980.4
Duboisine	971.1	E855.4	E941.1	E950.4	E962.0	E980.4
Dulcolax	973.1	E858.4	E943.1	E950.4	E962.0	E980.4
Duponol (C) (EP)	976.2	E858.7	E946.2	E950.4	E962.0	E980.4
Durabolin	962.1	E858.0	E932.1	E950.4	E962.0	E980.4
Dyclone	968.5	E855.2	E938.5	E950.4	E962.0	E980.4
Dyclonine	968.5	E855.2	E938.5	E950.4	E962.0	E980.4
Dydrogesterone	962.2	E858.0	E932.2	E950.4	E962.0	E980.4
Dyes NEC	989.89	E866.8	—	E950.9	E962.1	E980.9
diagnostic agents	977.8	E858.8	E947.8	E950.4	E962.0	E980.4
pharmaceutical NEC	977.4	E858.8	E947.4	E950.4	E962.0	E980.4
Dyfols	971.0	E855.3	E941.0	E950.4	E962.0	E980.4
Dymelor	962.3	E858.0	E932.3	E950.4	E962.0	E980.4
Dynamite	989.89	E866.8	—	E950.9	E962.1	E980.9
fumes	987.8	E869.8	—	E952.8	E962.2	E982.8
Dyphylline	975.1	E858.6	E945.1	E950.4	E962.0	E980.4
Ear preparations	976.6	E858.7	E946.6	E950.4	E962.0	E980.4
Echothiopate, ecothiopate	971.0	E855.3	E941.0	E950.4	E962.0	E980.4
Ecstasy	969.7	E854.2	E939.7	E950.3	E962.0	E980.3
Ectylurea	967.8	E852.8	E937.8	E950.2	E962.0	E980.2
Edathamil disodium	963.8	E858.1	E933.8	E950.4	E962.0	E980.4
Edecrin	974.4	E858.5	E944.4	E950.4	E962.0	E980.4
Edetate, disodium (calcium)	963.8	E858.1	E933.8	E950.4	E962.0	E980.4
Edrophonium	971.0	E855.3	E941.0	E950.4	E962.0	E980.4
Elase	976.8	E858.7	E946.8	E950.4	E962.0	E980.4
Elaterium	973.1	E858.4	E943.1	E950.4	E962.0	E980.4
Elder	988.2	E865.4	—	E950.9	E962.1	E980.9
berry (unripe)	988.2	E865.3	—	E950.9	E962.1	E980.9
Electrolytes NEC	974.5	E858.5	E944.5	E950.4	E962.0	E980.4
Electrolytic agent NEC	974.5	E858.5	E944.5	E950.4	E962.0	E980.4
Embramine	963.0	E858.1	E933.0	E950.4	E962.0	E980.4
Emetics	973.6	E858.4	E943.6	E950.4	E962.0	E980.4
Emetine (hydrochloride)	961.5	E857	E931.5	E950.4	E962.0	E980.4
Emollients	976.3	E858.7	E946.3	E950.4	E962.0	E980.4
Emylcamate	969.5	E853.8	E939.5	E950.3	E962.0	E980.3
Encyprate	969.0	E854.0	E939.0	E950.3	E962.0	E980.3
Endocaine	968.5	E855.2	E938.5	E950.4	E962.0	E980.4
Endrin	989.2	E863.0	—	E950.6	E962.1	E980.7
Enflurane	968.2	E855.1	E938.2	E950.4	E962.0	E980.4
Enovid	962.2	E858.0	E932.2	E950.4	E962.0	E980.4
ENT preparations (anti-infectives)	976.6	E858.7	E946.6	E950.4	E962.0	E980.4
Enzodase	963.4	E858.1	E933.4	E950.4	E962.0	E980.4

		External Cause (E-Code)				
	Poisoning	Accident	Therapeutic Use	Suicide Attempt	Assault	Undetermined
Enzymes NEC	963.4	E858.1	E933.4	E950.4	E962.0	E980.4
Epanutin	966.1	E855.0	E936.1	E950.4	E962.0	E980.4
Ephedra (tincture)	971.2	E855.5	E941.2	E950.4	E962.0	E980.4
Ephedrine	971.2	E855.5	E941.2	E950.4	E962.0	E980.4
Epiestriol	962.2	E858.0	E932.2	E950.4	E962.0	E980.4
Epilim — *see* Sodium valproate						
Epinephrine	971.2	E855.5	E941.2	E950.4	E962.0	E980.4
Epsom salt	973.3	E858.4	E943.3	E950.4	E962.0	E980.4
Equanil	969.5	E853.8	E939.5	E950.3	E962.0	E980.3
Equisetum (diuretic)	974.4	E858.5	E944.4	E950.4	E962.0	E980.4
Ergometrine	975.0	E858.6	E945.0	E950.4	E962.0	E980.4
Ergonovine	975.0	E858.6	E945.0	E950.4	E962.0	E980.4
Ergot NEC	988.2	E865.4	—	E950.9	E962.1	E980.9
medicinal (alkaloids)	975.0	E858.6	E945.0	E950.4	E962.0	E980.4
Ergotamine (tartrate) (for migraine) NEC	972.9	E858.3	E942.9	E950.4	E962.0	E980.4
Ergotrate	975.0	E858.6	E945.0	E950.4	E962.0	E980.4
Erythrityl tetranitrate	972.4	E858.3	E942.4	E950.4	E962.0	E980.4
Erythrol tetranitrate	972.4	E858.3	E942.4	E950.4	E962.0	E980.4
Erythromycin	960.3	E856	E930.3	E950.4	E962.0	E980.4
ophthalmic preparation	976.5	E858.7	E946.5	E950.4	E962.0	E980.4
topical NEC	976.0	E858.7	E946.0	E950.4	E962.0	E980.4
Eserine	971.0	E855.3	E941.0	E950.4	E962.0	E980.4
Eskabarb	967.0	E851	E937.0	E950.1	E962.0	E980.1
Eskalith	969.8	E855.8	E939.8	E950.3	E962.0	E980.3
Estradiol (cypionate) (dipropionate) (valerate)	962.2	E858.0	E932.2	E950.4	E962.0	E980.4
Estriol	962.2	E858.0	E932.2	E950.4	E962.0	E980.4
Estrogens (with progestogens)	962.2	E858.0	E932.2	E950.4	E962.0	E980.4
Estrone	962.2	E858.0	E932.2	E950.4	E962.0	E980.4
Etafedrine	971.2	E855.5	E941.2	E950.4	E962.0	E980.4
Ethacrynate sodium	974.4	E858.5	E944.4	E950.4	E962.0	E980.4
Ethacrynic acid	974.4	E858.5	E944.4	E950.4	E962.0	E980.4
Ethambutol	961.8	E857	E931.8	E950.4	E962.0	E980.4
Ethamide	974.2	E858.5	E944.2	E950.4	E962.0	E980.4
Ethamivan	970.0	E854.3	E940.0	E950.4	E962.0	E980.4
Ethamsylate	964.5	E858.2	E934.5	E950.4	E962.0	E980.4
Ethanol	980.0	E860.1	—	E950.9	E962.1	E980.9
beverage	980.0	E860.0	—	E950.9	E962.1	E980.9
Ethchlorvynol	967.8	E852.8	E937.8	E950.2	E962.0	E980.2
Ethebenecid	974.7	E858.5	E944.7	E950.4	E962.0	E980.4
Ether(s) (diethyl) (ethyl) (vapor)	987.8	E869.8	—	E952.8	E962.2	E982.8
anesthetic	968.2	E855.1	E938.2	E950.4	E962.0	E980.4
petroleum — *see* Ligroin						
solvent	982.8	E862.4	—	E950.9	E962.1	E980.9
Ethidine chloride (vapor)	987.8	E869.8	—	E952.8	E962.2	E982.8
liquid (solvent)	982.3	E862.4	—	E950.9	E962.1	E980.9
Ethinamate	967.8	E852.8	E937.8	E950.2	E962.0	E980.2
Ethinylestradiol	962.2	E858.0	E932.2	E950.4	E962.0	E980.4
Ethionamide	961.8	E857	E931.8	E950.4	E962.0	E980.4
Ethisterone	962.2	E858.0	E932.2	E950.4	E962.0	E980.4
Ethobral	967.0	E851	E937.0	E950.1	E962.0	E980.1
Ethocaine (infiltration) (topical)	968.5	E855.2	E938.5	E950.4	E962.0	E980.4
nerve block (peripheral) (plexus)	968.6	E855.2	E938.6	E950.4	E962.0	E980.4
spinal	968.7	E855.2	E938.7	E950.4	E962.0	E980.4
Ethoheptazine (citrate)	965.7	E850.7	E935.7	E950.0	E962.0	E980.0
Ethopropazine	966.4	E855.0	E936.4	E950.4	E962.0	E980.4
Ethosuximide	966.2	E855.0	E936.2	E950.4	E962.0	E980.4
Ethotoin	966.1	E855.0	E936.1	E950.4	E962.0	E980.4
Ethoxazene	961.9	E857	E931.9	E950.4	E962.0	E980.4
Ethoxzolamide	974.2	E858.5	E944.2	E950.4	E962.0	E980.4
Ethyl						
acetate (vapor)	982.8	E862.4	—	E950.9	E962.1	E980.9
alcohol	980.0	E860.1	—	E950.9	E962.1	E980.9
beverage	980.0	E860.0	—	E950.9	E962.1	E980.9
aldehyde (vapor)	987.8	E869.8	—	E952.8	E962.2	E982.8
liquid	989.89	E866.8	—	E950.9	E962.1	E980.9
aminobenzoate	968.5	E855.2	E938.5	E950.4	E962.0	E980.4
biscoumacetate	964.2	E858.2	E934.2	E950.4	E962.0	E980.4
bromide (anesthetic)	968.2	E855.1	E938.2	E950.4	E962.0	E980.4
carbamate (antineoplastic)	963.1	E858.1	E933.1	E950.4	E962.0	E980.4
carbinol	980.3	E860.4	—	E950.9	E962.1	E980.9
chaulmoograte	961.8	E857	E931.8	E950.4	E962.0	E980.4
chloride (vapor)	987.8	E869.8	—	E952.8	E962.2	E982.8
anesthetic (local)	968.5	E855.2	E938.5	E950.4	E962.0	E980.4
inhaled	968.2	E855.1	E938.2	E950.4	E962.0	E980.4
solvent	982.3	E862.4	—	E950.9	E962.1	E980.9

	Poisoning	External Cause (E-Code)				
		Accident	Therapeutic Use	Suicide Attempt	Assault	Undetermined
Ethyl — *continued*						
estranol	962.1	E858.0	E932.1	E950.4	E962.0	E980.4
ether — *see* Ether(s)						
formate (solvent) NEC	982.8	E862.4	—	E950.9	E962.1	E980.9
iodoacetate	987.5	E869.3	—	E952.8	E962.2	E982.8
lactate (solvent) NEC	982.8	E862.4	—	E950.9	E962.1	E980.9
methylcarbinol	980.8	E860.8	—	E950.9	E962.1	E980.9
morphine	965.09	E850.2	E935.2	E950.0	E962.0	E980.0
Ethylene (gas)	987.1	E869.8	—	E952.8	E962.2	E982.8
anesthetic (general)	968.2	E855.1	E938.2	E950.4	E962.0	E980.4
chlorohydrin (vapor)	982.3	E862.4	—	E950.9	E962.1	E980.9
dichloride (vapor)	982.3	E862.4	—	E950.9	E962.1	E980.9
glycol(s) (any) (vapor)	982.8	E862.4	—	E950.9	E962.1	E980.9
Ethylidene						
chloride NEC	982.3	E862.4	—	E950.9	E962.1	E980.9
diethyl ether	982.8	E862.4	—	E950.9	E962.1	E980.9
Ethynodiol	962.2	E858.0	E932.2	E950.4	E962.0	E980.4
Etidocaine	968.9	E855.2	E938.9	E950.4	E962.0	E980.4
infiltration (subcutaneous)	968.5	E855.2	E938.5	E950.4	E962.0	E980.4
nerve (peripheral) (plexus)	968.6	E855.2	E938.6	E950.4	E962.0	E980.4
Etilfen	967.0	E851	E937.0	E950.1	E962.0	E980.1
Etomide	965.7	E850.7	E935.7	E950.0	E962.0	E980.0
Etorphine	965.09	E850.2	E935.2	E950.0	E962.0	E980.0
Etoval	967.0	E851	E937.0	E950.1	E962.0	E980.1
Etryptamine	969.0	E854.0	E939.0	E950.3	E962.0	E980.3
Eucaine	968.5	E855.2	E938.5	E950.4	E962.0	E980.4
Eucalyptus (oil) NEC	975.5	E858.6	E945.5	E950.4	E962.0	E980.4
Eucatropine	971.1	E855.4	E941.1	E950.4	E962.0	E980.4
Eucodal	965.09	E850.2	E935.2	E950.0	E962.0	E980.0
Euneryl	967.0	E851	E937.0	E950.1	E962.0	E980.1
Euphthalmine	971.1	E855.4	E941.1	E950.4	E962.0	E980.4
Eurax	976.0	E858.7	E946.0	E950.4	E962.0	E980.4
Euresol	976.4	E858.7	E946.4	E950.4	E962.0	E980.4
Euthroid	962.7	E858.0	E932.7	E950.4	E962.0	E980.4
Evans blue	977.8	E858.8	E947.8	E950.4	E962.0	E980.4
Evipal	967.0	E851	E937.0	E950.1	E962.0	E980.1
sodium	968.3	E855.1	E938.3	E950.4	E962.0	E980.4
Evipan	967.0	E851	E937.0	E950.1	E962.0	E980.1
sodium	968.3	E855.1	E938.3	E950.4	E962.0	E980.4
Exalgin	965.4	E850.4	E935.4	E950.0	E962.0	E980.0
Excipients, pharmaceutical	977.4	E858.8	E947.4	E950.4	E962.0	E980.4
Exhaust gas — *see* Carbon, monoxide						
Ex-Lax (phenolphthalein)	973.1	E858.4	E943.1	E950.4	E962.0	E980.4
Expectorants	975.5	E858.6	E945.5	E950.4	E962.0	E980.4
External medications (skin) (mucous membrane)	976.9	E858.7	E946.9	E950.4	E962.0	E980.4
dental agent	976.7	E858.7	E946.7	E950.4	E962.0	E980.4
ENT agent	976.6	E858.7	E946.6	E950.4	E962.0	E980.4
ophthalmic preparation	976.5	E858.7	E946.5	E950.4	E962.0	E980.4
specified NEC	976.8	E858.7	E946.8	E950.4	E962.0	E980.4
Eye agents (anti-infective)	976.5	E858.7	E946.5	E950.4	E962.0	E980.4
Factor IX complex (human)	964.5	E858.2	E934.5	E950.4	E962.0	E980.4
Fecal softeners	973.2	E858.4	E943.2	E950.4	E962.0	E980.4
Fenbutrazate	977.0	E858.8	E947.0	E950.4	E962.0	E980.4
Fencamfamin	970.8	E854.3	E940.8	E950.4	E962.0	E980.4
Fenfluramine	977.0	E858.8	E947.0	E950.4	E962.0	E980.4
Fenoprofen	965.61	E850.6	E935.6	E950.0	E962.0	E980.0
Fentanyl	965.09	E850.2	E935.2	E950.0	E962.0	E980.0
Fentazin	969.1	E853.0	E939.1	E950.3	E962.0	E980.3
Fenticlor, fentichlor	976.0	E858.7	E946.0	E950.4	E962.0	E980.4
Fer de lance (bite) (venom)	989.5	E905.0	—	E950.9	E962.1	E980.9
Ferric — *see* Iron						
Ferrocholinate	964.0	E858.2	E934.0	E950.4	E962.0	E980.4
Ferrous fumerate, gluconate, lactate, salt NEC, sulfate (medicinal)	964.0	E858.2	E934.0	E950.4	E962.0	E980.4
Ferrum — *see* Iron						
Fertilizers NEC	989.89	E866.5	—	E950.9	E962.1	E980.4
with herbicide mixture	989.4	E863.5	—	E950.6	E962.1	E980.7
Fibrinogen (human)	964.7	E858.2	E934.7	E950.4	E962.0	E980.4
Fibrinolysin	964.4	E858.2	E934.4	E950.4	E962.0	E980.4
Fibrinolysis-affecting agents	964.4	E858.2	E934.4	E950.4	E962.0	E980.4
Filix mas	961.6	E857	E931.6	E950.4	E962.0	E980.4
Fiorinal	965.1	E850.3	E935.3	E950.0	E962.0	E980.0
Fire damp	987.1	E869.8	—	E952.8	E962.2	E982.8
Fish, nonbacterial or noxious	988.0	E865.2	—	E950.9	E962.1	E980.9
shell	988.0	E865.1	—	E950.9	E962.1	E980.9
Flagyl	961.5	E857	E931.5	E950.4	E962.0	E980.4

	Poisoning	External Cause (E-Code)				
		Accident	Therapeutic Use	Suicide Attempt	Assault	Undetermined
Flavoxate	975.1	E858.6	E945.1	E950.4	E962.0	E980.4
Flaxedil	975.2	E858.6	E945.2	E950.4	E962.0	E980.4
Flaxseed (medicinal)	976.3	E858.7	E946.3	E950.4	E962.0	E980.4
Florantyrone	973.4	E858.4	E943.4	E950.4	E962.0	E980.4
Floraquin	961.3	E857	E931.3	E950.4	E962.0	E980.4
Florinef	962.0	E858.0	E932.0	E950.4	E962.0	E980.4
ENT agent	976.6	E858.7	E946.6	E950.4	E962.0	E980.4
ophthalmic preparation	976.5	E858.7	E946.5	E950.4	E962.0	E980.4
topical NEC	976.0	E858.7	E946.0	E950.4	E962.0	E980.4
Flowers of sulfur	976.4	E858.7	E946.4	E950.4	E962.0	E980.4
Floxuridine	963.1	E858.1	E933.1	E950.4	E962.0	E980.4
Flucytosine	961.9	E857	E931.9	E950.4	E962.0	E980.4
Fludrocortisone	962.0	E858.0	E932.0	E950.4	E962.0	E980.4
ENT agent	976.6	E858.7	E946.6	E950.4	E962.0	E980.4
ophthalmic preparation	976.5	E858.7	E946.5	E950.4	E962.0	E980.4
topical NEC	976.0	E858.7	E946.0	E950.4	E962.0	E980.4
Flumethasone	976.0	E858.7	E946.0	E950.4	E962.0	E980.4
Flumethiazide	974.3	E858.5	E944.3	E950.4	E962.0	E980.4
Flumidin	961.7	E857	E931.7	E950.4	E962.0	E980.4
Flunitrazepam	969.4	E853.2	E939.4	E950.3	E962.0	E980.3
Fluocinolone	976.0	E858.7	E946.0	E950.4	E962.0	E980.4
Fluocortolone	962.0	E858.0	E932.0	E950.4	E962.0	E980.4
Fluohydrocortisone	962.0	E858.0	E932.0	E950.4	E962.0	E980.4
ENT agent	976.6	E858.7	E946.6	E950.4	E962.0	E980.4
ophthalmic preparation	976.5	E858.7	E946.5	E950.4	E962.0	E980.4
topical NEC	976.0	E858.7	E946.0	E950.4	E962.0	E980.4
Fluonid	976.0	E858.7	E946.0	E950.4	E962.0	E980.4
Fluopromazine	969.1	E853.0	E939.1	E950.3	E962.0	E980.3
Fluoracetate	989.4	E863.7	—	E950.6	E962.1	E980.7
Fluorescein (sodium)	977.8	E858.8	E947.8	E950.4	E962.0	E980.4
Fluoride(s) (pesticides) (sodium) NEC	989.4	E863.4	—	E950.6	E962.1	E980.7
hydrogen — *see* Hydrofluoric acid						
medicinal	976.7	E858.7	E946.7	E950.4	E962.0	E980.4
not pesticide NEC	983.9	E864.4	—	E950.7	E962.1	E980.6
stannous	976.7	E858.7	E946.7	E950.4	E962.0	E980.4
Fluorinated corticosteroids	962.0	E858.0	E932.0	E950.4	E962.0	E980.4
Fluorine (compounds) (gas)	987.8	E869.8	—	E952.8	E962.2	E982.8
salt — *see* Fluoride(s)						
Fluoristan	976.7	E858.7	E946.7	E950.4	E962.0	E980.4
Fluoroacetate	989.4	E863.7	—	E950.6	E962.1	E980.7
Fluorodeoxyuridine	963.1	E858.1	E933.1	E950.4	E962.0	E980.4
Fluorometholone (topical) NEC	976.0	E858.7	E946.0	E950.4	E962.0	E980.4
ophthalmic preparation	976.5	E858.7	E946.5	E950.4	E962.0	E980.4
Fluorouracil	963.1	E858.1	E933.1	E950.4	E962.0	E980.4
Fluothane	968.1	E855.1	E938.1	E950.4	E962.0	E980.4
Fluoxetine hydrochloride	969.0	E854.0	E939.0	E950.3	E962.0	E980.3
Fluoxymesterone	962.1	E858.0	E932.1	E950.4	E962.0	E980.4
Fluphenazine	969.1	E853.0	E939.1	E950.3	E962.0	E980.3
Fluprednisolone	962.0	E858.0	E932.0	E950.4	E962.0	E980.4
Flurandrenolide	976.0	E858.7	E946.0	E950.4	E962.0	E980.4
Flurazepam (hydrochloride)	969.4	E853.2	E939.4	E950.3	E962.0	E980.3
Flurbiprofen	965.61	E850.6	E935.6	E950.0	E962.0	E980.0
Flurobate	976.0	E858.7	E946.0	E950.4	E962.0	E980.4
Flurothyl	969.8	E855.8	E939.8	E950.3	E962.0	E980.3
Fluroxene	968.2	E855.1	E938.2	E950.4	E962.0	E980.4
Folacin	964.1	E858.2	E934.1	E950.4	E962.0	E980.4
Folic acid	964.1	E858.2	E934.1	E950.4	E962.0	E980.4
Follicle stimulating hormone	962.4	E858.0	E932.4	E950.4	E962.0	E980.4
Food, foodstuffs, nonbacterial or noxious	988.9	E865.9	—	E950.9	E962.1	E980.9
berries, seeds	988.2	E865.3	—	E950.9	E962.1	E980.9
fish	988.0	E865.2	—	E950.9	E962.1	E980.9
mushrooms	988.1	E865.5	—	E950.9	E962.1	E980.9
plants	988.2	E865.9	—	E950.9	E962.1	E980.9
specified type NEC	988.2	E865.4	—	E950.9	E962.1	E980.9
shellfish	988.0	E865.1	—	E950.9	E962.1	E980.9
specified NEC	988.8	E865.8	—	E950.9	E962.1	E980.9
Fool's parsley	988.2	E865.4	—	E950.9	E962.1	E980.9
Formaldehyde (solution)	989.89	E861.4	—	E950.9	E962.1	E980.9
fungicide	989.4	E863.6	—	E950.6	E962.1	E980.7
gas or vapor	987.8	E869.8	—	E952.8	E962.2	E982.8
Formalin	989.89	E861.4	—	E950.9	E962.1	E980.9
fungicide	989.4	E863.6	—	E950.6	E962.1	E980.7
vapor	987.8	E869.8	—	E952.8	E962.2	E982.8
Formic acid	983.1	E864.1	—	E950.7	E962.1	E980.6
vapor	987.8	E869.8	—	E952.8	E962.2	E982.8

☑ Additional Digit Required — Refer to the Tabular List (Numeric Code Section) for Additional Digit Selection
▶◀ Revised Text ● New Line ▲ Revised Code

		External Cause (E-Code)				
	Poisoning	Accident	Therapeutic Use	Suicide Attempt	Assault	Undetermined
Fowler's solution	985.1	E866.3	—	E950.8	E962.1	E980.8
Foxglove	988.2	E865.4	—	E950.9	E962.1	E980.9
Fox green	977.8	E858.8	E947.8	E950.4	E962.0	E980.4
Framycetin	960.8	E856	E930.8	E950.4	E962.0	E980.4
Frangula (extract)	973.1	E858.4	E943.1	E950.4	E962.0	E980.4
Frei antigen	977.8	E858.8	E947.8	E950.4	E962.0	E980.4
Freons	987.4	E869.2	—	E952.8	E962.2	E982.8
Fructose	974.5	E858.5	E944.5	E950.4	E962.0	E980.4
Frusemide	974.4	E858.5	E944.4	E950.4	E962.0	E980.4
FSH	962.4	E858.0	E932.4	E950.4	E962.0	E980.4
Fuel						
automobile	981	E862.1	—	E950.9	E962.1	E980.9
exhaust gas, not in transit	986	E868.2	—	E952.0	E962.2	E982.0
vapor NEC	987.1	E869.8	—	E952.8	E962.2	E982.8
gas (domestic use) — *see also* Carbon, monoxide, fuel						
utility	987.1	E868.1	—	E951.8	E962.2	E981.8
incomplete combustion of — *see* Carbon, monoxide, fuel, utility						
in mobile container	987.0	E868.0	—	E951.1	E962.2	E981.1
piped (natural)	987.1	E867	—	E951.0	E962.2	E981.0
industrial, incomplete combustion	986	E868.3	—	E952.1	E962.2	E982.1
Fugillin	960.8	E856	E930.8	E950.4	E962.0	E980.4
Fulminate of mercury	985.0	E866.1	—	E950.9	E962.1	E980.9
Fulvicin	960.1	E856	E930.1	E950.4	E962.0	E980.4
Fumadil	960.8	E856	E930.8	E950.4	E962.0	E980.4
Fumagillin	960.8	E856	E930.8	E950.4	E962.0	E980.4
Fumes (from)	987.9	E869.9	—	E952.9	E962.2	E982.9
carbon monoxide — *see* Carbon, monoxide						
charcoal (domestic use)	986	E868.3	—	E952.1	E962.2	E982.1
chloroform — *see* Chloroform						
coke (in domestic stoves, fireplaces)	986	E868.3	—	E952.1	E962.2	E982.1
corrosive NEC	987.8	E869.8	—	E952.8	E962.2	E982.8
ether — *see* Ether(s)						
freons	987.4	E869.2	—	E952.8	E962.2	E982.8
hydrocarbons	987.1	E869.8	—	E952.8	E962.2	E982.8
petroleum (liquefied)	987.0	E868.0	—	E951.1	E962.2	E981.1
distributed through pipes (pure or mixed with air)	987.0	E867	—	E951.0	E962.2	E981.0
lead — *see* Lead						
metals — *see* specified metal						
nitrogen dioxide	987.2	E869.0	—	E952.8	E962.2	E982.8
pesticides — *see* Pesticides						
petroleum (liquefied)	987.0	E868.0	—	E951.1	E962.2	E981.1
distributed through pipes (pure or mixed with air)	987.0	E867	—	E951.0	E962.2	E981.0
polyester	987.8	E869.8	—	E952.8	E962.2	E982.8
specified, source other (*see also* substance specified)	987.8	E869.8	—	E952.8	E962.2	E982.8
sulfur dioxide	987.3	E869.1	—	E952.8	E962.2	E982.8
Fumigants	989.4	E863.8	—	E950.6	E962.1	E980.7
Fungi, noxious, used as food	988.1	E865.5	—	E950.9	E962.1	E980.9
Fungicides (*see also* Antifungals)	989.4	E863.6	—	E950.6	E962.1	E980.7
Fungizone	960.1	E856	E930.1	E950.4	E962.0	E980.4
topical	976.0	E858.7	E946.0	E950.4	E962.0	E980.4
Furacin	976.0	E858.7	E946.0	E950.4	E962.0	E980.4
Furadantin	961.9	E857	E931.9	E950.4	E962.0	E980.4
Furazolidone	961.9	E857	E931.9	E950.4	E962.0	E980.4
Furnace (coal burning) (domestic), gas from	986	E868.3	—	E952.1	E962.2	E982.1
industrial	986	E868.8	—	E952.1	E962.2	E982.1
Furniture polish	989.89	E861.2	—	E950.9	E962.1	E980.9
Furosemide	974.4	E858.5	E944.4	E950.4	E962.0	E980.4
Furoxone	961.9	E857	E931.9	E950.4	E962.0	E980.4
Fusel oil (amyl) (butyl) (propyl)	980.3	E860.4	—	E950.9	E962.1	E980.9
Fusidic acid	960.8	E856	E930.8	E950.4	E962.0	E980.4
Gallamine	975.2	E858.6	E945.2	E950.4	E962.0	E980.4
Gallotannic acid	976.2	E858.7	E946.2	E950.4	E962.0	E980.4
Gamboge	973.1	E858.4	E943.1	E950.4	E962.0	E980.4
Gamimune	964.6	E858.2	E934.6	E950.4	E962.0	E980.4
Gamma-benzene hexachloride (vapor)	989.2	E863.0	—	E950.6	E962.1	E980.7
Gamma globulin	964.6	E858.2	E934.6	E950.4	E962.0	E980.4
Gamma hydroxy butyrate (GHB)	968.4	E855.1	E938.4	E950.4	E962.0	E980.4
Gamulin	964.6	E858.2	E934.6	E950.4	E962.0	E980.4
Ganglionic blocking agents	972.3	E858.3	E942.3	E950.4	E962.0	E980.4
Ganja	969.6	E854.1	E939.6	E950.3	E962.0	E980.3
Garamycin	960.8	E856	E930.8	E950.4	E962.0	E980.4
ophthalmic preparation	976.5	E858.7	E946.5	E950.4	E962.0	E980.4
topical NEC	976.0	E858.7	E946.0	E950.4	E962.0	E980.4
Gardenal	967.0	E851	E937.0	E950.1	E962.0	E980.1
Gardepanyl	967.0	E851	E937.0	E950.1	E962.0	E980.1
Gas	987.9	E869.9	—	E952.9	E962.2	E982.9
acetylene	987.1	E868.1	—	E951.8	E962.2	E981.8
incomplete combustion of — *see* Carbon, monoxide, fuel, utility						
air contaminants, source or type not specified	987.9	E869.9	—	E952.9	E962.2	E982.9
anesthetic (general) NEC	968.2	E855.1	E938.2	E950.4	E962.0	E980.4
blast furnace	986	E868.8	—	E952.1	E962.2	E982.1
butane — *see* Butane						
carbon monoxide — *see* Carbon, monoxide						
chlorine	987.6	E869.8	—	E952.8	E962.2	E982.8
coal — *see* Carbon, monoxide, coal						
cyanide	987.7	E869.8	—	E952.8	E962.2	E982.8
dicyanogen	987.8	E869.8	—	E952.8	E962.2	E982.8
domestic — *see* Gas, utility						
exhaust — *see* Carbon, monoxide, exhaust gas						
from wood- or coal-burning stove or fireplace	986	E868.3	—	E952.1	E962.2	E982.1
fuel (domestic use) — *see also* Carbon, monoxide, fuel						
industrial use	986	E868.8	—	E952.1	E962.2	E982.1
utility	987.1	E868.1	—	E951.8	E962.2	E981.8
incomplete combustion of — *see* Carbon, monoxide, fuel, utility						
in mobile container	987.0	E868.0	—	E951.1	E962.2	E981.1
piped (natural)	987.1	E867	—	E951.0	E962.2	E981.0
garage	986	E868.2	—	E952.0	E962.2	E982.0
hydrocarbon NEC	987.1	E869.8	—	E952.8	E962.2	E982.8
incomplete combustion of — *see* Carbon, monoxide, fuel, utility						
liquefied (mobile container)	987.0	E868.0	—	E951.1	E962.2	E981.1
piped	987.0	E867	—	E951.0	E962.2	E981.0
hydrocyanic acid	987.7	E869.8	—	E952.8	E962.2	E982.8
illuminating — *see* Gas, utility						
incomplete combustion, any — *see* Carbon, monoxide						
kiln	986	E868.8	—	E952.1	E962.2	E982.1
lacrimogenic	987.5	E869.3	—	E952.8	E962.2	E982.8
marsh	987.1	E869.8	—	E952.8	E962.2	E982.8
motor exhaust, not in transit	986	E868.8	—	E952.1	E962.2	E982.1
mustard — *see* Mustard, gas						
natural	987.1	E867	—	E951.0	E962.2	E981.0
nerve (war)	987.9	E869.9	—	E952.9	E962.2	E982.9
oils	981	E862.1	—	E950.9	E962.1	E980.9
petroleum (liquefied) (distributed in mobile containers)	987.0	E868.0	—	E951.1	E962.2	E981.1
piped (pure or mixed with air)	987.0	E867	—	E951.1	E962.2	E981.1
piped (manufactured) (natural) NEC	987.1	E867	—	E951.0	E962.2	E981.0

		External Cause (E-Code)				
	Poisoning	Accident	Therapeutic Use	Suicide Attempt	Assault	Undetermined
Gas — *continued*						
producer	986	E868.8	—	E952.1	E962.2	E982.1
propane — *see* Propane						
refrigerant (freon)	987.4	E869.2	—	E952.8	E962.2	E982.8
not freon	987.9	E869.9	—	E952.9	E962.2	E982.9
sewer	987.8	E869.8	—	E952.8	E962.2	E982.8
specified source NEC (*see also* substance specified)	987.8	E869.8	—	E952.8	E962.2	E982.8
stove — *see* Gas, utility						
tear	987.5	E869.3	—	E952.8	E962.2	E982.8
utility (for cooking, heating, or lighting) (piped) NEC	987.1	E868.1	—	E951.8	E962.2	E981.8
incomplete combustion of — *see* Carbon, monoxide, fuel, utilty						
in mobile container	987.0	E868.0	—	E951.1	E962.2	E981.1
piped (natural)	987.1	E867	—	E951.0	E962.2	E981.0
water	987.1	E868.1	—	E951.8	E962.2	E981.8
incomplete combustion of — *see* Carbon, monoxide, fuel, utility						
Gaseous substance — *see* Gas						
Gasoline, gasolene	981	E862.1	—	E950.9	E962.1	E980.9
vapor	987.1	E869.8	—	E952.8	E962.2	E982.8
Gastric enzymes	973.4	E858.4	E943.4	E950.4	E962.0	E980.4
Gastrografin	977.8	E858.8	E947.8	E950.4	E962.0	E980.4
Gastrointestinal agents	973.9	E858.4	E943.9	E950.4	E962.0	E980.4
specified NEC	973.8	E858.4	E943.8	E950.4	E962.0	E980.4
Gaultheria procumbens	988.2	E865.4	—	E950.9	E962.1	E980.9
Gelatin (intravenous)	964.8	E858.2	E934.8	E950.4	E962.0	E980.4
absorbable (sponge)	964.5	E858.2	E934.5	E950.4	E962.0	E980.4
Gelfilm	976.8	E858.7	E946.8	E950.4	E962.0	E980.4
Gelfoam	964.5	E858.2	E934.5	E950.4	E962.0	E980.4
Gelsemine	970.8	E854.3	E940.8	E950.4	E962.0	E980.4
Gelsemium (sempervirens)	988.2	E865.4	—	E950.9	E962.1	E980.9
Gemonil	967.0	E851	E937.0	E950.1	E962.0	E980.1
Gentamicin	960.8	E856	E930.8	E950.4	E962.0	E980.4
ophthalmic preparation	976.5	E858.7	E946.5	E950.4	E962.0	E980.4
topical NEC	976.0	E858.7	E946.0	E950.4	E962.0	E980.4
Gentian violet	976.0	E858.7	E946.0	E950.4	E962.0	E980.4
Gexane	976.0	E858.7	E946.0	E950.4	E962.0	E980.4
Gila monster (venom)	989.5	E905.0	—	E950.9	E962.1	E980.9
Ginger, Jamaica	989.89	E866.8	—	E950.9	E962.1	E980.9
Gitalin	972.1	E858.3	E942.1	E950.4	E962.0	E980.4
Gitoxin	972.1	E858.3	E942.1	E950.4	E962.0	E980.4
Glandular extract (medicinal) NEC	977.9	E858.9	E947.9	E950.5	E962.0	E980.5
Glaucarubin	961.5	E857	E931.5	E950.4	E962.0	E980.4
Globin zinc insulin	962.3	E858.0	E932.3	E950.4	E962.0	E980.4
Glucagon	962.3	E858.0	E932.3	E950.4	E962.0	E980.4
Glucochloral	967.1	E852.0	E937.1	E950.2	E962.0	E980.2
Glucocorticoids	962.0	E858.0	E932.0	E950.4	E962.0	E980.4
Glucose	974.5	E858.5	E944.5	E950.4	E962.0	E980.4
oxidase reagent	977.8	E858.8	E947.8	E950.4	E962.0	E980.4
Glucosulfone sodium	961.8	E857	E931.8	E950.4	E962.0	E980.4
Glue(s)	989.89	E866.6	—	E950.9	E962.1	E980.9
Glutamic acid (hydrochloride)	973.4	E858.4	E943.4	E950.4	E962.0	E980.4
Glutaraldehyde	989.89	E861.4	—	E950.9	E962.1	E980.9
Glutathione	963.8	E858.1	E933.8	E950.4	E962.0	E980.4
Glutethimide (group)	967.5	E852.4	E937.5	E950.2	E962.0	E980.2
Glycerin (lotion)	976.3	E858.7	E946.3	E950.4	E962.0	E980.4
Glycerol (topical)	976.3	E858.7	E946.3	E950.4	E962.0	E980.4
Glyceryl						
guaiacolate	975.5	E858.6	E945.5	E950.4	E962.0	E980.4
triacetate (topical)	976.0	E858.7	E946.0	E950.4	E962.0	E980.4
trinitrate	972.4	E858.3	E942.4	E950.4	E962.0	E980.4
Glycine	974.5	E858.5	E944.5	E950.4	E962.0	E980.4
Glycobiarsol	961.1	E857	E931.1	E950.4	E962.0	E980.4
Glycols (ether)	982.8	E862.4	—	E950.9	E962.1	E980.9
Glycopyrrolate	971.1	E855.4	E941.1	E950.4	E962.0	E980.4
Glymidine	962.3	E858.0	E932.3	E950.4	E962.0	E980.4
Gold (compounds) (salts)	965.69	E850.6	E935.6	E950.0	E962.0	E980.0
Golden sulfide of antimony	985.4	E866.2	—	E950.9	E962.1	E980.9
Goldylocks	988.2	E865.4	—	E950.9	E962.1	E980.9
Gonadal tissue extract	962.9	E858.0	E932.9	E950.4	E962.0	E980.4
female	962.2	E858.0	E932.2	E950.4	E962.0	E980.4
male	962.1	E858.0	E932.1	E950.4	E962.0	E980.4

		External Cause (E-Code)				
	Poisoning	Accident	Therapeutic Use	Suicide Attempt	Assault	Undetermined
Gonadotropin	962.4	E858.0	E932.4	E950.4	E962.0	E980.4
Grain alcohol	980.0	E860.1	—	E950.9	E962.1	E980.9
beverage	980.0	E860.0	—	E950.9	E962.1	E980.9
Gramicidin	960.8	E856	E930.8	E950.4	E962.0	E980.4
Gratiola officinalis	988.2	E865.4	—	E950.9	E962.1	E980.9
Grease	989.89	E866.8	—	E950.9	E962.1	E980.9
Green hellebore	988.2	E865.4	—	E950.9	E962.1	E980.9
Green soap	976.2	E858.7	E946.2	E950.4	E962.0	E980.4
Grifulvin	960.1	E856	E930.1	E950.4	E962.0	E980.4
Griseofulvin	960.1	E856	E930.1	E950.4	E962.0	E980.4
Growth hormone	962.4	E858.0	E932.4	E950.4	E962.0	E980.4
Guaiacol	975.5	E858.6	E945.5	E950.4	E962.0	E980.4
Guaiac reagent	977.8	E858.8	E947.8	E950.4	E962.0	E980.4
Guaifenesin	975.5	E858.6	E945.5	E950.4	E962.0	E980.4
Guaiphenesin	975.5	E858.6	E945.5	E950.4	E962.0	E980.4
Guanatol	961.4	E857	E931.4	E950.4	E962.0	E980.4
Guanethidine	972.6	E858.3	E942.6	E950.4	E962.0	E980.4
Guano	989.89	E866.5	—	E950.9	E962.1	E980.9
Guanochlor	972.6	E858.3	E942.6	E950.4	E962.0	E980.4
Guanoctine	972.6	E858.3	E942.6	E950.4	E962.0	E980.4
Guanoxan	972.6	E858.3	E942.6	E950.4	E962.0	E980.4
Hair treatment agent NEC	976.4	E858.7	E946.4	E950.4	E962.0	E980.4
Halcinonide	976.0	E858.7	E946.0	E950.4	E962.0	E980.4
Halethazole	976.0	E858.7	E946.0	E950.4	E962.0	E980.4
Hallucinogens	969.6	E854.1	E939.6	E950.3	E962.0	E980.3
Haloperidol	969.2	E853.1	E939.2	E950.3	E962.0	E980.3
Haloprogin	976.0	E858.7	E946.0	E950.4	E962.0	E980.4
Halotex	976.0	E858.7	E946.0	E950.4	E962.0	E980.4
Halothane	968.1	E855.1	E938.1	E950.4	E962.0	E980.4
Halquinols	976.0	E858.7	E946.0	E950.4	E962.0	E980.4
Harmonyl	972.6	E858.3	E942.6	E950.4	E962.0	E980.4
Hartmann's solution	974.5	E858.5	E944.5	E950.4	E962.0	E980.4
Hashish	969.6	E854.1	E939.6	E950.3	E962.0	E980.3
Hawaiian wood rose seeds	969.6	E854.1	E939.6	E950.3	E962.0	E980.3
Headache cures, drugs, powders NEC	977.9	E858.9	E947.9	E950.5	E962.0	E980.9
Heavenly Blue (morning glory)	969.6	E854.1	E939.6	E950.3	E962.0	E980.3
Heavy metal antagonists	963.8	E858.1	E933.8	E950.4	E962.0	E980.4
anti-infectives	961.2	E857	E931.2	E950.4	E962.0	E980.4
Hedaquinium	976.0	E858.7	E946.0	E950.4	E962.0	E980.4
Hedge hyssop	988.2	E865.4	—	E950.9	E962.1	E980.9
Heet	976.8	E858.7	E946.8	E950.4	E962.0	E980.4
Helenin	961.6	E857	E931.6	E950.4	E962.0	E980.4
Hellebore (black) (green) (white)	988.2	E865.4	—	E950.9	E962.1	E980.9
Hemlock	988.2	E865.4	—	E950.9	E962.1	E980.9
Hemostatics	964.5	E858.2	E934.5	E950.4	E962.0	E980.4
capillary active drugs	972.8	E858.3	E942.8	E950.4	E962.0	E980.4
Henbane	988.2	E865.4	—	E950.9	E962.1	E980.9
Heparin (sodium)	964.2	E858.2	E934.2	E950.4	E962.0	E980.4
Heptabarbital, heptabarbitone	967.0	E851	E937.0	E950.1	E962.0	E980.1
Heptachlor	989.2	E863.0	—	E950.6	E962.1	E980.7
Heptalgin	965.09	E850.2	E935.2	E950.0	E962.0	E980.0
Herbicides	989.4	E863.5	—	E950.6	E962.1	E980.7
Heroin	965.01	E850.0	E935.0	E950.0	E962.0	E980.0
Herplex	976.5	E858.7	E946.5	E950.4	E962.0	E980.4
HES	964.8	E858.2	E934.8	E950.4	E962.0	E980.4
Hetastarch	964.8	E858.2	E934.8	E950.4	E962.0	E980.4
Hexachlorocyclohexane	989.2	E863.0	—	E950.6	E962.1	E980.7
Hexachlorophene	976.2	E858.7	E946.2	E950.4	E962.0	E980.4
Hexadimethrine (bromide)	964.5	E858.2	E934.5	E950.4	E962.0	E980.4
Hexafluorenium	975.2	E858.6	E945.2	E950.4	E962.0	E980.4
Hexa-germ	976.2	E858.7	E946.2	E950.4	E962.0	E980.4
Hexahydrophenol	980.8	E860.8	—	E950.9	E962.1	E980.9
Hexalin	980.8	E860.8	—	E950.9	E962.1	E980.9
Hexamethonium	972.3	E858.3	E942.3	E950.4	E962.0	E980.4
Hexamethyleneamine	961.9	E857	E931.9	E950.4	E962.0	E980.4
Hexamine	961.9	E857	E931.9	E950.4	E962.0	E980.4
Hexanone	982.8	E862.4	—	E950.9	E962.1	E980.9
Hexapropymate	967.8	E852.8	E937.8	E950.2	E962.0	E980.2
Hexestrol	962.2	E858.0	E932.2	E950.4	E962.0	E980.4
Hexethal (sodium)	967.0	E851	E937.0	E950.1	E962.0	E980.1
Hexetidine	976.0	E858.7	E946.0	E950.4	E962.0	E980.4
Hexobarbital, hexobarbitone	967.0	E851	E937.0	E950.1	E962.0	E980.1
sodium (anesthetic)	968.3	E855.1	E938.3	E950.4	E962.0	E980.4
soluble	968.3	E855.1	E938.3	E950.4	E962.0	E980.4
Hexocyclium	971.1	E855.4	E941.1	E950.4	E962.0	E980.4
Hexoestrol	962.2	E858.0	E932.2	E950.4	E962.0	E980.4

		External Cause (E-Code)				
	Poisoning	Accident	Therapeutic Use	Suicide Attempt	Assault	Undetermined
Hexone	982.8	E862.4	—	E950.9	E962.1	E980.9
Hexylcaine	968.5	E855.2	E938.5	E950.4	E962.0	E980.4
Hexylresorcinol	961.6	E857	E931.6	E950.4	E962.0	E980.4
Hinkle's pills	973.1	E858.4	E943.1	E950.4	E962.0	E980.4
Histalog	977.8	E858.8	E947.8	E950.4	E962.0	E980.4
Histamine (phosphate)	972.5	E858.3	E942.5	E950.4	E962.0	E980.4
Histoplasmin	977.8	E858.8	E947.8	E950.4	E962.0	E980.4
Holly berries	988.2	E865.3	—	E950.9	E962.1	E980.9
Homatropine	971.1	E855.4	E941.1	E950.4	E962.0	E980.4
Homo-tet	964.6	E858.2	E934.6	E950.4	E962.0	E980.4
Hormones (synthetic substitute) NEC	962.9	E858.0	E932.9	E950.4	E962.0	E980.4
adrenal cortical steroids	962.0	E858.0	E932.0	E950.4	E962.0	E980.4
antidiabetic agents	962.3	E858.0	E932.3	E950.4	E962.0	E980.4
follicle stimulating	962.4	E858.0	E932.4	E950.4	E962.0	E980.4
gonadotropic	962.4	E858.0	E932.4	E950.4	E962.0	E980.4
growth	962.4	E858.0	E932.4	E950.4	E962.0	E980.4
ovarian (substitutes)	962.2	E858.0	E932.2	E950.4	E962.0	E980.4
parathyroid (derivatives)	962.6	E858.0	E932.6	E950.4	E962.0	E980.4
pituitary (posterior)	962.5	E858.0	E932.5	E950.4	E962.0	E980.4
anterior	962.4	E858.0	E932.4	E950.4	E962.0	E980.4
thyroid (derivative)	962.7	E858.0	E932.7	E950.4	E962.0	E980.4
Hornet (sting)	989.5	E905.3	—	E950.9	E962.1	E980.9
Horticulture agent NEC	989.4	E863.9	—	E950.6	E962.1	E980.7
Hyaluronidase	963.4	E858.1	E933.4	E950.4	E962.0	E980.4
Hyazyme	963.4	E858.1	E933.4	E950.4	E962.0	E980.4
Hycodan	965.09	E850.2	E935.2	E950.0	E962.0	E980.0
Hydantoin derivatives	966.1	E855.0	E936.1	E950.4	E962.0	E980.4
Hydeltra	962.0	E858.0	E932.0	E950.4	E962.0	E980.4
Hydergine	971.3	E855.6	E941.3	E950.4	E962.0	E980.4
Hydrabamine penicillin	960.0	E856	E930.0	E950.4	E962.0	E980.4
Hydralazine, hydrallazine	972.6	E858.3	E942.6	E950.4	E962.0	E980.4
Hydrargaphen	976.0	E858.7	E946.0	E950.4	E962.0	E980.4
Hydrazine	983.9	E864.3	—	E950.7	E962.1	E980.6
Hydriodic acid	975.5	E858.6	E945.5	E950.4	E962.0	E980.4
Hydrocarbon gas	987.1	E869.8	—	E952.8	E962.2	E982.8
incomplete combustion of — *see* Carbon, monoxide, fuel, utility						
liquefied (mobile container)	987.0	E868.0	—	E951.1	E962.2	E981.1
piped (natural)	987.0	E867	—	E951.0	E962.2	E981.0
Hydrochloric acid (liquid)	983.1	E864.1	—	E950.7	E962.1	E980.6
medicinal	973.4	E858.4	E943.4	E950.4	E962.0	E980.4
vapor	987.8	E869.8	—	E952.8	E962.2	E982.8
Hydrochlorothiazide	974.3	E858.5	E944.3	E950.4	E962.0	E980.4
Hydrocodone	965.09	E850.2	E935.2	E950.0	E962.0	E980.0
Hydrocortisone	962.0	E858.0	E932.0	E950.4	E962.0	E980.4
ENT agent	976.6	E858.7	E946.6	E950.4	E962.0	E980.4
ophthalmic preparation	976.5	E858.7	E946.5	E950.4	E962.0	E980.4
topical NEC	976.0	E858.7	E946.0	E950.4	E962.0	E980.4
Hydrocortone	962.0	E858.0	E932.0	E950.4	E962.0	E980.4
ENT agent	976.6	E858.7	E946.6	E950.4	E962.0	E980.4
ophthalmic preparation	976.5	E858.7	E946.5	E950.4	E962.0	E980.4
topical NEC	976.0	E858.7	E946.0	E950.4	E962.0	E980.4
Hydrocyanic acid — *see* Cyanide(s)						
Hydroflumethiazide	974.3	E858.5	E944.3	E950.4	E962.0	E980.4
Hydrofluoric acid (liquid)	983.1	E864.1	—	E950.7	E962.1	E980.6
vapor	987.8	E869.8	—	E952.8	E962.2	E982.8
Hydrogen	987.8	E869.8	—	E952.8	E962.2	E982.8
arsenide	985.1	E866.3	—	E950.8	E962.1	E980.8
arseniureted	985.1	E866.3	—	E950.8	E962.1	E980.8
cyanide (salts)	989.0	E866.8	—	E950.9	E962.1	E980.9
gas	987.7	E869.8	—	E952.8	E962.2	E982.8
fluoride (liquid)	983.1	E864.1	—	E950.7	E962.1	E980.6
vapor	987.8	E869.8	—	E952.8	E962.2	E982.8
peroxide (solution)	976.6	E858.7	E946.6	E950.4	E962.0	E980.4
phosphureted	987.8	E869.8	—	E952.8	E962.2	E982.8
sulfide (gas)	987.8	E869.8	—	E952.8	E962.2	E982.8
arseniureted	985.1	E866.3	—	E950.8	E962.1	E980.8
sulfureted	987.8	E869.8	—	E952.8	E962.2	E982.8
Hydromorphinol	965.09	E850.2	E935.2	E950.0	E962.0	E980.0
Hydromorphinone	965.09	E850.2	E935.2	E950.0	E962.0	E980.0
Hydromorphone	965.09	E850.2	E935.2	E950.0	E962.0	E980.0
Hydromox	974.3	E858.5	E944.3	E950.4	E962.0	E980.4
Hydrophilic lotion	976.3	E858.7	E946.3	E950.4	E962.0	E980.4
Hydroquinone	983.0	E864.0	—	E950.7	E962.1	E980.6
vapor	987.8	E869.8	—	E952.8	E962.2	E982.8
Hydrosulfuric acid (gas)	987.8	E869.8	—	E952.8	E962.2	E982.8
Hydrous wool fat (lotion)	976.3	E858.7	E946.3	E950.4	E962.0	E980.4
Hydroxide, caustic	983.2	E864.2	—	E950.7	E962.1	E980.6
Hydroxocobalamin	964.1	E858.2	E934.1	E950.4	E962.0	E980.4
Hydroxyamphetamine	971.2	E855.5	E941.2	E950.4	E962.0	E980.4
Hydroxychloroquine	961.4	E857	E931.4	E950.4	E962.0	E980.4
Hydroxydihydrocodeinone	965.09	E850.2	E935.2	E950.0	E962.0	E980.0
Hydroxyethyl starch	964.8	E858.2	E934.8	E950.4	E962.0	E980.4
Hydroxyphenamate	969.5	E853.8	E939.5	E950.3	E962.0	E980.3
Hydroxyphenylbutazone	965.5	E850.5	E935.5	E950.0	E962.0	E980.0
Hydroxyprogesterone	962.2	E858.0	E932.2	E950.4	E962.0	E980.4
Hydroxyquinoline derivatives	961.3	E857	E931.3	E950.4	E962.0	E980.4
Hydroxystilbamidine	961.5	E857	E931.5	E950.4	E962.0	E980.4
Hydroxyurea	963.1	E858.1	E933.1	E950.4	E962.0	E980.4
Hydroxyzine	969.5	E853.8	E939.5	E950.3	E962.0	E980.3
Hyoscine (hydrobromide)	971.1	E855.4	E941.1	E950.4	E962.0	E980.4
Hyoscyamine	971.1	E855.4	E941.1	E950.4	E962.0	E980.4
Hyoscyamus (albus) (niger)	988.2	E865.4	—	E950.9	E962.1	E980.9
Hypaque	977.8	E858.8	E947.8	E950.4	E962.0	E980.4
Hypertussis	964.6	E858.2	E934.6	E950.4	E962.0	E980.4
Hypnotics NEC	967.9	E852.9	E937.9	E950.2	E962.0	E980.2
Hypochlorites — *see* Sodium, hypochlorite						
Hypotensive agents NEC	972.6	E858.3	E942.6	E950.4	E962.0	E980.4
Ibufenac	965.69	E850.6	E935.6	E950.0	E962.0	E980.0
Ibuprofen	965.61	E850.6	E935.6	E950.0	E962.0	E980.0
ICG	977.8	E858.8	E947.8	E950.4	E962.0	E980.4
Ichthammol	976.4	E858.7	E946.4	E950.4	E962.0	E980.4
Ichthyol	976.4	E858.7	E946.4	E950.4	E962.0	E980.4
Idoxuridine	976.5	E858.7	E946.5	E950.4	E962.0	E980.4
IDU	976.5	E858.7	E946.5	E950.4	E962.0	E980.4
Iletin	962.3	E858.0	E932.3	E950.4	E962.0	E980.4
Ilex	988.2	E865.4	—	E950.9	E962.1	E980.9
Illuminating gas — *see* Gas, utility						
Ilopan	963.5	E858.1	E933.5	E950.4	E962.0	E980.4
Ilotycin	960.3	E856	E930.3	E950.4	E962.0	E980.4
ophthalmic preparation	976.5	E858.7	E946.5	E950.4	E962.0	E980.4
topical NEC	976.0	E858.7	E946.0	E950.4	E962.0	E980.4
Imipramine	969.0	E854.0	E939.0	E950.3	E962.0	E980.3
Immu-G	964.6	E858.2	E934.6	E950.4	E962.0	E980.4
Immuglobin	964.6	E858.2	E934.6	E950.4	E962.0	E980.4
Immune serum globulin	964.6	E858.2	E934.6	E950.4	E962.0	E980.4
Immunosuppressive agents	963.1	E858.1	E933.1	E950.4	E962.0	E980.4
Immu-tetanus	964.6	E858.2	E934.6	E950.4	E962.0	E980.4
Indandione (derivatives)	964.2	E858.2	E934.2	E950.4	E962.0	E980.4
Inderal	972.0	E858.3	E942.0	E950.4	E962.0	E980.4
Indian						
hemp	969.6	E854.1	E939.6	E950.3	E962.0	E980.3
tobacco	988.2	E865.4	—	E950.9	E962.1	E980.9
Indigo carmine	977.8	E858.8	E947.8	E950.4	E962.0	E980.4
Indocin	965.69	E850.6	E935.6	E950.0	E962.0	E980.0
Indocyanine green	977.8	E858.8	E947.8	E950.4	E962.0	E980.4
Indomethacin	965.69	E850.6	E935.6	E950.0	E962.0	E980.0
Industrial						
alcohol	980.9	E860.9	—	E950.9	E962.1	E980.9
fumes	987.8	E869.8	—	E952.8	E962.2	E982.8
solvents (fumes) (vapors)	982.8	E862.9	—	E950.9	E962.1	E980.9
Influenza vaccine	979.6	E858.8	E949.6	E950.4	E962.0	E982.8
Ingested substances NEC	989.9	E866.9	—	E950.9	E962.1	E980.9
INH (isoniazid)	961.8	E857	E931.8	E950.4	E962.0	E980.4
Inhalation, gas (noxious) — *see* Gas						
Ink	989.89	E866.8	—	E950.9	E962.1	E980.9
Innovar	967.6	E852.5	E937.6	E950.2	E962.0	E980.2
Inositol niacinate	972.2	E858.3	E942.2	E950.4	E962.0	E980.4
Inproquone	963.1	E858.1	E933.1	E950.4	E962.0	E980.4
Insect (sting), venomous	989.5	E905.5	—	E950.9	E962.1	E980.9
Insecticides (*see also* Pesticides)	989.4	E863.4	—	E950.6	E962.1	E980.7
chlorinated	989.2	E863.0	—	E950.6	E962.1	E980.7
mixtures	989.4	E863.3	—	E950.6	E962.1	E980.7
organochlorine (compounds)	989.2	E863.0	—	E950.6	E962.1	E980.7
organophosphorus (compounds)	989.3	E863.1	—	E950.6	E962.1	E980.7
Insular tissue extract	962.3	E858.0	E932.3	E950.4	E962.0	E980.4
Insulin (amorphous) (globin) (isophane) (Lente) (NPH) (protamine) (Semilente) (Ultralente) (zinc)	962.3	E858.0	E932.3	E950.4	E962.0	E980.4
Intranarcon	968.3	E855.1	E938.3	E950.4	E962.0	E980.4
Inulin	977.8	E858.8	E947.8	E950.4	E962.0	E980.4
Invert sugar	974.5	E858.5	E944.5	E950.4	E962.0	E980.4

☑ Additional Digit Required — Refer to the Tabular List (Numeric Code Section) for Additional Digit Selection

▶◀ Revised Text ● New Line ▲ Revised Code

	Poisoning	External Cause (E-Code)				
		Accident	Therapeutic Use	Suicide Attempt	Assault	Undetermined
Inza — *see* Naproxen						
Iodide NEC (*see also* Iodine)	976.0	E858.7	E946.0	E950.4	E962.0	E980.4
mercury (ointment)	976.0	E858.7	E946.0	E950.4	E962.0	E980.4
methylate	976.0	E858.7	E946.0	E950.4	E962.0	E980.4
potassium (expectorant) NEC	975.5	E858.6	E945.5	E950.4	E962.0	E980.4
Iodinated glycerol	975.5	E858.6	E945.5	E950.4	E962.0	E980.4
Iodine (antiseptic, external) (tincture) NEC	976.0	E858.7	E946.0	E950.4	E962.0	E980.4
diagnostic	977.8	E858.8	E947.8	E950.4	E962.0	E980.4
for thyroid conditions (antithyroid)	962.8	E858.0	E932.8	E950.4	E962.0	E980.4
vapor	987.8	E869.8	—	E952.8	E962.2	E982.8
Iodized oil	977.8	E858.8	E947.8	E950.4	E962.0	E980.4
Iodobismitol	961.2	E857	E931.2	E950.4	E962.0	E980.4
Iodochlorhydroxyquin	961.3	E857	E931.3	E950.4	E962.0	E980.4
topical	976.0	E858.7	E946.0	E950.4	E962.0	E980.4
Iodoform	976.0	E858.7	E946.0	E950.4	E962.0	E980.4
Iodopanoic acid	977.8	E858.8	E947.8	E950.4	E962.0	E980.4
Iodophthalein	977.8	E858.8	E947.8	E950.4	E962.0	E980.4
Ion exchange resins	974.5	E858.5	E944.5	E950.4	E962.0	E980.4
Iopanoic acid	977.8	E858.8	E947.8	E950.4	E962.0	E980.4
Iophendylate	977.8	E858.8	E947.8	E950.4	E962.0	E980.4
Iothiouracil	962.8	E858.0	E932.8	E950.4	E962.0	E980.4
Ipecac	973.6	E858.4	E943.6	E950.4	E962.0	E980.4
Ipecacuanha	973.6	E858.4	E943.6	E950.4	E962.0	E980.4
Ipodate	977.8	E858.8	E947.8	E950.4	E962.0	E980.4
Ipral	967.0	E851	E937.0	E950.1	E962.0	E980.1
Ipratropium	975.1	E858.6	E945.1	E950.4	E962.0	E980.4
Iproniazid	969.0	E854.0	E939.0	E950.3	E962.0	E980.3
Iron (compounds) (medicinal) (preparations)	964.0	E858.2	E934.0	E950.4	E962.0	E980.4
dextran	964.0	E858.2	E934.0	E950.4	E962.0	E980.4
nonmedicinal (dust) (fumes) NEC	985.8	E866.4	—	E950.9	E962.1	E980.9
Irritant drug	977.9	E858.9	E947.9	E950.5	E962.0	E980.5
Ismelin	972.6	E858.3	E942.6	E950.4	E962.0	E980.4
Isoamyl nitrite	972.4	E858.3	E942.4	E950.4	E962.0	E980.4
Isobutyl acetate	982.8	E862.4	—	E950.9	E962.1	E980.9
Isocarboxazid	969.0	E854.0	E939.0	E950.3	E962.0	E980.3
Isoephedrine	971.2	E855.5	E941.2	E950.4	E962.0	E980.4
Isoetharine	971.2	E855.5	E941.2	E950.4	E962.0	E980.4
Isofluorophate	971.0	E855.3	E941.0	E950.4	E962.0	E980.4
Isoniazid (INH)	961.8	E857	E931.8	E950.4	E962.0	E980.4
Isopentaquine	961.4	E857	E931.4	E950.4	E962.0	E980.4
Isophane insulin	962.3	E858.0	E932.3	E950.4	E962.0	E980.4
Isopregnenone	962.2	E858.0	E932.2	E950.4	E962.0	E980.4
Isoprenaline	971.2	E855.5	E941.2	E950.4	E962.0	E980.4
Isopropamide	971.1	E855.4	E941.1	E950.4	E962.0	E980.4
Isopropanol	980.2	E860.3	—	E950.9	E962.1	E980.9
topical (germicide)	976.0	E858.7	E946.0	E950.4	E962.0	E980.4
Isopropyl						
acetate	982.8	E862.4	—	E950.9	E962.1	E980.9
alcohol	980.2	E860.3	—	E950.9	E962.1	E980.9
topical (germicide)	976.0	E858.7	E946.0	E950.4	E962.0	E980.4
ether	982.8	E862.4	—	E950.9	E962.1	E980.9
Isoproterenol	971.2	E855.5	E941.2	E950.4	E962.0	E980.4
Isosorbide dinitrate	972.4	E858.3	E942.4	E950.4	E962.0	E980.4
Isothipendyl	963.0	E858.1	E933.0	E950.4	E962.0	E980.4
Isoxazolyl penicillin	960.0	E856	E930.0	E950.4	E962.0	E980.4
Isoxsuprine hydrochloride	972.5	E858.3	E942.5	E950.4	E962.0	E980.4
I-thyroxine sodium	962.7	E858.0	E932.7	E950.4	E962.0	E980.4
Jaborandi (pilocarpus) (extract)	971.0	E855.3	E941.0	E950.4	E962.0	E980.4
Jalap	973.1	E858.4	E943.1	E950.4	E962.0	E980.4
Jamaica						
dogwood (bark)	965.7	E850.7	E935.7	E950.0	E962.0	E980.0
ginger	989.89	E866.8	—	E950.9	E962.1	E980.9
Jatropha	988.2	E865.4	—	E950.9	E962.1	E980.9
curcas	988.2	E865.3	—	E950.9	E962.1	E980.9
Jectofer	964.0	E858.2	E934.0	E950.4	E962.0	E980.4
Jellyfish (sting)	989.5	E905.6	—	E950.9	E962.1	E980.9
Jequirity (bean)	988.2	E865.3	—	E950.9	E962.1	E980.9
Jimson weed	988.2	E865.4	—	E950.9	E962.1	E980.9
seeds	988.2	E865.3	—	E950.9	E962.1	E980.9
Juniper tar (oil) (ointment)	976.4	E858.7	E946.4	E950.4	E962.0	E980.4
Kallikrein	972.5	E858.3	E942.5	E950.4	E962.0	E980.4
Kanamycin	960.6	E856	E930.6	E950.4	E962.0	E980.4
Kantrex	960.6	E856	E930.6	E950.4	E962.0	E980.4
Kaolin	973.5	E858.4	E943.5	E950.4	E962.0	E980.4
Karaya (gum)	973.3	E858.4	E943.3	E950.4	E962.0	E980.4
Kemithal	968.3	E855.1	E938.3	E950.4	E962.0	E980.4

	Poisoning	External Cause (E-Code)				
		Accident	Therapeutic Use	Suicide Attempt	Assault	Undetermined
Kenacort	962.0	E858.0	E932.0	E950.4	E962.0	E980.4
Keratolytics	976.4	E858.7	E946.4	E950.4	E962.0	E980.4
Keratoplastics	976.4	E858.7	E946.4	E950.4	E962.0	E980.4
Kerosene, kerosine (fuel) (solvent) NEC	981	E862.1	—	E950.9	E962.1	E980.9
insecticide	981	E863.4	—	E950.6	E962.1	E980.7
vapor	987.1	E869.8	—	E952.8	E962.2	E982.8
Ketamine	968.3	E855.1	E938.3	E950.4	E962.0	E980.4
Ketobemidone	965.09	E850.2	E935.2	E950.0	E962.0	E980.0
Ketols	982.8	E862.4	—	E950.9	E962.1	E980.9
Ketone oils	982.8	E862.4	—	E950.9	E962.1	E980.9
Ketoprofen	965.61	E850.6	E935.6	E950.0	E962.0	E980.0
Kiln gas or vapor (carbon monoxide)	986	E868.8	—	E952.1	E962.2	E982.1
Konsyl	973.3	E858.4	E943.3	E950.4	E962.0	E980.4
Kosam seed	988.2	E865.3	—	E950.9	E962.1	E980.9
Krait (venom)	989.5	E905.0	—	E950.9	E962.1	E980.9
Kwell (insecticide)	989.2	E863.0	—	E950.6	E962.1	E980.7
anti-infective (topical)	976.0	E858.7	E946.0	E950.4	E962.0	E980.4
Laburnum (flowers) (seeds)	988.2	E865.3	—	E950.9	E962.1	E980.9
leaves	988.2	E865.4	—	E950.9	E962.1	E980.9
Lacquers	989.89	E861.6	—	E950.9	E962.1	E980.9
Lacrimogenic gas	987.5	E869.3	—	E952.8	E962.2	E982.8
Lactic acid	983.1	E864.1	—	E950.7	E962.1	E980.6
Lactobacillus acidophilus	973.5	E858.4	E943.5	E950.4	E962.0	E980.4
Lactoflavin	963.5	E858.1	E933.5	E950.4	E962.0	E980.4
Lactuca (virosa) (extract)	967.8	E852.8	E937.8	E950.2	E962.0	E980.2
Lactucarium	967.8	E852.8	E937.8	E950.2	E962.0	E980.2
Laevulose	974.5	E858.5	E944.5	E950.4	E962.0	E980.4
Lanatoside (C)	972.1	E858.3	E942.1	E950.4	E962.0	E980.4
Lanolin (lotion)	976.3	E858.7	E946.3	E950.4	E962.0	E980.4
Largactil	969.1	E853.0	E939.1	E950.3	E962.0	E980.3
Larkspur	988.2	E865.3	—	E950.9	E962.1	E980.9
Laroxyl	969.0	E854.0	E939.0	E950.3	E962.0	E980.3
Lasix	974.4	E858.5	E944.4	E950.4	E962.0	E980.4
Latex	989.82	E866.8	—	E950.9	E962.1	E980.9
Lathyrus (seed)	988.2	E865.3	—	E950.9	E962.1	E980.9
Laudanum	965.09	E850.2	E935.2	E950.0	E962.0	E980.0
Laudexium	975.2	E858.6	E945.2	E950.4	E962.0	E980.4
Laurel, black or cherry	988.2	E865.4	—	E950.9	E962.1	E980.9
Laurolinium	976.0	E858.7	E946.0	E950.4	E962.0	E980.4
Lauryl sulfoacetate	976.2	E858.7	E946.2	E950.4	E962.0	E980.4
Laxatives NEC	973.3	E858.4	E943.3	E950.4	E962.0	E980.4
emollient	973.2	E858.4	E943.2	E950.4	E962.0	E980.4
L-dopa	966.4	E855.0	E936.4	E950.4	E962.0	E980.4
Lead (dust) (fumes) (vapor) NEC	984.9	E866.0	—	E950.9	E962.1	E980.9
acetate (dust)	984.1	E866.0	—	E950.9	E962.1	E980.9
anti-infectives	961.2	E857	E931.2	E950.4	E962.0	E980.4
antiknock compound (tetraethyl)	984.1	E862.1	—	E950.9	E962.1	E980.9
arsenate, arsenite (dust) (insecticide) (vapor)	985.1	E863.4	—	E950.8	E962.1	E980.8
herbicide	985.1	E863.5	—	E950.8	E962.1	E980.8
carbonate	984.0	E866.0	—	E950.9	E962.1	E980.9
paint	984.0	E861.5	—	E950.9	E962.1	E980.9
chromate	984.0	E866.0	—	E950.9	E962.1	E980.9
paint	984.0	E861.5	—	E950.9	E962.1	E980.9
dioxide	984.0	E866.0	—	E950.9	E962.1	E980.9
inorganic (compound)	984.0	E866.0	—	E950.9	E962.1	E980.9
paint	984.0	E861.5	—	E950.9	E962.1	E980.9
iodide	984.0	E866.0	—	E950.9	E962.1	E980.9
pigment (paint)	984.0	E861.5	—	E950.9	E962.1	E980.9
monoxide (dust)	984.0	E866.0	—	E950.9	E962.1	E980.9
paint	984.0	E861.5	—	E950.9	E962.1	E980.9
organic	984.1	E866.0	—	E950.9	E962.1	E980.9
oxide	984.0	E866.0	—	E950.9	E962.1	E980.9
paint	984.0	E861.5	—	E950.9	E962.1	E980.9
paint	984.0	E861.5	—	E950.9	E962.1	E980.9
salts	984.0	E866.0	—	E950.9	E962.1	E980.9
specified compound NEC	984.8	E866.0	—	E950.9	E962.1	E980.9
tetra-ethyl	984.1	E862.1	—	E950.9	E962.1	E980.9
Lebanese red	969.6	E854.1	E939.6	E950.3	E962.0	E980.3
Lente Iletin (insulin)	962.3	E858.0	E932.3	E950.4	E962.0	E980.4
Leptazol	970.0	E854.3	E940.0	E950.4	E962.0	E980.4
Leritine	965.09	E850.2	E935.2	E950.0	E962.0	E980.0
Letter	962.7	E858.0	E932.7	E950.4	E962.0	E980.4
Lettuce opium	967.8	E852.8	E937.8	E950.2	E962.0	E980.2
Leucovorin (factor)	964.1	E858.2	E934.1	E950.4	E962.0	E980.4
Leukeran	963.1	E858.1	E933.1	E950.4	E962.0	E980.4
Levalbuterol	975.7	E858.6	E945.7	E950.4	E962.0	E980.4

		External Cause (E-Code)				
	Poisoning	**Accident**	**Therapeutic Use**	**Suicide Attempt**	**Assault**	**Undetermined**
Levallorphan	970.1	E854.3	E940.1	E950.4	E962.0	E980.4
Levanil	967.8	E852.8	E937.8	E950.2	E962.0	E980.2
Levarterenol	971.2	E855.5	E941.2	E950.4	E962.0	E980.4
Levodopa	966.4	E855.0	E936.4	E950.4	E962.0	E980.4
Levo-dromoran	965.09	E850.2	E935.2	E950.0	E962.0	E980.0
Levoid	962.7	E858.0	E932.7	E950.4	E962.0	E980.4
Levo-iso-methadone	965.02	E850.1	E935.1	E950.0	E962.0	E980.0
Levomepromazine	967.8	E852.8	E937.8	E950.2	E962.0	E980.2
Levoprome	967.8	E852.8	E937.8	E950.2	E962.0	E980.2
Levopropoxyphene	975.4	E858.6	E945.4	E950.4	E962.0	E980.4
Levorphan, levophanol	965.09	E850.2	E935.2	E950.0	E962.0	E980.0
Levothyroxine (sodium)	962.7	E858.0	E932.7	E950.4	E962.0	E980.4
Levsin	971.1	E855.4	E941.1	E950.4	E962.0	E980.4
Levulose	974.5	E858.5	E944.5	E950.4	E962.0	E980.4
Lewisite (gas)	985.1	E866.3	—	E950.8	E962.1	E980.8
Librium	969.4	E853.2	E939.4	E950.3	E962.0	E980.3
Lidex	976.0	E858.7	E946.0	E950.4	E962.0	E980.4
Lidocaine (infiltration) (topical)	968.5	E855.2	E938.5	E950.4	E962.0	E980.4
nerve block (peripheral) (plexus)	968.6	E855.2	E938.6	E950.4	E962.0	E980.4
spinal	968.7	E855.2	E938.7	E950.4	E962.0	E980.4
Lighter fluid	981	E862.1	—	E950.9	E962.1	E980.9
Lignocaine (infiltration) (topical)	968.5	E855.2	E938.5	E950.4	E962.0	E980.4
nerve block (peripheral) (plexus)	968.6	E855.2	E938.6	E950.4	E962.0	E980.4
spinal	968.7	E855.2	E938.7	E950.4	E962.0	E980.4
Ligroin(e) (solvent)	981	E862.0	—	E950.9	E962.1	E980.9
vapor	987.1	E869.8	—	E952.8	E962.2	E982.8
Ligustrum vulgare	988.2	E865.3	—	E950.9	E962.1	E980.9
Lily of the valley	988.2	E865.4	—	E950.9	E962.1	E980.9
Lime (chloride)	983.2	E864.2	—	E950.7	E962.1	E980.6
solution, sulferated	976.4	E858.7	E946.4	E950.4	E962.0	E980.4
Limonene	982.8	E862.4	—	E950.9	E962.1	E980.9
Lincomycin	960.8	E856	E930.8	E950.4	E962.0	E980.4
Lindane (insecticide) (vapor)	989.2	E863.0	—	E950.6	E962.1	E980.7
anti-infective (topical)	976.0	E858.7	E946.0	E950.4	E962.0	E980.4
Liniments NEC	976.9	E858.7	E946.9	E950.4	E962.0	E980.4
Linoleic acid	972.2	E858.3	E942.2	E950.4	E962.0	E980.4
Liothyronine	962.7	E858.0	E932.7	E950.4	E962.0	E980.4
Liotrix	962.7	E858.0	E932.7	E950.4	E962.0	E980.4
Lipancreatin	973.4	E858.4	E943.4	E950.4	E962.0	E980.4
Lipo-Lutin	962.2	E858.0	E932.2	E950.4	E962.0	E980.4
Lipotropic agents	977.1	E858.8	E947.1	E950.4	E962.0	E980.4
Liquefied petroleum gases	987.0	E868.0	—	E951.1	E962.2	E981.1
piped (pure or mixed with air)	987.0	E867	—	E951.0	E962.2	E981.0
Liquid petrolatum	973.2	E858.4	E943.2	E950.4	E962.0	E980.4
substance	989.9	E866.9	—	E950.9	E962.1	E980.9
specified NEC	989.89	E866.8	—	E950.9	E962.1	E980.9
Lirugen	979.4	E858.8	E949.4	E950.4	E962.0	E980.4
Lithane	969.8	E855.8	E939.8	E950.3	E962.0	E980.3
Lithium	985.8	E866.4	—	E950.9	E962.1	E980.9
carbonate	969.8	E855.8	E939.8	E950.3	E962.0	E980.3
Lithonate	969.8	E855.8	E939.8	E950.3	E962.0	E980.3
Liver (extract) (injection) (preparations)	964.1	E858.2	E934.1	E950.4	E962.0	E980.4
Lizard (bite) (venom)	989.5	E905.0	—	E950.9	E962.1	E980.9
LMD	964.8	E858.2	E934.8	E950.4	E962.0	E980.4
Lobelia	988.2	E865.4	—	E950.9	E962.1	E980.9
Lobeline	970.0	E854.3	E940.0	E950.4	E962.0	E980.4
Locorten	976.0	E858.7	E946.0	E950.4	E962.0	E980.4
Lolium temulentum	988.2	E865.3	—	E950.9	E962.1	E980.9
Lomotil	973.5	E858.4	E943.5	E950.4	E962.0	E980.4
Lomustine	963.1	E858.1	E933.1	E950.4	E962.0	E980.4
Lophophora williamsii	969.6	E854.1	E939.6	E950.3	E962.0	E980.3
Lorazepam	969.4	E853.2	E939.4	E950.3	E962.0	E980.3
Lotions NEC	976.9	E858.7	E946.9	E950.4	E962.0	E980.4
Lotronex	973.8	E858.4	E943.8	E950.4	E962.0	E980.4
Lotusate	967.0	E851	E937.0	E950.1	E962.0	E980.1
Lowila	976.2	E858.7	E946.2	E950.4	E962.0	E980.4
Loxapine	969.3	E853.8	E939.3	E950.3	E962.0	E980.3
Lozenges (throat)	976.6	E858.7	E946.6	E950.4	E962.0	E980.4
LSD (25)	969.6	E854.1	E939.6	E950.3	E962.0	E980.3
L-Tryptophan — *see* amino acid						
Lubricating oil NEC	981	E862.2	—	E950.9	E962.1	E980.9
Lucanthone	961.6	E857	E931.6	E950.4	E962.0	E980.4
Luminal	967.0	E851	E937.0	E950.1	E962.0	E980.1
Lung irritant (gas) NEC	987.9	E869.9	—	E952.9	E962.2	E982.9
Lutocylol	962.2	E858.0	E932.2	E950.4	E962.0	E980.4
Lutromone	962.2	E858.0	E932.2	E950.4	E962.0	E980.4
Lututrin	975.0	E858.6	E945.0	E950.4	E962.0	E980.4
Lye (concentrated)	983.2	E864.2	—	E950.7	E962.1	E980.6
Lygranum (skin test)	977.8	E858.8	E947.8	E950.4	E962.0	E980.4
Lymecycline	960.4	E856	E930.4	E950.4	E962.0	E980.4
Lymphogranuloma venereum antigen	977.8	E858.8	E947.8	E950.4	E962.0	E980.4
Lynestrenol	962.2	E858.0	E932.2	E950.4	E962.0	E980.4
Lyovac Sodium Edecrin	974.4	E858.5	E944.4	E950.4	E962.0	E980.4
Lypressin	962.5	E858.0	E932.5	E950.4	E962.0	E980.4
Lysergic acid (amide) (diethylamide)	969.6	E854.1	E939.6	E950.3	E962.0	E980.3
Lysergide	969.6	E854.1	E939.6	E950.3	E962.0	E980.3
Lysine vasopressin	962.5	E858.0	E932.5	E950.4	E962.0	E980.4
Lysol	983.0	E864.0	—	E950.7	E962.1	E980.6
Lytta (vitatta)	976.8	E858.7	E946.8	E950.4	E962.0	E980.4
Mace	987.5	E869.3	—	E952.8	E962.2	E982.8
Macrolides (antibiotics)	960.3	E856	E930.3	E950.4	E962.0	E980.4
Mafenide	976.0	E858.7	E946.0	E950.4	E962.0	E980.4
Magaldrate	973.0	E858.4	E943.0	E950.4	E962.0	E980.4
Magic mushroom	969.6	E854.1	E939.6	E950.3	E962.0	E980.3
Magnamycin	960.8	E856	E930.8	E950.4	E962.0	E980.4
Magnesia magma	973.0	E858.4	E943.0	E950.4	E962.0	E980.4
Magnesium (compounds) (fumes) NEC	985.8	E866.4	—	E950.9	E962.1	E980.9
antacid	973.0	E858.4	E943.0	E950.4	E962.0	E980.4
carbonate	973.0	E858.4	E943.0	E950.4	E962.0	E980.4
cathartic	973.3	E858.4	E943.3	E950.4	E962.0	E980.4
citrate	973.3	E858.4	E943.3	E950.4	E962.0	E980.4
hydroxide	973.0	E858.4	E943.0	E950.4	E962.0	E980.4
oxide	973.0	E858.4	E943.0	E950.4	E962.0	E980.4
sulfate (oral)	973.3	E858.4	E943.3	E950.4	E962.0	E980.4
intravenous	966.3	E855.0	E936.3	E950.4	E962.0	E980.4
trisilicate	973.0	E858.4	E943.0	E950.4	E962.0	E980.4
Malathion (insecticide)	989.3	E863.1	—	E950.6	E962.1	E980.7
Male fern (oleoresin)	961.6	E857	E931.6	E950.4	E962.0	E980.4
Mandelic acid	961.9	E857	E931.9	E950.4	E962.0	E980.4
Manganese compounds (fumes) NEC	985.2	E866.4	—	E950.9	E962.1	E980.9
Mannitol (diuretic) (medicinal) NEC	974.4	E858.5	E944.4	E950.4	E962.0	E980.4
hexanitrate	972.4	E858.3	E942.4	E950.4	E962.0	E980.4
mustard	963.1	E858.1	E933.1	E950.4	E962.0	E980.4
Mannomustine	963.1	E858.1	E933.1	E950.4	E962.0	E980.4
MAO inhibitors	969.0	E854.0	E939.0	E950.3	E962.0	E980.3
Mapharsen	961.1	E857	E931.1	E950.4	E962.0	E980.4
Marcaine	968.9	E855.2	E938.9	E950.4	E962.0	E980.4
infiltration (subcutaneous)	968.5	E855.2	E938.5	E950.4	E962.0	E980.4
nerve block (peripheral) (plexus)	968.6	E855.2	E938.6	E950.4	E962.0	E980.4
Marezine	963.0	E858.1	E933.0	E950.4	E962.0	E980.4
Marihuana, marijuana (derivatives)	969.6	E854.1	E939.6	E950.3	E962.0	E980.3
Marine animals or plants (sting)	989.5	E905.6	—	E950.9	E962.1	E980.9
Marplan	969.0	E854.0	E939.0	E950.3	E962.0	E980.3
Marsh gas	987.1	E869.8	—	E952.8	E962.2	E982.8
Marsilid	969.0	E854.0	E939.0	E950.3	E962.0	E980.3
Matulane	963.1	E858.1	E933.1	E950.4	E962.0	E980.4
Mazindol	977.0	E858.8	E947.0	E950.4	E962.0	E980.4
MDMA	969.7	E854.2	E939.7	E950.3	E962.0	E980.3
Meadow saffron	988.2	E865.3	—	E950.9	E962.1	E980.9
Measles vaccine	979.4	E858.8	E949.4	E950.4	E962.0	E980.4
Meat, noxious or nonbacterial	988.8	E865.0	—	E950.9	E962.1	E980.9
Mebanazine	969.0	E854.0	E939.0	E950.3	E962.0	E980.3
Mebaral	967.0	E851	E937.0	E950.1	E962.0	E980.1
Mebendazole	961.6	E857	E931.6	E950.4	E962.0	E980.4
Mebeverine	975.1	E858.6	E945.1	E950.4	E962.0	E980.4
Mebhydroline	963.0	E858.1	E933.0	E950.4	E962.0	E980.4
Mebrophenhydramine	963.0	E858.1	E933.0	E950.4	E962.0	E980.4
Mebutamate	969.5	E853.8	E939.5	E950.3	E962.0	E980.3
Mecamylamine (chloride)	972.3	E858.3	E942.3	E950.4	E962.0	E980.4
Mechlorethamine hydrochloride	963.1	E858.1	E933.1	E950.4	E962.0	E980.4
Meclizene (hydrochloride)	963.0	E858.1	E933.0	E950.4	E962.0	E980.4
Meclofenoxate	970.0	E854.3	E940.0	E950.4	E962.0	E980.4
Meclozine (hydrochloride)	963.0	E858.1	E933.0	E950.4	E962.0	E980.4
Medazepam	969.4	E853.2	E939.4	E950.3	E962.0	E980.3

	Poisoning	External Cause (E-Code): Accident	Therapeutic Use	Suicide Attempt	Assault	Undetermined
Medicine, medicinal substance	977.9	E858.9	E947.9	E950.5	E962.0	E980.5
specified NEC	977.8	E858.8	E947.8	E950.4	E962.0	E980.4
Medinal	967.0	E851	E937.0	E950.1	E962.0	E980.1
Medomin	967.0	E851	E937.0	E950.1	E962.0	E980.1
Medroxyprogesterone	962.2	E858.0	E932.2	E950.4	E962.0	E980.4
Medrysone	976.5	E858.7	E946.5	E950.4	E962.0	E980.4
Mefenamic acid	965.7	E850.7	E935.7	E950.0	E962.0	E980.0
Megahallucinogen	969.6	E854.1	E939.6	E950.3	E962.0	E980.3
Megestrol	962.2	E858.0	E932.2	E950.4	E962.0	E980.4
Meglumine	977.8	E858.8	E947.8	E950.4	E962.0	E980.4
Meladinin	976.3	E858.7	E946.3	E950.4	E962.0	E980.4
Melanizing agents	976.3	E858.7	E946.3	E950.4	E962.0	E980.4
Melarsoprol	961.1	E857	E931.1	E950.4	E962.0	E980.4
Melia azedarach	988.2	E865.3	—	E950.9	E962.1	E980.9
Mellaril	969.1	E853.0	E939.1	E950.3	E962.0	E980.3
Meloxine	976.3	E858.7	E946.3	E950.4	E962.0	E980.4
Melphalan	963.1	E858.1	E933.1	E950.4	E962.0	E980.4
Menadiol sodium diphosphate	964.3	E858.2	E934.3	E950.4	E962.0	E980.4
Menadione (sodium bisulfite)	964.3	E858.2	E934.3	E950.4	E962.0	E980.4
Menaphthone	964.3	E858.2	E934.3	E950.4	E962.0	E980.4
Meningococcal vaccine	978.8	E858.8	E948.8	E950.4	E962.0	E980.4
Menningovax-C	978.8	E858.8	E948.8	E950.4	E962.0	E980.4
Menotropins	962.4	E858.0	E932.4	E950.4	E962.0	E980.4
Menthol NEC	976.1	E858.7	E946.1	E950.4	E962.0	E980.4
Mepacrine	961.3	E857	E931.3	E950.4	E962.0	E980.4
Meparfynol	967.8	E852.8	E937.8	E950.2	E962.0	E980.2
Mepazine	969.1	E853.0	E939.1	E950.3	E962.0	E980.3
Mepenzolate	971.1	E855.4	E941.1	E950.4	E962.0	E980.4
Meperidine	965.09	E850.2	E935.2	E950.0	E962.0	E980.0
Mephenamin(e)	966.4	E855.0	E936.4	E950.4	E962.0	E980.4
Mephenesin (carbamate)	968.0	E855.1	E938.0	E950.4	E962.0	E980.4
Mephenoxalone	969.5	E853.8	E939.5	E950.3	E962.0	E980.3
Mephentermine	971.2	E855.5	E941.2	E950.4	E962.0	E980.4
Mephenytoin	966.1	E855.0	E936.1	E950.4	E962.0	E980.4
Mephobarbital	967.0	E851	E937.0	E950.1	E962.0	E980.1
Mepiperphenidol	971.1	E855.4	E941.1	E950.4	E962.0	E980.4
Mepivacaine	968.9	E855.2	E938.9	E950.4	E962.0	E980.4
infiltration (subcutaneous)	968.5	E855.2	E938.5	E950.4	E962.0	E980.4
nerve block (peripheral) (plexus)	968.6	E855.2	E938.6	E950.4	E962.0	E980.4
topical (surface)	968.5	E855.2	E938.5	E950.4	E962.0	E980.4
Meprednisone	962.0	E858.0	E932.0	E950.4	E962.0	E980.4
Meprobam	969.5	E853.8	E939.5	E950.3	E962.0	E980.3
Meprobamate	969.5	E853.8	E939.5	E950.3	E962.0	E980.3
Mepyramine (maleate)	963.0	E858.1	E933.0	E950.4	E962.0	E980.4
Meralluride	974.0	E858.5	E944.0	E950.4	E962.0	E980.4
Merbaphen	974.0	E858.5	E944.0	E950.4	E962.0	E980.4
Merbromin	976.0	E858.7	E946.0	E950.4	E962.0	E980.4
Mercaptomerin	974.0	E858.5	E944.0	E950.4	E962.0	E980.4
Mercaptopurine	963.1	E858.1	E933.1	E950.4	E962.0	E980.4
Mercumatilin	974.0	E858.5	E944.0	E950.4	E962.0	E980.4
Mercuramide	974.0	E858.5	E944.0	E950.4	E962.0	E980.4
Mercuranin	976.0	E858.7	E946.0	E950.4	E962.0	E980.4
Mercurochrome	976.0	E858.7	E946.0	E950.4	E962.0	E980.4
Mercury, mercuric, mercurous (compounds) (cyanide) (fumes) (nonmedicinal) (vapor) NEC	985.0	E866.1	—	E950.9	E962.1	E980.9
ammoniated	976.0	E858.7	E946.0	E950.4	E962.0	E980.4
anti-infective	961.2	E857	E931.2	E950.4	E962.0	E980.4
topical	976.0	E858.7	E946.0	E950.4	E962.0	E980.4
chloride (antiseptic) NEC	976.0	E858.7	E946.0	E950.4	E962.0	E980.4
fungicide	985.0	E863.6	—	E950.6	E962.1	E980.7
diuretic compounds	974.0	E858.5	E944.0	E950.4	E962.0	E980.4
fungicide	985.0	E863.6	—	E950.6	E962.1	E980.7
organic (fungicide)	985.0	E863.6	—	E950.6	E962.1	E980.7
Merethoxylline	974.0	E858.5	E944.0	E950.4	E962.0	E980.4
Mersalyl	974.0	E858.5	E944.0	E950.4	E962.0	E980.4
Merthiolate (topical)	976.0	E858.7	E946.0	E950.4	E962.0	E980.4
ophthalmic preparation	976.5	E858.7	E946.5	E950.4	E962.0	E980.4
Meruvax	979.4	E858.8	E949.4	E950.4	E962.0	E980.4
Mescal buttons	969.6	E854.1	E939.6	E950.3	E962.0	E980.3
Mescaline (salts)	969.6	E854.1	E939.6	E950.3	E962.0	E980.3
Mesoridazine besylate	969.1	E853.0	E939.1	E950.3	E962.0	E980.3
Mestanolone	962.1	E858.0	E932.1	E950.4	E962.0	E980.4
Mestranol	962.2	E858.0	E932.2	E950.4	E962.0	E980.4
Metacresylacetate	976.0	E858.7	E946.0	E950.4	E962.0	E980.4
Metaldehyde (snail killer) NEC	989.4	E863.4	—	E950.6	E962.1	E980.7
Metals (heavy) (nonmedicinal) NEC	985.9	E866.4	—	E950.9	E962.1	E980.9
dust, fumes, or vapor NEC	985.9	E866.4	—	E950.9	E962.1	E980.9
light NEC	985.9	E866.4	—	E950.9	E962.1	E980.9
dust, fumes, or vapor NEC	985.9	E866.4	—	E950.9	E962.1	E980.9
pesticides (dust) (vapor)	985.9	E863.4	—	E950.6	E962.1	E980.7
Metamucil	973.3	E858.4	E943.3	E950.4	E962.0	E980.4
Metaphen	976.0	E858.7	E946.0	E950.4	E962.0	E980.4
Metaproterenol	975.1	E858.6	E945.1	E950.4	E962.0	E980.4
Metaraminol	972.8	E858.3	E942.8	E950.4	E962.0	E980.4
Metaxalone	968.0	E855.1	E938.0	E950.4	E962.0	E980.4
Metformin	962.3	E858.0	E932.3	E950.4	E962.0	E980.4
Methacycline	960.4	E856	E930.4	E950.4	E962.0	E980.4
Methadone	965.02	E850.1	E935.1	E950.0	E962.0	E980.0
Methallenestril	962.2	E858.0	E932.2	E950.4	E962.0	E980.4
Methamphetamine	969.7	E854.2	E939.7	E950.3	E962.0	E980.3
Methandienone	962.1	E858.0	E932.1	E950.4	E962.0	E980.4
Methandriol	962.1	E858.0	E932.1	E950.4	E962.0	E980.4
Methandrostenolone	962.1	E858.0	E932.1	E950.4	E962.0	E980.4
Methane gas	987.1	E869.8	—	E952.8	E962.2	E982.8
Methanol	980.1	E860.2	—	E950.9	E962.1	E980.9
vapor	987.8	E869.8	—	E952.8	E962.2	E982.8
Methantheline	971.1	E855.4	E941.1	E950.4	E962.0	E980.4
Methaphenilene	963.0	E858.1	E933.0	E950.4	E962.0	E980.4
Methapyrilene	963.0	E858.1	E933.0	E950.4	E962.0	E980.4
Methaqualone (compounds)	967.4	E852.3	E937.4	E950.2	E962.0	E980.2
Metharbital, metharbitone	967.0	E851	E937.0	E950.1	E962.0	E980.1
Methazolamide	974.2	E858.5	E944.2	E950.4	E962.0	E980.4
Methdilazine	963.0	E858.1	E933.0	E950.4	E962.0	E980.4
Methedrine	969.7	E854.2	E939.7	E950.3	E962.0	E980.3
Methenamine (mandelate)	961.9	E857	E931.9	E950.4	E962.0	E980.4
Methenolone	962.1	E858.0	E932.1	E950.4	E962.0	E980.4
Methergine	975.0	E858.6	E945.0	E950.4	E962.0	E980.4
Methiacil	962.8	E858.0	E932.8	E950.4	E962.0	E980.4
Methicillin (sodium)	960.0	E856	E930.0	E950.4	E962.0	E980.4
Methimazole	962.8	E858.0	E932.8	E950.4	E962.0	E980.4
Methionine	977.1	E858.8	E947.1	E950.4	E962.0	E980.4
Methisazone	961.7	E857	E931.7	E950.4	E962.0	E980.4
Methitural	967.0	E851	E937.0	E950.1	E962.0	E980.1
Methixene	971.1	E855.4	E941.1	E950.4	E962.0	E980.4
Methobarbital, methobarbitone	967.0	E851	E937.0	E950.1	E962.0	E980.1
Methocarbamol	968.0	E855.1	E938.0	E950.4	E962.0	E980.4
Methohexital, methohexitone (sodium)	968.3	E855.1	E938.3	E950.4	E962.0	E980.4
Methoin	966.1	E855.0	E936.1	E950.4	E962.0	E980.4
Methopholine	965.7	E850.7	E935.7	E950.0	E962.0	E980.0
Methorate	975.4	E858.6	E945.4	E950.4	E962.0	E980.4
Methoserpidine	972.6	E858.3	E942.6	E950.4	E962.0	E980.4
Methotrexate	963.1	E858.1	E933.1	E950.4	E962.0	E980.4
Methotrimeprazine	967.8	E852.8	E937.8	E950.2	E962.0	E980.2
Methoxa-Dome	976.3	E858.7	E946.3	E950.4	E962.0	E980.4
Methoxamine	971.2	E855.5	E941.2	E950.4	E962.0	E980.4
Methoxsalen	976.3	E858.7	E946.3	E950.4	E962.0	E980.4
Methoxybenzyl penicillin	960.0	E856	E930.0	E950.4	E962.0	E980.4
Methoxychlor	989.2	E863.0	—	E950.6	E962.1	E980.7
Methoxyflurane	968.2	E855.1	E938.2	E950.4	E962.0	E980.4
Methoxyphenamine	971.2	E855.5	E941.2	E950.4	E962.0	E980.4
Methoxypromazine	969.1	E853.0	E939.1	E950.3	E962.0	E980.3
Methoxypsoralen	976.3	E858.7	E946.3	E950.4	E962.0	E980.4
Methscopolamine (bromide)	971.1	E855.4	E941.1	E950.4	E962.0	E980.4
Methsuximide	966.2	E855.0	E936.2	E950.4	E962.0	E980.4
Methyclothiazide	974.3	E858.5	E944.3	E950.4	E962.0	E980.4
Methyl						
acetate	982.8	E862.4	—	E950.9	E962.1	E980.9
acetone	982.8	E862.4	—	E950.9	E962.1	E980.9
alcohol	980.1	E860.2	—	E950.9	E962.1	E980.9
amphetamine	969.7	E854.2	E939.7	E950.3	E962.0	E980.3
androstanolone	962.1	E858.0	E932.1	E950.4	E962.0	E980.4
atropine	971.1	E855.4	E941.1	E950.4	E962.0	E980.4
benzene	982.0	E862.4	—	E950.9	E962.1	E980.9
bromide (gas)	987.8	E869.8	—	E952.8	E962.2	E982.8
fumigant	987.8	E863.8	—	E950.6	E962.2	E980.7
butanol	980.8	E860.8	—	E950.9	E962.1	E980.9
carbinol	980.1	E860.2	—	E950.9	E962.1	E980.9
cellosolve	982.8	E862.4	—	E950.9	E962.1	E980.9
cellulose	973.3	E858.4	E943.3	E950.4	E962.0	E980.4
chloride (gas)	987.8	E869.8	—	E952.8	E962.2	E982.8

☑ Additional Digit Required — Refer to the Tabular List (Numeric Code Section) for Additional Digit Selection

▶◀ Revised Text ● New Line ▲ Revised Code

	Poisoning	External Cause (E-Code) Accident	Therapeutic Use	Suicide Attempt	Assault	Undetermined
Methyl — *continued*						
cyclohexane	982.8	E862.4	—	E950.9	E962.1	E980.9
cyclohexanone	982.8	E862.4	—	E950.9	E962.1	E980.9
dihydromorphinone	965.09	E850.2	E935.2	E950.0	E962.0	E980.0
ergometrine	975.0	E858.6	E945.0	E950.4	E962.0	E980.4
ergonovine	975.0	E858.6	E945.0	E950.4	E962.0	E980.4
ethyl ketone	982.8	E862.4	—	E950.9	E962.1	E980.9
hydrazine	983.9	E864.3	—	E950.7	E962.1	E980.6
isobutyl ketone	982.8	E862.4	—	E950.9	E962.1	E980.9
morphine NEC	965.09	E850.2	E935.2	E950.0	E962.0	E980.0
parafynol	967.8	E852.8	E937.8	E950.2	E962.0	E980.2
parathion	989.3	E863.1	—	E950.6	E962.1	E980.7
pentynol NEC	967.8	E852.8	E937.8	E950.2	E962.0	E980.2
peridol	969.2	E853.1	E939.2	E950.3	E962.0	E980.3
phenidate	969.7	E854.2	E939.7	E950.3	E962.0	E980.3
prednisolone	962.0	E858.0	E932.0	E950.4	E962.0	E980.4
ENT agent	976.6	E858.7	E946.6	E950.4	E962.0	E980.4
ophthalmic preparation	976.5	E858.7	E946.5	E950.4	E962.0	E980.4
topical NEC	976.0	E858.7	E946.0	E950.4	E962.0	E980.4
propylcarbinol	980.8	E860.8	—	E950.9	E962.1	E980.9
rosaniline NEC	976.0	E858.7	E946.0	E950.4	E962.0	E980.4
salicylate NEC	976.3	E858.7	E946.3	E950.4	E962.0	E980.4
sulfate (fumes)	987.8	E869.8	—	E952.8	E962.2	E982.8
liquid	983.9	E864.3	—	E950.7	E962.1	E980.6
sulfonal	967.8	E852.8	E937.8	E950.2	E962.0	E980.2
testosterone	962.1	E858.0	E932.1	E950.4	E962.0	E980.4
thiouracil	962.8	E858.0	E932.8	E950.4	E962.0	E980.4
Methylated spirit	980.0	E860.1	—	E950.9	E962.1	E980.9
Methyldopa	972.6	E858.3	E942.6	E950.4	E962.0	E980.4
Methylene						
blue	961.9	E857	E931.9	E950.4	E962.0	E980.4
chloride or dichloride (solvent) NEC	982.3	E862.4	—	E950.9	E962.1	E980.9
Methylhexabital	967.0	E851	E937.0	E950.1	E962.0	E980.1
Methylparaben (ophthalmic)	976.5	E858.7	E946.5	E950.4	E962.0	E980.4
Methyprylon	967.5	E852.4	E937.5	E950.2	E962.0	E980.2
Methysergide	971.3	E855.6	E941.3	E950.4	E962.0	E980.4
Metoclopramide	963.0	E858.1	E933.0	E950.4	E962.0	E980.4
Metofoline	965.7	E850.7	E935.7	E950.0	E962.0	E980.0
Metopon	965.09	E850.2	E935.2	E950.0	E962.0	E980.0
Metronidazole	961.5	E857	E931.5	E950.4	E962.0	E980.4
Metycaine	968.9	E855.2	E938.9	E950.4	E962.0	E980.4
infiltration (subcutaneous)	968.5	E855.2	E938.5	E950.4	E962.0	E980.4
nerve block (peripheral) (plexus)	968.6	E855.2	E938.6	E950.4	E962.0	E980.4
topical (surface)	968.5	E855.2	E938.5	E950.4	E962.0	E980.4
Metyrapone	977.8	E858.8	E947.8	E950.4	E962.0	E980.4
Mevinphos	989.3	E863.1	—	E950.6	E962.1	E980.7
Mezereon (berries)	988.2	E865.3	—	E950.9	E962.1	E980.9
Micatin	976.0	E858.7	E946.0	E950.4	E962.0	E980.4
Miconazole	976.0	E858.7	E946.0	E950.4	E962.0	E980.4
Midol	965.1	E850.3	E935.3	E950.0	E962.0	E980.0
Mifepristone	962.9	E858.0	E932.9	E950.4	E962.0	E980.4
Milk of magnesia	973.0	E858.4	E943.0	E950.4	E962.0	E980.4
Millipede (tropical) (venomous)	989.5	E905.4	—	E950.9	E962.1	E980.9
Miltown	969.5	E853.8	E939.5	E950.3	E962.0	E980.3
Mineral						
oil (medicinal)	973.2	E858.4	E943.2	E950.4	E962.0	E980.4
nonmedicinal	981	E862.1	—	E950.9	E962.1	E980.9
topical	976.3	E858.7	E946.3	E950.4	E962.0	E980.4
salts NEC	974.6	E858.5	E944.6	E950.4	E962.0	E980.4
spirits	981	E862.0	—	E950.9	E962.1	E980.9
Minocycline	960.4	E856	E930.4	E950.4	E962.0	E980.4
Mithramycin (antineoplastic)	960.7	E856	E930.7	E950.4	E962.0	E980.4
Mitobronitol	963.1	E858.1	E933.1	E950.4	E962.0	E980.4
Mitomycin (antineoplastic)	960.7	E856	E930.7	E950.4	E962.0	E980.4
Mitotane	963.1	E858.1	E933.1	E950.4	E962.0	E980.4
Moderil	972.6	E858.3	E942.6	E950.4	E962.0	E980.4
Mogadon — *see* Nitrazepam						
Molindone	969.3	E853.8	E939.3	E950.3	E962.0	E980.3
Monistat	976.0	E858.7	E946.0	E950.4	E962.0	E980.4
Monkshood	988.2	E865.4	—	E950.9	E962.1	E980.9
Monoamine oxidase inhibitors	969.0	E854.0	E939.0	E950.3	E962.0	E980.3
Monochlorobenzene	982.0	E862.4	—	E950.9	E962.1	E980.9
Monosodium glutamate	989.89	E866.8	—	E950.9	E962.1	E980.9
Monoxide, carbon — *see* Carbon, monoxide						
Moperone	969.2	E853.1	E939.2	E950.3	E962.0	E980.3
Morning glory seeds	969.6	E854.1	E939.6	E950.3	E962.0	E980.3

	Poisoning	External Cause (E-Code) Accident	Therapeutic Use	Suicide Attempt	Assault	Undetermined
Moroxydine (hydrochloride)	961.7	E857	E931.7	E950.4	E962.0	E980.4
Morphazinamide	961.8	E857	E931.8	E950.4	E962.0	E980.4
Morphinans	965.09	E850.2	E935.2	E950.0	E962.0	E980.0
Morphine NEC	965.09	E850.2	E935.2	E950.0	E962.0	E980.0
antagonists	970.1	E854.3	E940.1	E950.4	E962.0	E980.4
Morpholinylethylmorphine	965.09	E850.2	E935.2	E950.0	E962.0	E980.0
Morrhuate sodium	972.7	E858.3	E942.7	E950.4	E962.0	E980.4
Moth balls (*see also* Pesticides)	989.4	E863.4	—	E950.6	E962.1	E980.7
naphthalene	983.0	E863.4	—	E950.7	E962.1	E980.6
Motor exhaust gas — *see* Carbon, monoxide, exhaust gas						
Mouth wash	976.6	E858.7	E946.6	E950.4	E962.0	E980.4
Mucolytic agent	975.5	E858.6	E945.5	E950.4	E962.0	E980.4
Mucomyst	975.5	E858.6	E945.5	E950.4	E962.0	E980.4
Mucous membrane agents (external)	976.9	E858.7	E946.9	E950.4	E962.0	E980.4
specified NEC	976.8	E858.7	E946.8	E950.4	E962.0	E980.4
Mumps						
immune globulin (human)	964.6	E858.2	E934.6	E950.4	E962.0	E980.4
skin test antigen	977.8	E858.8	E947.8	E950.4	E962.0	E980.4
vaccine	979.6	E858.8	E949.6	E950.4	E962.0	E980.4
Mumpsvax	979.6	E858.8	E949.6	E950.4	E962.0	E980.4
Muriatic acid — *see* Hydrochloric acid						
Muscarine	971.0	E855.3	E941.0	E950.4	E962.0	E980.4
Muscle affecting agents NEC	975.3	E858.6	E945.3	E950.4	E962.0	E980.4
oxytocic	975.0	E858.6	E945.0	E950.4	E962.0	E980.4
relaxants	975.3	E858.6	E945.3	E950.4	E962.0	E980.4
central nervous system	968.0	E855.1	E938.0	E950.4	E962.0	E980.4
skeletal	975.2	E858.6	E945.2	E950.4	E962.0	E980.4
smooth	975.1	E858.6	E945.1	E950.4	E962.0	E980.4
Mushrooms, noxious	988.1	E865.5	—	E950.9	E962.1	E980.9
Mussel, noxious	988.0	E865.1	—	E950.9	E962.1	E980.9
Mustard (emetic)	973.6	E858.4	E943.6	E950.4	E962.0	E980.4
gas	987.8	E869.8	—	E952.8	E962.2	E982.8
nitrogen	963.1	E858.1	E933.1	E950.4	E962.0	E980.4
Mustine	963.1	E858.1	E933.1	E950.4	E962.0	E980.4
M-vac	979.4	E858.8	E949.4	E950.4	E962.0	E980.4
Mycifradin	960.8	E856	E930.8	E950.4	E962.0	E980.4
topical	976.0	E858.7	E946.0	E950.4	E962.0	E980.4
Mycitracin	960.8	E856	E930.8	E950.4	E962.0	E980.4
ophthalmic preparation	976.5	E858.7	E946.5	E950.4	E962.0	E980.4
Mycostatin	960.1	E856	E930.1	E950.4	E962.0	E980.4
topical	976.0	E858.7	E946.0	E950.4	E962.0	E980.4
Mydriacyl	971.1	E855.4	E941.1	E950.4	E962.0	E980.4
Myelobromal	963.1	E858.1	E933.1	E950.4	E962.0	E980.4
Myleran	963.1	E858.1	E933.1	E950.4	E962.0	E980.4
Myochrysin(e)	965.69	E850.6	E935.6	E950.0	E962.0	E980.0
Myoneural blocking agents	975.2	E858.6	E945.2	E950.4	E962.0	E980.4
Myristica fragrans	988.2	E865.3	—	E950.9	E962.1	E980.9
Myristicin	988.2	E865.3	—	E950.9	E962.1	E980.9
Mysoline	966.3	E855.0	E936.3	E950.4	E962.0	E980.4
Nafcillin (sodium)	960.0	E856	E930.0	E950.4	E962.0	E980.4
Nail polish remover	982.8	E862.4	—	E950.9	E962.1	E908.9
Nalidixic acid	961.9	E857	E931.9	E950.4	E962.0	E980.4
Nalorphine	970.1	E854.3	E940.1	E950.4	E962.0	E980.4
Naloxone	970.1	E854.3	E940.1	E950.4	E962.0	E980.4
Nandrolone (decanoate) (phenproprioate)	962.1	E858.0	E932.1	E950.4	E962.0	E980.4
Naphazoline	971.2	E855.5	E941.2	E950.4	E962.0	E980.4
Naphtha (painter's) (petroleum)	981	E862.0	—	E950.9	E962.1	E980.9
solvent	981	E862.0	—	E950.9	E962.1	E980.9
vapor	987.1	E869.8	—	E952.8	E962.2	E982.8
Naphthalene (chlorinated)	983.0	E864.0	—	E950.7	E962.1	E980.6
insecticide or moth repellent	983.0	E863.4	—	E950.7	E962.1	E980.6
vapor	987.8	E869.8	—	E952.8	E962.2	E982.8
Naphthol	983.0	E864.0	—	E950.7	E962.1	E980.6
Naphthylamine	983.0	E864.0	—	E950.7	E962.1	E980.6
Naprosyn — *see* Naproxen						
Naproxen	965.61	E850.6	E935.6	E950.0	E962.0	E980.0
Narcotic (drug)	967.9	E852.9	E937.9	E950.2	E962.0	E980.2
analgesic NEC	965.8	E850.8	E935.8	E950.0	E962.0	E980.0
antagonist	970.1	E854.3	E940.1	E950.4	E962.0	E980.4
specified NEC	967.8	E852.8	E937.8	E950.2	E962.0	E980.2
Narcotine	975.4	E858.6	E945.4	E950.4	E962.0	E980.4
Nardil	969.0	E854.0	E939.0	E950.3	E962.0	E980.3

☑ Additional Digit Required — Refer to the Tabular List (Numeric Code Section) for Additional Digit Selection

▶◀ Revised Text ● New Line ▲ Revised Code

		External Cause (E-Code)				
	Poisoning	Accident	Therapeutic Use	Suicide Attempt	Assault	Undeter-mined
Natrium cyanide — *see* Cyanide(s)						
Natural						
blood (product)	964.7	E858.2	E934.7	E950.4	E962.0	E980.4
gas (piped)	987.1	E867	—	E951.0	E962.2	E981.0
incomplete combustion	986	E867	—	E951.0	E962.2	E981.0
Nealbarbital, nealbarbitone	967.0	E851	E937.0	E950.1	E962.0	E980.1
Nectadon	975.4	E858.6	E945.4	E950.4	E962.0	E980.4
Nematocyst (sting)	989.5	E905.6	—	E950.9	E962.1	E980.9
Nembutal	967.0	E851	E937.0	E950.1	E962.0	E980.1
Neoarsphenamine	961.1	E857	E931.1	E950.4	E962.0	E980.4
Neocinchophen	974.7	E858.5	E944.7	E950.4	E962.0	E980.4
Neomycin	960.8	E856	E930.8	E950.4	E962.0	E980.4
ENT agent	976.6	E858.7	E946.6	E950.4	E962.0	E980.4
ophthalmic preparation	976.5	E858.7	E946.5	E950.4	E962.0	E980.4
topical NEC	976.0	E858.7	E946.0	E950.4	E962.0	E980.4
Neonal	967.0	E851	E937.0	E950.1	E962.0	E980.1
Neoprontosil	961.0	E857	E931.0	E950.4	E962.0	E980.4
Neosalvarsan	961.1	E857	E931.1	E950.4	E962.0	E980.4
Neosilversalvarsan	961.1	E857	E931.1	E950.4	E962.0	E980.4
Neosporin	960.8	E856	E930.8	E950.4	E962.0	E980.4
ENT agent	976.6	E858.7	E946.6	E950.4	E962.0	E980.4
opthalmic preparation	976.5	E858.7	E946.5	E950.4	E962.0	E980.4
topical NEC	976.0	E858.7	E946.0	E950.4	E962.0	E980.4
Neostigmine	971.0	E855.3	E941.0	E950.4	E962.0	E980.4
Neraval	967.0	E851	E937.0	E950.1	E962.0	E980.1
Neravan	967.0	E851	E937.0	E950.1	E962.0	E980.1
Nerium oleander	988.2	E865.4	—	E950.9	E962.1	E980.9
Nerve gases (war)	987.9	E869.9	—	E952.9	E962.2	E982.9
Nesacaine	968.9	E855.2	E938.9	E950.4	E962.0	E980.4
infiltration (subcutaneous)	968.5	E855.2	E938.5	E950.4	E962.0	E980.4
nerve block (peripheral) (plexus)	968.6	E855.2	E938.6	E950.4	E962.0	E980.4
Neurobarb	967.0	E851	E937.0	E950.1	E962.0	E980.1
Neuroleptics NEC	969.3	E853.8	E939.3	E950.3	E962.0	E980.3
Neuroprotective agent	977.8	E858.8	E947.8	E950.4	E962.0	E980.4
Neutral spirits	980.0	E860.1	—	E950.9	E962.1	E980.9
beverage	980.0	E860.0	—	E950.9	E962.1	E980.9
Niacin, niacinamide	972.2	E858.3	E942.2	E950.4	E962.0	E980.4
Nialamide	969.0	E854.0	E939.0	E950.3	E962.0	E980.3
Nickle (carbonyl) (compounds) (fumes) (tetracarbonyl) (vapor)	985.8	E866.4	—	E950.9	E962.1	E980.9
Niclosamide	961.6	E857	E931.6	E950.4	E962.0	E980.4
Nicomorphine	965.09	E850.2	E935.2	E950.0	E962.0	E980.0
Nicotinamide	972.2	E858.3	E942.2	E950.4	E962.0	E980.4
Nicotine (insecticide) (spray) (sulfate) NEC	989.4	E863.4	—	E950.6	E962.1	E980.7
not insecticide	989.89	E866.8	—	E950.9	E962.1	E980.9
Nicotinic acid (derivatives)	972.2	E858.3	E942.2	E950.4	E962.0	E980.4
Nicotinyl alcohol	972.2	E858.3	E942.2	E950.4	E962.0	E980.4
Nicoumalone	964.2	E858.2	E934.2	E950.4	E962.0	E980.4
Nifenazone	965.5	E850.5	E935.5	E950.0	E962.0	E980.0
Nifuraldezone	961.9	E857	E931.9	E950.4	E962.0	E980.4
Nightshade (deadly)	988.2	E865.4	—	E950.9	E962.1	E980.9
Nikethamide	970.0	E854.3	E940.0	E950.4	E962.0	E980.4
Nilstat	960.1	E856	E930.1	E950.4	E962.0	E980.4
topical	976.0	E858.7	E946.0	E950.4	E962.0	E980.4
Nimodipine	977.8	E858.8	E947.8	E950.4	E962.0	E980.4
Niridazole	961.6	E857	E931.6	E950.4	E962.0	E980.4
Nisentil	965.09	E850.2	E935.2	E950.0	E962.0	E980.0
Nitrates	972.4	E858.3	E942.4	E950.4	E962.0	E980.4
Nitrazepam	969.4	E853.2	E939.4	E950.3	E962.0	E980.3
Nitric						
acid (liquid)	983.1	E864.1	—	E950.7	E962.1	E980.6
vapor	987.8	E869.8	—	E952.8	E962.2	E982.8
oxide (gas)	987.2	E869.0	—	E952.8	E962.2	E982.8
Nitrite, amyl (medicinal) (vapor)	972.4	E858.3	E942.4	E950.4	E962.0	E980.4
Nitroaniline	983.0	E864.0	—	E950.7	E962.1	E980.6
vapor	987.8	E869.8	—	E952.8	E962.2	E982.8
Nitrobenzene, nitrobenzol	983.0	E864.0	—	E950.7	E962.1	E980.6
vapor	987.8	E869.8	—	E952.8	E962.2	E982.8
Nitrocellulose	976.3	E858.7	E946.3	E950.4	E962.0	E980.4
Nitrofuran derivatives	961.9	E857	E931.9	E950.4	E962.0	E980.4
Nitrofurantoin	961.9	E857	E931.9	E950.4	E962.0	E980.4
Nitrofurazone	976.0	E858.7	E946.0	E950.4	E962.0	E980.4
Nitrogen (dioxide) (gas) (oxide)	987.2	E869.0	—	E952.8	E962.2	E982.8
mustard (antineoplastic)	963.1	E858.1	E933.1	E950.4	E962.0	E980.4
Nitroglycerin, nitroglycerol (medicinal)	972.4	E858.3	E942.4	E950.4	E962.0	E980.4
nonmedicinal	989.89	E866.8	—	E950.9	E962.1	E980.9
fumes	987.8	E869.8	—	E952.8	E962.2	E982.8
Nitrohydrochloric acid	983.1	E864.1	—	E950.7	E962.1	E980.6
Nitromersol	976.0	E858.7	E946.0	E950.4	E962.0	E980.4
Nitronaphthalene	983.0	E864.0	—	E950.7	E962.2	E980.6
Nitrophenol	983.0	E864.0	—	E950.7	E962.2	E980.6
Nitrothiazol	961.6	E857	E931.6	E950.4	E962.0	E980.4
Nitrotoluene, nitrotoluol	983.0	E864.0	—	E950.7	E962.1	E980.6
vapor	987.8	E869.8	—	E952.8	E962.2	E982.8
Nitrous	968.2	E855.1	E938.2	E950.4	E962.0	E980.4
acid (liquid)	983.1	E864.1	—	E950.7	E962.1	E980.6
fumes	987.2	E869.0	—	E952.8	E962.2	E982.8
oxide (anesthetic) NEC	968.2	E855.1	E938.2	E950.4	E962.0	E980.4
Nitrozone	976.0	E858.7	E946.0	E950.4	E962.0	E980.4
Noctec	967.1	E852.0	E937.1	E950.2	E962.0	E980.2
Noludar	967.5	E852.4	E937.5	E950.2	E962.0	E980.2
Noptil	967.0	E851	E937.0	E950.1	E962.0	E980.1
Noradrenalin	971.2	E855.5	E941.2	E950.4	E962.0	E980.4
Noramidopyrine	965.5	E850.5	E935.5	E950.0	E962.0	E980.0
Norepinephrine	971.2	E855.5	E941.2	E950.4	E962.0	E980.4
Norethandrolone	962.1	E858.0	E932.1	E950.4	E962.0	E980.4
Norethindrone	962.2	E858.0	E932.2	E950.4	E962.0	E980.4
Norethisterone	962.2	E858.0	E932.2	E950.4	E962.0	E980.4
Norethynodrel	962.2	E858.0	E932.2	E950.4	E962.0	E980.4
Norlestrin	962.2	E858.0	E932.2	E950.4	E962.0	E980.4
Norlutin	962.2	E858.0	E932.2	E950.4	E962.0	E980.4
Normison — *see* Benzodiazepines						
Normorphine	965.09	E850.2	E935.2	E950.0	E962.0	E980.0
Nortriptyline	969.0	E854.0	E939.0	E950.3	E962.0	E980.3
Noscapine	975.4	E858.6	E945.4	E950.4	E962.0	E980.4
Nose preparations	976.6	E858.7	E946.6	E950.4	E962.0	E980.4
Novobiocin	960.8	E856	E930.8	E950.4	E962.0	E980.4
Novocain (infiltration) (topical)	968.5	E855.2	E938.5	E950.4	E962.0	E980.4
nerve block (peripheral) (plexus)	968.6	E855.2	E938.6	E950.4	E962.0	E980.4
spinal	968.7	E855.2	E938.7	E950.4	E962.0	E980.4
Noxythiolin	961.9	E857	E931.9	E950.4	E962.0	E980.4
NPH Iletin (insulin)	962.3	E858.0	E932.3	E950.4	E962.0	E980.4
Numorphan	965.09	E850.2	E935.2	E950.0	E962.0	E980.0
Nunol	967.0	E851	E937.0	E950.1	E962.0	E980.1
Nupercaine (spinal anesthetic)	968.7	E855.2	E938.7	E950.4	E962.0	E980.4
topical (surface)	968.5	E855.2	E938.5	E950.4	E962.0	E980.4
Nutmeg oil (liniment)	976.3	E858.7	E946.3	E950.4	E962.0	E980.4
Nux vomica	989.1	E863.7	—	E950.6	E962.1	E980.7
Nydrazid	961.8	E857	E931.8	E950.4	E962.0	E980.4
Nylidrin	971.2	E855.5	E941.2	E950.4	E962.0	E980.4
Nystatin	960.1	E856	E930.1	E950.4	E962.0	E980.4
topical	976.0	E858.7	E946.0	E950.4	E962.0	E980.4
Nytol	963.0	E858.1	E933.0	E950.4	E962.0	E980.4
Oblivion	967.8	E852.8	E937.8	E950.2	E962.0	E980.2
Octyl nitrite	972.4	E858.3	E942.4	E950.4	E962.0	E980.4
Oestradiol (cypionate) (dipropionate) (valerate)	962.2	E858.0	E932.2	E950.4	E962.0	E980.4
Oestriol	962.2	E858.0	E932.2	E950.4	E962.0	E980.4
Oestrone	962.2	E858.0	E932.2	E950.4	E962.0	E980.4
Oil (of) NEC	989.89	E866.8	—	E950.9	E962.1	E980.9
bitter almond	989.0	E866.8	—	E950.9	E962.1	E980.9
camphor	976.1	E858.7	E946.1	E950.4	E962.0	E980.4
colors	989.89	E861.6	—	E950.9	E962.1	E980.9
fumes	987.8	E869.8	—	E952.8	E962.2	E982.8
lubricating	981	E862.2	—	E950.9	E962.1	E980.9
specified source, other — *see* substance specified						
vitriol (liquid)	983.1	E864.1	—	E950.7	E962.1	E980.6
fumes	987.8	E869.8	—	E952.8	E962.2	E982.8
wintergreen (bitter) NEC	976.3	E858.7	E946.3	E950.4	E962.0	E980.4
Ointments NEC	976.9	E858.7	E946.9	E950.4	E962.0	E980.4
Oleander	988.2	E865.4	—	E950.9	E962.1	E980.9
Oleandomycin	960.3	E856	E930.3	E950.4	E962.0	E980.4
Oleovitamin A	963.5	E858.1	E933.5	E950.4	E962.0	E980.4
Oleum ricini	973.1	E858.4	E943.1	E950.4	E962.0	E980.4
Olive oil (medicinal) NEC	973.2	E858.4	E943.2	E950.4	E962.0	E980.4
OMPA	989.3	E863.1	—	E950.6	E962.1	E980.7

☑ Additional Digit Required — Refer to the Tabular List (Numeric Code Section) for Additional Digit Selection

▶◀ Revised Text ● New Line ▲ Revised Code

		External Cause (E-Code)				
	Poisoning	Accident	Therapeutic Use	Suicide Attempt	Assault	Undetermined
Oncovin	963.1	E858.1	E933.1	E950.4	E962.0	E980.4
Ophthaine	968.5	E855.2	E938.5	E950.4	E962.0	E980.4
Ophthetic	968.5	E855.2	E938.5	E950.4	E962.0	E980.4
Opiates, opioids, opium NEC	965.00	E850.2	E935.2	E950.0	E962.0	E980.0
antagonists	970.1	E854.3	E940.1	E950.4	E962.0	E980.4
Oracon	962.2	E858.0	E932.2	E950.4	E962.0	E980.4
Oragrafin	977.8	E858.8	E947.8	E950.4	E962.0	E980.4
Oral contraceptives	962.2	E858.0	E932.2	E950.4	E962.0	E980.4
Orciprenaline	975.1	E858.6	E945.1	E950.4	E962.0	E980.4
Organidin	975.5	E858.6	E945.5	E950.4	E962.0	E980.4
Organophosphates	989.3	E863.1	—	E950.6	E962.1	E980.7
Orimune	979.5	E858.8	E949.5	E950.4	E962.0	E980.4
Orinase	962.3	E858.0	E932.3	E950.4	E962.0	E980.4
Orphenadrine	966.4	E855.0	E936.4	E950.4	E962.0	E980.4
Ortal (sodium)	967.0	E851	E937.0	E950.1	E962.0	E980.1
Orthoboric acid	976.0	E858.7	E946.0	E950.4	E962.0	E980.4
ENT agent	976.6	E858.7	E946.6	E950.4	E962.0	E980.4
ophthalmic preparation	976.5	E858.7	E946.5	E950.4	E962.0	E980.4
Orthocaine	968.5	E855.2	E938.5	E950.4	E962.0	E980.4
Ortho-Novum	962.2	E858.0	E932.2	E950.4	E962.0	E980.4
Orthotolidine (reagent)	977.8	E858.8	E947.8	E950.4	E962.0	E980.4
Osmic acid (liquid)	983.1	E864.1	—	E950.7	E962.1	E980.6
fumes	987.8	E869.8	—	E952.8	E962.2	E982.8
Osmotic diuretics	974.4	E858.5	E944.4	E950.4	E962.0	E980.4
Ouabain	972.1	E858.3	E942.1	E950.4	E962.0	E980.4
Ovarian hormones (synthetic substitutes)	962.2	E858.0	E932.2	E950.4	E962.0	E980.4
Ovral	962.2	E858.0	E932.2	E950.4	E962.0	E980.4
Ovulation suppressants	962.2	E858.0	E932.2	E950.4	E962.0	E980.4
Ovulen	962.2	E858.0	E932.2	E950.4	E962.0	E980.4
Oxacillin (sodium)	960.0	E856	E930.0	E950.4	E962.0	E980.4
Oxalic acid	983.1	E864.1	—	E950.7	E962.1	E980.6
Oxanamide	969.5	E853.8	E939.5	E950.3	E962.0	E980.3
Oxandrolone	962.1	E858.0	E932.1	E950.4	E962.0	E980.4
Oxaprozin	965.61	E850.6	E935.6	E950.0	E962.0	E980.0
Oxazepam	969.4	E853.2	E939.4	E950.3	E962.0	E980.3
Oxazolidine derivatives	966.0	E855.0	E936.0	E950.4	E962.0	E980.4
Ox bile extract	973.4	E858.4	E943.4	E950.4	E962.0	E980.4
Oxedrine	971.2	E855.5	E941.2	E950.4	E962.0	E980.4
Oxeladin	975.4	E858.6	E945.4	E950.4	E962.0	E980.4
Oxethazaine NEC	968.5	E855.2	E938.5	E950.4	E962.0	E980.4
Oxidizing agents NEC	983.9	E864.3	—	E950.7	E962.1	E980.6
Oxolinic acid	961.3	E857	E931.3	E950.4	E962.0	E980.4
Oxophenarsine	961.1	E857	E931.1	E950.4	E962.0	E980.4
Oxsoralen	976.3	E858.7	E946.3	E950.4	E962.0	E980.4
Oxtriphylline	975.7	E858.6	E945.7	E950.4	E962.0	E980.4
Oxybuprocaine	968.5	E855.2	E938.5	E950.4	E962.0	E980.4
Oxybutynin	975.1	E858.6	E945.1	E950.4	E962.0	E980.4
Oxycodone	965.09	E850.2	E935.2	E950.0	E962.0	E980.0
Oxygen	987.8	E869.8	—	E952.8	E962.2	E982.8
Oxylone	976.0	E858.7	E946.0	E950.4	E962.0	E980.4
ophthalmic preparation	976.5	E858.7	E946.5	E950.4	E962.0	E980.4
Oxymesterone	962.1	E858.0	E932.1	E950.4	E962.0	E980.4
Oxymetazoline	971.2	E855.5	E941.2	E950.4	E962.0	E980.4
Oxymetholone	962.1	E858.0	E932.1	E950.4	E962.0	E980.4
Oxymorphone	965.09	E850.2	E935.2	E950.0	E962.0	E980.0
Oxypertine	969.0	E854.0	E939.0	E950.3	E962.0	E980.3
Oxyphenbutazone	965.5	E850.5	E935.5	E950.0	E962.0	E980.0
Oxyphencyclimine	971.1	E855.4	E941.1	E950.4	E962.0	E980.4
Oxyphenisatin	973.1	E858.4	E943.1	E950.4	E962.0	E980.4
Oxyphenonium	971.1	E855.4	E941.1	E950.4	E962.0	E980.4
Oxyquinoline	961.3	E857	E931.3	E950.4	E962.0	E980.4
Oxytetracycline	960.4	E856	E930.4	E950.4	E962.0	E980.4
Oxytocics	975.0	E858.6	E945.0	E950.4	E962.0	E980.4
Oxytocin	975.0	E858.6	E945.0	E950.4	E962.0	E980.4
Ozone	987.8	E869.8	—	E952.8	E962.2	E982.8
PABA	976.3	E858.7	E946.3	E950.4	E962.0	E980.4
Packed red cells	964.7	E858.2	E934.7	E950.4	E962.0	E980.4
Paint NEC	989.89	E861.6	—	E950.9	E962.1	E980.9
cleaner	982.8	E862.9	—	E950.9	E962.1	E980.9
fumes NEC	987.8	E869.8	—	E952.8	E962.1	E982.8
lead (fumes)	984.0	E861.5	—	E950.9	E962.1	E980.9
solvent NEC	982.8	E862.9	—	E950.9	E962.1	E980.9
stripper	982.8	E862.9	—	E950.9	E962.1	E980.9
Palfium	965.09	E850.2	E935.2	E950.0	E962.0	E980.0
Palivizumab	979.9	E858.8	E949.6	E950.4	E962.0	E980.4
Paludrine	961.4	E857	E931.4	E950.4	E962.0	E980.4
PAM	977.2	E855.8	E947.2	E950.4	E962.0	E980.4
Pamaquine (naphthoate)	961.4	E857	E931.4	E950.4	E962.0	E980.4
Pamprin	965.1	E850.3	E935.3	E950.0	E962.0	E980.0
Panadol	965.4	E850.4	E935.4	E950.0	E962.0	E980.0
Pancreatic dornase (mucolytic)	963.4	E858.1	E933.4	E950.4	E962.0	E980.4
Pancreatin	973.4	E858.4	E943.4	E950.4	E962.0	E980.4
Pancrelipase	973.4	E858.4	E943.4	E950.4	E962.0	E980.4
Pangamic acid	963.5	E858.1	E933.5	E950.4	E962.0	E980.4
Panthenol	963.5	E858.1	E933.5	E950.4	E962.0	E980.4
topical	976.8	E858.7	E946.8	E950.4	E962.0	E980.4
Pantopaque	977.8	E858.8	E947.8	E950.4	E962.0	E980.4
Pantopon	965.00	E850.2	E935.2	E950.0	E962.0	E980.0
Pantothenic acid	963.5	E858.1	E933.5	E950.4	E962.0	E980.4
Panwarfin	964.2	E858.2	E934.2	E950.4	E962.0	E980.4
Papain	973.4	E858.4	E943.4	E950.4	E962.0	E980.4
Papaverine	972.5	E858.3	E942.5	E950.4	E962.0	E980.4
Para-aminobenzoic acid	976.3	E858.7	E946.3	E950.4	E962.0	E980.4
Para-aminophenol derivatives	965.4	E850.4	E935.4	E950.0	E962.0	E980.0
Para-aminosalicylic acid (derivatives)	961.8	E857	E931.8	E950.4	E962.0	E980.4
Paracetaldehyde (medicinal)	967.2	E852.1	E937.2	E950.2	E962.0	E980.2
Paracetamol	965.4	E850.4	E935.4	E950.0	E962.0	E980.0
Paracodin	965.09	E850.2	E935.2	E950.0	E962.0	E980.0
Paradione	966.0	E855.0	E936.0	E950.4	E962.0	E980.4
Paraffin(s) (wax)	981	E862.3	—	E950.9	E962.1	E980.9
liquid (medicinal)	973.2	E858.4	E943.2	E950.4	E962.0	E980.4
nonmedicinal (oil)	981	E962.1	—	E950.9	E962.1	E980.9
Paraldehyde (medicinal)	967.2	E852.1	E937.2	E950.2	E962.0	E980.2
Paramethadione	966.0	E855.0	E936.0	E950.4	E962.0	E980.4
Paramethasone	962.0	E858.0	E932.0	E950.4	E962.0	E980.4
Paraquat	989.4	E863.5	—	E950.6	E962.1	E980.7
Parasympatholytics	971.1	E855.4	E941.1	E950.4	E962.0	E980.4
Parasympathomimetics	971.0	E855.3	E941.0	E950.4	E962.0	E980.4
Parathion	989.3	E863.1	—	E950.6	E962.1	E980.7
Parathormone	962.6	E858.0	E932.6	E950.4	E962.0	E980.4
Parathyroid (derivatives)	962.6	E858.0	E932.6	E950.4	E962.0	E980.4
Paratyphoid vaccine	978.1	E858.8	E948.1	E950.4	E962.0	E980.4
Paredrine	971.2	E855.5	E941.2	E950.4	E962.0	E980.4
Paregoric	965.00	E850.2	E935.2	E950.0	E962.0	E980.0
Pargyline	972.3	E858.3	E942.3	E950.4	E962.0	E980.4
Paris green	985.1	E866.3	—	E950.8	E962.1	E980.8
insecticide	985.1	E863.4	—	E950.8	E962.1	E980.8
Parnate	969.0	E854.0	E939.0	E950.3	E962.0	E980.3
Paromomycin	960.8	E856	E930.8	E950.4	E962.0	E980.4
Paroxypropione	963.1	E858.1	E933.1	E950.4	E962.0	E980.4
Parzone	965.09	E850.2	E935.2	E950.0	E962.0	E980.0
PAS	961.8	E857	E931.8	E950.4	E962.0	E980.4
PCBs	981	E862.3	—	E950.9	E962.1	E980.9
PCP (pentachlorophenol)	989.4	E863.6	—	E950.6	E962.1	E980.7
herbicide	989.4	E863.5	—	E950.6	E962.1	E980.7
insecticide	989.4	E863.4	—	E950.6	E962.1	E980.7
phencyclidine	968.3	E855.1	E938.3	E950.4	E962.0	E980.4
Peach kernel oil (emulsion)	973.2	E858.4	E943.2	E950.4	E962.0	E980.4
Peanut oil (emulsion) NEC	973.2	E858.4	E943.2	E950.4	E962.0	E980.4
topical	976.3	E858.7	E946.3	E950.4	E962.0	E980.4
Pearly Gates (morning glory seeds)	969.6	E854.1	E939.6	E950.3	E962.0	E980.3
Pecazine	969.1	E853.0	E939.1	E950.3	E962.0	E980.3
Pecilocin	960.1	E856	E930.1	E950.4	E962.0	E980.4
Pectin (with kaolin) NEC	973.5	E858.4	E943.5	E950.4	E962.0	E980.4
Pelletierine tannate	961.6	E857	E931.6	E950.4	E962.0	E980.4
Pemoline	969.7	E854.2	E939.7	E950.3	E962.0	E980.3
Pempidine	972.3	E858.3	E942.3	E950.4	E962.0	E980.4
Penamecillin	960.0	E856	E930.0	E950.4	E962.0	E980.4
Penethamate hydriodide	960.0	E856	E930.0	E950.4	E962.0	E980.4
Penicillamine	963.8	E858.1	E933.8	E950.4	E962.0	E980.4
Penicillin (any type)	960.0	E856	E930.0	E950.4	E962.0	E980.4
Penicillinase	963.4	E858.1	E933.4	E950.4	E962.0	E980.4
Pentachlorophenol (fungicide)	989.4	E863.6	—	E950.6	E962.1	E980.7
herbicide	989.4	E863.5	—	E950.6	E962.1	E980.7
insecticide	989.4	E863.4	—	E950.6	E962.1	E980.7
Pentaerythritol	972.4	E858.3	E942.4	E950.4	E962.0	E980.4
chloral	967.1	E852.0	E937.1	E950.2	E962.0	E980.2
tetranitrate NEC	972.4	E858.3	E942.4	E950.4	E962.0	E980.4
Pentagastrin	977.8	E858.8	E947.8	E950.4	E962.0	E980.4
Pentalin	982.3	E862.4	—	E950.9	E962.1	E980.9
Pentamethonium (bromide)	972.3	E858.3	E942.3	E950.4	E962.0	E980.4
Pentamidine	961.5	E857	E931.5	E950.4	E962.0	E980.4
Pentanol	980.8	E860.8	—	E950.9	E962.1	E980.9
Pentaquine	961.4	E857	E931.4	E950.4	E962.0	E980.4
Pentazocine	965.8	E850.8	E935.8	E950.0	E962.0	E980.0

☑ Additional Digit Required — Refer to the Tabular List (Numeric Code Section) for Additional Digit Selection

▶◀ Revised Text ● New Line ▲ Revised Code

	Poisoning	External Cause (E-Code)				
		Accident	Therapeutic Use	Suicide Attempt	Assault	Undetermined
Penthienate	971.1	E855.4	E941.1	E950.4	E962.0	E980.4
Pentobarbital, pentobarbitone (sodium)	967.0	E851	E937.0	E950.1	E962.0	E980.1
Pentolinium (tartrate)	972.3	E858.3	E942.3	E950.4	E962.0	E980.4
Pentothal	968.3	E855.1	E938.3	E950.4	E962.0	E980.4
Pentylenetetrazol	970.0	E854.3	E940.0	E950.4	E962.0	E980.4
Pentylsalicylamide	961.8	E857	E931.8	E950.4	E962.0	E980.4
Pepsin	973.4	E858.4	E943.4	E950.4	E962.0	E980.4
Peptavlon	977.8	E858.8	E947.8	E950.4	E962.0	E980.4
Percaine (spinal)	968.7	E855.2	E938.7	E950.4	E962.0	E980.4
topical (surface)	968.5	E855.2	E938.5	E950.4	E962.0	E980.4
Perchloroethylene (vapor)	982.3	E862.4	—	E950.9	E962.1	E980.9
medicinal	961.6	E857	E931.6	E950.4	E962.0	E980.4
Percodan	965.09	E850.2	E935.2	E950.0	E962.0	E980.0
Percogesic	965.09	E850.2	E935.2	E950.0	E962.0	E980.0
Percorten	962.0	E858.0	E932.0	E950.4	E962.0	E980.4
Pergonal	962.4	E858.0	E932.4	E950.4	E962.0	E980.4
Perhexiline	972.4	E858.3	E942.4	E950.4	E962.0	E980.4
Periactin	963.0	E858.1	E933.0	E950.4	E962.0	E980.4
Periclor	967.1	E852.0	E937.1	E950.2	E962.0	E980.2
Pericyazine	969.1	E853.0	E939.1	E950.3	E962.0	E980.3
Peritrate	972.4	E858.3	E942.4	E950.4	E962.0	E980.4
Permanganates NEC	983.9	E864.3	—	E950.7	E962.1	E980.6
potassium (topical)	976.0	E858.7	E946.0	E950.4	E962.0	E980.4
Pernocton	967.0	E851	E937.0	E950.1	E962.0	E980.1
Pernoston	967.0	E851	E937.0	E950.1	E962.0	E980.1
Peronin(e)	965.09	E850.2	E935.2	E950.0	E962.0	E980.0
Perphenazine	969.1	E853.0	E939.1	E950.3	E962.0	E980.3
Pertofrane	969.0	E854.0	E939.0	E950.3	E962.0	E980.3
Pertussis						
immune serum (human)	964.6	E858.2	E934.6	E950.4	E962.0	E980.4
vaccine (with diphtheria toxoid) (with tetanus toxoid)	978.6	E858.8	E948.6	E950.4	E962.0	E980.4
Peruvian balsam	976.8	E858.7	E946.8	E950.4	E962.0	E980.4
Pesticides (dust) (fumes) (vapor)	989.4	E863.4	—	E950.6	E962.1	E980.7
arsenic	985.1	E863.4	—	E950.8	E962.1	E980.8
chlorinated	989.2	E863.0	—	E950.6	E962.1	E980.7
cyanide	989.0	E863.4	—	E950.6	E962.1	E980.7
kerosene	981	E863.4	—	E950.6	E962.1	E980.7
mixture (of compounds)	989.4	E863.3	—	E950.6	E962.1	E980.7
naphthalene	983.0	E863.4	—	E950.7	E962.1	E980.6
organochlorine (compounds)	989.2	E863.0	—	E950.6	E962.1	E980.7
petroleum (distillate) (products) NEC	981	E863.4	—	E950.6	E962.1	E980.7
specified ingredient NEC	989.4	E863.4	—	E950.6	E962.1	E980.7
strychnine	989.1	E863.4	—	E950.6	E962.1	E980.7
thallium	985.8	E863.7	—	E950.6	E962.1	E980.7
Pethidine (hydrochloride)	965.09	E850.2	E935.2	E950.0	E962.0	E980.0
Petrichloral	967.1	E852.0	E937.1	E950.2	E962.0	E980.2
Petrol	981	E862.1	—	E950.9	E962.1	E980.9
vapor	987.1	E869.8	—	E952.8	E962.2	E982.8
Petrolatum (jelly) (ointment)	976.3	E858.7	E946.3	E950.4	E962.0	E980.4
hydrophilic	976.3	E858.7	E946.3	E950.4	E962.0	E980.4
liquid	973.2	E858.4	E943.2	E950.4	E962.0	E980.4
topical	976.3	E858.7	E946.3	E950.4	E962.0	E980.4
nonmedicinal	981	E862.1	—	E950.9	E962.1	E980.9
Petroleum (cleaners) (fuels) (products) NEC	981	E862.1	—	E950.9	E962.1	E980.9
benzin(e) — *see* Ligroin						
ether — *see* Ligroin						
jelly — *see* Petrolatum						
naphtha — *see* Ligroin						
pesticide	981	E863.4	—	E950.6	E962.1	E980.7
solids	981	E862.3	—	E950.9	E962.1	E980.9
solvents	981	E862.0	—	E950.9	E962.1	E980.9
vapor	987.1	E869.8	—	E952.8	E962.2	E982.8
Peyote	969.6	E854.1	E939.6	E950.3	E962.0	E980.3
Phanodorm, phanodorn	967.0	E851	E937.0	E950.1	E962.0	E980.1
Phanquinone, phanquone	961.5	E857	E931.5	E950.4	E962.0	E980.4
Pharmaceutical excipient or adjunct	977.4	E858.8	E947.4	E950.4	E962.0	E980.4
Phenacemide	966.3	E855.0	E936.3	E950.4	E962.0	E980.4
Phenacetin	965.4	E850.4	E935.4	E950.0	E962.0	E980.0
Phenadoxone	965.09	E850.2	E935.2	E950.0	E962.0	E980.0
Phenaglycodol	969.5	E853.8	E939.5	E950.3	E962.0	E980.3
Phenantoin	966.1	E855.0	E936.1	E950.4	E962.0	E980.4
Phenaphthazine reagent	977.8	E858.8	E947.8	E950.4	E962.0	E980.4
Phenazocine	965.09	E850.2	E935.2	E950.0	E962.0	E980.0

	Poisoning	External Cause (E-Code)				
		Accident	Therapeutic Use	Suicide Attempt	Assault	Undetermined
Phenazone	965.5	E850.5	E935.5	E950.0	E962.0	E980.0
Phenazopyridine	976.1	E858.7	E946.1	E950.4	E962.0	E980.4
Phenbenicillin	960.0	E856	E930.0	E950.4	E962.0	E980.4
Phenbutrazate	977.0	E858.8	E947.0	E950.4	E962.0	E980.4
Phencyclidine	968.3	E855.1	E938.3	E950.4	E962.0	E980.4
Phendimetrazine	977.0	E858.8	E947.0	E950.4	E962.0	E980.4
Phenelzine	969.0	E854.0	E939.0	E950.3	E962.0	E980.3
Phenergan	967.8	E852.8	E937.8	E950.2	E962.0	E980.2
Phenethicillin (potassium)	960.0	E856	E930.0	E950.4	E962.0	E980.4
Phenetsal	965.1	E850.3	E935.3	E950.0	E962.0	E980.0
Pheneturide	966.3	E855.0	E936.3	E950.4	E962.0	E980.4
Phenformin	962.3	E858.0	E932.3	E950.4	E962.0	E980.4
Phenglutarimide	971.1	E855.4	E941.1	E950.4	E962.0	E980.4
Phenicarbazide	965.8	E850.8	E935.8	E950.0	E962.0	E980.0
Phenindamine (tartrate)	963.0	E858.1	E933.0	E950.4	E962.0	E980.4
Phenindione	964.2	E858.2	E934.2	E950.4	E962.0	E980.4
Pheniprazine	969.0	E854.0	E939.0	E950.3	E962.0	E980.3
Pheniramine (maleate)	963.0	E858.1	E933.0	E950.4	E962.0	E980.4
Phenmetrazine	977.0	E858.8	E947.0	E950.4	E962.0	E980.4
Phenobal	967.0	E851	E937.0	E950.1	E962.0	E980.1
Phenobarbital	967.0	E851	E937.0	E950.1	E962.0	E980.1
Phenobarbitone	967.0	E851	E937.0	E950.1	E962.0	E980.1
Phenoctide	976.0	E858.7	E946.0	E950.4	E962.0	E980.4
Phenol (derivatives) NEC	983.0	E864.0	—	E950.7	E962.1	E980.6
disinfectant	983.0	E864.0	—	E950.7	E962.1	E980.6
pesticide	989.4	E863.4	—	E950.6	E962.1	E980.7
red	977.8	E858.8	E947.8	E950.4	E962.0	E980.4
Phenolphthalein	973.1	E858.4	E943.1	E950.4	E962.0	E980.4
Phenolsulfonphthalein	977.8	E858.8	E947.8	E950.4	E962.0	E980.4
Phenomorphan	965.09	E850.2	E935.2	E950.0	E962.0	E980.0
Phenonyl	967.0	E851	E937.0	E950.1	E962.0	E980.1
Phenoperidine	965.09	E850.2	E935.2	E950.0	E962.0	E980.0
Phenoquin	974.7	E858.5	E944.7	E950.4	E962.0	E980.4
Phenothiazines (tranquilizers) NEC	969.1	E853.0	E939.1	E950.3	E962.0	E980.3
insecticide	989.3	E863.4	—	E950.6	E962.1	E980.7
Phenoxybenzamine	971.3	E855.6	E941.3	E950.4	E962.0	E980.4
Phenoxymethyl penicillin	960.0	E856	E930.0	E950.4	E962.0	E980.4
Phenprocoumon	964.2	E858.2	E934.2	E950.4	E962.0	E980.4
Phensuximide	966.2	E855.0	E936.2	E950.4	E962.0	E980.4
Phentermine	977.0	E858.8	E947.0	E950.4	E962.0	E980.4
Phentolamine	971.3	E855.6	E941.3	E950.4	E962.0	E980.4
Phenyl						
butazone	965.5	E850.5	E935.5	E950.0	E962.0	E980.0
enediamine	983.0	E864.0	—	E950.7	E962.1	E980.6
hydrazine	983.0	E864.0	—	E950.7	E962.1	E980.6
antineoplastic	963.1	E858.1	E933.1	E950.4	E962.0	E980.4
mercuric compounds — *see* Mercury						
salicylate	976.3	E858.7	E946.3	E950.4	E962.0	E980.4
Phenylephrin	971.2	E855.5	E941.2	E950.4	E962.0	E980.4
Phenylethylbiguanide	962.3	E858.0	E932.3	E950.4	E962.0	E980.4
Phenylpropanolamine	971.2	E855.5	E941.2	E950.4	E962.0	E980.4
Phenylsulfthion	989.3	E863.1	—	E950.6	E962.1	E980.7
Phenyramidol, phenyramidon	965.7	E850.7	E935.7	E950.0	E962.0	E980.0
Phenytoin	966.1	E855.0	E936.1	E950.4	E962.0	E980.4
pHisoHex	976.2	E858.7	E946.2	E950.4	E962.0	E980.4
Pholcodine	965.09	E850.2	E935.2	E950.0	E962.0	E980.0
Phorate	989.3	E863.1	—	E950.6	E962.1	E980.7
Phosdrin	989.3	E863.1	—	E950.6	E962.1	E980.7
Phosgene (gas)	987.8	E869.8	—	E952.8	E962.2	E982.8
Phosphate (tricresyl)	989.89	E866.8	—	E950.9	E962.1	E980.9
organic	989.3	E863.1	—	E950.6	E962.1	E980.7
solvent	982.8	E862.4	—	E950.9	E926.1	E980.9
Phosphine	987.8	E869.8	—	E952.8	E962.2	E982.8
fumigant	987.8	E863.8	—	E950.6	E962.2	E980.7
Phospholine	971.0	E855.3	E941.0	E950.4	E962.0	E980.4
Phosphoric acid	983.1	E864.1	—	E950.7	E962.1	E980.6
Phosphorus (compounds) NEC	983.9	E864.3	—	E950.7	E962.1	E980.6
rodenticide	983.9	E863.7	—	E950.7	E962.1	E980.6
Phthalimidoglutarimide	967.8	E852.8	E937.8	E950.2	E962.0	E980.2
Phthalylsulfathiazole	961.0	E857	E931.0	E950.4	E962.0	E980.4
Phylloquinone	964.3	E858.2	E934.3	E950.4	E962.0	E980.4
Physeptone	965.02	E850.1	E935.1	E950.0	E962.0	E980.0
Physostigma venenosum	988.2	E865.4	—	E950.9	E962.1	E980.9
Physostigmine	971.0	E855.3	E941.0	E950.4	E962.0	E980.4
Phytolacca decandra	988.2	E865.4	—	E950.9	E962.1	E980.9
Phytomenadione	964.3	E858.2	E934.3	E950.4	E962.0	E980.4
Phytonadione	964.3	E858.2	E934.3	E950.4	E962.0	E980.4

		External Cause (E-Code)				
	Poisoning	Accident	Therapeutic Use	Suicide Attempt	Assault	Undetermined
Picric (acid)	983.0	E864.0	—	E950.7	E962.1	E980.6
Picrotoxin	970.0	E854.3	E940.0	E950.4	E962.0	E980.4
Pilocarpine	971.0	E855.3	E941.0	E950.4	E962.0	E980.4
Pilocarpus (jaborandi) extract	971.0	E855.3	E941.0	E950.4	E962.0	E980.4
Pimaricin	960.1	E856	E930.1	E950.4	E962.0	E980.4
Piminodine	965.09	E850.2	E935.2	E950.0	E962.0	E980.0
Pine oil, pinesol (disinfectant)	983.9	E861.4	—	E950.7	E962.1	E980.6
Pinkroot	961.6	E857	E931.6	E950.4	E962.0	E980.4
Pipadone	965.09	E850.2	E935.2	E950.0	E962.0	E980.0
Pipamazine	963.0	E858.1	E933.0	E950.4	E962.0	E980.4
Pipazethate	975.4	E858.6	E945.4	E950.4	E962.0	E980.4
Pipenzolate	971.1	E855.4	E941.1	E950.4	E962.0	E980.4
Piperacetazine	969.1	E853.0	E939.1	E950.3	E962.0	E980.3
Piperazine NEC	961.6	E857	E931.6	E950.4	E962.0	E980.4
estrone sulfate	962.2	E858.0	E932.2	E950.4	E962.0	E980.4
Piper cubeba	988.2	E865.4	—	E950.9	E962.1	E980.9
Piperidione	975.4	E858.6	E945.4	E950.4	E962.0	E980.4
Piperidolate	971.1	E855.4	E941.1	E950.4	E962.0	E980.4
Piperocaine	968.9	E855.2	E938.9	E950.4	E962.0	E980.4
infiltration (subcutaneous)	968.5	E855.2	E938.5	E950.4	E962.0	E980.4
nerve block (peripheral) (plexus)	968.6	E855.2	E938.6	E950.4	E962.0	E980.4
topical (surface)	968.5	E855.2	E938.5	E950.4	E962.0	E980.4
Pipobroman	963.1	E858.1	E933.1	E950.4	E962.0	E980.4
Pipradrol	970.8	E854.3	E940.8	E950.4	E962.0	E980.4
Piscidia (bark) (erythrina)	965.7	E850.7	E935.7	E950.0	E962.0	E980.0
Pitch	983.0	E864.0	—	E950.7	E962.1	E980.6
Pitkin's solution	968.7	E855.2	E938.7	E950.4	E962.0	E980.4
Pitocin	975.0	E858.6	E945.0	E950.4	E962.0	E980.4
Pitressin (tannate)	962.5	E858.0	E932.5	E950.4	E962.0	E980.4
Pituitary extracts (posterior)	962.5	E858.0	E932.5	E950.4	E962.0	E980.4
anterior	962.4	E858.0	E932.4	E950.4	E962.0	E980.4
Pituitrin	962.5	E858.0	E932.5	E950.4	E962.0	E980.4
Placental extract	962.9	E858.0	E932.9	E950.4	E962.0	E980.4
Placidyl	967.8	E852.8	E937.8	E950.2	E962.0	E980.2
Plague vaccine	978.3	E858.8	E948.3	E950.4	E962.0	E980.4
Plant foods or fertilizers NEC	989.89	E866.5	—	E950.9	E962.1	E980.9
mixed with herbicides	989.4	E863.5	—	E950.6	E962.1	E980.7
Plants, noxious, used as food	988.2	E865.9	—	E950.9	E962.1	E980.9
berries and seeds	988.2	E865.3	—	E950.9	E962.1	E980.9
specified type NEC	988.2	E865.4	—	E950.9	E962.1	E980.9
Plasma (blood)	964.7	E858.2	E934.7	E950.4	E962.0	E980.4
expanders	964.8	E858.2	E934.8	E950.4	E962.0	E980.4
Plasmanate	964.7	E858.2	E934.7	E950.4	E962.0	E980.4
Plegicil	969.1	E853.0	E939.1	E950.3	E962.0	E980.3
Podophyllin	976.4	E858.7	E946.4	E950.4	E962.0	E980.4
Podophyllum resin	976.4	E858.7	E946.4	E950.4	E962.0	E980.4
Poison NEC	989.9	E866.9	—	E950.9	E962.1	E980.9
Poisonous berries	988.2	E865.3	—	E950.9	E962.1	E980.9
Pokeweed (any part)	988.2	E865.4	—	E950.9	E962.1	E980.9
Poldine	971.1	E855.4	E941.1	E950.4	E962.0	E980.4
Poliomyelitis vaccine	979.5	E858.8	E949.5	E950.4	E962.0	E980.4
Poliovirus vaccine	979.5	E858.8	E949.5	E950.4	E962.0	E980.4
Polish (car) (floor) (furniture) (metal) (silver)	989.89	E861.2	—	E950.9	E962.1	E980.9
abrasive	989.89	E861.3	—	E950.9	E962.1	E980.9
porcelain	989.89	E861.3	—	E950.9	E962.1	E980.9
Poloxalkol	973.2	E858.4	E943.2	E950.4	E962.0	E980.4
Polyaminostyrene resins	974.5	E858.5	E944.5	E950.4	E962.0	E980.4
Polychlorinated biphenyl — *see* PCBs						
Polycycline	960.4	E856	E930.4	E950.4	E962.0	E980.4
Polyester resin hardener	982.8	E862.4	—	E950.9	E962.1	E980.9
fumes	987.8	E869.8	—	E952.8	E962.2	E982.8
Polyestradiol (phosphate)	962.2	E858.0	E932.2	E950.4	E962.0	E980.4
Polyethanolamine alkyl sulfate	976.2	E858.7	E946.2	E950.4	E962.0	E980.4
Polyethylene glycol	976.3	E858.7	E946.3	E950.4	E962.0	E980.4
Polyferose	964.0	E858.2	E934.0	E950.4	E962.0	E980.4
Polymyxin B	960.8	E856	E930.8	E950.4	E962.0	E980.4
ENT agent	976.6	E858.7	E946.6	E950.4	E962.0	E980.4
ophthalmic preparation	976.5	E858.7	E946.5	E950.4	E962.0	E980.4
topical NEC	976.0	E858.7	E946.0	E950.4	E962.0	E980.4
Polynoxylin(e)	976.0	E858.7	E946.0	E950.4	E962.0	E980.4
Polyoxymethyleneurea	976.0	E858.7	E946.0	E950.4	E962.0	E980.4
Polytetrafluoroethylene (inhaled)	987.8	E869.8	—	E952.8	E962.2	E982.8

		External Cause (E-Code)				
	Poisoning	Accident	Therapeutic Use	Suicide Attempt	Assault	Undetermined
Polythiazide	974.3	E858.5	E944.3	E950.4	E962.0	E980.4
Polyvinylpyrrolidone	964.8	E858.2	E934.8	E950.4	E962.0	E980.4
Pontocaine (hydrochloride) (infiltration) (topical)	968.5	E855.2	E938.5	E950.4	E962.0	E980.4
nerve block (peripheral) (plexus)	968.6	E855.2	E938.6	E950.4	E962.0	E980.4
spinal	968.7	E855.2	E938.7	E950.4	E962.0	E980.4
Pot	969.6	E854.1	E939.6	E950.3	E962.0	E980.3
Potash (caustic)	983.2	E864.2	—	E950.7	E962.1	E980.6
Potassic saline injection (lactated)	974.5	E858.5	E944.5	E950.4	E962.0	E980.4
Potassium (salts) NEC	974.5	E858.5	E944.5	E950.4	E962.0	E980.4
aminosalicylate	961.8	E857	E931.8	E950.4	E962.0	E980.4
arsenite (solution)	985.1	E866.3	—	E950.8	E962.1	E980.8
bichromate	983.9	E864.3	—	E950.7	E962.1	E980.6
bisulfate	983.9	E864.3	—	E950.7	E962.1	E980.6
bromide (medicinal) NEC	967.3	E852.2	E937.3	E950.2	E962.0	E980.2
carbonate	983.2	E864.2	—	E950.7	E962.1	E980.6
chlorate NEC	983.9	E864.3	—	E950.7	E962.1	E980.6
cyanide — *see* Cyanide						
hydroxide	983.2	E864.2	—	E950.7	E962.1	E980.6
iodide (expectorant) NEC	975.5	E858.6	E945.5	E950.4	E962.0	E980.4
nitrate	989.89	E866.8	—	E950.9	E962.1	E980.9
oxalate	983.9	E864.3	—	E950.7	E962.1	E980.6
perchlorate NEC	977.8	E858.8	E947.8	E950.4	E962.0	E980.4
antithyroid	962.8	E858.0	E932.8	E950.4	E962.0	E980.4
permanganate	976.0	E858.7	E946.0	E950.4	E962.0	E980.4
nonmedicinal	983.9	E864.3	—	E950.7	E962.1	E980.6
Povidone-iodine (anti-infective) NEC	976.0	E858.7	E946.0	E950.4	E962.0	E980.4
Practolol	972.0	E858.3	E942.0	E950.4	E962.0	E980.4
Pralidoxime (chloride)	977.2	E858.8	E947.2	E950.4	E962.0	E980.4
Pramoxine	968.5	E855.2	E938.5	E950.4	E962.0	E980.4
Prazosin	972.6	E858.3	E942.6	E950.4	E962.0	E980.4
Prednisolone	962.0	E858.0	E932.0	E950.4	E962.0	E980.4
ENT agent	976.6	E858.7	E946.6	E950.4	E962.0	E980.4
ophthalmic preparation	976.5	E858.7	E946.5	E950.4	E962.0	E980.4
topical NEC	976.0	E858.7	E946.0	E950.4	E962.0	E980.4
Prednisone	962.0	E858.0	E932.0	E950.4	E962.0	E980.4
Pregnanediol	962.2	E858.0	E932.2	E950.4	E962.0	E980.4
Pregneninolone	962.2	E858.0	E932.2	E950.4	E962.0	E980.4
Preludin	977.0	E858.8	E947.0	E950.4	E962.0	E980.4
Premarin	962.2	E858.0	E932.2	E950.4	E962.0	E980.4
Prenylamine	972.4	E858.3	E942.4	E950.4	E962.0	E980.4
Preparation H	976.8	E858.7	E946.8	E950.4	E962.0	E980.4
Preservatives	989.89	E866.8	—	E950.9	E962.1	E980.9
Pride of China	988.2	E865.3	—	E950.9	E962.1	E980.9
Prilocaine	968.9	E855.2	E938.9	E950.4	E962.0	E980.4
infiltration (subcutaneous)	968.5	E855.2	E938.5	E950.4	E962.0	E980.4
nerve block (peripheral) (plexus)	968.6	E855.2	E938.6	E950.4	E962.0	E980.4
Primaquine	961.4	E857	E931.4	E950.4	E962.0	E980.4
Primidone	966.3	E855.0	E936.3	E950.4	E962.0	E980.4
Primula (veris)	988.2	E865.4	—	E950.9	E962.1	E980.9
Prinadol	965.09	E850.2	E935.2	E950.0	E962.0	E980.0
Priscol, Priscoline	971.3	E855.6	E941.3	E950.4	E962.0	E980.4
Privet	988.2	E865.4	—	E950.9	E962.1	E980.9
Privine	971.2	E855.5	E941.2	E950.4	E962.0	E980.4
Pro-Banthine	971.1	E855.4	E941.1	E950.4	E962.0	E980.4
Probarbital	967.0	E851	E937.0	E950.1	E962.0	E980.1
Probenecid	974.7	E858.5	E944.7	E950.4	E962.0	E980.4
Procainamide (hydrochloride)	972.0	E858.3	E942.0	E950.4	E962.0	E980.4
Procaine (hydrochloride) (infiltration) (topical)	968.5	E855.2	E938.5	E950.4	E962.0	E980.4
nerve block (peripheral) (plexus)	968.6	E855.2	E938.6	E950.4	E962.0	E980.4
penicillin G	960.0	E856	E930.0	E950.4	E962.0	E980.4
spinal	968.7	E855.2	E938.7	E950.4	E962.0	E980.4
Procalmidol	969.5	E853.8	E939.5	E950.3	E962.0	E980.3
Procarbazine	963.1	E858.1	E933.1	E950.4	E962.0	E980.4
Prochlorperazine	969.1	E853.0	E939.1	E950.3	E962.0	E980.3
Procyclidine	966.4	E855.0	E936.4	E950.4	E962.0	E980.4
Producer gas	986	E868.8	—	E952.1	E962.2	E982.1
Profenamine	966.4	E855.0	E936.4	E950.4	E962.0	E980.4
Profenil	975.1	E858.6	E945.1	E950.4	E962.0	E980.4
Progesterones	962.2	E858.0	E932.2	E950.4	E962.0	E980.4
Progestin	962.2	E858.0	E932.2	E950.4	E962.0	E980.4
Progestogens (with estrogens)	962.2	E858.0	E932.2	E950.4	E962.0	E980.4
Progestone	962.2	E858.0	E932.2	E950.4	E962.0	E980.4
Proguanil	961.4	E857	E931.4	E950.4	E962.0	E980.4

☑ Additional Digit Required — Refer to the Tabular List (Numeric Code Section) for Additional Digit Selection

▶◀ Revised Text ● New Line ▲ Revised Code

	Poisoning	External Cause (E-Code)				
		Accident	Therapeutic Use	Suicide Attempt	Assault	Undetermined
Prolactin	962.4	E858.0	E932.4	E950.4	E962.0	E980.4
Proloid	962.7	E858.0	E932.7	E950.4	E962.0	E980.4
Proluton	962.2	E858.0	E932.2	E950.4	E962.0	E980.4
Promacetin	961.8	E857	E931.8	E950.4	E962.0	E980.4
Promazine	969.1	E853.0	E939.1	E950.3	E962.0	E980.3
Promedol	965.09	E850.2	E935.2	E950.0	E962.0	E980.0
Promethazine	967.8	E852.8	E937.8	E950.2	E962.0	E980.2
Promin	961.8	E857	E931.8	E950.4	E962.0	E980.4
Pronestyl (hydrochloride)	972.0	E858.3	E942.0	E950.4	E962.0	E980.4
Pronetalol, pronethalol	972.0	E858.3	E942.0	E950.4	E962.0	E980.4
Prontosil	961.0	E857	E931.0	E950.4	E962.0	E980.4
Propamidine isethionate	961.5	E857	E931.5	E950.4	E962.0	E980.4
Propanal (medicinal)	967.8	E852.8	E937.8	E950.2	E962.0	E980.2
Propane (gas) (distributed in mobile container)	987.0	E868.0	—	E951.1	E962.2	E981.1
distributed through pipes	987.0	E867	—	E951.0	E962.2	E981.0
incomplete combustion of — *see* Carbon monoxide, Propane						
Propanidid	968.3	E855.1	E938.3	E950.4	E962.0	E980.4
Propanol	980.3	E860.4	—	E950.9	E962.1	E980.9
Propantheline	971.1	E855.4	E941.1	E950.4	E962.0	E980.4
Proparacaine	968.5	E855.2	E938.5	E950.4	E962.0	E980.4
Propatyl nitrate	972.4	E858.3	E942.4	E950.4	E962.0	E980.4
Propicillin	960.0	E856	E930.0	E950.4	E962.0	E980.4
Propiolactone (vapor)	987.8	E869.8	—	E952.8	E962.2	E982.8
Propiomazine	967.8	E852.8	E937.8	E950.2	E962.0	E980.2
Propionaldehyde (medicinal)	967.8	E852.8	E937.8	E950.2	E962.0	E980.2
Propionate compound	976.0	E858.7	E946.0	E950.4	E962.0	E980.4
Propion gel	976.0	E858.7	E946.0	E950.4	E962.0	E980.4
Propitocaine	968.9	E855.2	E938.9	E950.4	E962.0	E980.4
infiltration (subcutaneous)	968.5	E855.2	E938.5	E950.4	E962.0	E980.4
nerve block (peripheral) (plexus)	968.6	E855.2	E938.6	E950.4	E962.0	E980.4
Propoxur	989.3	E863.2	—	E950.6	E962.1	E980.7
Propoxycaine	968.9	E855.2	E938.9	E950.4	E962.0	E980.4
infiltration (subcutaneous)	968.5	E855.2	E938.5	E950.4	E962.0	E980.4
nerve block (peripheral) (plexus)	968.6	E855.2	E938.6	E950.4	E962.0	E980.4
topical (surface)	968.5	E855.2	E938.5	E950.4	E962.0	E980.4
Propoxyphene (hydrochloride)	965.8	E850.8	E935.8	E950.0	E962.0	E980.0
Propranolol	972.0	E858.3	E942.0	E950.4	E962.0	E980.4
Propyl						
alcohol	980.3	E860.4	—	E950.9	E962.1	E980.9
carbinol	980.3	E860.4	—	E950.9	E962.1	E980.9
hexadrine	971.2	E855.5	E941.2	E950.4	E962.0	E980.4
iodone	977.8	E858.8	E947.8	E950.4	E962.0	E980.4
thiouracil	962.8	E858.0	E932.8	E950.4	E962.0	E980.4
Propylene	987.1	E869.8	—	E952.8	E962.2	E982.8
Propylparaben (ophthalmic)	976.5	E858.7	E946.5	E950.4	E962.0	E980.4
Proscillaridin	972.1	E858.3	E942.1	E950.4	E962.0	E980.4
Prostaglandins	975.0	E858.6	E945.0	E950.4	E962.0	E980.4
Prostigmin	971.0	E855.3	E941.0	E950.4	E962.0	E980.4
Protamine (sulfate)	964.5	E858.2	E934.5	E950.4	E962.0	E980.4
zinc insulin	962.3	E858.0	E932.3	E950.4	E962.0	E980.4
Protectants (topical)	976.3	E858.7	E946.3	E950.4	E962.0	E980.4
Protein hydrolysate	974.5	E858.5	E944.5	E950.4	E962.0	E980.4
Prothiaden — *see* Dothiepin hydrochloride						
Prothionamide	961.8	E857	E931.8	E950.4	E962.0	E980.4
Prothipendyl	969.5	E853.8	E939.5	E950.3	E962.0	E980.3
Protokylol	971.2	E855.5	E941.2	E950.4	E962.0	E980.4
Protopam	977.2	E858.8	E947.2	E950.4	E962.0	E980.4
Protoveratrine(s) (A) (B)	972.6	E858.3	E942.6	E950.4	E962.0	E980.4
Protriptyline	969.0	E854.0	E939.0	E950.3	E962.0	E980.3
Provera	962.2	E858.0	E932.2	E950.4	E962.0	E980.4
Provitamin A	963.5	E858.1	E933.5	E950.4	E962.0	E980.4
Proxymetacaine	968.5	E855.2	E938.5	E950.4	E962.0	E980.4
Proxyphylline	975.1	E858.6	E945.1	E950.4	E962.0	E980.4
Prozac — *see* Fluoxetine hydrochloride						
Prunus						
laurocerasus	988.2	E865.4	—	E950.9	E962.1	E980.9
virginiana	988.2	E865.4	—	E950.9	E962.1	E980.9
Prussic acid	989.0	E866.8	—	E950.9	E962.1	E980.9
vapor	987.7	E869.8	—	E952.8	E962.2	E982.8
Pseudoephedrine	971.2	E855.5	E941.2	E950.4	E962.0	E980.4
Psilocin	969.6	E854.1	E939.6	E950.3	E962.0	E980.3
Psilocybin	969.6	E854.1	E939.6	E950.3	E962.0	E980.3
PSP	977.8	E858.8	E947.8	E950.4	E962.0	E980.4
Psychedelic agents	969.6	E854.1	E939.6	E950.3	E962.0	E980.3

	Poisoning	External Cause (E-Code)				
		Accident	Therapeutic Use	Suicide Attempt	Assault	Undetermined
Psychodysleptics	969.6	E854.1	E939.6	E950.3	E962.0	E980.3
Psychostimulants	969.7	E854.2	E939.7	E950.3	E962.0	E980.3
Psychotherapeutic agents	969.9	E855.9	E939.9	E950.3	E962.0	E980.3
antidepressants	969.0	E854.0	E939.0	E950.3	E962.0	E980.3
specified NEC	969.8	E855.8	E939.8	E950.3	E962.0	E980.3
tranquilizers NEC	969.5	E853.9	E939.5	E950.3	E962.0	E980.3
Psychotomimetic agents	969.6	E854.1	E939.6	E950.3	E962.0	E980.3
Psychotropic agents	969.9	E854.8	E939.9	E950.3	E962.0	E980.3
specified NEC	969.8	E854.8	E939.8	E950.3	E962.0	E980.3
Psyllium	973.3	E858.4	E943.3	E950.4	E962.0	E980.4
Pteroylglutamic acid	964.1	E858.2	E934.1	E950.4	E962.0	E980.4
Pteroyltriglutamate	963.1	E858.1	E933.1	E950.4	E962.0	E980.4
PTFE	987.8	E869.8	—	E952.8	E962.2	E982.8
Pulsatilla	988.2	E865.4	—	E950.9	E962.1	E980.9
Purex (bleach)	983.9	E864.3	—	E950.7	E962.1	E980.6
Purine diuretics	974.1	E858.5	E944.1	E950.4	E962.0	E980.4
Purinethol	963.1	E858.1	E933.1	E950.4	E962.0	E980.4
PVP	964.8	E858.2	E934.8	E950.4	E962.0	E980.4
Pyrabital	965.7	E850.7	E935.7	E950.0	E962.0	E980.0
Pyramidon	965.5	E850.5	E935.5	E950.0	E962.0	E980.0
Pyrantel (pamoate)	961.6	E857	E931.6	E950.4	E962.0	E980.4
Pyrathiazine	963.0	E858.1	E933.0	E950.4	E962.0	E980.4
Pyrazinamide	961.8	E857	E931.8	E950.4	E962.0	E980.4
Pyrazinoic acid (amide)	961.8	E857	E931.8	E950.4	E962.0	E980.4
Pyrazole (derivatives)	965.5	E850.5	E935.5	E950.0	E962.0	E980.0
Pyrazolone (analgesics)	965.5	E850.5	E935.5	E950.0	E962.0	E980.0
Pyrethrins, pyrethrum	989.4	E863.4	—	E950.6	E962.1	E980.7
Pyribenzamine	963.0	E858.1	E933.0	E950.4	E962.0	E980.4
Pyridine (liquid) (vapor)	982.0	E862.4	—	E950.9	E962.1	E980.9
aldoxime chloride	977.2	E858.8	E947.2	E950.4	E962.0	E980.4
Pyridium	976.1	E858.7	E946.1	E950.4	E962.0	E980.4
Pyridostigmine	971.0	E855.3	E941.0	E950.4	E962.0	E980.4
Pyridoxine	963.5	E858.1	E933.5	E950.4	E962.0	E980.4
Pyrilamine	963.0	E858.1	E933.0	E950.4	E962.0	E980.4
Pyrimethamine	961.4	E857	E931.4	E950.4	E962.0	E980.4
Pyrogallic acid	983.0	E864.0	—	E950.7	E962.1	E980.6
Pyroxylin	976.3	E858.7	E946.3	E950.4	E962.0	E980.4
Pyrrobutamine	963.0	E858.1	E933.0	E950.4	E962.0	E980.4
Pyrrocitine	968.5	E855.2	E938.5	E950.4	E962.0	E980.4
Pyrvinium (pamoate)	961.6	E857	E931.6	E950.4	E962.0	E980.4
PZI	962.3	E858.0	E932.3	E950.4	E962.0	E980.4
Quaalude	967.4	E852.3	E937.4	E950.2	E962.0	E980.2
Quaternary ammonium derivatives	971.1	E855.4	E941.1	E950.4	E962.0	E980.4
Quicklime	983.2	E864.2	—	E950.7	E962.1	E980.6
Quinacrine	961.3	E857	E931.3	E950.4	E962.0	E980.4
Quinaglute	972.0	E858.3	E942.0	E950.4	E962.0	E980.4
Quinalbarbitone	967.0	E851	E937.0	E950.1	E962.0	E980.1
Quinestradiol	962.2	E858.0	E932.2	E950.4	E962.0	E980.4
Quinethazone	974.3	E858.5	E944.3	E950.4	E962.0	E980.4
Quinidine (gluconate) (polygalacturonate) (salts) (sulfate)	972.0	E858.3	E942.0	E950.4	E962.0	E980.4
Quinine	961.4	E857	E931.4	E950.4	E962.0	E980.4
Quiniobine	961.3	E857	E931.3	E950.4	E962.0	E980.4
Quinolines	961.3	E857	E931.3	E950.4	E962.0	E980.4
Quotane	968.5	E855.2	E938.5	E950.4	E962.0	E980.4
Rabies						
immune globulin (human)	964.6	E858.2	E934.6	E950.4	E962.0	E980.4
vaccine	979.1	E858.8	E949.1	E950.4	E962.0	E980.4
Racemoramide	965.09	E850.2	E935.2	E950.0	E962.0	E980.0
Racemorphan	965.09	E850.2	E935.2	E950.0	E962.0	E980.0
Radiator alcohol	980.1	E860.2	—	E950.9	E962.1	E980.9
Radio-opaque (drugs) (materials)	977.8	E858.8	E947.8	E950.4	E962.0	E980.4
Ranunculus	988.2	E865.4	—	E950.9	E962.1	E980.9
Rat poison	989.4	E863.7	—	E950.6	E962.1	E980.7
Rattlesnake (venom)	989.5	E905.0	—	E950.9	E962.1	E980.9
Raudixin	972.6	E858.3	E942.6	E950.4	E962.0	E980.4
Rautensin	972.6	E858.3	E942.6	E950.4	E962.0	E980.4
Rautina	972.6	E858.3	E942.6	E950.4	E962.0	E980.4
Rautotal	972.6	E858.3	E942.6	E950.4	E962.0	E980.4
Rauwiloid	972.6	E858.3	E942.6	E950.4	E962.0	E980.4
Rauwoldin	972.6	E858.3	E942.6	E950.4	E962.0	E980.4
Rauwolfia (alkaloids)	972.6	E858.3	E942.6	E950.4	E962.0	E980.4
Realgar	985.1	E866.3	—	E950.8	E962.1	E980.8
Red cells, packed	964.7	E858.2	E934.7	E950.4	E962.0	E980.4
Reducing agents, industrial NEC	983.9	E864.3	—	E950.7	E962.1	E980.6
Refrigerant gas (freon)	987.4	E869.2	—	E952.8	E962.2	E982.8
not freon	987.9	E869.9	—	E952.9	E962.2	E982.9

☑ Additional Digit Required — Refer to the Tabular List (Numeric Code Section) for Additional Digit Selection

▶◀ Revised Text ● New Line ▲ Revised Code

	Poisoning	External Cause (E-Code) Accident	Therapeutic Use	Suicide Attempt	Assault	Undetermined
Regroton	974.4	E858.5	E944.4	E950.4	E962.0	E980.4
Rela	968.0	E855.1	E938.0	E950.4	E962.0	E980.4
Relaxants, skeletal muscle (autonomic)	975.2	E858.6	E945.2	E950.4	E962.0	E980.4
central nervous system	968.0	E855.1	E938.0	E950.4	E962.0	E980.4
Renese	974.3	E858.5	E944.3	E950.4	E962.0	E980.4
Renografin	977.8	E858.8	E947.8	E950.4	E962.0	E980.4
Replacement solutions	974.5	E858.5	E944.5	E950.4	E962.0	E980.4
Rescinnamine	972.6	E858.3	E942.6	E950.4	E962.0	E980.4
Reserpine	972.6	E858.3	E942.6	E950.4	E962.0	E980.4
Resorcin, resorcinol	976.4	E858.7	E946.4	E950.4	E962.0	E980.4
Respaire	975.5	E858.6	E945.5	E950.4	E962.0	E980.4
Respiratory agents NEC	975.8	E858.6	E945.8	E950.4	E962.0	E980.4
Retinoic acid	976.8	E858.7	E946.8	E950.4	E962.0	E980.4
Retinol	963.5	E858.1	E933.5	E950.4	E962.0	E980.4
Rh (D) immune globulin (human)	964.6	E858.2	E934.6	E950.4	E962.0	E980.4
Rhodine	965.1	E850.3	E935.3	E950.0	E962.0	E980.0
RhoGAM	964.6	E858.2	E934.6	E950.4	E962.0	E980.4
Riboflavin	963.5	E858.1	E933.5	E950.4	E962.0	E980.4
Ricin	989.89	E866.8	—	E950.9	E962.1	E980.9
Ricinus communis	988.2	E865.3	—	E950.9	E962.1	E980.9
Rickettsial vaccine NEC	979.6	E858.8	E949.6	E950.4	E962.0	E980.4
with viral and bacterial vaccine	979.7	E858.8	E949.7	E950.4	E962.0	E980.4
Rifampin	960.6	E856	E930.6	E950.4	E962.0	E980.4
Rimifon	961.8	E857	E931.8	E950.4	E962.0	E980.4
Ringer's injection (lactated)	974.5	E858.5	E944.5	E950.4	E962.0	E980.4
Ristocetin	960.8	E856	E930.8	E950.4	E962.0	E980.4
Ritalin	969.7	E854.2	E939.7	E950.3	E962.0	E980.3
Roach killers — *see* Pesticides						
Rocky Mountain spotted fever vaccine	979.6	E858.8	E949.6	E950.4	E962.0	E980.4
Rodenticides	989.4	E863.7	—	E950.6	E962.1	E980.7
Rohypnol	969.4	E853.2	E939.4	E950.3	E962.0	E980.3
Rolaids	973.0	E858.4	E943.0	E950.4	E962.0	E980.4
Rolitetracycline	960.4	E856	E930.4	E950.4	E962.0	E980.4
Romilar	975.4	E858.6	E945.4	E950.4	E962.0	E980.4
Rose water ointment	976.3	E858.7	E946.3	E950.4	E962.0	E980.4
Rotenone	989.4	E863.7	—	E950.6	E962.1	E980.7
Rotoxamine	963.0	E858.1	E933.0	E950.4	E962.0	E980.4
Rough-on-rats	989.4	E863.7	—	E950.6	E962.1	E980.7
RU486	962.9	E858.0	E932.9	E950.4	E962.0	E980.4
Rubbing alcohol	980.2	E860.3	—	E950.9	E962.1	E980.9
Rubella virus vaccine	979.4	E858.8	E949.4	E950.4	E962.0	E980.4
Rubelogen	979.4	E858.8	E949.4	E950.4	E962.0	E980.4
Rubeovax	979.4	E858.8	E949.4	E950.4	E962.0	E980.4
Rubidomycin	960.7	E856	E930.7	E950.4	E962.0	E980.4
Rue	988.2	E865.4	—	E950.9	E962.1	E980.9
Ruta	988.2	E865.4	—	E950.9	E962.1	E980.9
Sabadilla (medicinal)	976.0	E858.7	E946.0	E950.4	E962.0	E980.4
pesticide	989.4	E863.4	—	E950.6	E962.1	E980.7
Sabin oral vaccine	979.5	E858.8	E949.5	E950.4	E962.0	E980.4
Saccharated iron oxide	964.0	E858.2	E934.0	E950.4	E962.0	E980.4
Saccharin	974.5	E858.5	E944.5	E950.4	E962.0	E980.4
Safflower oil	972.2	E858.3	E942.2	E950.4	E962.0	E980.4
Salbutamol sulfate	975.7	E858.6	E945.7	E950.4	E962.0	E980.4
Salicylamide	965.1	E850.3	E935.3	E950.0	E962.0	E980.0
Salicylate(s)	965.1	E850.3	E935.3	E950.0	E962.0	E980.0
methyl	976.3	E858.7	E946.3	E950.4	E962.0	E980.4
theobromine calcium	974.1	E858.5	E944.1	E950.4	E962.0	E980.4
Salicylazosulfapyridine	961.0	E857	E931.0	E950.4	E962.0	E980.4
Salicylhydroxamic acid	976.0	E858.7	E946.0	E950.4	E962.0	E980.4
Salicylic acid (keratolytic) NEC	976.4	E858.7	E946.4	E950.4	E962.0	E980.4
congeners	965.1	E850.3	E935.3	E950.0	E962.0	E980.0
salts	965.1	E850.3	E935.3	E950.0	E962.0	E980.0
Saliniazid	961.8	E857	E931.8	E950.4	E962.0	E980.4
Salol	976.3	E858.7	E946.3	E950.4	E962.0	E980.4
Salt (substitute) NEC	974.5	E858.5	E944.5	E950.4	E962.0	E980.4
Saluretics	974.3	E858.5	E944.3	E950.4	E962.0	E980.4
Saluron	974.3	E858.5	E944.3	E950.4	E962.0	E980.4
Salvarsan 606 (neosilver) (silver)	961.1	E857	E931.1	E950.4	E962.0	E980.4
Sambucus canadensis	988.2	E865.4	—	E950.9	E962.1	E980.9
berry	988.2	E865.3	—	E950.9	E962.1	E980.9
Sandril	972.6	E858.3	E942.6	E950.4	E962.0	E980.4
Sanguinaria canadensis	988.2	E865.4	—	E950.9	E962.1	E980.9
Saniflush (cleaner)	983.9	E861.3	—	E950.7	E962.1	E980.6
Santonin	961.6	E857	E931.6	E950.4	E962.0	E980.4
Santyl	976.8	E858.7	E946.8	E950.4	E962.0	E980.4

	Poisoning	External Cause (E-Code) Accident	Therapeutic Use	Suicide Attempt	Assault	Undetermined
Sarkomycin	960.7	E856	E930.7	E950.4	E962.0	E980.4
Saroten	969.0	E854.0	E939.0	E950.3	E962.0	E980.3
Saturnine — *see* Lead						
Savin (oil)	976.4	E858.7	E946.4	E950.4	E962.0	E980.4
Scammony	973.1	E858.4	E943.1	E950.4	E962.0	E980.4
Scarlet red	976.8	E858.7	E946.8	E950.4	E962.0	E980.4
Scheele's green	985.1	E866.3	—	E950.8	E962.1	E980.8
insecticide	985.1	E863.4	—	E950.8	E962.1	E980.8
Schradan	989.3	E863.1	—	E950.6	E962.1	E980.7
Schweinfurt(h) green	985.1	E866.3	—	E950.8	E962.1	E980.8
insecticide	985.1	E863.4	—	E950.8	E962.1	E980.8
Scilla — *see* Squill						
Sclerosing agents	972.7	E858.3	E942.7	E950.4	E962.0	E980.4
Scopolamine	971.1	E855.4	E941.1	E950.4	E962.0	E980.4
Scouring powder	989.89	E861.3	—	E950.9	E962.1	E980.9
Sea						
anemone (sting)	989.5	E905.6	—	E950.9	E962.1	E980.9
cucumber (sting)	989.5	E905.6	—	E950.9	E962.1	E980.9
snake (bite) (venom)	989.5	E905.0	—	E950.9	E962.1	E980.9
urchin spine (puncture)	989.5	E905.6	—	E950.9	E962.1	E980.9
Secbutabarbital	967.0	E851	E937.0	E950.1	E962.0	E980.1
Secbutabarbitone	967.0	E851	E937.0	E950.1	E962.0	E980.1
Secobarbital	967.0	E851	E937.0	E950.1	E962.0	E980.1
Seconal	967.0	E851	E937.0	E950.1	E962.0	E980.1
Secretin	977.8	E858.8	E947.8	E950.4	E962.0	E980.4
Sedatives, nonbarbiturate	967.9	E852.9	E937.9	E950.2	E962.0	E980.2
specified NEC	967.8	E852.8	E937.8	E950.2	E962.0	E980.2
Sedormid	967.8	E852.8	E937.8	E950.2	E962.0	E980.2
Seed (plant)	988.2	E865.3	—	E950.9	E962.1	E980.9
disinfectant or dressing	989.89	E866.5	—	E950.9	E962.1	E980.9
Selenium (fumes) NEC	985.8	E866.4	—	E950.9	E962.1	E980.9
disulfide or sulfide	976.4	E858.7	E946.4	E950.4	E962.0	E980.4
Selsun	976.4	E858.7	E946.4	E950.4	E962.0	E980.4
Senna	973.1	E858.4	E943.1	E950.4	E962.0	E980.4
Septisol	976.2	E858.7	E946.2	E950.4	E962.0	E980.4
Serax	969.4	E853.2	E939.4	E950.3	E962.0	E980.3
Serenesil	967.8	E852.8	E937.8	E950.2	E962.0	E980.2
Serenium (hydrochloride)	961.9	E857	E931.9	E950.4	E962.0	E980.4
Serepax — *see* Oxazepam						
Sernyl	968.3	E855.1	E938.3	E950.4	E962.0	E980.4
Serotonin	977.8	E858.8	E947.8	E950.4	E962.0	E980.4
Serpasil	972.6	E858.3	E942.6	E950.4	E962.0	E980.4
Sewer gas	987.8	E869.8	—	E952.8	E962.2	E982.8
Shampoo	989.6	E861.0	—	E950.9	E962.1	E980.9
Shellfish, nonbacterial or noxious	988.0	E865.1	—	E950.9	E962.1	E980.9
Silicones NEC	989.83	E866.8	E947.8	E950.9	E962.1	E980.9
Silvadene	976.0	E858.7	E946.0	E950.4	E962.0	E980.4
Silver (compound) (medicinal) NEC	976.0	E858.7	E946.0	E950.4	E962.0	E980.4
anti-infectives	976.0	E858.7	E946.0	E950.4	E962.0	E980.4
arsphenamine	961.1	E857	E931.1	E950.4	E962.0	E980.4
nitrate	976.0	E858.7	E946.0	E950.4	E962.0	E980.4
ophthalmic preparation	976.5	E858.7	E946.5	E950.4	E962.0	E980.4
toughened (keratolytic)	976.4	E858.7	E946.4	E950.4	E962.0	E980.4
nonmedicinal (dust)	985.8	E866.4	—	E950.9	E962.1	E980.9
protein (mild) (strong)	976.0	E858.7	E946.0	E950.4	E962.0	E980.4
salvarsan	961.1	E857	E931.1	E950.4	E962.0	E980.4
Simethicone	973.8	E858.4	E943.8	E950.4	E962.0	E980.4
Sinequan	969.0	E854.0	E939.0	E950.3	E962.0	E980.3
Singoserp	972.6	E858.3	E942.6	E950.4	E962.0	E980.4
Sintrom	964.2	E858.2	E934.2	E950.4	E962.0	E980.4
Sitosterols	972.2	E858.3	E942.2	E950.4	E962.0	E980.4
Skeletal muscle relaxants	975.2	E858.6	E945.2	E950.4	E962.0	E980.4
Skin						
agents (external)	976.9	E858.7	E946.9	E950.4	E962.0	E980.4
specified NEC	976.8	E858.7	E946.8	E950.4	E962.0	E980.4
test antigen	977.8	E858.8	E947.8	E950.4	E962.0	E980.4
Sleep-eze	963.0	E858.1	E933.0	E950.4	E962.0	E980.4
Sleeping draught (drug) (pill) (tablet)	967.9	E852.9	E937.9	E950.2	E962.0	E980.2
Smallpox vaccine	979.0	E858.8	E949.0	E950.4	E962.0	E980.4
Smelter fumes NEC	985.9	E866.4	—	E950.9	E962.1	E980.9
Smog	987.3	E869.1	—	E952.8	E962.2	E982.8
Smoke NEC	987.9	E869.9	—	E952.9	E962.2	E982.9
Smooth muscle relaxant	975.1	E858.6	E945.1	E950.4	E962.0	E980.4
Snail killer	989.4	E863.4	—	E950.6	E962.1	E980.7
Snake (bite) (venom)	989.5	E905.0	—	E950.9	E962.1	E980.9
Snuff	989.89	E866.8	—	E950.9	E962.1	E980.9
Soap (powder) (product)	989.6	E861.1	—	E950.9	E962.1	E980.9
medicinal, soft	976.2	E858.7	E946.2	E950.4	E962.0	E980.4

☑ Additional Digit Required — Refer to the Tabular List (Numeric Code Section) for Additional Digit Selection

▶◀ Revised Text ● New Line ▲ Revised Code

	Poisoning	External Cause (E-Code)				
		Accident	Therapeutic Use	Suicide Attempt	Assault	Undetermined
Soda (caustic)	983.2	E864.2	—	E950.7	E962.1	E980.6
bicarb	963.3	E858.1	E933.3	E950.4	E962.0	E980.4
chlorinated — *see* Sodium, hypochlorite						
Sodium						
acetosulfone	961.8	E857	E931.8	E950.4	E962.0	E980.4
acetrizoate	977.8	E858.8	E947.8	E950.4	E962.0	E980.4
amytal	967.0	E851	E937.0	E950.1	E962.0	E980.1
arsenate — *see* Arsenic						
bicarbonate	963.3	E858.1	E933.3	E950.4	E962.0	E980.4
bichromate	983.9	E864.3	—	E950.7	E962.1	E980.6
biphosphate	963.2	E858.1	E933.2	E950.4	E962.0	E980.4
bisulfate	983.9	E864.3	—	E950.7	E962.1	E980.6
borate (cleanser)	989.6	E861.3	—	E950.9	E962.1	E980.9
bromide NEC	967.3	E852.2	E937.3	E950.2	E962.0	E980.2
cacodylate (nonmedicinal) NEC	978.8	E858.8	E948.8	E950.4	E962.0	E980.4
anti-infective	961.1	E857	E931.1	E950.4	E962.0	E980.4
herbicide	989.4	E863.5	—	E950.6	E962.1	E980.7
calcium edetate	963.8	E858.1	E933.8	E950.4	E962.0	E980.4
carbonate NEC	983.2	E864.2	—	E950.7	E962.1	E980.6
chlorate NEC	983.9	E864.3	—	E950.7	E962.1	E980.6
herbicide	983.9	E863.5	—	E950.7	E962.1	E980.6
chloride NEC	974.5	E858.5	E944.5	E950.4	E962.0	E980.4
chromate	983.9	E864.3	—	E950.7	E962.1	E980.6
citrate	963.3	E858.1	E933.3	E950.4	E962.0	E980.4
cyanide — *see* Cyanide(s)						
cyclamate	974.5	E858.5	E944.5	E950.4	E962.0	E980.4
diatrizoate	977.8	E858.8	E947.8	E950.4	E962.0	E980.4
dibunate	975.4	E858.6	E945.4	E950.4	E962.0	E980.4
dioctyl sulfosuccinate	973.2	E858.4	E943.2	E950.4	E962.0	E980.4
edetate	963.8	E858.1	E933.8	E950.4	E962.0	E980.4
ethacrynate	974.4	E858.5	E944.4	E950.4	E962.0	E980.4
fluoracetate (dust) (rodenticide)	989.4	E863.7	—	E950.6	E962.1	E980.7
fluoride — *see* Fluoride(s)						
free salt	974.5	E858.5	E944.5	E950.4	E962.0	E980.4
glucosulfone	961.8	E857	E931.8	E950.4	E962.0	E980.4
hydroxide	983.2	E864.2	—	E950.7	E962.1	E980.6
hypochlorite (bleach) NEC	983.9	E864.3	—	E950.7	E962.1	E980.6
disinfectant	983.9	E861.4	—	E950.7	E962.1	E980.6
medicinal (anti-infective) (external)	976.0	E858.7	E946.0	E950.4	E962.0	E980.4
vapor	987.8	E869.8	—	E952.8	E962.2	E982.8
hyposulfite	976.0	E858.7	E946.0	E950.4	E962.0	E980.4
indigotindisulfonate	977.8	E858.8	E947.8	E950.4	E962.0	E980.4
iodide	977.8	E858.8	E947.8	E950.4	E962.0	E980.4
iothalamate	977.8	E858.8	E947.8	E950.4	E962.0	E980.4
iron edetate	964.0	E858.2	E934.0	E950.4	E962.0	E980.4
lactate	963.3	E858.1	E933.3	E950.4	E962.0	E980.4
lauryl sulfate	976.2	E858.7	E946.2	E950.4	E962.0	E980.4
L-triiodothyronine	962.7	E858.0	E932.7	E950.4	E962.0	E980.4
metrizoate	977.8	E858.8	E947.8	E950.4	E962.0	E980.4
monofluoracetate (dust) (rodenticide)	989.4	E863.7	—	E950.6	E962.1	E980.7
morrhuate	972.7	E858.3	E942.7	E950.4	E962.0	E980.4
nafcillin	960.0	E856	E930.0	E950.4	E962.0	E980.4
nitrate (oxidizing agent)	983.9	E864.3	—	E950.7	E962.1	E980.6
nitrite (medicinal)	972.4	E858.3	E942.4	E950.4	E962.0	E980.4
nitroferricyanide	972.6	E858.3	E942.6	E950.4	E962.0	E980.4
nitroprusside	972.6	E858.3	E942.6	E950.4	E962.0	E980.4
para-aminohippurate	977.8	E858.8	E947.8	E950.4	E962.0	E980.4
perborate (nonmedicinal) NEC	989.89	E866.8	—	E950.9	E962.1	E980.9
medicinal	976.6	E858.7	E946.6	E950.4	E962.0	E980.4
soap	989.6	E861.1	—	E950.9	E962.1	E980.9
percarbonate — *see* Sodium, perborate						
phosphate	973.3	E858.4	E943.3	E950.4	E962.0	E980.4
polystyrene sulfonate	974.5	E858.5	E944.5	E950.4	E962.0	E980.4
propionate	976.0	E858.7	E946.0	E950.4	E962.0	E980.4
psylliate	972.7	E858.3	E942.7	E950.4	E962.0	E980.4
removing resins	974.5	E858.5	E944.5	E950.4	E962.0	E980.4
salicylate	965.1	E850.3	E935.3	E950.0	E962.0	E980.0
sulfate	973.3	E858.4	E943.3	E950.4	E962.0	E980.4
sulfoxone	961.8	E857	E931.8	E950.4	E962.0	E980.4
tetradecyl sulfate	972.7	E858.3	E942.7	E950.4	E962.0	E980.4
thiopental	968.3	E855.1	E938.3	E950.4	E962.0	E980.4
thiosalicylate	965.1	E850.3	E935.3	E950.0	E962.0	E980.0
thiosulfate	976.0	E858.7	E946.0	E950.4	E962.0	E980.4
tolbutamide	977.8	E858.8	E947.8	E950.4	E962.0	E980.4
Sodium — *continued*						
tyropanoate	977.8	E858.8	E947.8	E950.4	E962.0	E980.4
valproate	966.3	E855.0	E936.3	E950.4	E962.0	E980.4
Solanine	977.8	E858.8	E947.8	E950.4	E962.0	E980.4
Solanum dulcamara	988.2	E865.4	—	E950.9	E962.1	E980.9
Solapsone	961.8	E857	E931.8	E950.4	E962.0	E980.4
Solasulfone	961.8	E857	E931.8	E950.4	E962.0	E980.4
Soldering fluid	983.1	E864.1	—	E950.7	E962.1	E980.6
Solid substance	989.9	E866.9	—	E950.9	E962.1	E980.9
specified NEC	989.9	E866.8	—	E950.9	E962.1	E980.9
Solvents, industrial	982.8	E862.9	—	E950.9	E962.1	E980.9
naphtha	981	E862.0	—	E950.9	E962.1	E980.9
petroleum	981	E862.0	—	E950.9	E962.1	E980.9
specified NEC	982.8	E862.4	—	E950.9	E962.1	E980.9
Soma	968.0	E855.1	E938.0	E950.4	E962.0	E980.4
Somatotropin	962.4	E858.0	E932.4	E950.4	E962.0	E980.4
Sominex	963.0	E858.1	E933.0	E950.4	E962.0	E980.4
Somnos	967.1	E852.0	E937.1	E950.2	E962.0	E980.2
Somonal	967.0	E851	E937.0	E950.1	E962.0	E980.1
Soneryl	967.0	E851	E937.0	E950.1	E962.0	E980.1
Soothing syrup	977.9	E858.9	E947.9	E950.5	E962.0	E980.5
Sopor	967.4	E852.3	E937.4	E950.2	E962.0	E980.2
Soporific drug	967.9	E852.9	E937.9	E950.2	E962.0	E980.2
specified type NEC	967.8	E852.8	E937.8	E950.2	E962.0	E980.2
Sorbitol NEC	977.4	E858.8	E947.4	E950.4	E962.0	E980.4
Sotradecol	972.7	E858.3	E942.7	E950.4	E962.0	E980.4
Spacoline	975.1	E858.6	E945.1	E950.4	E962.0	E980.4
Spanish fly	976.8	E858.7	E946.8	E950.4	E962.0	E980.4
Sparine	969.1	E853.0	E939.1	E950.3	E962.0	E980.3
Sparteine	975.0	E858.6	E945.0	E950.4	E962.0	E980.4
Spasmolytics	975.1	E858.6	E945.1	E950.4	E962.0	E980.4
anticholinergics	971.1	E855.4	E941.1	E950.4	E962.0	E980.4
Spectinomycin	960.8	E856	E930.8	E950.4	E962.0	E980.4
Speed	969.7	E854.2	E939.7	E950.3	E962.0	E980.3
Spermicides	976.8	E858.7	E946.8	E950.4	E962.0	E980.4
Spider (bite) (venom)	989.5	E905.1	—	E950.9	E962.1	E980.9
antivenin	979.9	E858.8	E949.9	E950.4	E962.0	E980.4
Spigelia (root)	961.6	E857	E931.6	E950.4	E962.0	E980.4
Spiperone	969.2	E853.1	E939.2	E950.3	E962.0	E980.3
Spiramycin	960.3	E856	E930.3	E950.4	E962.0	E980.4
Spirilene	969.5	E853.8	E939.5	E950.3	E962.0	E980.3
Spirit(s) (neutral) NEC	980.0	E860.1	—	E950.9	E962.1	E980.9
beverage	980.0	E860.0	—	E950.9	E962.1	E980.9
industrial	980.9	E860.9	—	E950.9	E962.1	E980.9
mineral	981	E862.0	—	E950.9	E962.1	E980.9
of salt — *see* Hydrochloric acid						
surgical	980.9	E860.9	—	E950.9	E962.1	E980.9
Spironolactone	974.4	E858.5	E944.4	E950.4	E962.0	E980.4
Sponge, absorbable (gelatin)	964.5	E858.2	E934.5	E950.4	E962.0	E980.4
Sporostacin	976.0	E858.7	E946.0	E950.4	E962.0	E980.4
Sprays (aerosol)	989.89	E866.8	—	E950.9	E962.1	E980.9
cosmetic	989.89	E866.7	—	E950.9	E962.1	E980.9
medicinal NEC	977.9	E858.9	E947.9	E950.5	E962.0	E980.5
pesticides — *see* Pesticides						
specified content — *see* substance specified						
Spurge flax	988.2	E865.4	—	E950.9	E962.1	E980.9
Spurges	988.2	E865.4	—	E950.9	E962.1	E980.9
Squill (expectorant) NEC	975.5	E858.6	E945.5	E950.4	E962.0	E980.4
rat poison	989.4	E863.7	—	E950.6	E962.1	E980.7
Squirting cucumber (cathartic)	973.1	E858.4	E943.1	E950.4	E962.0	E980.4
Stains	989.89	E866.8	—	E950.9	E962.1	E980.9
Stannous — *see also* Tin						
fluoride	976.7	E858.7	E946.7	E950.4	E962.0	E980.4
Stanolone	962.1	E858.0	E932.1	E950.4	E962.0	E980.4
Stanozolol	962.1	E858.0	E932.1	E950.4	E962.0	E980.4
Staphisagria or stavesacre (pediculicide)	976.0	E858.7	E946.0	E950.4	E962.0	E980.4
Stelazine	969.1	E853.0	E939.1	E950.3	E962.0	E980.3
Stemetil	969.1	E853.0	E939.1	E950.3	E962.0	E980.3
Sterculia (cathartic) (gum)	973.3	E858.4	E943.3	E950.4	E962.0	E980.4
Sternutator gas	987.8	E869.8	—	E952.8	E962.2	E982.8
Steroids NEC	962.0	E858.0	E932.0	E950.4	E962.0	E980.4
ENT agent	976.6	E858.7	E946.6	E950.4	E962.0	E980.4
ophthalmic preparation	976.5	E858.7	E946.5	E950.4	E962.0	E980.4
topical NEC	976.0	E858.7	E946.0	E950.4	E962.0	E980.4
Stibine	985.8	E866.4	—	E950.9	E962.1	E980.9
Stibophen	961.2	E857	E931.2	E950.4	E962.0	E980.4
Stilbamide, stilbamidine	961.5	E857	E931.5	E950.4	E962.0	E980.4

		External Cause (E-Code)				
	Poisoning	Accident	Therapeutic Use	Suicide Attempt	Assault	Undetermined
Stilbestrol	962.2	E858.0	E932.2	E950.4	E962.0	E980.4
Stimulants (central nervous system)	970.9	E854.3	E940.9	E950.4	E962.0	E980.4
analeptics	970.0	E854.3	E940.0	E950.4	E962.0	E980.4
opiate antagonist	970.1	E854.3	E940.1	E950.4	E962.0	E980.4
psychotherapeutic NEC	969.0	E854.0	E939.0	E950.3	E962.0	E980.3
specified NEC	970.8	E854.3	E940.8	E950.4	E962.0	E980.4
Storage batteries (acid) (cells)	983.1	E864.1	—	E950.7	E962.1	E980.6
Stovaine	968.9	E855.2	E938.9	E950.4	E962.0	E980.4
infiltration (subcutaneous)	968.5	E855.2	E938.5	E950.4	E962.0	E980.4
nerve block (peripheral) (plexus)	968.6	E855.2	E938.6	E950.4	E962.0	E980.4
spinal	968.7	E855.2	E938.7	E950.4	E962.0	E980.4
topical (surface)	968.5	E855.2	E938.5	E950.4	E962.0	E980.4
Stovarsal	961.1	E857	E931.1	E950.4	E962.0	E980.4
Stove gas — *see* Gas, utility						
Stoxil	976.5	E858.7	E946.5	E950.4	E962.0	E980.4
STP	969.6	E854.1	E939.6	E950.3	E962.0	E980.3
Stramonium (medicinal) NEC	971.1	E855.4	E941.1	E950.4	E962.0	E980.4
natural state	988.2	E865.4	—	E950.9	E962.1	E980.9
Streptodornase	964.4	E858.2	E934.4	E950.4	E962.0	E980.4
Streptoduocin	960.6	E856	E930.6	E950.4	E962.0	E980.4
Streptokinase	964.4	E858.2	E934.4	E950.4	E962.0	E980.4
Streptomycin	960.6	E856	E930.6	E950.4	E962.0	E980.4
Streptozocin	960.7	E856	E930.7	E950.4	E962.0	E980.4
Stripper (paint) (solvent)	982.8	E862.9	—	E950.9	E962.1	E980.9
Strobane	989.2	E863.0	—	E950.6	E962.1	E980.7
Strophanthin	972.1	E858.3	E942.1	E950.4	E962.0	E980.4
Strophanthus hispidus or kombe	988.2	E865.4	—	E950.9	E962.1	E980.9
Strychnine (rodenticide) (salts)	989.1	E863.7	—	E950.6	E962.1	E980.7
medicinal NEC	970.8	E854.3	E940.8	E950.4	E962.0	E980.4
Strychnos (ignatii) — *see* Strychnine						
Styramate	968.0	E855.1	E938.0	E950.4	E962.0	E980.4
Styrene	983.0	E864.0	—	E950.7	E962.1	E980.6
Succinimide (anticonvulsant)	966.2	E855.0	E936.2	E950.4	E962.0	E980.4
mercuric — *see* Mercury						
Succinylcholine	975.2	E858.6	E945.2	E950.4	E962.0	E980.4
Succinylsulfathiazole	961.0	E857	E931.0	E950.4	E962.0	E980.4
Sucrose	974.5	E858.5	E944.5	E950.4	E962.0	E980.4
Sulfacetamide	961.0	E857	E931.0	E950.4	E962.0	E980.4
ophthalmic preparation	976.5	E858.7	E946.5	E950.4	E962.0	E980.4
Sulfachlorpyridazine	961.0	E857	E931.0	E950.4	E962.0	E980.4
Sulfacytine	961.0	E857	E931.0	E950.4	E962.0	E980.4
Sulfadiazine	961.0	E857	E931.0	E950.4	E962.0	E980.4
silver (topical)	976.0	E858.7	E946.0	E950.4	E962.0	E980.4
Sulfadimethoxine	961.0	E857	E931.0	E950.4	E962.0	E980.4
Sulfadimidine	961.0	E857	E931.0	E950.4	E962.0	E980.4
Sulfaethidole	961.0	E857	E931.0	E950.4	E962.0	E980.4
Sulfafurazole	961.0	E857	E931.0	E950.4	E962.0	E980.4
Sulfaguanidine	961.0	E857	E931.0	E950.4	E962.0	E980.4
Sulfamerazine	961.0	E857	E931.0	E950.4	E962.0	E980.4
Sulfameter	961.0	E857	E931.0	E950.4	E962.0	E980.4
Sulfamethizole	961.0	E857	E931.0	E950.4	E962.0	E980.4
Sulfamethoxazole	961.0	E857	E931.0	E950.4	E962.0	E980.4
Sulfamethoxydiazine	961.0	E857	E931.0	E950.4	E962.0	E980.4
Sulfamethoxypyridazine	961.0	E857	E931.0	E950.4	E962.0	E980.4
Sulfamethylthiazole	961.0	E857	E931.0	E950.4	E962.0	E980.4
Sulfamylon	976.0	E858.7	E946.0	E950.4	E962.0	E980.4
Sulfan blue (diagnostic dye)	977.8	E858.8	E947.8	E950.4	E962.0	E980.4
Sulfanilamide	961.0	E857	E931.0	E950.4	E962.0	E980.4
Sulfanilylguanidine	961.0	E857	E931.0	E950.4	E962.0	E980.4
Sulfaphenazole	961.0	E857	E931.0	E950.4	E962.0	E980.4
Sulfaphenylthiazole	961.0	E857	E931.0	E950.4	E962.0	E980.4
Sulfaproxyline	961.0	E857	E931.0	E950.4	E962.0	E980.4
Sulfapyridine	961.0	E857	E931.0	E950.4	E962.0	E980.4
Sulfapyrimidine	961.0	E857	E931.0	E950.4	E962.0	E980.4
Sulfarsphenamine	961.1	E857	E931.1	E950.4	E962.0	E980.4
Sulfasalazine	961.0	E857	E931.0	E950.4	E962.0	E980.4
Sulfasomizole	961.0	E857	E931.0	E950.4	E962.0	E980.4
Sulfasuxidine	961.0	E857	E931.0	E950.4	E962.0	E980.4
Sulfinpyrazone	974.7	E858.5	E944.7	E950.4	E962.0	E980.4
Sulfisoxazole	961.0	E857	E931.0	E950.4	E962.0	E980.4
ophthalmic preparation	976.5	E858.7	E946.5	E950.4	E962.0	E980.4
Sulfomyxin	960.8	E856	E930.8	E950.4	E962.0	E980.4
Sulfonal	967.8	E852.8	E937.8	E950.2	E962.0	E980.2
Sulfonamides (mixtures)	961.0	E857	E931.0	E950.4	E962.0	E980.4
Sulfones	961.8	E857	E931.8	E950.4	E962.0	E980.4

		External Cause (E-Code)				
	Poisoning	Accident	Therapeutic Use	Suicide Attempt	Assault	Undetermined
Sulfonethylmethane	967.8	E852.8	E937.8	E950.2	E962.0	E980.2
Sulfonmethane	967.8	E852.8	E937.8	E950.2	E962.0	E980.2
Sulfonphthal, sulfonphthol	977.8	E858.8	E947.8	E950.4	E962.0	E980.4
Sulfonylurea derivatives, oral	962.3	E858.0	E932.3	E950.4	E962.0	E980.4
Sulfoxone	961.8	E857	E931.8	E950.4	E962.0	E980.4
Sulfur, sulfureted, sulfuric, sulfurous, sulfuryl (compounds) NEC	989.89	E866.8	—	E950.9	E962.1	E980.9
acid	983.1	E864.1	—	E950.7	E962.1	E980.6
dioxide	987.3	E869.1	—	E952.8	E962.2	E982.8
ether — *see* Ether(s)						
hydrogen	987.8	E869.8	—	E952.8	E962.2	E982.8
medicinal (keratolytic) (ointment) NEC	976.4	E858.7	E946.4	E950.4	E962.0	E980.4
pesticide (vapor)	989.4	E863.4	—	E950.6	E962.1	E980.7
vapor NEC	987.8	E869.8	—	E952.8	E962.2	E982.8
Sulkowitch's reagent	977.8	E858.8	E947.8	E950.4	E962.0	E980.4
Sulph — *see also* Sulf-						
Sulphadione	961.8	E857	E931.8	E950.4	E962.0	E980.4
Sulthiame, sultiame	966.3	E855.0	E936.3	E950.4	E962.0	E980.4
Superinone	975.5	E858.6	E945.5	E950.4	E962.0	E980.4
Suramin	961.5	E857	E931.5	E950.4	E962.0	E980.4
Surfacaine	968.5	E855.2	E938.5	E950.4	E962.0	E980.4
Surital	968.3	E855.1	E938.3	E950.4	E962.0	E980.4
Sutilains	976.8	E858.7	E946.8	E950.4	E962.0	E980.4
Suxamethonium (bromide) (chloride) (iodide)	975.2	E858.6	E945.2	E950.4	E962.0	E980.4
Suxethonium (bromide)	975.2	E858.6	E945.2	E950.4	E962.0	E980.4
Sweet oil (birch)	976.3	E858.7	E946.3	E950.4	E962.0	E980.4
Sym-dichloroethyl ether	982.3	E862.4	—	E950.9	E962.1	E980.9
Sympatholytics	971.3	E855.6	E941.3	E950.4	E962.0	E980.4
Sympathomimetics	971.2	E855.5	E941.2	E950.4	E962.0	E980.4
Synagis	979.6	E858.8	E949.6	E950.4	E962.0	E980.4
Synalar	976.0	E858.7	E946.0	E950.4	E962.0	E980.4
Synthroid	962.7	E858.0	E932.7	E950.4	E962.0	E980.4
Syntocinon	975.0	E858.6	E945.0	E950.4	E962.0	E950.4
Syrosingopine	972.6	E858.3	E942.6	E950.4	E962.0	E980.4
Systemic agents (primarily)	963.9	E858.1	E933.9	E950.4	E962.0	E980.4
specified NEC	963.8	E858.1	E933.8	E950.4	E962.0	E980.4
Tablets (*see also* specified substance)	977.9	E858.9	E947.9	E950.5	E962.0	E980.5
Tace	962.2	E858.0	E932.2	E950.4	E962.0	E980.4
Tacrine	971.0	E855.3	E941.0	E950.4	E962.0	E980.4
Talbutal	967.0	E851	E937.0	E950.1	E962.0	E980.1
Talc	976.3	E858.7	E946.3	E950.4	E962.0	E980.4
Talcum	976.3	E858.7	E946.3	E950.4	E962.0	E980.4
Tandearil, tanderil	965.5	E850.5	E935.5	E950.0	E962.0	E980.0
Tannic acid	983.1	E864.1	—	E950.7	E962.1	E980.6
medicinal (astringent)	976.2	E858.7	E946.2	E950.4	E962.0	E980.4
Tannin — *see* Tannic acid						
Tansy	988.2	E865.4	—	E950.9	E962.1	E980.9
TAO	960.3	E856	E930.3	E950.4	E962.0	E980.4
Tapazole	962.8	E858.0	E932.8	E950.4	E962.0	E980.4
Tar NEC	983.0	E864.0	—	E950.7	E962.1	E980.6
camphor — *see* Naphthalene						
fumes	987.8	E869.8	—	E952.8	E962.2	E982.8
Taractan	969.3	E853.8	E939.3	E950.3	E962.0	E980.3
Tarantula (venomous)	989.5	E905.1	—	E950.9	E962.1	E980.9
Tartar emetic (anti-infective)	961.2	E857	E931.2	E950.4	E962.0	E980.4
Tartaric acid	983.1	E864.1	—	E950.7	E962.1	E980.6
Tartrated antimony (anti-infective)	961.2	E857	E931.2	E950.4	E962.0	E980.4
TCA — *see* Trichloroacetic acid						
TDI	983.0	E864.0	—	E950.7	E962.1	E980.6
vapor	987.8	E869.8	—	E952.8	E962.2	E982.8
Tear gas	987.5	E869.3	—	E952.8	E962.2	E982.8
Teclothiazide	974.3	E858.5	E944.3	E950.4	E962.0	E980.4
Tegretol	966.3	E855.0	E936.3	E950.4	E962.0	E980.4
Telepaque	977.8	E858.8	E947.8	E950.4	E962.0	E980.4
Tellurium	985.8	E866.4	—	E950.9	E962.1	E980.9
fumes	985.8	E866.4	—	E950.9	E962.1	E980.9
TEM	963.1	E858.1	E933.1	E950.4	E962.0	E980.4
Temazepan — *see* Benzodiazepines						
TEPA	963.1	E858.1	E933.1	E950.4	E962.0	E980.4
TEPP	989.3	E863.1	—	E950.6	E962.1	E980.7
Terbutaline	971.2	E855.5	E941.2	E950.4	E962.0	E980.4
Teroxalene	961.6	E857	E931.6	E950.4	E962.0	E980.4
Terpin hydrate	975.5	E858.6	E945.5	E950.4	E962.0	E980.4
Terramycin	960.4	E856	E930.4	E950.4	E962.0	E980.4

		External Cause (E-Code)				
	Poisoning	Accident	Therapeutic Use	Suicide Attempt	Assault	Undetermined
Tessalon	975.4	E858.6	E945.4	E950.4	E962.0	E980.4
Testosterone	962.1	E858.0	E932.1	E950.4	E962.0	E980.4
Tetanus (vaccine)	978.4	E858.8	E948.4	E950.4	E962.0	E980.4
antitoxin	979.9	E858.8	E949.9	E950.4	E962.0	E980.4
immune globulin (human)	964.6	E858.2	E934.6	E950.4	E962.0	E980.4
toxoid	978.4	E858.8	E948.4	E950.4	E962.0	E980.4
with diphtheria toxoid	978.9	E858.8	E948.9	E950.4	E962.0	E980.4
with pertussis	978.6	E858.8	E948.6	E950.4	E962.0	E980.4
Tetrabenazine	969.5	E853.8	E939.5	E950.3	E962.0	E980.3
Tetracaine (infiltration) (topical)	968.5	E855.2	E938.5	E950.4	E962.0	E980.4
nerve block (peripheral) (plexus)	968.6	E855.2	E938.6	E950.4	E962.0	E980.4
spinal	968.7	E855.2	E938.7	E950.4	E962.0	E980.4
Tetrachlorethylene — *see* Tetrachloroethylene						
Tetrachlormethiazide	974.3	E858.5	E944.3	E950.4	E962.0	E980.4
Tetrachloroethane (liquid) (vapor)	982.3	E862.4	—	E950.9	E962.1	E980.9
paint or varnish	982.3	E861.6	—	E950.9	E962.1	E980.9
Tetrachloroethylene (liquid) (vapor)	982.3	E862.4	—	E950.9	E962.1	E980.9
medicinal	961.6	E857	E931.6	E950.4	E962.0	E980.4
Tetrachloromethane — *see* Carbon, tetrachloride						
Tetracycline	960.4	E856	E930.4	E950.4	E962.0	E980.4
ophthalmic preparation	976.5	E858.7	E946.5	E950.4	E962.0	E980.4
topical NEC	976.0	E858.7	E946.0	E950.4	E962.0	E980.4
Tetraethylammonium chloride	972.3	E858.3	E942.3	E950.4	E962.0	E980.4
Tetraethyl lead (antiknock compound)	984.1	E862.1	—	E950.9	E962.1	E980.9
Tetraethyl pyrophosphate	989.3	E863.1	—	E950.6	E962.1	E980.7
Tetraethylthiuram disulfide	977.3	E858.8	E947.3	E950.4	E962.0	E980.4
Tetrahydroaminoacridine	971.0	E855.3	E941.0	E950.4	E962.0	E980.4
Tetrahydrocannabinol	969.6	E854.1	E939.6	E950.3	E962.0	E980.3
Tetrahydronaphthalene	982.0	E862.4	—	E950.9	E962.1	E980.9
Tetrahydrozoline	971.2	E855.5	E941.2	E950.4	E962.0	E980.4
Tetralin	982.0	E862.4	—	E950.9	E962.1	E980.9
Tetramethylthiuram (disulfide) NEC	989.4	E863.6	—	E950.6	E962.1	E980.7
medicinal	976.2	E858.7	E946.2	E950.4	E962.0	E980.4
Tetronal	967.8	E852.8	E937.8	E950.2	E962.0	E980.2
Tetryl	983.0	E864.0	—	E950.7	E962.1	E980.6
Thalidomide	967.8	E852.8	E937.8	E950.2	E962.0	E980.2
Thallium (compounds) (dust) NEC	985.8	E866.4	—	E950.9	E962.1	E980.9
pesticide (rodenticide)	985.8	E863.7	—	E950.6	E962.1	E980.7
THC	969.6	E854.1	E939.6	E950.3	E962.0	E980.3
Thebacon	965.09	E850.2	E935.2	E950.0	E962.0	E980.0
Thebaine	965.09	E850.2	E935.2	E950.0	E962.0	E980.0
Theobromine (calcium salicylate)	974.1	E858.5	E944.1	E950.4	E962.0	E980.4
Theophylline (diuretic)	974.1	E858.5	E944.1	E950.4	E962.0	E980.4
ethylenediamine	975.7	E858.6	E945.7	E950.4	E962.0	E980.4
Thiabendazole	961.6	E857	E931.6	E950.4	E962.0	E980.4
Thialbarbital, thialbarbitone	968.3	E855.1	E938.3	E950.4	E962.0	E980.4
Thiamine	963.5	E858.1	E933.5	E950.4	E962.0	E980.4
Thiamylal (sodium)	968.3	E855.1	E938.3	E950.4	E962.0	E980.4
Thiazesim	969.0	E854.0	E939.0	E950.3	E962.0	E980.3
Thiazides (diuretics)	974.3	E858.5	E944.3	E950.4	E962.0	E980.4
Thiethylperazine	963.0	E858.1	E933.0	E950.4	E962.0	E980.4
Thimerosal (topical)	976.0	E858.7	E946.0	E950.4	E962.0	E980.4
ophthalmic preparation	976.5	E858.7	E946.5	E950.4	E962.0	E980.4
Thioacetazone	961.8	E857	E931.8	E950.4	E962.0	E980.4
Thiobarbiturates	968.3	E855.1	E938.3	E950.4	E962.0	E980.4
Thiobismol	961.2	E857	E931.2	E950.4	E962.0	E980.4
Thiocarbamide	962.8	E858.0	E932.8	E950.4	E962.0	E980.4
Thiocarbarsone	961.1	E857	E931.1	E950.4	E962.0	E980.4
Thiocarlide	961.8	E857	E931.8	E950.4	E962.0	E980.4
Thioguanine	963.1	E858.1	E933.1	E950.4	E962.0	E980.4
Thiomercaptomerin	974.0	E858.5	E944.0	E950.4	E962.0	E980.4
Thiomerin	974.0	E858.5	E944.0	E950.4	E962.0	E980.4
Thiopental, thiopentone (sodium)	968.3	E855.1	E938.3	E950.4	E962.0	E980.4
Thiopropazate	969.1	E853.0	E939.1	E950.3	E962.0	E980.3
Thioproperazine	969.1	E853.0	E939.1	E950.3	E962.0	E980.3
Thioridazine	969.1	E853.0	E939.1	E950.3	E962.0	E980.3
Thio-TEPA, thiotepa	963.1	E858.1	E933.1	E950.4	E962.0	E980.4
Thiothixene	969.3	E853.8	E939.3	E950.3	E962.0	E980.3
Thiouracil	962.8	E858.0	E932.8	E950.4	E962.0	E980.4
Thiourea	962.8	E858.0	E932.8	E950.4	E962.0	E980.4
Thiphenamil	971.1	E855.4	E941.1	E950.4	E962.0	E980.4
Thiram NEC	989.4	E863.6	—	E950.6	E962.1	E980.7
medicinal	976.2	E858.7	E946.2	E950.4	E962.0	E980.4
Thonzylamine	963.0	E858.1	E933.0	E950.4	E962.0	E980.4
Thorazine	969.1	E853.0	E939.1	E950.3	E962.0	E980.3
Thornapple	988.2	E865.4	—	E950.9	E962.1	E980.9
Throat preparation (lozenges) NEC	976.6	E858.7	E946.6	E950.4	E962.0	E980.4
Thrombin	964.5	E858.2	E934.5	E950.4	E962.0	E980.4
Thrombolysin	964.4	E858.2	E934.4	E950.4	E962.0	E980.4
Thymol	983.0	E864.0	—	E950.7	E962.1	E980.6
Thymus extract	962.9	E858.0	E932.9	E950.4	E962.0	E980.4
Thyroglobulin	962.7	E858.0	E932.7	E950.4	E962.0	E980.4
Thyroid (derivatives) (extract)	962.7	E858.0	E932.7	E950.4	E962.0	E980.4
Thyrolar	962.7	E858.0	E932.7	E950.4	E962.0	E980.4
Thyrothrophin, thyrotropin	977.8	E858.8	E947.8	E950.4	E962.0	E980.4
Thyroxin(e)	962.7	E858.0	E932.7	E950.4	E962.0	E980.4
Tigan	963.0	E858.1	E933.0	E950.4	E962.0	E980.4
Tigloidine	968.0	E855.1	E938.0	E950.4	E962.0	E980.4
Tin (chloride) (dust) (oxide) NEC	985.8	E866.4	—	E950.9	E962.1	E980.9
anti-infectives	961.2	E857	E931.2	E950.4	E962.0	E980.4
Tinactin	976.0	E858.7	E946.0	E950.4	E962.0	E980.4
Tincture, iodine — *see* Iodine						
Tindal	969.1	E853.0	E939.1	E950.3	E962.0	E980.3
Titanium (compounds) (vapor)	985.8	E866.4	—	E950.9	E962.1	E980.9
ointment	976.3	E858.7	E946.3	E950.4	E962.0	E980.4
Titroid	962.7	E858.0	E932.7	E950.4	E962.0	E980.4
TMTD — *see* Tetramethylthiuram disulfide						
TNT	989.89	E866.8	—	E950.9	E962.1	E980.9
fumes	987.8	E869.8	—	E952.8	E962.2	E982.8
Toadstool	988.1	E865.5	—	E950.9	E962.1	E980.9
Tobacco NEC	989.84	E866.8	—	E950.9	E962.1	E980.9
Indian	988.2	E865.4	—	E950.9	E962.1	E980.9
smoke, second-hand	987.8	E869.4	—	—	—	—
Tocopherol	963.5	E858.1	E933.5	E950.4	E962.0	E980.4
Tocosamine	975.0	E858.6	E945.0	E950.4	E962.0	E980.4
Tofranil	969.0	E854.0	E939.0	E950.3	E962.0	E980.3
Toilet deodorizer	989.89	E866.8	—	E950.9	E962.1	E980.9
Tolazamide	962.3	E858.0	E932.3	E950.4	E962.0	E980.4
Tolazoline	971.3	E855.6	E941.3	E950.4	E962.0	E980.4
Tolbutamide	962.3	E858.0	E932.3	E950.4	E962.0	E980.4
sodium	977.8	E858.8	E947.8	E950.4	E962.0	E980.4
Tolmetin	965.69	E850.6	E935.6	E950.0	E962.0	E980.0
Tolnaftate	976.0	E858.7	E946.0	E950.4	E962.0	E980.4
Tolpropamine	976.1	E858.7	E946.1	E950.4	E962.0	E980.4
Tolserol	968.0	E855.1	E938.0	E950.4	E962.0	E980.4
Toluene (liquid) (vapor)	982.0	E862.4	—	E950.9	E962.1	E980.9
diisocyanate	983.0	E864.0	—	E950.7	E962.1	E980.6
Toluidine	983.0	E864.0	—	E950.7	E962.1	E980.6
vapor	987.8	E869.8	—	E952.8	E962.2	E982.8
Toluol (liquid) (vapor)	982.0	E862.4	—	E950.9	E962.1	E980.9
Tolylene-2, 4-diisocyanate	983.0	E864.0	—	E950.7	E962.1	E980.6
Tonics, cardiac	972.1	E858.3	E942.1	E950.4	E962.0	E980.4
Toxaphene (dust) (spray)	989.2	E863.0	—	E950.6	E962.1	E980.7
Toxoids NEC	978.8	E858.8	E948.8	E950.4	E962.0	E980.4
Tractor fuel NEC	981	E862.1	—	E950.9	E962.1	E980.9
Tragacanth	973.3	E858.4	E943.3	E950.4	E962.0	E980.4
Tramazoline	971.2	E855.5	E941.2	E950.4	E962.0	E980.4
Tranquilizers	969.5	E853.9	E939.5	E950.3	E962.0	E980.3
benzodiazepine-based	969.4	E853.2	E939.4	E950.3	E962.0	E980.3
butyrophenone-based	969.2	E853.1	E939.2	E950.3	E962.0	E980.3
major NEC	969.3	E853.8	E939.3	E950.3	E962.0	E980.3
phenothiazine-based	969.1	E853.0	E939.1	E950.3	E962.0	E980.3
specified NEC	969.5	E853.8	E939.5	E950.3	E962.0	E980.3
Trantoin	961.9	E857	E931.9	E950.4	E962.0	E980.4
Tranxene	969.4	E853.2	E939.4	E950.3	E962.0	E980.3
Tranylcypromine (sulfate)	969.0	E854.0	E939.0	E950.3	E962.0	E980.3
Trasentine	975.1	E858.6	E945.1	E950.4	E962.0	E980.4
Travert	974.5	E858.5	E944.5	E950.4	E962.0	E980.4
Trecator	961.8	E857	E931.8	E950.4	E962.0	E980.4
Tretinoin	976.8	E858.7	E946.8	E950.4	E962.0	E980.4
Triacetin	976.0	E858.7	E946.0	E950.4	E962.0	E980.4
Triacetyloleandomycin	960.3	E856	E930.3	E950.4	E962.0	E980.4
Triamcinolone	962.0	E858.0	E932.0	E950.4	E962.0	E980.4
ENT agent	976.6	E858.7	E946.6	E950.4	E962.0	E980.4
ophthalmic preparation	976.5	E858.7	E946.5	E950.4	E962.0	E980.4
topical NEC	976.0	E858.7	E946.0	E950.4	E962.0	E980.4

☑ Additional Digit Required — Refer to the Tabular List (Numeric Code Section) for Additional Digit Selection

▶◀ Revised Text ● New Line ▲ Revised Code

		External Cause (E-Code)				
	Poisoning	Accident	Therapeutic Use	Suicide Attempt	Assault	Undetermined
Triamterene	974.4	E858.5	E944.4	E950.4	E962.0	E980.4
Triaziquone	963.1	E858.1	E933.1	E950.4	E962.0	E980.4
Tribromacetaldehyde	967.3	E852.2	E937.3	E950.2	E962.0	E980.2
Tribromoethanol	968.2	E855.1	E938.2	E950.4	E962.0	E980.4
Tribromomethane	967.3	E852.2	E937.3	E950.2	E962.0	E980.2
Trichlorethane	982.3	E862.4	—	E950.9	E962.1	E980.9
Trichlormethiazide	974.3	E858.5	E944.3	E950.4	E962.0	E980.4
Trichloroacetic acid	983.1	E864.1	—	E950.7	E962.1	E980.6
medicinal (keratolytic)	976.4	E858.7	E946.4	E950.4	E962.0	E980.4
Trichloroethanol	967.1	E852.0	E937.1	E950.2	E962.0	E980.2
Trichloroethylene (liquid) (vapor)	982.3	E862.4	—	E950.9	E962.1	E980.9
anesthetic (gas)	968.2	E855.1	E938.2	E950.4	E962.0	E980.4
Trichloroethyl phosphate	967.1	E852.0	E937.1	E950.2	E962.0	E980.2
Trichlorofluoromethane NEC	987.4	E869.2	—	E952.8	E962.2	E982.8
Trichlorotriethylamine	963.1	E858.1	E933.1	E950.4	E962.0	E980.4
Trichomonacides NEC	961.5	E857	E931.5	E950.4	E962.0	E980.4
Trichomycin	960.1	E856	E930.1	E950.4	E962.0	E980.4
Triclofos	967.1	E852.0	E937.1	E950.2	E962.0	E980.2
Tricresyl phosphate	989.89	E866.8	—	E950.9	E962.1	E980.9
solvent	982.8	E862.4	—	E950.9	E962.1	E980.9
Tricyclamol	966.4	E855.0	E936.4	E950.4	E962.0	E980.4
Tridesilon	976.0	E858.7	E946.0	E950.4	E962.0	E980.4
Tridihexethyl	971.1	E855.4	E941.1	E950.4	E962.0	E980.4
Tridione	966.0	E855.0	E936.0	E950.4	E962.0	E980.4
Triethanolamine NEC	983.2	E864.2	—	E950.7	E962.1	E980.6
detergent	983.2	E861.0	—	E950.7	E962.1	E980.6
trinitrate	972.4	E858.3	E942.4	E950.4	E962.0	E980.4
Triethanomelamine	963.1	E858.1	E933.1	E950.4	E962.0	E980.4
Triethylene melamine	963.1	E858.1	E933.1	E950.4	E962.0	E980.4
Triethylenephosphoramide	963.1	E858.1	E933.1	E950.4	E962.0	E980.4
Triethylenethiophosphoramide	963.1	E858.1	E933.1	E950.4	E962.0	E980.4
Trifluoperazine	969.1	E853.0	E939.1	E950.3	E962.0	E980.3
Trifluperidol	969.2	E853.1	E939.2	E950.3	E962.0	E980.3
Triflupromazine	969.1	E853.0	E939.1	E950.3	E962.0	E980.3
Trihexyphenidyl	971.1	E855.4	E941.1	E950.4	E962.0	E980.4
Triiodothyronine	962.7	E858.0	E932.7	E950.4	E962.0	E980.4
Trilene	968.2	E855.1	E938.2	E950.4	E962.0	E980.4
Trimeprazine	963.0	E858.1	E933.0	E950.4	E962.0	E980.4
Trimetazidine	972.4	E858.3	E942.4	E950.4	E962.0	E980.4
Trimethadione	966.0	E855.0	E936.0	E950.4	E962.0	E980.4
Trimethaphan	972.3	E858.3	E942.3	E950.4	E962.0	E980.4
Trimethidinium	972.3	E858.3	E942.3	E950.4	E962.0	E980.4
Trimethobenzamide	963.0	E858.1	E933.0	E950.4	E962.0	E980.4
Trimethylcarbinol	980.8	E860.8	—	E950.9	E962.1	E980.9
Trimethylpsoralen	976.3	E858.7	E946.3	E950.4	E962.0	E980.4
Trimeton	963.0	E858.1	E933.0	E950.4	E962.0	E980.4
Trimipramine	969.0	E854.0	E939.0	E950.3	E962.0	E980.3
Trimustine	963.1	E858.1	E933.1	E950.4	E962.0	E980.4
Trinitrin	972.4	E858.3	E942.4	E950.4	E962.0	E980.4
Trinitrophenol	983.0	E864.0	—	E950.7	E962.1	E980.6
Trinitrotoluene	989.89	E866.8	—	E950.9	E962.1	E980.9
fumes	987.8	E869.8	—	E952.8	E962.2	E982.8
Trional	967.8	E852.8	E937.8	E950.2	E962.0	E980.2
Trioxide of arsenic — *see* Arsenic						
Trioxsalen	976.3	E858.7	E946.3	E950.4	E962.0	E980.4
Tripelennamine	963.0	E858.1	E933.0	E950.4	E962.0	E980.4
Triperidol	969.2	E853.1	E939.2	E950.3	E962.0	E980.3
Triprolidine	963.0	E858.1	E933.0	E950.4	E962.0	E980.4
Trisoralen	976.3	E858.7	E946.3	E950.4	E962.0	E980.4
Troleandomycin	960.3	E856	E930.3	E950.4	E962.0	E980.4
Trolnitrate (phosphate)	972.4	E858.3	E942.4	E950.4	E962.0	E980.4
Trometamol	963.3	E858.1	E933.3	E950.4	E962.0	E980.4
Tromethamine	963.3	E858.1	E933.3	E950.4	E962.0	E980.4
Tronothane	968.5	E855.2	E938.5	E950.4	E962.0	E980.4
Tropicamide	971.1	E855.4	E941.1	E950.4	E962.0	E980.4
Troxidone	966.0	E855.0	E936.0	E950.4	E962.0	E980.4
Tryparsamide	961.1	E857	E931.1	E950.4	E962.0	E980.4
Trypsin	963.4	E858.1	E933.4	E950.4	E962.0	E980.4
Tryptizol	969.0	E854.0	E939.0	E950.3	E962.0	E980.3
Tuaminoheptane	971.2	E855.5	E941.2	E950.4	E962.0	E980.4
Tuberculin (old)	977.8	E858.8	E947.8	E950.4	E962.0	E980.4
Tubocurare	975.2	E858.6	E945.2	E950.4	E962.0	E980.4
Tubocurarine	975.2	E858.6	E945.2	E950.4	E962.0	E980.4
Turkish green	969.6	E854.1	E939.6	E950.3	E962.0	E980.3
Turpentine (spirits of) (liquid) (vapor)	982.8	E862.4	—	E950.9	E962.1	E980.9
Tybamate	969.5	E853.8	E939.5	E950.3	E962.0	E980.3
Tyloxapol	975.5	E858.6	E945.5	E950.4	E962.0	E980.4
Tymazoline	971.2	E855.5	E941.2	E950.4	E962.0	E980.4
Typhoid vaccine	978.1	E858.8	E948.1	E950.4	E962.0	E980.4
Typhus vaccine	979.2	E858.8	E949.2	E950.4	E962.0	E980.4
Tyrothricin	976.0	E858.7	E946.0	E950.4	E962.0	E980.4
ENT agent	976.6	E858.7	E946.6	E950.4	E962.0	E980.4
ophthalmic preparation	976.5	E858.7	E946.5	E950.4	E962.0	E980.4
Undecenoic acid	976.0	E858.7	E946.0	E950.4	E962.0	E980.4
Undecylenic acid	976.0	E858.7	E946.0	E950.4	E962.0	E980.4
Unna's boot	976.3	E858.7	E946.3	E950.4	E962.0	E980.4
Uracil mustard	963.1	E858.1	E933.1	E950.4	E962.0	E980.4
Uramustine	963.1	E858.1	E933.1	E950.4	E962.0	E980.4
Urari	975.2	E858.6	E945.2	E950.4	E962.0	E980.4
Urea	974.4	E858.5	E944.4	E950.4	E962.0	E980.4
topical	976.8	E858.7	E946.8	E950.4	E962.0	E980.4
Urethan(e) (antineoplastic)	963.1	E858.1	E933.1	E950.4	E962.0	E980.4
Urginea (maritima) (scilla) — *see* Squill						
Uric acid metabolism agents NEC	974.7	E858.5	E944.7	E950.4	E962.0	E980.4
Urokinase	964.4	E858.2	E934.4	E950.4	E962.0	E980.4
Urokon	977.8	E858.8	E947.8	E950.4	E962.0	E980.4
Urotropin	961.9	E857	E931.9	E950.4	E962.0	E980.4
Urtica	988.2	E865.4	—	E950.9	E962.1	E980.9
Utility gas — *see* Gas, utility						
Vaccine NEC	979.9	E858.8	E949.9	E950.4	E962.0	E980.4
bacterial NEC	978.8	E858.8	E948.8	E950.4	E962.0	E980.4
with						
other bacterial component	978.9	E858.8	E948.9	E950.4	E962.0	E980.4
pertussis component	978.6	E858.8	E948.6	E950.4	E962.0	E980.4
viral-rickettsial component	979.7	E858.8	E949.7	E950.4	E962.0	E980.4
mixed NEC	978.9	E858.8	E948.9	E950.4	E962.0	E980.4
BCG	978.0	E858.8	E948.0	E950.4	E962.0	E980.4
cholera	978.2	E858.8	E948.2	E950.4	E962.0	E980.4
diphtheria	978.5	E858.8	E948.5	E950.4	E962.0	E980.4
influenza	979.6	E858.8	E949.6	E950.4	E962.0	E980.4
measles	979.4	E858.8	E949.4	E950.4	E962.0	E980.4
meningococcal	978.8	E858.8	E948.8	E950.4	E962.0	E980.4
mumps	979.6	E858.8	E949.6	E950.4	E962.0	E980.4
paratyphoid	978.1	E858.8	E948.1	E950.4	E962.0	E980.4
pertussis (with diphtheria toxoid) (with tetanus toxoid)	978.6	E858.8	E948.6	E950.4	E962.0	E980.4
plague	978.3	E858.8	E948.3	E950.4	E962.0	E980.4
poliomyelitis	979.5	E858.8	E949.5	E950.4	E962.0	E980.4
poliovirus	979.5	E858.8	E949.5	E950.4	E962.0	E980.4
rabies	979.1	E858.8	E949.1	E950.4	E962.0	E980.4
respiratory syncytial virus	979.6	E858.8	E949.6	E950.4	E962.0	E980.4
rickettsial NEC	979.6	E858.8	E949.6	E950.4	E962.0	E980.4
with						
bacterial component	979.7	E858.8	E949.7	E950.4	E962.0	E980.4
pertussis component	978.6	E858.8	E948.6	E950.4	E962.0	E980.4
viral component	979.7	E858.8	E949.7	E950.4	E962.0	E980.4
Rocky mountain spotted fever	979.6	E858.8	E949.6	E950.4	E962.0	E980.4
rotavirus	979.6	E858.8	E949.6	E950.4	E962.0	E980.4
rubella virus	979.4	E858.8	E949.4	E950.4	E962.0	E980.4
sabin oral	979.5	E858.8	E949.5	E950.4	E962.0	E980.4
smallpox	979.0	E858.8	E949.0	E950.4	E962.0	E980.4
tetanus	978.4	E858.8	E948.4	E950.4	E962.0	E980.4
typhoid	978.1	E858.8	E948.1	E950.4	E962.0	E980.4
typhus	979.2	E858.8	E949.2	E950.4	E962.0	E980.4
viral NEC	979.6	E858.8	E949.6	E950.4	E962.0	E980.4
with						
bacterial component	979.7	E858.8	E949.7	E950.4	E962.0	E980.4
pertussis component	978.6	E858.8	E948.6	E950.4	E962.0	E980.4
rickettsial component	979.7	E858.8	E949.7	E950.4	E962.0	E980.4
yellow fever	979.3	E858.8	E949.3	E950.4	E962.0	E980.4
Vaccinia immune globulin (human)	964.6	E858.2	E934.6	E950.4	E962.0	E980.4
Vaginal contraceptives	976.8	E858.7	E946.8	E950.4	E962.0	E980.4
Valethamate	971.1	E855.4	E941.1	E950.4	E962.0	E980.4

☑ Additional Digit Required — Refer to the Tabular List (Numeric Code Section) for Additional Digit Selection

▶◀ Revised Text ● New Line ▲ Revised Code

	Poisoning	External Cause (E-Code) Accident	Therapeutic Use	Suicide Attempt	Assault	Undetermined
Valisone	976.0	E858.7	E946.0	E950.4	E962.0	E980.4
Valium	969.4	E853.2	E939.4	E950.3	E962.0	E980.3
Valmid	967.8	E852.8	E937.8	E950.2	E962.0	E980.2
Vanadium	985.8	E866.4	—	E950.9	E962.1	E980.9
Vancomycin	960.8	E856	E930.8	E950.4	E962.0	E980.4
Vapor (*see also* Gas)	987.9	E869.9	—	E952.9	E962.2	E982.9
kiln (carbon monoxide)	986	E868.8	—	E952.1	E962.2	E982.1
lead — *see* Lead						
specified source NEC (*see also* specific substance)	987.8	E869.8	—	E952.8	E962.2	E982.8
Varidase	964.4	E858.2	E934.4	E950.4	E962.0	E980.4
Varnish	989.89	E861.6	—	E950.9	E962.1	E980.9
cleaner	982.8	E862.9	—	E950.9	E962.1	E980.9
Vaseline	976.3	E858.7	E946.3	E950.4	E962.0	E980.4
Vasodilan	972.5	E858.3	E942.5	E950.4	E962.0	E980.4
Vasodilators NEC	972.5	E858.3	E942.5	E950.4	E962.0	E980.4
coronary	972.4	E858.3	E942.4	E950.4	E962.0	E980.4
Vasopressin	962.5	E858.0	E932.5	E950.4	E962.0	E980.4
Vasopressor drugs	962.5	E858.0	E932.5	E950.4	E962.0	E980.4
Venom, venomous (bite) (sting)	989.5	E905.9	—	E950.9	E962.1	E980.9
arthropod NEC	989.5	E905.5	—	E950.9	E962.1	E980.9
bee	989.5	E905.3	—	E950.9	E962.1	E980.9
centipede	989.5	E905.4	—	E950.9	E962.1	E980.9
hornet	989.5	E905.3	—	E950.9	E962.1	E980.9
lizard	989.5	E905.0	—	E950.9	E962.1	E980.9
marine animals or plants	989.5	E905.6	—	E950.9	E962.1	E980.9
millipede (tropical)	989.5	E905.4	—	E950.9	E962.1	E980.9
plant NEC	989.5	E905.7	—	E950.9	E962.1	E980.9
marine	989.5	E905.6	—	E950.9	E962.1	E980.9
scorpion	989.5	E905.2	—	E950.9	E962.1	E980.9
snake	989.5	E905.0	—	E950.9	E962.1	E980.9
specified NEC	989.5	E905.8	—	E950.9	E962.1	E980.9
spider	989.5	E905.1	—	E950.9	E962.1	E980.9
wasp	989.5	E905.3	—	E950.9	E962.1	E980.9
Veramon	967.0	E851	E937.0	E950.1	E962.0	E980.1
Veratrum						
album	988.2	E865.4	—	E950.9	E962.1	E980.9
alkaloids	972.6	E858.3	E942.6	E950.4	E962.0	E980.4
viride	988.2	E865.4	—	E950.9	E962.1	E980.9
Verdigris (*see also* Copper)	985.8	E866.4	—	E950.9	E962.1	E980.9
Veronal	967.0	E851	E937.0	E950.1	E962.0	E980.1
Veroxil	961.6	E857	E931.6	E950.4	E962.0	E980.4
Versidyne	965.7	E850.7	E935.7	E950.0	E962.0	E980.0
Viagra	972.5	E858.3	E942.5	E950.4	E962.0	E980.4
Vienna						
green	985.1	E866.3	—	E950.8	E962.1	E980.8
insecticide	985.1	E863.4	—	E950.6	E962.1	E980.7
red	989.89	E866.8	—	E950.9	E962.1	E980.9
pharmaceutical dye	977.4	E858.8	E947.4	E950.4	E962.0	E980.4
Vinbarbital, vinbarbitone	967.0	E851	E937.0	E950.1	E962.0	E980.1
Vinblastine	963.1	E858.1	E933.1	E950.4	E962.0	E980.4
Vincristine	963.1	E858.1	E933.1	E950.4	E962.0	E980.4
Vinesthene, vinethene	968.2	E855.1	E938.2	E950.4	E962.0	E980.4
Vinyl						
bital	967.0	E851	E937.0	E950.1	E962.0	E980.1
ether	968.2	E855.1	E938.2	E950.4	E962.0	E980.4
Vioform	961.3	E857	E931.3	E950.4	E962.0	E980.4
topical	976.0	E858.7	E946.0	E950.4	E962.0	E980.4
Viomycin	960.6	E856	E930.6	E950.4	E962.0	E980.4
Viosterol	963.5	E858.1	E933.5	E950.4	E962.0	E980.4
Viper (venom)	989.5	E905.0	—	E950.9	E962.1	E980.9
Viprynium (embonate)	961.6	E857	E931.6	E950.4	E962.0	E980.4
Virugon	961.7	E857	E931.7	E950.4	E962.0	E980.4
Visine	976.5	E858.7	E946.5	E950.4	E962.0	E980.4
Vitamins NEC	963.5	E858.1	E933.5	E950.4	E962.0	E980.4
B_{12}	964.1	E858.2	E934.1	E950.4	E962.0	E980.4
hematopoietic	964.1	E858.2	E934.1	E950.4	E962.0	E980.4
K	964.3	E858.2	E934.3	E950.4	E962.0	E980.4
Vleminckx's solution	976.4	E858.7	E946.4	E950.4	E962.0	E980.4
Voltaren — *see* Diclofenac sodium						
Ventolin — *see* Salbutamol sulfate						
Warfarin (potassium) (sodium)	964.2	E858.2	E934.2	E950.4	E962.0	E980.4
rodenticide	989.4	E863.7	—	E950.6	E962.1	E980.7
Wasp (sting)	989.5	E905.3	—	E950.9	E962.1	E980.9
Water						
balance agents NEC	974.5	E858.5	E944.5	E950.4	E962.0	E980.4
Water — *continued*						
gas	987.1	E868.1	—	E951.8	E962.2	E981.8
incomplete combustion of — *see* Carbon, monoxide, fuel, utility						
hemlock	988.2	E865.4	—	E950.9	E962.1	E980.9
moccasin (venom)	989.5	E905.0	—	E950.9	E962.1	E980.9
Wax (paraffin) (petroleum)	981	E862.3	—	E950.9	E962.1	E980.9
automobile	989.89	E861.2	—	E950.9	E962.1	E980.9
floor	981	E862.0	—	E950.9	E962.1	E980.9
Weed killers NEC	989.4	E863.5	—	E950.6	E962.1	E980.7
Welldorm	967.1	E852.0	E937.1	E950.2	E962.0	E980.2
White						
arsenic — *see* Arsenic						
hellebore	988.2	E865.4	—	E950.9	E962.1	E980.9
lotion (keratolytic)	976.4	E858.7	E946.4	E950.4	E962.0	E980.4
spirit	981	E862.0	—	E950.9	E962.1	E980.9
Whitewashes	989.89	E861.6	—	E950.9	E962.1	E980.9
Whole blood	964.7	E858.2	E934.7	E950.4	E962.0	E980.4
Wild						
black cherry	988.2	E865.4	—	E950.9	E962.1	E980.9
poisonous plants NEC	988.2	E865.4	—	E950.9	E962.1	E980.9
Window cleaning fluid	989.89	E861.3	—	E950.9	E962.1	E980.9
Wintergreen (oil)	976.3	E858.7	E946.3	E950.4	E962.0	E980.4
Witch hazel	976.2	E858.7	E946.2	E950.4	E962.0	E980.4
Wood						
alcohol	980.1	E860.2	—	E950.9	E962.1	E980.9
spirit	980.1	E860.2	—	E950.9	E962.1	E980.9
Woorali	975.2	E858.6	E945.2	E950.4	E962.0	E980.4
Wormseed, American	961.6	E857	E931.6	E950.4	E962.0	E980.4
Xanthine diuretics	974.1	E858.5	E944.1	E950.4	E962.0	E980.4
Xanthocillin	960.0	E856	E930.0	E950.4	E962.0	E980.4
Xanthotoxin	976.3	E858.7	E946.3	E950.4	E962.0	E980.4
Xigris	964.2	E858.2	E934.2	E950.4	E962.0	E980.4
Xylene (liquid) (vapor)	982.0	E862.4	—	E950.9	E962.1	E980.9
Xylocaine (infiltration) (topical)	968.5	E855.2	E938.5	E950.4	E962.0	E980.4
nerve block (peripheral) (plexus)	968.6	E855.2	E938.6	E950.4	E962.0	E980.4
spinal	968.7	E855.2	E938.7	E950.4	E962.0	E980.4
Xylol (liquid) (vapor)	982.0	E862.4	—	E950.9	E962.1	E980.9
Xylometazoline	971.2	E855.5	E941.2	E950.4	E962.0	E980.4
Yellow						
fever vaccine	979.3	E858.8	E949.3	E950.4	E962.0	E980.4
jasmine	988.2	E865.4	—	E950.9	E962.1	E980.9
Yew	988.2	E865.4	—	E950.9	E962.1	E980.9
Zactane	965.7	E850.7	E935.7	E950.0	E962.0	E980.0
Zaroxolyn	974.3	E858.5	E944.3	E950.4	E962.0	E980.4
Zephiran (topical)	976.0	E858.7	E946.0	E950.4	E962.0	E980.4
ophthalmic preparation	976.5	E858.7	E946.5	E950.4	E962.0	E980.4
Zerone	980.1	E860.2	—	E950.9	E962.1	E980.9
Zinc (compounds) (fumes) (salts) (vapor) NEC	985.8	E866.4	—	E950.9	E962.1	E980.9
anti-infectives	976.0	E858.7	E946.0	E950.4	E962.0	E980.4
antivaricose	972.7	E858.3	E942.7	E950.4	E962.0	E980.4
bacitracin	976.0	E858.7	E946.0	E950.4	E962.0	E980.4
chloride	976.2	E858.7	E946.2	E950.4	E962.0	E980.4
gelatin	976.3	E858.7	E946.3	E950.4	E962.0	E980.4
oxide	976.3	E858.7	E946.3	E950.4	E962.0	E980.4
peroxide	976.0	E858.7	E946.0	E950.4	E962.0	E980.4
pesticides	985.8	E863.4	—	E950.6	E962.1	E980.7
phosphide (rodenticide)	985.8	E863.7	—	E950.6	E962.1	E980.7
stearate	976.3	E858.7	E946.3	E950.4	E962.0	E980.4
sulfate (antivaricose)	972.7	E858.3	E942.7	E950.4	E962.0	E980.4
ENT agent	976.6	E858.7	E946.6	E950.4	E962.0	E980.4
ophthalmic solution	976.5	E858.7	E946.5	E950.4	E962.0	E980.4
topical NEC	976.0	E858.7	E946.0	E950.4	E962.0	E980.4
undecylenate	976.0	E858.7	E946.0	E950.4	E962.0	E980.4
Zovant	964.2	E858.2	E934.2	E950.4	E962.0	E980.4
Zoxazolamine	968.0	E855.1	E938.0	E950.4	E962.0	E980.4
Zygadenus (venenosus)	988.2	E865.4	—	E950.9	E962.1	E980.9

SECTION 3

Alphabetic Index to External Causes of Injury and Poisoning (E Code)

This section contains the index to the codes which classify environmental events, circumstances, and other conditions as the cause of injury and other adverse effects. Where a code from the section Supplementary Classification of External Causes of Injury and Poisoning (E800-E999) is applicable, it is intended that the E code shall be used in addition to a code from the main body of the classification, Chapters 1 to 17.

The alphabetic index to the E codes is organized by main terms which describe the *accident, circumstance, event,* or *specific agent* which caused the injury or other adverse effect.

Note — Transport accidents (E800-E848) include accidents involving:

aircraft and spacecraft (E840-E845)

watercraft (E830-E838)

motor vehicle (E810-E825)

railway (E800-E807)

other road vehicles (E826-E829)

For definitions and examples related to transport accidents — see Volume 1 code categories E800-E848.

The fourth-digit subdivisions for use with categories E800-E848 to identify the injured person are found at the end of this section.

For identifying the place in which an accident or poisoning occurred (circumstances classifiable to categories E850-E869 and E880-E928) — see the listing in this section under "Accident, occurring."

See the Table of Drugs and Chemicals (Section 2 of this volume) for identifying the specific agent involved in drug overdose or a wrong substance given or taken in error, and for intoxication or poisoning by a drug or other chemical substance.

The specific adverse effect, reaction, or localized toxic effect to a correct drug or substance properly administered in therapeutic or prophylactic dosage should be classified according to the nature of the adverse effect (e.g., allergy, dermatitis, tachycardia) listed in Section 1 of this volume.

A

- **Abandonment**
  - causing exposure to weather conditions — *see* Exposure
  - child, with intent to injure or kill E968.4
  - helpless person, infant, newborn E904.0
    - with intent to injure or kill E968.4
- **Abortion, criminal, injury to child** E968.8
- **Abuse** (alleged) (suspected)
  - adult
    - by
      - child E967.4
      - ex-partner E967.3
      - ex-spouse E967.3
      - father E967.0
      - grandchild E967.7
      - grandparent E967.6
      - mother E967.2
      - non-related caregiver E967.8
      - other relative E967.7
      - other specified person E967.1
      - partner E967.3
      - sibling E967.5
      - spouse E967.3
      - stepfather E967.0
      - stepmother E967.2
      - unspecified person E967.9
  - child
    - by
      - boyfriend of parent or guardian E967.0
      - child E967.4
      - father E967.0
      - female partner of parent or guardian E967.2
      - girlfriend of parent or guardian E967.2
      - grandchild E967.7
      - grandparent E967.6
      - male partner of parent or guardian E967.0
      - mother E967.2
      - non-related caregiver E967.8
      - other relative E967.7
      - other specified person(s) E967.1
      - sibling E967.5
      - stepfather E967.0
      - stepmother E967.2
      - unspecified person E967.9
- **Accident (to)** E928.9
  - aircraft (in transit) (powered) E841 ☑
    - at landing, take-off E840 ☑
    - due to, caused by cataclysm — *see* categories E908 ☑, E909 ☑
    - late effect of E929.1
    - unpowered (*see also* Collision, aircraft, unpowered) E842 ☑
    - while alighting, boarding E843 ☑
  - amphibious vehicle
    - on
      - land — *see* Accident, motor vehicle
      - water — *see* Accident, watercraft
  - animal, ridden NEC E828 ☑
  - animal-drawn vehicle NEC E827 ☑
  - balloon (*see also* Collision, aircraft, unpowered) E842 ☑
  - caused by, due to
    - abrasive wheel (metalworking) E919.3
    - animal NEC E906.9
      - being ridden (in sport or transport) E828 ☑
    - avalanche NEC E909.2
    - band saw E919.4
    - bench saw E919.4
    - bore, earth-drilling or mining (land) (seabed) E919.1
    - bulldozer E919.7
    - cataclysmic
      - earth surface movement or eruption E909.9
      - storm E908.9
    - chain
      - hoist E919.2
        - agricultural operations E919.0
        - mining operations E919.1
      - saw E920.1
    - circular saw E919.4

Accident (to) — *continued*
  - caused by, due to — *continued*
    - cold (excessive) (*see also* Cold, exposure to) E901.9
    - combine E919.0
    - conflagration — *see* Conflagration
    - corrosive liquid, substance NEC E924.1
    - cotton gin E919.8
    - crane E919.2
      - agricultural operations E919.0
      - mining operations E919.1
    - cutting or piercing instrument (*see also* Cut) E920.9
    - dairy equipment E919.8
    - derrick E919.2
      - agricultural operations E919.0
      - mining operations E919.1
    - drill E920.1
      - earth (land) (seabed) E919.1
      - hand (powered) E920.1
        - not powered E920.4
      - metalworking E919.3
      - woodworking E919.4
    - earth(-)
      - drilling machine E919.1
      - moving machine E919.7
      - scraping machine E919.7
    - electric
      - current (*see also* Electric shock) E925.9
      - motor — *see also* Accident, machine, by type of machine
        - current (of) — *see* Electric shock
    - elevator (building) (grain) E919.2
      - agricultural operations E919.0
      - mining operations E919.1
    - environmental factors NEC E928.9
    - excavating machine E919.7
    - explosive material (*see also* Explosion) E923.9
    - farm machine E919.0
    - fire, flames — *see also* Fire
      - conflagration — *see* Conflagration
    - firearm missile — *see* Shooting
    - forging (metalworking) machine E919.3
    - forklift (truck) E919.2
      - agricultural operations E919.0
      - mining operations E919.1
    - gas turbine E919.5
    - harvester E919.0
    - hay derrick, mower, or rake E919.0
    - heat (excessive) (*see also* Heat) E900.9
    - hoist (*see also* Accident, caused by, due to, lift) E919.2
      - chain — *see* Accident, caused by, due to, chain
      - shaft E919.1
    - hot
      - liquid E924.0
        - caustic or corrosive E924.1
      - object (not producing fire or flames) E924.8
      - substance E924.9
        - caustic or corrosive E924.1
        - liquid (metal) NEC E924.0
        - specified type NEC E924.8
    - human bite E928.3
    - ignition — *see* Ignition
    - internal combustion engine E919.5
    - landslide NEC E909.2
    - lathe (metalworking) E919.3
      - turnings E920.8
      - woodworking E919.4
    - lift, lifting (appliances) E919.2
      - agricultural operations E919.0
      - mining operations E919.1
      - shaft E919.1
    - lightning NEC E907
    - machine, machinery — *see also* Accident, machine
      - drilling, metal E919.3
      - manufacturing, for manufacture of
        - beverages E919.8
        - clothing E919.8
        - foodstuffs E919.8
        - paper E919.8
        - textiles E919.8

Accident (to) — *continued*
  - caused by, due to — *continued*
    - machine, machinery — *see also* Accident, machine — *continued*
      - milling, metal E919.3
      - moulding E919.4
      - power press, metal E919.3
      - printing E919.8
      - rolling mill, metal E919.3
      - sawing, metal E919.3
      - specified type NEC E919.8
      - spinning E919.8
      - weaving E919.8
    - natural factor NEC E928.9
    - overhead plane E919.4
    - plane E920.4
      - overhead E919.4
    - powered
      - hand tool NEC E920.1
      - saw E919.4
        - hand E920.1
    - printing machine E919.8
    - pulley (block) E919.2
      - agricultural operations E919.0
      - mining operations E919.1
      - transmission E919.6
    - radial saw E919.4
    - radiation — *see* Radiation
    - reaper E919.0
    - road scraper E919.7
      - when in transport under its own power — *see* categories E810-E825 ☑
    - roller coaster E919.8
    - sander E919.4
    - saw E920.4
      - band E919.4
      - bench E919.4
      - chain E920.1
      - circular E919.4
      - hand E920.4
        - powered E920.1
      - powered, except hand E919.4
      - radial E919.4
    - sawing machine, metal E919.3
    - shaft
      - hoist E919.1
      - lift E919.1
      - transmission E919.6
    - shears E920.4
      - hand E920.4
        - powered E920.1
      - mechanical E919.3
    - shovel E920.4
      - steam E919.7
    - spinning machine E919.8
    - steam — *see also* Burning, steam
      - engine E919.5
      - shovel E919.7
    - thresher E919.0
    - thunderbolt NEC E907
    - tractor E919.0
      - when in transport under its own power — *see* categories E810-E825 ☑
    - transmission belt, cable, chain, gear, pinion, pulley, shaft E919.6
    - turbine (gas) (water driven) E919.5
    - under-cutter E919.1
    - weaving machine E919.8
    - winch E919.2
      - agricultural operations E919.0
      - mining operations E919.1
  - diving E883.0
    - with insufficient air supply E913.2
  - glider (hang) (*see also* Collision, aircraft, unpowered) E842 ☑
  - hovercraft
    - on
      - land — *see* Accident, motor vehicle
      - water — *see* Accident, watercraft
  - ice yacht (*see also* Accident, vehicle NEC) E848
  - in
    - medical, surgical procedure
      - as, or due to misadventure — *see* Misadventure

- **Accident (to)** — *continued*
  - in — *continued*
    - medical, surgical procedure — *continued*
      - causing an abnormal reaction or later complication without mention of misadventure — *see* Reaction, abnormal
  - kite carrying a person (*see also* Collision, involving aircraft, unpowered) E842 ☑
  - land yacht (*see also* Accident, vehicle NEC) E848
  - late effect of — *see* Late effect
  - launching pad E845 ☑
  - machine, machinery (*see also* Accident, caused by, due to, by specific type of machine) E919.9
    - agricultural including animal-powered E919.0
    - earth-drilling E919.1
    - earth moving or scraping E919.7
    - excavating E919.7
    - involving transport under own power on highway or transport vehicle — *see* categories E810-E825 ☑, E840-E845 ☑
    - lifting (appliances) E919.2
    - metalworking E919.3
    - mining E919.1
    - prime movers, except electric motors E919.5
      - electric motors — *see* Accident, machine, by specific type of machine
    - recreational E919.8
    - specified type NEC E919.8
    - transmission E919.6
    - watercraft (deck) (engine room) (galley) (laundry) (loading) E836 ☑
    - woodworking or forming E919.4
  - motor vehicle (on public highway) (traffic) E819 ☑
    - due to cataclysm — *see* categories E908 ☑, E909 ☑
    - involving
      - collision (*see also* Collision, motor vehicle) E812 ☑
    - nontraffic, not on public highway — *see* categories E820-E825 ☑
    - not involving collision — *see* categories E816-E819 ☑
  - nonmotor vehicle NEC E829 ☑
    - nonroad — *see* Accident, vehicle NEC
    - road, except pedal cycle, animal-drawn vehicle, or animal being ridden E829 ☑
  - nonroad vehicle NEC — *see* Accident, vehicle NEC
  - not elsewhere classifiable involving
    - cable car (not on rails) E847
      - on rails E829 ☑
    - coal car in mine E846
    - hand truck — *see* Accident, vehicle NEC
    - logging car E846
    - sled(ge), meaning snow or ice vehicle E848
    - tram, mine or quarry E846
    - truck
      - mine or quarry E846
      - self-propelled, industrial E846
      - station baggage E846
    - tub, mine or quarry E846
    - vehicle NEC E848
      - snow and ice E848
      - used only on industrial premises E846
    - wheelbarrow E848
  - occurring (at) (in)
    - apartment E849.0
    - baseball field, diamond E849.4
    - construction site, any E849.3
    - dock E849.8
      - yard E849.3
    - dormitory E849.7
    - factory (building) (premises) E849.3
    - farm E849.1
      - buildings E849.1
      - house E849.0
    - football field E849.4
    - forest E849.8
    - garage (place of work) E849.3
      - private (home) E849.0

- **Accident (to)** — *continued*
  - occurring (at) (in) — *continued*
    - gravel pit E849.2
    - gymnasium E849.4
    - highway E849.5
    - home (private) (residential) E849.0
      - institutional E849.7
    - hospital E849.7
    - hotel E849.6
    - house (private) (residential) E849.0
      - movie E849.6
      - public E849.6
    - institution, residential E849.7
    - jail E849.7
    - mine E849.2
    - motel E849.6
    - movie house E849.6
    - office (building) E849.6
    - orphanage E849.7
    - park (public) E849.4
      - mobile home E849.8
      - trailer E849.8
    - parking lot or place E849.8
    - place
      - industrial NEC E849.3
      - parking E849.8
      - public E849.8
        - specified place NEC E849.5
      - recreational NEC E849.4
      - sport NEC E849.4
    - playground (park) (school) E849.4
    - prison E849.6
    - public building NEC E849.6
    - quarry E849.2
    - railway
      - line NEC E849.8
      - yard E849.3
    - residence
      - home (private) E849.0
    - resort (beach) (lake) (mountain) (seashore) (vacation) E849.4
    - restaurant E849.6
    - sand pit E849.2
    - school (building) (private) (public) (state) E849.6
      - reform E849.7
      - riding E849.4
    - seashore E849.8
      - resort E849.4
    - shop (place of work) E849.3
      - commercial E849.6
    - skating rink E849.4
    - sports palace E849.4
    - stadium E849.4
    - store E849.6
    - street E849.5
    - swimming pool (public) E849.4
      - private home or garden E849.0
    - tennis court (public) E849.4
    - theatre, theater E849.6
    - trailer court E849.8
    - tunnel E849.8
      - under construction E849.2
    - warehouse E849.3
    - yard
      - dock E849.3
      - industrial E849.3
      - private (home) E849.0
      - railway E849.3
  - off-road type motor vehicle (not on public highway) NEC E821 ☑
    - on public highway — *see* categories E810-E819 ☑
  - pedal cycle E826 ☑
  - railway E807 ☑
    - due to cataclysm — *see* categories E908 ☑, E909 ☑
    - involving
      - avalanche E909.2
      - burning by engine, locomotive, train (*see also* Explosion, railway engine) E803 ☑
      - collision (*see also* Collision, railway) E800 ☑
      - derailment (*see also* Derailment, railway) E802 ☑

- **Accident (to)** — *continued*
  - railway — *continued*
    - involving — *continued*
      - explosion (*see also* Explosion, railway engine) E803 ☑
      - fall (*see also* Fall, from, railway rolling stock) E804 ☑
      - fire (*see also* Explosion, railway engine) E803 ☑
      - hitting by, being struck by
        - object falling in, on, from, rolling stock, train, vehicle E806 ☑
        - rolling stock, train, vehicle E805 ☑
      - overturning, railway rolling stock, train, vehicle (*see also* Derailment, railway) E802 ☑
      - running off rails, railway (*see also* Derailment, railway) E802 ☑
      - specified circumstances NEC E806 ☑
      - train or vehicle hit by
        - avalanche E909.2
        - falling object (earth, rock, tree) E806 ☑
          - due to cataclysm — *see* categories E908 ☑, E909 ☑
        - landslide E909.2
  - roller skate E885.1
  - scooter (nonmotorized) E885.0
  - skateboard E885.2
  - ski(ing) E885.3
    - jump E884.9
    - lift or tow (with chair or gondola) E847
  - snow vehicle, motor driven (not on public highway) E820 ☑
    - on public highway — *see* categories E810-E819 ☑
  - snowboard E885.4
  - spacecraft E845 ☑
  - specified cause NEC E928.8
  - street car E829 ☑
  - traffic NEC E819 ☑
  - vehicle NEC (with pedestrian) E848
    - battery powered
      - airport passenger vehicle E846
      - truck (baggage) (mail) E846
    - powered commercial or industrial (with other vehicle or object within commercial or industrial premises) E846
  - watercraft E838 ☑
    - with
      - drowning or submersion resulting from
        - accident other than to watercraft E832 ☑
        - accident to watercraft E830 ☑
      - injury, except drowning or submersion, resulting from
        - accident other than to watercraft — *see* categories E833-E838 ☑
        - accident to watercraft E831 ☑
    - due to, caused by cataclysm — *see* categories E908 ☑, E909 ☑
    - machinery E836 ☑
- **Acid throwing** E961
- **Acosta syndrome** E902.0
- **Aeroneurosis** E902.1
- **Aero-otitis media** — *see* Effects of, air pressure
- **Aerosinusitis** — *see* Effects of, air pressure
- **After-effect, late** — *see* Late effect
- **Air**
  - blast
    - in
      - terrorism E979.2
      - war operations E993
  - embolism (traumatic) NEC E928.9
    - in
      - infusion or transfusion E874.1
      - perfusion E874.2
  - sickness E903
- **Alpine sickness** E902.0
- **Altitude sickness** — *see* Effects of, air pressure
- **Anaphylactic shock, anaphylaxis** (*see also* Table of Drugs and Chemicals) E947.9
  - due to bite or sting (venomous) — *see* Bite, venomous
- **Andes disease** E902.0

☑ Additional Digit Required — Refer to the Tabular List (Numeric Code Section) for Additional Digit Selection

▶◀ Revised Text ● New Line ▲ Revised Code

- **Collision** — *continued*
  - railway — *continued*
    - and — *continued*
      - object (fallen) (fixed) (movable) (moving) not falling from, set in motion by, aircraft or motor vehicle NEC E801 ☑
      - pedal cycle E801 ☑
      - pedestrian (conveyance) E805 ☑
      - person (using pedestrian conveyance) E805 ☑
      - platform E801 ☑
      - rock on railway E801 ☑
      - street car E801 ☑
  - snow vehicle, motor-driven (not on public highway) E820 ☑
    - and
      - animal (being ridden) (-drawn vehicle) E820 ☑
      - another off-road motor vehicle E820 ☑
      - other motor vehicle, not on public highway E820 ☑
      - other object or vehicle NEC, fixed or movable, not set in motion by aircraft or motor vehicle on highway E820 ☑
      - pedal cycle E820 ☑
      - pedestrian (conveyance) E820 ☑
      - railway train E820 ☑
    - on public highway — *see* Collision, motor vehicle
  - street car(s) E829 ☑
    - and
      - animal, herded, not being ridden, unattended E829 ☑
      - nonmotor road vehicle NEC E829 ☑
      - object (fallen) (fixed) (movable) (moving) not falling from or set in motion by aircraft, animal-drawn vehicle, animal being ridden, motor vehicle, pedal cycle, or railway train E829 ☑
      - pedestrian (conveyance) E829 ☑
      - person (using pedestrian conveyance) E829 ☑
  - vehicle
    - animal-drawn — *see* Collision, animal-drawn vehicle
    - motor — *see* Collision, motor vehicle
    - nonmotor
      - nonroad E848
        - and
          - another nonmotor, nonroad vehicle E848
          - object (fallen) (fixed) (movable) (moving) not falling from or set in motion by aircraft, animal-drawn vehicle, animal being ridden, motor vehicle, nonmotor road vehicle, pedal cycle, railway train, or streetcar E848
      - road, except animal being ridden, animal-drawn vehicle, or pedal cycle E829 ☑
        - and
          - animal, herded, not being ridden, unattended E829 ☑
          - another nonmotor road vehicle, except animal being ridden, animal-drawn vehicle, or pedal cycle E829 ☑
          - object (fallen) (fixed) (movable) (moving) not falling from or set in motion by, aircraft, animal-drawn vehicle, animal being ridden, motor vehicle, pedal cycle, or railway train E829 ☑
          - pedestrian (conveyance) E829 ☑
          - person (using pedestrian conveyance) E829 ☑
          - vehicle, nonmotor, nonroad E829 ☑

- **Collision** — *continued*
  - watercraft E838 ☑
    - and
      - person swimming or water skiing E838 ☑
    - causing
      - drowning, submersion E830 ☑
      - injury except drowning, submersion E831 ☑
- **Combustion, spontaneous** — *see* Ignition
- **Complication of medical or surgical procedure or treatment**
  - as an abnormal reaction — *see* Reaction, abnormal
  - delayed, without mention of misadventure — *see* Reaction, abnormal
  - due to misadventure — *see* Misadventure
- **Compression**
  - divers' squeeze E902.2
  - trachea by
    - food E911
    - foreign body, except food E912
- **Conflagration**
  - building or structure, except private dwelling (barn) (church) (convalescent or residential home) (factory) (farm outbuilding) (hospital) (hotel) (institution) (educational) (domitory) (residential) (school) (shop) (store) (theater) E891.9
    - with or causing (injury due to)
      - accident or injury NEC E891.9
        - specified circumstance NEC E891.8
      - burns, burning E891.3
      - carbon monoxide E891.2
      - fumes E891.2
        - polyvinylchloride (PVC) or similar material E891.1
      - smoke E891.2
    - causing explosion E891.0
    - in terrorism E979.3
  - not in building or structure E892
  - private dwelling (apartment) (boarding house) (camping place) (caravan) (farmhouse) (home (private)) (house) (lodging house) (private garage) (rooming house) (tenement) E890.9
    - with or causing (injury due to)
      - accident or injury NEC E890.9
        - specified circumstance NEC E890.8
      - burns, burning E890.3
      - carbon monoxide E890.2
      - fumes E890.2
        - polyvinylchloride (PVC) or similar material E890.1
      - smoke E890.2
    - causing explosion E890.0
- **Constriction, external**
  - caused by
    - hair E928.4
    - other object E928.5
- **Contact with**
  - dry ice E901.1
  - liquid air, hydrogen, nitrogen E901.1
- **Cramp(s)**
  - Heat — *see* Heat
  - swimmers (*see also* category E910 ☑) E910.2
    - not in recreation or sport E910.3
- **Cranking** (car) (truck) (bus) (engine), injury by E917.9
- **Crash**
  - aircraft (in transit) (powered) E841 ☑
    - at landing, take-off E840 ☑
    - in
      - terrorism E979.1
      - war operations E994
    - on runway NEC E840 ☑
    - stated as
      - homicidal E968.8
      - suicidal E958.6
      - undetermined whether accidental or intentional E988.6
    - unpowered E842 ☑
  - glider E842 ☑

- **Crash** — *continued*
  - motor vehicle — *see also* Accident, motor vehicle
    - homicidal E968.5
    - suicidal E958.5
    - undetermined whether accidental or intentional E988.5
- **Crushed** (accidentally) E928.9
  - between
    - boat(s), ship(s), watercraft (and dock or pier) (without accident to watercraft) E838 ☑
      - after accident to, or collision, watercraft E831 ☑
    - objects (moving) (stationary and moving) E918
  - by
    - avalanche NEC E909.2
    - boat, ship, watercraft after accident to, collision, watercraft E831 ☑
    - cave-in E916
      - with asphyxiation or suffocation (*see also* Suffocation, due to, cave-in) E913.3
    - crowd, human stampede E917.1
    - falling
      - aircraft (*see also* Accident, aircraft) E841 ☑
        - in
          - terrorism E979.1
          - war operations E994
      - earth, material E916
        - with asphyxiation or suffocation (*see also* Suffocation, due to, cave-in) E913.3
      - object E916
        - on ship, watercraft E838 ☑
        - while loading, unloading watercraft E838 ☑
    - landslide NEC E909.2
    - lifeboat after abandoning ship E831 ☑
    - machinery — *see* Accident, machine
    - railway rolling stock, train, vehicle (part of) E805 ☑
    - street car E829 ☑
    - vehicle NEC — *see* Accident, vehicle NEC
  - in
    - machinery — *see* Accident, machine
    - object E918
    - transport accident — *see* categories E800-E848 ☑
  - late effect of NEC E929.9
- **Cut, cutting** (any part of body) (accidental) E920.9
  - by
    - arrow E920.8
    - axe E920.4
    - bayonet (*see also* Bayonet wound) E920.3
    - blender E920.2
    - broken glass E920.8
      - following fall E888.0
    - can opener E920.4
      - powered E920.2
    - chisel E920.4
    - circular saw E919.4
    - cutting or piercing instrument — *see also* category E920 ☑
      - following fall E888.0
      - late effect of E929.8
    - dagger E920.3
    - dart E920.8
    - drill — *see* Accident, caused by drill
    - edge of stiff paper E920.8
    - electric
      - beater E920.2
      - fan E920.2
      - knife E920.2
      - mixer E920.2
    - fork E920.4
    - garden fork E920.4
    - hand saw or tool (not powered) E920.4
      - powered E920.1
    - hedge clipper E920.4
      - powered E920.1
    - hoe E920.4
    - ice pick E920.4

- **Hit, hitting** by — *continued*
  - object — *continued*
    - set in motion by
      - compressed air or gas, spring, striking, throwing — *see* Striking against, object
      - explosion — *see* Explosion
    - thrown into, on, or towards
      - motor vehicle (in motion) (on public highway) E818 ☑
        - not on public highway E825 ☑
      - nonmotor road vehicle NEC E829 ☑
      - pedal cycle E826 ☑
      - street car E829 ☑
  - off-road type motor vehicle (not on public highway) E821 ☑
    - on public highway E814 ☑
  - other person(s) E917.9
    - with blunt or thrown object E917.9
      - in sports E917.0
        - with subsequent fall E917.5
      - intentionally, homicidal E968.2
    - as, or caused by, a crowd E917.1
      - with subsequent fall E917.6
    - in sports E917.0
  - pedal cycle E826 ☑
  - police (on duty) E975
    - with blunt object (baton) (nightstick) (stave) (truncheon) E973
  - railway, rolling stock, train, vehicle (part of) E805 ☑
  - shot — *see* Shooting
  - snow vehicle, motor-driven (not on public highway) E820 ☑
    - on public highway E814 ☑
  - street car E829 ☑
  - vehicle NEC — *see* Accident, vehicle NEC
- **Homicide, homicidal** (attempt) (justifiable) (*see also* Assault) E968.9
- **Hot**
  - liquid, object, substance, accident caused by — *see also* Accident, caused by, hot, by type of substance
    - late effect of E929.8
  - place, effects — *see* Heat
  - weather, effects E900.0
- **Humidity, causing problem** E904.3
- **Hunger** E904.1
  - resulting from
    - abandonment or neglect E904.0
    - transport accident — *see* categories E800-E848 ☑
- **Hurricane** (any injury) E908.0
- **Hypobarism, hypobaropathy** — *see* Effects of, air pressure
- **Hypothermia** — *see* Cold, exposure to

I

- **Ictus**
  - caloris — *see* Heat
  - solaris E900.0
- **Ignition** (accidental)
  - anesthetic gas in operating theatre E923.2
  - bedclothes
    - with
      - conflagration — *see* Conflagration
      - ignition (of)
        - clothing — *see* Ignition, clothes
        - highly inflammable material (benzine) (fat) (gasoline) (kerosene) (paraffin) (petrol) E894
  - benzine E894
  - clothes, clothing (from controlled fire) (in building) E893.9
    - with conflagration — *see* Conflagration
    - from
      - bonfire E893.2
      - highly inflammable material E894
      - sources or material as listed in E893.8
      - trash fire E893.2
      - uncontrolled fire — *see* Conflagration
    - in
      - private dwelling E893.0
      - specified building or structure, except private dwelling E893.1
- **Ignition** — *continued*
  - clothes, clothing — *continued*
    - not in building or structure E893.2
  - explosive material — *see* Explosion
  - fat E894
  - gasoline E894
  - kerosene E894
  - material
    - explosive — *see* Explosion
    - highly inflammable E894
      - with conflagration — *see* Conflagration
      - with explosion E923.2
  - nightdress — *see* Ignition, clothes
  - paraffin E894
  - petrol E894
- **Immersion** — *see* Submersion
- **Implantation of quills of porcupine** E906.8
- **Inanition** (from) E904.9
  - hunger — *see* Lack of, food
  - resulting from homicidal intent E968.4
  - thirst — *see* Lack of, water
- **Inattention after, at birth** E904.0
  - homicidal, infanticidal intent E968.4
- **Infanticide** (*see also* Assault)
- **Ingestion**
  - foreign body (causing injury) (with obstruction) — *see* Foreign body, alimentary canal
  - poisonous substance NEC — *see* Table of Drugs and Chemicals
- **Inhalation**
  - excessively cold substance, manmade E901.1
  - foreign body — *see* Foreign body, aspiration
  - liquid air, hydrogen, nitrogen E901.1
  - mucus, not of newborn (with asphyxia, obstruction respiratory passage, suffocation) E912
  - phlegm (with asphyxia, obstruction respiratory passage, suffocation) E912
  - poisonous gas — *see* Table of Drugs and Chemicals
  - smoke from, due to
    - fire — *see* Fire
    - tobacco, second-hand E869.4
  - vomitus (with asphyxia, obstruction respiratory passage, suffocation) E911
- **Injury, injured** (accidental(ly)) NEC E928.9
  - by, caused by, from
    - air rifle (BB gun) E922.4
    - animal (not being ridden) NEC E906.9
      - being ridden (in sport or transport) E828 ☑
    - assault (*see also* Assault) E968.9
    - avalanche E909.2
    - bayonet (*see also* Bayonet wound) E920.3
    - being thrown against some part of, or object in
      - motor vehicle (in motion) (on public highway) E818 ☑
        - not on public highway E825 ☑
      - nonmotor road vehicle NEC E829 ☑
      - off-road motor vehicle NEC E821 ☑
      - railway train E806 ☑
      - snow vehicle, motor-driven E820 ☑
      - street car E829 ☑
    - bending E927
    - bite, human E928.3
    - broken glass E920.8
    - bullet — *see* Shooting
    - cave-in (*see also* Suffocation, due to, cave-in) E913.3
      - without asphyxiation or suffocation E916
      - earth surface movement or eruption E909.9
      - storm E908.9
    - cloudburst E908.8
    - cutting or piercing instrument (*see also* Cut) E920.9
    - cyclone E908.1
    - earth surface movement or eruption E909.9
    - earthquake E909.0
    - electric current (*see also* Electric shock) E925.9
- **Injury, injured** — *continued*
  - by, caused by, from — *continued*
    - explosion (*see also* Explosion) E923.9
    - fire — *see* Fire
    - flare, Verey pistol E922.8
    - flood E908.2
    - foreign body — *see* Foreign body
    - hailstones E904.3
    - hurricane E908.0
    - landslide E909.2
    - law-enforcing agent, police, in course of legal intervention — *see* Legal intervention
    - lightning E907
    - live rail or live wire — *see* Electric shock
    - machinery — *see also* Accident, machine
      - aircraft, without accident to aircraft E844 ☑
      - boat, ship, watercraft (deck) (engine room) (galley) (laundry) (loading) E836 ☑
    - missile
      - explosive E923.8
      - firearm — *see* Shooting
      - in
        - terrorism — *see* Terrorism, missile
        - war operations — *see* War operations, missile
    - moving part of motor vehicle (in motion) (on public highway) E818 ☑
      - not on public highway, nontraffic accident E825 ☑
      - while alighting, boarding, entering, leaving — *see* Fall, from, motor vehicle, while alighting, boarding
    - nail E920.8
    - needle (sewing) E920.4
      - hypodermic E920.5
    - noise E928.1
    - object
      - fallen on
        - motor vehicle (in motion) (on public highway) E818 ☑
          - not on public highway E825 ☑
      - falling — *see* Hit by, object, falling
    - paintball gun E922.5
    - radiation — *see* Radiation
    - railway rolling stock, train, vehicle (part of) E805 ☑
      - door or window E806 ☑
    - rotating propeller, aircraft E844 ☑
    - rough landing of off-road type motor vehicle (after leaving ground or rough terrain) E821 ☑
      - snow vehicle E820 ☑
    - saber (*see also* Wound, saber) E920.3
    - shot — *see* Shooting
    - sound waves E928.1
    - splinter or sliver, wood E920.8
    - straining E927
    - street car (door) E829 ☑
    - suicide (attempt) E958.9
    - sword E920.3
    - terrorism — *see* Terrorism
    - third rail — *see* Electric shock
    - thunderbolt E907
    - tidal wave E909.4
      - caused by storm E908.0
    - tornado E908.1
    - torrential rain E908.2
    - twisting E927
    - vehicle NEC — *see* Accident, vehicle NEC
    - vibration E928.2
    - volcanic eruption E909.1
    - weapon burst, in war operations E993
    - weightlessness (in spacecraft, real or simulated) E928.0
    - wood splinter or sliver E920.8
  - due to
    - civil insurrection — *see* War operations
      - occurring after cessation of hostilities E998
    - terrorism — *see* Terrorism
    - war operations — *see* War operations
      - occurring after cessation of hostilities E998

J

K

L

Late effect of — *continued*
natural or environmental factor, accident due to (accident classifiable to E900-E909) E929.5
poisoning, accidental (accident classifiable to E850-E858, E860-E869) E929.2
suicide, attempt (any means) E959
transport accident NEC (accident classifiable to E800-E807, E826-E838, E840-E848) E929.1
war operations, injury due to (injury classifiable to E990-E998) E999.0
Launching pad accident E845 ☑
Legal
execution, any method E978
intervention (by) (injury from) E976
baton E973
bayonet E974
blow E975
blunt object (baton) (nightstick) (stave) (truncheon) E973
cutting or piercing instrument E974
dynamite E971
execution, any method E973
explosive(s) (shell) E971
firearm(s) E970
gas (asphyxiation) (poisoning) (tear) E972
grenade E971
late effect of E977
machine gun E970
manhandling E975
mortar bomb E971
nightstick E973
revolver E970
rifle E970
specified means NEC E975
stabbing E974
stave E973
truncheon E973
Lifting, injury in E927
Lightning (shock) (stroke) (struck by) E907
Liquid (noncorrosive) in eye E914
corrosive E924.1
Loss of control
motor vehicle (on public highway) (without antecedent collision) E816 ☑
with
antecedent collision on public highway — *see* Collision, motor vehicle
involving any object, person or vehicle not on public highway E816 ☑
on public highway — *see* Collision, motor vehicle
not on public highway, nontraffic accident E825 ☑
with antecedent collision — *see* Collision, motor vehicle, not on public highway
off-road type motor vehicle (not on public highway) E821 ☑
on public highway — *see* Loss of control, motor vehicle
snow vehicle, motor-driven (not on public highway) E820 ☑
on public highway — *see* Loss of control, motor vehicle
Lost at sea E832 ☑
with accident to watercraft E830 ☑
in war operations E995
Low
pressure, effects — *see* Effects of, air pressure
temperature, effects — *see* Cold, exposure to
Lying before train, vehicle or other moving object (unspecified whether accidental or intentional) E988.0
stated as intentional, purposeful, suicidal (attempt) E958.0
Lynching (*see also* Assault) E968.9

M

Malfunction, atomic power plant in water transport E838 ☑
Mangled (accidentally) NEC E928.9
Manhandling (in brawl, fight) E960.0
legal intervention E975
Manslaughter (nonaccidental) — *see* Assault
Marble in nose E912
Mauled by animal E906.8
Medical procedure, complication of
delayed or as an abnormal reaction without mention of misadventure — *see* Reaction, abnormal
due to or as a result of misadventure — *see* Misadventure
Melting of fittings and furniture in burning
in terrorism E979.3
Minamata disease E865.2
Misadventure(s) to patient(s) during surgical or medical care E876.9
contaminated blood, fluid, drug or biological substance (presence of agents and toxins as listed in E875) E875.9
administered (by) NEC E875.9
infusion E875.0
injection E875.1
specified means NEC E875.2
transfusion E875.0
vaccination E875.1
cut, cutting, puncture, perforation or hemorrhage (accidental) (inadvertent) (inappropriate) (during) E870.9
aspiration of fluid or tissue (by puncture or catheterization, except heart) E870.5
biopsy E870.8
needle (aspirating) E870.5
blood sampling E870.5
catheterization E870.5
heart E870.6
dialysis (kidney) E870.2
endoscopic examination E870.4
enema E870.7
infusion E870.1
injection E870.3
lumbar puncture E870.5
needle biopsy E870.5
paracentesis, abdominal E870.5
perfusion E870.2
specified procedure NEC E870.8
surgical operation E870.0
thoracentesis E870.5
transfusion E870.1
vaccination E870.3
excessive amount of blood or other fluid during transfusion or infusion E873.0
failure
in dosage E873.9
electroshock therapy E873.4
inappropriate temperature (too hot or too cold) in local application and packing E873.5
infusion
excessive amount of fluid E873.0
incorrect dilution of fluid E873.1
insulin-shock therapy E873.4
nonadministration of necessary drug or medicinal E873.6
overdose — *see also* Overdose
radiation, in therapy E873.2
radiation
inadvertent exposure of patient (receiving radiation for test or therapy) E873.3
not receiving radiation for test or therapy — *see* Radiation
overdose E873.2
specified procedure NEC E873.8
transfusion
excessive amount of blood E873.0
mechanical, of instrument or apparatus (during procedure) E874.9
aspiration of fluid or tissue (by puncture or catheterization, except of heart) E874.4
biopsy E874.8
needle (aspirating) E874.4
blood sampling E874.4
catheterization E874.4
heart E874.5

Misadventure(s) to patient(s) during surgical or medical care — *continued*
failure — *continued*
mechanical, of instrument or apparatus — *continued*
dialysis (kidney) E874.2
endoscopic examination E874.3
enema E874.8
infusion E874.1
injection E874.8
lumbar puncture E874.4
needle biopsy E874.4
paracentesis, abdominal E874.4
perfusion E874.2
specified procedure NEC E874.8
surgical operation E874.0
thoracentesis E874.4
transfusion E874.1
vaccination E874.8
sterile precautions (during procedure) E872.9
aspiration of fluid or tissue (by puncture or catheterization, except heart) E872.5
biopsy E872.8
needle (aspirating) E872.5
blood sampling E872.5
catheterization E872.5
heart E872.6
dialysis (kidney) E872.2
endoscopic examination E872.4
enema E872.8
infusion E872.1
injection E872.3
lumbar puncture E872.5
needle biopsy E872.5
paracentesis, abdominal E872.5
perfusion E872.2
removal of catheter or packing E872.8
specified procedure NEC E872.8
surgical operation E872.0
thoracentesis E872.5
transfusion E872.1
vaccination E872.3
suture or ligature during surgical procedure E876.2
to introduce or to remove tube or instrument E876.4
foreign object left in body — *see* Misadventure, foreign object
foreign object left in body (during procedure) E871.9
aspiration of fluid or tissue (by puncture or catheterization, except heart) E871.5
biopsy E871.8
needle (aspirating) E871.5
blood sampling E871.5
catheterization E871.5
heart E871.6
dialysis (kidney) E871.2
endoscopic examination E871.4
enema E871.8
infusion E871.1
injection E871.3
lumbar puncture E871.5
needle biopsy E871.5
paracentesis, abdominal E871.5
perfusion E871.2
removal of catheter or packing E871.7
specified procedure NEC E871.8
surgical operation E871.0
thoracentesis E871.5
transfusion E871.1
vaccination E871.3
hemorrhage — *see* Misadventure, cut
inadvertent exposure of patient to radiation (being received for test or therapy) E873.3
inappropriate
operation performed E876.5
temperature (too hot or too cold) in local application or packing E873.5
infusion — *see also* Misadventure, by specific type, infusion
excessive amount of fluid E873.0
incorrect dilution of fluid E873.1
wrong fluid E876.1
mismatched blood in transfusion E876.0

Misadventure(s) to patient(s) during surgical or medical care — *continued*
- nonadministration of necessary drug or medicinal E873.6
- overdose — *see also* Overdose
  - radiation, in therapy E873.2
- perforation — *see* Misadventure, cut
- performance of inappropriate operation E876.5
- puncture — *see* Misadventure, cut
- specified type NEC E876.8
  - failure
    - suture or ligature during surgical operation E876.2
    - to introduce or to remove tube or instrument E876.4
      - foreign object left in body E871.9
  - infusion of wrong fluid E876.1
  - performance of inappropriate operation E876.5
  - transfusion of mismatched blood E876.0
  - wrong
    - fluid in infusion E876.1
    - placement of endotracheal tube during anesthetic procedure E876.3
- transfusion — *see also* Misadventure, by specific type, transfusion
  - excessive amount of blood E873.0
  - mismatched blood E876.0
- wrong
  - drug given in error — *see* Table of Drugs and Chemicals
  - fluid in infusion E876.1
  - placement of endotracheal tube during anesthetic procedure E876.3

Motion (effects) E903
- sickness E903

Mountain sickness E902.0

Mucus aspiration or inhalation, not of newborn (with asphyxia, obstruction respiratory passage, suffocation) E912

Mudslide of cataclysmic nature E909.2

Murder (attempt) (*see also* Assault) E968.9

N

Nail, injury by E920.8

Needlestick (sewing needle) E920.4
- hypodermic E920.5

Neglect — *see also* Privation
- criminal E968.4
- homicidal intent E968.4

Noise (causing injury) (pollution) E928.1

O

Object
- falling
  - from, in, on, hitting
    - aircraft E844 ☑
      - due to accident to aircraft — *see* categories E840-E842 ☑
    - machinery — *see also* Accident, machine
      - not in operation E916
    - motor vehicle (in motion) (on public highway) E818 ☑
      - not on public highway E825 ☑
      - stationary E916
    - nonmotor road vehicle NEC E829 ☑
    - pedal cycle E826 ☑
    - person E916
    - railway rolling stock, train, vehicle E806 ☑
    - street car E829 ☑
    - watercraft E838 ☑
      - due to accident to watercraft E831 ☑
- set in motion by
  - accidental explosion of pressure vessel — *see* category E921 ☑
  - firearm — *see* category E922 ☑
  - machine(ry) — *see* Accident, machine
  - transport vehicle — *see* categories E800-E848 ☑

Object — *continued*
- thrown from, in, on, towards
  - aircraft E844 ☑
  - cable car (not on rails) E847
    - on rails E829 ☑
  - motor vehicle (in motion) (on public highway) E818 ☑
    - not on public highway E825 ☑
  - nonmotor road vehicle NEC E829 ☑
  - pedal cycle E826 ☑
  - street car E829 ☑
  - vehicle NEC — *see* Accident, vehicle NEC

Obstruction
- air passages, larynx, respiratory passages
  - by
    - external means NEC — *see* Suffocation
    - food, any type (regurgitated) (vomited) E911
    - material or object, except food E912
    - mucus E912
    - phlegm E912
    - vomitus E911
- digestive tract, except mouth or pharynx
  - by
    - food, any type E915
    - foreign body (any) E915
- esophagus
  - food E911
  - foreign body, except food E912
  - without asphyxia or obstruction of respiratory passage E915
- mouth or pharynx
  - by
    - food, any type E911
    - material or object, except food E912
- respiration — *see* Obstruction, air passages

Oil in eye E914

Overdose
- anesthetic (drug) — *see* Table of Drugs and Chemicals
- drug — *see* Table of Drugs and Chemicals

Overexertion (lifting) (pulling) (pushing) E927

Overexposure (accidental) (to)
- cold (*see also* Cold, exposure to) E901.9
  - due to manmade conditions E901.1
- heat (*see also* Heat) E900.9
- radiation — *see* Radiation
- radioactivity — *see* Radiation
- sun, except sunburn E900.0
- weather — *see* Exposure
- wind — *see* Exposure

Overheated (*see also* Heat) E900.9

Overlaid E913.0

Overturning (accidental)
- animal-drawn vehicle E827 ☑
- boat, ship, watercraft
  - causing
    - drowning, submersion E830 ☑
    - injury except drowning, submersion E831 ☑
- machinery — *see* Accident, machine
- motor vehicle (*see also* Loss of control, motor vehicle) E816 ☑
  - with antecedent collision on public highway — *see* Collision, motor vehicle
  - not on public highway, nontraffic accident E825 ☑
    - with antecedent collision — *see* Collision, motor vehicle, not on public highway
- nonmotor road vehicle NEC E829 ☑
- off-road type motor vehicle — *see* Loss of control, off-road type motor vehicle
- pedal cycle E826 ☑
- railway rolling stock, train, vehicle (*see also* Derailment, railway) E802 ☑
- street car E829 ☑
- vehicle NEC — *see* Accident, vehicle NEC

P

Palsy, divers' E902.2

Parachuting (voluntary) (without accident to aircraft) E844 ☑

Parachuting — *continued*
- due to accident to aircraft — *see* categories E840-E842 ☑

Paralysis
- divers' E902.2
- lead or saturnine E866.0
  - from pesticide NEC E863.4

Pecked by bird E906.8

Phlegm aspiration or inhalation (with asphyxia, obstruction respiratory passage, suffocation) E912

Piercing (*see also* Cut) E920.9

Pinched
- between objects (moving) (stationary and moving) E918
- in object E918

Pinned under
- machine(ry) — *see* Accident, machine

Place of occurrence of accident — *see* Accident (to), occurring (at) (in)

Plumbism E866.0
- from insecticide NEC E863.4

Poisoning (accidental) (by) — *see also* Table of Drugs and Chemicals
- carbon monoxide
  - generated by
    - aircraft in transit E844 ☑
    - motor vehicle
      - in motion (on public highway) E818 ☑
        - not on public highway E825 ☑
    - watercraft (in transit) (not in transit) E838 ☑
- caused by injection of poisons or toxins into or through skin by plant thorns, spines, or other mechanism E905.7
  - marine or sea plants E905.6
- fumes or smoke due to
  - conflagration — *see* Conflagration
  - explosion or fire — *see* Fire
  - ignition — *see* Ignition
- gas
  - in legal intervention E972
  - legal execution, by E978
  - on watercraft E838 ☑
  - used as anesthetic — *see* Table of Drugs and Chemicals
- in
  - terrorism (chemical weapons) E979.7
  - war operations E997.2
- late effect of — *see* Late effect
- legal
  - execution E978
  - intervention
    - by gas E972

Pressure, external, causing asphyxia, suffocation (*see also* Suffocation) E913.9

Privation E904.9
- food (*see also* Lack of, food) E904.1
- helpless person, infant, newborn due to abandonment or neglect E904.0
- late effect of NEC E929.5
- resulting from transport accident — *see* categories E800-E848 ☑
- water (*see also* Lack of, water) E904.2

Projected objects, striking against or struck by — *see* Striking against, object

Prolonged stay in
- high altitude (causing conditions as listed in E902.0) E902.0
- weightless environment E928.0

Prostration
- heat — *see* Heat

Pulling, injury in E927

Puncture, puncturing (*see also* Cut) E920.9
- by
  - plant thorns or spines E920.8
    - toxic reaction E905.7
      - marine or sea plants E905.6
  - sea-urchin spine E905.6

- **Scald, scalding** — *continued*
  - inflicted by other person
    - stated as
      - intentional or homicidal E968.3
      - undetermined whether accidental or intentional E988.2
  - late effect of NEC E929.8
  - liquid (boiling) (hot) E924.0
  - local application of externally applied substance in medical or surgical care E873.5
  - molten metal E924.0
  - self-inflicted (unspecified whether accidental or intentional) E988.2
    - stated as intentional, purposeful E958.2
  - stated as undetermined whether accidental or intentional E988.2
  - steam E924.0
  - tap water (boiling) E924.2
  - transport accident — *see* categories E800-E848
  - vapor E924.0
- **Scratch, cat** E906.8
- **Sea**
  - sickness E903
- **Self-mutilation** — *see* Suicide
- **Sequelae (of)**
  - in
    - terrorism E999.1
    - war operations E999.0
- **Shock**
  - anaphylactic (*see also* Table of Drugs and Chemicals) E947.9
    - due to
      - bite (venomous) — *see* Bite, venomous NEC
      - sting — *see* Sting
  - electric (*see also* Electric shock) E925.9
  - from electric appliance or current (*see also* Electric shock) E925.9
- **Shooting, shot** (accidental(ly)) E922.9
  - air gun E922.4
  - BB gun E922.4
  - hand gun (pistol) (revolver) E922.0
  - himself (*see also* Shooting, self-inflicted) E985.4
    - hand gun (pistol) (revolver) E985.0
    - military firearm, except hand gun E985.3
      - hand gun (pistol) (revolver) E985.0
    - rifle (hunting) E985.2
      - military E985.3
    - shotgun (automatic) E985.1
    - specified firearm NEC E985.4
    - Verey pistol E985.4
  - homicide (attempt) E965.4
    - air gun E968.6
    - BB gun E968.6
    - hand gun (pistol) (revolver) E965.0
    - military firearm, except hand gun E965.3
      - hand gun (pistol) (revolver) E965.0
    - paintball gun E965.4
    - rifle (hunting) E965.2
      - military E965.3
    - shotgun (automatic) E965.1
    - specified firearm NEC E965.4
    - Verey pistol E965.4
  - inflicted by other person
    - in accidental circumstances E922.9
      - hand gun (pistol) (revolver) E922.0
      - military firearm, except hand gun E922.3
        - hand gun (pistol) (revolver) E922.0
      - rifle (hunting) E922.2
        - military E922.3
      - shotgun (automatic) E922.1
      - specified firearm NEC E922.8
      - Verey pistol E922.8
    - stated as
      - intentional, homicidal E965.4
        - hand gun (pistol) (revolver) E965.0
        - military firearm, except hand gun E965.3
          - hand gun (pistol) (revolver) E965.0
        - paintball gun E965.4
        - rifle (hunting) E965.2
          - military E965.3
        - shotgun (automatic) E965.1
        - specified firearm E965.4
- **Shooting, shot** — *continued*
  - inflicted by other person — *continued*
    - stated as — *continued*
      - intentional, homicidal — *continued*
        - Verey pistol E965.4
      - undetermined whether accidental or intentional E985.4
        - air gun E985.6
        - BB gun E985.6
        - hand gun (pistol) (revolver) E985.0
        - military firearm, except hand gun E985.3
          - hand gun (pistol) (revolver) E985.0
        - paintball gun E985.7
        - rifle (hunting) E985.2
        - shotgun (automatic) E985.1
        - specified firearm NEC E985.4
        - Verey pistol E985.4
  - in
    - terrorism — *see* Terrorism, shooting
    - war operations — *see* War operations, shooting
  - legal
    - execution E978
    - intervention E970
  - military firearm, except hand gun E922.3
    - hand gun (pistol) (revolver) E922.0
  - paintball gun E922.5
  - rifle (hunting) E922.2
    - military E922.3
  - self-inflicted (unspecified whether accidental or intentional) E985.4
    - air gun E985.6
    - BB gun E985.6
    - hand gun (pistol) (revolver) E985.0
    - military firearm, except hand gun E985.3
      - hand gun (pistol) (revolver) E985.0
    - paintball gun E985.7
    - rifle (hunting) E985.2
      - military E985.3
    - shotgun (automatic) E985.1
    - specified firearm NEC E985.4
    - stated as
      - accidental E922.9
        - hand gun (pistol) (revolver) E922.0
        - military firearm, except hand gun E922.3
          - hand gun (pistol) (revolver) E922.0
        - paintball gun E922.5
        - rifle (hunting) E922.2
          - military E922.3
        - shotgun (automatic) E922.1
        - specified firearm NEC E922.8
        - Verey pistol E922.8
      - intentional, purposeful E955.4
        - hand gun (pistol) (revolver) E955.0
        - military firearm, except hand gun E955.3
          - hand gun (pistol) (revolver) E955.0
        - paintball gun E955.7
        - rifle (hunting) E955.2
          - military E955.3
        - shotgun (automatic) E955.1
        - specified firearm NEC E955.4
        - Verey pistol E955.4
  - shotgun (automatic) E922.1
  - specified firearm NEC E922.8
  - stated as undetermined whether accidental or intentional E985.4
    - hand gun (pistol) (revolver) E985.0
    - military firearm, except hand gun E985.3
      - hand gun (pistol) (revolver) E985.0
    - paintball gun E985.7
    - rifle (hunting) E985.2
      - military E985.3
    - shotgun (automatic) E985.1
    - specified firearm NEC E985.4
    - Verey pistol E985.4
  - suicidal (attempt) E955.4
    - air gun E955.6
    - BB gun E955.6
    - hand gun (pistol) (revolver) E955.0
    - military firearm, except hand gun E955.3
      - hand gun (pistol) (revolver) E955.0
    - paintball gun E955.7
    - rifle (hunting) E955.2
      - military E955.3
- **Shooting, shot** — *continued*
  - suicidal — *continued*
    - shotgun (automatic) E955.1
    - specified firearm NEC E955.4
    - Verey pistol E955.4
  - Verey pistol E922.8
- **Shoving** (accidentally) by other person (*see also* Pushing by other person) E917.9
- **Sickness**
  - air E903
  - alpine E902.0
  - car E903
  - motion E903
  - mountain E902.0
  - sea E903
  - travel E903
- **Sinking** (accidental)
  - boat, ship, watercraft (causing drowning, submersion) E830 ☑
    - causing injury except drowning, submersion E831 ☑
- **Siriasis** E900.0
- **Skydiving** E844 ☑
- **Slashed wrists** (*see also* Cut, self-inflicted) E986
- **Slipping** (accidental)
  - on
    - deck (of boat, ship, watercraft) (icy) (oily) (wet) E835 ☑
    - ice E885.9
    - ladder of ship E833 ☑
      - due to accident to watercraft E831 ☑
    - mud E885.9
    - oil E885.9
    - snow E885.9
    - stairs of ship E833 ☑
      - due to accident to watercraft E831 ☑
    - surface
      - slippery E885 ☑
      - wet E885 ☑
- **Sliver, wood, injury by** E920.8
- **Smouldering building or structure in terrorism** E979.3
- **Smothering, smothered** (*see also* Suffocation) E913.9
- **Sodomy** (assault) E960.1
- **Solid substance in eye** (any part) or adnexa E914
- **Sound waves** (causing injury) E928.1
- **Splinter, injury by** E920.8
- **Stab, stabbing** E966
  - accidental — *see* Cut
- **Starvation** E904.1
  - helpless person, infant, newborn — *see* Lack of food
  - homicidal intent E968.4
  - late effect of NEC E929.5
  - resulting from accident connected with transport — *see* categories E800-E848
- **Stepped on**
  - by
    - animal (not being ridden) E906.8
      - being ridden (in sport or transport) E828 ☑
    - crowd E917.1
    - person E917.9
      - in sports E917.0
  - in sports E917.0
- **Stepping on**
  - object (moving) E917.9
    - in sports E917.0
      - with subsequent fall E917.5
    - stationary E917.4
      - with subsequent fall E917.8
  - person E917.9
    - as, or caused by a crowd E917.1
      - with subsequent fall E917.6
    - in sports E917.0
- **Sting** E905.9
  - ant E905.5
  - bee E905.3
  - caterpillar E905.5
  - coral E905.6
  - hornet E905.3
  - insect NEC E905.5
  - jellyfish E905.6

T

Railway Accidents (E800-E807)

The following fourth-digit subdivisions are for use with categories E800-E807 to identify the injured person:

.0 **Railway employee**
Any person who by virtue of his employment in connection with a railway, whether by the railway company or not, is at increased risk of involvement in a railway accident, such as:
catering staff on train
postal staff on train
driver
railway fireman
guard
shunter
porter
sleeping car attendant

.1 **Passenger on railway**
Any authorized person traveling on a train, except a railway employee
EXCLUDES intending passenger waiting at station (.8)
unauthorized rider on railway vehicle (.8)

.2 **Pedestrian** See definition (r), E-Codes-2

.3 **Pedal cyclist** See definition (p), E-Codes-2

.8 **Other specified person** Intending passenger waiting at station
Unauthorized rider on railway vehicle

.9 **Unspecified person**

Motor Vehicle Traffic and Nontraffic Accidents (E810-E825)

The following fourth-digit subdivisions are for use with categories E810-E819 and E820-E825 to identify the injured person:

.0 **Driver of motor vehicle other than motorcycle** See definition (1), E-Codes-2

.1 **Passenger in motor vehicle other than motorcycle** See definition (1), E-Codes-2

.2 **Motorcyclist** See definition (1), E-Codes-2

.3 **Passenger on motorcycle** See definition (1), E-Codes-2

.4 **Occupant of streetcar**

.5 **Rider of animal; occupant of animal-drawn vehicle**

.6 **Pedal cyclist** See definition (p), E-Codes-2

.7 **Pedestrian** See definition (r), E-Codes-2

.8 **Other specified person**
Occupant of vehicle other than above
Person in railway train involved in accident
Unauthorized rider of motor vehicle

.9 **Unspecified person**

Other Road Vehicle Accidents (E826-E829)

(animal-drawn vehicle, streetcar, pedal cycle, and other nonmotor road vehicle accidents)

The following fourth-digit subdivisions are for use with categories E826-E829 to identify the injured person:

.0 **Pedestrian** See definition (r), E-Codes-2

.1 **Pedal cyclist** (does not apply to codes E827, E828, E829) See definition (p), E-Codes-2

.2 **Rider of animal** (does not apply to code E829)

.3 **Occupant of animal-drawn vehicle** (does not apply to codes E828, E829)

.4 **Occupant of streetcar**

.8 **Other specified person**

.9 **Unspecified person**

Water Transport Accidents (E830-E838)

The following fourth-digit subdivisions are for use with categories E830-E838 to identify the injured person:

.0 **Occupant of small boat, unpowered**

.1 **Occupant of small boat, powered** See definition (t), E-Codes-2
EXCLUDES water skier (.4)

.2 **Occupant of other watercraft — crew**
Persons:
engaged in operation of watercraft
providing passenger services [cabin attendants, ship's physician, catering personnel]
working on ship during voyage in other capacity [musician in band, operators of shops and beauty parlors]

.3 **Occupant of other watercraft — other than crew**
Passenger
Occupant of lifeboat, other than crew, after abandoning ship

.4 **Water skier**

.5 **Swimmer**

.6 **Dockers, stevedores**
Longshoreman employed on the dock in loading and unloading ships

.8 **Other specified person**
Immigration and custom officials on board ship
Persons:
accompanying passenger or member of crew visiting boat
Pilot (guiding ship into port)

.9 **Unspecified person**

Air and Space Transport Accidents (E840-E845)

The following fourth-digit subdivisions are for use with categories E840-E845 to identify the injured person:

.0 **Occupant of spacecraft**

Crew
Passenger (civilian)
(military)
Troops
} in military aircraft [air force] [army] [national guard] [navy]

.1 **Occupant of military aircraft, any**
EXCLUDES occupants of aircraft operated under jurisdiction of police departments (.5) parachutist (.7)

.2 **Crew of commercial aircraft (powered) in surface to surface transport**

.3 **Other occupant of commercial aircraft (powered) in surface to surface transport**
Flight personnel:
not part of crew
on familiarization flight
Passenger on aircraft

.4 **Occupant of commercial aircraft (powered) in surface to air transport**
Occupant [crew] [passenger] of aircraft (powered) engaged in activities, such as:
air drops of emergency supplies
air drops of parachutists, except from military craft
crop dusting
lowering of construction material [bridge or telephone pole]
sky writing

.5 **Occupant of other powered aircraft**
Occupant [crew] [passenger] of aircraft (powered) engaged in activities, such as:
aerial spraying (crops) (fire retardants)
aerobatic flying
aircraft racing
rescue operation
storm surveillance
traffic suveillance
Occupant of private plane NOS

.6 **Occupant of unpowered aircraft, except parachutist**
Occupant of aircraft classifiable to E842

.7 **Parachutist (military) (other)**
Person making voluntary descent
person making descent after accident to aircraft (.1-.6)

.8 **Ground crew, airline employee**
Persons employed at airfields (civil) (military) or launching pads, not occupants of aircraft

.9 **Other person**

1. INFECTIOUS AND PARASITIC DISEASES (001-139)

Note: Categories for "late effects" of infectious and parasitic diseases are to be found at 137-139.

INCLUDES diseases generally recognized as communicable or transmissible as well as a few diseases of unknown but possibly infectious origin

EXCLUDES *acute respiratory infections (460-466)*
carrier or suspected carrier of infectious organism (V02.0-V02.9)
certain localized infections
influenza (487.0-487.8)

INTESTINAL INFECTIOUS DISEASES (001-009)

EXCLUDES *helminthiases (120.0-129)*

✓4th **001 Cholera**

DEF: An acute infectious enteritis caused by a potent enterotoxin elaborated by *Vibrio cholerae*; the vibrio produces a toxin in the intestinal tract that changes the permeability of the mucosa leading to diarrhea and dehydration.

001.0 Due to Vibrio cholerae
001.1 Due to Vibrio cholerae el tor
001.9 Cholera, unspecified

✓4th **002 Typhoid and paratyphoid fevers**

DEF: Typhoid fever: an acute generalized illness caused by *Salmonella typhi*; notable clinical features are fever, headache, abdominal pain, cough, toxemia, leukopenia, abnormal pulse, rose spots on the skin, bacteremia, hyperplasia of intestinal lymph nodes, mesenteric lymphadenopathy, and Peyer's patches in the intestines.

DEF: Paratyphoid fever: a prolonged febrile illness, much like typhoid but usually less severe; caused by salmonella serotypes other than *S. typhi*, especially *S. enteritidis* serotypes paratyphi A and B and *S. choleraesuis*.

002.0 Typhoid fever
Typhoid (fever) (infection) [any site]
002.1 Paratyphoid fever A
002.2 Paratyphoid fever B
002.3 Paratyphoid fever C
002.9 Paratyphoid fever, unspecified

✓4th **003 Other salmonella infections**

INCLUDES infection or food poisoning by Salmonella [any serotype]

DEF: Infections caused by a genus of gram-negative, anaerobic bacteria of the family *Enterobacteriaceae*; affecting warm-blooded animals, like humans; major symptoms are enteric fevers, acute gastroenteritis and septicemia.

003.0 Salmonella gastroenteritis
Salmonellosis
003.1 Salmonella septicemia
✓5th **003.2 Localized salmonella infections**
003.20 Localized salmonella infection, unspecified
003.21 Salmonella meningitis
003.22 Salmonella pneumonia
003.23 Salmonella arthritis
003.24 Salmonella osteomyelitis
003.29 Other
003.8 Other specified salmonella infections
003.9 Salmonella infection, unspecified

✓4th **004 Shigellosis**

INCLUDES bacillary dysentery

DEF: Acute infectious dysentery caused by the genus *Shigella*, of the family *Enterobacteriaceae*; affecting the colon causing the release of blood-stained stools with accompanying tenesmus, abdominal cramps and fever.

004.0 Shigella dysenteriae
Infection by group A Shigella (Schmitz) (Shiga)
004.1 Shigella flexneri
Infection by group B Shigella
004.2 Shigella boydii
Infection by group C Shigella
004.3 Shigella sonnei
Infection by group D Shigella
004.8 Other specified Shigella infections
004.9 Shigellosis, unspecified

✓4th **005 Other food poisoning (bacterial)**

EXCLUDES *salmonella infections (003.0-003.9)*
toxic effect of:
food contaminants (989.7)
noxious foodstuffs (988.0-988.9)

DEF: Enteritis caused by ingesting contaminated foods and characterized by diarrhea, abdominal pain, vomiting; symptoms may be mild or life threatening.

005.0 Staphylococcal food poisoning
Staphylococcal toxemia specified as due to food
005.1 Botulism
Food poisoning due to Clostridium botulinum
005.2 Food poisoning due to Clostridium perfringens [C. welchii]
Enteritis necroticans
005.3 Food poisoning due to other Clostridia
005.4 Food poisoning due to Vibrio parahaemolyticus
✓5th **005.8 Other bacterial food poisoning**
EXCLUDES *salmonella food poisoning (003.0-003.9)*
005.81 Food poisoning due to Vibrio vulnificus
005.89 Other bacterial food poisoning
Food poisoning due to Bacillus cereus
005.9 Food poisoning, unspecified

✓4th **006 Amebiasis**

INCLUDES infection due to Entamoeba histolytica
EXCLUDES *amebiasis due to organisms other than Entamoeba histolytica (007.8)*

DEF: Infection of the large intestine caused by *Entamoeba histolytica*; usually asymptomatic but symptoms may range from mild diarrhea to profound life-threatening dysentery. Extraintestinal complications include hepatic abscess, which may rupture into the lung, pericardium or abdomen, causing life-threatening infections.

006.0 Acute amebic dysentery without mention of abscess
Acute amebiasis
006.1 Chronic intestinal amebiasis without mention of abscess
Chronic: amebiasis
Chronic: amebic dysentery
006.2 Amebic nondysenteric colitis
DEF: *Entamoeba histolytica* infection with inflamed colon but no dysentery.
006.3 Amebic liver abscess
Hepatic amebiasis
006.4 Amebic lung abscess
Amebic abscess of lung (and liver)
006.5 Amebic brain abscess
Amebic abscess of brain (and liver) (and lung)
006.6 Amebic skin ulceration
Cutaneous amebiasis
006.8 Amebic infection of other sites
Amebic: appendicitis, balanitis
Ameboma
EXCLUDES *specific infections by free-living amebae (136.2)*
006.9 Amebiasis, unspecified
Amebiasis NOS

✓4th **007 Other protozoal intestinal diseases**

INCLUDES protozoal: colitis, diarrhea
protozoal: dysentery

007.0 Balantidiasis
Infection by Balantidium coli
007.1 Giardiasis
Infection by Giardia lamblia
Lambliasis

007.2 Coccidiosis
Infection by Isospora belli and Isospora hominis
Isosporiasis

007.3 Intestinal trichomoniasis
DEF: Colitis, diarrhea, or dysentery caused by the protozoa *Trichomonas.*

007.4 Cryptosporidiosis
AHA: 4Q, '97, 30
DEF: An intestinal infection by protozoan parasites causing intractable diarrhea in patients with AIDS and other immunosuppressed individuals.

007.5 Cyclosporiasis
AHA: 4Q, '00, 38
DEF: An infection of the small intestine by the protozoal organism, *Cyclospora caytenanesis,* spread to humans though ingestion of contaminated water or food. Symptoms include watery diarrhea with frequent explosive bowel movements, loss of appetite, loss of weight, bloating, increased gas, stomach cramps, nausea, vomiting, muscle aches, low grade fever, and fatigue.

007.8 Other specified protozoal intestinal diseases
Amebiasis due to organisms other than Entamoeba histolytica

007.9 Unspecified protozoal intestinal disease
Flagellate diarrhea
Protozoal dysentery NOS

✓4th **008 Intestinal infections due to other organisms**
INCLUDES any condition classifiable to 009.0-009.3 with mention of the responsible organisms
EXCLUDES *food poisoning by these organisms (005.0-005.9)*

✓5th **008.0 Escherichia coli [E. coli]**
AHA: 4Q, '92, 17

008.00 E. coli, unspecified
E. coli enteritis NOS

008.01 Enteropathogenic E. coli
DEF: E. coli causing inflammation of intestines.

008.02 Enterotoxigenic E. coli
DEF: A toxic reaction to E. coli of the intestinal mucosa, causing voluminous watery secretions.

008.03 Enteroinvasive E. coli
DEF: E. coli infection penetrating intestinal mucosa.

008.04 Enterohemorrhagic E. coli
DEF: E. coli infection penetrating the intestinal mucosa, producing microscopic ulceration and bleeding.

008.09 Other intestinal E. coli infections

008.1 Arizona group of paracolon bacilli

008.2 Aerobacter aerogenes
Enterobacter aeogenes

008.3 Proteus (mirabilis) (morganii)

✓5th **008.4 Other specified bacteria**
AHA: 4Q, '92, 18

008.41 Staphylococcus
Staphylococcal enterocolitis

008.42 Pseudomonas
AHA: 2Q, '89, 10

008.43 Campylobacter

008.44 Yersinia enterocolitica

008.45 Clostridium difficile
Pseudomembranous colitis
DEF: An overgrowth of a species of bacterium that is a part of the normal colon flora in human infants and sometimes in adults; produces a toxin that causes pseudomembranous enterocolitis; typically is seen in patients undergoing antibiotic therapy.

008.46 Other anaerobes
Anaerobic enteritis NOS
Bacteroides (fragilis)
Gram-negative anaerobes

008.47 Other gram-negative bacteria
Gram-negative enteritis NOS
EXCLUDES *gram-negative anaerobes (008.46)*

008.49 Other
AHA: 2Q, '89, 10; 1Q, '88, 6

008.5 Bacterial enteritis, unspecified

✓5th **008.6 Enteritis due to specified virus**
AHA: 4Q, '92, 18

008.61 Rotavirus

008.62 Adenovirus

008.63 Norwalk virus
Norwalk-like agent

008.64 Other small round viruses [SRVs]
Small round virus NOS

008.65 Calicivirus
DEF: Enteritis due to a subgroup of *Picornaviruses.*

008.66 Astrovirus

008.67 Enterovirus NEC
Coxsackie virus Echovirus
EXCLUDES *poliovirus (045.0-045.9)*

008.69 Other viral enteritis
Torovirus
AHA: 1Q, '03,10

008.8 Other organism, not elsewhere classified
Viral:
enteritis NOS
gastroenteritis
EXCLUDES *influenza with involvement of gastrointestinal tract (487.8)*

✓4th **009 Ill-defined intestinal infections**
EXCLUDES *diarrheal disease or intestinal infection due to specified organism (001.0-008.8)*
diarrhea following gastrointestinal surgery (564.4)
intestinal malabsorption (579.0-579.9)
ischemic enteritis (557.0-557.9)
other noninfectious gastroenteritis and colitis (558.1-558.9)
regional enteritis (555.0-555.9)
ulcerative colitis (556)

009.0 Infectious colitis, enteritis, and gastroenteritis
Colitis } septic
Enteritis } septic
Gastroenteritis } septic

Dysentery:
NOS
catarrhal
hemorrhagic
AHA: 3Q, '99, 4
DEF: Colitis: An inflammation of mucous membranes of the colon.
DEF: Enteritis: An inflammation of mucous membranes of the small intestine.
DEF: Gastroenteritis: An inflammation of mucous membranes of stomach and intestines.

009.1 Colitis, enteritis, and gastroenteritis of presumed infectious origin
EXCLUDES *colitis NOS (558.9)*
enteritis NOS (558.9)
gastroenteritis NOS (558.9)
AHA: 3Q, '99, 6

009.2 Infectious diarrhea
Diarrhea:
dysenteric
epidemic
Infectious diarrheal disease NOS

009.3 Diarrhea of presumed infectious origin
EXCLUDES *diarrhea NOS (787.91)*
AHA: N-D, '87, 7

TUBERCULOSIS (010-018)

INCLUDES infection by Mycobacterium tuberculosis (human) (bovine)

EXCLUDES *congenital tuberculosis (771.2)*
late effects of tuberculosis (137.0-137.4)

The following fifth-digit subclassification is for use with categories 010-018:
- **0 unspecified**
- **1 bacteriological or histological examination not done**
- **2 bacteriological or histological examination unknown (at present)**
- **3 tubercle bacilli found (in sputum) by microscopy**
- **4 tubercle bacilli not found (in sputum) by microscopy, but found by bacterial culture**
- **5 tubercle bacilli not found by bacteriological examination, but tuberculosis confirmed histologically**
- **6 tubercle bacilli not found by bacteriological or histological examination but tuberculosis confirmed by other methods [inoculation of animals]**

DEF: An infection by *Mycobacterium tuberculosis* causing the formation of small, rounded nodules, called tubercles, that can disseminate throughout the body via lymph and blood vessels. Localized tuberculosis is most often seen in the lungs.

✓4th **010 Primary tuberculous infection**
DEF: Tuberculosis of the lungs occurring when the patient is first infected.

✓5th **010.0 Primary tuberculous infection**
EXCLUDES *nonspecific reaction to tuberculin skin test without active tuberculosis (795.5)*
positive PPD (795.5)
positive tuberculin skin test without active tuberculosis (795.5)
DEF: Hilar or paratracheal lymph node enlargement in pulmonary tuberculosis.

✓5th **010.1 Tuberculous pleurisy in primary progressive tuberculosis**
DEF: Inflammation and exudation in the lining of the tubercular lung.

✓5th **010.8 Other primary progressive tuberculosis**
EXCLUDES *tuberculous erythema nodosum (017.1)*

✓5th **010.9 Primary tuberculous infection, unspecified**

✓4th **011 Pulmonary tuberculosis**
Use additional code to identify any associated silicosis (502)

✓5th **011.0 Tuberculosis of lung, infiltrative**

✓5th **011.1 Tuberculosis of lung, nodular**

✓5th **011.2 Tuberculosis of lung with cavitation**

✓5th **011.3 Tuberculosis of bronchus**
EXCLUDES *isolated bronchial tuberculosis (012.2)*

✓5th **011.4 Tuberculous fibrosis of lung**

✓5th **011.5 Tuberculous bronchiectasis**

✓5th **011.6 Tuberculous pneumonia [any form]**
DEF: Inflammatory pulmonary reaction to tuberculous cells.

✓5th **011.7 Tuberculous pneumothorax**
DEF: Spontaneous rupture of damaged tuberculous pulmonary tissue.

✓5th **011.8 Other specified pulmonary tuberculosis**

✓5th **011.9 Pulmonary tuberculosis, unspecified**
Respiratory tuberculosis NOS
Tuberculosis of lung NOS

✓4th **012 Other respiratory tuberculosis**
EXCLUDES *respiratory tuberculosis, unspecified (011.9)*

✓5th **012.0 Tuberculous pleurisy**
Tuberculosis of pleura
Tuberculous empyema
Tuberculous hydrothorax
EXCLUDES *pleurisy with effusion without mention of cause (511.9)*
tuberculous pleurisy in primary progressive tuberculosis (010.1)
DEF: Inflammation and exudation in the lining of the tubercular lung.

✓5th **012.1 Tuberculosis of intrathoracic lymph nodes**
Tuberculosis of lymph nodes:
hilar
mediastinal
tracheobronchial
Tuberculous tracheobronchial adenopathy
EXCLUDES *that specified as primary (010.0-010.9)*

✓5th **012.2 Isolated tracheal or bronchial tuberculosis**

✓5th **012.3 Tuberculous laryngitis**
Tuberculosis of glottis

✓5th **012.8 Other specified respiratory tuberculosis**
Tuberculosis of:
mediastinum
nasopharynx
Tuberculosis of:
nose (septum)
sinus [any nasal]

✓4th **013 Tuberculosis of meninges and central nervous system**

✓5th **013.0 Tuberculous meningitis**
Tuberculosis of meninges (cerebral) (spinal)
Tuberculous:
leptomeningitis
meningoencephalitis
EXCLUDES *tuberculoma of meninges (013.1)*

✓5th **013.1 Tuberculoma of meninges**

✓5th **013.2 Tuberculoma of brain**
Tuberculosis of brain (current disease)

✓5th **013.3 Tuberculous abscess of brain**

✓5th **013.4 Tuberculoma of spinal cord**

✓5th **013.5 Tuberculous abscess of spinal cord**

✓5th **013.6 Tuberculous encephalitis or myelitis**

✓5th **013.8 Other specified tuberculosis of central nervous system**

✓5th **013.9 Unspecified tuberculosis of central nervous system**
Tuberculosis of central nervous system NOS

✓4th **014 Tuberculosis of intestines, peritoneum, and mesenteric glands**

✓5th **014.0 Tuberculous peritonitis**
Tuberculous ascites
DEF: Tuberculous inflammation of the membrane lining the abdomen.

✓5th **014.8 Other**
Tuberculosis (of):
anus
intestine (large) (small)
mesenteric glands
rectum
retroperitoneal (lymph nodes)
Tuberculous enteritis

4th 015 Tuberculosis of bones and joints

Use additional code to identify manifestation, as:
tuberculous:
arthropathy (711.4)
necrosis of bone (730.8)
osteitis (730.8)
osteomyelitis (730.8)
synovitis (727.01)
tenosynovitis (727.01)

§ 5th **015.0 Vertebral column**
Pott's disease
Use additional code to identify manifestation, as:
curvature of spine [Pott's] (737.4)
kyphosis (737.4)
spondylitis (720.81)

§ 5th **015.1 Hip**

§ 5th **015.2 Knee**

§ 5th **015.5 Limb bones**
Tuberculous dactylitis

§ 5th **015.6 Mastoid**
Tuberculous mastoiditis

§ 5th **015.7 Other specified bone**

§ 5th **015.8 Other specified joint**

§ 5th **015.9 Tuberculosis of unspecified bones and joints**

4th 016 Tuberculosis of genitourinary system

§ 5th **016.0 Kidney**
Renal tuberculosis
Use additional code to identify manifestation, as:
tuberculous:
nephropathy (583.81)
pyelitis (590.81)
pyelonephritis (590.81)

§ 5th **016.1 Bladder**

§ 5th **016.2 Ureter**

§ 5th **016.3 Other urinary organs**

§ 5th **016.4 Epididymis** ♂

§ 5th **016.5 Other male genital organs** ♂
Use additional code to identify manifestation, as:
tuberculosis of:
prostate (601.4)
seminal vesicle (608.81)
testis (608.81)

§ 5th **016.6 Tuberculous oophoritis and salpingitis** ♀

§ 5th **016.7 Other female genital organs** ♀
Tuberculous:
cervicitis
endometritis

§ 5th **016.9 Genitourinary tuberculosis, unspecified**

4th 017 Tuberculosis of other organs

§ 5th **017.0 Skin and subcutaneous cellular tissue**
Lupus:
exedens
vulgaris
Scrofuloderma
Tuberculosis:
colliquativa
cutis
lichenoides
papulonecrotica
verrucosa cutis

EXCLUDES *lupus erythematosus (695.4)*
disseminated (710.0)
lupus NOS (710.0)
nonspecific reaction to tuberculin skin test without active tuberculosis (795.5)
positive PPD (795.5)
positive tuberculin skin test without active tuberculosis (795.5)

§ 5th **017.1 Erythema nodosum with hypersensitivity reaction in tuberculosis**
Bazin's disease
Erythema:
induratum
nodosum, tuberculous
Tuberculosis indurativa

EXCLUDES *erythema nodosum NOS (695.2)*

DEF: Tender, inflammatory, bilateral nodules appearing on the shins and thought to be an allergic reaction to tuberculotoxin.

§ 5th **017.2 Peripheral lymph nodes**
Scrofula
Scrofulous abscess
Tuberculous adenitis

EXCLUDES *tuberculosis of lymph nodes:*
bronchial and mediastinal (012.1)
mesenteric and retroperitoneal (014.8)
tuberculous tracheobronchial adenopathy (012.1)

DEF: Scrofula: Old name for tuberculous cervical lymphadenitis.

§ 5th **017.3 Eye**
Use additional code to identify manifestation, as:
tuberculous:
chorioretinitis, disseminated (363.13)
episcleritis (379.09)
interstitial keratitis (370.59)
iridocyclitis, chronic (364.11)
keratoconjunctivitis (phlyctenular) (370.31)

§ 5th **017.4 Ear**
Tuberculosis of ear
Tuberculous otitis media

EXCLUDES *tuberculous mastoiditis (015.6)*

§ 5th **017.5 Thyroid gland**

§ 5th **017.6 Adrenal glands**
Addison's disease, tuberculous

§ 5th **017.7 Spleen**

§ 5th **017.8 Esophagus**

§ 5th **017.9 Other specified organs**
Use additional code to identify manifestation, as:
tuberculosis of:
endocardium [any valve] (424.91)
myocardium (422.0)
pericardium (420.0)

4th 018 Miliary tuberculosis

INCLUDES tuberculosis:
disseminated
generalized
miliary, whether of a single specified site, multiple sites, or unspecified site
polyserositis

DEF: A form of tuberculosis caused by caseous material carried through the bloodstream planting seedlike tubercles in various body organs.

§ 5th **018.0 Acute miliary tuberculosis**

§ 5th **018.8 Other specified miliary tuberculosis**

§ 5th **018.9 Miliary tuberculosis, unspecified**

ZOONOTIC BACTERIAL DISEASES (020-027)

4th 020 Plague

INCLUDES infection by Yersinia [Pasteurella] pestis

020.0 Bubonic
DEF: Most common acute and severe form of plague characterized by lymphadenopathy (buboes), chills, fever and headache.

020.1 Cellulocutaneous
DEF: Plague characterized by inflammation and necrosis of skin.

020.2 Septicemic
DEF: Plague characterized by massive infection in the bloodstream.

§ Requires fifth-digit. See beginning of section 010–018 for codes and definitions.

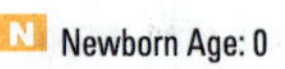 Newborn Age: 0
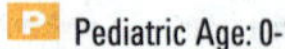 Pediatric Age: 0-17
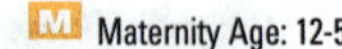 Maternity Age: 12-55
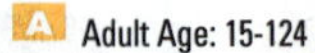 Adult Age: 15-124
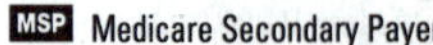 Medicare Secondary Payer

020.3 Primary pneumonic
DEF: Plague characterized by massive pulmonary infection.

020.4 Secondary pneumonic
DEF: Lung infection as a secondary complication of plague.

020.5 Pneumonic, unspecified

020.8 Other specified types of plague
Abortive plague
Ambulatory plague
Pestis minor

020.9 Plague, unspecified

✓4th **021 Tularemia**

INCLUDES deerfly fever
infection by Francisella [Pasteurella] tularensis
rabbit fever

DEF: A febrile disease transmitted by the bites of deer flies, fleas and ticks, by inhalations of aerosolized *F. tulairensis* or by ingestion of contaminated food or water; patients quickly develop fever, chills, weakness, headache, backache and malaise.

021.0 Ulceroglandular tularemia
DEF: Lesions occur at the site *Francisella tularensis;* organism enters body, usually the fingers or hands.

021.1 Enteric tularemia
Tularemia:
cryptogenic
intestinal
Tularemia:
typhoidal

021.2 Pulmonary tularemia
Bronchopneumonic tularemia

021.3 Oculoglandular tularemia
DEF: Painful conjunctival infection by *Francisella tularensis* organism with possible corneal, preauricular lymph, or lacrimal involvement.

021.8 Other specified tularemia
Tularemia:
generalized or disseminated
glandular

021.9 Unspecified tularemia

✓4th **022 Anthrax**
AHA: 4Q '02, 70

DEF: An infectious bacterial disease usually transmitted by contact with infected animals or their discharges or products; it is classified by primary routes of inoculation as cutaneous, gastrointestinal and by inhalation.

022.0 Cutaneous anthrax
Malignant pustule

022.1 Pulmonary anthrax
Respiratory anthrax
Wool-sorters' disease

022.2 Gastrointestinal anthrax

022.3 Anthrax septicemia

022.8 Other specified manifestations of anthrax

022.9 Anthrax, unspecified

✓4th **023 Brucellosis**

INCLUDES fever:
Malta
Mediterranean
undulant

DEF: An infectious disease caused by gram-negative, *aerobic coccobacilli* organisms; it is transmitted to humans through contact with infected tissue or dairy products; fever, sweating, weakness and aching are symptoms of the disease.

023.0 Brucella melitensis
DEF: Infection from direct or indirect contact with infected sheep or goats.

023.1 Brucella abortus
DEF: Infection from direct or indirect contact with infected cattle.

023.2 Brucella suis
DEF: Infection from direct or indirect contact with infected swine.

023.3 Brucella canis
DEF: Infection from direct or indirect contact with infected dogs.

023.8 Other brucellosis
Infection by more than one organism

023.9 Brucellosis, unspecified

024 Glanders
Infection by:
Actinobacillus mallei
Malleomyces mallei
Pseudomonas mallei
Farcy
Malleus

DEF: Equine infection causing mucosal inflammation and skin ulcers in humans.

025 Melioidosis
Infection by:
Malleomyces pseudomallei
Pseudomonas pseudomallei
Whitmore's bacillus
Pseudoglanders

DEF: Rare infection caused by *Pseudomonas pseudomallei*; clinical symptoms range from localized infection to fatal septicemia.

✓4th **026 Rat-bite fever**

026.0 Spirillary fever
Rat-bite fever due to Spirillum minor [S. minus]
Sodoku

026.1 Streptobacillary fever
Epidemic arthritic erythema
Haverhill fever
Rat-bite fever due to Streptobacillus moniliformis

026.9 Unspecified rat-bite fever

✓4th **027 Other zoonotic bacterial diseases**

027.0 Listeriosis
Infection } by Listeria monocytogenes
Septicemia }

Use additional code to identify manifestation, as meningitis (320.7)

EXCLUDES *congenital listeriosis (771.2)*

027.1 Erysipelothrix infection
Erysipeloid (of Rosenbach)
Infection } by Erysipelothrix insidiosa [E. rhusiopathiae]
Septicemia }

DEF: Usually associated with handling of fish, meat, or poultry; symptoms range from localized inflammation to septicemia.

027.2 Pasteurellosis
Pasteurella pseudotuberculosis infection
Mesenteric adenitis } by Pasteurella multocida [P. septica]
Septic infection (cat bite) }
(dog bite) }

EXCLUDES *infection by:*
Francisella [Pasteurella] tularensis (021.0-021.9)
Yersinia [Pasteurella] pestis (020.0-020.9)

DEF: Swelling, abscesses, or septicemia from *Pasteurella multocida*, commonly transmitted to humans by a dog or cat scratch.

027.8 Other specified zoonotic bacterial diseases

027.9 Unspecified zoonotic bacterial disease

OTHER BACTERIAL DISEASES (030-041)

EXCLUDES *bacterial venereal diseases (098.0-099.9)*
bartonellosis (088.0)

✓4th **030 Leprosy**

INCLUDES Hansen's disease
infection by Mycobacterium leprae

030.0 Lepromatous [type L]
Lepromatous leprosy (macular) (diffuse) (infiltrated) (nodular) (neuritic)

DEF: Infectious disseminated leprosy bacilli with lesions and deformities.

030.1 Tuberculoid [type T]
Tuberculoid leprosy (macular) (maculoanesthetic) (major) (minor) (neuritic)

DEF: Relatively benign, self-limiting leprosy with neuralgia and scales.

030.2 Indeterminate [group I]
Indeterminate [uncharacteristic] leprosy (macular) (neuritic)

DEF: Uncharacteristic leprosy, frequently an early manifestation.

030.3 Borderline [group B]
Borderline or dimorphous leprosy (infiltrated) (neuritic)

DEF: Transitional form of leprosy, neither lepromatous nor tuberculoid.

030.8 Other specified leprosy

030.9 Leprosy, unspecified

✓4th **031 Diseases due to other mycobacteria**

031.0 Pulmonary
Battey disease
Infection by Mycobacterium:
avium
intracellulare [Battey bacillus]
kansasii

031.1 Cutaneous
Buruli ulcer
Infection by Mycobacterium:
marinum [M. balnei]
ulcerans

031.2 Disseminated
Disseminated mycobacterium avium-intracellulare complex (DMAC)
Mycobacterium avium-intracellulare complex (MAC) bacteremia

AHA: 4Q, '97, 31

DEF: Disseminated mycobacterium avium-intracellulare complex (DMAC): A serious systemic form of MAC commonly observed in patients in the late course of AIDS.

DEF: Mycobacterium avium-intracellulare complex (MAC) bacterium: Human pulmonary disease, lymphadenitis in children and systemic disease in immunocompromised individuals caused by a slow growing, gram-positive, aerobic organism.

031.8 Other specified mycobacterial diseases

031.9 Unspecified diseases due to mycobacteria
Atypical mycobacterium infection NOS

✓4th **032 Diphtheria**

INCLUDES infection by Corynebacterium diphtheriae

032.0 Faucial diphtheria
Membranous angina, diphtheritic

DEF: Diphtheria of the throat.

032.1 Nasopharyngeal diphtheria

032.2 Anterior nasal diphtheria

032.3 Laryngeal diphtheria
Laryngotracheitis, diphtheritic

✓5th **032.8 Other specified diphtheria**

032.81 Conjunctival diphtheria
Pseudomembranous diphtheritic conjunctivitis

032.82 Diphtheritic myocarditis

032.83 Diphtheritic peritonitis

032.84 Diphtheritic cystitis

032.85 Cutaneous diphtheria

032.89 Other

032.9 Diphtheria, unspecified

✓4th **033 Whooping cough**

INCLUDES pertussis

Use additional code to identify any associated pneumonia (484.3)

DEF: An acute, highly contagious respiratory tract infection caused by *Bordetella pertussis* and *B. bronchiseptica*; characteristic paroxysmal cough.

033.0 Bordetella pertussis [B. pertussis]

033.1 Bordetella parapertussis [B. parapertussis]

033.8 Whooping cough due to other specified organism
Bordetella bronchiseptica [B. bronchiseptica]

033.9 Whooping cough, unspecified organism

✓4th **034 Streptococcal sore throat and scarlet fever**

034.0 Streptococcal sore throat
Septic:
angina
sore throat
Streptococcal:
angina
Streptococcal:
laryngitis
pharyngitis
tonsillitis

034.1 Scarlet fever
Scarlatina

EXCLUDES *parascarlatina (057.8)*

DEF: Streptococcal infection and fever with red rash spreading from trunk.

035 Erysipelas

EXCLUDES *postpartum or puerperal erysipelas (670)*

DEF: An acute superficial cellulitis involving the dermal lymphatics; it is often caused by group A streptococci.

✓4th **036 Meningococcal infection**

036.0 Meningococcal meningitis
Cerebrospinal fever (meningococcal)
Meningitis:
cerebrospinal
epidemic

036.1 Meningococcal encephalitis

036.2 Meningococcemia
Meningococcal septicemia

036.3 Waterhouse-Friderichsen syndrome, meningococcal
Meningococcal hemorrhagic adrenalitis
Meningococcic adrenal syndrome
Waterhouse-Friderichsen syndrome NOS

✓5th **036.4 Meningococcal carditis**

036.40 Meningococcal carditis, unspecified

036.41 Meningococcal pericarditis

DEF: Meningococcal infection of the outer membrane of the heart.

036.42 Meningococcal endocarditis

DEF: Meningococcal infection of the membranes lining the cavities of the heart.

036.43 Meningococcal myocarditis

DEF: Meningococcal infection of the muscle of the heart.

✓5th **036.8 Other specified meningococcal infections**

036.81 Meningococcal optic neuritis

036.82 Meningococcal arthropathy

036.89 Other

036.9 Meningococcal infection, unspecified
Meningococcal infection NOS

037 Tetanus

EXCLUDES *tetanus:*
complicating:
abortion (634-638 with .0, 639.0)
ectopic or molar pregnancy (639.0)
neonatorum (771.3)
puerperal (670)

DEF: An acute, often fatal, infectious disease caused by the anaerobic, spore-forming bacillus *Clostridium tetani*; the bacillus most often enters the body through a contaminated wound, burns, surgical wounds, or cutaneous ulcers. Symptoms include lockjaw, spasms, seizures, and paralysis.

✓4th **038 Septicemia**

Use additional code for systemic inflammatory response syndrome (SIRS) (995.91-995.92)

EXCLUDES *bacteremia (790.7)*
during labor (659.3)
following ectopic or molar pregnancy (639.0)
following infusion, injection, transfusion, or vaccination (999.3)
postpartum, puerperal (670)
septicemia (sepsis) of newborn (771.81)
that complicating abortion (634-638 with .0, 639.0)

AHA: 2Q, '04, 16; 4Q, '88, 10; 3Q, '88, 12

DEF: A systemic disease associated with the presence and persistence of pathogenic microorganisms or their toxins in the blood.

038.0 Streptococcal septicemia
AHA: 4Q, '03, 79; 2Q, '96. 5

✓5th **038.1 Staphylococcal septicemia**
AHA: 4Q, '97, 32

038.10 Staphylococcal septicemia, unspecified

038.11 Staphylococcus aureus septicemia
AHA: ▶1Q, '05, 7;◀ 2Q, '00, 5; 4Q, '98, 42

038.19 Other staphylococcal septicemia
AHA: 2Q, '00, 5

038.2 Pneumococcal septicemia [Streptococcus pneumoniae septicemia]
AHA: 2Q, '96, 5; 1Q, '91, 13

038.3 Septicemia due to anaerobes
Septicemia due to bacteroides

EXCLUDES *gas gangrene (040.0)*
that due to anaerobic streptococci (038.0)

DEF: Infection of blood by microorganisms that thrive without oxygen.

✓5th **038.4 Septicemia due to other gram-negative organisms**

DEF: Infection of blood by microorganisms categorized as gram-negative by Gram's method of staining for identification of bacteria.

038.40 Gram-negative organism, unspecified
Gram-negative septicemia NOS

038.41 Hemophilus influenzae [H. influenzae]

038.42 Escherichia coli [E. coli]
AHA: 4Q, '03, 73

038.43 Pseudomonas

038.44 Serratia

038.49 Other

038.8 Other specified septicemias

EXCLUDES *septicemia (due to):*
anthrax (022.3)
gonococcal (098.89)
herpetic (054.5)
meningococcal (036.2)
septicemic plague (020.2)

038.9 Unspecified septicemia
Septicemia NOS

EXCLUDES *bacteremia NOS (790.7)*

AHA: 2Q, '04, 16; 4Q, '03, 79; 2Q, '00, 3; 3Q, '99. 5. 9; 1Q, '98, 5; 3Q, '96, 16; 2Q, '96, 6

✓4th **039 Actinomycotic infections**

INCLUDES actinomycotic mycetoma
infection by Actinomycetales, such as species of Actinomyces, Actinomadura, Nocardia, Streptomyces
maduromycosis (actinomycotic)
schizomycetoma (actinomycotic)

DEF: Inflammatory lesions and abscesses at site of infection by *Actinomyces israelii*.

039.0 Cutaneous
Erythrasma
Trichomycosis axillaris

039.1 Pulmonary
Thoracic actinomycosis

039.2 Abdominal

039.3 Cervicofacial

039.4 Madura foot

EXCLUDES *madura foot due to mycotic infection (117.4)*

039.8 Of other specified sites

039.9 Of unspecified site
Actinomycosis NOS
Nocardiosis NOS
Maduromycosis NOS

✓4th **040 Other bacterial diseases**

EXCLUDES *bacteremia NOS (790.7)*
bacterial infection NOS (041.9)

040.0 Gas gangrene
Gas bacillus infection or gangrene
Infection by Clostridium:
histolyticum
oedematiens
perfringens [welchii]
septicum
sordellii
Malignant edema
Myonecrosis, clostridial
Myositis, clostridial

AHA: 1Q, '95, 11

040.1 Rhinoscleroma

DEF: Growths on the nose and nasopharynx caused by *Klebsiella rhinoscleromatis*.

040.2 Whipple's disease
Intestinal lipodystrophy

040.3 Necrobacillosis

DEF: Infection with *Fusobacterium necrophorum* causing abscess or necrosis.

✓5th **040.8 Other specified bacterial diseases**

040.81 Tropical pyomyositis

040.82 Toxic shock syndrome
Use additional code to identify the organism
AHA: 4Q, '02, 44

DEF: Syndrome caused by staphylococcal exotoxin that may rapidly progress to severe and intractable shock; symptoms include characteristic sunburn-like rash with peeling of skin on palms and soles, sudden onset high fever, vomiting, diarrhea, malagia, and hypotension.

040.89 Other
AHA: N-D, '86, 7

✓4th **041 Bacterial infection in conditions classified elsewhere and of unspecified site**

Note: This category is provided to be used as an additional code to identify the bacterial agent in diseases classified elsewhere. This category will also be used to classify bacterial infections of unspecified nature or site.

EXCLUDES *bacteremia NOS (790.7)*
septicemia (038.0-038.9)

AHA: 2Q, '01, 12; J-A, '84, 19

Infectious and Parasitic Diseases 037–041

✓4th ✓5th Additional Digit Required | Unspecified Code | Other Specified Code | Manifestation Code | ▶◀ Revised Text | ● New Code | ▲ Revised Code Title

✓5th **041.0 Streptococcus**
- **041.00 Streptococcus, unspecified**
- **041.01 Group A**
  AHA: 1Q, '02, 3
- **041.02 Group B**
- **041.03 Group C**
- **041.04 Group D [Enterococcus]**
- **041.05 Group G**
- **041.09 Other Streptococcus**

✓5th **041.1 Staphylococcus**
- **041.10 Staphylococcus, unspecified**
- **041.11 Staphylococcus aureus**
  AHA: 4Q, '03, 104, 106; 2Q, '01, 11; 4Q, '98, 42, 54;4Q, '97, 32
- **041.19 Other Staphylococcus**

041.2 Pneumococcus

041.3 Friedländer's bacillus
Infection by Klebsiella pneumoniae

041.4 Escherichia coli [E. coli]

041.5 Hemophilus influenzae [H. influenzae]

041.6 Proteus (mirabilis) (morganii)

041.7 Pseudomonas
AHA: 4Q, '02, 45

✓5th **041.8 Other specified bacterial infections**
- **041.81 Mycoplasma**
  Eaton's agent
  Pleuropneumonia-like organisms [PPLO]
- **041.82 Bacteroides fragilis**
  DEF: Anaerobic gram-negative bacilli of the gastrointestinal tract; frequently implicated in intra-abdominal infection; commonly resistant to antibiotics.
- **041.83 Clostridium perfringens**
- **041.84 Other anaerobes**
  Gram-negative anaerobes
  EXCLUDES *Helicobacter pylori (041.86)*
- **041.85 Other gram-negative organisms**
  Aerobacter aerogenes
  Gram-negative bacteria NOS
  Mima polymorpha
  Serratia
  EXCLUDES *gram-negative anaerobes (041.84)*
  AHA: 1Q, 95, 18
- **041.86 Helicobacter pylori (H. pylori)**
  AHA: 4Q, '95, 60
- **041.89 Other specified bacteria**
  AHA: 2Q, '03, 7

041.9 Bacterial infection, unspecified
AHA: 2Q, '91, 9

HUMAN IMMUNODEFICIENCY VIRUS (HIV) INFECTION (042)

042 Human immunodeficiency virus [HIV] disease
Acquired immune deficiency syndrome
Acquired immunodeficiency syndrome
AIDS
AIDS-like syndrome
AIDS-related complex
ARC
HIV infection, symptomatic
Use additional code(s) to identify all manifestations of HIV.
Use additional code to identify HIV-2 infection (079.53)
EXCLUDES *asymptomatic HIV infection status (V08)*
exposure to HIV virus (V01.79)
nonspecific serologic evidence of HIV (795.71)
AHA: ►1Q, '05, 7;◄ 2Q, '04, 11; 1Q, '04, 5; 1Q, '03, 15; 1Q, '99, 14, 4Q, '97, 30, 31; 1Q, '93, 21; 2Q, '92, 11; 3Q, '90, 17; J-A, '87, 8

POLIOMYELITIS AND OTHER NON-ARTHROPOD-BORNE VIRAL DISEASES OF CENTRAL NERVOUS SYSTEM (045-049)

✓4th **045 Acute poliomyelitis**
EXCLUDES *late effects of acute poliomyelitis (138)*

The following fifth-digit subclassification is for use with category 045:
- **0 poliovirus, unspecified type**
- **1 poliovirus type I**
- **2 poliovirus type II**
- **3 poliovirus type III**

✓5th **045.0 Acute paralytic poliomyelitis specified as bulbar**
Infantile paralysis (acute) } specified as bulbar
Poliomyelitis (acute) (anterior) } specified as bulbar
Polioencephalitis (acute) (bulbar)
Polioencephalomyelitis (acute) (anterior) (bulbar)
DEF: Acute paralytic infection occurring where the brain merges with the spinal cord; affecting breathing, swallowing, and heart rate.

✓5th **045.1 Acute poliomyelitis with other paralysis**
Paralysis:
- acute atrophic, spinal
- infantile, paralytic

Poliomyelitis (acute) anterior epidemic } with paralysis except bulbar
DEF: Paralytic infection affecting peripheral or spinal nerves.

✓5th **045.2 Acute nonparalytic poliomyelitis**
Poliomyelitis (acute) anterior epidemic } specified as nonparalytic
DEF: Nonparalytic infection causing pain, stiffness, and paresthesias.

✓5th **045.9 Acute poliomyelitis, unspecified**
Infantile paralysis
Poliomyelitis (acute) anterior epidemic } unspecified whether paralytic or nonparalytic

✓4th **046 Slow virus infection of central nervous system**

046.0 Kuru
DEF: A chronic, progressive, fatal nervous system disorder; clinical symptoms include cerebellar ataxia, trembling, spasticity and progressive dementia.

046.1 Jakob-Creutzfeldt disease
Subacute spongiform encephalopathy
DEF: Communicable, progressive spongiform encephalopathy thought to be caused by an infectious particle known as a "prion" (proteinaceous infection particle). This is a progressive, fatal disease manifested principally by mental deterioration.

046.2 Subacute sclerosing panencephalitis
Dawson's inclusion body encephalitis
Van Bogaert's sclerosing leukoencephalitis
DEF: Progressive viral infection causing cerebral dysfunction, blindness, dementia, and death (SSPE).

046.3 Progressive multifocal leukoencephalopathy
Multifocal leukoencephalopathy NOS
DEF: Infection affecting cerebral cortex in patients with weakened immune systems.

046.8 Other specified slow virus infection of central nervous system

046.9 Unspecified slow virus infection of central nervous system

✓4th 047 Meningitis due to enterovirus

INCLUDES meningitis:
- abacterial
- aseptic
- viral

EXCLUDES *meningitis due to:*
- *adenovirus (049.1)*
- *arthropod-borne virus (060.0-066.9)*
- *leptospira (100.81)*
- *virus of:*
  - *herpes simplex (054.72)*
  - *herpes zoster (053.0)*
  - *lymphocytic choriomeningitis (049.0)*
  - *mumps (072.1)*
  - *poliomyelitis (045.0-045.9)*
- *any other infection specifically classified elsewhere*

AHA: J-F, '87, 6

047.0 Coxsackie virus

047.1 ECHO virus

Meningo-eruptive syndrome

047.8 Other specified viral meningitis

047.9 Unspecified viral meningitis

Viral meningitis NOS

048 Other enterovirus diseases of central nervous system

Boston exanthem

✓4th 049 Other non-arthropod-borne viral diseases of central nervous system

EXCLUDES *late effects of viral encephalitis (139.0)*

049.0 Lymphocytic choriomeningitis

Lymphocytic:
- meningitis (serous) (benign)
- meningoencephalitis (serous) (benign)

049.1 Meningitis due to adenovirus

DEF: Inflammation of lining of brain caused by Arenaviruses and usually occurring in adults in fall and winter months.

049.8 Other specified non-arthropod-borne viral diseases of central nervous system

Encephalitis:
- acute:
  - inclusion body
  - necrotizing
- epidemic
- lethargica
- Rio Bravo

von Economo's disease

049.9 Unspecified non-arthropod-borne viral diseases of central nervous system

Viral encephalitis NOS

VIRAL DISEASES ACCOMPANIED BY EXANTHEM (050-057)

EXCLUDES *arthropod-borne viral diseases (060.0-066.9)*
Boston exanthem (048)

✓4th 050 Smallpox

050.0 Variola major

Hemorrhagic (pustular) smallpox
Malignant smallpox
Purpura variolosa

DEF: Form of smallpox known for its high mortality; exists only in laboratories.

050.1 Alastrim

Variola minor

DEF: Mild form of smallpox known for its low mortality rate.

050.2 Modified smallpox

Varioloid

DEF: Mild form occurring in patients with history of infection or vaccination.

050.9 Smallpox, unspecified

✓4th 051 Cowpox and paravaccinia

051.0 Cowpox

Vaccinia not from vaccination

EXCLUDES *vaccinia (generalized) (from vaccination) (999.0)*

DEF: A disease contracted by milking infected cows; vesicles usually appear on the fingers, may spread to hands and adjacent areas and usually disappear without scarring; other associated features of the disease may include local edema, lymphangitis and regional lymphadenitis with or without fever.

051.1 Pseudocowpox

Milkers' node

DEF: Hand lesions and mild fever in dairy workers caused by exposure to paravaccinia.

051.2 Contagious pustular dermatitis

Ecthyma contagiosum
Orf

DEF: Skin eruptions caused by exposure to poxvirus-infected sheep or goats.

051.9 Paravaccinia, unspecified

✓4th 052 Chickenpox

DEF: Contagious infection by varicella-zoster virus causing rash with pustules and fever.

052.0 Postvaricella encephalitis

Postchickenpox encephalitis

052.1 Varicella (hemorrhagic) pneumonitis

052.7 With other specified complications

AHA: 1Q, '02, 3

052.8 With unspecified complication

052.9 Varicella without mention of complication

Chickenpox NOS
Varicella NOS

✓4th 053 Herpes zoster

INCLUDES shingles
zona

DEF: Self-limiting infection by varicella-zoster virus causing unilateral eruptions and neuralgia along affected nerves.

053.0 With meningitis

DEF: Varicella-zoster virus infection causing inflammation of the lining of the brain and/or spinal cord.

✓5th 053.1 With other nervous system complications

053.10 With unspecified nervous system complication

053.11 Geniculate herpes zoster

Herpetic geniculate ganglionitis

DEF: Unilateral eruptions and neuralgia along the facial nerve geniculum affecting face and outer and middle ear.

053.12 Postherpetic trigeminal neuralgia

DEF: Severe oral or nasal pain following a herpes zoster infection.

053.13 Postherpetic polyneuropathy

DEF: Multiple areas of pain following a herpes zoster infection.

053.19 Other

✓5th 053.2 With ophthalmic complications

053.20 Herpes zoster dermatitis of eyelid

Herpes zoster ophthalmicus

053.21 Herpes zoster keratoconjunctivitis

053.22 Herpes zoster iridocyclitis

053.29 Other

✓5th 053.7 With other specified complications

053.71 Otitis externa due to herpes zoster

053.79 Other

053.8 With unspecified complication

053.9 **Herpes zoster without mention of complication**
Herpes zoster NOS

✓4th 054 **Herpes simplex**
EXCLUDES *congenital herpes simplex (771.2)*

054.0 **Eczema herpeticum**
Kaposi's varicelliform eruption
DEF: Herpes simplex virus invading site of preexisting skin inflammation.

✓5th 054.1 **Genital herpes**
AHA: J-F, '87, 15, 16

054.10 **Genital herpes, unspecified**
Herpes progenitalis

054.11 **Herpetic vulvovaginitis** ♀
054.12 **Herpetic ulceration of vulva** ♀
054.13 **Herpetic infection of penis** ♂
054.19 **Other**

054.2 **Herpetic gingivostomatitis**
054.3 **Herpetic meningoencephalitis**
Herpes encephalitis
Simian B disease
DEF: Inflammation of the brain and its lining; caused by infection of herpes simplex 1 in adults and simplex 2 in newborns.

✓5th 054.4 **With ophthalmic complications**
054.40 **With unspecified ophthalmic complication**
054.41 **Herpes simplex dermatitis of eyelid**
054.42 **Dendritic keratitis**
054.43 **Herpes simplex disciform keratitis**
054.44 **Herpes simplex iridocyclitis**
054.49 **Other**

054.5 **Herpetic septicemia**
AHA: 2Q, '00, 5

054.6 **Herpetic whitlow**
Herpetic felon
DEF: A primary infection of the terminal segment of a finger by herpes simplex; intense itching and pain start the disease, vesicles form, and tissue ultimately is destroyed.

✓5th 054.7 **With other specified complications**
054.71 **Visceral herpes simplex**
054.72 **Herpes simplex meningitis**
054.73 **Herpes simplex otitis externa**
054.79 **Other**

054.8 **With unspecified complication**
054.9 **Herpes simplex without mention of complication**

✓4th 055 **Measles**
INCLUDES morbilli
rubeola

055.0 **Postmeasles encephalitis**
055.1 **Postmeasles pneumonia**
055.2 **Postmeasles otitis media**

✓5th 055.7 **With other specified complications**
055.71 **Measles keratoconjunctivitis**
Measles keratitis
055.79 **Other**

055.8 **With unspecified complication**
055.9 **Measles without mention of complication**

✓4th 056 **Rubella**
INCLUDES German measles
EXCLUDES *congenital rubella (771.0)*
DEF: Acute but usually benign togavirus infection causing fever, sore throat, and rash; associated with complications to fetus as a result of maternal infection.

✓5th 056.0 **With neurological complications**
056.00 **With unspecified neurological complication**
056.01 **Encephalomyelitis due to rubella**
Encephalitis } due to rubella
Meningoencephalitis } due to rubella
056.09 **Other**

✓5th 056.7 **With other specified complications**
056.71 **Arthritis due to rubella**
056.79 **Other**

056.8 **With unspecified complications**
056.9 **Rubella without mention of complication**

✓4th 057 **Other viral exanthemata**
DEF: Skin eruptions or rashes and fever caused by viruses, including poxviruses.

057.0 **Erythema infectiosum [fifth disease]**
DEF: A moderately contagious, benign, epidemic disease, usually seen in children, and of probable viral etiology; a red macular rash appears on the face and may spread to the limbs and trunk.

057.8 **Other specified viral exanthemata**
Dukes (-Filatow) disease
Exanthema subitum [sixth disease]
Fourth disease
Parascarlatina
Pseudoscarlatina
Roseola infantum

057.9 **Viral exanthem, unspecified**

ARTHROPOD-BORNE VIRAL DISEASES (060-066)

Use additional code to identify any associated meningitis (321.2)
EXCLUDES *late effects of viral encephalitis (139.0)*

✓4th 060 **Yellow fever**
DEF: Fever and jaundice from infection by mosquito-borne virus of genus Flavivirus.

060.0 **Sylvatic**
Yellow fever:
jungle
sylvan
DEF: Yellow fever transmitted from animal to man, via mosquito.

060.1 **Urban**
DEF: Yellow fever transmitted from man to man, via mosquito.

060.9 **Yellow fever, unspecified**

061 **Dengue**
Breakbone fever
EXCLUDES *hemorrhagic fever caused by dengue virus (065.4)*
DEF: Acute, self-limiting infection by mosquito-borne virus characterized by fever and generalized aches

✓4th 062 **Mosquito-borne viral encephalitis**
062.0 **Japanese encephalitis**
Japanese B encephalitis
DEF: Flavivirus causing inflammation of the brain with a wide range of clinical manifestations

062.1 **Western equine encephalitis**
DEF: Alphavirus WEE infection causing inflammation of the brain, found in areas west of the Mississippi; transmitted horse to mosquito to man.

062.2 **Eastern equine encephalitis**
EXCLUDES *Venezuelan equine encephalitis (066.2)*
DEF: Alphavirus EEE causing inflammation of the brain and spinal cord, found as far north as Canada and south into South America and Mexico; transmitted horse to mosquito to man.

062.3 St. Louis encephalitis
DEF: Epidemic form caused by Flavivirus and transmitted by mosquito, and characterized by fever, difficulty in speech, and headache.

062.4 Australian encephalitis
Australian arboencephalitis
Australian X disease
Murray Valley encephalitis
DEF: Flavivirus causing inflammation of the brain, occurring in Australia and New Guinea.

062.5 California virus encephalitis
Encephalitis:
California
La Crosse
Tahyna fever
DEF: Bunya virus causing inflammation of the brain.

062.8 Other specified mosquito-borne viral encephalitis
Encephalitis by Ilheus virus
EXCLUDES *West Nile virus (066.40-066.49)*

062.9 Mosquito-borne viral encephalitis, unspecified

4th **063 Tick-borne viral encephalitis**
INCLUDES diphasic meningoencephalitis

063.0 Russian spring-summer [taiga] encephalitis

063.1 Louping ill
DEF: Inflammation of brain caused by virus transmitted sheep to tick to man; incidence usually limited to British Isles.

063.2 Central European encephalitis
DEF: Inflammation of brain caused by virus transmitted by tick; limited to central Europe and presenting with two distinct phases.

063.8 Other specified tick-borne viral encephalitis
Langat encephalitis
Powassan encephalitis

063.9 Tick-borne viral encephalitis, unspecified

064 Viral encephalitis transmitted by other and unspecified arthropods
Arthropod-borne viral encephalitis, vector unknown
Negishi virus encephalitis
EXCLUDES *viral encephalitis NOS (049.9)*

4th **065 Arthropod-borne hemorrhagic fever**

065.0 Crimean hemorrhagic fever [CHF Congo virus]
Central Asian hemorrhagic fever

065.1 Omsk hemorrhagic fever

065.2 Kyasanur Forest disease

065.3 Other tick-borne hemorrhagic fever

065.4 Mosquito-borne hemorrhagic fever
Chikungunya hemorrhagic fever
Dengue hemorrhagic fever
EXCLUDES *Chikungunya fever (066.3)*
dengue (061)
yellow fever (060.0-060.9)

065.8 Other specified arthropod-borne hemorrhagic fever
Mite-borne hemorrhagic fever

065.9 Arthropod-borne hemorrhagic fever, unspecified
Arbovirus hemorrhagic fever NOS

4th **066 Other arthropod-borne viral diseases**

066.0 Phlebotomus fever
Changuinola fever
Sandfly fever
DEF: Sandfly-borne viral infection occurring in Asia, Middle East and South America.

066.1 Tick-borne fever
Nairobi sheep disease
Tick fever:
American mountain
Colorado
Kemerovo
Quaranfil

066.2 Venezuelan equine fever
Venezuelan equine encephalitis
DEF: Alphavirus VEE infection causing inflammation of the brain, usually limited to South America, Mexico, and Florida; transmitted horse to mosquito to man.

066.3 Other mosquito-borne fever
Fever (viral):
Bunyamwera
Bwamba
Chikungunya
Guama
Mayaro
Mucambo
O'Nyong-Nyong
Oropouche
Pixuna
Rift valley
Ross river
Wesselsbron
Zika
EXCLUDES *dengue (061)*
yellow fever (060.0-060.9)

5th **066.4 West Nile fever**
AHA: 4Q, '02, 44
DEF: Mosquito-borne fever causing fatal inflammation of the brain, the lining of the brain, or of the lining of the brain and spinal cord.

066.40 West Nile fever, unspecified
West Nile fever NOS
West Nile fever without complications
West Nile virus NOS

066.41 West Nile fever with encephalitis
West Nile encephalitis
West Nile encephalomyelitis
AHA: ▶4Q, '04, 51◀

066.42 West Nile fever with other neurologic manifestation
Use additional code to specify the neurologic manifestation
AHA: ▶4Q, '04, 51◀

066.49 West Nile fever with other complications
Use additional code to specify the other conditions

066.8 Other specified arthropod-borne viral diseases
Chandipura fever
Piry fever

066.9 Arthropod-borne viral disease, unspecified
Arbovirus infection NOS

OTHER DISEASES DUE TO VIRUSES AND CHLAMYDIAE (070-079)

4th **070 Viral hepatitis**
INCLUDES viral hepatitis (acute) (chronic)
EXCLUDES *cytomegalic inclusion virus hepatitis (078.5)*

The following fifth-digit subclassification is for use with categories 070.2 and 070.3:
0 acute or unspecified, without mention of hepatitis delta
1 acute or unspecified, with hepatitis delta
2 chronic, without mention of hepatitis delta
3 chronic, with hepatitis delta

DEF: Hepatitis A: HAV infection is self-limiting with flu like symptoms; transmission, fecal-oral.
DEF: Hepatitis B: HBV infection can be chronic and systemic; transmission, bodily fluids.
DEF: Hepatitis C: HCV infection can be chronic and systemic; transmission, blood transfusion and unidentified agents.
DEF: Hepatitis D (delta): HDV occurs only in the presence of hepatitis B virus.
DEF: Hepatitis E: HEV is epidemic form; transmission and nature under investigation.

070.0 Viral hepatitis A with hepatic coma

070.1 Viral hepatitis A without mention of hepatic coma
Infectious hepatitis

5th **070.2 Viral hepatitis B with hepatic coma**
AHA: 4Q, '91, 28

5th **070.3 Viral hepatitis B without mention of hepatic coma**
Serum hepatitis
AHA: 1Q, '93, 28; 4Q, '91, 28

5th **070.4 Other specified viral hepatitis with hepatic coma**
AHA: 4Q, '91, 28

070.41 Acute hepatitis C with hepatic coma

Infectious and Parasitic Diseases 062.3–070.41

4th 5th Additional Digit Required | Unspecified Code | Other Specified Code | Manifestation Code | ▶◀ Revised Text | ● New Code | ▲ Revised Code Title

070.42 **Hepatitis delta without mention of active hepatitis B disease with hepatic coma**
Hepatitis delta with hepatitis B carrier state

070.43 **Hepatitis E with hepatic coma**

070.44 **Chronic hepatitis C with hepatic coma**

070.49 **Other specified viral hepatitis with hepatic coma**

✓5th 070.5 **Other specified viral hepatitis without mention of hepatic coma**
AHA: 4Q, '91, 28

070.51 **Acute hepatitis C without mention of hepatic coma**

070.52 **Hepatitis delta without mention of active hepatititis B disease or hepatic coma**

070.53 **Hepatitis E without mention of hepatic coma**

070.54 **Chronic hepatitis C without mention of hepatic coma**

070.59 **Other specified viral hepatitis without mention of hepatic coma**

070.6 **Unspecified viral hepatitis with hepatic coma**
EXCLUDES *unspecified viral hepatitis C with hepatic coma (070.71)*

✓5th 070.7 **Unspecified viral hepatitis C**

070.70 **Unspecified viral hepatitis C without hepatic coma**
Unspecified viral hepatitis C NOS
AHA: ▶4Q, '04, 52◀

070.71 **Unspecified viral hepatitis C with hepatic coma**
AHA: ▶4Q, '04, 52◀

070.9 **Unspecified viral hepatitis without mention of hepatic coma**
Viral hepatitis NOS
EXCLUDES *unspecified viral hepatitis C without hepatic coma (070.70)*

071 **Rabies**
Hydrophobia
Lyssa

DEF: Acute infectious disease of the CNS caused by a rhabdovirus; usually spread by virus-laden saliva from bites by infected animals; it progresses from fever, restlessness, and extreme excitability, to hydrophobia, seizures, confusion and death.

✓4th 072 **Mumps**

DEF: Acute infectious disease caused by paramyxovirus; usually seen in children less than 15 years of age; salivary glands are typically enlarged, and other organs, such as testes, pancreas and meninges, are often involved.

072.0 **Mumps orchitis** ♂

072.1 **Mumps meningitis**

072.2 **Mumps encephalitis**
Mumps meningoencephalitis

072.3 **Mumps pancreatitis**

✓5th 072.7 **Mumps with other specified complications**

072.71 **Mumps hepatitis**

072.72 **Mumps polyneuropathy**

072.79 **Other**

072.8 **Mumps with unspecified complication**

072.9 **Mumps without mention of complication**
Epidemic parotitis
Infectious parotitis

✓4th 073 **Ornithosis**
INCLUDES parrot fever
psittacosis

DEF: *Chlamydia psittaci* infection often transmitted from birds to humans.

073.0 **With pneumonia**
Lobular pneumonitis due to ornithosis

073.7 **With other specified complications**

073.8 **With unspecified complication**

073.9 **Ornithosis, unspecified**

✓4th 074 **Specific diseases due to Coxsackie virus**
EXCLUDES *Coxsackie virus:*
infection NOS (079.2)
meningitis (047.0)

074.0 **Herpangina**
Vesicular pharyngitis

DEF: Acute infectious coxsackie virus infection causing throat lesions, fever, and vomiting; generally affects children in summer.

074.1 **Epidemic pleurodynia**
Bornholm disease
Devil's grip
Epidemic:
myalgia
myositis

DEF: Paroxysmal pain in chest, accompanied by fever and usually limited to children and young adults; caused by coxsackie virus.

✓5th 074.2 **Coxsackie carditis**

074.20 **Coxsackie carditis, unspecified**

074.21 **Coxsackie pericarditis**

DEF: Coxsackie infection of the outer lining of the heart.

074.22 **Coxsackie endocarditis**

DEF: Coxsackie infection within the heart's cavities.

074.23 **Coxsackie myocarditis**
Aseptic myocarditis of newborn

DEF: Coxsackie infection of the muscle of the heart.

074.3 **Hand, foot, and mouth disease**
Vesicular stomatitis and exanthem

DEF: Mild coxsackie infection causing lesions on hands, feet and oral mucosa; most commonly seen in preschool children.

074.8 **Other specified diseases due to Coxsackie virus**
Acute lymphonodular pharyngitis

075 **Infectious mononucleosis**
Glandular fever
Monocytic angina
Pfeiffer's disease
AHA: 3Q, '01, 13; M-A, '87, 8

DEF: Acute infection by Epstein-Barr virus causing fever, sore throat, enlarged lymph glands and spleen, and fatigue; usually seen in teens and young adults.

✓4th 076 **Trachoma**
EXCLUDES *late effect of trachoma (139.1)*

DEF: A chronic infectious disease of the cornea and conjunctiva caused by a strain of the bacteria *Chlamydia trachomatis*; the infection can cause photophobia, pain, excessive tearing and sometimes blindness.

076.0 **Initial stage**
Trachoma dubium

076.1 **Active stage**
Granular conjunctivitis (trachomatous)
Trachomatous
follicular conjunctivitis
pannus

076.9 **Trachoma, unspecified**
Trachoma NOS

✓4th 077 **Other diseases of conjunctiva due to viruses and Chlamydiae**
EXCLUDES *ophthalmic complications of viral diseases classified elsewhere*

077.0 **Inclusion conjunctivitis**
Paratrachoma
Swimming pool conjunctivitis
EXCLUDES *inclusion blennorrhea (neonatal) (771.6)*

DEF: Pus in conjunctiva caused by *Chlamydiae trachomatis* infection.

077.1 **Epidemic keratoconjunctivitis**
Shipyard eye

DEF: Highly contagious corneal or conjunctival infection caused by adenovirus type 8; symptoms include inflammation and corneal infiltrates.

077.2 **Pharyngoconjunctival fever**
Viral pharyngoconjunctivitis

077.3 Other adenoviral conjunctivitis
Acute adenoviral follicular conjunctivitis

077.4 Epidemic hemorrhagic conjunctivitis
Apollo:
conjunctivitis
disease
Conjunctivitis due to enterovirus type 70
Hemorrhagic conjunctivitis (acute) (epidemic)

077.8 Other viral conjunctivitis
Newcastle conjunctivitis

✓5th **077.9 Unspecified diseases of conjunctiva due to viruses and Chlamydiae**

077.98 Due to Chlamydiae

077.99 Due to viruses
Viral conjunctivitis NOS

✓4th **078 Other diseases due to viruses and Chlamydiae**
EXCLUDES *viral infection NOS (079.0-079.9)*
viremia NOS (790.8)

078.0 Molluscum contagiosum
DEF: Benign poxvirus infection causing small bumps on the skin or conjunctiva; transmitted by close contact.

✓5th **078.1 Viral warts**
Viral warts due to human papilloma virus
AHA: 2Q, '97, 9; 4Q, '93, 22
DEF: A keratotic papilloma of the epidermis caused by the human papilloma virus; the superficial vegetative lesions last for varying durations and eventually regress spontaneously.

078.10 Viral warts, unspecified
Condyloma NOS
Verruca:
NOS
Vulgaris
Warts (infectious)

078.11 Condyloma acuminatum
DEF: Clusters of mucosa or epidermal lesions on external genitalia; viral infection is sexually transmitted.

078.19 Other specified viral warts
Genital warts NOS
Verruca:
plana
Verruca:
plantaris

078.2 Sweating fever
Miliary fever
Sweating disease
DEF: A viral infection characterized by profuse sweating; various papular, vesicular and other eruptions cause the blockage of sweat glands.

078.3 Cat-scratch disease
Benign lymphoreticulosis (of inoculation)
Cat-scratch fever

078.4 Foot and mouth disease
Aphthous fever
Epizootic:
aphthae
Epizootic:
stomatitis
DEF: Ulcers on oral mucosa, legs, and feet after exposure to infected animal.

078.5 Cytomegaloviral disease
Cytomegalic inclusion disease
Salivary gland virus disease
Use additional code to identify manifestation, as:
cytomegalic inclusion virus:
hepatitis (573.1)
pneumonia (484.1)
EXCLUDES *congenital cytomegalovirus infection (771.1)*
AHA: 1Q, '03 ,10; 3Q, '98, 4; 2Q, '93, 11; 1Q, '89, 9
DEF: A herpes virus inclusion associated with serious disease morbidity including fever, leukopenia, pneumonia, retinitis, hepatitis and organ transplant; often leads to syndromes such as hepatomegaly, splenomegaly and thrombocytopenia; a common post-transplant complication for organ transplant recipients.

078.6 Hemorrhagic nephrosonephritis
Hemorrhagic fever:
epidemic
Korean
Russian
with renal syndrome
DEF: Viral infection causing kidney dysfunction and bleeding disorders.

078.7 Arenaviral hemorrhagic fever
Hemorrhagic fever:
Argentine
Bolivian
Junin virus
Machupo virus

✓5th **078.8 Other specified diseases due to viruses and Chlamydiae**
EXCLUDES *epidemic diarrhea (009.2)*
lymphogranuloma venereum (099.1)

078.81 Epidemic vertigo

078.82 Epidemic vomiting syndrome
Winter vomiting disease

078.88 Other specified diseases due to Chlamydiae
AHA: 4Q, '96, 22

078.89 Other specified diseases due to viruses
Epidemic cervical myalgia
Marburg disease
Tanapox

✓4th **079 Viral and chlamydial infection in conditions classified elsewhere and of unspecified site**
Note: This category is provided to be used as an additional code to identify the viral agent in diseases classifiable elsewhere. This category will also be used to classify virus infection of unspecified nature or site.

079.0 Adenovirus

079.1 ECHO virus
DEF: An "orphan" enteric RNA virus, certain serotypes of which are associated with human disease, especially aseptic meningitis.

079.2 Coxsackie virus
DEF: A heterogenous group of viruses associated with aseptic meningitis, myocarditis, pericarditis, and acute onset juvenile diabetes.

079.3 Rhinovirus
DEF: Rhinoviruses affect primarily the upper respiratory tract. Over 100 distinct types infect humans.

079.4 Human papillomavirus
AHA: 2Q, '97, 9; 4Q, '93, 22
DEF: Viral infection caused by the genus *Papillomavirus* causing cutaneous and genital warts, including verruca vulgaris and condyloma acuminatum; certain types are associated with cervical dysplasia, cancer and other genital malignancies.

✓5th **079.5 Retrovirus**
EXCLUDES *human immunodeficiency virus, type 1 [HIV-1] (042)*
human T-cell lymphotrophic virus, type III [HTLV-III] (042)
lymphadenopathy-associated virus [LAV] (042)
AHA: 4Q, '93, 22, 23
DEF: A large group of RNA viruses that carry reverse transcriptase and include the leukoviruses and lentiviruses.

079.50 Retrovirus, unspecified

079.51 Human T-cell lymphotrophic virus, type I [HTLV-I]

079.52 Human T-cell lymphotrophic virus, type II [HTLV-II]

✓4th ✓5th Additional Digit Required | Unspecified Code | Other Specified Code | Manifestation Code | ▶◀ Revised Text | ● New Code | ▲ Revised Code Title

079.53 **Human immunodeficiency virus, type 2 [HIV-2]**

079.59 **Other specified retrovirus**

079.6 **Respiratory syncytial virus (RSV)**

AHA: 4Q, '96, 27, 28

DEF: The major respiratory pathogen of young children, causing severe bronchitis and bronchopneumonia, and minor infection in adults.

✓5th 079.8 **Other specified viral and chlamydial infections**

AHA: 1Q, '88, 12

079.81 **Hantavirus**

AHA: 4Q, '95, 60

DEF: An infection caused by the Muerto Canyon virus whose primary rodent reservoir is the deer mouse Peromyscus maniculatus; commonly characterized by fever, myalgias, headache, cough and rapid respiratory failure.

079.82 **SARS-associated coronavirus**

AHA: 4Q, '03, 46

DEF: A life-threatening respiratory disease described as severe acute respiratory syndrome (SARS); etiology coronavirus; most common presenting symptoms may range from mild to more severe forms of flu-like conditions; fever, chills, cough, headache, myalgia; diagnosis of SARS is based upon clinical, laboratory, and epidemiological criteria.x

079.88 **Other specified chlamydial infection**

079.89 **Other specified viral infection**

✓5th 079.9 **Unspecified viral and chlamydial infections**

EXCLUDES *viremia NOS (790.8)*

AHA: 2Q, '91, 8

079.98 **Unspecified chlamydial infection**

Chlamydial infections NOS

079.99 **Unspecified viral infection**

Viral infections NOS

RICKETTSIOSES AND OTHER ARTHROPOD-BORNE DISEASES (080-088)

EXCLUDES *arthropod-borne viral diseases (060.0-066.9)*

080 Louse-borne [epidemic] typhus

Typhus (fever):
- classical
- epidemic

Typhus (fever):
- exanthematic NOS
- louse-borne

DEF: *Rickettsia prowazekii*; causes severe headache, rash, high fever.

✓4th **081 Other typhus**

081.0 **Murine [endemic] typhus**

Typhus (fever):
- endemic

Typhus (fever):
- flea-borne

DEF: Milder typhus caused by *Rickettsia typhi (mooseri)*; transmitted by rat flea.

081.1 **Brill's disease**

Brill-Zinsser disease
Recrudescent typhus (fever)

081.2 **Scrub typhus**

Japanese river fever
Kedani fever
Mite-borne typhus
Tsutsugamushi

DEF: Typhus caused by *Rickettsia tsutsugamushi* transmitted by chigger.

081.9 **Typhus, unspecified**

Typhus (fever) NOS

✓4th **082 Tick-borne rickettsioses**

082.0 **Spotted fevers**

Rocky mountain spotted fever
Sao Paulo fever

082.1 **Boutonneuse fever**

African tick typhus
India tick typhus
Kenya tick typhus
Marseilles fever
Mediterranean tick fever

082.2 **North Asian tick fever**

Siberian tick typhus

082.3 **Queensland tick typhus**

✓5th 082.4 **Ehrlichiosis**

AHA: 4Q, '00, 38

082.40 **Ehrlichiosis, unspecified**

082.41 **Ehrlichiosis chaffeensis [E. chaffeensis]**

DEF: A febrile illness caused by bacterial infection, also called human monocytic ehrlichiosis (HME). Causal organism is *Ehrlichia chaffeensis*, transmitted by the Lone Star tick, *Amblyomma americanum.* Symptoms include fever, chills, myalgia, nausea, vomiting, diarrhea, confusion, and severe headache occurring one week after a tick bite. Clinical findings are lymphadenopathy, rash, thrombocytopenia, leukopenia, and abnormal liver function tests

082.49 **Other ehrlichiosis**

082.8 **Other specified tick-borne rickettsioses**

Lone star fever

AHA: 4Q, '99, 19

082.9 **Tick-borne rickettsiosis, unspecified**

Tick-borne typhus NOS

✓4th **083 Other rickettsioses**

083.0 **Q fever**

DEF: Infection of *Coxiella burnetii* usually acquired through airborne organisms.

083.1 **Trench fever**

Quintan fever
Wolhynian fever

083.2 **Rickettsialpox**

Vesicular rickettsiosis

DEF: Infection of *Rickettsia akari* usually acquired through a mite bite.

083.8 **Other specified rickettsioses**

083.9 **Rickettsiosis, unspecified**

✓4th **084 Malaria**

Note: Subcategories 084.0-084.6 exclude the listed conditions with mention of pernicious complications (084.8-084.9).

EXCLUDES *congenital malaria (771.2)*

DEF: Mosquito-borne disease causing high fever and prostration and cataloged by species of *Plasmodium: P. falciparum, P. malariae, P. ovale*, and *P. vivax.*

084.0 **Falciparum malaria [malignant tertian]**

Malaria (fever):
- by Plasmodium falciparum
- subtertian

084.1 **Vivax malaria [benign tertian]**

Malaria (fever) by Plasmodium vivax

084.2 **Quartan malaria**

Malaria (fever) by Plasmodium malariae
Malariae malaria

084.3 **Ovale malaria**

Malaria (fever) by Plasmodium ovale

084.4 **Other malaria**

Monkey malaria

084.5 **Mixed malaria**

Malaria (fever) by more than one parasite

084.6 **Malaria, unspecified**

Malaria (fever) NOS

084.7 **Induced malaria**

Therapeutically induced malaria

EXCLUDES *accidental infection from syringe, blood transfusion, etc. (084.0-084.6, above, according to parasite species)*
transmission from mother to child during delivery (771.2)

084.8 Blackwater fever
Hemoglobinuric:
fever (bilious)
malaria
Malarial hemoglobinuria

DEF: Severe hemic and renal complication of *Plasmodium falciparum* infection.

084.9 Other pernicious complications of malaria
Algid malaria
Cerebral malaria
Use additional code to identify complication, as:
malarial:
hepatitis (573.2)
nephrosis (581.81)

✓4th **085 Leishmaniasis**

085.0 Visceral [kala-azar]
Dumdum fever
Infection by Leishmania:
donovani
infantum
Leishmaniasis:
dermal, post-kala-azar
Mediterranean
visceral (Indian)

085.1 Cutaneous, urban
Aleppo boil
Baghdad boil
Delhi boil
Infection by Leishmania tropica (minor)
Leishmaniasis, cutaneous:
dry form
late
recurrent
ulcerating
Oriental sore

085.2 Cutaneous, Asian desert
Infection by Leishmania tropica major
Leishmaniasis, cutaneous:
acute necrotizing
rural
wet form
zoonotic form

085.3 Cutaneous, Ethiopian
Infection by Leishmania ethiopica
Leishmaniasis, cutaneous:
diffuse
lepromatous

085.4 Cutaneous, American
Chiclero ulcer
Infection by Leishmania mexicana
Leishmaniasis tegumentaria diffusa

085.5 Mucocutaneous (American)
Espundia
Infection by Leishmania braziliensis
Uta

085.9 Leishmaniasis, unspecified

✓4th **086 Trypanosomiasis**
Use additional code to identify manifestations, as:
trypanosomiasis:
encephalitis (323.2)
meningitis (321.3)

086.0 Chagas' disease with heart involvement
American trypanosomiasis } with heart involvement
Infection by Trypanosoma cruzi } with heart involvement
Any condition classifiable to 086.2 with heart involvement

086.1 Chagas' disease with other organ involvement
American trypanosomiasis } with involvement of organ other than heart
Infection by Trypanosoma cruzi } with involvement of organ other than heart
Any condition classifiable to 086.2 with involvement of organ other than heart

086.2 Chagas' disease without mention of organ involvement
American trypanosomiasis
Infection by Trypanosoma cruzi

086.3 Gambian trypanosomiasis
Gambian sleeping sickness
Infection by Trypanosoma gambiense

086.4 Rhodesian trypanosomiasis
Infection by Trypanosoma rhodesiense
Rhodesian sleeping sickness

086.5 African trypanosomiasis, unspecified
Sleeping sickness NOS

086.9 Trypanosomiasis, unspecified

✓4th **087 Relapsing fever**
INCLUDES recurrent fever

DEF: Infection by *Borrelia*; symptoms are episodic and include fever and arthralgia.

087.0 Louse-borne

087.1 Tick-borne

087.9 Relapsing fever, unspecified

✓4th **088 Other arthropod-borne diseases**

088.0 Bartonellosis
Carrión's disease
Oroya fever
Verruga peruana

✓5th **088.8 Other specified arthropod-borne diseases**

088.81 Lyme disease
Erythema chronicum migrans
AHA: 4Q, '91, 15; 3Q, '90, 14; 2Q, '89, 10

DEF: A recurrent multisystem disorder caused by the spirochete *Borrelia burgdorferi* with the carrier being the tick *Ixodes dammini*; the disease begins with lesions of erythema chronicum migrans; it is followed by arthritis of the large joints, myalgia, malaise, and neurological and cardiac manifestations.

088.82 Babesiosis
Babesiasis
AHA: 4Q, '93, 23

DEF: A tick-borne disease caused by infection of *Babesia*, characterized by fever, malaise, listlessness, severe anemia and hemoglobinuria.

088.89 Other

088.9 Arthropod-borne disease, unspecified

SYPHILIS AND OTHER VENEREAL DISEASES (090-099)

EXCLUDES *nonvenereal endemic syphilis (104.0)*
urogenital trichomoniasis (131.0)

✓4th **090 Congenital syphilis**

DEF: Infection by spirochete *Treponema pallidum* acquired in utero from the infected mother.

090.0 Early congenital syphilis, symptomatic
Congenital syphilitic:
choroiditis
coryza (chronic)
hepatomegaly
mucous patches
periostitis
Congenital syphilitic:
splenomegaly
Syphilitic (congenital):
epiphysitis
osteochondritis
pemphigus
Any congenital syphilitic condition specified as early or manifest less than two years after birth

090.1 Early congenital syphilis, latent
Congenital syphilis without clinical manifestations, with positive serological reaction and negative spinal fluid test, less than two years after birth

090.2 Early congenital syphilis, unspecified
Congenital syphilis NOS, less than two years after birth

090.3 Syphilitic interstitial keratitis
Syphilitic keratitis:
parenchymatous
punctata profunda
EXCLUDES *interstitial keratitis NOS (370.50)*

✓5th **090.4 Juvenile neurosyphilis**
Use additional code to identify any associated mental disorder
DEF: *Treponema pallidum* infection involving the nervous system.

090.40 Juvenile neurosyphilis, unspecified
Congenital neurosyphilis
Dementia paralytica juvenilis
Juvenile:
general paresis
tabes
taboparesis

090.41 Congenital syphilitic encephalitis
DEF: Congenital *Treponema pallidum* infection involving the brain.

090.42 Congenital syphilitic meningitis
DEF: Congenital *Treponema pallidum* infection involving the lining of the brain and/or spinal cord.

090.49 Other

090.5 Other late congenital syphilis, symptomatic
Gumma due to congenital syphilis
Hutchinson's teeth
Syphilitic saddle nose
Any congenital syphilitic condition specified as late or manifest two years or more after birth

090.6 Late congenital syphilis, latent
Congenital syphilis without clinical manifestations, with positive serological reaction and negative spinal fluid test, two years or more after birth

090.7 Late congenital syphilis, unspecified
Congenital syphilis NOS, two years or more after birth

090.9 Congenital syphilis, unspecified

✓4th **091 Early syphilis, symptomatic**
EXCLUDES *early cardiovascular syphilis (093.0-093.9)*
early neurosyphilis (094.0-094.9)

091.0 Genital syphilis (primary)
Genital chancre
DEF: Genital lesion at the site of initial infection by *Treponema pallidum.*

091.1 Primary anal syphilis
DEF: Anal lesion at the site of initial infection by *Treponema pallidum.*

091.2 Other primary syphilis
Primary syphilis of:
breast
fingers
lip
tonsils
DEF: Lesion at the site of initial infection by *Treponema pallidum.*

091.3 Secondary syphilis of skin or mucous membranes
Condyloma latum
Secondary syphilis of:
anus
mouth
pharynx
skin
tonsils
vulva
DEF: Transitory or chronic lesions following initial syphilis infection.

091.4 Adenopathy due to secondary syphilis
Syphilitic adenopathy (secondary)
Syphilitic lymphadenitis (secondary)

✓5th **091.5 Uveitis due to secondary syphilis**

091.50 Syphilitic uveitis, unspecified

091.51 Syphilitic chorioretinitis (secondary)
DEF: Inflammation of choroid and retina as a secondary infection.

091.52 Syphilitic iridocyclitis (secondary)
DEF: Inflammation of iris and ciliary body as a secondary infection.

✓5th **091.6 Secondary syphilis of viscera and bone**

091.61 Secondary syphilitic periostitis
DEF: Inflammation of outer layers of bone as a secondary infection.

091.62 Secondary syphilitic hepatitis
Secondary syphilis of liver

091.69 Other viscera

091.7 Secondary syphilis, relapse
Secondary syphilis, relapse (treated) (untreated)

✓5th **091.8 Other forms of secondary syphilis**

091.81 Acute syphilitic meningitis (secondary)
DEF: Sudden, severe inflammation of the lining of the brain and/or spinal cord as a secondary infection.

091.82 Syphilitic alopecia
DEF: Hair loss following initial syphilis infection.

091.89 Other

091.9 Unspecified secondary syphilis

✓4th **092 Early syphilis, latent**
INCLUDES syphilis (acquired) without clinical manifestations, with positive serological reaction and negative spinal fluid test, less than two years after infection

092.0 Early syphilis, latent, serological relapse after treatment

092.9 Early syphilis, latent, unspecified

✓4th **093 Cardiovascular syphilis**

093.0 Aneurysm of aorta, specified as syphilitic
Dilatation of aorta, specified as syphilitic

093.1 Syphilitic aortitis
DEF: Inflammation of the aorta - the main artery leading from the heart.

✓5th **093.2 Syphilitic endocarditis**
DEF: Inflammation of the tissues lining the cavities of the heart.

093.20 Valve, unspecified
Syphilitic ostial coronary disease

093.21 Mitral valve

093.22 Aortic valve
Syphilitic aortic incompetence or stenosis

093.23 Tricuspid valve

093.24 Pulmonary valve

✓5th **093.8 Other specified cardiovascular syphilis**

093.81 Syphilitic pericarditis
DEF: Inflammation of the outer lining of the heart.

093.82 Syphilitic myocarditis
DEF: Inflammation of the muscle of the heart.

093.89 Other

093.9 Cardiovascular syphilis, unspecified

✓4th **094 Neurosyphilis**
Use additional code to identify any associated mental disorder

094.0 Tabes dorsalis
Locomotor ataxia (progressive)
Posterior spinal sclerosis (syphilitic)
Tabetic neurosyphilis
Use additional code to identify manifestation, as:
neurogenic arthropathy [Charcot's joint disease] (713.5)
DEF: Progressive degeneration of nerves associated with long-term syphilis; causing pain, wasting away, incontinence, and ataxia.

094.1 General paresis
Dementia paralytica
General paralysis (of the insane) (progressive)
Paretic neurosyphilis
Taboparesis
DEF: Degeneration of brain associated with long-term syphilis, causing loss of brain function, progressive dementia, and paralysis.

094.2 Syphilitic meningitis
Meningovascular syphilis
EXCLUDES *acute syphilitic meningitis (secondary) (091.81)*
DEF: Inflammation of the lining of the brain and/or spinal cord.

094.3 Asymptomatic neurosyphilis

✓5th **094.8 Other specified neurosyphilis**

094.81 Syphilitic encephalitis

094.82 Syphilitic Parkinsonism
DEF: Decreased motor function, tremors, and muscular rigidity.

094.83 Syphilitic disseminated retinochoroiditis
DEF: Inflammation of retina and choroid due to neurosyphilis.

094.84 Syphilitic optic atrophy
DEF: Degeneration of the eye and its nerves due to neurosyphilis.

094.85 Syphilitic retrobulbar neuritis
DEF: Inflammation of the posterior optic nerve due to neurosyphilis.

094.86 Syphilitic acoustic neuritis
DEF: Inflammation of acoustic nerve due to neurosyphilis.

094.87 Syphilitic ruptured cerebral aneurysm

094.89 Other

094.9 Neurosyphilis, unspecified
Gumma (syphilitic)
Syphilis (early) (late)
Syphiloma
} of central nervous system NOS

✓4th **095 Other forms of late syphilis, with symptoms**
INCLUDES gumma (syphilitic)
syphilis, late, tertiary, or unspecified stage

095.0 Syphilitic episcleritis

095.1 Syphilis of lung

095.2 Syphilitic peritonitis

095.3 Syphilis of liver

095.4 Syphilis of kidney

095.5 Syphilis of bone

095.6 Syphilis of muscle
Syphilitic myositis

095.7 Syphilis of synovium, tendon, and bursa
Syphilitic:
bursitis
Syphilitic:
synovitis

095.8 Other specified forms of late symptomatic syphilis
EXCLUDES *cardiovascular syphilis (093.0-093.9)*
neurosyphilis (094.0-094.9)

095.9 Late symptomatic syphilis, unspecified

096 Late syphilis, latent
Syphilis (acquired) without clinical manifestations, with positive serological reaction and negative spinal fluid test, two years or more after infection

✓4th **097 Other and unspecified syphilis**

097.0 Late syphilis, unspecified

097.1 Latent syphilis, unspecified
Positive serological reaction for syphilis

097.9 Syphilis, unspecified
Syphilis (acquired) NOS
EXCLUDES *syphilis NOS causing death under two years of age (090.9)*

✓4th **098 Gonococcal infections**
DEF: *Neisseria gonorrhoeae* infection generally acquired in utero or in sexual congress.

098.0 Acute, of lower genitourinary tract
Gonococcal:
Bartholinitis (acute)
urethritis (acute)
vulvovaginitis (acute)
Gonorrhea (acute):
NOS
genitourinary (tract) NOS

✓5th **098.1 Acute, of upper genitourinary tract**

098.10 Gonococcal infection (acute) of upper genitourinary tract, site unspecified

098.11 Gonococcal cystitis (acute)
Gonorrhea (acute) of bladder

098.12 Gonococcal prostatitis (acute) ♂

098.13 Gonococcal epididymo-orchitis (acute) ♂
Gonococcal orchitis (acute)
DEF: Acute inflammation of the testes.

098.14 Gonococcal seminal vesiculitis (acute) ♂
Gonorrhea (acute) of seminal vesicle

098.15 Gonococcal cervicitis (acute) ♀
Gonorrhea (acute) of cervix

098.16 Gonococcal endometritis (acute) ♀
Gonorrhea (acute) of uterus

098.17 Gonococcal salpingitis, specified as acute ♀
DEF: Acute inflammation of the fallopian tubes.

098.19 Other

098.2 Chronic, of lower genitourinary tract
Gonococcal:
Bartholinitis
urethritis
vulvovaginitis
Gonorrhea:
NOS
genitourinary (tract)
} specified as chronic or with duration of two months or more

Any condition classifiable to 098.0 specified as chronic or with duration of two months or more

✓5th **098.3 Chronic, of upper genitourinary tract**
INCLUDES any condition classifiable to 098.1 stated as chronic or with a duration of two months or more

098.30 Chronic gonococcal infection of upper genitourinary tract, site unspecified

098.31 Gonococcal cystitis, chronic
Any condition classifiable to 098.11, specified as chronic
Gonorrhea of bladder, chronic

098.32 Gonococcal prostatitis, chronic ♂
Any condition classifiable to 098.12, specified as chronic

098.33 Gonococcal epididymo-orchitis, chronic ♂
Any condition classifiable to 098.13, specified as chronic
Chronic gonococcal orchitis
DEF: Chronic inflammation of the testes.

098.34 Gonococcal seminal vesiculitis, chronic ♂
Any condition classifiable to 098.14, specified as chronic
Gonorrhea of seminal vesicle, chronic

098.35 Gonococcal cervicitis, chronic ♀
Any condition classifiable to 098.15, specified as chronic
Gonorrhea of cervix, chronic

098.36 Gonococcal endometritis, chronic ♀
Any condition classifiable to 098.16, specified as chronic
DEF: Chronic inflammation of the uterus.

098.37 Gonococcal salpingitis (chronic) ♀

DEF: Chronic inflammation of the fallopian tubes.

098.39 Other

✓5th **098.4 Gonococcal infection of eye**

098.40 Gonococcal conjunctivitis (neonatorum)

Gonococcal ophthalmia (neonatorum)

DEF: Inflammation and infection of conjunctiva present at birth.

098.41 Gonococcal iridocyclitis

DEF: Inflammation and infection of iris and ciliary body.

098.42 Gonococcal endophthalmia

DEF: Inflammation and infection of the contents of the eyeball.

098.43 Gonococcal keratitis

DEF: Inflammation and infection of the cornea.

098.49 Other

✓5th **098.5 Gonococcal infection of joint**

098.50 Gonococcal arthritis

Gonococcal infection of joint NOS

098.51 Gonococcal synovitis and tenosynovitis

098.52 Gonococcal bursitis

DEF: Inflammation of the sac-like cavities in a joint.

098.53 Gonococcal spondylitis

098.59 Other

Gonococcal rheumatism

098.6 Gonococcal infection of pharynx

098.7 Gonococcal infection of anus and rectum

Gonococcal proctitis

✓5th **098.8 Gonococcal infection of other specified sites**

098.81 Gonococcal keratosis (blennorrhagica)

DEF: Pustular skin lesions caused by *Neisseria gonorrhoeae.*

098.82 Gonococcal meningitis

DEF: Inflammation of the lining of the brain and/or spinal cord.

098.83 Gonococcal pericarditis

DEF: Inflammation of the outer lining of the heart.

098.84 Gonococcal endocarditis

DEF: Inflammation of the tissues lining the cavities of the heart.

098.85 Other gonococcal heart disease

098.86 Gonococcal peritonitis

DEF: Inflammation of the membrane lining the abdomen.

098.89 Other

Gonococcemia

✓4th **099 Other venereal diseases**

099.0 Chancroid

Bubo (inguinal):
- chancroidal
- due to Hemophilus ducreyi

Chancre:
- Ducrey's
- simple
- soft

Ulcus molle (cutis) (skin)

DEF: A sexually transmitted disease caused by *Haemophilus ducreyi*; it is identified by a painful primary ulcer at the site of inoculation (usually on the external genitalia) with related lymphadenitis.

099.1 Lymphogranuloma venereum

Climatic or tropical bubo
(Durand-) Nicolas-Favre disease
Esthiomene
Lymphogranuloma inguinale

DEF: Sexually transmitted infection of *Chlamydia trachomatis* causing skin lesions.

099.2 Granuloma inguinale

Donovanosis
Granuloma pudendi (ulcerating)
Granuloma venereum
Pudendal ulcer

DEF: Chronic, sexually transmitted infection of *Calymmatobacterium granulomatis*, resulting in progressive, anogenital skin ulcers.

099.3 Reiter's disease

Reiter's syndrome
Use additional code for associated:
- arthropathy (711.1)
- conjunctivitis (372.33)

DEF: A symptom complex of unknown etiology consisting of urethritis, conjunctivitis, arthritis and myocutaneous lesions. It occurs most commonly in young men and patients with HIV and may precede or follow AIDS. Also a form of reactive arthritis.

✓5th **099.4 Other nongonococcal urethritis [NGU]**

099.40 Unspecified

Nonspecific urethritis

099.41 Chlamydia trachomatis

099.49 Other specified organism

✓5th **099.5 Other venereal diseases due to Chlamydia trachomatis**

EXCLUDES *Chlamydia trachomatis infection of conjunctiva (076.0-076.9, 077.0, 077.9)*
Lymphogranuloma venereum (099.1)

DEF: Venereal diseases caused by *Chlamydia trachomatis* at other sites besides the urethra (e.g., pharynx, anus and rectum, conjunctiva and peritoneum).

099.50 Unspecified site

099.51 Pharynx

099.52 Anus and rectum

099.53 Lower genitourinary sites

EXCLUDES *urethra (099.41)*

Use additional code to specify site of infection, such as:
- bladder (595.4)
- cervix (616.0)
- vagina and vulva (616.11)

099.54 Other genitourinary sites

Use additional code to specify site of infection, such as:
- pelvic inflammatory disease NOS (614.9)
- testis and epididymis (604.91)

099.55 Unspecified genitourinary site

099.56 Peritoneum

Perihepatitis

099.59 Other specified site

099.8 Other specified venereal diseases

099.9 Venereal disease, unspecified

OTHER SPIROCHETAL DISEASES (100-104)

✓4th **100 Leptospirosis**

DEF: An infection of any spirochete of the genus Leptospire in blood. This zoonosis is transmitted to humans most often by exposure with contaminated animal tissues or water and less often by contact with urine. Patients present with flulike symptoms, the most common being muscle aches involving the thighs and low back. Treatment is with hydration and antibiotics.

100.0 Leptospirosis icterohemorrhagica

Leptospiral or spirochetal jaundice (hemorrhagic)
Weil's disease

✓5th **100.8 Other specified leptospiral infections**

100.81 Leptospiral meningitis (aseptic)

100.89 Other

Fever:
- Fort Bragg
- pretibial
- swamp

Infection by Leptospira:
- australis
- bataviae
- pyrogenes

100.9 Leptospirosis, unspecified

101 Vincent's angina

Acute necrotizing ulcerative:
 gingivitis
 stomatitis
Fusospirochetal pharyngitis
Spirochetal stomatitis
Trench mouth
Vincent's:
 gingivitis
 infection [any site]

DEF: Painful ulceration with edema and hypermic patches of the oropharyngeal and throat membranes; it is caused by spreading of acute ulcerative gingivitis.

✓4th **102 Yaws**

INCLUDES frambesia
 pian

DEF: An infectious, endemic, tropical disease caused by *Treponema pertenue;* it usually affects persons 15 years old or younger; a primary cutaneous lesion develops, then a granulomatous skin eruption, and occasionally lesions that destroy skin and bone.

102.0 Initial lesions
Chancre of yaws
Frambesia, initial or primary
Initial frambesial ulcer
Mother yaw

102.1 Multiple papillomata and wet crab yaws
Butter yaws
Frambesioma
Pianoma
Plantar or palmar papilloma of yaws

102.2 Other early skin lesions
Cutaneous yaws, less than five years after infection
Early yaws (cutaneous) (macular) (papular) (maculopapular) (micropapular)
Frambeside of early yaws

102.3 Hyperkeratosis
Ghoul hand
Hyperkeratosis, palmar or plantar (early) (late) due to yaws
Worm-eaten soles

DEF: Overgrowth of the skin of the palms or bottoms of the feet, due to yaws.

102.4 Gummata and ulcers
Gummatous frambeside
Nodular late yaws (ulcerated)

DEF: Rubbery lesions and areas of dead skin caused by yaws.

102.5 Gangosa
Rhinopharyngitis mutilans

DEF: Massive, mutilating lesions of the nose and oral cavity caused by yaws.

102.6 Bone and joint lesions
Goundou
Gumma, bone
Gummatous osteitis or periostitis
} of yaws (late)

Hydrarthrosis
Osteitis
Periostitis (hypertrophic)
} of yaws (early) (late)

102.7 Other manifestations
Juxta-articular nodules of yaws
Mucosal yaws

102.8 Latent yaws
Yaws without clinical manifestations, with positive serology

102.9 Yaws, unspecified

✓4th **103 Pinta**

DEF: A chronic form of treponematosis, endemic in areas of tropical America; it is identified by the presence of red, violet, blue, coffee-colored or white spots on the skin.

103.0 Primary lesions
Chancre (primary)
Papule (primary)
Pintid
} of pinta [carate]

103.1 Intermediate lesions
Erythematous plaques
Hyperchromic lesions
Hyperkeratosis
} of pinta [carate]

103.2 Late lesions
Cardiovascular lesions
Skin lesions:
 achromic
 cicatricial
 dyschromic
Vitiligo
} of pinta [carate]

103.3 Mixed lesions
Achromic and hyperchromic skin lesions of pinta [carate]

103.9 Pinta, unspecified

✓4th **104 Other spirochetal infection**

104.0 Nonvenereal endemic syphilis
Bejel
Njovera

DEF: *Treponema pallidum, T. pertenue,* or *T. carateum* infection transmitted non-sexually, causing lesions on mucosa and skin.

104.8 Other specified spirochetal infections

EXCLUDES *relapsing fever (087.0-087.9)*
 syphilis (090.0-097.9)

104.9 Spirochetal infection, unspecified

MYCOSES (110-118)

Use additional code to identify manifestation as:
 arthropathy (711.6)
 meningitis (321.0-321.1)
 otitis externa (380.15)

EXCLUDES *infection by Actinomycetales, such as species of Actinomyces, Actinomadura, Nocardia, Streptomyces (039.0-039.9)*

✓4th **110 Dermatophytosis**

INCLUDES infection by species of Epidermophyton, Microsporum, and Trichophyton
 tinea, any type except those in 111

DEF: Superficial infection of the skin caused by a parasitic fungus.

110.0 Of scalp and beard
Kerion
Sycosis, mycotic
Trichophytic tinea [black dot tinea], scalp

110.1 Of nail
Dermatophytic onychia
Onychomycosis
Tinea unguium

110.2 Of hand
Tinea manuum

110.3 Of groin and perianal area
Dhobie itch
Eczema marginatum
Tinea cruris

110.4 Of foot
Athlete's foot
Tinea pedis

110.5 Of the body
Herpes circinatus
Tinea imbricata [Tokelau]

110.6 Deep seated dermatophytosis
Granuloma trichophyticum
Majocchi's granuloma

110.8 Of other specified sites

110.9 Of unspecified site
Favus NOS
Microsporic tinea NOS
Ringworm NOS

✓4th **111 Dermatomycosis, other and unspecified**

111.0 Pityriasis versicolor
Infection by Malassezia [Pityrosporum] furfur
Tinea flava
Tinea versicolor

111.1 Tinea nigra
Infection by Cladosporium species
Keratomycosis nigricans
Microsporosis nigra
Pityriasis nigra
Tinea palmaris nigra

111.2 Tinea blanca
Infection by Trichosporon (beigelii) cutaneum
White piedra

111.3 Black piedra
Infection by Piedraia hortai

111.8 Other specified dermatomycoses

111.9 Dermatomycosis, unspecified

✓4th **112 Candidiasis**

INCLUDES infection by Candida species
moniliasis

EXCLUDES *neonatal monilial infection (771.7)*

DEF: Fungal infection caused by *Candida*; usually seen in mucous membranes or skin.

112.0 Of mouth
Thrush (oral)

112.1 Of vulva and vagina ♀
Candidal vulvovaginitis
Monilial vulvovaginitis

112.2 Of other urogenital sites
Candidal balanitis
AHA: 4Q, '03, 105; 4Q, '96, 33

112.3 Of skin and nails
Candidal intertrigo
Candidal onychia
Candidal perionyxis [paronychia]

112.4 Of lung
Candidal pneumonia
AHA: 2Q, '98, 7

112.5 Disseminated
Systemic candidiasis
AHA: 2Q, '00, 5; 2Q, '89, 10

✓5th **112.8 Of other specified sites**

112.81 Candidal endocarditis

112.82 Candidal otitis externa
Otomycosis in moniliasis

112.83 Candidal meningitis

112.84 Candidal esophagitis
AHA: 4Q, '92, 19

112.85 Candidal enteritis
AHA: 4Q, '92, 19

112.89 Other
AHA: 1Q, '92, 17; 3Q, '91, 20

112.9 Of unspecified site

✓4th **114 Coccidioidomycosis**

INCLUDES infection by Coccidioides (immitis)
Posada-Wernicke disease

AHA: 4Q. '93, 23

DEF: A fungal disease caused by inhalation of dust particles containing arthrospores of *Coccidiodes immitis*; a self-limited respiratory infection; the primary form is known as San Joaquin fever, desert fever or valley fever.

114.0 Primary coccidioidomycosis (pulmonary)
Acute pulmonary coccidioidomycosis
Coccidioidomycotic pneumonitis
Desert rheumatism
Pulmonary coccidioidomycosis
San Joaquin Valley fever

DEF: Acute, self-limiting *Coccidioides immitis* infection of the lung.

114.1 Primary extrapulmonary coccidioidomycosis
Chancriform syndrome
Primary cutaneous coccidioidomycosis

DEF: Acute, self-limiting *Coccidioides immitis* infection in nonpulmonary site.

114.2 Coccidioidal meningitis

DEF: *Coccidioides immitis* infection of the lining of the brain and/or spinal cord.

114.3 Other forms of progressive coccidioidomycosis
Coccidioidal granuloma
Disseminated coccidioidomycosis

114.4 Chronic pulmonary coccidioidomycosis

114.5 Pulmonary coccidioidomycosis, unspecified

114.9 Coccidioidomycosis, unspecified

✓4th **115 Histoplasmosis**

The following fifth-digit subclassification is for use with category 115:

0 without mention of manifestation
1 meningitis
2 retinitis
3 pericarditis
4 endocarditis
5 pneumonia
9 other

✓5th **115.0 Infection by Histoplasma capsulatum**
American histoplasmosis
Darling's disease
Reticuloendothelial cytomycosis
Small form histoplasmosis

DEF: Infection resulting from inhalation of fungal spores, causing acute pneumonia, an influenza-like illness, or a disseminated disease of the reticuloendothelial system. In immunocompromised patients it can reactivate, affecting lungs, meninges, heart, peritoneum and adrenals.

✓5th **115.1 Infection by Histoplasma duboisii**
African histoplasmosis
Large form histoplasmosis

✓5th **115.9 Histoplasmosis, unspecified**
Histoplasmosis NOS

✓4th **116 Blastomycotic infection**

116.0 Blastomycosis
Blastomycotic dermatitis
Chicago disease
Cutaneous blastomycosis
Disseminated blastomycosis
Gilchrist's disease
Infection by Blastomyces [Ajellomyces] dermatitidis
North American blastomycosis
Primary pulmonary blastomycosis

116.1 Paracoccidioidomycosis
Brazilian blastomycosis
Infection by Paracoccidioides [Blastomyces] brasiliensis
Lutz-Splendore-Almeida disease
Mucocutaneous-lymphangitic paracoccidioidomycosis
Pulmonary paracoccidioidomycosis
South American blastomycosis
Visceral paracoccidioidomycosis

116.2 Lobomycosis
Infections by Loboa [Blastomyces] loboi
Keloidal blastomycosis
Lobo's disease

✓4th **117 Other mycoses**

117.0 Rhinosporidiosis
Infection by Rhinosporidium seeberi

117.1 Sporotrichosis
Cutaneous sporotrichosis
Disseminated sporotrichosis
Infection by Sporothrix [Sporotrichum] schenckii
Lymphocutaneous sporotrichosis
Pulmonary sporotrichosis
Sporotrichosis of the bones

117.2 Chromoblastomycosis
Chromomycosis
Infection by Cladosporidium carrionii, Fonsecaea compactum, Fonsecaea pedrosoi, Phialophora verrucosa

117.3 Aspergillosis
Infection by Aspergillus species, mainly A. fumigatus, A. flavus group, A. terreus group
AHA: 4Q, '97, 40

117.4 Mycotic mycetomas
Infection by various genera and species of Ascomycetes and Deuteromycetes, such as Acremonium [Cephalosporium] falciforme, Neotestudina rosatii, Madurella grisea, Madurella mycetomii, Pyrenochaeta romeroi, Zopfia [Leptosphaeria] senegalensis
Madura foot, mycotic
Maduromycosis, mycotic
EXCLUDES *actinomycotic mycetomas (039.0-039.9)*

117.5 Cryptococcosis
Busse-Buschke's disease
European cryptococcosis
Infection by Cryptococcus neoformans
Pulmonary cryptococcosis
Systemic cryptococcosis
Torula

117.6 Allescheriosis [Petriellidosis]
Infections by Allescheria [Petriellidium] boydii [Monosporium apiospermum]
EXCLUDES *mycotic mycetoma (117.4)*

117.7 Zygomycosis [Phycomycosis or Mucormycosis]
Infection by species of Absidia, Basidiobolus, Conidiobolus, Cunninghamella, Entomophthora, Mucor, Rhizopus, Saksenaea

117.8 Infection by dematiacious fungi, [Phaehyphomycosis]
Infection by dematiacious fungi, such as Cladosporium trichoides [bantianum], Dreschlera hawaiiensis, Phialophora gougerotii, Phialophora jeanselmi

117.9 Other and unspecified mycoses

118 Opportunistic mycoses
Infection of skin, subcutaneous tissues, and/or organs by a wide variety of fungi generally considered to be pathogenic to compromised hosts only (e.g., infection by species of Alternaria, Dreschlera, Fusarium)

HELMINTHIASES (120-129)

✓4th **120 Schistosomiasis [bilharziasis]**
DEF: Infection caused by *Schistosoma*, a genus of flukes or trematode parasites.

120.0 Schistosoma haematobium
Vesical schistosomiasis NOS

120.1 Schistosoma mansoni
Intestinal schistosomiasis NOS

120.2 Schistosoma japonicum
Asiatic schistosomiasis NOS
Katayama disease or fever

120.3 Cutaneous
Cercarial dermatitis
Infection by cercariae of Schistosoma
Schistosome dermatitis
Swimmers' itch

120.8 Other specified schistosomiasis
Infection by Schistosoma:
bovis
intercalatum
mattheii
spindale
Schistosomiasis chestermani

120.9 Schistosomiasis, unspecified
Blood flukes NOS
Hemic distomiasis

✓4th **121 Other trematode infections**

121.0 Opisthorchiasis
Infection by:
cat liver fluke
Opisthorchis (felineus) (tenuicollis) (viverrini)

121.1 Clonorchiasis
Biliary cirrhosis due to clonorchiasis
Chinese liver fluke disease
Hepatic distomiasis due to Clonorchis sinensis
Oriental liver fluke disease

121.2 Paragonimiasis
Infection by Paragonimus
Lung fluke disease (oriental)
Pulmonary distomiasis

121.3 Fascioliasis
Infection by Fasciola:
gigantica
hepatica
Liver flukes NOS
Sheep liver fluke infection

121.4 Fasciolopsiasis
Infection by Fasciolopsis (buski)
Intestinal distomiasis

121.5 Metagonimiasis
Infection by Metagonimus yokogawai

121.6 Heterophyiasis
Infection by:
Heterophyes heterophyes
Stellantchasmus falcatus

121.8 Other specified trematode infections
Infection by:
Dicrocoelium dendriticum
Echinostoma ilocanum
Gastrodiscoides hominis

121.9 Trematode infection, unspecified
Distomiasis NOS
Fluke disease NOS

✓4th **122 Echinococcosis**
INCLUDES echinococciasis
hydatid disease
hydatidosis

DEF: Infection caused by larval forms of tapeworms of the genus *Echinococcus*.

122.0 Echinococcus granulosus infection of liver
122.1 Echinococcus granulosus infection of lung
122.2 Echinococcus granulosus infection of thyroid
122.3 Echinococcus granulosus infection, other
122.4 Echinococcus granulosus infection, unspecified
122.5 Echinococcus multilocularis infection of liver
122.6 Echinococcus multilocularis infection, other
122.7 Echinococcus multilocularis infection, unspecified
122.8 Echinococcosis, unspecified, of liver
122.9 Echinococcosis, other and unspecified

✓4th **123 Other cestode infection**

123.0 Taenia solium infection, intestinal form
Pork tapeworm (adult) (infection)

123.1 Cysticercosis
Cysticerciasis
Infection by Cysticercus cellulosae [larval form of Taenia solium]
AHA: 2Q, '97, 8

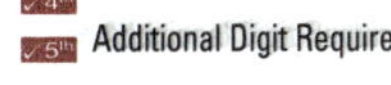 Additional Digit Required | Unspecified Code | Other Specified Code | Manifestation Code | ▶◀ Revised Text | ● New Code | ▲ Revised Code Title

123.2 Taenia saginata infection
Beef tapeworm (infection)
Infection by Taeniarhynchus saginatus

123.3 Taeniasis, unspecified

123.4 Diphyllobothriasis, intestinal
Diphyllobothrium (adult) (latum) (pacificum) infection
Fish tapeworm (infection)

123.5 Sparganosis [larval diphyllobothriasis]
Infection by:
Diphyllobothrium larvae
Sparganum (mansoni) (proliferum)
Spirometra larvae

123.6 Hymenolepiasis
Dwarf tapeworm (infection)
Hymenolepis (diminuta) (nana) infection
Rat tapeworm (infection)

123.8 Other specified cestode infection
Diplogonoporus (grandis) infection
Dipylidium (caninum) infection
Dog tapeworm (infection)

123.9 Cestode infection, unspecified
Tapeworm (infection) NOS

124 Trichinosis
Trichinella spiralis infection
Trichinellosis
Trichiniasis

DEF: Infection by *Trichinella spiralis,* the smallest of the parasitic nematodes.

✓4th **125 Filarial infection and dracontiasis**

125.0 Bancroftian filariasis
Chyluria due to Wuchereria bancrofti
Elephantiasis due to Wuchereria bancrofti
Infection due to Wuchereria bancrofti
Lymphadenitis due to Wuchereria bancrofti
Lymphangitis due to Wuchereria bancrofti
Wuchereriasis

125.1 Malayan filariasis
Brugia filariasis due to Brugia [Wuchereria] malayi
Chyluria due to Brugia [Wuchereria] malayi
Elephantiasis due to Brugia [Wuchereria] malayi
Infection due to Brugia [Wuchereria] malayi
Lymphadenitis due to Brugia [Wuchereria] malayi
Lymphangitis due to Brugia [Wuchereria] malayi

125.2 Loiasis
Eyeworm disease of Africa
Loa loa infection

125.3 Onchocerciasis
Onchocerca volvulus infection
Onchocercais

125.4 Dipetalonemiasis
Infection by:
Acanthocheilonema perstans
Dipetalonema perstans

125.5 Mansonella ozzardi infection
Filariasis ozzardi

125.6 Other specified filariasis
Dirofilaria infection
Infection by:
Acanthocheilonema streptocerca
Dipetalonema streptocerca

125.7 Dracontiasis
Guinea-worm infection
Infection by Dracunculus medinensis

125.9 Unspecified filariasis

✓4th **126 Ancylostomiasis and necatoriasis**

INCLUDES cutaneous larva migrans due to Ancylostoma
hookworm (disease) (infection)
uncinariasis

126.0 Ancylostoma duodenale

126.1 Necator americanus

126.2 Ancylostoma braziliense

126.3 Ancylostoma ceylanicum

126.8 Other specified Ancylostoma

126.9 Ancylostomiasis and necatoriasis, unspecified
Creeping eruption NOS
Cutaneous larva migrans NOS

✓4th **127 Other intestinal helminthiases**

127.0 Ascariasis
Ascaridiasis
Infection by Ascaris lumbricoides
Roundworm infection

127.1 Anisakiasis
Infection by Anisakis larva

127.2 Strongyloidiasis
Infection by Strongyloides stercoralis
EXCLUDES *trichostrongyliasis (127.6)*

127.3 Trichuriasis
Infection by Trichuris trichiuria
Trichocephaliasis
Whipworm (disease) (infection)

127.4 Enterobiasis
Infection by Enterobius vermicularis
Oxyuriasis
Oxyuris vermicularis infection
Pinworm (disease) (infection)
Threadworm infection

127.5 Capillariasis
Infection by Capillaria philippinensis
EXCLUDES *infection by Capillaria hepatica (128.8)*

127.6 Trichostrongyliasis
Infection by Trichostrongylus species

127.7 Other specified intestinal helminthiasis
Infection by:
Oesophagostomum apiostomum and related species
Ternidens diminutus
other specified intestinal helminth
Physalopteriasis

127.8 Mixed intestinal helminthiasis
Infection by intestinal helminths classified to more than one of the categories 120.0-127.7
Mixed helminthiasis NOS

127.9 Intestinal helminthiasis, unspecified

✓4th **128 Other and unspecified helminthiases**

128.0 Toxocariasis
Larva migrans visceralis
Toxocara (canis) (cati) infection
Visceral larva migrans syndrome

128.1 Gnathostomiasis
Infection by Gnathostoma spinigerum and related species

128.8 Other specified helminthiasis
Infection by:
Angiostrongylus cantonensis
Capillaria hepatica
other specified helminth

128.9 Helminth infection, unspecified
Helminthiasis NOS
Worms NOS

129 Intestinal parasitism, unspecified

OTHER INFECTIOUS AND PARASITIC DISEASES (130–136)

✓4th **130 Toxoplasmosis**

INCLUDES infection by toxoplasma gondii
toxoplasmosis (acquired)

EXCLUDES *congenital toxoplasmosis (771.2)*

130.0 Meningoencephalitis due to toxoplasmosis
Encephalitis due to acquired toxoplasmosis

130.1 Conjunctivitis due to toxoplasmosis

130.2 Chorioretinitis due to toxoplasmosis
Focal retinochoroiditis due to acquired toxoplasmosis

N Newborn Age: 0 P Pediatric Age: 0-17 M Maternity Age: 12-55 A Adult Age: 15-124 MSP Medicare Secondary Payer

130.3 Myocarditis due to toxoplasmosis
130.4 Pneumonitis due to toxoplasmosis
130.5 Hepatitis due to toxoplasmosis
130.7 Toxoplasmosis of other specified sites
130.8 Multisystemic disseminated toxoplasmosis
Toxoplasmosis of multiple sites
130.9 Toxoplasmosis, unspecified

✓4th **131 Trichomoniasis**
INCLUDES infection due to Trichomonas (vaginalis)

✓5th **131.0 Urogenital trichomoniasis**
131.00 Urogenital trichomoniasis, unspecified
Fluor (vaginalis) / Leukorrhea (vaginalis) } trichomonal or due to Trichomonas (vaginalis)

DEF: *Trichomonas vaginalis* infection of reproductive and urinary organs, transmitted through coitus.

131.01 Trichomonal vulvovaginitis ♀
Vaginitis, trichomonal or due to Trichomonas (vaginalis)

DEF: *Trichomonas vaginalis* infection of vulva and vagina; often asymptomatic, transmitted through coitus.

131.02 Trichomonal urethritis

DEF: *Trichomonas vaginalis* infection of the urethra.

131.03 Trichomonal prostatitis ♂

DEF: *Trichomonas vaginalis* infection of the prostate.

131.09 Other
131.8 Other specified sites
EXCLUDES *intestinal (007.3)*
131.9 Trichomoniasis, unspecified

✓4th **132 Pediculosis and phthirus infestation**
132.0 Pediculus capitis [head louse]
132.1 Pediculus corporis [body louse]
132.2 Phthirus pubis [pubic louse]
Pediculus pubis
132.3 Mixed infestation
Infestation classifiable to more than one of the categories 132.0-132.2
132.9 Pediculosis, unspecified

✓4th **133 Acariasis**
133.0 Scabies
Infestation by Sarcoptes scabiei
Norwegian scabies
Sarcoptic itch
133.8 Other acariasis
Chiggers
Infestation by:
- Demodex folliculorum
- Trombicula

133.9 Acariasis, unspecified
Infestation by mites NOS

✓4th **134 Other infestation**
134.0 Myiasis
Infestation by:
- Dermatobia (hominis)
- fly larvae
- Gasterophilus (intestinalis)
- maggots
- Oestrus ovis

134.1 Other arthropod infestation
Infestation by:
- chigoe
- sand flea

Tunga penetrans
Jigger disease
Tungiasis
Scarabiasis

134.2 Hirudiniasis
Hirudiniasis (external) (internal)
Leeches (aquatic) (land)
134.8 Other specified infestations
134.9 Infestation, unspecified
Infestation (skin) NOS
Skin parasites NOS

135 Sarcoidosis
Besnier-Boeck-Schaumann disease
Lupoid (miliary) of Boeck
Lupus pernio (Besnier)
Lymphogranulomatosis, benign (Schaumann's)
Sarcoid (any site):
- NOS
- Boeck
- Darier-Roussy

Uveoparotid fever

DEF: A chronic, granulomatous reticulosis (abnormal increase in cells), affecting any organ or tissue; acute form has high rate of remission; chronic form is progressive.

✓4th **136 Other and unspecified infectious and parasitic diseases**
136.0 Ainhum
Dactylolysis spontanea

DEF: A disease affecting the toes, especially the fifth digit, and sometimes the fingers, especially seen in black adult males; it is characterized by a linear constriction around the affected digit leading to spontaneous amputation of the distal part of the digit.

136.1 Behçet's syndrome

DEF: A chronic inflammatory disorder of unknown etiology involving the small blood vessels; it is characterized by recurrent aphthous ulceration of the oral and pharyngeal mucous membranes and the genitalia, skin lesions, severe uvetis, retinal vascularitis and optic atrophy.

136.2 Specific infections by free-living amebae
Meningoencephalitis due to Naegleria
136.3 Pneumocystosis
Pneumonia due to Pneumocystis carinii
AHA: ▶1Q, '05, 7;◀ 1Q, '03, 15; N-D, '87, 5, 6

DEF: *Pneumocystis carinii* fungus causing pneumonia in immunocompromised patients; a leading cause of death among AIDS patients.

136.4 Psorospermiasis
136.5 Sarcosporidiosis
Infection by Sarcocystis lindemanni

DEF: Sarcocystis infection causing muscle cysts of intestinal inflammation.

136.8 Other specified infectious and parasitic diseases
Candiru infection
136.9 Unspecified infectious and parasitic diseases
Infectious disease NOS
Parasitic disease NOS
AHA: 2Q, '91, 8

LATE EFFECTS OF INFECTIOUS AND PARASITIC DISEASES (137-139)

✓4th **137 Late effects of tuberculosis**
Note: This category is to be used to indicate conditions classifiable to 010-018 as the cause of late effects, which are themselves classified elsewhere. The "late effects" include those specified as such, as sequelae, or as due to old or inactive tuberculosis, without evidence of active disease.
137.0 Late effects of respiratory or unspecified tuberculosis
137.1 Late effects of central nervous system tuberculosis
137.2 Late effects of genitourinary tuberculosis
137.3 Late effects of tuberculosis of bones and joints
137.4 Late effects of tuberculosis of other specified organs

138 Late effects of acute poliomyelitis

Note: This category is to be used to indicate conditions classifiable to 045 as the cause of late effects, which are themselves classified elsewhere. The "late effects" include conditions specified as such, or as sequelae, or as due to old or inactive poliomyelitis, without evidence of active disease.

✓4th **139 Late effects of other infectious and parasitic diseases**

Note: This category is to be used to indicate conditions classifiable to categories 001-009, 020-041, 046-136 as the cause of late effects, which are themselves classified elsewhere. The "late effects" include conditions specified as such; they also include sequela of diseases classifiable to the above categories if there is evidence that the disease itself is no longer present.

139.0 Late effects of viral encephalitis

Late effects of conditions classifiable to 049.8-049.9, 062-064

139.1 Late effects of trachoma

Late effects of conditions classifiable to 076

139.8 Late effects of other and unspecified infectious and parasitic diseases

AHA: 4Q, '91, 15; 3Q, '90, 14; M-A, '87, 8

2. NEOPLASMS (140-239)

Notes:

1. Content

This chapter contains the following broad groups:

140-195	Malignant neoplasms, stated or presumed to be primary, of specified sites, except of lymphatic and hematopoietic tissue
196-198	Malignant neoplasms, stated or presumed to be secondary, of specified sites
199	Malignant neoplasms, without specification of site
200-208	Malignant neoplasms, stated or presumed to be primary, of lymphatic and hematopoietic tissue
210-229	Benign neoplasms
230-234	Carcinoma in situ
235-238	Neoplasms of uncertain behavior [see Note at beginning of section]
239	Neoplasms of unspecified nature

2. Functional activity

All neoplasms are classified in this chapter, whether or not functionally active. An additional code from Chapter 3 may be used to identify such functional activity associated with any neoplasm, e.g.:

catecholamine-producing malignant pheochromocytoma of adrenal:

code 194.0, additional code 255.6

basophil adenoma of pituitary with Cushing's syndrome:

code 227.3, additional code 255.0

3. Morphology [Histology]

For those wishing to identify the histological type of neoplasms, a comprehensive coded nomenclature, which comprises the morphology rubrics of the ICD-Oncology, is given in Appendix A.

4. Malignant neoplasms overlapping site boundaries

Categories 140-195 are for the classification of primary malignant neoplasms according to their point of origin. A malignant neoplasm that overlaps two or more subcategories within a three-digit rubric and whose point of origin cannot be determined should be classified to the subcategory .8 "Other."

For example, "carcinoma involving tip and ventral surface of tongue" should be assigned to 141.8. On the other hand, "carcinoma of tip of tongue, extending to involve the ventral surface" should be coded to 141.2, as the point of origin, the tip, is known. Three subcategories (149.8, 159.8, 165.8) have been provided for malignant neoplasms that overlap the boundaries of three-digit rubrics within certain systems.

Overlapping malignant neoplasms that cannot be classified as indicated above should be assigned to the appropriate subdivision of category 195 (Malignant neoplasm of other and ill-defined sites).

AHA: 2Q, '90, 7

DEF: An abnormal growth, such as a tumor. Morphology determines behavior, i.e., whether it will remain intact (benign) or spread to adjacent tissue (malignant). The term mass is not synonymous with neoplasm, as it is often used to describe cysts and thickenings such as those occurring with hematoma or infection.

MALIGNANT NEOPLASM OF LIP, ORAL CAVITY, AND PHARYNX (140-149)

EXCLUDES *carcinoma in situ (230.0)*

✓4th **140 Malignant neoplasm of lip**

EXCLUDES *skin of lip (173.0)*

140.0 Upper lip, vermilion border
Upper lip:
NOS
external
Upper lip:
lipstick area

Lip

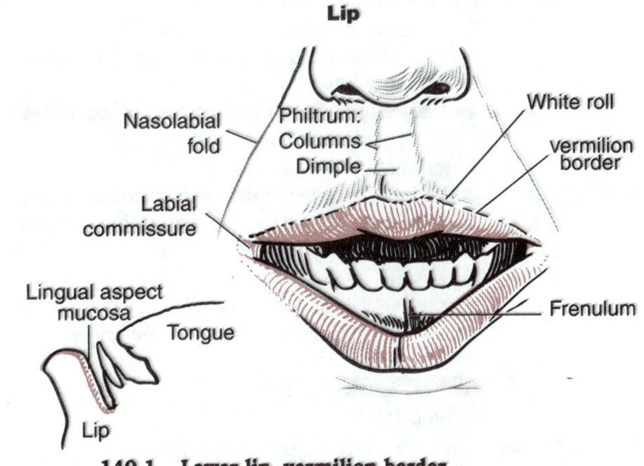

140.1 Lower lip, vermilion border
Lower lip:
NOS
external
Lower lip:
lipstick area

140.3 Upper lip, inner aspect
Upper lip:
buccal aspect
frenulum
Upper lip:
mucosa
oral aspect

140.4 Lower lip, inner aspect
Lower lip:
buccal aspect
frenulum
Lower lip:
mucosa
oral aspect

140.5 Lip, unspecified, inner aspect
Lip, not specified whether upper or lower:
buccal aspect
frenulum
mucosa
oral aspect

140.6 Commissure of lip
Labial commissure

140.8 Other sites of lip
Malignant neoplasm of contiguous or overlapping sites of lip whose point of origin cannot be determined

140.9 Lip, unspecified, vermilion border
Lip, not specified as upper or lower:
NOS
external
lipstick area

✓4th **141 Malignant neoplasm of tongue**

141.0 Base of tongue
Dorsal surface of base of tongue
Fixed part of tongue NOS

141.1 Dorsal surface of tongue
Anterior two-thirds of tongue, dorsal surface
Dorsal tongue NOS
Midline of tongue

EXCLUDES *dorsal surface of base of tongue (141.0)*

Tongue

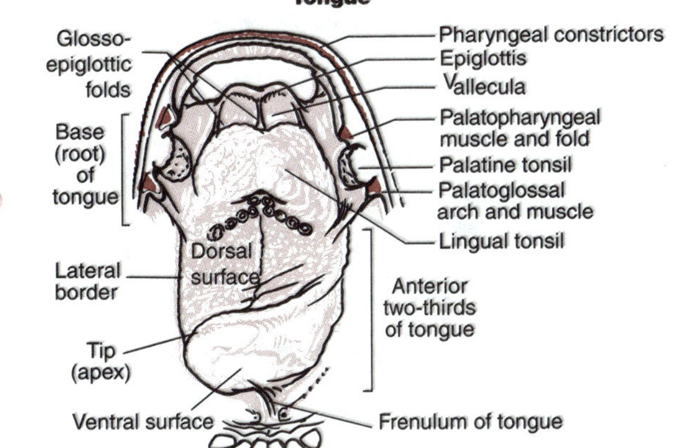

141.2 Tip and lateral border of tongue

141.3 Ventral surface of tongue
Anterior two-thirds of tongue, ventral surface
Frenulum linguae

141.4 Anterior two-thirds of tongue, part unspecified
Mobile part of tongue NOS

141.5 Junctional zone
Border of tongue at junction of fixed and mobile parts at insertion of anterior tonsillar pillar

141.6 Lingual tonsil

141.8 Other sites of tongue
Malignant neoplasm of contiguous or overlapping sites of tongue whose point of origin cannot be determined

141.9 Tongue, unspecified
Tongue NOS

✓4th **142 Malignant neoplasm of major salivary glands**

INCLUDES salivary ducts

EXCLUDES *malignant neoplasm of minor salivary glands:*
NOS (145.9)
buccal mucosa (145.0)
soft palate (145.3)
tongue (141.0-141.9)
tonsil, palatine (146.0)

142.0 Parotid gland

142.1 Submandibular gland
Submaxillary gland

142.2 Sublingual gland

142.8 Other major salivary glands
Malignant neoplasm of contiguous or overlapping sites of salivary glands and ducts whose point of origin cannot be determined

142.9 Salivary gland, unspecified
Salivary gland (major) NOS

✓4th **143 Malignant neoplasm of gum**

INCLUDES alveolar (ridge) mucosa
gingiva (alveolar) (marginal)
interdental papillae

EXCLUDES *malignant odontogenic neoplasms (170.0-170.1)*

143.0 Upper gum

143.1 Lower gum

143.8 Other sites of gum
Malignant neoplasm of contiguous or overlapping sites of gum whose point of origin cannot be determined

143.9 Gum, unspecified

✓4th **144 Malignant neoplasm of floor of mouth**

144.0 Anterior portion
Anterior to the premolar-canine junction

144.1 Lateral portion

Main Salivary Glands

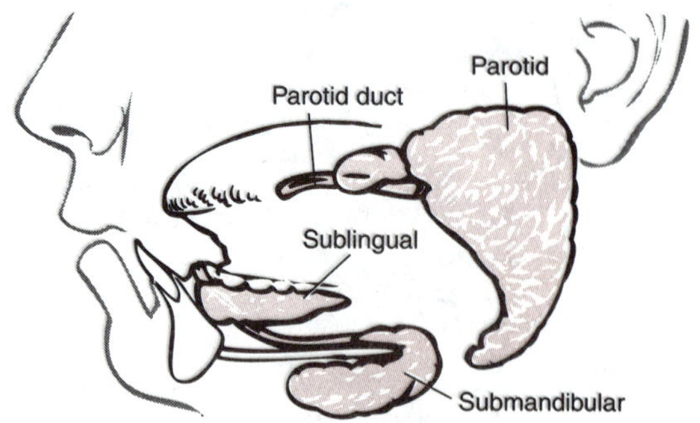

Mouth

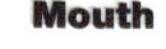

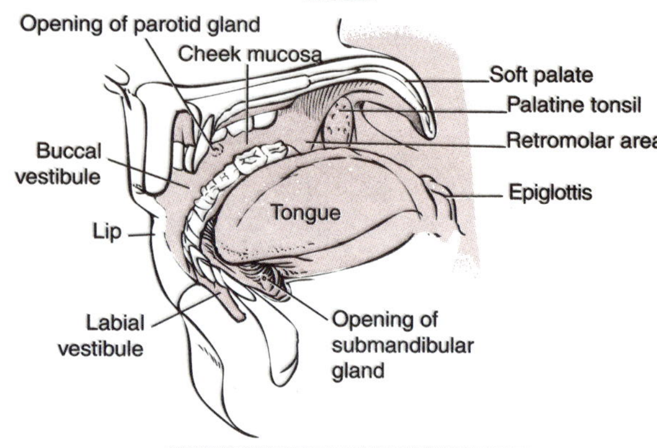

144.8 Other sites of floor of mouth
Malignant neoplasm of contiguous or overlapping sites of floor of mouth whose point of origin cannot be determined

144.9 Floor of mouth, part unspecified

✓4th **145 Malignant neoplasm of other and unspecified parts of mouth**

EXCLUDES *mucosa of lips (140.0-140.9)*

145.0 Cheek mucosa
Buccal mucosa
Cheek, inner aspect

145.1 Vestibule of mouth
Buccal sulcus (upper) (lower)
Labial sulcus (upper) (lower)

145.2 Hard palate

145.3 Soft palate

EXCLUDES *nasopharyngeal [posterior] [superior] surface of soft palate (147.3)*

145.4 Uvula

145.5 Palate, unspecified
Junction of hard and soft palate
Roof of mouth

145.6 Retromolar area

145.8 Other specified parts of mouth
Malignant neoplasm of contiguous or overlapping sites of mouth whose point of origin cannot be determined

145.9 Mouth, unspecified
Buccal cavity NOS
Minor salivary gland, unspecified site
Oral cavity NOS

✓4th **146 Malignant neoplasm of oropharynx**

146.0 Tonsil
Tonsil:
NOS
faucial
palatine

EXCLUDES *lingual tonsil (141.6)*
pharyngeal tonsil (147.1)

AHA: S-O, '87, 8

146.1 Tonsillar fossa

146.2 Tonsillar pillars (anterior) (posterior)
Faucial pillar
Glossopalatine fold
Palatoglossal arch
Palatopharyngeal arch

146.3 Vallecula
Anterior and medial surface of the pharyngoepiglottic fold

146.4 Anterior aspect of epiglottis
Epiglottis, free border [margin]
Glossoepiglottic fold(s)

EXCLUDES *epiglottis:*
NOS (161.1)
suprahyoid portion (161.1)

Oropharynx

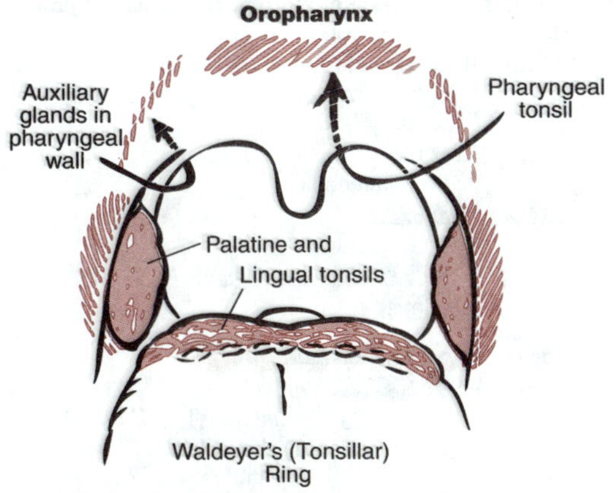

146.5 Junctional region
Junction of the free margin of the epiglottis, the aryepiglottic fold, and the pharyngoepiglottic fold

146.6 Lateral wall of oropharynx

146.7 Posterior wall of oropharynx

146.8 Other specified sites of oropharynx
Branchial cleft
Malignant neoplasm of contiguous or overlapping sites of oropharynx whose point of origin cannot be determined

146.9 Oropharynx, unspecified
AHA: 2Q, '02, 6

✓4th **147 Malignant neoplasm of nasopharynx**

147.0 Superior wall
Roof of nasopharynx

147.1 Posterior wall
Adenoid
Pharyngeal tonsil

147.2 Lateral wall
Fossa of Rosenmüller
Opening of auditory tube
Pharyngeal recess

147.3 Anterior wall
Floor of nasopharynx
Nasopharyngeal [posterior] [superior] surface of soft palate
Posterior margin of nasal septum and choanae

147.8 Other specified sites of nasopharynx
Malignant neoplasm of contiguous or overlapping sites of nasopharynx whose point of origin cannot be determined

147.9 Nasopharynx, unspecified
Nasopharyngeal wall NOS

✓4th **148 Malignant neoplasm of hypopharynx**

148.0 Postcricoid region

148.1 Pyriform sinus
Pyriform fossa

Nasopharynx

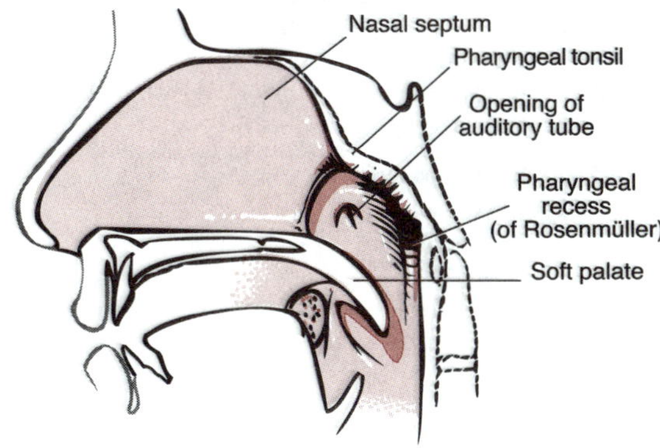

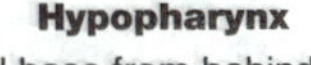

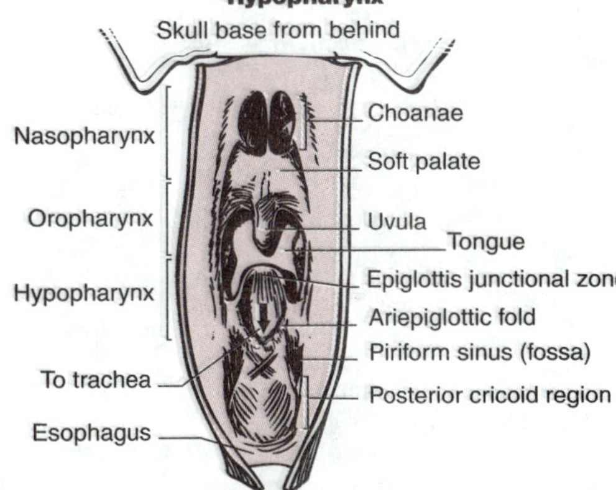

148.2 Aryepiglottic fold, hypopharyngeal aspect
Aryepiglottic fold or interarytenoid fold:
NOS
marginal zone
EXCLUDES *aryepiglottic fold or interarytenoid fold, laryngeal aspect (161.1)*

148.3 Posterior hypopharyngeal wall

148.8 Other specified sites of hypopharynx
Malignant neoplasm of contiguous or overlapping sites of hypopharynx whose point of origin cannot be determined

148.9 Hypopharynx, unspecified
Hypopharyngeal wall NOS
Hypopharynx NOS

✓4th **149 Malignant neoplasm of other and ill-defined sites within the lip, oral cavity, and pharynx**

149.0 Pharynx, unspecified

149.1 Waldeyer's ring

149.8 Other
Malignant neoplasms of lip, oral cavity, and pharynx whose point of origin cannot be assigned to any one of the categories 140-148
EXCLUDES *"book leaf" neoplasm [ventral surface of tongue and floor of mouth] (145.8)*

149.9 Ill-defined

MALIGNANT NEOPLASM OF DIGESTIVE ORGANS AND PERITONEUM (150-159)

EXCLUDES *carcinoma in situ (230.1-230.9)*

✓4th **150 Malignant neoplasm of esophagus**

150.0 Cervical esophagus

150.1 Thoracic esophagus

150.2 Abdominal esophagus
EXCLUDES *adenocarcinoma (151.0)*
cardio-esophageal junction (151.0)

150.3 Upper third of esophagus
Proximal third of esophagus

150.4 Middle third of esophagus

150.5 Lower third of esophagus
Distal third of esophagus
EXCLUDES *adenocarcinoma (151.0)*
cardio-esophageal junction (151.0)

150.8 Other specified part
Malignant neoplasm of contiguous or overlapping sites of esophagus whose point of origin cannot be determined

150.9 Esophagus, unspecified

✓4th **151 Malignant neoplasm of stomach**

151.0 Cardia
Cardiac orifice
Cardio-esophageal junction
EXCLUDES *squamous cell carcinoma (150.2, 150.5)*

Colon

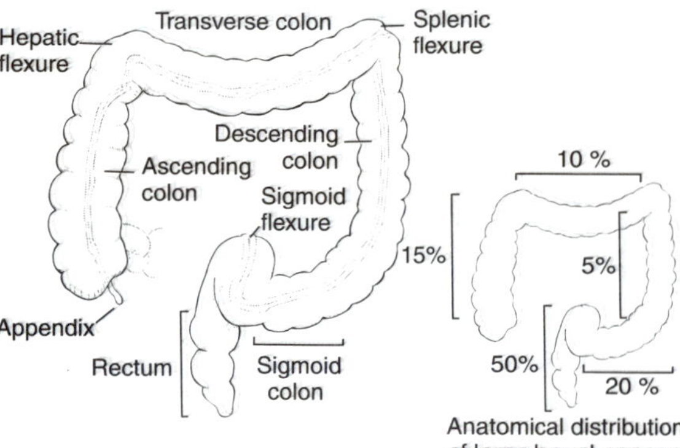

151.1 Pylorus
Prepylorus
Pyloric canal

151.2 Pyloric antrum
Antrum of stomach NOS

151.3 Fundus of stomach

151.4 Body of stomach

151.5 Lesser curvature, unspecified
Lesser curvature, not classifiable to 151.1-151.4

151.6 Greater curvature, unspecified
Greater curvature, not classifiable to 151.0-151.4

151.8 Other specified sites of stomach
Anterior wall, not classifiable to 151.0-151.4
Posterior wall, not classifiable to 151.0-151.4
Malignant neoplasm of contiguous or overlapping sites of stomach whose point of origin cannot be determined

151.9 Stomach, unspecified
Carcinoma ventriculi
Gastric cancer
AHA: 2Q, '01, 17

✓4th 152 Malignant neoplasm of small intestine, including duodenum

152.0 Duodenum

152.1 Jejunum

152.2 Ileum
EXCLUDES *ileocecal valve (153.4)*

152.3 Meckel's diverticulum

152.8 Other specified sites of small intestine
Duodenojejunal junction
Malignant neoplasm of contiguous or overlapping sites of small intestine whose point of origin cannot be determined

152.9 Small intestine, unspecified

✓4th 153 Malignant neoplasm of colon

153.0 Hepatic flexure

153.1 Transverse colon

153.2 Descending colon
Left colon

153.3 Sigmoid colon
Sigmoid (flexure)
EXCLUDES *rectosigmoid junction (154.0)*

153.4 Cecum
Ileocecal valve

153.5 Appendix

153.6 Ascending colon
Right colon

153.7 Splenic flexure

153.8 Other specified sites of large intestine
Malignant neoplasm of contiguous or overlapping sites of colon whose point of origin cannot be determined
EXCLUDES *ileocecal valve (153.4)*
rectosigmoid junction (154.0)

153.9 Colon, unspecified
Large intestine NOS

✓4th 154 Malignant neoplasm of rectum, rectosigmoid junction, and anus

154.0 Rectosigmoid junction
Colon with rectum
Rectosigmoid (colon)

154.1 Rectum
Rectal ampulla

154.2 Anal canal
Anal sphincter
EXCLUDES *skin of anus (172.5, 173.5)*
AHA: 1Q, '01, 8

154.3 Anus, unspecified
EXCLUDES *anus:*
margin (172.5, 173.5)
skin (172.5, 173.5)
perianal skin (172.5, 173.5)

154.8 Other
Anorectum
Cloacogenic zone
Malignant neoplasm of contiguous or overlapping sites of rectum, rectosigmoid junction, and anus whose point of origin cannot be determined

✓4th 155 Malignant neoplasm of liver and intrahepatic bile ducts

155.0 Liver, primary
Carcinoma:
hepatocellular
liver cell
liver, specified as primary
Hepatoblastoma

155.1 Intrahepatic bile ducts
Canaliculi biliferi
Interlobular:
bile ducts
biliary canals
Intrahepatic:
biliary passages
canaliculi
gall duct
EXCLUDES *hepatic duct (156.1)*

155.2 Liver, not specified as primary or secondary

✓4th 156 Malignant neoplasm of gallbladder and extrahepatic bile ducts

156.0 Gallbladder

156.1 Extrahepatic bile ducts
Biliary duct or passage NOS
Common bile duct
Cystic duct
Hepatic duct
Sphincter of Oddi

156.2 Ampulla of Vater
DEF: Malignant neoplasm in the area of dilation at the juncture of the common bile and pancreatic ducts near the opening into the lumen of the duodenum.

156.8 Other specified sites of gallbladder and extrahepatic bile ducts
Malignant neoplasm of contiguous or overlapping sites of gallbladder and extrahepatic bile ducts whose point of origin cannot be determined

156.9 Biliary tract, part unspecified
Malignant neoplasm involving both intrahepatic and extrahepatic bile ducts

✓4th 157 Malignant neoplasm of pancreas

157.0 Head of pancreas
AHA: 4Q, '00, 40

157.1 Body of pancreas

157.2 Tail of pancreas

157.3 Pancreatic duct
Duct of:
Santorini
Wirsung

Retroperitoneum and Peritoneum

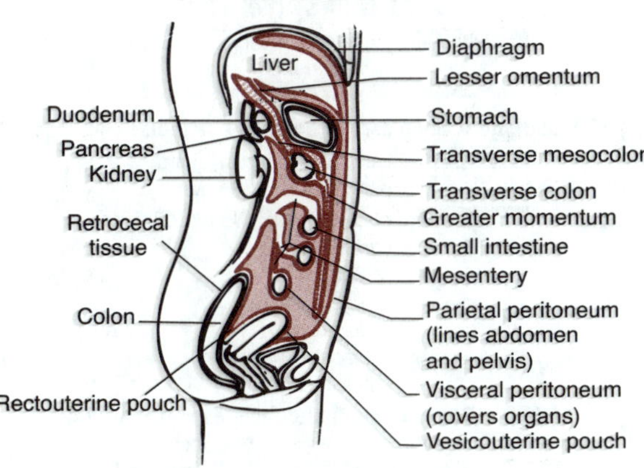

157.4 Islets of Langerhans
Islets of Langerhans, any part of pancreas
Use additional code to identify any functional activity

DEF: Malignant neoplasm within the structures of the pancreas that produce insulin, somatostatin and glucagon.

157.8 Other specified sites of pancreas
Ectopic pancreatic tissue
Malignant neoplasm of contiguous or overlapping sites of pancreas whose point of origin cannot be determined

157.9 Pancreas, part unspecified
AHA: 4Q, '89, 11

✓4th **158 Malignant neoplasm of retroperitoneum and peritoneum**

158.0 Retroperitoneum
Periadrenal tissue
Perinephric tissue
Perirenal tissue
Retrocecal tissue

158.8 Specified parts of peritoneum
Cul-de-sac (of Douglas)
Mesentery
Mesocolon
Omentum
Peritoneum:
parietal
pelvic
Rectouterine pouch
Malignant neoplasm of contiguous or overlapping sites of retroperitoneum and peritoneum whose point of origin cannot be determined

158.9 Peritoneum, unspecified

✓4th **159 Malignant neoplasm of other and ill-defined sites within the digestive organs and peritoneum**

159.0 Intestinal tract, part unspecified
Intestine NOS

159.1 Spleen, not elsewhere classified
Angiosarcoma } of spleen
Fibrosarcoma } of spleen

EXCLUDES *Hodgkin's disease (201.0-201.9)*
lymphosarcoma (200.1)
reticulosarcoma (200.0)

159.8 Other sites of digestive system and intra-abdominal organs
Malignant neoplasm of digestive organs and peritoneum whose point of origin cannot be assigned to any one of the categories 150-158

EXCLUDES *anus and rectum (154.8)*
cardio-esophageal junction (151.0)
colon and rectum (154.0)

159.9 Ill-defined
Alimentary canal or tract NOS
Gastrointestinal tract NOS

EXCLUDES *abdominal NOS (195.2)*
intra-abdominal NOS (195.2)

MALIGNANT NEOPLASM OF RESPIRATORY AND INTRATHORACIC ORGANS (160-165)

EXCLUDES *carcinoma in situ (231.0-231.9)*

✓4th **160 Malignant neoplasm of nasal cavities, middle ear, and accessory sinuses**

160.0 Nasal cavities
Cartilage of nose
Conchae, nasal
Internal nose
Septum of nose
Vestibule of nose

EXCLUDES *nasal bone (170.0)*
nose NOS (195.0)
olfactory bulb (192.0)
posterior margin of septum and choanae (147.3)
skin of nose (172.3, 173.3)
turbinates (170.0)

160.1 Auditory tube, middle ear, and mastoid air cells
Antrum tympanicum
Eustachian tube
Tympanic cavity

EXCLUDES *auditory canal (external) (172.2, 173.2)*
bone of ear (meatus) (170.0)
cartilage of ear (171.0)
ear (external) (skin) (172.2, 173.2)

160.2 Maxillary sinus
Antrum (Highmore) (maxillary)

160.3 Ethmoidal sinus

160.4 Frontal sinus

160.5 Sphenoidal sinus

160.8 Other
Malignant neoplasm of contiguous or overlapping sites of nasal cavities, middle ear, and accessory sinuses whose point of origin cannot be determined

160.9 Accessory sinus, unspecified

✓4th **161 Malignant neoplasm of larynx**

161.0 Glottis
Intrinsic larynx
Laryngeal commissure (anterior) (posterior)
True vocal cord
Vocal cord NOS

161.1 Supraglottis
Aryepiglottic fold or interarytenoid fold, laryngeal aspect
Epiglottis (suprahyoid portion) NOS
Extrinsic larynx
False vocal cords
Posterior (laryngeal) surface of epiglottis
Ventricular bands

EXCLUDES *anterior aspect of epiglottis (146.4)*
aryepiglottic fold or interarytenoid fold:
NOS (148.2)
hypopharyngeal aspect (148.2)
marginal zone (148.2)

161.2 Subglottis

161.3 Laryngeal cartilages
Cartilage:
arytenoid
cricoid
Cartilage:
cuneiform
thyroid

161.8 Other specified sites of larynx
Malignant neoplasm of contiguous or overlapping sites of larynx whose point of origin cannot be determined

161.9 Larynx, unspecified

✓4th 162 Malignant neoplasm of trachea, bronchus, and lung

162.0 Trachea

Cartilage } of trachea
Mucosa }

162.2 Main bronchus

Carina
Hilus of lung

162.3 Upper lobe, bronchus or lung

AHA: 1Q, '04, 4

162.4 Middle lobe, bronchus or lung

162.5 Lower lobe, bronchus or lung

162.8 Other parts of bronchus or lung

Malignant neoplasm of contiguous or overlapping sites of bronchus or lung whose point of origin cannot be determined

162.9 Bronchus and lung, unspecified

AHA: 2Q, '97, 3; 4Q, '96, 48

✓4th 163 Malignant neoplasm of pleura

163.0 Parietal pleura

163.1 Visceral pleura

163.8 Other specified sites of pleura

Malignant neoplasm of contiguous or overlapping sites of pleura whose point of origin cannot be determined

163.9 Pleura, unspecified

✓4th 164 Malignant neoplasm of thymus, heart, and mediastinum

164.0 Thymus

164.1 Heart

Endocardium
Epicardium
Myocardium
Pericardium

EXCLUDES *great vessels (171.4)*

164.2 Anterior mediastinum

164.3 Posterior mediastinum

164.8 Other

Malignant neoplasm of contiguous or overlapping sites of thymus, heart, and mediastinum whose point of origin cannot be determined

164.9 Mediastinum, part unspecified

✓4th 165 Malignant neoplasm of other and ill-defined sites within the respiratory system and intrathoracic organs

165.0 Upper respiratory tract, part unspecified

165.8 Other

Malignant neoplasm of respiratory and intrathoracic organs whose point of origin cannot be assigned to any one of the categories 160-164

165.9 Ill-defined sites within the respiratory system

Respiratory tract NOS

EXCLUDES *intrathoracic NOS (195.1)*
thoracic NOS (195.1)

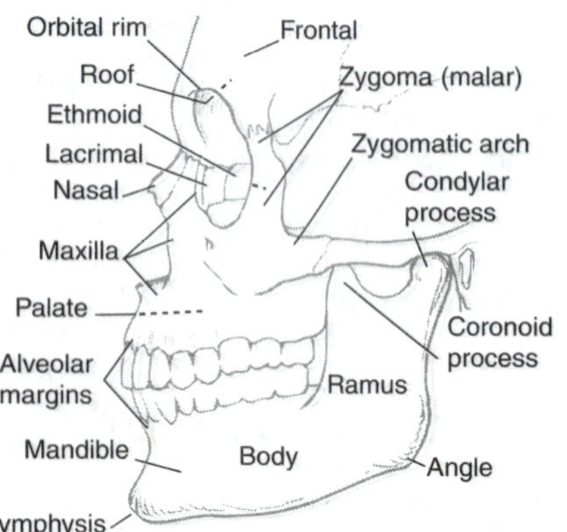

MALIGNANT NEOPLASM OF BONE, CONNECTIVE TISSUE, SKIN, AND BREAST (170-176)

EXCLUDES *carcinoma in situ:*
breast (233.0)
skin (232.0-232.9)

✓4th 170 Malignant neoplasm of bone and articular cartilage

INCLUDES cartilage (articular) (joint)
periosteum

EXCLUDES *bone marrow NOS (202.9)*
cartilage:
ear (171.0)
eyelid (171.0)
larynx (161.3)
nose (160.0)
synovia (171.0-171.9)

170.0 Bones of skull and face, except mandible

Bone:
ethmoid
frontal
malar
nasal
occipital
orbital
parietal

Bone:
sphenoid
temporal
zygomatic
Maxilla (superior)
Turbinate
Upper jaw bone
Vomer

EXCLUDES *carcinoma, any type except intraosseous or odontogenic:*
maxilla, maxillary (sinus) (160.2)
upper jaw bone (143.0)
jaw bone (lower) (170.1)

170.1 Mandible

Inferior maxilla
Jaw bone NOS
Lower jaw bone

EXCLUDES *carcinoma, any type except intraosseous or odontogenic:*
jaw bone NOS (143.9)
lower (143.1)
upper jaw bone (170.0)

170.2 Vertebral column, excluding sacrum and coccyx

Spinal column
Spine
Vertebra

EXCLUDES *sacrum and coccyx (170.6)*

170.3 Ribs, sternum, and clavicle

Costal cartilage
Costovertebral joint
Xiphoid process

170.4 Scapula and long bones of upper limb

Acromion
Bones NOS of upper limb
Humerus
Radius
Ulna

AHA: 2Q, '99, 9

170.5 Short bones of upper limb

Carpal
Cuneiform, wrist
Metacarpal
Navicular, of hand
Phalanges of hand
Pisiform
Scaphoid (of hand)
Semilunar or lunate
Trapezium
Trapezoid
Unciform

170.6 Pelvic bones, sacrum, and coccyx

Coccygeal vertebra
Ilium
Ischium
Pubic bone
Sacral vertebra

170.7 Long bones of lower limb

Bones NOS of lower limb
Femur
Fibula
Tibia

170.8 Short bones of lower limb

Astragalus [talus]
Calcaneus
Cuboid
Cuneiform, ankle
Metatarsal
Navicular (of ankle)
Patella
Phalanges of foot
Tarsal

170.9 Bone and articular cartilage, site unspecified

✓4th **171 Malignant neoplasm of connective and other soft tissue**

INCLUDES blood vessel
bursa
fascia
fat
ligament, except uterine
muscle
peripheral, sympathetic, and parasympathetic nerves and ganglia
synovia
tendon (sheath)

EXCLUDES *cartilage (of):*
articular (170.0-170.9)
larynx (161.3)
nose (160.0)
connective tissue:
breast (174.0-175.9)
internal organs—code to malignant neoplasm of the site [e.g., leiomyosarcoma of stomach, 151.9]
heart (164.1)
uterine ligament (183.4)

171.0 Head, face, and neck

Cartilage of: ear
Cartilage of: eyelid

AHA: 2Q, '99, 6

171.2 Upper limb, including shoulder

Arm
Finger
Forearm
Hand

171.3 Lower limb, including hip

Foot
Leg
Popliteal space
Thigh
Toe

171.4 Thorax

Axilla
Diaphragm
Great vessels

EXCLUDES *heart (164.1)*
mediastinum (164.2-164.9)
thymus (164.0)

171.5 Abdomen

Abdominal wall
Hypochondrium

EXCLUDES *peritoneum (158.8)*
retroperitoneum (158.0)

171.6 Pelvis

Buttock
Groin
Inguinal region
Perineum

EXCLUDES *pelvic peritoneum (158.8)*
retroperitoneum (158.0)
uterine ligament, any (183.3-183.5)

171.7 Trunk, unspecified

Back NOS
Flank NOS

171.8 Other specified sites of connective and other soft tissue

Malignant neoplasm of contiguous or overlapping sites of connective tissue whose point of origin cannot be determined

171.9 Connective and other soft tissue, site unspecified

✓4th **172 Malignant melanoma of skin**

INCLUDES melanocarcinoma
melanoma (skin) NOS

EXCLUDES *skin of genital organs (184.0-184.9, 187.1-187.9)*
sites other than skin—code to malignant neoplasm of the site

DEF: Malignant neoplasm of melanocytes; most common in skin, may involve oral cavity, esophagus, anal canal, vagina, leptomeninges or conjunctiva.

172.0 Lip

EXCLUDES *vermilion border of lip (140.0-140.1, 140.9)*

172.1 Eyelid, including canthus

172.2 Ear and external auditory canal

Auricle (ear)
Auricular canal, external
External [acoustic] meatus
Pinna

172.3 Other and unspecified parts of face

Cheek (external)
Chin
Eyebrow
Forehead
Nose, external
Temple

172.4 Scalp and neck

172.5 Trunk, except scrotum

Axilla
Breast
Buttock
Groin
Perianal skin
Perineum
Umbilicus

EXCLUDES *anal canal (154.2)*
anus NOS (154.3)
scrotum (187.7)

172.6 Upper limb, including shoulder

Arm
Finger
Forearm
Hand

172.7 Lower limb, including hip

Ankle
Foot
Heel
Knee
Leg
Popliteal area
Thigh
Toe

172.8 Other specified sites of skin

Malignant melanoma of contiguous or overlapping sites of skin whose point of origin cannot be determined

172.9 Melanoma of skin, site unspecified

✓4th **173 Other malignant neoplasm of skin**

INCLUDES malignant neoplasm of:
sebaceous glands
sudoriferous, sudoriparous glands
sweat glands

EXCLUDES *Kaposi's sarcoma (176.0-176.9)*
malignant melanoma of skin (172.0-172.9)
skin of genital organs (184.0-184.9, 187.1-187.9)

AHA: 1Q, '00, 18; 2Q, '96, 12

173.0 Skin of lip

EXCLUDES *vermilion border of lip (140.0-140.1, 140.9)*

173.1 Eyelid, including canthus

EXCLUDES *cartilage of eyelid (171.0)*

173.2 Skin of ear and external auditory canal

Auricle (ear)
Auricular canal, external
External meatus
Pinna

EXCLUDES *cartilage of ear (171.0)*

173.3 Skin of other and unspecified parts of face

Cheek, external
Chin
Eyebrow
Forehead
Nose, external
Temple

AHA: 1Q, '00, 3

Female Breast

Upper outer quadrant
Upper inner quadrant
Midline
Areola
Nipple
Axillary tail
Mammary gland
Right Breast
Lower outer quadrant
Lower inner quadrant

173.4 Scalp and skin of neck

173.5 Skin of trunk, except scrotum

Axillary fold
Perianal skin
Skin of:
abdominal wall
anus
back
breast
Skin of:
buttock
chest wall
groin
perineum
Umbilicus

EXCLUDES *anal canal (154.2)*
anus NOS (154.3)
skin of scrotum (187.7)

AHA: 1Q, '01, 8

173.6 Skin of upper limb, including shoulder

Arm
Finger
Forearm
Hand

173.7 Skin of lower limb, including hip

Ankle
Foot
Heel
Knee
Leg
Popliteal area
Thigh
Toe

173.8 Other specified sites of skin

Malignant neoplasm of contiguous or overlapping sites of skin whose point of origin cannot be determined

173.9 Skin, site unspecified

✓4th **174 Malignant neoplasm of female breast**

INCLUDES breast (female)
connective tissue
soft parts
Paget's disease of:
breast
nipple

EXCLUDES *skin of breast (172.5, 173.5)*

AHA: 3Q, '97, 8; 4Q, '89, 11

174.0 Nipple and areola ♀

174.1 Central portion ♀

174.2 Upper-inner quadrant ♀

174.3 Lower-inner quadrant ♀

174.4 Upper-outer quadrant ♀

AHA: 1Q, '04, 3

174.5 Lower-outer quadrant ♀

174.6 Axillary tail ♀

174.8 Other specified sites of female breast ♀

Ectopic sites
Inner breast
Lower breast
Malignant neoplasm of contiguous or overlapping sites of breast whose point of origin cannot be determined
Midline of breast
Outer breast
Upper breast

174.9 Breast (female), unspecified ♀

✓4th **175 Malignant neoplasm of male breast**

EXCLUDES *skin of breast (172.5,173.5)*

175.0 Nipple and areola ♂

175.9 Other and unspecified sites of male breast ♂

Ectopic breast tissue, male

✓4th **176 Kaposi's sarcoma**

AHA: 4Q, '91, 24

176.0 Skin

176.1 Soft tissue

Blood vessel
Connective tissue
Fascia
Ligament
Lymphatic(s) NEC
Muscle

EXCLUDES *lymph glands and nodes (176.5)*

176.2 Palate

176.3 Gastrointestinal sites

176.4 Lung

176.5 Lymph nodes

176.8 Other specified sites

Oral cavity NEC

176.9 Unspecified

Viscera NOS

MALIGNANT NEOPLASM OF GENITOURINARY ORGANS (179-189)

EXCLUDES *carcinoma in situ (233.1-233.9)*

179 Malignant neoplasm of uterus, part unspecified ♀

✓4th **180 Malignant neoplasm of cervix uteri**

INCLUDES invasive malignancy [carcinoma]

EXCLUDES *carcinoma in situ (233.1)*

180.0 Endocervix ♀

Cervical canal NOS
Endocervical canal
Endocervical gland

180.1 Exocervix ♀

180.8 Other specified sites of cervix ♀

Cervical stump
Squamocolumnar junction of cervix
Malignant neoplasm of contiguous or overlapping sites of cervix uteri whose point of origin cannot be determined

180.9 Cervix uteri, unspecified ♀

181 Malignant neoplasm of placenta ♀

Choriocarcinoma NOS
Chorioepithelioma NOS

EXCLUDES *chorioadenoma (destruens) (236.1)*
hydatidiform mole (630)
malignant (236.1)
invasive mole (236.1)
male choriocarcinoma NOS (186.0-186.9)

✓4th **182 Malignant neoplasm of body of uterus**

EXCLUDES *carcinoma in situ (233.2)*

182.0 Corpus uteri, except isthmus ♀

Cornu
Endometrium
Fundus
Myometrium

182.1 Isthmus ♀

Lower uterine segment

182.8 Other specified sites of body of uterus ♀

Malignant neoplasm of contiguous or overlapping sites of body of uterus whose point of origin cannot be determined

EXCLUDES *uterus NOS (179)*

N Newborn Age: 0   P Pediatric Age: 0-17   M Maternity Age: 12-55   A Adult Age: 15-124   MSP Medicare Secondary Payer

✓4th 183 Malignant neoplasm of ovary and other uterine adnexa

EXCLUDES *Douglas' cul-de-sac (158.8)*

183.0 Ovary ♀

Use additional code to identify any functional activity

183.2 Fallopian tube ♀

Oviduct
Uterine tube

183.3 Broad ligament ♀

Mesovarium
Parovarian region

183.4 Parametrium ♀

Uterine ligament NOS
Uterosacral ligament

183.5 Round ligament ♀

AHA: 3Q, '99, 5

183.8 Other specified sites of uterine adnexa ♀

Tubo-ovarian
Utero-ovarian
Malignant neoplasm of contiguous or overlapping sites of ovary and other uterine adnexa whose point of origin cannot be determined

183.9 Uterine adnexa, unspecified ♀

✓4th 184 Malignant neoplasm of other and unspecified female genital organs

EXCLUDES *carcinoma in situ (233.3)*

184.0 Vagina ♀

Gartner's duct
Vaginal vault

184.1 Labia majora ♀

Greater vestibular [Bartholin's] gland

184.2 Labia minora ♀

184.3 Clitoris ♀

184.4 Vulva, unspecified ♀

External female genitalia NOS
Pudendum

184.8 Other specified sites of female genital organs ♀

Malignant neoplasm of contiguous or overlapping sites of female genital organs whose point of origin cannot be determined

184.9 Female genital organ, site unspecified ♀

Female genitourinary tract NOS

185 Malignant neoplasm of prostate ♂

EXCLUDES *seminal vesicles (187.8)*

AHA: 3Q, '03, 13; 3Q, '99, 5; 3Q, '92, 7

✓4th 186 Malignant neoplasm of testis

Use additional code to identify any functional activity

186.0 Undescended testis ♂

Ectopic testis
Retained testis

186.9 Other and unspecified testis ♂

Testis:
NOS
descended
Testis:
scrotal

✓4th 187 Malignant neoplasm of penis and other male genital organs

187.1 Prepuce ♂

Foreskin

187.2 Glans penis ♂

187.3 Body of penis ♂

Corpus cavernosum

187.4 Penis, part unspecified ♂

Skin of penis NOS

187.5 Epididymis ♂

187.6 Spermatic cord ♂

Vas deferens

187.7 Scrotum ♂

Skin of scrotum

187.8 Other specified sites of male genital organs ♂

Seminal vesicle
Tunica vaginalis
Malignant neoplasm of contiguous or overlapping sites of penis and other male genital organs whose point of origin cannot be determined

187.9 Male genital organ, site unspecified ♂

Male genital organ or tract NOS

✓4th 188 Malignant neoplasm of bladder

EXCLUDES *carcinoma in situ (233.7)*

188.0 Trigone of urinary bladder

188.1 Dome of urinary bladder

188.2 Lateral wall of urinary bladder

188.3 Anterior wall of urinary bladder

188.4 Posterior wall of urinary bladder

188.5 Bladder neck

Internal urethral orifice

188.6 Ureteric orifice

188.7 Urachus

188.8 Other specified sites of bladder

Malignant neoplasm of contiguous or overlapping sites of bladder whose point of origin cannot be determined

188.9 Bladder, part unspecified

Bladder wall NOS

AHA: 1Q, '00, 5

✓4th 189 Malignant neoplasm of kidney and other and unspecified urinary organs

189.0 Kidney, except pelvis

Kidney NOS
Kidney parenchyma

AHA: ►2Q, '04, 4◄

189.1 Renal pelvis

Renal calyces
Ureteropelvic junction

189.2 Ureter

EXCLUDES *ureteric orifice of bladder (188.6)*

189.3 Urethra

EXCLUDES *urethral orifice of bladder (188.5)*

189.4 Paraurethral glands

189.8 Other specified sites of urinary organs

Malignant neoplasm of contiguous or overlapping sites of kidney and other urinary organs whose point of origin cannot be determined

189.9 Urinary organ, site unspecified

Urinary system NOS

MALIGNANT NEOPLASM OF OTHER AND UNSPECIFIED SITES (190-199)

EXCLUDES *carcinoma in situ (234.0-234.9)*

✓4th 190 Malignant neoplasm of eye

EXCLUDES *carcinoma in situ (234.0)*
eyelid (skin) (172.1, 173.1)
cartilage (171.0)
optic nerve (192.0)
orbital bone (170.0)

190.0 Eyeball, except conjunctiva, cornea, retina, and choroid

Ciliary body
Crystalline lens
Iris
Sclera
Uveal tract

190.1 Orbit

Connective tissue of orbit
Extraocular muscle
Retrobulbar

EXCLUDES *bone of orbit (170.0)*

190.2 Lacrimal gland

190.3 Conjunctiva

190.4 Cornea

190.5 Retina

190.6 Choroid

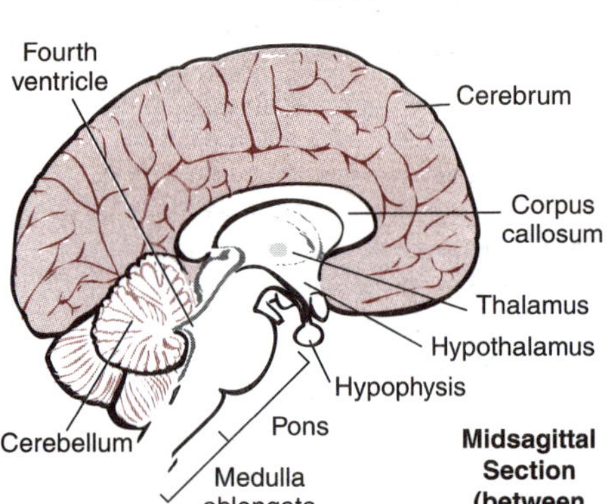

190.7 Lacrimal duct
Lacrimal sac | Nasolacrimal duct

190.8 Other specified sites of eye
Malignant neoplasm of contiguous or overlapping sites of eye whose point of origin cannot be determined

190.9 Eye, part unspecified

✓4th **191 Malignant neoplasm of brain**
EXCLUDES *cranial nerves (192.0)*
retrobulbar area (190.1)

191.0 Cerebrum, except lobes and ventricles
Basal ganglia | Globus pallidus
Cerebral cortex | Hypothalamus
Corpus striatum | Thalamus

191.1 Frontal lobe

191.2 Temporal lobe
Hippocampus | Uncus

191.3 Parietal lobe

191.4 Occipital lobe

191.5 Ventricles
Choroid plexus | Floor of ventricle

191.6 Cerebellum NOS
Cerebellopontine angle

191.7 Brain stem
Cerebral peduncle | Midbrain
Medulla oblongata | Pons

191.8 Other parts of brain
Corpus callosum
Tapetum
Malignant neoplasm of contiguous or overlapping sites of brain whose point of origin cannot be determined

191.9 Brain, unspecified
Cranial fossa NOS

✓4th **192 Malignant neoplasm of other and unspecified parts of nervous system**
EXCLUDES *peripheral, sympathetic, and parasympathetic nerves and ganglia (171.0-171.9)*

192.0 Cranial nerves
Olfactory bulb

192.1 Cerebral meninges
Dura (mater) | Meninges NOS
Falx (cerebelli) (cerebri) | Tentorium

192.2 Spinal cord
Cauda equina

192.3 Spinal meninges

192.8 Other specified sites of nervous system
Malignant neoplasm of contiguous or overlapping sites of other parts of nervous system whose point of origin cannot be determined

192.9 Nervous system, part unspecified
Nervous system (central) NOS
EXCLUDES *meninges NOS (192.1)*

193 Malignant neoplasm of thyroid gland
Sipple's syndrome
Thyroglossal duct
Use additional code to identify any functional activity

✓4th **194 Malignant neoplasm of other endocrine glands and related structures**
Use additional code to identify any functional activity
EXCLUDES *islets of Langerhans (157.4)*
ovary (183.0)
testis (186.0-186.9)
thymus (164.0)

194.0 Adrenal gland
Adrenal cortex | Suprarenal gland
Adrenal medulla

194.1 Parathyroid gland

194.3 Pituitary gland and craniopharyngeal duct
Craniobuccal pouch | Rathke's pouch
Hypophysis | Sella turcica
AHA: J-A, '85, 9

194.4 Pineal gland

194.5 Carotid body

194.6 Aortic body and other paraganglia
Coccygeal body | Para-aortic body
Glomus jugulare

194.8 Other
Pluriglandular involvement NOS
Note: If the sites of multiple involvements are known, they should be coded separately.

194.9 Endocrine gland, site unspecified

✓4th **195 Malignant neoplasm of other and ill-defined sites**
INCLUDES malignant neoplasms of contiguous sites, not elsewhere classified, whose point of origin cannot be determined
EXCLUDES *malignant neoplasm:*
lymphatic and hematopoietic tissue (200.0-208.9)
secondary sites (196.0-198.8)
unspecified site (199.0-199.1)

195.0 Head, face, and neck
Cheek NOS | Nose NOS
Jaw NOS | Supraclavicular region NOS
AHA: 4Q, '03, 107

195.1 Thorax
Axilla | Intrathoracic NOS
Chest (wall) NOS

195.2 Abdomen
Intra-abdominal NOS
AHA: 2Q, '97, 3

195.3 Pelvis
Groin
Inguinal region NOS
Presacral region
Sacrococcygeal region
Sites overlapping systems within pelvis, as:
rectovaginal (septum)
rectovesical (septum)

195.4 Upper limb

195.5 Lower limb

195.8 Other specified sites
Back NOS | Trunk NOS
Flank NOS

✓4th **196 Secondary and unspecified malignant neoplasm of lymph nodes**
EXCLUDES *any malignant neoplasm of lymph nodes, specified as primary (200.0-202.9)*
Hodgkin's disease (201.0-201.9)
lymphosarcoma (200.1)
reticulosarcoma (200.0)
other forms of lymphoma (202.0-202.9)
AHA: 2Q, '92, 3; M-J, '85, 3

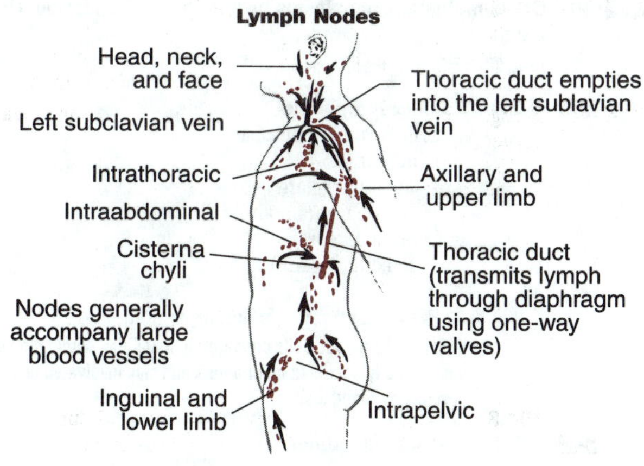

196.0 Lymph nodes of head, face, and neck
Cervical
Cervicofacial
Scalene
Supraclavicular

196.1 Intrathoracic lymph nodes
Bronchopulmonary
Intercostal
Mediastinal
Tracheobronchial

196.2 Intra-abdominal lymph nodes
Intestinal
Mesenteric
Retroperitoneal
AHA: 4Q, '03, 111

196.3 Lymph nodes of axilla and upper limb
Brachial
Epitrochlear
Infraclavicular
Pectoral

196.5 Lymph nodes of inguinal region and lower limb
Femoral
Groin
Popliteal
Tibial

196.6 Intrapelvic lymph nodes
Hypogastric
Iliac
Obturator
Parametrial

196.8 Lymph nodes of multiple sites

196.9 Site unspecified
Lymph nodes NOS

4th **197 Secondary malignant neoplasm of respiratory and digestive systems**
EXCLUDES *lymph node metastasis (196.0-196.9)*
AHA: M-J, '85, 3

197.0 Lung
Bronchus
AHA: 2Q, '99, 9

197.1 Mediastinum

197.2 Pleura
AHA: 4Q, '03, 110; 4Q, '89, 11

197.3 Other respiratory organs
Trachea

197.4 Small intestine, including duodenum

197.5 Large intestine and rectum

197.6 Retroperitoneum and peritoneum
AHA: ►2Q, '04, 4;◄ 4Q, '89, 11

197.7 Liver, specified as secondary

197.8 Other digestive organs and spleen
AHA: 2Q, '97, 3; 2Q, '92, 3

4th **198 Secondary malignant neoplasm of other specified sites**
EXCLUDES *lymph node metastasis (196.0-196.9)*
AHA: M-J, '85, 3

198.0 Kidney

198.1 Other urinary organs

198.2 Skin
Skin of breast

198.3 Brain and spinal cord
AHA: 3Q, '99, 7

198.4 Other parts of nervous system
Meninges (cerebral) (spinal)
AHA: J-F, '87, 7

198.5 Bone and bone marrow
AHA: 4Q, '03, 110; 3Q, '99, 5; 2Q, '92, 3; 1Q, '91, 16; 4Q, '89, 10

198.6 Ovary ♀

198.7 Adrenal gland
Suprarenal gland

5th **198.8 Other specified sites**

198.81 Breast
EXCLUDES *skin of breast (198.2)*

198.82 Genital organs

198.89 Other
EXCLUDES *retroperitoneal lymph nodes (196.2)*
AHA: 2Q, '97, 4

4th **199 Malignant neoplasm without specification of site**

199.0 Disseminated
Carcinomatosis
Generalized:
cancer
malignancy
Multiple cancer
} unspecified site (primary) (secondary)
AHA: 4Q, '89, 10

199.1 Other
Cancer
Carcinoma
Malignancy
} unspecified site (primary) (secondary)

MALIGNANT NEOPLASM OF LYMPHATIC AND HEMATOPOIETIC TISSUE (200-208)

EXCLUDES *secondary neoplasm of:*
bone marrow (198.5)
spleen (197.8)
secondary and unspecified neoplasm of lymph nodes (196.0-196.9)

The following fifth-digit subclassification is for use with categories 200-202:
0 unspecified site, extranodal and solid organ sites
1 lymph nodes of head, face, and neck
2 intrathoracic lymph nodes
3 intra-abdominal lymph nodes
4 lymph nodes of axilla and upper limb
5 lymph nodes of inguinal region and lower limb
6 intrapelvic lymph nodes
7 spleen
8 lymph nodes of multiple sites

4th **200 Lymphosarcoma and reticulosarcoma**
AHA: 2Q, '92, 3; N-D, '86, 5

5th **200.0 Reticulosarcoma**
Lymphoma (malignant):
histiocytic (diffuse):
nodular
pleomorphic cell type
reticulum cell type
Reticulum cell sarcoma:
NOS
pleomorphic cell type
AHA: For Code 200.03: 3Q, '01, 12

DEF: Malignant lymphoma of primarily histolytic cells; commonly originates in reticuloendothelium of lymph nodes.

4th 5th Additional Digit Required   Unspecified Code   Other Specified Code   Manifestation Code   ►◄ Revised Text   ● New Code   ▲ Revised Code Title

§ ✓5th **200.1 Lymphosarcoma**
Lymphoblastoma (diffuse)
Lymphoma (malignant):
lymphoblastic (diffuse)
lymphocytic (cell type) (diffuse)
lymphosarcoma type
Lymphosarcoma:
NOS
diffuse NOS
lymphoblastic (diffuse)
lymphocytic (diffuse)
prolymphocytic

EXCLUDES *lymphosarcoma:*
follicular or nodular (202.0)
mixed cell type (200.8)
lymphosarcoma cell leukemia (207.8)

DEF: Malignant lymphoma created from anaplastic lymphoid cells resembling lymphocytes or lymphoblasts.

§ ✓5th **200.2 Burkitt's tumor or lymphoma**
Malignant lymphoma, Burkitt's type
DEF: Large osteolytic lesion most common in jaw or as abdominal mass; usually found in central Africa but reported elsewhere.

§ ✓5th **200.8 Other named variants**
Lymphoma (malignant):
lymphoplasmacytoid type
mixed lymphocytic-histiocytic (diffuse)
Lymphosarcoma, mixed cell type (diffuse)
Reticulolymphosarcoma (diffuse)

✓4th **201 Hodgkin's disease**
AHA: 2Q, '92, 3; N-D, '86, 5
DEF: Painless, progressive enlargement of lymph nodes, spleen and general lymph tissue; symptoms include anorexia, lassitude, weight loss, fever, pruritis, night sweats, anemia.

§ ✓5th **201.0 Hodgkin's paragranuloma**

§ ✓5th **201.1 Hodgkin's granuloma**
AHA: 2Q, '99, 7

§ ✓5th **201.2 Hodgkin's sarcoma**

§ ✓5th **201.4 Lymphocytic-histiocytic predominance**

§ ✓5th **201.5 Nodular sclerosis**
Hodgkin's disease, nodular sclerosis:
NOS
cellular phase

§ ✓5th **201.6 Mixed cellularity**

§ ✓5th **201.7 Lymphocytic depletion**
Hodgkin's disease, lymphocytic depletion:
NOS
diffuse fibrosis
reticular type

§ ✓5th **201.9 Hodgkin's disease, unspecified**
Hodgkin's:
disease NOS
lymphoma NOS
Malignant:
lymphogranuloma
lymphogranulomatosis

✓4th **202 Other malignant neoplasms of lymphoid and histiocytic tissue**
AHA: 2Q, '92, 3; N-D, '86, 5

§ ✓5th **202.0 Nodular lymphoma**
Brill-Symmers disease
Lymphoma:
follicular (giant)
lymphocytic, nodular
Lymphosarcoma:
follicular (giant)
nodular
Reticulosarcoma, follicular or nodular
DEF: Lymphomatous cells clustered into nodules within the lymph node; usually occurs in older adults and may involve all nodes and possibly extranodal sites.

§ ✓5th **202.1 Mycosis fungoides**
AHA: 2Q, '92, 4
DEF: Type of cutaneous T-cell lymphoma; may evolve into generalized lymphoma; formerly thought to be of fungoid origin.

§ ✓5th **202.2 Sézary's disease**
AHA: 2Q, '99, 7
DEF: Type of cutaneous T-cell lymphoma with erythroderma, intense pruritus, peripheral lymphadenopathy, abnormal hyperchromatic mononuclear cells in skin, lymph nodes and peripheral blood.

§ ✓5th **202.3 Malignant histiocytosis**
Histiocytic medullary reticulosis
Malignant:
reticuloendotheliosis
reticulosis

§ ✓5th **202.4 Leukemic reticuloendotheliosis**
Hairy-cell leukemia
DEF: Chronic leukemia with large, mononuclear cells with "hairy" appearance in marrow, spleen, liver, blood.

§ ✓5th **202.5 Letterer-Siwe disease**
Acute:
differentiated progressive histiocytosis
histiocytosis X (progressive)
infantile reticuloendotheliosis
reticulosis of infancy

EXCLUDES *Hand-Schüller-Christian disease (277.89)*
histiocytosis (acute) (chronic) (277.89)
histiocytosis X (chronic) (277.89)

DEF: A recessive reticuloendotheliosis of early childhood, with a hemorrhagic tendency, eczema-like skin eruption, hepatosplenomegaly, including lymph node enlargement, and progressive anemia; it is often a fatal disease with no established cause.

§ ✓5th **202.6 Malignant mast cell tumors**
Malignant:
mastocytoma
mastocytosis
Mast cell sarcoma
Systemic tissue mast cell disease

EXCLUDES *mast cell leukemia (207.8)*

§ ✓5th **202.8 Other lymphomas**
Lymphoma (malignant):
NOS
diffuse

EXCLUDES *benign lymphoma (229.0)*

AHA: 2Q, '92, 4

§ ✓5th **202.9 Other and unspecified malignant neoplasms of lymphoid and histiocytic tissue**
Follicular dendritic cell sarcoma
Interdigitating dendritic cell sarcoma
Langerhans cell sarcom
Malignant neoplasm of bone marrow NOS

§ Requires fifth-digit. See beginning of section 200–208 for codes and definitions.

✓4th 203 Multiple myeloma and immunoproliferative neoplasms

The following fifth-digit subclassification is for use with category 203:
0 without mention of remission
1 in remission

✓5th 203.0 Multiple myeloma
Kahler's disease
Myelomatosis
EXCLUDES *solitary myeloma (238.6)*
AHA: 1Q, '96, 16; 4Q, '91, 26

✓5th 203.1 Plasma cell leukemia
Plasmacytic leukemia
AHA: 4Q, '90, 26; S-O, '86, 12

✓5th 203.8 Other immunoproliferative neoplasms
AHA: 4Q, '90, 26; S-O, '86, 12

✓4th 204 Lymphoid leukemia
INCLUDES leukemia:
lymphatic
lymphoblastic
lymphocytic
lymphogenous
AHA: 3Q, '93, 4

The following fifth-digit subclassification is for use with category 204:
0 without mention of remission
1 in remission

✓5th 204.0 Acute
EXCLUDES *acute exacerbation of chronic lymphoid leukemia (204.1)*
AHA: 3Q, '99, 6

✓5th 204.1 Chronic

✓5th 204.2 Subacute

✓5th 204.8 Other lymphoid leukemia
Aleukemic leukemia:
lymphatic
lymphocytic
Aleukemic leukemia:
lymphoid

✓5th 204.9 Unspecified lymphoid leukemia

✓4th 205 Myeloid leukemia
INCLUDES leukemia:
granulocytic
myeloblastic
myelocytic
myelogenous
myelomonocytic
myelosclerotic
myelosis
AHA: 3Q, '93, 3; 4Q, '91, 26; 4Q, '90, 3; M-J, '85, 18

The following fifth-digit subclassification is for use with category 205:
0 without mention of remission
1 in remission

✓5th 205.0 Acute
Acute promyelocytic leukemia
EXCLUDES *acute exacerbation of chronic myeloid leukemia (205.1)*

✓5th 205.1 Chronic
Eosinophilic leukemia
Neutrophilic leukemia
AHA: 1Q, 00, 6; J-A, '85, 13

✓5th 205.2 Subacute

✓5th 205.3 Myeloid sarcoma
Chloroma
Granulocytic sarcoma

✓5th 205.8 Other myeloid leukemia
Aleukemic leukemia:
granulocytic
myelogenous
Aleukemic leukemia:
myeloid
Aleukemic myelosis

✓5th 205.9 Unspecified myeloid leukemia

✓4th 206 Monocytic leukemia
INCLUDES leukemia:
histiocytic
monoblastic
monocytoid

The following fifth-digit subclassification is for use with category 206:
0 without mention of remission
1 in remission

✓5th 206.0 Acute
EXCLUDES *acute exacerbation of chronic monocytic leukemia (206.1)*

✓5th 206.1 Chronic

✓5th 206.2 Subacute

✓5th 206.8 Other monocytic leukemia
Aleukemic:
monocytic leukemia
Aleukemic:
monocytoid leukemia

✓5th 206.9 Unspecified monocytic leukemia

✓4th 207 Other specified leukemia
EXCLUDES *leukemic reticuloendotheliosis (202.4)*
plasma cell leukemia (203.1)

The following fifth-digit subclassification is for use with category 207:
0 without mention of remission
1 in remission

✓5th 207.0 Acute erythremia and erythroleukemia
Acute erythremic myelosis
Di Guglielmo's disease
Erythremic myelosis

DEF: Erythremia: polycythemia vera.

DEF: Erythroleukemia: a malignant blood dyscrasia (a myeloproliferative disorder).

✓5th 207.1 Chronic erythremia
Heilmeyer-Schöner disease

✓5th 207.2 Megakaryocytic leukemia
Megakaryocytic myelosis
Thrombocytic leukemia

✓5th 207.8 Other specified leukemia
Lymphosarcoma cell leukemia

✓4th 208 Leukemia of unspecified cell type

The following fifth-digit subclassification is for use with category 208:
0 without mention of remission
1 in remission

✓5th 208.0 Acute
Acute leukemia NOS
Blast cell leukemia
Stem cell leukemia
EXCLUDES *acute exacerbation of chronic unspecified leukemia (208.1)*

✓5th 208.1 Chronic
Chronic leukemia NOS

✓5th 208.2 Subacute
Subacute leukemia NOS

✓5th 208.8 Other leukemia of unspecified cell type

✓5th 208.9 Unspecified leukemia
Leukemia NOS

BENIGN NEOPLASMS (210-229)

✓4th **210 Benign neoplasm of lip, oral cavity, and pharynx**

EXCLUDES *cyst (of):*
jaw (526.0-526.2,526.89)
oral soft tissue (528.4)
radicular (522.8)

210.0 Lip
Frenulum labii
Lip (inner aspect) (mucosa) (vermilion border)
EXCLUDES *labial commissure (210.4)*
skin of lip (216.0)

210.1 Tongue
Lingual tonsil

210.2 Major salivary glands
Gland:
parotid
sublingual
submandibular
EXCLUDES *benign neoplasms of minor salivary glands:*
NOS (210.4)
buccal mucosa (210.4)
lips (210.0)
palate (hard) (soft) (210.4)
tongue (210.1)
tonsil, palatine (210.5)

210.3 Floor of mouth

210.4 Other and unspecified parts of mouth
Gingiva
Gum (upper) (lower)
Labial commissure
Oral cavity NOS
Oral mucosa
Palate (hard) (soft)
Uvula
EXCLUDES *benign odontogenic neoplasms of bone (213.0-213.1)*
developmental odontogenic cysts (526.0)
mucosa of lips (210.0)
nasopharyngeal [posterior] [superior] surface of soft palate (210.7)

210.5 Tonsil
Tonsil (faucial) (palatine)
EXCLUDES *lingual tonsil (210.1)*
pharyngeal tonsil (210.7)
tonsillar:
fossa (210.6)
pillars (210.6)

210.6 Other parts of oropharynx
Branchial cleft or vestiges
Epiglottis, anterior aspect
Fauces NOS
Mesopharynx NOS
Tonsillar:
fossa
pillars
Vallecula
EXCLUDES *epiglottis:*
NOS (212.1)
suprahyoid portion (212.1)

210.7 Nasopharynx
Adenoid tissue
Lymphadenoid tissue
Pharyngeal tonsil
Posterior nasal septum

210.8 Hypopharynx
Arytenoid fold
Laryngopharynx
Postcricoidregion
Pyriform fossa

210.9 Pharynx, unspecified
Throat NOS

✓4th **211 Benign neoplasm of other parts of digestive system**

211.0 Esophagus

211.1 Stomach
Body, Cardia, Fundus } of stomach
Cardiac orifice
Pylorus

211.2 Duodenum, jejunum, and ileum
Small intestine NOS
EXCLUDES *ampulla of Vater (211.5)*
ileocecal valve (211.3)

211.3 Colon
Appendix
Cecum
Ileocecal valve
Large intestine NOS
EXCLUDES *rectosigmoid junction (211.4)*
AHA: 4Q, '01, 56

211.4 Rectum and anal canal
Anal canal or sphincter
Anus NOS
Rectosigmoid junction
EXCLUDES *anus:*
margin (216.5)
skin (216.5)
perianal skin (216.5)

211.5 Liver and biliary passages
Ampulla of Vater
Common bile duct
Cystic duct
Gallbladder
Hepatic duct
Sphincter of Oddi

211.6 Pancreas, except islets of Langerhans

211.7 Islets of Langerhans
Islet cell tumor
Use additional code to identify any functional activity

211.8 Retroperitoneum and peritoneum
Mesentery
Mesocolon
Omentum
Retroperitoneal tissue

211.9 Other and unspecified site
Alimentary tract NOS
Digestive system NOS
Gastrointestinal tract NOS
Intestinal tract NOS
Intestine NOS
Spleen, not elsewhere classified

✓4th **212 Benign neoplasm of respiratory and intrathoracic organs**

212.0 Nasal cavities, middle ear, and accessory sinuses
Cartilage of nose
Eustachian tube
Nares
Septum of nose
Sinus:
ethmoidal
frontal
maxillary
sphenoidal
EXCLUDES *auditory canal (external) (216.2)*
bone of:
ear (213.0)
nose [turbinates] (213.0)
cartilage of ear (215.0)
ear (external) (skin) (216.2)
nose NOS (229.8)
skin (216.3)
olfactory bulb (225.1)
polyp of:
accessory sinus (471.8)
ear (385.30-385.35)
nasal cavity (471.0)
posterior margin of septum and choanae (210.7)

212.1 Larynx
Cartilage:
arytenoid
cricoid
cuneiform
thyroid
Epiglottis (suprahyoid portion) NOS
Glottis
Vocal cords (false) (true)
EXCLUDES *epiglottis, anterior aspect (210.6)*
polyp of vocal cord or larynx (478.4)

212.2 Trachea

212.3 Bronchus and lung
Carina
Hilus of lung

212.4 Pleura

212.5 Mediastinum

212.6 Thymus

212.7 Heart

EXCLUDES *great vessels (215.4)*

212.8 Other specified sites

212.9 Site unspecified

Respiratory organ NOS
Upper respiratory tract NOS

EXCLUDES *intrathoracic NOS (229.8)*
thoracic NOS (229.8)

✓4th 213 Benign neoplasm of bone and articular cartilage

INCLUDES cartilage (articular) (joint)
periosteum

EXCLUDES *cartilage of:*
ear (215.0)
eyelid (215.0)
larynx (212.1)
nose (212.0)
exostosis NOS (726.91)
synovia (215.0-215.9)

213.0 Bones of skull and face

EXCLUDES *lower jaw bone (213.1)*

213.1 Lower jaw bone

213.2 Vertebral column, excluding sacrum and coccyx

213.3 Ribs, sternum, and clavicle

213.4 Scapula and long bones of upper limb

213.5 Short bones of upper limb

213.6 Pelvic bones, sacrum, and coccyx

213.7 Long bones of lower limb

213.8 Short bones of lower limb

213.9 Bone and articular cartilage, site unspecified

✓4th 214 Lipoma

INCLUDES angiolipoma
fibrolipoma
hibernoma
lipoma (fetal) (infiltrating) (intramuscular)
myelolipoma
myxolipoma

DEF: Benign tumor frequently composed of mature fat cells; may occasionally be composed of fetal fat cells.

214.0 Skin and subcutaneous tissue of face

214.1 Other skin and subcutaneous tissue

214.2 Intrathoracic organs

214.3 Intra-abdominal organs

214.4 Spermatic cord ♂

214.8 Other specified sites

AHA: 3Q, '94, 7

214.9 Lipoma, unspecified site

✓4th 215 Other benign neoplasm of connective and other soft tissue

INCLUDES blood vessel
bursa
fascia
ligament
muscle
peripheral, sympathetic, and parasympathetic nerves and ganglia
synovia
tendon (sheath)

EXCLUDES *cartilage:*
articular (213.0-213.9)
larynx (212.1)
nose (212.0)
connective tissue of:
breast (217)
internal organ, except lipoma and hemangioma—code to benign neoplasm of the site
lipoma (214.0-214.9)

215.0 Head, face, and neck

215.2 Upper limb, including shoulder

215.3 Lower limb, including hip

215.4 Thorax

EXCLUDES *heart (212.7)*
mediastinum (212.5)
thymus (212.6)

215.5 Abdomen

Abdominal wall
Hypochondrium

215.6 Pelvis

Buttock
Groin
Inguinal region
Perineum

EXCLUDES *uterine:*
leiomyoma (218.0-218.9)
ligament, any (221.0)

215.7 Trunk, unspecified

Back NOS
Flank NOS

215.8 Other specified sites

215.9 Site unspecified

✓4th 216 Benign neoplasm of skin

INCLUDES blue nevus
dermatofibroma
hydrocystoma
pigmented nevus
syringoadenoma
syringoma

EXCLUDES *skin of genital organs (221.0-222.9)*

AHA: 1Q, '00, 21

216.0 Skin of lip

EXCLUDES *vermilion border of lip (210.0)*

216.1 Eyelid, including canthus

EXCLUDES *cartilage of eyelid (215.0)*

216.2 Ear and external auditory canal

Auricle (ear)
Auricular canal, external
External meatus
Pinna

EXCLUDES *cartilage of ear (215.0)*

216.3 Skin of other and unspecified parts of face

Cheek, external
Eyebrow
Nose, external
Temple

216.4 Scalp and skin of neck

AHA: 3Q, '91, 12

216.5 Skin of trunk, except scrotum

Axillary fold
Perianal skin
Skin of:
abdominal wall
anus
back
breast
Skin of:
buttock
chest wall
groin
perineum
Umbilicus

EXCLUDES *anal canal (211.4)*
anus NOS (211.4)
skin of scrotum (222.4)

216.6 Skin of upper limb, including shoulder

216.7 Skin of lower limb, including hip

216.8 Other specified sites of skin

216.9 Skin, site unspecified

217 Benign neoplasm of breast

Breast (male) (female):
connective tissue
glandular tissue
Breast (male) (female):
soft parts

EXCLUDES *adenofibrosis (610.2)*
benign cyst of breast (610.0)
fibrocystic disease (610.1)
skin of breast (216.5)

AHA: 1Q, '00, 4

✓4th **218 Uterine leiomyoma**

INCLUDES fibroid (bleeding) (uterine)
uterine:
fibromyoma
myoma

DEF: Benign tumor primarily derived from uterine smooth muscle tissue; may contain fibrous, fatty, or epithelial tissue; also called uterine fibroid or myoma.

218.0 Submucous leiomyoma of uterus ♀

218.1 Intramural leiomyoma of uterus ♀
Interstitial leiomyoma of uterus

218.2 Subserous leiomyoma of uterus ♀

218.9 Leiomyoma of uterus, unspecified ♀
AHA: 1Q, '03, 4

✓4th **219 Other benign neoplasm of uterus**

219.0 Cervix uteri ♀

219.1 Corpus uteri ♀
Endometrium
Fundus
Myometrium

219.8 Other specified parts of uterus ♀

219.9 Uterus, part unspecified ♀

220 Benign neoplasm of ovary ♀
Use additional code to identify any functional activity (256.0-256.1)

EXCLUDES *cyst:*
corpus albicans (620.2)
corpus luteum (620.1)
endometrial (617.1)
follicular (atretic) (620.0)
graafian follicle (620.0)
ovarian NOS (620.2)
retention (620.2)

✓4th **221 Benign neoplasm of other female genital organs**

INCLUDES adenomatous polyp
benign teratoma

EXCLUDES *cyst:*
epoophoron (752.11)
fimbrial (752.11)
Gartner's duct (752.11)
parovarian (752.11)

221.0 Fallopian tube and uterine ligaments ♀
Oviduct
Parametruim
Uterine ligament (broad) (round) (uterosacral)
Uterine tube

221.1 Vagina ♀

221.2 Vulva ♀
Clitoris
External female genitalia NOS
Greater vestibular [Bartholin's] gland
Labia (majora) (minora)
Pudendum

EXCLUDES *Bartholin's (duct) (gland) cyst (616.2)*

Eyeball

221.8 Other specified sites of female genital organs ♀

221.9 Female genital organ, site unspecified ♀
Female genitourinary tract NOS

✓4th **222 Benign neoplasm of male genital organs**

222.0 Testis ♂
Use additional code to identify any functional activity

222.1 Penis ♂
Corpus cavernosum
Glans penis
Prepuce

222.2 Prostate ♂

EXCLUDES *adenomatous hyperplasia of prostate (600.20-600.21)*
prostatic:
adenoma (600.20-600.21)
enlargement (600.00-600.01)
hypertrophy (600.00-600.01)

222.3 Epididymis ♂

222.4 Scrotum ♂
Skin of scrotum

222.8 Other specified sites of male genital organs ♂
Seminal vesicle
Spermatic cord

222.9 Male genital organ, site unspecified ♂
Male genitourinary tract NOS

✓4th **223 Benign neoplasm of kidney and other urinary organs**

223.0 Kidney, except pelvis
Kidney NOS

EXCLUDES *renal:*
calyces (223.1)
pelvis (223.1)

223.1 Renal pelvis

223.2 Ureter

EXCLUDES *ureteric orifice of bladder (223.3)*

223.3 Bladder

✓5th **223.8 Other specified sites of urinary organs**

223.81 Urethra

EXCLUDES *urethral orifice of bladder (223.3)*

223.89 Other
Paraurethral glands

223.9 Urinary organ, site unspecified
Urinary system NOS

✓4th **224 Benign neoplasm of eye**

EXCLUDES *cartilage of eyelid (215.0)*
eyelid (skin) (216.1)
optic nerve (225.1)
orbital bone (213.0)

224.0 Eyeball, except conjunctiva, cornea, retina, and choroid
Ciliary body
Iris
Sclera
Uveal tract

224.1 Orbit

EXCLUDES *bone of orbit (213.0)*

224.2 Lacrimal gland

224.3 Conjunctiva

224.4 Cornea

224.5 Retina

EXCLUDES *hemangioma of retina (228.03)*

224.6 Choroid

224.7 Lacrimal duct
Lacrimal sac
Nasolacrimal duct

224.8 Other specified parts of eye

224.9 Eye, part unspecified

N Newborn Age: 0 P Pediatric Age: 0-17 M Maternity Age: 12-55 A Adult Age: 15-124 MSP Medicare Secondary Payer

✓4th **225 Benign neoplasm of brain and other parts of nervous system**

EXCLUDES *hemangioma (228.02)*
neurofibromatosis (237.7)
peripheral, sympathetic, and parasympathetic nerves and ganglia (215.0-215.9)
retrobulbar (224.1)

225.0 Brain

225.1 Cranial nerves
AHA: ►4Q, '04, 113◄

225.2 Cerebral meninges
Meninges NOS
Meningioma (cerebral)

225.3 Spinal cord
Cauda equina

225.4 Spinal meninges
Spinal meningioma

225.8 Other specified sites of nervous system

225.9 Nervous system, part unspecified
Nervous system (central) NOS
EXCLUDES *meninges NOS (225.2)*

226 Benign neoplasm of thyroid glands
Use additional code to identify any functional activity

✓4th **227 Benign neoplasm of other endocrine glands and related structures**
Use additional code to identify any functional activity
EXCLUDES *ovary (220)*
pancreas (211.6)
testis (222.0)

227.0 Adrenal gland
Suprarenal gland

227.1 Parathyroid gland

227.3 Pituitary gland and craniopharyngeal duct (pouch)
Craniobuccal pouch
Hypophysis
Rathke's pouch
Sella turcica

227.4 Pineal gland
Pineal body

227.5 Carotid body

227.6 Aortic body and other paraganglia
Coccygeal body
Glomus jugulare
Para-aortic body
AHA: N-D, '84, 17

227.8 Other

227.9 Endocrine gland, site unspecified

✓4th **228 Hemangioma and lymphangioma, any site**

INCLUDES angioma (benign) (cavernous) (congenital) NOS
cavernous nevus
glomus tumor
hemangioma (benign) (congenital)

EXCLUDES *benign neoplasm of spleen, except hemangioma and lymphangioma (211.9)*
glomus jugulare (227.6)
nevus:
NOS (216.0-216.9)
blue or pigmented (216.0-216.9)
vascular (757.32)

AHA: 1Q, '00, 21

✓5th **228.0 Hemangioma, any site**
AHA: J-F, '85, 19

DEF: A common benign tumor usually occurring in infancy; composed of newly formed blood vessels due to malformation of angioblastic tissue.

228.00 Of unspecified site

228.01 Of skin and subcutaneous tissue

228.02 Of intracranial structures

228.03 Of retina

228.04 Of intra-abdominal structures
Peritoneum
Retroperitoneal tissue

228.09 Of other sites
Systemic angiomatosis
AHA: 3Q, '91, 20

228.1 Lymphangioma, any site
Congenital lymphangioma
Lymphatic nevus

✓4th **229 Benign neoplasm of other and unspecified sites**

229.0 Lymph nodes
EXCLUDES *lymphangioma (228.1)*

229.8 Other specified sites
Intrathoracic NOS
Thoracic NOS

229.9 Site unspecified

CARCINOMA IN SITU (230-234)

INCLUDES Bowen's disease
erythroplasia
Queyrat's erythroplasia

EXCLUDES *leukoplakia—see Alphabetic Index*

DEF: A neoplastic type; with tumor cells confined to epithelium of origin; without further invasion.

✓4th **230 Carcinoma in situ of digestive organs**

230.0 Lip, oral cavity, and pharynx
Gingiva
Hypopharynx
Mouth [any part]
Nasopharynx
Oropharynx
Salivary gland or duct
Tongue

EXCLUDES *aryepiglottic fold or interarytenoid fold, laryngeal aspect (231.0)*
epiglottis:
NOS (231.0)
suprahyoid portion (231.0)
skin of lip (232.0)

230.1 Esophagus

230.2 Stomach
Body, Cardia, Fundus } of stomach
Cardiac orifice
Pylorus

230.3 Colon
Appendix
Cecum
Ileocecal valve
Large intestine NOS
EXCLUDES *rectosigmoid junction (230.4)*

230.4 Rectum
Rectosigmoid junction

230.5 Anal canal
Anal sphincter

230.6 Anus, unspecified
EXCLUDES *anus:*
margin (232.5)
skin (232.5)
perianal skin (232.5)

230.7 Other and unspecified parts of intestine
Duodenum
Ileum
Jejunum
Small intestine NOS
EXCLUDES *ampulla of Vater (230.8)*

230.8 Liver and biliary system
Ampulla of Vater
Common bile duct
Cystic duct
Gallbladder
Hepatic duct
Sphincter of Oddi

230.9 Other and unspecified digestive organs
Digestive organ NOS
Gastrointestinal tract NOS
Pancreas
Spleen

✓4th **231 Carcinoma in situ of respiratory system**

231.0 Larynx

Cartilage:
- arytenoid
- cricoid
- cuneiform
- thyroid

Epiglottis:
- NOS
- posterior surface
- suprahyoid portion

Vocal cords (false) (true)

EXCLUDES *aryepiglottic fold or interarytenoid fold:*
NOS (230.0)
hypopharyngeal aspect (230.0)
marginal zone (230.0)

231.1 Trachea

231.2 Bronchus and lung

Carina
Hilus of lung

231.8 Other specified parts of respiratory system

Accessory sinuses
Middle ear
Nasal cavities
Pleura

EXCLUDES *ear (external) (skin) (232.2)*
nose NOS (234.8)
skin (232.3)

231.9 Respiratory system, part unspecified

Respiratory organ NOS

✓4th **232 Carcinoma in situ of skin**

INCLUDES pigment cells

232.0 Skin of lip

EXCLUDES *vermilion border of lip (230.0)*

232.1 Eyelid, including canthus

232.2 Ear and external auditory canal

232.3 Skin of other and unspecified parts of face

232.4 Scalp and skin of neck

232.5 Skin of trunk, except scrotum

Anus, margin
Axillary fold
Perianal skin
Skin of:
- abdominal wall
- anus
- back
- breast
- buttock
- chest wall
- groin
- perineum

Umbilicus

EXCLUDES *anal canal (230.5)*
anus NOS (230.6)
skin of genital organs (233.3, 233.5-233.6)

232.6 Skin of upper limb, including shoulder

232.7 Skin of lower limb, including hip

232.8 Other specified sites of skin

232.9 Skin, site unspecified

✓4th **233 Carcinoma in situ of breast and genitourinary system**

233.0 Breast

EXCLUDES *Paget's disease (174.0-174.9)*
skin of breast (232.5)

233.1 Cervix uteri ♀

Cervical intraepithelial neoplasia III [CIN III]
Severe dysplasia of cervix

EXCLUDES *cervical intraepithelial neoplasia II [CIN II] (622.12)*
cytologic evidence of malignancy without histologic confirmation (795.04)
high grade squamous intraepithelial lesion (HGSIL) (795.04)
moderate dysplasia of cervix (622.12)

AHA: 3Q, '92, 7; 3Q, '92, 8; 1Q, '91, 11

233.2 Other and unspecified parts of uterus ♀

233.3 Other and unspecified female genital organs ♀

233.4 Prostate ♂

233.5 Penis ♂

233.6 Other and unspecified male genital organs ♂

233.7 Bladder

233.9 Other and unspecified urinary organs

✓4th **234 Carcinoma in situ of other and unspecified sites**

234.0 Eye

EXCLUDES *cartilage of eyelid (234.8)*
eyelid (skin) (232.1)
optic nerve (234.8)
orbital bone (234.8)

234.8 Other specified sites

Endocrine gland [any]

234.9 Site unspecified

Carcinoma in situ NOS

NEOPLASMS OF UNCERTAIN BEHAVIOR (235-238)

Note: Categories 235–238 classify by site certain histomorphologically well-defined neoplasms, the subsequent behavior of which cannot be predicted from the present appearance.

✓4th **235 Neoplasm of uncertain behavior of digestive and respiratory systems**

235.0 Major salivary glands

Gland:
- parotid
- sublingual
- submandibular

EXCLUDES *minor salivary glands (235.1)*

235.1 Lip, oral cavity, and pharynx

Gingiva
Hypopharynx
Minor salivary glands
Mouth
Nasopharynx
Oropharynx
Tongue

EXCLUDES *aryepiglottic fold or interarytenoid fold, laryngeal aspect (235.6)*
epiglottis:
NOS (235.6)
suprahyoid portion (235.6)
skin of lip (238.2)

235.2 Stomach, intestines, and rectum

235.3 Liver and biliary passages

Ampulla of Vater
Bile ducts [any]
Gallbladder
Liver

235.4 Retroperitoneum and peritoneum

235.5 Other and unspecified digestive organs

Anal:
- canal
- sphincter

Anus NOS
Esophagus
Pancreas
Spleen

EXCLUDES *anus:*
margin (238.2)
skin (238.2)
perianal skin (238.2)

235.6 Larynx

EXCLUDES *aryepiglottic fold or interarytenoid fold:*
NOS (235.1)
hypopharyngeal aspect (235.1)
marginal zone (235.1)

235.7 Trachea, bronchus, and lung

235.8 Pleura, thymus, and mediastinum

235.9 Other and unspecified respiratory organs

Accessory sinuses
Middle ear
Nasal cavities
Respiratory organ NOS

EXCLUDES *ear (external) (skin) (238.2)*
nose (238.8)
skin (238.2)

✓4th **236 Neoplasm of uncertain behavior of genitourinary organs**

236.0 Uterus ♀

236.1 Placenta ♀

Chorioadenoma (destruens)
Invasive mole
Malignant hydatid(iform) mole

236.2 Ovary ♀

Use additional code to identify any functional activity

236.3 Other and unspecified female genital organs ♀

236.4 Testis ♂
Use additional code to identify any functional activity

236.5 Prostate ♂

236.6 Other and unspecified male genital organs ♂

236.7 Bladder

✓5th **236.9 Other and unspecified urinary organs**

236.90 Urinary organ, unspecified

236.91 Kidney and ureter

236.99 Other

✓4th **237 Neoplasm of uncertain behavior of endocrine glands and nervous system**

237.0 Pituitary gland and craniopharyngeal duct
Use additional code to identify any functional activity

237.1 Pineal gland

237.2 Adrenal gland
Suprarenal gland
Use additional code to identify any functional activity

237.3 Paraganglia
Aortic body
Carotid body
Coccygeal body
Glomus jugulare
AHA: N-D, '84, 17

237.4 Other and unspecified endocrine glands
Parathyroid gland
Thyroid gland

237.5 Brain and spinal cord

237.6 Meninges
Meninges:
NOS
cerebral
spinal

✓5th **237.7 Neurofibromatosis**
von Recklinghausen's disease
DEF: An inherited condition with developmental changes in the nervous system, muscles, bones and skin; multiple soft tumors (neurofibromas) distributed over the entire body.

237.70 Neurofibromatosis, unspecified

237.71 Neurofibromatosis, type 1 [von Recklinghausen's disease]

237.72 Neurofibromatosis, type 2 [acoustic neurofibromatosis]
DEF: Inherited condition with cutaneous lesions, benign tumors of peripheral nerves and bilateral 8th nerve masses.

237.9 Other and unspecified parts of nervous system
Cranial nerves
EXCLUDES *peripheral, sympathetic, and parasympathetic nerves and ganglia (238.1)*

✓4th **238 Neoplasm of uncertain behavior of other and unspecified sites and tissues**

238.0 Bone and articular cartilage
EXCLUDES *cartilage:*
ear (238.1)
eyelid (238.1)
larynx (235.6)
nose (235.9)
synovia (238.1)
AHA: 4Q, '04, 128

238.1 Connective and other soft tissue
Peripheral, sympathetic, and parasympathetic nerves and ganglia
EXCLUDES *cartilage (of):*
articular (238.0)
larynx (235.6)
nose (235.9)
connective tissue of breast (238.3)

238.2 Skin
EXCLUDES *anus NOS (235.5)*
skin of genital organs (236.3, 236.6)
vermilion border of lip (235.1)

238.3 Breast
EXCLUDES *skin of breast (238.2)*

238.4 Polycythemia vera
DEF: Abnormal proliferation of all bone marrow elements, increased red cell mass and total blood volume; unknown etiology, frequently associated with splenomegaly, leukocytosis, and thrombocythemia.

238.5 Histiocytic and mast cells
Mast cell tumor NOS
Mastocytoma NOS

238.6 Plasma cells
Plasmacytoma NOS
Solitary myeloma

238.7 Other lymphatic and hematopoietic tissues
Disease:
lymphoproliferative (chronic) NOS
myeloproliferative (chronic) NOS
Idiopathic thrombocythemia
Megakaryocytic myelosclerosis
Myelodysplastic syndrome
Myelosclerosis with myeloid metaplasia
Panmyelosis (acute)
▶Refractory anemia◀
EXCLUDES *myelofibrosis (289.89)*
myelosclerosis NOS (289.89)
myelosis:
NOS (205.9)
megakaryocytic (207.2)
AHA: 3Q, '01, 13; 1Q, '97, 5; 2Q, '89, 8

238.8 Other specified sites
Eye
Heart
EXCLUDES *eyelid (skin) (238.2)*
cartilage (238.1)

238.9 Site unspecified

NEOPLASMS OF UNSPECIFIED NATURE (239)

✓4th **239 Neoplasms of unspecified nature**
Note: Category 239 classifies by site neoplasms of unspecified morphology and behavior. The term "mass,"unless otherwise stated, is not to be regarded as a neoplastic growth.
INCLUDES "growth" NOS
neoplasm NOS
new growth NOS
tumor NOS

239.0 Digestive system
EXCLUDES *anus:*
margin (239.2)
skin (239.2)
perianal skin (239.2)

239.1 Respiratory system

239.2 Bone, soft tissue, and skin
EXCLUDES *anal canal (239.0)*
anus NOS (239.0)
bone marrow (202.9)
cartilage:
larynx (239.1)
nose (239.1)
connective tissue of breast (239.3)
skin of genital organs (239.5)
vermilion border of lip (239.0)

239.3 Breast
EXCLUDES *skin of breast (239.2)*

239.4 Bladder

239.5 Other genitourinary organs

239.6 Brain

EXCLUDES *cerebral meninges (239.7)*
cranial nerves (239.7)

239.7 Endocrine glands and other parts of nervous system

EXCLUDES *peripheral, sympathetic, and parasympathetic nerves and ganglia (239.2)*

239.8 Other specified sites

EXCLUDES *eyelid (skin) (239.2)*
cartilage (239.2)
great vessels (239.2)
optic nerve (239.7)

239.9 Site unspecified

Endocrine System

Hypothalamus
Pituitary (Hypophysis) gland
Thyroid gland
Thymus gland
Pineal gland
Parathyoid glands
Adrenal (Suprarenal) glands
Pancreas
Ovaries
Testes

3. ENDOCRINE, NUTRITIONAL AND METABOLIC DISEASES, AND IMMUNITY DISORDERS (240-279)

EXCLUDES *endocrine and metabolic disturbances specific to the fetus and newborn (775.0-775.9)*

Note: All neoplasms, whether functionally active or not, are classified in Chapter 2. Codes in Chapter 3 (i.e., 242.8, 246.0, 251-253, 255-259) may be used to identify such functional activity associated with any neoplasm, or by ectopic endocrine tissue.

DISORDERS OF THYROID GLAND (240-246)

✓4th **240 Simple and unspecified goiter**

DEF: An enlarged thyroid gland often caused by an inadequate dietary intake of iodine.

240.0 Goiter, specified as simple

Any condition classifiable to 240.9, specified as simple

240.9 Goiter, unspecified

Enlargement of thyroid
Goiter or struma:
- NOS
- diffuse colloid
- endemic

Goiter or struma:
- hyperplastic
- nontoxic (diffuse)
- parenchymatous
- sporadic

EXCLUDES *congenital (dyshormonogenic) goiter (246.1)*

✓4th **241 Nontoxic nodular goiter**

EXCLUDES *adenoma of thyroid (226)*
cystadenoma of thyroid (226)

241.0 Nontoxic uninodular goiter

Thyroid nodule
Uninodular goiter (nontoxic)

DEF: Enlarged thyroid, commonly due to decreased thyroid production, with single nodule; no clinical hypothyroidism.

241.1 Nontoxic multinodular goiter

Multinodular goiter (nontoxic)

DEF: Enlarged thyroid, commonly due to decreased thyroid production with multiple nodules; no clinical hypothyroidism.

241.9 Unspecified nontoxic nodular goiter

Adenomatous goiter
Nodular goiter (nontoxic) NOS
Struma nodosa (simplex)

✓4th **242 Thyrotoxicosis with or without goiter**

EXCLUDES *neonatal thyrotoxicosis (775.3)*

The following fifth-digit subclassification is for use with category 242:

0 without mention of thyrotoxic crisis or storm
1 with mention of thyrotoxic crisis or storm

DEF: A condition caused by excess quantities of thyroid hormones being introduced into the tissues.

✓5th **242.0 Toxic diffuse goiter**

Basedow's disease
Exophthalmic or toxic goiter NOS
Graves' disease
Primary thyroid hyperplasia

DEF: Diffuse thyroid enlargement accompanied by hyperthyroidism, bulging eyes, and dermopathy.

✓5th **242.1 Toxic uninodular goiter**

Thyroid nodule } toxic or with hyperthyroidism
Uninodular goiter } toxic or with hyperthyroidism

DEF: Symptomatic hyperthyroidism with a single nodule on the enlarged thyroid gland. Abrupt onset of symptoms; including extreme nervousness, insomnia, weight loss, tremors, and psychosis or coma.

✓5th **242.2 Toxic multinodular goiter**

Secondary thyroid hyperplasia

DEF: Symptomatic hyperthyroidism with multiple nodules on the enlarged thyroid gland. Abrupt onset of symptoms; including extreme nervousness, insomnia, weight loss, tremors, and psychosis or coma.

✓5th **242.3 Toxic nodular goiter, unspecified**

Adenomatous goiter } toxic or with hyperthyroidism
Nodular goiter } toxic or with hyperthyroidism
Struma nodosa } toxic or with hyperthyroidism

Any condition classifiable to 241.9 specified as toxic or with hyperthyroidism

✓5th **242.4 Thyrotoxicosis from ectopic thyroid nodule**

✓5th **242.8 Thyrotoxicosis of other specified origin**

Overproduction of thyroid-stimulating hormone [TSH]
Thyrotoxicosis:
- factitia from ingestion of excessive thyroid material

Use additional E code to identify cause, if drug-induced

✓5th **242.9 Thyrotoxicosis without mention of goiter or other cause**

Hyperthyroidism NOS
Thyrotoxicosis NOS

243 Congenital hypothyroidism

Congenital thyroid insufficiency
Cretinism (athyrotic) (endemic)
Use additional code to identify associated mental retardation

EXCLUDES *congenital (dyshormonogenic) goiter (246.1)*

DEF: Underproduction of thyroid hormone present from birth.

✓4th **244 Acquired hypothyroidism**

INCLUDES athyroidism (acquired)
hypothyroidism (acquired)
myxedema (adult) (juvenile)
thyroid (gland) insufficiency (acquired)

244.0 Postsurgical hypothyroidism

DEF: Underproduction of thyroid hormone due to surgical removal of all or part of the thyroid gland.

244.1 Other postablative hypothyroidism

Hypothyroidism following therapy, such as irradiation

244.2 Iodine hypothyroidism

Hypothyroidism resulting from administration or ingestion of iodide
Use additional E code to identify drug

244.3 Other iatrogenic hypothyroidism

Hypothyroidism resulting from:
- P-aminosalicylic acid [PAS]
- Phenylbutazone
- Resorcinol

Iatrogenic hypothyroidism NOS
Use additional E code to identify drug

244.8 Other specified acquired hypothyroidism
Secondary hypothyroidism NEC
AHA: J-A, '85, 9

244.9 Unspecified hypothyroidism
Hypothyroidism } primary or NOS
Myxedema } primary or NOS
AHA: 3Q, '99, 19; 4Q, '96, 29

✓4th **245 Thyroiditis**

245.0 Acute thyroiditis
Abscess of thyroid
Thyroiditis:
- nonsuppurative, acute
- pyogenic
- suppurative

Use additional code to identify organism
DEF: Inflamed thyroid caused by infection, with abscess and liquid puris.

245.1 Subacute thyroiditis
Thyroiditis:
- de Quervain's
- giant cell
- granulomatous
- viral

DEF: Inflammation of the thyroid, characterized by fever and painful enlargement of the thyroid gland, with granulomas in the gland.

245.2 Chronic lymphocytic thyroiditis
Hashimoto's disease
Struma lymphomatosa
Thyroiditis:
- autoimmune
- lymphocytic (chronic)

DEF: Autoimmune disease of thyroid; lymphocytes infiltrate the gland and thyroid antibodies are produced; women more often affected.

245.3 Chronic fibrous thyroiditis
Struma fibrosa
Thyroiditis:
- invasive (fibrous)
- ligneous
- Riedel's

DEF: Persistent fibrosing inflammation of thyroid with adhesions to nearby structures; rare condition.

245.4 Iatrogenic thyroiditis
Use additional code to identify cause
DEF: Thyroiditis resulting from treatment or intervention by physician or in a patient intervention setting.

245.8 Other and unspecified chronic thyroiditis
Chronic thyroiditis: NOS
Chronic thyroiditis: nonspecific

245.9 Thyroiditis, unspecified
Thyroiditis NOS

✓4th **246 Other disorders of thyroid**

246.0 Disorders of thyrocalcitonin secretion
Hypersecretion of calcitonin or thyrocalcitonin

246.1 Dyshormonogenic goiter
Congenital (dyshormonogenic) goiter
Goiter due to enzyme defect in synthesis of thyroid hormone
Goitrous cretinism (sporadic)

246.2 Cyst of thyroid
EXCLUDES *cystadenoma of thyroid (226)*

246.3 Hemorrhage and infarction of thyroid

246.8 Other specified disorders of thyroid
Abnormality of thyroid-binding globulin
Atrophy of thyroid
Hyper-TBG-nemia
Hypo-TBG-nemia

246.9 Unspecified disorder of thyroid

DISEASES OF OTHER ENDOCRINE GLANDS (250-259)

✓4th **250 Diabetes mellitus**
EXCLUDES *gestational diabetes (648.8)*
hyperglycemia NOS (790.6)
neonatal diabetes mellitus (775.1)
nonclinical diabetes (790.29

The following fifth-digit subclassification is for use with category 250:

0 type II or unspecified type, not stated as uncontrolled
Fifth-digit 0 is for use for type II patients, even if the patient requires insulin
Use additional code, if applicable, for associated long-term (current) insulin use V58.67

1 type I [juvenile type], not stated as uncontrolled

2 type II or unspecified type, uncontrolled
Fifth-digit 2 is for use for type II patients, even if the patient requires insulin
Use additional code, if applicable, for associated long-term (current) insulin use V58.67

3 type I [juvenile type], uncontrolled

AHA: 4Q, '04, 56; 2Q, '04, 17; 2Q, '02, 13; 2Q,'01, 16; 2Q,'98, 15; 4Q, '97, 32; 2Q, '97, 14; 3Q, '96, 5; 4Q, '93, 19; 2Q, '92, 5; 3Q, '91, 3; 2Q, '90, 22; N-D, '85, 11

DEF: Diabetes mellitus: Inability to metabolize carbohydrates, proteins, and fats with insufficient secretion of insulin. Symptoms may be unremarkable, with long-term complications, involving kidneys, nerves, blood vessels, and eyes.

DEF: Uncontrolled diabetes: A nonspecific term indicating that the current treatment regimen does not keep the blood sugar level of a patient within acceptable levels.

✓5th **250.0 Diabetes mellitus without mention of complication**
Diabetes mellitus without mention of complication or manifestation classifiable to 250.1-250.9
Diabetes (mellitus) NOS
AHA: 4Q, '97, 32; 3Q, '91, 3, 12; N-D, '85, 11; **For code 250.00:** ▶1Q, '05, 15;◀ 4Q, '04, 55; 4Q, '03, 105, 108; 2Q, '03, 16; 1Q, '02, 7, 11; **For code: 250.01:** 4Q, '04, 55; 4Q, '03, 110; 2Q, '03, 6; **For code: 250.02:** 1Q, '03, 5

✓5th **250.1 Diabetes with ketoacidosis**
Diabetic:
- acidosis } without mention of coma
- ketosis } without mention of coma

AHA: 3Q, '91, 6; **For code 250.11:** 4Q, '03, 82
DEF: Diabetic hyperglycemic crisis causing ketone presence in body fluids.

✓5th **250.2 Diabetes with hyperosmolarity**
Hyperosmolar (nonketotic) coma
AHA: 4Q, '93, 19; 3Q, '91, 7

✓5th **250.3 Diabetes with other coma**
Diabetic coma (with ketoacidosis)
Diabetic hypoglycemic coma
Insulin coma NOS
EXCLUDES *diabetes with hyperosmolar coma (250.2)*
AHA: 3Q, '91, 7,12
DEF: Coma (not hyperosmolar) caused by hyperglycemia or hypoglycemia as complication of diabetes.

✓5th **250.4 Diabetes with renal manifestations**
Use additional code to identify manifestation, as:
▶chronic kidney disease (585.1-585.9)◀
diabetic:
- nephropathy NOS (583.81)
- nephrosis (581.81)

intercapillary glomerulosclerosis (581.81)
Kimmelstiel-Wilson syndrome (581.81)
AHA: 3Q, '91, 8,12; S-O, '87, 9; S-O, '84, 3; **For code: 250.40:** 1Q, '03, 20

N Newborn Age: 0 | P Pediatric Age: 0-17 | M Maternity Age: 12-55 | A Adult Age: 15-124 | MSP Medicare Secondary Payer

✓5th **250.5 Diabetes with ophthalmic manifestations**
Use additional code to identify manifestation, as:
diabetic:
blindness (369.00-369.9)
cataract (366.41)
glaucoma (365.44)
▶macular edema (362.07)◀
retinal edema ▶(362.07)◀
retinopathy ▶(362.01-362.07)◀
AHA: 3Q, '91, 8; S-O, '85, 11

✓5th **250.6 Diabetes with neurological manifestations**
Use additional code to identify manifestation, as:
diabetic:
amyotrophy (358.1)
gastroparalysis (536.3)
gastroparesis (536.3)
mononeuropathy (354.0-355.9)
neurogenic arthropathy (713.5)
peripheral autonomic neuropathy (337.1)
polyneuropathy (357.2)
AHA: 2Q, '93, 6; 2Q, '92, 15; 3Q, '91, 9; N-D, '84, 9; **For code 250.60:** 4Q, '03, 105; **For code 250.61:** 2Q, '04, 7

✓5th **250.7 Diabetes with peripheral circulatory disorders**
Use additional code to identify manifestation, as:
diabetic:
gangrene (785.4)
peripheral angiopathy (443.81)
DEF: Blood vessel damage or disease, usually in the feet, legs, or hands, as a complication of diabetes.
AHA 1Q, '96, 10; 3Q, '94, 5; 2Q, '94, 17; 3Q, '91, 10, 12; 3Q, '90, 15; **For code 250.70:** 1Q, '04, 14

✓5th **250.8 Diabetes with other specified manifestations**
Diabetic hypoglycemia
Hypoglycemic shock
Use additional code to identify manifestation, as:
any associated ulceration (707.10-707.9)
diabetic bone changes (731.8)
Use additional E code to identify cause, if drug-induced
AHA: 4Q, '00, 44; 4Q, '97, 43; 2Q, '97, 16; 4Q, '93, 20; 3Q, '91, 10; **For code 250.80:** 1Q, '04, 14

✓5th **250.9 Diabetes with unspecified complication**
AHA: 2Q, '92, 15; 3Q, '91, 7, 12

✓4th **251 Other disorders of pancreatic internal secretion**

251.0 Hypoglycemic coma
Iatrogenic hyperinsulinism
Non-diabetic insulin coma
Use additional E code to identify cause, if drug-induced
EXCLUDES *hypoglycemic coma in diabetes mellitus (250.3)*
AHA: M-A, '85, 8
DEF: Coma induced by low blood sugar in non-diabetic patient.

251.1 Other specified hypoglycemia
Hyperinsulinism:
NOS
ectopic
functional
Hyperplasia of pancreatic islet beta cells NOS
EXCLUDES *hypoglycemia:*
in diabetes mellitus (250.8)
in infant of diabetic mother (775.0)
neonatal hypoglycemia (775.6)
hypoglycemic coma (251.0)
Use additional E code to identify cause, if drug-induced.
DEF: Excessive production of insulin by the pancreas; associated with obesity and insulin-producing tumors.
AHA: 1Q, '03, 10

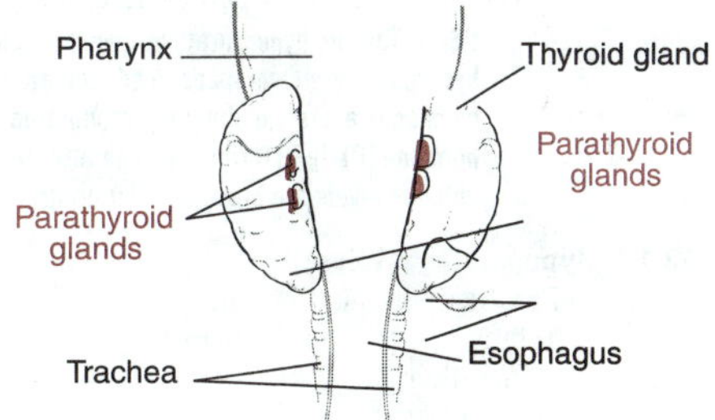

251.2 Hypoglycemia, unspecified
Hypoglycemia:
NOS
reactive
spontaneous
EXCLUDES *hypoglycemia:*
with coma (251.0)
in diabetes mellitus (250.8)
leucine-induced (270.3)
AHA: M-A, '85, 8

251.3 Postsurgical hypoinsulinemia
Hypoinsulinemia following complete or partial pancreatectomy
Postpancreatectomy hyperglycemia
AHA: 3Q, '91, 6

251.4 Abnormality of secretion of glucagon
Hyperplasia of pancreatic islet alpha cells with glucagon excess
DEF: Production malfunction of a pancreatic hormone secreted by cells of the islets of Langerhans

251.5 Abnormality of secretion of gastrin
Hyperplasia of pancreatic alpha cells with gastrin excess
Zollinger-Ellison syndrome

251.8 Other specified disorders of pancreatic internal secretion
AHA: 2Q, '98, 15; 3Q, '91, 6

251.9 Unspecified disorder of pancreatic internal secretion
Islet cell hyperplasia NOS

✓4th **252 Disorders of parathyroid gland**

✓5th **252.0 Hyperparathyroidism**
EXCLUDES *ectopic hyperparathyroidism (259.3)*
DEF: Abnormally high secretion of parathyroid hormones causing bone deterioration, reduced renal function, kidney stones.

252.00 Hyperparathyroidism, unspecified

252.01 Primary hyperparathyroidism
Hyperplasia of parathyroid
DEF: Parathyroid dysfunction commonly caused by hyperplasia of two or more glands; characteristic hypercalcemia and increased parathyroid hormone levels.

252.02 Secondary hyperparathyroidism, non-renal
EXCLUDES *secondary hyperparathyroidism (of renal origin) (588.81)*
AHA: 4Q, '04, 57-59
DEF: Underlying disease of nonrenal origin decreases blood levels of calcium causing the parathyroid to release increased levels of parathyroid hormone; parathyroid hormone levels return to normal once underlying condition is treated and blood calcium levels are normal.

252.08 Other hyperparathyroidism

Tertiary hyperparathyroidism

DEF: ▶Tertiary hyperparathyroidism: chronic secondary hyperparathyroidism leads to adenomatous parathyroid causing irreversible abnormal production of parathyroid hormone (PTH); PTH remains high after the serum calcium levels are brought under control.◀

252.1 Hypoparathyroidism

Parathyroiditis (autoimmune)
Tetany:
parathyroid
parathyroprival

EXCLUDES *pseudohypoparathyroidism (275.4)*
pseudopseudohypoparathyroidism (275.4)
tetany NOS (781.7)
transitory neonatal hypoparathyroidism (775.4)

DEF: Abnormally low secretion of parathyroid hormones which causes decreased calcium and increased phosphorus in the blood. Resulting in muscle cramps, tetany, urinary frequency and cataracts.

252.8 Other specified disorders of parathyroid gland

Cyst } of parathyroid gland
Hemorrhage } of parathyroid gland

252.9 Unspecified disorder of parathyroid gland

✓4th **253 Disorders of the pituitary gland and its hypothalamic control**

INCLUDES the listed conditions whether the disorder is in the pituitary or the hypothalamus

EXCLUDES *Cushing's syndrome (255.0)*

253.0 Acromegaly and gigantism

Overproduction of growth hormone

DEF: Acromegaly: chronic, beginning in middle age; caused by hypersecretion of the pituitary growth hormone; produces enlarged parts of skeleton, especially the nose, ears, jaws, fingers and toes.

DEF: Gigantism: pituitary gigantism caused by excess growth of short flat bones; men may grow 78 to 80 inches tall.

253.1 Other and unspecified anterior pituitary hyperfunction

Forbes-Albright syndrome

EXCLUDES *overproduction of:*
ACTH (255.3)
thyroid-stimulating hormone [TSH] (242.8)

AHA: J-A, '85, 9

DEF: Spontaneous galactorrhea-amenorrhea syndrome unrelated to pregnancy; usually related to presence of pituitary tumor.

253.2 Panhypopituitarism

Cachexia, pituitary
Necrosis of pituitary (postpartum)
Pituitary insufficiency NOS
Sheehan's syndrome
Simmonds' disease

EXCLUDES *iatrogenic hypopituitarism (253.7)*

DEF: Damage to or absence of pituitary gland leading to impaired sexual function, weight loss, fatigue, bradycardia, hypotension, pallor, depression, and impaired growth in children; called Simmonds' disease if cachexia is prominent.

253.3 Pituitary dwarfism

Isolated deficiency of (human) growth hormone [HGH]
Lorain-Levi dwarfism

DEF: Dwarfism with infantile physical characteristics due to abnormally low secretion of growth hormone and gonadotropin deficiency.

253.4 Other anterior pituitary disorders

Isolated or partial deficiency of an anterior pituitary hormone, other than growth hormone
Prolactin deficiency

AHA: J-A, '85, 9

253.5 Diabetes insipidus

Vasopressin deficiency

EXCLUDES *nephrogenic diabetes insipidus (588.1)*

DEF: Metabolic disorder causing insufficient antidiuretic hormone release; symptoms include frequent urination, thirst, ravenous hunger, loss of weight, fatigue.

253.6 Other disorders of neurohypophysis

Syndrome of inappropriate secretion of antidiuretic hormone [ADH]

EXCLUDES *ectopic antidiuretic hormone secretion (259.3)*

253.7 Iatrogenic pituitary disorders

Hypopituitarism:
hormone-induced
hypophysectomy-induced
Hypopituitarism:
postablative
radiotherapy-induced

Use additional E code to identify cause

DEF: Pituitary dysfunction that results from drug therapy, radiation therapy, or surgery, causing mild to severe symptoms.

253.8 Other disorders of the pituitary and other syndromes of diencephalohypophyseal origin

Abscess of pituitary
Adiposogenital dystrophy
Cyst of Rathke's pouch
Fröhlich's syndrome

EXCLUDES *craniopharyngioma (237.0)*

253.9 Unspecified

Dyspituitarism

✓4th **254 Diseases of thymus gland**

EXCLUDES *aplasia or dysplasia with immunodeficiency (279.2)*
hypoplasia with immunodeficiency (279.2)
myasthenia gravis (358.00-358.01)

254.0 Persistent hyperplasia of thymus

Hypertrophy of thymus

DEF: Continued abnormal growth of the twin lymphoid lobes that produce T lymphocytes.

254.1 Abscess of thymus

254.8 Other specified diseases of thymus gland

Atrophy } of thymus
Cyst } of thymus

EXCLUDES *thymoma (212.6)*

254.9 Unspecified disease of thymus gland

✓4th **255 Disorders of adrenal glands**

INCLUDES the listed conditions whether the basic disorder is in the adrenals or is pituitary-induced

255.0 Cushing's syndrome

Adrenal hyperplasia due to excess ACTH
Cushing's syndrome:
NOS
iatrogenic
idiopathic
pituitary-dependent
Ectopic ACTH syndrome
Iatrogenic syndrome of excess cortisol
Overproduction of cortisol
Use additional E code to identify cause, if drug-induced

EXCLUDES *congenital adrenal hyperplasia (255.2)*

DEF: Due to adrenal cortisol oversecretion or glucocorticoid medications; may cause fatty tissue of the face, neck and body, osteoporosis and curvature of spine, hypertension, diabetes mellitus, female genitourinary problems, male impotence, degeneration of muscle tissues, weakness.

✓5th **255.1 Hyperaldosteronism**

AHA: 4Q, '03, 48

DEF: Oversecretion of aldosterone causing fluid retention, hypertension.

255.10 Primary aldosteronism

Aldosteronism NOS
Hyperaldosteronism, unspecified

EXCLUDES *Conn's syndrome (255.12)*

255.11 Glucocorticoid-remediable aldosteronism
Familial aldosteronism type I
EXCLUDES *Conn's syndrome (255.12)*
DEF: A rare autosomal dominant familial form of primary aldosteronism in which the secretion of aldosterone is under the influence of adrenocortiotrophic hormone (ACTH) rather than the renin-angiotensin mechanism; characterized by moderate hypersecretion of aldosterone and suppressed plasma renin activity rapidly reversed by administration of glucosteroids; symptoms include hypertension and mild hypokalemia.

255.12 Conn's syndrome
DEF: A type of primary aldosteronism caused by an adenoma of the glomerulosa cells in the adrenal cortex; presence of hypertension.

255.13 Bartter's syndrome
DEF: A cluster of symptoms caused by a defect in the ability of the kidney to reabsorb potassium; signs include alkalosis (hypokalemic alkalosis), increased aldosterone, increased plasma renin, and normal blood pressure; symptoms include muscle cramping, weakness, constipation, frequency of urination, and failure to grow; also known as urinary potassium wasting or juxtaglomerular cell hyperplasia.

255.14 Other secondary aldosteronism

255.2 Adrenogenital disorders
Achard-Thiers syndrome
Adrenogenital syndromes, virilizing or feminizing, whether acquired or associated with congenital adrenal hyperplasia consequent on inborn enzyme defects in hormone synthesis
Congenital adrenal hyperplasia
Female adrenal pseudohermaphroditism
Male:
  macrogenitosomia praecox
  sexual precocity with adrenal hyperplasia
Virilization (female) (suprarenal)
EXCLUDES *adrenal hyperplasia due to excess ACTH (255.0)*
isosexual virilization (256.4)

255.3 Other corticoadrenal overactivity
Acquired benign adrenal androgenic overactivity
Overproduction of ACTH

255.4 Corticoadrenal insufficiency
Addisonian crisis
Addison's disease NOS
Adrenal:
  atrophy (autoimmune)
  calcification
  crisis
  hemorrhage
  infarction
  insufficiency NOS
EXCLUDES *tuberculous Addison's disease (017.6)*
DEF: Underproduction of adrenal hormones causing low blood pressure.

255.5 Other adrenal hypofunction
Adrenal medullary insufficiency
EXCLUDES *Waterhouse-Friderichsen syndrome (meningococcal) (036.3)*

255.6 Medulloadrenal hyperfunction
Catecholamine secretion by pheochromocytoma

255.8 Other specified disorders of adrenal glands
Abnormality of cortisol-binding globulin

255.9 Unspecified disorder of adrenal glands

✓4th **256 Ovarian dysfunction**
AHA: 4Q, '00, 51

256.0 Hyperestrogenism ♀
DEF: Excess secretion of estrogen by the ovaries; characterized by ovaries containing multiple follicular cysts filled with serous fluid.

256.1 Other ovarian hyperfunction ♀
Hypersecretion of ovarian androgens
AHA: 3Q, '95, 15

256.2 Postablative ovarian failure ♀
Ovarian failure:
  iatrogenic
  postirradiation
  postsurgical
Use additional code for states associated with artificial menopause (627.4)
EXCLUDES *acquired absence of ovary (V45.77)*
asymptomatic age-related (natural) postmenopausal status (V49.81)
AHA: 2Q, '02, 12
DEF: Failed ovarian function after medical or surgical intervention.

✓5th **256.3 Other ovarian failure**
Use additional code for states associated with natural menopause (627.2)
EXCLUDES *asymptomatic age-related (natural) postmenopausal status (V49.81)*
AHA: 4Q, '01, 41

256.31 Premature menopause A ♀
DEF: Permanent cessation of ovarian function before the age of 40 occurring naturally of unknown cause.

256.39 Other ovarian failure ♀
Delayed menarche
Ovarian hypofunction
Primary ovarian failure NOS

256.4 Polycystic ovaries ♀
Isosexual virilization
Stein-Leventhal syndrome
DEF: Multiple serous filled cysts of ovary; symptoms of infertility, hirsutism, oligomenorrhea or amenorrhea.

256.8 Other ovarian dysfunction ♀

256.9 Unspecified ovarian dysfunction ♀

✓4th **257 Testicular dysfunction**

257.0 Testicular hyperfunction ♂
Hypersecretion of testicular hormones

257.1 Postablative testicular hypofunction ♂
Testicular hypofunction:
  iatrogenic
  postirradiation
  postsurgical

257.2 Other testicular hypofunction
Defective biosynthesis of testicular androgen
Eunuchoidism:
  NOS
  hypogonadotropic
Failure:
  Leydig's cell, adult
  seminiferous tubule, adult
Testicular hypogonadism
EXCLUDES *azoospermia (606.0)*

257.8 Other testicular dysfunction
EXCLUDES ▶ *androgen insensitivity syndrome (259.5)*◀

257.9 Unspecified testicular dysfunction ♂

✓4th **258 Polyglandular dysfunction and related disorders**

258.0 Polyglandular activity in multiple endocrine adenomatosis
Wermer's syndrome
DEF: Wermer's syndrome: A rare hereditary condition characterized by the presence of adenomas or hyperplasia in more than one endocrine gland causing premature aging.

258.1 Other combinations of endocrine dysfunction
Lloyd's syndrome
Schmidt's syndrome

258.8 Other specified polyglandular dysfunction

258.9 Polyglandular dysfunction, unspecified

✓4th 259 Other endocrine disorders

259.0 Delay in sexual development and puberty, not elsewhere classified
Delayed puberty

259.1 Precocious sexual development and puberty, not elsewhere classified P
Sexual precocity: NOS, constitutional
Sexual precocity: cryptogenic, idiopathic

259.2 Carcinoid syndrome
Hormone secretion by carcinoid tumors
DEF: Presence of carcinoid tumors that spread to liver; characterized by cyanotic flushing of skin, diarrhea, bronchospasm, acquired tricuspid and pulmonary stenosis, sudden drops in blood pressure, edema, ascites.

259.3 Ectopic hormone secretion, not elsewhere classified
Ectopic:
antidiuretic hormone secretion [ADH]
hyperparathyroidism
EXCLUDES *ectopic ACTH syndrome (255.0)*
AHA: N-D, '85, 4

259.4 Dwarfism, not elsewhere classified
Dwarfism:
NOS
constitutional
EXCLUDES *dwarfism:*
achondroplastic (756.4)
intrauterine (759.7)
nutritional (263.2)
pituitary (253.3)
renal (588.0)
progeria (259.8)

● **259.5 Androgen insensitivity syndrome**
Partial androgen insensitivity
Reifenstein syndrome

259.8 Other specified endocrine disorders
Pineal gland dysfunction
Progeria
Werner's syndrome

259.9 Unspecified endocrine disorder
Disturbance: endocrine NOS, hormone NOS
Infantilism NOS

NUTRITIONAL DEFICIENCIES (260-269)

EXCLUDES *deficiency anemias (280.0-281.9)*

260 Kwashiorkor
Nutritional edema with dyspigmentation of skin and hair
DEF: Syndrome, particularly of children; excessive carbohydrate with inadequate protein intake, inhibited growth potential, anomalies in skin and hair pigmentation, edema and liver disease.

261 Nutritional marasmus
Nutritional atrophy
Severe calorie deficiency
Severe malnutrition NOS
DEF: Protein-calorie malabsorption or malnutrition of children; characterized by tissue wasting, dehydration, and subcutaneous fat depletion; may occur with infectious disease; also called infantile atrophy.

262 Other severe, protein-calorie malnutrition
Nutritional edema without mention of dyspigmentation of skin and hair
AHA: 4Q, '92, 24; J-A, '85, 12

✓4th 263 Other and unspecified protein-calorie malnutrition
AHA: 4Q, '92, 24

263.0 Malnutrition of moderate degree
AHA: J-A, '85, 1
DEF: Malnutrition characterized by biochemical changes in electrolytes, lipids, blood plasma.

263.1 Malnutrition of mild degree
AHA: J-A, '85, 1

263.2 Arrested development following protein-calorie malnutrition
Nutritional dwarfism
Physical retardation due to malnutrition

263.8 Other protein-calorie malnutrition

263.9 Unspecified protein-calorie malnutrition
Dystrophy due to malnutrition
Malnutrition (calorie) NOS
EXCLUDES *nutritional deficiency NOS (269.9)*
AHA: 4Q, '03, 109; N-D, '84, 19

✓4th 264 Vitamin A deficiency

264.0 With conjunctival xerosis
DEF: Vitamin A deficiency with conjunctival dryness.

264.1 With conjunctival xerosis and Bitot's spot
Bitot's spot in the young child
DEF: Vitamin A deficiency with conjunctival dryness, superficial spots of keratinized epithelium.

264.2 With corneal xerosis
DEF: Vitamin A deficiency with corneal dryness.

264.3 With corneal ulceration and xerosis
DEF: Vitamin A deficiency with corneal dryness, epithelial ulceration.

264.4 With keratomalacia
DEF: Vitamin A deficiency creating corneal dryness; progresses to corneal insensitivity, softness, necrosis; usually bilateral.

264.5 With night blindness
DEF: Vitamin A deficiency causing vision failure in dim light.

264.6 With xerophthalmic scars of cornea
DEF: Vitamin A deficiency with corneal scars from dryness.

264.7 Other ocular manifestations of vitamin A deficiency
Xerophthalmia due to vitamin A deficiency

264.8 Other manifestations of vitamin A deficiency
Follicular keratosis } due to vitamin A deficiency
Xeroderma }

264.9 Unspecified vitamin A deficiency
Hypovitaminosis A NOS

✓4th 265 Thiamine and niacin deficiency states

265.0 Beriberi
DEF: Inadequate vitamin B_1 (thiamine) intake, affects heart and peripheral nerves; individual may become edematous and develop cardiac disease due to the excess fluid; alcoholics and people with a diet of excessive polished rice prone to the disease.

265.1 Other and unspecified manifestations of thiamine deficiency
Other vitamin B_1 deficiency states

265.2 Pellagra
Deficiency: niacin (-tryptophan), nicotinamide, nicotinic acid
Deficiency: vitamin PP
Pellagra (alcoholic)
DEF: Niacin deficiency causing dermatitis, inflammation of mucous membranes, diarrhea, and psychic disturbances.

✓4th 266 Deficiency of B-complex components

266.0 Ariboflavinosis
Riboflavin [vitamin B_2] deficiency
AHA: S-O, '86, 10
DEF: Vitamin B_2 (riboflavin) deficiency marked by swollen lips and tongue fissures, corneal vascularization, scaling lesions, and anemia.

266.1 Vitamin B_6 deficiency
Deficiency:
pyridoxal
pyridoxamine
Deficiency:
pyridoxine
Vitamin B_6 deficiency syndrome
EXCLUDES *vitamin B_6-responsive sideroblastic anemia (285.0)*
DEF: Vitamin B_6 deficiency causing skin, lip, and tongue disturbances, peripheral neuropathy; and convulsions in infants.

266.2 Other B-complex deficiencies
Deficiency:
cyanocobalamin
folic acid
Deficiency:
vitamin B_{12}
EXCLUDES *combined system disease with anemia (281.0-281.1)*
deficiency anemias (281.0-281.9)
subacute degeneration of spinal cord with anemia (281.0-281.1)

266.9 Unspecified vitamin B deficiency

267 Ascorbic acid deficiency
Deficiency of vitamin C
Scurvy
EXCLUDES *scorbutic anemia (281.8)*
DEF: Vitamin C deficiency causing swollen gums, myalgia, weight loss, and weakness.

✓4th **268 Vitamin D deficiency**
EXCLUDES *vitamin D-resistant:*
osteomalacia (275.3)
rickets (275.3)

268.0 Rickets, active
EXCLUDES *celiac rickets (579.0)*
renal rickets (588.0)
DEF: Inadequate vitamin D intake, usually in pediatrics, that affects bones most involved with muscular action; may cause nodules on ends and sides of bones; delayed closure of fontanels in infants; symptoms may include muscle soreness, and profuse sweating.

268.1 Rickets, late effect
Any condition specified as due to rickets and stated to be a late effect or sequela of rickets
Use additional code to identify the nature of late effect
DEF: Distorted or demineralized bones as a result of vitamin D deficiency.

268.2 Osteomalacia, unspecified
DEF: Softening of bones due to decrease in calcium; marked by pain, tenderness, muscular weakness, anorexia, and weight loss.

268.9 Unspecified vitamin D deficiency
Avitaminosis D

✓4th **269 Other nutritional deficiencies**

269.0 Deficiency of vitamin K
EXCLUDES *deficiency of coagulation factor due to vitamin K deficiency (286.7)*
vitamin K deficiency of newborn (776.0)

269.1 Deficiency of other vitamins
Deficiency:
vitamin E
Deficiency:
vitamin P

269.2 Unspecified vitamin deficiency
Multiple vitamin deficiency NOS

269.3 Mineral deficiency, not elsewhere classified
Deficiency:
calcium, dietary
Deficiency:
iodine
EXCLUDES *deficiency:*
calcium NOS (275.4)
potassium (276.8)
sodium (276.1)

269.8 Other nutritional deficiency
EXCLUDES *adult failure to thrive (783.7)*
failure to thrive in childhood (783.41)
feeding problems (783.3)
newborn (779.3)

269.9 Unspecified nutritional deficiency

OTHER METABOLIC AND IMMUNITY DISORDERS (270-279)

Use additional code to identify any associated mental retardation

✓4th **270 Disorders of amino-acid transport and metabolism**
EXCLUDES *abnormal findings without manifest disease (790.0-796.9)*
disorders of purine and pyrimidine metabolism (277.1-277.2)
gout (274.0-274.9)

270.0 Disturbances of amino-acid transport
Cystinosis
Cystinuria
Fanconi (-de Toni) (-Debré) syndrome
Glycinuria (renal)
Hartnup disease

270.1 Phenylketonuria [PKU]
Hyperphenylalaninemia
DEF: Inherited metabolic condition causing excess phenylpyruvic and other acids in urine; results in mental retardation, neurological manifestations, including spasticity and tremors, light pigmentation, eczema, and mousy odor.

270.2 Other disturbances of aromatic amino-acid metabolism
Albinism
Alkaptonuria
Alkaptonuric ochronosis
Disturbances of metabolism of tyrosine and tryptophan
Homogentisic acid defects
Hydroxykynureninuria
Hypertyrosinemia
Indicanuria
Kynureninase defects
Oasthouse urine disease
Ochronosis
Tyrosinosis
Tyrosinuria
Waardenburg syndrome
EXCLUDES *vitamin B_6-deficiency syndrome (266.1)*
AHA: 3Q, '99, 20

270.3 Disturbances of branched-chain amino-acid metabolism
Disturbances of metabolism of leucine, isoleucine, and valine
Hypervalinemia
Intermittent branched-chain ketonuria
Leucine-induced hypoglycemia
Leucinosis
Maple syrup urine disease
AHA: 3Q, '00, 8

270.4 Disturbances of sulphur-bearing amino-acid metabolism
Cystathioninemia
Cystathioninuria
Disturbances of metabolism of methionine, homocystine, and cystathionine
Homocystinuria
Hypermethioninemia
Methioninemia
AHA: 1Q, '04, 6

270.5 Disturbances of histidine metabolism
Carnosinemia
Histidinemia
Hyperhistidinemia
Imidazole aminoaciduria

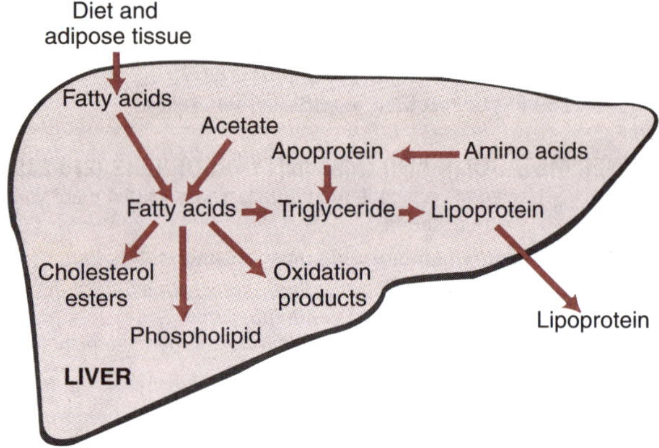

270.6 Disorders of urea cycle metabolism
Argininosuccinic aciduria
Citrullinemia
Disorders of metabolism of ornithine, citrulline, argininosuccinic acid, arginine, and ammonia
Hyperammonemia
Hyperomithinemia

270.7 Other disturbances of straight-chain amino-acid metabolism
Glucoglycinuria
Glycinemia (with methyl-malonic acidemia)
Hyperglycinemia
Hyperlysinemia
Other disturbances of metabolism of glycine, threonine, serine, glutamine, and lysine
Pipecolic acidemia
Saccharopinuria

AHA: 3Q, '00, 8

270.8 Other specified disorders of amino-acid metabolism
Alaninemia
Ethanolaminuria
Glycoprolinuria
Hydroxyprolinemia
Hyperprolinemia
Iminoacidopathy
Prolinemia
Prolinuria
Sarcosinemia

270.9 Unspecified disorder of amino-acid metabolism

✓4th **271 Disorders of carbohydrate transport and metabolism**

EXCLUDES *abnormality of secretion of glucagon (251.4)*
diabetes mellitus (250.0-250.9)
hypoglycemia NOS (251.2)
mucopolysaccharidosis (277.5)

271.0 Glycogenosis
Amylopectinosis
Glucose-6-phosphatase deficiency
Glycogen storage disease
McArdle's disease
Pompe's disease
von Gierke's disease

AHA: 1Q, '98, 5

DEF: Excess glycogen storage; rare inherited trait affects liver, kidneys; causes various symptoms depending on type, though often weakness, and muscle cramps.

271.1 Galactosemia
Galactose-1-phosphate uridyl transferase deficiency
Galactosuria

DEF: Any of three genetic disorders due to defective galactose metabolism; symptoms include failure to thrive in infancy, jaundice, liver and spleen damage, cataracts, and mental retardation.

271.2 Hereditary fructose intolerance
Essential benign fructosuria
Fructosemia

DEF: Chromosome recessive disorder of carbohydrate metabolism; in infants, occurs after dietary sugar introduced; characterized by enlarged spleen, yellowish cast to skin, and progressive inability to thrive.

271.3 Intestinal disaccharidase deficiencies and disaccharide malabsorption
Intolerance or malabsorption (congenital) (of):
- glucose-galactose
- lactose
- sucrose-isomaltose

271.4 Renal glycosuria
Renal diabetes

DEF: Persistent abnormal levels of glucose in urine, with normal blood glucose levels; caused by failure of the renal tubules to reabsorb glucose.

271.8 Other specified disorders of carbohydrate transport and metabolism
Essential benign pentosuria
Fucosidosis
Glycolic aciduria
Hyperoxaluria (primary)
Mannosidosis
Oxalosis
Xylosuria
Xylulosuria

271.9 Unspecified disorder of carbohydrate transport and metabolism

✓4th **272 Disorders of lipoid metabolism**

EXCLUDES *localized cerebral lipidoses (330.1)*

272.0 Pure hypercholesterolemia
Familial hypercholesterolemia
Fredrickson Type IIa hyperlipoproteinemia
Hyperbetalipoproteinemia
Hyperlipidemia, Group A
Low-density-lipoid-type [LDL] hyperlipoproteinemia

272.1 Pure hyperglyceridemia
Endogenous hyperglyceridemia
Fredrickson Type IV hyperlipoproteinemia
Hyperlipidemia, Group B
Hyperprebetalipoproteinemia
Hypertriglyceridemia, essential
Very-low-density-lipoid-type [VLDL] hyperlipoproteinemia

272.2 Mixed hyperlipidemia
Broad- or floating-betalipoproteinemia
Fredrickson Type IIb or III hyperlipoproteinemia
Hypercholesterolemia with endogenous hyperglyceridemia
Hyperbetalipoproteinemia with prebetalipoproteinemia
Tubo-eruptive xanthoma
Xanthoma tuberosum

DEF: Elevated levels of lipoprotein, a complex of fats and proteins, in blood due to inherited metabolic disorder.

272.3 Hyperchylomicronemia
Bürger-Grütz syndrome
Fredrickson type I or V hyperlipoproteinemia
Hyperlipidemia, Group D
Mixed hyperglyceridemia

272.4 Other and unspecified hyperlipidemia
Alpha-lipoproteinemia
Combined hyperlipidemia
Hyperlipidemia NOS
Hyperlipoproteinemia NOS

AHA: ►1Q, '05, 17◄

DEF: Hyperlipoproteinemia: elevated levels of transient chylomicrons in the blood which are a form of lipoproteins which transport dietary cholesterol and triglycerides from the small intestine to the blood.

272.5 Lipoprotein deficiencies
Abetalipoproteinemia
Bassen-Kornzweig syndrome
High-density lipoid deficiency (familial)
Hypoalphalipoproteinemia
Hypobetalipoproteinemia
DEF: Abnormally low levels of lipoprotein, a complex of fats and protein, in the blood.

272.6 Lipodystrophy
Barraquer-Simons disease
Progressive lipodystrophy
Use additional E code to identify cause, if iatrogenic
EXCLUDES *intestinal lipodystrophy (040.2)*
DEF: Disturbance of fat metabolism resulting in loss of fatty tissue in some areas of the body.

272.7 Lipidoses
Chemically-induced lipidosis
Disease:
- Anderson's
- Fabry's
- Gaucher's
- I cell [mucolipidosis I]
- lipoid storage NOS
- Niemann-Pick
- pseudo-Hurler's or mucolipdosis III
- triglyceride storage, Type I or II
- Wolman's or triglyceride storage, Type III

Mucolipidosis II
Primary familial xanthomatosis
EXCLUDES *cerebral lipidoses (330.1)*
Tay-Sachs disease (330.1)
DEF: Lysosomal storage diseases marked by an abnormal amount of lipids in reticuloendothelial cells.

272.8 Other disorders of lipoid metabolism
Hoffa's disease or liposynovitis prepatellaris
Launois-Bensaude's lipomatosis
Lipoid dermatoarthritis

272.9 Unspecified disorder of lipoid metabolism

✓4th **273 Disorders of plasma protein metabolism**
EXCLUDES *agammaglobulinemia and hypogammaglobulinemia (279.0-279.2)*
coagulation defects (286.0-286.9)
hereditary hemolytic anemias (282.0-282.9)

273.0 Polyclonal hypergammaglobulinemia
Hypergammaglobulinemic purpura:
- benign primary
- Waldenström's

DEF: Elevated blood levels of gamma globulins, frequently found in patients with chronic infectious diseases.

273.1 Monoclonal paraproteinemia
Benign monoclonal hypergammaglobulinemia [BMH]
Monoclonal gammopathy:
- NOS
- associated with lymphoplasmacytic dyscrasias
- benign

Paraproteinemia:
- benign (familial)
- secondary to malignant or inflammatory disease

DEF: Elevated blood levels of macroglobulins (plasma globulins of high weight); characterized by malignant neoplasms of bone marrow, spleen, liver, or lymph nodes; symptoms include weakness, fatigue, bleeding disorders, and vision problems.

273.2 Other paraproteinemias
Cryoglobulinemic:
- purpura
- vasculitis

Mixed cryoglobulinemia

273.3 Macroglobulinemia
Macroglobulinemia (idiopathic) (primary)
Waldenström's macroglobulinemia

273.4 Alpha-1-antitrypsin deficiency
AAT deficiency
DEF: ▶Disorder of plasma protein metabolism that results in a deficiency of Alpha-1-antitrypsin, an acute-phase reactive protein, released into the blood in response to infection or injury to protect tissue against the harmful effect of enzymes.◀

273.8 Other disorders of plasma protein metabolism
Abnormality of transport protein
Bisalbuminemia
AHA: 2Q, '98, 11

273.9 Unspecified disorder of plasma protein metabolism

✓4th **274 Gout**
EXCLUDES *lead gout (984.0-984.9)*
AHA: 2Q, '95, 4
DEF: Purine and pyrimidine metabolic disorders; manifested by hyperuricemia and recurrent acute inflammatory arthritis; monosodium urate or monohydrate crystals may be deposited in and around the joints, leading to joint destruction, and severe crippling.

274.0 Gouty arthropathy

✓5th **274.1 Gouty nephropathy**

274.10 Gouty nephropathy, unspecified
AHA: N-D, '85, 15

274.11 Uric acid nephrolithiasis
DEF: Sodium urate stones in the kidney.

274.19 Other

✓5th **274.8 Gout with other specified manifestations**

274.81 Gouty tophi of ear
DEF: Chalky sodium urate deposit in the ear due to gout; produces chronic inflammation of external ear.

274.82 Gouty tophi of other sites
Gouty tophi of heart

274.89 Other
Use additional code to identify manifestations, as:
gouty:
- iritis (364.11)
- neuritis (357.4)

274.9 Gout, unspecified

✓4th **275 Disorders of mineral metabolism**
EXCLUDES *abnormal findings without manifest disease (790.0-796.9)*

275.0 Disorders of iron metabolism
Bronzed diabetes
Hemochromatosis
Pigmentary cirrhosis (of liver)
EXCLUDES *anemia:*
- *iron deficiency (280.0-280.9)*
- *sideroblastic (285.0)*

AHA: 2Q, '97, 11

275.1 Disorders of copper metabolism
Hepatolenticular degeneration
Wilson's disease

275.2 Disorders of magnesium metabolism
Hypermagnesemia
Hypomagnesemia

275.3 Disorders of phosphorus metabolism
Familial hypophosphatemia
Hypophosphatasia
Vitamin D-resistant:
- osteomalacia
- rickets

✓5th **275.4 Disorders of calcium metabolism**
EXCLUDES *parathyroid disorders (252.00-252.9)*
vitamin D deficiency (268.0-268.9)
AHA: 4Q, '97, 33

275.40 Unspecified disorder of calcium metabolism

275.41 Hypocalcemia

DEF: Abnormally decreased blood calcium level; symptoms include hyperactive deep tendon reflexes, muscle, abdominal cramps, and carpopedal spasm.

275.42 Hypercalcemia

AHA: 4Q, '03, 110

DEF: Abnormally increased blood calcium level; symptoms include muscle weakness, fatigue, nausea, depression, and constipation.

275.49 Other disorders of calcium metabolism

Nephrocalcinosis
Pseudohypoparathyroidism
Pseudopseudohypoparathryoidism

DEF: Nephrocalcinosis: calcium phosphate deposits in the tubules of the kidney with resultant renal insufficiency.

DEF: Pseudohypoparathyroidism: inherited disorder with signs and symptoms of hypoparathyroidism; caused by inadequate response to parathyroid hormone, not hormonal deficiency. Symptoms include muscle cramps, tetany, urinary frequency, blurred vision due to cataracts, and dry scaly skin.

DEF: Pseudopseudohypoparathyroidism: clinical manifestations of hypoparathyroidism without affecting blood calcium levels.

275.8 Other specified disorders of mineral metabolism

275.9 Unspecified disorder of mineral metabolism

✓4th **276 Disorders of fluid, electrolyte, and acid-base balance**

EXCLUDES *diabetes insipidus (253.5)*
familial periodic paralysis (359.3)

276.0 Hyperosmolality and/or hypernatremia

Sodium [Na] excess
Sodium [Na] overload

276.1 Hyposmolality and/or hyponatremia

Sodium [Na] deficiency

276.2 Acidosis

Acidosis:
NOS
lactic
metabolic
respiratory

EXCLUDES *diabetic acidosis (250.1)*

AHA: J-F, '87, 15

DEF: Disorder involves decrease of pH (hydrogen ion) concentration in blood and cellular tissues; caused by increase in acid and decrease in bicarbonate.

276.3 Alkalosis

Alkalosis:
NOS
metabolic
respiratory

DEF: Accumulation of base (non-acid part of salt), or loss of acid without relative loss of base in body fluids; caused by increased arterial plasma bicarbonate concentration or loss of carbon dioxide due to hyperventilation.

276.4 Mixed acid-base balance disorder

Hypercapnia with mixed acid-base disorder

✓5th **276.5 Volume depletion**

EXCLUDES *hypovolemic shock:*
postoperative (998.0)
traumatic (958.4)

AHA: 1Q, '03, 5, 22; 3Q, '02, 21; 4Q, '97, 30; 2Q, '88, 9

● **276.50 Volume depletion, unspecified**

● **276.51 Dehydration**

● **276.52 Hypovolemia**

Depletion of volume of plasma

276.6 Fluid overload

Fluid retention

EXCLUDES *ascites (789.5)*
localized edema (782.3)

276.7 Hyperpotassemia

Hyperkalemia
Potassium [K]:
excess
intoxication
overload

AHA: ▶1Q, '05, 9;◀ 2Q,'01, 12

DEF: Elevated blood levels of potassium; symptoms include abnormal EKG readings, weakness; related to defective renal excretion.

276.8 Hypopotassemia

Hypokalemia
Potassium [K] deficiency

DEF: Decreased blood levels of potassium; symptoms include neuromuscular disorders.

276.9 Electrolyte and fluid disorders not elsewhere classified

Electrolyte imbalance
Hyperchloremia
Hypochloremia

EXCLUDES *electrolyte imbalance:*
associated with hyperemesis gravidarum (643.1)
complicating labor and delivery (669.0)
following abortion and ectopic or molar pregnancy (634-638 with .4, 639.4)

AHA: J-F, '87, 15

✓4th **277 Other and unspecified disorders of metabolism**

✓5th **277.0 Cystic fibrosis**

Fibrocystic disease of the pancreas
Mucoviscidosis

DEF: Generalized, genetic disorder of infants, children, and young adults marked by exocrine gland dysfunction; characterized by chronic pulmonary disease with excess mucus production, pancreatic deficiency, high levels of electrolytes in the sweat.

AHA: 4Q, '90, 16; 3Q, '90, 18

277.00 Without mention of meconium ileus

Cystic fibrosis NOS

AHA: 2Q, '03, 12

277.01 With meconium ileus N

Meconium:
ileus (of newborn)
obstruction of intestine in mucoviscidosis

277.02 With pulmonary manifestations

Cystic fibrosis with pulmonary exacerbation
Use additional code to identify any infectious organism present, such as:
pseudomonas (041.7)

AHA: 4Q, '02, 45, 46

277.03 With gastrointestinal manifestations

EXCLUDES *with meconium ileus (277.01)*

AHA: 4Q, '02, 45

277.09 With other manifestations

277.1 Disorders of porphyrin metabolism

Hematoporphyria
Hematoporphyrinuria
Hereditary coproporphyria
Porphyria
Porphyrinuria
Protocoproporphyria
Protoporphyria
Pyrroloporphyria

277.2 Other disorders of purine and pyrimidine metabolism

Hypoxanthine-guanine-phosphoribosyltransferase deficiency [HG-PRT deficiency]
Lesch-Nyhan syndrome
Xanthinuria

EXCLUDES *gout (274.0-274.9)*
orotic aciduric anemia (281.4)

N Newborn Age: 0 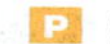 Pediatric Age: 0-17 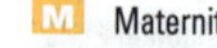 Maternity Age: 12-55 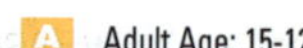 Adult Age: 15-124 MSP Medicare Secondary Payer

277.3 Amyloidosis
Amyloidosis:
NOS
inherited systemic
nephropathic
neuropathic (Portuguese) (Swiss)
secondary
Benign paroxysmal peritonitis
Familial Mediterranean fever
Hereditary cardiac amyloidosis
AHA: 1Q, '96, 16
DEF: Conditions of diverse etiologies characterized by the accumulation of insoluble fibrillar proteins (amyloid) in various organs and tissues of the body, compromising vital functions.

277.4 Disorders of bilirubin excretion
Hyperbilirubinemia:
congenital
constitutional
Syndrome:
Crigler-Najjar
Syndrome:
Dubin-Johnson
Gilbert's
Rotor's
EXCLUDES *hyperbilirubinemias specific to the perinatal period (774.0-774.7)*

277.5 Mucopolysaccharidosis
Gargoylism
Hunter's syndrome
Hurler's syndrome
Lipochondrodystrophy
Maroteaux-Lamy syndrome
Morquio-Brailsford disease
Osteochondrodystrophy
Sanfilippo's syndrome
Scheie's syndrome
DEF: Metabolism disorders evidenced by excretion of various mucopolysaccharides in urine and infiltration of these substances into connective tissue, with resulting various defects of bone, cartilage and connective tissue.

277.6 Other deficiencies of circulating enzymes
Hereditary angioedema

277.7 Dysmetabolic syndrome X
Use additional code for associated manifestation, such as:
cardiovascular disease (414.00-414.07)
obesity (278.00-278.01)
AHA: 4Q, '01, 42
DEF: A specific group of metabolic disorders that are related to the state of insulin resistance (decreased cellular response to insulin) without elevated blood sugars; often related to elevated cholesterol and triglycerides, obesity, cardiovascular disease, and high blood pressure.

✓5th **277.8 Other specified disorders of metabolism**
AHA: 4Q, '03, 50; 2Q, '01, 18; S-O, '87, 9

277.81 Primary carnitine deficiency

277.82 Carnitine deficiency due to inborn errors of metabolism

277.83 Iatrogenic carnitine deficiency
Carnitine deficiency due to:
hemodialysis
valproic acid therapy

277.84 Other secondary carnitine deficiency

277.85 Disorders of fatty acid oxidation
Carnitine palmitoyltransferase deficiencies (CPT1, CPT2)
Glutaric aciduria type II (type IIA, IIB, IIC)
Long chain 3-hydroxyacyl CoA dehydrogenase deficiency (LCHAD)
Long chain/very long chain acyl CoA dehydrogenase deficiency (LCAD, VLCAD)
Medium chain acyl CoA dehydrogenase deficiency (MCAD)
Short chain acyl CoA dehydrogenase deficiency (SCAD)
EXCLUDES *primary carnitine deficiency (277.81)*

277.86 Peroxisomal disorders
Adrenomyeloneuropathy
Neonatal adrenoleukodystrophy
Rhizomelic chrondrodysplasia punctata
X-linked adrenoleukodystrophy
Zellweger syndrome
EXCLUDES *infantile Refsum disease (356.3)*

277.87 Disorders of mitochondrial metabolism
Kearns-Sayre syndrome
Mitochondrial Encephalopathy, Lactic Acidosis and Stroke-like episodes (MELAS syndrome)
Mitochondrial Neurogastrointestinal Encephalopathy syndrome (MNGIE)
Myoclonus with Epilepsy and with Ragged Red Fibers (MERRF syndrome)
Neuropathy, Ataxia and Retinitis Pigmentosa (NARP syndrome)
Use additional code for associated conditions
EXCLUDES *disorders of pyruvate metabolism (271.8)*
Leber's optic atrophy (377.16)
Leigh's subacute necrotizing encephalopathy (330.8)
Reye's syndrome (331.81)
AHA: 4Q, '04, 62

277.89 Other specified disorders of metabolism
Hand-Schüller-Christian disease
Histiocytosis (acute) (chronic)
Histiocytosis X (chronic)
EXCLUDES *histiocytosis:*
acute differentiated progressive (202.5)
X, acute (progressive) (202.5)

277.9 Unspecified disorder of metabolism
Enzymopathy NOS

▲ ✓4th **278 Overweight, obesity and other hyperalimentation**
EXCLUDES *hyperalimentation NOS (783.6)*
poisoning by vitamins NOS (963.5)
polyphagia (783.6)

▲ ✓5th **278.0 Overweight and obesity**
▶Use additional code to identify Body Mass Index (BMI), if known (V85.21- V85.4)◀
EXCLUDES *adiposogenital dystrophy (253.8)*
obesity of endocrine origin NOS (259.9)

278.00 Obesity, unspecified
Obesity NOS
AHA: 4Q, '01, 42;1Q, '99, 5, 6

278.01 Morbid obesity
Severe obesity
AHA: 3Q, '03, 6-8
DEF: Increased weight beyond limits of skeletal and physical requirements (125 percent or more over ideal body weight), as a result of excess fat in subcutaneous connective tissues.

● **278.02 Overweight**

278.1 Localized adiposity
Fat pad

278.2 Hypervitaminosis A

278.3 Hypercarotinemia
DEF: Elevated blood carotene level due to ingesting excess carotenoids or the inability to convert carotenoids to vitamin A.

278.4 Hypervitaminosis D
DEF: Weakness, fatigue, loss of weight, and other symptoms resulting from ingesting excessive amounts of vitamin D.

278.8 Other hyperalimentation

✓4th **279 Disorders involving the immune mechanism**

✓5th **279.0 Deficiency of humoral immunity**

DEF: Inadequate immune response to bacterial infections with potential reinfection by viruses due to lack of circulating immunoglobulins (acquired antibodies).

279.00 Hypogammaglobulinemia, unspecified
Agammaglobulinemia NOS

279.01 Selective IgA immunodeficiency

279.02 Selective IgM immunodeficiency

279.03 Other selective immunoglobulin deficiencies
Selective deficiency of IgG

279.04 Congenital hypogammaglobulinemia
Agammaglobulinemia:
- Bruton's type
- X-linked

279.05 Immunodeficiency with increased IgM
Immunodeficiency with hyper-IgM:
- autosomal recessive
- X-linked

279.06 Common variable immunodeficiency
Dysgammaglobulinemia (acquired) (congenital) (primary)
Hypogammaglobulinemia:
- acquired primary
- congenital non-sex-linked
- sporadic

279.09 Other
Transient hypogammaglobulinemia of infancy

✓5th **279.1 Deficiency of cell-mediated immunity**

279.10 Immunodeficiency with predominant T-cell defect, unspecified
AHA: S-O, '87, 10

279.11 DiGeorge's syndrome
Pharyngeal pouch syndrome
Thymic hypoplasia

DEF: Congenital disorder due to defective development of the third and fourth pharyngeal pouches; results in hypoplasia or aplasia of the thymus, parathyroid glands; related to congenital heart defects, anomalies of the great vessels, esophageal atresia, and abnormalities of facial structures.

279.12 Wiskott-Aldrich syndrome

DEF: A disease characterized by chronic conditions, such as eczema, suppurative otitis media and anemia; it results from an X-linked recessive gene and is classified as an immune deficiency syndrome.

279.13 Nezelof's syndrome
Cellular immunodeficiency with abnormal immunoglobulin deficiency

DEF: Immune system disorder characterized by a pathological deficiency in cellular immunity and humoral antibodies resulting in inability to fight infectious diseases.

279.19 Other
EXCLUDES *ataxia-telangiectasia (334.8)*

279.2 Combined immunity deficiency
Agammaglobulinemia:
- autosomal recessive
- Swiss-type
- x-linked recessive

Severe combined immunodeficiency [SCID]
Thymic:
- alymophoplasia
- aplasia or dysplasia with immunodeficiency

EXCLUDES *thymic hypoplasia (279.11)*

DEF: Agammaglobulinemia: no immunoglobulins in the blood.

DEF: Thymic alymphoplasia: severe combined immunodeficiency; result of failed lymphoid tissue development.

279.3 Unspecified immunity deficiency

279.4 Autoimmune disease, not elsewhere classified
Autoimmune disease NOS
EXCLUDES *transplant failure or rejection (996.80-996.89)*

279.8 Other specified disorders involving the immune mechanism
Single complement [C1-C9] deficiency or dysfunction

279.9 Unspecified disorder of immune mechanism
AHA: 3Q, '92, 13

4. DISEASES OF THE BLOOD AND BLOOD-FORMING ORGANS (280-289)

EXCLUDES *anemia complicating pregnancy or the puerperium (648.2)*

✓4th 280 Iron deficiency anemias

INCLUDES anemia:
- asiderotic
- hypochromic-microcytic
- sideropenic

EXCLUDES *familial microcytic anemia (282.49)*

280.0 Secondary to blood loss (chronic)
Normocytic anemia due to blood loss
EXCLUDES *acute posthemorrhagic anemia (285.1)*
AHA: 4Q, '93, 34

280.1 Secondary to inadequate dietary iron intake

280.8 Other specified iron deficiency anemias
Paterson-Kelly syndrome
Plummer-Vinson syndrome
Sideropenic dysphagia

280.9 Iron deficiency anemia, unspecified
Anemia:
- achlorhydric
- chlorotic
- idiopathic hypochromic
- iron [Fe] deficiency NOS

✓4th 281 Other deficiency anemias

281.0 Pernicious anemia
Anemia:
- Addison's
- Biermer's
- congenital pernicious

Congenital intrinsic factor [Castle's] deficiency
EXCLUDES *combined system disease without mention of anemia (266.2)*
subacute degeneration of spinal cord without mention of anemia (266.2)
AHA: N-D, '84, 1; S-O, '84, 16
DEF: Chronic progressive anemia due to Vitamin B_{12} malabsorption; caused by lack of a secretion known as intrinsic factor, which is produced by the gastric mucosa of the stomach.

281.1 Other vitamin B_{12} deficiency anemia
Anemia:
- vegan's
- vitamin B_{12} deficiency (dietary)
- due to selective vitamin B_{12} malabsorption with proteinuria

Syndrome:
- Imerslund's
- Imerslund-Gräsbeck

EXCLUDES *combined system disease without mention of anemia (266.2)*
subacute degeneration of spinal cord without mention of anemia (266.2)

281.2 Folate-deficiency anemia
Congenital folate malabsorption
Folate or folic acid deficiency anemia:
- NOS
- dietary
- drug-induced

Goat's milk anemia
Nutritional megaloblastic anemia (of infancy)
Use additional E code to identify drug
DEF: Macrocytic anemia resembles pernicious anemia but without absence of hydrochloric acid secretions; responsive to folic acid therapy.

281.3 Other specified megaloblastic anemias not elsewhere classified
Combined B_{12} and folate-deficiency anemia
Refractory megaloblastic anemia
DEF: Megaloblasts predominant in bone marrow with few normoblasts; rare familial type associated with proteinuria and genitourinary tract anomalies.

281.4 Protein-deficiency anemia
Amino-acid-deficiency anemia

281.8 Anemia associated with other specified nutritional deficiency
Scorbutic anemia

281.9 Unspecified deficiency anemia
Anemia:
- dimorphic
- macrocytic
- megaloblastic NOS
- nutritional NOS
- simple chronic

✓4th 282 Hereditary hemolytic anemias

DEF: Escalated rate of erythrocyte destruction; similar to all anemias, occurs when imbalance exists between blood loss and blood production.

282.0 Hereditary spherocytosis
Acholuric (familial) jaundice
Congenital hemolytic anemia (spherocytic)
Congenital spherocytosis
Minkowski-Chauffard syndrome
Spherocytosis (familial)
EXCLUDES *hemolytic anemia of newborn (773.0-773.5)*
DEF: Hereditary, chronic illness marked by abnormal red blood cell membrane; symptoms include enlarged spleen, jaundice; and anemia in severe cases.

282.1 Hereditary elliptocytosis
Elliptocytosis (congenital)
Ovalocytosis (congenital) (hereditary)
DEF: Genetic hemolytic anemia characterized by malformed, elliptical erythrocytes; there is increased destruction of red cells with resulting anemia.

282.2 Anemias due to disorders of glutathione metabolism
Anemia:
- 6-phosphogluconic dehydrogenase deficiency
- enzyme deficiency, drug-induced
- erythrocytic glutathione deficiency
- glucose-6-phosphate dehydrogenase [G-6-PD] deficiency
- glutathione-reductase deficiency
- hemolytic nonspherocytic (hereditary), type I

Disorder of pentose phosphate pathway
Favism

282.3 Other hemolytic anemias due to enzyme deficiency
Anemia:
- hemolytic nonspherocytic (hereditary), type II
- hexokinase deficiency
- pyruvate kinase [PK] deficiency
- triosephosphate isomerase deficiency

✓5th 282.4 Thalassemias
EXCLUDES *sickle-cell:*
disease (282.60-282.69)
trait (282.5)
AHA: 4Q, '03, 51
DEF: A group of inherited hemolytic disorders characterized by decreased production of at least one of the four polypeptide globin chains which results in defective hemoglobin synthesis; symptoms include severe anemia, expanded marrow spaces, transfusional and absorptive iron overload, impaired growth rate, thickened cranial bones, and pathologic fractures.

282.41 Sickle-cell thalassemia without crisis
Sickle-cell thalassemia NOS
Thalassemia Hb-S disease without crisis

282.42 Sickle-cell thalassemia with crisis
Sickle-cell thalassemia with vaso-occlusive pain
Thalassemia Hb-S disease with crisis
Use additional code for type of crisis, such as:
acute chest syndrome (517.3)
splenic sequestration (289.52)

282.49 Other thalassemia
Cooley's anemia
▶Hb-Bart's disease◀
Hereditary leptocytosis
Mediterranean anemia (with other hemoglobinopathy)
Microdrepanocytosis
Thalassemia (alpha) (beta) (intermedia) (major) (minima) (minor) (mixed) (trait) (with other hemoglobinopathy)
Thalassemia NOS

282.5 Sickle-cell trait
Hb-AS genotype
Hemoglobin S [Hb-S] trait
Heterozygous:
hemoglobin S
Hb-S

EXCLUDES *that with other hemoglobinopathy (282.60-282.69)*
that with thalassemia (282.49)

DEF: Heterozygous genetic makeup characterized by one gene for normal hemoglobin and one for sickle-cell hemoglobin; clinical disease rarely present.

✓5th **282.6 Sickle-cell disease**
Sickle-cell anemia

EXCLUDES *sickle-cell thalassemia (282.41-282.42)*
sickle-cell trait (282.5)

DEF: Inherited blood disorder; sickle-shaped red blood cells are hard and pointed, clogging blood flow; anemia characterized by, periodic episodes of pain, acute abdominal discomfort, skin ulcerations of the legs, increased infections; occurs primarily in persons of African descent.

282.60 Sickle-cell disease, unspecified
Sickle-cell anemia NOS
AHA: 2Q, '97, 11

282.61 Hb-SS disease without crisis

282.62 Hb-SS disease with crisis
Hb-SS disease with vaso-occlusive pain
Sickle-cell crisis NOS
Use additional code for type of crisis, such as:
acute chest syndrome (517.3)
splenic sequestration (289.52)
AHA: 4Q, '03, 56; 2Q, '98, 8; 2Q, '91, 15

282.63 Sickle-cell/Hb-C disease without crisis
Hb-S/Hb-C disease without crisis

282.64 Sickle-cell/Hb-C disease with crisis
Hb-S/Hb-C disease with crisis
Sickle-cell/Hb-C disease with vaso-occlusive pain
Use additional code for type of crisis, such as:
acute chest syndrome (517.3)
splenic sequestration (289.52)
AHA: 4Q, '03, 51

282.68 Other sickle-cell disease without crisis
Hb-S/Hb-D, Hb-S/Hb-E, Sickle-cell/Hb-D, Sickle-cell/Hb-E } disease without crisis
AHA: 4Q, '03, 51

282.69 Other sickle-cell disease with crisis
Hb-S/Hb-D, Hb-S/Hb-E, Sickle-cell/Hb-D, Sickle-cell/Hb-E } disease with crisis
Other sickle-cell disease with vaso-occlusive pain
Use additional code for type of crisis, such as:
acute chest syndrome (517.3)
splenic sequestration (289.52)

282.7 Other hemoglobinopathies
Abnormal hemoglobin NOS
Congenital Heinz-body anemia
Disease:
hemoglobin C [Hb-C]
hemoglobin D [Hb-D]
hemoglobin E [Hb-E]
hemoglobin Zurich [Hb-Zurich]
Hemoglobinopathy NOS
Hereditary persistence of fetal hemoglobin [HPFH]
Unstable hemoglobin hemolytic disease

EXCLUDES *familial polycythemia (289.6)*
hemoglobin M [Hb-M] disease (289.7)
high-oxygen-affinity hemoglobin (289.0)

DEF: Any disorder of hemoglobin due to alteration of molecular structure; may include overt anemia.

282.8 Other specified hereditary hemolytic anemias
Stomatocytosis

282.9 Hereditary hemolytic anemia, unspecified
Hereditary hemolytic anemia NOS

✓4th **283 Acquired hemolytic anemias**
AHA: N-D, '84, 1

DEF: Non-heriditary anemia characterized by premature destruction of red blood cells; caused by infectious organisms, poisons, and physical agents.

283.0 Autoimmune hemolytic anemias
Autoimmune hemolytic disease (cold type) (warm type)
Chronic cold hemagglutinin disease
Cold agglutinin disease or hemoglobinuria
Hemolytic anemia:
cold type (secondary) (symptomatic)
drug-induced
warm type (secondary) (symptomatic)
Use additional E code to identify cause, if drug-induced

EXCLUDES *Evans' syndrome ▶(287.32)◀*
hemolytic disease of newborn (773.0-773.5)

✓5th **283.1 Non-autoimmune hemolytic anemias**
Use additional E code to identify cause
AHA: 4Q, '93, 25

DEF: Hemolytic anemia and thrombocytopenia with acute renal failure; relatively rare condition; 50 percent of patients require renal dialysis.

283.10 Non-autoimmune hemolytic anemia, unspecified

283.11 Hemolytic-uremic syndrome

283.19 Other non-autoimmune hemolytic anemias
Hemolytic anemia:
mechanical
microangiopathic
toxic

283.2 Hemoglobinuria due to hemolysis from external causes
Acute intravascular hemolysis
Hemoglobinuria:
from exertion
march
paroxysmal (cold) (nocturnal)
due to other hemolysis
Marchiafava-Micheli syndrome
Use additional E code to identify cause

283.9 Acquired hemolytic anemia, unspecified
Acquired hemolytic anemia NOS
Chronic idiopathic hemolytic anemia

✓4th **284 Aplastic anemia**
AHA: 1Q, '91, 14; N-D, '84, 1; S-O, '84, 16

DEF: Bone marrow failure to produce the normal amount of blood components; generally non-responsive to usual therapy.

284.0 Constitutional aplastic anemia
Aplasia, (pure) red cell:
congenital
of infants
primary
Blackfan-Diamond syndrome
Familial hypoplastic anemia
Fanconi's anemia
Pancytopenia with malformations
AHA: 1Q, '91, 14

284.8 Other specified aplastic anemias
Aplastic anemia (due to):
chronic systemic disease
drugs
infection
radiation
toxic (paralytic)
Pancytopenia (acquired)
Red cell aplasia (acquired) (adult) (pure) (with thymoma)
Use additional E code to identify cause
AHA: 1Q, '97, 5; 1Q, '92, 15; 1Q, '91, 14

284.9 Aplastic anemia, unspecified
Anemia:
aplastic (idiopathic) NOS
aregenerative
hypoplastic NOS
nonregenerative
Medullary hypoplasia
EXCLUDES ▶ *refractory anemia (238.7)*◀

✓4th **285 Other and unspecified anemias**
AHA: 1Q, '91, 14; N-D, '84, 1

285.0 Sideroblastic anemia
Anemia:
hypochromic with iron loading
sideroachrestic
sideroblastic:
acquired
congenital
hereditary
primary
secondary (drug-induced) (due to disease)
sex-linked hypochromic
vitamin B_6-responsive
Pyridoxine-responsive (hypochromic) anemia
Use additional E code to identify cause, if drug induced
EXCLUDES ▶ *refractory sideroblastic anemia (238.7)*◀

DEF: Characterized by a disruption of final heme synthesis; results in iron overload of reticuloendothelial tissues.

285.1 Acute posthemorrhagic anemia
Anemia due to acute blood loss
EXCLUDES *anemia due to chronic blood loss (280.0)*
blood loss anemia NOS (280.0)
AHA: 2Q, '92, 15

✓5th **285.2 Anemia in chronic illness**
AHA: 4Q, '00, 39

▲ **285.21 Anemia in chronic kidney disease**
▶Anemia in end stage renal disease◀
Erythropoietin-resistant anemia (EPO resistant anemia)

285.22 Anemia in neoplastic disease

285.29 Anemia of other chronic illness

285.8 Other specified anemias
Anemia:
dyserythropoietic (congenital)
dyshematopoietic (congenital)
leukoerythroblastic
von Jaksch's
Infantile pseudoleukemia
AHA: 1Q, '91, 16

285.9 Anemia, unspecified
Anemia:
NOS
essential
normocytic, not due to blood loss
profound
progressive
secondary
Oligocythemia
EXCLUDES *anemia (due to):*
blood loss:
acute (285.1)
chronic or unspecified (280.0)
iron deficiency (280.0-280.9)
AHA: 1Q, '02, 14; 2Q, '92, 16; M-A, '85, 13; ND, '84, 1

✓4th **286 Coagulation defects**

286.0 Congenital factor VIII disorder
Antihemophilic globulin [AHG] deficiency
Factor VIII (functional) deficiency
Hemophilia:
NOS
A
classical
familial
hereditary
Subhemophilia
EXCLUDES *factor VIII deficiency with vascular defect (286.4)*

DEF: Hereditary, sex-linked, results in missing antihemophilic globulin (AHG) (factor VIII); causes abnormal coagulation characterized by increased tendency to bleeding, large bruises of skin, soft tissue; may also be bleeding in mouth, nose, gastrointestinal tract; after childhood, hemorrhages in joints, resulting in swelling and impaired function.

286.1 Congenital factor IX disorder
Christmas disease
Deficiency:
factor IX (functional)
plasma thromboplastin component [PTC]
Hemophilia B

DEF: Deficiency of plasma thromboplastin component (PTC) (factor IX) and plasma thromboplastin antecedent (PTA); PTC deficiency clinically indistinguishable from classical hemophilia; PTA deficiency found in both sexes.

286.2 Congenital factor XI deficiency
Hemophilia C
Plasma thromboplastin antecedent [PTA] deficiency
Rosenthal's disease

286.3 Congenital deficiency of other clotting factors
Congenital afibrinogenemia
Deficiency:
AC globulin factor:
I [fibrinogen]
II [prothrombin]
V [labile]
VII [stable]
X [Stuart-Prower]
XII [Hageman]
XIII [fibrin stabilizing]
Laki-Lorand factor
proaccelerin
Disease
Owren's
Stuart-Prower
Dysfibrinogenemia (congenital)
Dysprothrombinemia (constitutional)
Hypoproconvertinemia
Hypoprothrmbinemia (hereditary)
Parahemophilia

286.4 von Willebrand's disease
Angiohemophilia (A) (B)
Constitutional thrombopathy
Factor VIII deficiency with vascular defect
Pseudohemophilia type B
Vascular hemophilia
von Willebrand's (-Jürgens') disease
EXCLUDES *factor VIII deficiency:*
NOS (286.0)
with functional defect (286.0)
hereditary capillary fragility (287.8)

DEF: Abnormal blood coagulation caused by deficient blood Factor VII; congenital; symptoms include excess or prolonged bleeding, such as hemorrhage during menstruation, following birthing, or after surgical procedure.

286.5 Hemorrhagic disorder due to intrinsic circulating anticoagulants
Antithrombinemia
Antithromboplastinemia
Antithromboplastino-genemia
Hyperheparinemia
Increase in:
anti-VIIIa
anti-IXa
anti-Xa
anti-XIa
antithrombin
Secondary hemophilia
Systemic lupus erythematosus [SLE] inhibitor
AHA: 3Q, '92, 15; 3Q, '90, 14

286.6 Defibrination syndrome
Afibrinogenemia, acquired
Consumption coagulopathy
Diffuse or disseminated intravascular coagulation [DIC syndrome]
Fibrinolytic hemorrhage, acquired
Hemorrhagic fibrinogenolysis
Pathologic fibrinolysis
Purpura:
fibrinolytic
fulminans
EXCLUDES *that complicating:*
abortion (634-638 with .1, 639.1)
pregnancy or the puerperium (641.3, 666.3)
disseminated intravascular coagulation in newborn (776.2)
AHA: 4Q, '93, 29

DEF: Characterized by destruction of circulating fibrinogen; often precipitated by other conditions, such as injury, causing release of thromboplastic particles in blood stream.

286.7 Acquired coagulation factor deficiency
Deficiency of coagulation factor due to:
liver disease
vitamin K deficiency
Hypoprothrombinemia, acquired
Use additional E code to identify cause, if drug induced
EXCLUDES *vitamin K deficiency of newborn (776.0)*
AHA: 4Q, '93, 29

286.9 Other and unspecified coagulation defects
Defective coagulation NOS
Deficiency, coagulation factor NOS
Delay, coagulation
Disorder:
coagulation
hemostasis
EXCLUDES *abnormal coagulation profile (790.92)*
hemorrhagic disease of newborn (776.0)
that complicating:
abortion (634-638 with .1, 639.1)
pregnancy or the puerperium (641.3, 666.3)

✓4th **287 Purpura and other hemorrhagic conditions**
EXCLUDES *hemorrhagic thrombocythemia (238.7)*
purpura fulminans (286.6)
AHA: 1Q, '91, 14

287.0 Allergic purpura
Peliosis rheumatica
Purpura:
anaphylactoid
autoimmune
Henoch's
nonthrombocytopenic:
hemorrhagic
idiopathic
Purpura:
rheumatica
Schönlein-Henoch
vascular
Vasculitis, allergic
EXCLUDES *hemorrhagic purpura ▶(287.39)◀*
purpura annularis telangiectodes (709.1)

DEF: Any hemorrhagic condition, thrombocytic or nonthrombocytopenic in origin, caused by a presumed allergic reaction.

287.1 Qualitative platelet defects
Thrombasthenia (hemorrhagic) (hereditary)
Thrombocytasthenia
Thrombocytopathy (dystrophic)
Thrombopathy (Bernard-Soulier)
EXCLUDES *von Willebrand's disease (286.4)*

287.2 Other nonthrombocytopenic purpuras
Purpura:
NOS
senile
simplex

✓5th **287.3 Primary thrombocytopenia**
EXCLUDES *thrombotic thrombocytopenic purpura (446.6)*
transient thrombocytopenia of newborn (776.1)

DEF: Decrease in number of blood platelets in circulating blood and purpural skin hemorrhages.

● **287.30 Primary thrombocytopenia, unspecified**
Megakaryocytic hypoplasia

● **287.31 Immune thrombocytopenic purpura**
Idiopathic thrombocytopenic purpura
Tidal platelet dysgenesis

● **287.32 Evans' syndrome**

● **287.33 Congenital and hereditary thrombocytopenic purpura**
Congenital and hereditary thrombocytopenia
Thrombocytopenia with absent radii (TAR) syndrome
EXCLUDES *Wiskott-Aldrich syndrome (279.12)*

● **287.39 Other primary thrombocytopenia**

287.4 Secondary thrombocytopenia
Posttransfusion purpura
Thrombocytopenia (due to):
- dilutional
- drugs
- extracorporeal circulation of blood
- platelet alloimmunization

Use additional E code to identify cause
EXCLUDES *transient thrombocytopenia of newborn (776.1)*
AHA: 4Q, '99, 22; 4Q, '93, 29
DEF: Reduced number of platelets in circulating blood as consequence of an underlying disease or condition.

287.5 Thrombocytopenia, unspecified

287.8 Other specified hemorrhagic conditions
Capillary fragility (hereditary)
Vascular pseudohemophilia

287.9 Unspecified hemorrhagic conditions
Hemorrhagic diathesis (familial)

✓4th **288 Diseases of white blood cells**
EXCLUDES *leukemia (204.0-208.9)*
AHA: 1Q, '91, 14

288.0 Agranulocytosis
Infantile genetic agranulocytosis
Kostmann's syndrome
Neutropenia:
- NOS
- cyclic
- drug-induced
- immune
- periodic
- toxic

Neutropenic splenomegaly
Use additional E code to identify drug or other cause
EXCLUDES *transitory neonatal neutropenia (776.7)*
AHA: 3Q, '99, 6; 2Q, '99, 9; 3Q, '96, 16; 2Q, '96, 6
DEF: Sudden, severe condition characterized by reduced number of white blood cells; results in sores in the throat, stomach or skin; symptoms include chills, fever; some drugs can bring on condition.

288.1 Functional disorders of polymorphonuclear neutrophils
Chronic (childhood) granulomatous disease
Congenital dysphagocytosis
Job's syndrome
Lipochrome histiocytosis (familial)
Progressive septic granulomatosis

288.2 Genetic anomalies of leukocytes
Anomaly (granulation) (granulocyte) or syndrome:
- Alder's (-Reilly)
- Chédiak-Steinbrinck (-Higashi)
- Jordan's
- May-Hegglin
- Pelger-Huet

Hereditary:
- hypersegmentation
- hyposegmentation
- leukomelanopathy

288.3 Eosinophilia
Eosinophilia:
- allergic
- hereditary
- idiopathic
- secondary

Eosinophilic leukocytosis
EXCLUDES *Löffler's syndrome (518.3)*
pulmonary eosinophilia (518.3)
AHA: 3Q, '00, 11
DEF: Elevated number of eosinophils in the blood; characteristic of allergic states and various parasitic infections.

288.8 Other specified disease of white blood cells
Leukemoid reaction:
- lymphocytic
- monocytic
- myelocytic

Leukocytosis
Lymphocytopenia
Lymphocytosis (symptomatic)
Lymphopenia
Monocytosis (symptomatic)
Plasmacytosis
EXCLUDES *immunity disorders (279.0-279.9)*
AHA: M-A, '87, 12

288.9 Unspecified disease of white blood cells

✓4th **289 Other diseases of blood and blood-forming organs**

289.0 Polycythemia, secondary
High-oxygen-affinity hemoglobin
Polycythemia:
- acquired
- benign
- due to:
  - fall in plasma volume
  - high altitude
- emotional
- erythropoietin
- hypoxemic
- nephrogenous
- relative
- spurious
- stress

EXCLUDES *polycythemia:*
neonatal (776.4)
primary (238.4)
vera (238.4)
DEF: Elevated number of red blood cells in circulating blood as result of reduced oxygen supply to the tissues.

289.1 Chronic lymphadenitis
Chronic:
- adenitis } any lymph node, except mesenteric
- lymphadenitis }

EXCLUDES *acute lymphadenitis (683)*
mesenteric (289.2)
enlarged glands NOS (785.6)
DEF: Persistent inflammation of lymph node tissue; origin of infection is usually elsewhere.

289.2 Nonspecific mesenteric lymphadenitis
Mesenteric lymphadenitis (acute) (chronic)
DEF: Inflammation of the lymph nodes in peritoneal fold that encases abdominal organs; disease resembles acute appendicitis; unknown etiology.

289.3 Lymphadenitis, unspecified, except mesenteric
AHA: 2Q, '92, 8

289.4 Hypersplenism
"Big spleen" syndrome
Dyssplenism
Hypersplenia
EXCLUDES *primary splenic neutropenia (288.0)*
DEF: An overactive spleen; it causes a deficiency of the peripheral blood components, an increase in bone marrow cells and sometimes a notable increase in the size of the spleen.

✓5th **289.5 Other diseases of spleen**

289.50 Disease of spleen, unspecified

289.51 Chronic congestive splenomegaly

***289.52* Splenic sequestration**

Code first sickle-cell disease in crisis (282.42, 282.62, 282.64, 282.69)

AHA: 4Q, '03, 51

DEF: Blood is entrapped in the spleen due to vessel occlusion; most often associated with sickle-cell disease; spleen becomes enlarged and there is a sharp drop in hemoglobin.

289.59 Other

Lien migrans
Perisplenitis
Splenic:
  abscess
  atrophy
  cyst
Splenic:
  fibrosis
  infarction
  rupture, nontraumatic
Splenitis
Wandering spleen

EXCLUDES *bilharzial splenic fibrosis (120.0-120.9)*
hepatolienal fibrosis (571.5)
splenomegaly NOS (789.2)

289.6 Familial polycythemia

Familial:
  benign polycythemia
  erythrocytosis

DEF: Elevated number of red blood cells.

289.7 Methemoglobinemia

Congenital NADH [DPNH]-methemoglobin-reductase deficiency
Hemoglobin M [Hb-M] disease
Methemoglobinemia:
  NOS
  acquired (with sulfhemoglobinemia)
  hereditary
  toxic
Stokvis' disease
Sulfhemoglobinemia
Use additional E code to identify cause

DEF: Presence in the blood of methemoglobin, a chemically altered form of hemoglobin; causes cyanosis, headache, dizziness, ataxia dyspnea, tachycardia, nausea, stupor, coma, and, rarely, death.

✓5th **289.8 Other specified diseases of blood and blood-forming organs**

AHA: 4Q, '03, 56; 1Q, '02, 16; 2Q, '89, 8; M-A, '87, 12

DEF: Hypercoagulable states: a group of inherited or acquired abnormalities of specific proteins and anticoagulant factors; also called thromboembolic states or thrombotic disorders, these disorders result in the abnormal development of blood clots.

289.81 Primary hypercoagulable state

Activated protein C resistance
Antithrombin III deficiency
Factor V Leiden mutation
Lupus anticoagulant
Protein C deficiency
Protein S deficiency
Prothrombin gene mutation

DEF: Activated protein C resistance: decreased effectiveness of protein C to degrade factor V, necessary to inhibit clotting cascade; also called Factor V Leiden mutation.

DEF: Antithrombin III deficiency: deficiency in plasma antithrombin III one of six naturally occurring antithrombins that limit coagulation.

DEF: Factor V Leiden mutation: also called activated protein C resistance.

DEF: Lupus anticoagulant: deficiency in a circulating anticoagulant that inhibits the conversion of prothrombin into thrombin; autoimmune antibodies induce procoagulant surfaces in platelets; also called anti-phospholipid syndrome.

DEF: Protein C deficiency: deficiency of activated protein C which functions to bring the blood-clotting process into balance; same outcome as factor V Leiden mutation.

DEF: Protein S deficiency: similar to protein C deficiency; protein S is a vitamin K dependent cofactor in the activation of protein C.

DEF: Prothrombin gene mutation: increased levels of prothrombin, or factor II, a plasma protein that is converted to thrombin, which acts upon fibrinogen to form the fibrin.

289.82 Secondary hypercoagulable state

289.89 Other specified diseases of blood and blood-forming organs

Hypergammaglobulinemia
Myelofibrosis
Pseudocholinesterase deficiency

289.9 Unspecified diseases of blood and blood-forming organs

Blood dyscrasia NOS
Erythroid hyperplasia

AHA: M-A, '85, 14

5. MENTAL DISORDERS (290-319)

PSYCHOSES (290-299)

EXCLUDES *mental retardation (317-319)*

ORGANIC PSYCHOTIC CONDITIONS (290-294)

INCLUDES psychotic organic brain syndrome

EXCLUDES *nonpsychotic syndromes of organic etiology (310.0-310.9)*
psychoses classifiable to 295-298 and without impairment of orientation, comprehension, calculation, learning capacity, and judgment, but associated with physical disease, injury, or condition affecting the brain [eg., following childbirth] (295.0-298.8)

✓4th **290 Dementias**

Code first the associated neurological condition

EXCLUDES *dementia due to alcohol (291.0-291.2)*
dementia due to drugs (292.82)
dementia not classified as senile, presenile, or arteriosclerotic (294.10-294.11)
psychoses classifiable to 295-298 occurring in the senium without dementia or delirium (295.0-298.8)
senility with mental changes of nonpsychotic severity (310.1)
transient organic psychotic conditions (293.0-293.9)

290.0 Senile dementia, uncomplicated A

Senile dementia:
NOS
simple type

EXCLUDES *mild memory disturbances, not amounting to dementia, associated with senile brain disease (310.1)*
senile dementia with:
delirium or confusion (290.3)
delusional [paranoid] features (290.20)
depressive features (290.21)

AHA: 4Q, '99, 4

✓5th **290.1 Presenile dementia**

Brain syndrome with presenile brain disease

EXCLUDES *arteriosclerotic dementia (290.40-290.43)*
dementia associated with other cerebral conditions (294.10-294.11)

AHA: N-D, '84, 20

290.10 Presenile dementia, uncomplicated A

Presenile dementia: NOS
Presenile dementia: simple type

290.11 Presenile dementia with delirium A

Presenile dementia with acute confusional state

AHA: 1Q, '88, 3

290.12 Presenile dementia with delusional features A

Presenile dementia, paranoid type

290.13 Presenile dementia with depressive features A

Presenile dementia, depressed type

✓5th **290.2 Senile dementia with delusional or depressive features**

EXCLUDES *senile dementia:*
NOS (290.0)
with delirium and/or confusion (290.3)

290.20 Senile dementia with delusional features A

Senile dementia, paranoid type
Senile psychosis NOS

290.21 Senile dementia with depressive features A

290.3 Senile dementia with delirium A

Senile dementia with acute confusional state

EXCLUDES *senile:*
dementia NOS (290.0)
psychosis NOS (290.20)

✓5th **290.4 Vascular dementia**

Multi-infarct dementia or psychosis
Use additional code to identify cerebral atherosclerosis (437.0)

EXCLUDES *suspected cases with no clear evidence of arteriosclerosis (290.9)*

AHA: 1Q, '88, 3

290.40 Vascular dementia, uncomplicated A

Arteriosclerotic dementia:
NOS
simple type

290.41 Vascular dementia with delirium A

Arteriosclerotic dementia with acute confusional state

290.42 Vascular dementia with delusions A

Arteriosclerotic dementia, paranoid type

290.43 Vascular dementia with depressed mood A

Arteriosclerotic dementia, depressed type

290.8 Other specified senile psychotic conditions

Presbyophrenic psychosis

290.9 Unspecified senile psychotic condition A

✓4th **291 Alcohol induced mental disorders**

EXCLUDES *alcoholism without psychosis (303.0-303.9)*

AHA: 1Q, '88, 3; S-O, '86, 3

291.0 Alcohol withdrawal delirium

Alcoholic delirium
Delirium tremens

EXCLUDES *alcohol withdrawal (291.81)*

AHA: 2Q, '91, 11

291.1 Alcohol induced persisting amnestic disorder

Alcoholic polyneuritic psychosis
Korsakoff's psychosis, alcoholic
Wernicke-Korsakoff syndrome (alcoholic)

DEF: Prominent and lasting reduced memory span, disordered time appreciation and confabulation, occurring in alcoholics, as sequel to acute alcoholic psychosis.

291.2 Alcohol induced persisting dementia

Alcoholic dementia NOS
Alcoholism associated with dementia NOS
Chronic alcoholic brain syndrome

291.3 Alcohol induced psychotic disorder with hallucinations

Alcoholic:
hallucinosis (acute)
psychosis with hallucinosis

EXCLUDES *alcohol withdrawal with delirium (291.0)*
schizophrenia (295.0-295.9) and paranoid states (297.0-297.9) taking the form of chronic hallucinosis with clear consciousness in an alcoholic

AHA: 2Q, '91, 11

DEF: Psychosis lasting less than six months with slight or no clouding of consciousness in which auditory hallucinations predominate.

291.4 Idiosyncratic alcohol intoxication

Pathologic:
alcohol intoxication
drunkenness

EXCLUDES *acute alcohol intoxication (305.0)*
in alcoholism (303.0)
simple drunkenness (305.0)

DEF: Unique behavioral patterns, like belligerence, after intake of relatively small amounts of alcohol; behavior not due to excess consumption.

291.5 Alcohol induced psychotic disorder with delusions

Alcoholic:
paranoia

Alcoholic:
psychosis, paranoid type

EXCLUDES *nonalcoholic paranoid states (297.0-297.9)*
schizophrenia, paranoid type (295.3)

✓5th **291.8 Other specified alcohol induced mental disorders**

AHA: 3Q, '94, 13; J-A, '85, 10

291.81 Alcohol withdrawal

Alcohol:
abstinence syndrome or symptoms
withdrawal syndrome or symptoms

EXCLUDES *alcohol withdrawal:*
delirium (291.0)
hallucinosis (291.3)
delirium tremens (291.0)

AHA: 4Q, '96, 28; 2Q, '91, 11

● **291.82 Alcohol induced sleep disorders**

Alcohol induced circadian rhythm sleep disorders
Alcohol induced hypersomnia
Alcohol induced insomnia
Alcohol induced parasomnia

291.89 Other

Alcohol induced anxiety disorder
Alcohol induced mood disorder
Alcohol induced sexual dysfunction

291.9 Unspecified alcohol induced mental disorders

Alcoholic:
mania NOS
psychosis NOS
Alcoholism (chronic) with psychosis
Alcohol related disorder NOS

✓4th **292 Drug induced mental disorders**

INCLUDES organic brain syndrome associated with consumption of drugs

Use additional code for any associated drug dependence (304.0-304.9)

Use additional E code to identify drug

AHA: 3Q, '04, 8; 2Q, '91, 11; S-O, '86, 3

292.0 Drug withdrawal

Drug:
abstinence syndrome or symptoms
withdrawal syndrome or symptoms

AHA: 1Q, '97, 12; 1Q, '88, 3

✓5th **292.1 Drug induced psychotic disorders**

292.11 Drug induced psychotic disorder with delusions

Paranoid state induced by drugs

292.12 Drug induced psychotic disorder with hallucinations

Hallucinatory state induced by drugs

EXCLUDES *states following LSD or other hallucinogens, lasting only a few days or less ["bad trips"] (305.3)*

292.2 Pathological drug intoxication

Drug reaction: NOS, idiosyncratic, pathologic } resulting in brief psychotic states

EXCLUDES *expected brief psychotic reactions to hallucinogens ["bad trips"] (305.3)*
physiological side-effects of drugs (e.g., dystonias)

✓5th **292.8 Other specified drug induced mental disorders**

292.81 Drug induced delirium

AHA: 1Q, '88, 3

292.82 Drug induced persisting dementia

292.83 Drug induced persisting amnestic disorder

292.84 Drug induced mood disorder

Depressive state induced by drugs

● **292.85 Drug induced sleep disorders**

Drug induced circadian rhythm sleep disorder
Drug induced hypersomnia
Drug induced insomnia
Drug induced parasomnia

292.89 Other

Drug induced anxiety disorder
Drug induced organic personality syndrome
Drug induced sexual dysfunction
Drug intoxication

292.9 Unspecified drug induced mental disorder

Drug related disorder NOS
Organic psychosis NOS due to or associated with drugs

✓4th **293 Transient mental disorders due to conditions classified elsewhere**

INCLUDES transient organic mental disorders not associated with alcohol or drugs

Code first the associated physical or neurological condition

EXCLUDES *confusional state or delirium superimposed on senile dementia (290.3)*
dementia due to:
alcohol (291.0-291.9)
arteriosclerosis (290.40-290.43)
drugs (292.82)
senility (290.0)

293.0 Delirium due to conditions classified elsewhere

Acute:
confusional state
infective psychosis
organic reaction
posttraumatic organic psychosis
psycho-organic syndrome
Acute psychosis associated with endocrine, metabolic, or cerebrovascular disorder
Epileptic:
confusional state
twilight state

AHA: 1Q, '88, 3

293.1 Subacute delirium

Subacute:
confusional state
infective psychosis
organic reaction
posttraumatic organic psychosis
psycho-organic syndrome
psychosis associated with endocrine or metabolic disorder

✓5th **293.8 Other specified transient mental disorders due to conditions classified elsewhere**

293.81 Psychotic disorder with delusions in conditions classified elsewhere
Transient organic psychotic condition, paranoid type

293.82 Psychotic disorder with hallucinations in conditions classified elsewhere
Transient organic psychotic condition, hallucinatory type

293.83 Mood disorder in conditions classified elsewhere
Transient organic psychotic condition, depressive type

293.84 Anxiety disorder in conditions classified elsewhere
AHA: 4Q, '96, 29

293.89 Other
Catatonic disorder in conditions classified elsewhere

293.9 Unspecified transient mental disorder in conditions classified elsewhere
Organic psychosis:
- infective NOS
- posttraumatic NOS
- transient NOS

Psycho-organic syndrome

✓4th **294 Persistent mental disorders due to conditions classified elsewhere**
INCLUDES organic psychotic brain syndromes (chronic), not elsewhere classified
AHA: M-A, '85, 12

294.0 Amnestic disorder in conditions classified elsewhere
Korsakoff's psychosis or syndrome (nonalcoholic)
Code first underlying condition
EXCLUDES *alcoholic:*
amnestic syndrome (291.1)
Korsakoff's psychosis (291.1)

✓5th **294.1 Dementia in conditions classified elsewhere**
Dementia of the Alzheimer's type
Code first any underlying physical condition, as:
dementia in:
- Alzheimer's disease (331.0)
- cerebral lipidoses (330.1)
- dementia with Lewy bodies (331.82)
- dementia with Parkinsonism (331.82)
- epilepsy (345.0-345.9)
- frontal dementia (331.19)
- frontotemporal dementia (331.19)
- general paresis [syphilis] (094.1)
- hepatolenticular degeneration (275.1)
- Huntington's chorea (333.4)
- Jakob-Creutzfeldt disease (046.1)
- multiple sclerosis (340)
- Pick's disease of the brain (331.11)
- polyarteritis nodosa (446.0)
- syphilis (094.1)

EXCLUDES *dementia:*
arteriosclerotic (290.40-290.43)
presenile (290.10-290.13)
senile (290.0)
epileptic psychosis NOS (294.8)

AHA: 4Q, '00, 40; 1Q, '99, 14; N-D, '85, 5

294.10 Dementia in conditions classified elsewhere without behavioral disturbance
Dementia in conditions classified elsewhere NOS

294.11 Dementia in conditions classified elsewhere with behavioral disturbance
Aggressive behavior
Combative behavior
Violent behavior
Wandering off
AHA: 4Q, '00, 41

294.8 Other persistent mental disorders due to conditions classified elsewhere
Amnestic disorder NOS
Dementia NOS
Epileptic psychosis NOS
Mixed paranoid and affective organic psychotic states
Use additional code for associated epilepsy (345.0-345.9)
EXCLUDES *mild memory disturbances, not amounting to dementia (310.1)*
AHA: 3Q, '03, 14; 1Q, '88, 5

294.9 Unspecified persistent mental disorders due to conditions classified elsewhere
Cognitive disorder NOS
Organic psychosis (chronic)

OTHER PSYCHOSES (295-299)

Use additional code to identify any associated physical disease, injury, or condition affecting the brain with psychoses classifiable to 295-298

✓4th **295 Schizophrenic disorders**
INCLUDES schizophrenia of the types described in 295.0-295.9 occurring in children
EXCLUDES *childhood type schizophrenia (299.9)*
infantile autism (299.0)

The following fifth-digit subclassification is for use with category 295:
- **0 unspecified**
- **1 subchronic**
- **2 chronic**
- **3 subchronic with acute exacerbation**
- **4 chronic with acute exacerbation**
- **5 in remission**

DEF: Group of disorders with disturbances in thought (delusions, hallucinations), mood (blunted, flattened, inappropriate affect), sense of self, relationship to world; also bizarre, purposeless behavior, repetitious activity, or inactivity.

✓5th **295.0 Simple type**
Schizophrenia simplex
EXCLUDES *latent schizophrenia (295.5)*

✓5th **295.1 Disorganized type**
Hebephrenia
Hebephrenic type schizophrenia
DEF: Inappropriate behavior; results in extreme incoherence and disorganization of time, place and sense of social appropriateness; withdrawal from routine social interaction may occur.

✓5th **295.2 Catatonic type**
Catatonic (schizophrenia):
- agitation
- excitation
- excited type
- stupor
- withdrawn type

Schizophrenic:
- catalepsy
- catatonia
- flexibilitas cerea

DEF: Extreme changes in motor activity; one extreme is decreased response or reaction to the environment and the other is spontaneous activity.

§ ✓5th **295.3 Paranoid type**
Paraphrenic schizophrenia
EXCLUDES *involutional paranoid state (297.2)*
paranoia (297.1)
paraphrenia (297.2)

DEF: Preoccupied with delusional suspicions and auditory hallucinations related to single theme; usually hostile, grandiose, overly religious, occasionally hypochondriacal.

§ ✓5th **295.4 Schizophreniform disorder**
Oneirophrenia
Schizophreniform:
attack
Schizophreniform:
psychosis, confusional type
EXCLUDES *acute forms of schizophrenia of:*
catatonic type (295.2)
hebephrenic type (295.1)
paranoid type (295.3)
simple type (295.0)
undifferentiated type (295.8)

§ ✓5th **295.5 Latent schizophrenia**
Latent schizophrenic reaction
Schizophrenia:
borderline
incipient
prepsychotic
prodromal
pseudoneurotic
pseudopsychopathic
EXCLUDES *schizoid personality (301.20-301.22)*

§ ✓5th **295.6 Residual type**
Chronic undifferentiated schizophrenia
Restzustand (schizophrenic)
Schizophrenic residual state

§ ✓5th **295.7 Schizoaffective disorder**
Cyclic schizophrenia
Mixed schizophrenic and affective psychosis
Schizo-affective psychosis
Schizophreniform psychosis, affective type

§ ✓5th **295.8 Other specified types of schizophrenia**
Acute (undifferentiated) schizophrenia
Atypical schizophrenia
Cenesthopathic schizophrenia
EXCLUDES *infantile autism (299.0)*

§ ✓5th **295.9 Unspecified schizophrenia**
Schizophrenia:
NOS
mixed NOS
undifferentiated NOS
undifferentiated type
Schizophrenic reaction NOS
Schizophreniform psychosis NOS

AHA: 3Q, '95, 6

✓4th **296 Episodic mood disorders**
INCLUDES episodic affective disorders
EXCLUDES *neurotic depression (300.4)*
reactive depressive psychosis (298.0)
reactive excitation (298.1)

The following fifth-digit subclassification is for use with categories 296.0-296.6:
0 unspecified
1 mild
2 moderate
3 severe, without mention of psychotic behavior
4 severe, specified as with psychotic behavior
5 in partial or unspecified remission
6 in full remission

AHA: M-A, '85, 14

✓5th **296.0 Bipolar I disorder, single manic episode**
Hypomania (mild) NOS
Hypomanic psychosis
Mania (monopolar) NOS
Manic-depressive psychosis or reaction:
hypomanic
manic
} single episode or unspecified
EXCLUDES *circular type, if there was a previous attack of depression (296.4)*

DEF: Mood disorder identified by hyperactivity; may show extreme agitation or exaggerated excitability; speech and thought processes may be accelerated.

✓5th **296.1 Manic disorder, recurrent episode**
Any condition classifiable to 296.0, stated to be recurrent
EXCLUDES *circular type, if there was a previous attack of depression (296.4)*

✓5th **296.2 Major depressive disorder, single episode**
Depressive psychosis
Endogenous depression
Involutional melancholia
Manic-depressive psychosis or reaction, depressed type
Monopolar depression
Psychotic depression
} single episode or unspecified
EXCLUDES *circular type, if previous attack was of manic type (296.5)*
depression NOS (311)
reactive depression (neurotic) (300.4)
psychotic (298.0)

DEF: Mood disorder that produces depression; may exhibit as sadness, low self-esteem, or guilt feelings; other manifestations may be withdrawal from friends and family; interrupted normal sleep.

✓5th **296.3 Major depressive disorder, recurrent episode**
Any condition classifiable to 296.2, stated to be recurrent
EXCLUDES *circular type, if previous attack was of manic type (296.5)*
depression NOS (311)
reactive depression (neurotic) (300.4)
psychotic (298.0)

✓5th **296.4 Bipolar I disorder, most recent episode (or current) manic**
Bipolar disorder, now manic
Manic-depressive psychosis, circular type but currently manic
EXCLUDES *brief compensatory or rebound mood swings (296.99)*

✓5th **296.5 Bipolar I disorder, most recent episode (or current) depressed**
Bipolar disorder, now depressed
Manic-depressive psychosis, circular type but currently depressed
EXCLUDES *brief compensatory or rebound mood swings (296.99)*

✓5th **296.6 Bipolar I disorder, most recent episode (or current) mixed**
Manic-depressive psychosis, circular type, mixed

296.7 Bipolar I disorder, most recent episode (or current) unspecified
Atypical bipolar affective disorder NOS
Manic-depressive psychosis, circular type, current condition not specified as either manic or depressive

DEF: Manic-depressive disorder referred to as bipolar because of the mood range from manic to depressive.

§ Requires fifth-digit. See category 295 for codes and definitions.

N Newborn Age: 0 P Pediatric Age: 0-17 M Maternity Age: 12-55 A Adult Age: 15-124 MSP Medicare Secondary Payer

5th 296.8 **Other and unspecified bipolar disorders**

296.80 **Bipolar disorder, unspecified**
Bipolar disorder NOSx
Manic-depressive:
reaction NOS
syndrome NOS

296.81 **Atypical manic disorder**

296.82 **Atypical depressive disorder**

296.89 **Other**
Bipolar II disorder
Manic-depressive psychosis, mixed type

5th 296.9 **Other and unspecified episodic mood disorder**
EXCLUDES *psychogenic affective psychoses (298.0-298.8)*

296.90 **Unspecified episodic mood disorder**
Affective psychosis NOS
Melancholia NOS
Mood disorder NOS
AHA: M-A, '85, 14

296.99 **Other specified episodic mood disorder**
Mood swings:
brief compensatory
rebound

4th 297 **Delusional disorders**
INCLUDES paranoid disorders
EXCLUDES *acute paranoid reaction (298.3)*
alcoholic jealousy or paranoid state (291.5)
paranoid schizophrenia (295.3)

297.0 **Paranoid state, simple**

297.1 **Delusional disorder**
Chronic paranoid psychosis
Sander's disease
Systematized delusions
EXCLUDES *paranoid personality disorder (301.0)*

297.2 **Paraphrenia**
Involutional paranoid state
Late paraphrenia
Paraphrenia (involutional)
DEF: Paranoid schizophrenic disorder that persists over a prolonged period but does not distort personality despite persistent delusions.

297.3 **Shared psychotic disorder**
Folie à deux
Induced psychosis or paranoid disorder
DEF: Mental disorder two people share; first person with the delusional disorder convinces second person because of a close relationship and shared experiences to accept the delusions.

297.8 **Other specified paranoid states**
Paranoia querulans
Sensitiver Beziehungswahn
EXCLUDES *acute paranoid reaction or state (298.3)*
senile paranoid state (290.20)

297.9 **Unspecified paranoid state**
Paranoid:
disorder NOS
psychosis NOS
Paranoid:
reaction NOS
state NOS
AHA: J-A, '85, 9

4th 298 **Other nonorganic psychoses**
INCLUDES psychotic conditions due to or provoked by:
emotional stress
environmental factors as major part of etiology

298.0 **Depressive type psychosis**
Psychogenic depressive psychosis
Psychotic reactive depression
Reactive depressive psychosis
EXCLUDES *manic-depressive psychosis, depressed type (296.2-296.3)*
neurotic depression (300.4)
reactive depression NOS (300.4)

298.1 **Excitative type psychosis**
Acute hysterical psychosis
Psychogenic excitation
Reactive excitation
EXCLUDES *manic-depressive psychosis, manic type (296.0-296.1)*
DEF: Affective disorder similar to manic-depressive psychosis, in the manic phase, seemingly brought on by stress.

298.2 **Reactive confusion**
Psychogenic confusion
Psychogenic twilight state
EXCLUDES *acute confusional state (293.0)*
DEF: Confusion, disorientation, cloudiness in consciousness; brought on by severe emotional upheaval.

298.3 **Acute paranoid reaction**
Acute psychogenic paranoid psychosis
Bouffée délirante
EXCLUDES *paranoid states (297.0-297.9)*

298.4 **Psychogenic paranoid psychosis**
Protracted reactive paranoid psychosis

298.8 **Other and unspecified reactive psychosis**
Brief psychotic disorder
Brief reactive psychosis NOS
Hysterical psychosis
Psychogenic psychosis NOS
Psychogenic stupor
EXCLUDES *acute hysterical psychosis (298.1)*

298.9 **Unspecified psychosis**
Atypical psychosis
Psychosis NOS
Psychotic disorder NOS

4th 299 **Pervasive developmental disorders**
EXCLUDES *adult type psychoses occurring in childhood, as:*
affective disorders (296.0-296.9)
manic-depressive disorders (296.0-296.9)
schizophrenia (295.0-295.9)

The following fifth-digit subclassification is for use with category 299:
0 current or active state
1 residual state

5th 299.0 **Autistic disorder**
Childhood autism
Infantile psychosis
Kanner's syndrome
EXCLUDES *disintegrative psychosis (299.1)*
Heller's syndrome (299.1)
schizophrenic syndrome of childhood (299.9)
DEF: Severe mental disorder of children, results in impaired social behavior; abnormal development of communicative skills, appears to be unaware of the need for emotional support and offers little emotional response to family members.

5th 299.1 **Childhood disintegrative disorder**
Heller's syndrome
Use additional code to identify any associated neurological disorder
EXCLUDES *infantile autism (299.0)*
schizophrenic syndrome of childhood (299.9)
DEF: Mental disease of children identified by impaired development of reciprocal social skills, verbal and nonverbal communication skills, imaginative play.

5th 299.8 **Other specified pervasive developmental disorders**
Asperger's disorder
Atypical childhood psychosis
Borderline psychosis of childhood
EXCLUDES *simple stereotypes without psychotic disturbance (307.3)*

§ ✓5th **299.9 Unspecified pervasive developmental disorder**
Child psychosis NOS
Schizophrenia, childhood type NOS
Schizophrenic syndrome of childhood NOS
EXCLUDES *schizophrenia of adult type occurring in childhood (295.0-295.9)*

NEUROTIC DISORDERS, PERSONALITY DISORDERS, AND OTHER NONPSYCHOTIC MENTAL DISORDERS (300-316)

✓4th **300 Anxiety, dissociative and somatoform disorders**

✓5th **300.0 Anxiety states**
EXCLUDES *anxiety in:*
acute stress reaction (308.0)
transient adjustment reaction (309.24)
neurasthenia (300.5)
psychophysiological disorders (306.0-306.9)
separation anxiety (309.21)

DEF: Mental disorder characterized by anxiety and avoidance behavior not particularly related to any specific situation or stimulus; symptoms include emotional instability, apprehension, fatigue.

300.00 Anxiety state, unspecified
Anxiety:
neurosis
reaction
Anxiety:
state (neurotic)
Atypical anxiety disorder
AHA: 1Q, '02, 6

300.01 Panic disorder without agoraphobia
Panic:
attack
Panic:
state
EXCLUDES *panic disorder with agoraphobia (300.21)*

DEF: Neurotic disorder characterized by recurrent panic or anxiety, apprehension, fear or terror; symptoms include shortness of breath, palpitations, dizziness, faintness or shakiness; fear of dying may persist or fear of other morbid consequences.

300.02 Generalized anxiety disorder

300.09 Other

✓5th **300.1 Dissociative, conversion and factitious disorders**
EXCLUDES *adjustment reaction (309.0-309.9)*
anorexia nervosa (307.1)
gross stress reaction (308.0-308.9)
hysterical personality (301.50-301.59)
psychophysiologic disorders (306.0-306.9)

300.10 Hysteria, unspecified

300.11 Conversion disorder
Astasia-abasia, hysterical
Conversion hysteria or reaction
Hysterical
blindness
deafness
paralysis
AHA: N-D, '85, 15

DEF: Mental disorder that impairs physical functions with no physiological basis; sensory motor symptoms include seizures, paralysis, temporary blindness; increase in stress or avoidance of unpleasant responsibilities may precipitate.

300.12 Dissociative amnesia
Hysterical amnesia

300.13 Dissociative fugue
Hysterical fugue

DEF: Dissociative hysteria; identified by loss of memory, flight from familiar surroundings; conscious activity is not associated with perception of surroundings, no later memory of episode.

300.14 Dissociative identity disorder
Dissociative identity disorder

300.15 Dissociative disorder or reaction, unspecified

DEF: Hysterical neurotic episode; sudden but temporary changes in perceived identity, memory, consciousness, segregated memory patterns exist separate from dominant personality.

300.16 Factitious disorder with predominantly psychological signs and symptoms
Compensation neurosis
Ganser's syndrome, hysterical

DEF: A disorder characterized by the purposeful assumption of mental illness symptoms; the symptoms are not real, possibly representing what the patient imagines mental illness to be like, and are acted out more often when another person is present.

300.19 Other and unspecified factitious illness
Factitious disorder (with combined psychological and physical signs and symptoms) (with predominantly physical signs and symptoms) NOS
EXCLUDES *multiple operations or hospital addiction syndrome (301.51)*

✓5th **300.2 Phobic disorders**
EXCLUDES *anxiety state not associated with a specific situation or object (300.00-300.09)*
obsessional phobias (300.3)

300.20 Phobia, unspecified
Anxiety-hysteria NOS
Phobia NOS

300.21 Agoraphobia with panic disorder
Fear of:
open spaces }
streets } with panic attacks
travel }
Panic disorder with agoraphobia
EXCLUDES *agoraphobia without panic disorder (300.22)*
panic disorder without agoraphobia (300.01)

300.22 Agoraphobia without mention of panic attacks
Any condition classifiable to 300.21 without mention of panic attacks

300.23 Social phobia
Fear of:
eating in public
public speaking
Fear of:
washing in public

300.29 Other isolated or specific phobias
Acrophobia
Animal phobias
Claustrophobia
Fear of crowds

300.3 Obsessive-compulsive disorders
Anancastic neurosis
Compulsive neurosis
Obsessional phobia [any]
EXCLUDES *obsessive-compulsive symptoms occurring in:*
endogenous depression (296.2-296.3)
organic states (eg., encephalitis)
schizophrenia (295.0-295.9)

§ Requres fifth-digit. See category 299 for codes and definitions.

N Newborn Age: 0 P Pediatric Age: 0-17 M Maternity Age: 12-55 A Adult Age: 15-124 MSP Medicare Secondary Payer

300.4 Dysthymic disorder
Anxiety depression
Depression with anxiety
Depressive reaction
Neurotic depressive state
Reactive depression
EXCLUDES *adjustment reaction with depressive symptoms (309.0-309.1)*
depression NOS (311)
manic-depressive psychosis, depressed type (296.2-296.3)
reactive depressive psychosis (298.0)

DEF: Depression without psychosis; less severe depression related to personal change or unexpected circumstances; also referred to as "reactional depression."

300.5 Neurasthenia
Fatigue neurosis
Nervous debility
Psychogenic:
asthenia
general fatigue
Use additional code to identify any associated physical disorder
EXCLUDES *anxiety state (300.00-300.09)*
neurotic depression (300.4)
psychophysiological disorders (306.0-306.9)
specific nonpsychotic mental disorders following organic brain damage (310.0-310.9)

DEF: Physical and mental symptoms caused primarily by what is known as mental exhaustion; symptoms include chronic weakness, fatigue.

300.6 Depersonalization disorder
Derealization (neurotic)
Neurotic state with depersonalization episode
EXCLUDES *depersonalization associated with:*
anxiety (300.00-300.09)
depression (300.4)
manic-depressive disorder or psychosis (296.0-296.9)
schizophrenia (295.0-295.9)

DEF: Dissociative disorder characterized by feelings of strangeness about self or body image; symptoms include dizziness, anxiety, fear of insanity, loss of reality of surroundings.

300.7 Hypochondriasis
Body dysmorphic disorder
EXCLUDES *hypochondriasis in:*
hysteria (300.10-300.19)
manic-depressive psychosis, depressed type (296.2-296.3)
neurasthenia (300.5)
obsessional disorder (300.3)
schizophrenia (295.0-295.9)

✓5th **300.8 Somatoform disorders**

300.81 Somatization disorder
Briquet's disorder
Severe somatoform disorder

300.82 Undifferentiated somatoform disorder
Atypical somatoform disorder
Somatoform disorder NOS
AHA: 4Q, '96, 29

DEF: Disorders in which patients have symptoms that suggest an organic disease but no evidence of physical disorder after repeated testing.

300.89 Other somatoform disorders
Occupational neurosis, including writers' cramp
Psychasthenia
Psychasthenic neurosis

300.9 Unspecified nonpsychotic mental disorder
Psychoneurosis NOS

✓4th **301 Personality disorders**
INCLUDES character neurosis
Use additional code to identify any associated neurosis or psychosis, or physical condition
EXCLUDES *nonpsychotic personality disorder associated with organic brain syndromes (310.0-310.9)*

301.0 Paranoid personality disorder
Fanatic personality
Paranoid personality (disorder)
Paranoid traits
EXCLUDES *acute paranoid reaction (298.3)*
alcoholic paranoia (291.5)
paranoid schizophrenia (295.3)
paranoid states (297.0-297.9)
AHA: J-A, '85, 9

✓5th **301.1 Affective personality disorder**
EXCLUDES *affective psychotic disorders (296.0-296.9)*
neurasthenia (300.5)
neurotic depression (300.4)

301.10 Affective personality disorder, unspecified

301.11 Chronic hypomanic personality disorder
Chronic hypomanic disorder
Hypomanic personality

301.12 Chronic depressive personality disorder
Chronic depressive disorder
Depressive character or personality

301.13 Cyclothymic disorder
Cycloid personality
Cyclothymia
Cyclothymic personality

✓5th **301.2 Schizoid personality disorder**
EXCLUDES *schizophrenia (295.0-295.9)*

301.20 Schizoid personality disorder, unspecified

301.21 Introverted personality

301.22 Schizotypal personality disorder

301.3 Explosive personality disorder
Aggressive:
personality
reaction
Aggressiveness
Emotional instability (excessive)
Pathological emotionality
Quarrelsomeness
EXCLUDES *dyssocial personality (301.7)*
hysterical neurosis (300.10-300.19)

301.4 Obsessive-compulsive personality disorder
Anancastic personality
Obsessional personality
EXCLUDES *obsessive-compulsive disorder (300.3)*
phobic state (300.20-300.29)

✓5th **301.5 Histrionic personality disorder**
EXCLUDES *hysterical neurosis (300.10-300.19)*

DEF: Extreme emotional behavior, often theatrical; often concerned about own appeal; may demand attention, exhibit seductive behavior.

301.50 Histrionic personality disorder, unspecified
Hysterical personality NOS

301.51 Chronic factitious illness with physical symptoms
Hospital addiction syndrome
Multiple operations syndrome
Munchausen syndrome

301.59 Other histrionic personality disorder
Personality:
emotionally unstable
labile
psychoinfantile

301.6 Dependent personality disorder
Asthenic personality
Passive personality
Inadequate personality
EXCLUDES *neurasthenia (300.5)*
passive-aggressive personality (301.84)
DEF: Overwhelming feeling of helplessness; fears of abandonment may persist; difficulty in making personal decisions without confirmation by others; low self-esteem due to irrational sensitivity to criticism.

301.7 Antisocial personality disorder
Amoral personality
Asocial personality
Dyssocial personality
Personality disorder with predominantly sociopathic or asocial manifestation
EXCLUDES *disturbance of conduct without specifiable personality disorder (312.0-312.9)*
explosive personality (301.3)
AHA: S-0, '84, 16
DEF: Continuous antisocial behavior that violates rights of others; social traits include extreme aggression, total disregard for traditional social rules.

✓5th **301.8 Other personality disorders**

301.81 Narcissistic personality disorder
DEF: Grandiose fantasy or behavior, lack of social empathy, hypersensitive to the lack of others' judgment, exploits others; also sense of entitlement to have expectations met, need for continual admiration.

301.82 Avoidant personality disorder
DEF: Personality disorder marked by feelings of social inferiority; sensitivity to criticism, emotionally restrained due to fear of rejection.

301.83 Borderline personality disorder
DEF: Personality disorder characterized by unstable moods, self-image, and interpersonal relationships; uncontrolled anger, impulsive and self-destructive acts, fears of abandonment, feelings of emptiness and boredom, recurrent suicide threats or self-mutilation.

301.84 Passive-aggressive personality
DEF: Pattern of procrastination and refusal to meet standards; introduce own obstacles to success and exploit failure.

301.89 Other
Personality:
eccentric
"haltlose" type
immature
Personality:
masochistic
psychoneurotic
EXCLUDES *psychoinfantile personality (301.59)*

301.9 Unspecified personality disorder
Pathological personality NOS
Personality disorder NOS
Psychopathic:
constitutional state
personality (disorder)

✓4th **302 Sexual and gender identity disorders**
EXCLUDES *sexual disorder manifest in:*
organic brain syndrome (290.0-294.9, 310.0-310.9)
psychosis (295.0-298.9)

302.0 Ego-dystonic sexual orientation
Ego-dystonic lesbianism
Sexual orientation conflict disorder
EXCLUDES *homosexual pedophilia (302.2)*

302.1 Zoophilia
Bestiality
DEF: A sociodeviant disorder marked by engaging in sexual intercourse with animals.

302.2 Pedophilia
DEF: A sociodeviant condition of adults characterized by sexual activity with children.

302.3 Transvestic fetishism
EXCLUDES *trans-sexualism (302.5)*
DEF: The desire to dress in clothing of opposite sex.

302.4 Exhibitionism
DEF: Sexual deviant behavior; exposure of genitals to strangers; behavior prompted by intense sexual urges and fantasies.

✓5th **302.5 Trans-sexualism**
EXCLUDES *transvestism (302.3)*
DEF: Gender identity disturbance; overwhelming desire to change anatomic sex, due to belief that individual is a member of the opposite sex.

302.50 With unspecified sexual history
302.51 With asexual history
302.52 With homosexual history
302.53 With heterosexual history

302.6 Gender identity disorder in children
Feminism in boys
Gender identity disorder NOS
EXCLUDES *gender identity disorder in adult (302.85)*
trans-sexualism (302.50-302.53)
transvestism (302.3)

✓5th **302.7 Psychosexual dysfunction**
EXCLUDES *impotence of organic origin (607.84)*
normal transient symptoms from ruptured hymen
transient or occasional failures of erection due to fatigue, anxiety, alcohol, or drugs

302.70 Psychosexual dysfunction, unspecified
Sexual dysfunction NOS

302.71 Hypoactive sexual desire disorder
EXCLUDES *decreased sexual desire NOS (799.81)*

302.72 With inhibited sexual excitement
Female sexual arousal disorder
Frigidity
Impotence
Male erectile disorder

302.73 Female orgasmic disorder ♀
302.74 Male orgasmic disorder ♂
302.75 Premature ejaculation ♂
302.76 Dyspareunia, psychogenic ♀
Dyspareunia, psychogenic
DEF: Difficult or painful sex due to psychosomatic state.

302.79 With other specified psychosexual dysfunctions
Sexual aversion disorder

✓5th **302.8 Other specified psychosexual disorders**

302.81 Fetishism
DEF: Psychosexual disorder noted for intense sexual urges and arousal precipitated by fantasies; use of inanimate objects, such as clothing, to stimulate sexual arousal, orgasm.

302.82 Voyeurism
DEF: Psychosexual disorder characterized by uncontrollable impulse to observe others, without their knowledge, who are nude or engaged in sexual activity.

302.83 Sexual masochism
DEF: Psychosexual disorder noted for need to achieve sexual gratification through humiliating or hurtful acts inflicted on self.

302.84 Sexual sadism
DEF: Psychosexual disorder noted for need to achieve sexual gratification through humiliating or hurtful acts inflicted on someone else.

N Newborn Age: 0   P Pediatric Age: 0-17   M Maternity Age: 12-55   A Adult Age: 15-124   MSP Medicare Secondary Payer

302.85 **Gender identity disorder in adolescents or adults**
EXCLUDES *gender identity disorder NOS (302.6)*
gender identity disorder in children (302.6)

302.89 **Other**
Frotteurism
Nymphomania
Satyriasis

302.9 **Unspecified psychosexual disorder**
Paraphilia NOS
Pathologic sexuality NOS
Sexual deviation NOS
Sexual disorder NOS

✓4th **303 Alcohol dependence syndrome**
Use additional code to identify any associated condition, as:
alcoholic psychoses (291.0-291.9)
drug dependence (304.0-304.9)
physical complications of alcohol, such as:
cerebral degeneration (331.7)
cirrhosis of liver (571.2)
epilepsy (345.0-345.9)
gastritis (535.3)
hepatitis (571.1)
liver damage NOS (571.3)
EXCLUDES *drunkenness NOS (305.0)*

The following fifth-digit subclassification is for use with category 303:
0 **unspecified**
1 **continuous**
2 **episodic**
3 **in remission**

AHA: 3Q, '95, 6; 2Q, '91, 9; 4Q, '88, 8; S-O, '86, 3

✓5th 303.0 **Acute alcoholic intoxication**
Acute drunkenness in alcoholism

✓5th 303.9 **Other and unspecified alcohol dependence**
Chronic alcoholism
Dipsomania
AHA: 2Q, '02, 4; 2Q, '89, 9

✓4th **304 Drug dependence**
EXCLUDES *nondependent abuse of drugs (305.1-305.9)*

The following fifth-digit subclassification is for use with category 304:
0 **unspecified**
1 **continuous**
2 **episodic**
3 **in remission**

AHA: 2Q, '91, 10; 4Q, '88, 8; S-O, '86, 3

✓5th 304.0 **Opioid type dependence**
Heroin
Meperidine
Methadone
Morphine
Opium
Opium alkaloids and their derivatives
Synthetics with morphine-like effects

✓5th 304.1 **Sedative, hypnotic or anxiolytic dependence**
Barbiturates
Nonbarbiturate sedatives and tranquilizers with a similar effect:
chlordiazepoxide
diazepam
glutethimide
meprobamate
methaqualone

✓5th 304.2 **Cocaine dependence**
Coca leaves and derivatives

✓5th 304.3 **Cannabis dependence**
Hashish
Hemp
Marihuana

✓5th 304.4 **Amphetamine and other psychostimulant dependence**
Methylphenidate
Phenmetrazine

✓5th 304.5 **Hallucinogen dependence**
Dimethyltryptamine [DMT]
Lysergic acid diethylamide [LSD] and derivatives
Mescaline
Psilocybin

✓5th 304.6 **Other specified drug dependence**
Absinthe addiction
Glue sniffing
Inhalant dependence
Phencyclidine dependence
EXCLUDES *tobacco dependence (305.1)*

✓5th 304.7 **Combinations of opioid type drug with any other**
AHA: M-A, '86, 12

✓5th 304.8 **Combinations of drug dependence excluding opioid type drug**
AHA: M-A, '86, 12

✓5th 304.9 **Unspecified drug dependence**
Drug addiction NOS
Drug dependence NOS
AHA: For code 304.90: 4Q, '03, 103

✓4th **305 Nondependent abuse of drugs**
Note: Includes cases where a person, for whom no other diagnosis is possible, has come under medical care because of the maladaptive effect of a drug on which he is not dependent and that he has taken on his own initiative to the detriment of his health or social functioning.
EXCLUDES *alcohol dependence syndrome (303.0-303.9)*
drug dependence (304.0-304.9)
drug withdrawal syndrome (292.0)
poisoning by drugs or medicinal substances (960.0-979.9)

The following fifth-digit subclassification is for use with codes 305.0, 305.2-305.9:
0 **unspecified**
1 **continuous**
2 **episodic**
3 **in remission**

AHA: 2Q, '91, 10; 4Q, '88, 8; S-O, '86, 3

✓5th 305.0 **Alcohol abuse**
Drunkenness NOS
Excessive drinking of alcohol NOS
"Hangover" (alcohol)
Inebriety NOS
EXCLUDES *acute alcohol intoxication in alcoholism (303.0)*
alcoholic psychoses (291.0-291.9)
AHA: 3Q, '96, 16

305.1 **Tobacco use disorder**
Tobacco dependence
EXCLUDES *history of tobacco use (V15.82)*
AHA: 2Q, '96, 10; N-D, '84, 12

✓5th 305.2 **Cannabis abuse**

✓5th 305.3 **Hallucinogen abuse**
Acute intoxication from hallucinogens ["bad trips"]
LSD reaction

✓5th 305.4 **Sedative, hypnotic or anxiolytic abuse**

✓5th 305.5 **Opioid abuse**

✓5th 305.6 **Cocaine abuse**
AHA: 1Q, '93, 25 ►For code 305.60: 1Q, '05, 6◄

✓5th 305.7 **Amphetamine or related acting sympathomimetic abuse**
AHA: For code 305.70: 2Q, '03, 10-11

✓5th 305.8 **Antidepressant type abuse**

✓5th 305.9 **Other, mixed, or unspecified drug abuse**
Caffeine intoxication
Inhalant abuse
"Laxative habit"
Misuse of drugs NOS
Nonprescribed use of drugs or patent medicinals
Phencyclidine abuse
AHA: 3Q, '99, 20

✓4th **306 Physiological malfunction arising from mental factors**

INCLUDES psychogenic:
physical symptoms, physiological manifestations } not involving tissue damage

EXCLUDES *hysteria (300.11-300.19)*
physical symptoms secondary to a psychiatric disorder classified elsewhere
psychic factors associated with physical conditions involving tissue damage classified elsewhere (316)
specific nonpsychotic mental disorders following organic brain damage (310.0-310.9)

DEF: Functional disturbances or interruptions due to mental or psychological causes; no tissue damage sustained in these conditions.

306.0 Musculoskeletal
Psychogenic paralysis
Psychogenic torticollis
EXCLUDES *Gilles de la Tourette's syndrome (307.23)*
paralysis as hysterical or conversion reaction (300.11)
tics (307.20-307.22)

306.1 Respiratory
Psychogenic:
air hunger
cough
hiccough
hyperventilation
yawning
EXCLUDES *psychogenic asthma (316 and 493.9)*

306.2 Cardiovascular
Cardiac neurosis
Cardiovascular neurosis
Neurocirculatory asthenia
Psychogenic cardiovascular disorder
EXCLUDES *psychogenic paroxysmal tachycardia (316 and 427.2)*

AHA: J-A, '85, 14

DEF: Neurocirculatory asthenia: functional nervous and circulatory irregularities with palpitations, dyspnea, fatigue, rapid pulse, precordial pain, fear of effort, discomfort during exercise, anxiety; also called DaCosta's syndrome, Effort syndrome, Irritable or Soldier's Heart.

306.3 Skin
Psychogenic pruritus
EXCLUDES *psychogenic:*
alopecia (316 and 704.00)
dermatitis (316 and 692.9)
eczema (316 and 691.8 or 692.9)
urticaria (316 and 708.0-708.9)

306.4 Gastrointestinal
Aerophagy
Cyclical vomiting, psychogenic
Diarrhea, psychogenic
Nervous gastritis
Psychogenic dyspepsia
EXCLUDES *cyclical vomiting NOS (536.2)*
globus hystericus (300.11)
mucous colitis (316 and 564.9)
psychogenic:
cardiospasm (316 and 530.0)
duodenal ulcer (316 and 532.0-532.9)
gastric ulcer (316 and 531.0-531.9)
peptic ulcer NOS (316 and 533.0-533.9)
vomiting NOS (307.54)

AHA: 2Q, '89, 11

DEF: Aerophagy: excess swallowing of air, usually unconscious; related to anxiety; results in distended abdomen or belching, often interpreted by the patient as a physical disorder.

✓5th **306.5 Genitourinary**
EXCLUDES *enuresis, psychogenic (307.6)*
frigidity (302.72)
impotence (302.72)
psychogenic dyspareunia (302.76)

306.50 Psychogenic genitourinary malfunction, unspecified

306.51 Psychogenic vaginismus ♀
Functional vaginismus

DEF: Psychogenic response resulting in painful contractions of vaginal canal muscles; can be severe enough to prevent sexual intercourse.

306.52 Psychogenic dysmenorrhea ♀

306.53 Psychogenic dysuria

306.59 Other
AHA: M-A, '87, 11

306.6 Endocrine

306.7 Organs of special sense
EXCLUDES *hysterical blindness or deafness (300.11)*
psychophysical visual disturbances (368.16)

306.8 Other specified psychophysiological malfunction
Bruxism
Teeth grinding

306.9 Unspecified psychophysiological malfunction
Psychophysiologic disorder NOS
Psychosomatic disorder NOS

✓4th **307 Special symptoms or syndromes, not elsewhere classified**

Note: This category is intended for use if the psychopathology is manifested by a single specific symptom or group of symptoms which is not part of an organic illness or other mental disorder classifiable elsewhere.

EXCLUDES *those due to mental disorders classified elsewhere*
those of organic origin

307.0 Stuttering
EXCLUDES *dysphasia (784.5)*
lisping or lalling (307.9)
retarded development of speech (315.31-315.39)

307.1 Anorexia nervosa
EXCLUDES *eating disturbance NOS (307.50)*
feeding problem (783.3)
of nonorganic origin (307.59)
loss of appetite (783.0)
of nonorganic origin (307.59)

AHA: 4Q, '89, 11

✓5th **307.2 Tics**
EXCLUDES *nail-biting or thumb-sucking (307.9)*
stereotypes occurring in isolation (307.3)
tics of organic origin (333.3)

DEF: Involuntary muscle response usually confined to the face, shoulders.

307.20 Tic disorder, unspecified
Tic disorder NOS

307.21 Transient tic disorder

307.22 Chronic motor or vocal tic disorder

307.23 Tourette's disorder
Motor-verbal tic disorder

DEF: Syndrome of facial and vocal tics in childhood; progresses to spontaneous or involuntary jerking, obscene utterances, other uncontrollable actions considered inappropriate.

N Newborn Age: 0 P Pediatric Age: 0-17 M Maternity Age: 12-55 A Adult Age: 15-124 MSP Medicare Secondary Payer

307.3 Stereotypic movement disorder

Body-rocking
Head banging
Spasmus nutans
Stereotypes NOS

EXCLUDES *tics (307.20-307.23)*
of organic origin (333.3)

✓5th **307.4 Specific disorders of sleep of nonorganic origin**

EXCLUDES *narcolepsy (347.00-347.11)*
▶*organic hypersomnia (327.10-327.19)*
organic insomnia (327.00-327.09)◀
those of unspecified cause (780.50-780.59)

307.40 Nonorganic sleep disorder, unspecified

307.41 Transient disorder of initiating or maintaining sleep

▶Adjustment insomnia◀
Hyposomnia, Insomnia, Sleeplessness } associated with intermittent emotional reactions or conflicts

307.42 Persistent disorder of initiating or maintaining sleep

Hyposomnia, insomnia, or sleeplessness associated with:
anxiety
conditioned arousal
depression (major) (minor)
psychosis
▶Idiopathic insomnia
Paradoxical insomnia
Primary insomnia
Psychophysiological insomnia◀

307.43 Transient disorder of initiating or maintaining wakefulness

Hypersomnia associated with acute or intermittent emotional reactions or conflicts

307.44 Persistent disorder of initiating or maintaining wakefulness

Hypersomnia associated with depression (major) (minor)
▶Insufficient sleep syndrome
Primary hypersomnia◀

EXCLUDES ▶ *sleep deprivation (V69.4)*◀

▲ **307.45 Circadian rhythm sleep disorder of nonorganic origin**

307.46 Sleep arousal disorder

Night terror disorder
Night terrors
Sleep terror disorder
Sleepwalking
Somnambulism

DEF: Sleepwalking marked by extreme terror, panic, screaming, confusion; no recall of event upon arousal; term may refer to simply the act of sleepwalking.

307.47 Other dysfunctions of sleep stages or arousal from sleep

Nightmare disorder
Nightmares:
NOS
REM-sleep type
Sleep drunkenness

307.48 Repetitive intrusions of sleep

Repetitive intrusion of sleep with:
atypical polysomnographic features
environmental disturbances
repeated REM-sleep interruptions

307.49 Other

"Short-sleeper"
Subjective insomnia complaint

✓5th **307.5 Other and unspecified disorders of eating**

EXCLUDES *anorexia:*
nervosa (307.1)
of unspecified cause (783.0)
overeating, of unspecified cause (783.6)
vomiting:
NOS (787.0)
cyclical (536.2)
psychogenic (306.4)

307.50 Eating disorder, unspecified

Eating disorder NOS

307.51 Bulimia nervosa

Overeating of nonorganic origin

DEF: Mental disorder commonly characterized by binge eating followed by self-induced vomiting; perceptions of being fat; and fear the inability to stop eating voluntarily.

307.52 Pica

Perverted appetite of nonorganic origin

DEF: Compulsive eating disorder characterized by craving for substances, other than food; such as paint chips or dirt.

307.53 Rumination disorder

Regurgitation, of nonorganic origin, of food with reswallowing

EXCLUDES *obsessional rumination (300.3)*

307.54 Psychogenic vomiting

307.59 Other

▶Feeding disorder of infancy or early childhood of nonorganic origin◀
Infantile feeding disturbances, Loss of appetite } of nonorganic origin

307.6 Enuresis

Enuresis (primary) (secondary) of nonorganic origin

EXCLUDES *enuresis of unspecified cause (788.3)*

DEF: Involuntary urination past age of normal control; also called bedwetting; no trace to biological problem; focus on psychological issues.

307.7 Encopresis

Encopresis (continuous) (discontinuous) of nonorganic origin

EXCLUDES *encopresis of unspecified cause (787.6)*

DEF: Inability to control bowel movements; cause traced to psychological, not biological, problems.

✓5th **307.8 Pain disorders related to psychological factors**

307.80 Psychogenic pain, site unspecified

307.81 Tension headache

EXCLUDES *headache:*
NOS (784.0)
migraine (346.0-346.9)

AHA: N-D, '85, 16

307.89 Other

Code first to site of pain

EXCLUDES *pain disorder exclusively attributed to psychological factors (307.80)*
psychogenic pain (307.80)

307.9 Other and unspecified special symptoms or syndromes, not elsewhere classified

Communication disorder NOS
Hair plucking
Lalling
Lisping
Masturbation
Nail-biting
Thumb-sucking

✓4th **308 Acute reaction to stress**

INCLUDES catastrophic stress
combat fatigue
gross stress reaction (acute)
transient disorders in response to exceptional physical or mental stress which usually subside within hours or days

EXCLUDES *adjustment reaction or disorder (309.0-309.9)*
chronic stress reaction (309.1-309.9)

308.0 Predominant disturbance of emotions

Anxiety
Emotional crisis
Panic state
} as acute reaction to exceptional [gross] stress

308.1 Predominant disturbance of consciousness

Fugues as acute reaction to exceptional [gross] stress

308.2 Predominant psychomotor disturbance

Agitation states
Stupor
} as acute reaction to exceptional [gross] stress

308.3 Other acute reactions to stress

Acute situational disturbance
Acute stress disorder

EXCLUDES *prolonged posttraumatic emotional disturbance (309.81)*

308.4 Mixed disorders as reaction to stress

308.9 Unspecified acute reaction to stress

✓4th **309 Adjustment reaction**

INCLUDES adjustment disorders
reaction (adjustment) to chronic stress

EXCLUDES *acute reaction to major stress (308.0-308.9)*
neurotic disorders (300.0-300.9)

309.0 Adjustment disorder with depressed mood

Grief reaction

EXCLUDES *affective psychoses (296.0-296.9)*
neurotic depression (300.4)
prolonged depressive reaction (309.1)
psychogenic depressive psychosis (298.0)

309.1 Prolonged depressive reaction

EXCLUDES *affective psychoses (296.0-296.9)*
brief depressive reaction (309.0)
neurotic depression (300.4)
psychogenic depressive psychosis (298.0)

✓5th **309.2 With predominant disturbance of other emotions**

309.21 Separation anxiety disorder

DEF: Abnormal apprehension by a child when physically separated from support environment; byproduct of abnormal symbiotic child-parent relationship.

309.22 Emancipation disorder of adolescence and early adult life

DEF: Adjustment reaction of late adolescence; conflict over independence from parental supervision; symptoms include difficulty in making decisions, increased reliance on parental advice, deliberate adoption of values in opposition of parents.

309.23 Specific academic or work inhibition

309.24 Adjustment disorder with anxiety

309.28 Adjustment disorder with mixed anxiety and depressed mood

Adjustment reaction with anxiety and depression

309.29 Other

Culture shock

309.3 Adjustment disorder with disturbance of conduct

Conduct disturbance
Destructiveness
} as adjustment reaction

EXCLUDES *destructiveness in child (312.9)*
disturbance of conduct NOS (312.9)
dyssocial behavior without manifest psychiatric disorder (V71.01-V71.02)
personality disorder with predominantly sociopathic or asocial manifestations (301.7)

309.4 Adjustment disorder with mixed disturbance of emotions and conduct

✓5th **309.8 Other specified adjustment reactions**

309.81 Posttraumatic stress disorder

Chronic posttraumatic stress disorder
Concentration camp syndrome
Posttraumatic stress disorder NOS

EXCLUDES *acute stress disorder (308.3)*
posttraumatic brain syndrome:
nonpsychotic (310.2)
psychotic (293.0-293.9)

DEF: Preoccupation with traumatic events beyond normal experience; events such as rape, personal assault, combat, natural disasters, accidents, torture precipitate disorder; also recurring flashbacks of trauma; symptoms include difficulty remembering, sleeping, or concentrating, and guilt feelings for surviving.

309.82 Adjustment reaction with physical symptoms

309.83 Adjustment reaction with withdrawal

Elective mutism as adjustment reaction
Hospitalism (in children) NOS

309.89 Other

309.9 Unspecified adjustment reaction

Adaptation reaction NOS
Adjustment reaction NOS

✓4th **310 Specific nonpsychotic mental disorders due to brain damage**

EXCLUDES *neuroses, personality disorders, or other nonpsychotic conditions occurring in a form similar to that seen with functional disorders but in association with a physical condition (300.0-300.9, 301.0-301.9)*

310.0 Frontal lobe syndrome

Lobotomy syndrome
Postleucotomy syndrome [state]

EXCLUDES *postcontusion syndrome (310.2)*

310.1 Personality change due to conditions classified elsewhere

Cognitive or personality change of other type, of nonpsychotic severity
Organic psychosyndrome of nonpsychotic severity
Presbyophrenia NOS
Senility with mental changes of nonpsychotic severity

EXCLUDES *memory loss of unknown cause (780.93)*

DEF: Personality disorder caused by organic factors, such as brain lesions, head trauma, or cerebrovascular accident (CVA).

310.2 Postconcussion syndrome
Postcontusion syndrome or encephalopathy
Posttraumatic brain syndrome, nonpsychotic
Status postcommotio cerebri
EXCLUDES *frontal lobe syndrome (310.0)*
postencephalitic syndrome (310.8)
any organic psychotic conditions following head injury (293.0-294.0)

AHA: 4Q, '90, 24

DEF: Nonpsychotic disorder due to brain trauma, causes symptoms unrelated to any disease process; symptoms include amnesia, serial headaches, rapid heartbeat, fatigue, disrupted sleep patterns, inability to concentrate.

310.8 Other specified nonpsychotic mental disorders following organic brain damage
Mild memory disturbance
Postencephalitic syndrome
Other focal (partial) organic psychosyndromes

310.9 Unspecified nonpsychotic mental disorder following organic brain damage
AHA: 4Q, '03, 103

311 Depressive disorder, not elsewhere classified
Depressive disorder NOS
Depression NOS
Depressive state NOS
EXCLUDES *acute reaction to major stress with depressive symptoms (308.0)*
affective personality disorder (301.10-301.13)
affective psychoses (296.0-296.9)
brief depressive reaction (309.0)
depressive states associated with stressful events (309.0-309.1)
disturbance of emotions specific to childhood and adolescence, with misery and unhappiness (313.1)
mixed adjustment reaction with depressive symptoms (309.4)
neurotic depression (300.4)
prolonged depressive adjustment reaction (309.1)
psychogenic depressive psychosis (298.0)

AHA: 4Q, '03, 75

✓4th **312 Disturbance of conduct, not elsewhere classified**
EXCLUDES *adjustment reaction with disturbance of conduct (309.3)*
drug dependence (304.0-304.9)
dyssocial behavior without manifest psychiatric disorder (V71.01-V71.02)
personality disorder with predominantly sociopathic or asocial manifestations (301.7)
sexual deviations (302.0-302.9)

The following fifth-digit subclassification is for use with categories 312.0-312.2:
- **0 unspecified**
- **1 mild**
- **2 moderate**
- **3 severe**

✓5th **312.0 Undersocialized conduct disorder, aggressive type**
Aggressive outburst
Anger reaction
Unsocialized aggressive disorder

DEF: Mental condition identified by behaviors disrespectful of others' rights and of age-appropriate social norms or rules; symptoms include bullying, vandalism, verbal and physical abusiveness, lying, stealing, defiance.

✓5th **312.1 Undersocialized conduct disorder, unaggressive type**
Childhood truancy, unsocialized
Solitary stealing
Tantrums

✓5th **312.2 Socialized conduct disorder**
Childhood truancy, socialized
Group delinquency
EXCLUDES *gang activity without manifest psychiatric disorder (V71.01)*

✓5th **312.3 Disorders of impulse control, not elsewhere classified**
312.30 Impulse control disorder, unspecified
312.31 Pathological gambling
312.32 Kleptomania
312.33 Pyromania
312.34 Intermittent explosive disorder
312.35 Isolated explosive disorder
312.39 Other
Trichotillomania

312.4 Mixed disturbance of conduct and emotions
Neurotic delinquency
EXCLUDES *compulsive conduct disorder (312.3)*

✓5th **312.8 Other specified disturbances of conduct, not elsewhere classified**
312.81 Conduct disorder, childhood onset type
312.82 Conduct disorder, adolescent onset type
312.89 Other conduct disorder
Conduct disorder of unspecified onset

312.9 Unspecified disturbance of conduct
Delinquency (juvenile)
Disruptive behavior disorder NOS

✓4th **313 Disturbance of emotions specific to childhood and adolescence**
EXCLUDES *adjustment reaction (309.0-309.9)*
emotional disorder of neurotic type (300.0-300.9)
masturbation, nail-biting, thumbsucking, and other isolated symptoms (307.0-307.9)

313.0 Overanxious disorder
Anxiety and fearfulness } of childhood and adolescence
Overanxious disorder } of childhood and adolescence
EXCLUDES *abnormal separation anxiety (309.21)*
anxiety states (300.00-300.09)
hospitalism in children (309.83)
phobic state (300.20-300.29)

313.1 Misery and unhappiness disorder
EXCLUDES *depressive neurosis (300.4)*

✓5th **313.2 Sensitivity, shyness, and social withdrawal disorder**
EXCLUDES *infantile autism (299.0)*
schizoid personality (301.20-301.22)
schizophrenia (295.0-295.9)

313.21 Shyness disorder of childhood
Sensitivity reaction of childhood or adolescence

313.22 Introverted disorder of childhood
Social withdrawal } of childhood or adolescence
Withdrawal reaction } of childhood or adolescence

313.23 Selective mutism
EXCLUDES *elective mutism as adjustment reaction (309.83)*

313.3 Relationship problems
Sibling jealousy
EXCLUDES *relationship problems associated with aggression, destruction, or other forms of conduct disturbance (312.0-312.9)*

✓5th **313.8 Other or mixed emotional disturbances of childhood or adolescence**
313.81 Oppositional defiant disorder
DEF: Mental disorder of children noted for pervasive opposition, defiance of authority.

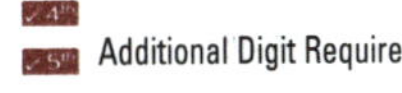
Additional Digit Required | Unspecified Code | Other Specified Code | Manifestation Code | ▶◀ Revised Text | ● New Code | ▲ Revised Code Title

313.82 Identity disorder
Identity problem
DEF: Distress of adolescents caused by inability to form acceptable self-identity; uncertainty about career choice, sexual orientation, moral values.

313.83 Academic underachievement disorder

313.89 Other P
Reactive attachment disorder of infancy or early childhood

313.9 Unspecified emotional disturbance of childhood or adolescence P
Mental disorder of infancy, childhood or adolescence NOS

✓4th **314 Hyperkinetic syndrome of childhood**
EXCLUDES *hyperkinesis as symptom of underlying disorder—code the underlying disorder*
DEF: A behavioral disorder usually diagnosed at an early age; characterized by the inability to focus attention for a normal period of time.

✓5th **314.0 Attention deficit disorder**
Adult
Child

314.00 Without mention of hyperactivity
Predominantly inattentive type
AHA: 1Q, '97, 8

314.01 With hyperactivity
Combined type
Overactivity NOS
Predominantly hyperactive/impulsive type
Simple disturbance of attention with overactivity
AHA: 1Q, '97, 8

314.1 Hyperkinesis with developmental delay
Developmental disorder of hyperkinesis
Use additional code to identify any associated neurological disorder

314.2 Hyperkinetic conduct disorder
Hyperkinetic conduct disorder without developmental delay
EXCLUDES *hyperkinesis with significant delays in specific skills (314.1)*

314.8 Other specified manifestations of hyperkinetic syndrome

314.9 Unspecified hyperkinetic syndrome
Hyperkinetic reaction of childhood or adolescence NOS
Hyperkinetic syndrome NOS

✓4th **315 Specific delays in development**
EXCLUDES *that due to a neurological disorder (320.0-389.9)*

✓5th **315.0 Specific reading disorder**

315.00 Reading disorder, unspecified

315.01 Alexia
DEF: Lack of ability to understand written language; manifestation of aphasia.

315.02 Developmental dyslexia
DEF: Serious impairment of reading skills unexplained in relation to general intelligence and teaching processes; it can be inherited or congenital.

315.09 Other
Specific spelling difficulty

315.1 Mathematics disorder
Dyscalculia

315.2 Other specific learning difficulties
Disorder of written expression
EXCLUDES *specific arithmetical disorder (315.1)*
specific reading disorder (315.00-315.09)

✓5th **315.3 Developmental speech or language disorder**

315.31 Expressive language disorder
Developmental aphasia
Word deafness
EXCLUDES *acquired aphasia (784.3)*
elective mutism (309.83, 313.0, 313.23)

315.32 Mixed receptive-expressive language disorder
AHA: 4Q, '96, 30

315.39 Other
Developmental articulation disorder
Dyslalia
Phonological disorder
EXCLUDES *lisping and lalling (307.9)*
stammering and stuttering (307.0)

315.4 Developmental coordination disorder
Clumsiness syndrome
Dyspraxia syndrome
Specific motor development disorder

315.5 Mixed development disorder
AHA: 2Q, '02, 11

315.8 Other specified delays in development

315.9 Unspecified delay in development
Developmental disorder NOS
Learning disorder NOS

316 Psychic factors associated with diseases classified elsewhere
Psychologic factors in physical conditions classified elsewhere
Use additional code to identify the associated physical condition, as:
psychogenic:
asthma (493.9)
dermatitis (692.9)
duodenal ulcer (532.0-532.9)
eczema (691.8, 692.9)
gastric ulcer (531.0-531.9)
mucous colitis (564.9)
paroxysmal tachycardia (427.2)
ulcerative colitis (556)
urticaria (708.0-708.9)
psychosocial dwarfism (259.4)
EXCLUDES *physical symptoms and physiological malfunctions, not involving tissue damage, of mental origin (306.0-306.9)*

MENTAL RETARDATION (317-319)

Use additional code(s) to identify any associated psychiatric or physical condition(s)

317 Mild mental retardation
High-grade defect
IQ 50-70
Mild mental subnormality

✓4th **318 Other specified mental retardation**

318.0 Moderate mental retardation
IQ 35-49
Moderate mental subnormality

318.1 Severe mental retardation
IQ 20-34
Severe mental subnormality

318.2 Profound mental retardation
IQ under 20
Profound mental subnormality

319 Unspecified mental retardation
Mental deficiency NOS
Mental subnormality NOS

6. NERVOUS SYSTEM AND SENSE ORGANS (320-389)

INFLAMMATORY DISEASES OF THE CENTRAL NERVOUS SYSTEM (320-326)

✓4th **320 Bacterial meningitis**

INCLUDES arachnoiditis, leptomeningitis, meningitis, meningoencephalitis, meningomyelitis, pachymeningitis } bacterial

AHA: J-F, '87, 6

DEF: Bacterial infection causing inflammation of the lining of the brain and/or spinal cord.

320.0 Hemophilus meningitis
Meningitis due to Hemophilus influenzae [H. influenzae]

320.1 Pneumococcal meningitis

320.2 Streptococcal meningitis

320.3 Staphylococcal meningitis

320.7 Meningitis in other bacterial diseases classified elsewhere
Code first underlying disease, as:
actinomycosis (039.8)
listeriosis (027.0)
typhoid fever (002.0)
whooping cough (033.0-033.9)

EXCLUDES *meningitis (in):*
epidemic (036.0)
gonococcal (098.82)
meningococcal (036.0)
salmonellosis (003.21)
syphilis:
NOS (094.2)
congenital (090.42)
meningovascular (094.2)
secondary (091.81)
tuberculous (013.0)

✓5th **320.8 Meningitis due to other specified bacteria**

320.81 Anaerobic meningitis
Bacteroides (fragilis)
Gram-negative anaerobes

320.82 Meningitis due to gram-negative bacteria, not elsewhere classified
Aerobacter aerogenes
Escherichia coli [E. coli]
Friedländer bacillus
Klebsiella pneumoniae
Proteus morganii
Pseudomonas

EXCLUDES *gram-negative anaerobes (320.81)*

320.89 Meningitis due to other specified bacteria
Bacillus pyocyaneus

320.9 Meningitis due to unspecified bacterium
Meningitis:
bacterial NOS
purulent NOS
pyogenic NOS
suppurative NOS

✓4th **321 Meningitis due to other organisms**

INCLUDES arachnoiditis, leptomeningitis, meningitis, pachymeningitis } due to organisms other than bacteria

AHA: J-F, '87, 6

DEF: Infection causing inflammation of the lining of the brain and/or spinal cord, due to organisms other than bacteria.

321.0 Cryptococcal meningitis
Code first underlying disease (117.5)

321.1 Meningitis in other fungal diseases
Code first underlying disease (110.0-118)

EXCLUDES *meningitis in:*
candidiasis (112.83)
coccidioidomycosis (114.2)
histoplasmosis (115.01, 115.11, 115.91)

321.2 Meningitis due to viruses not elsewhere classified
Code first underlying disease, as:
meningitis due to arbovirus (060.0-066.9)

EXCLUDES *meningitis (due to):*
abacterial (047.0-047.9)
adenovirus (049.1)
aseptic NOS (047.9)
Coxsackie (virus)(047.0)
ECHO virus (047.1)
enterovirus (047.0-047.9)
herpes simplex virus (054.72)
herpes zoster virus (053.0)
lymphocytic choriomeningitis virus (049.0)
mumps (072.1)
viral NOS (047.9)
meningo-eruptive syndrome (047.1)

AHA: ▶4Q, '04, 51◀

321.3 Meningitis due to trypanosomiasis
Code first underlying disease (086.0-086.9)

321.4 Meningitis in sarcoidosis
Code first underlying disease (135)

321.8 Meningitis due to other nonbacterial organisms classified elsewhere
Code first underlying disease

EXCLUDES *leptospiral meningitis (100.81)*

✓4th **322 Meningitis of unspecified cause**

INCLUDES arachnoiditis, leptomeningitis, meningitis, pachymeningitis } with no organism specified as cause

AHA: J-F, '87, 6

DEF: Infection causing inflammation of the lining of the brain and/or spinal cord, due to unspecified cause.

322.0 Nonpyogenic meningitis
Meningitis with clear cerebrospinal fluid

322.1 Eosinophilic meningitis

322.2 Chronic meningitis

322.9 Meningitis, unspecified

✓4th **323 Encephalitis, myelitis, and encephalomyelitis**

INCLUDES acute disseminated encephalomyelitis
meningoencephalitis, except bacterial
meningomyelitis, except bacterial
myelitis (acute):
ascending
transverse

EXCLUDES *bacterial:*
meningoencephalitis (320.0-320.9)
meningomyelitis (320.0-320.9)

DEF: Encephalitis: inflammation of brain tissues.
DEF: Myelitis: inflammation of the spinal cord.
DEF: Encephalomyelitis: inflammation of brain and spinal cord.

323.0 ***Encephalitis in viral diseases classified elsewhere***

Code first underlying disease, as:
- cat-scratch disease (078.3)
- infectious mononucleosis (075)
- ornithosis (073.7)

EXCLUDES *encephalitis (in):*
- *arthropod-borne viral (062.0-064)*
- *herpes simplex (054.3)*
- *mumps (072.2)*
- *other viral diseases of central nervous system (049.8-049.9)*
- *poliomyelitis (045.0-045.9)*
- *rubella (056.01)*
- *slow virus infections of central nervous system (046.0-046.9)*
- *viral NOS (049.9)*

323.1 ***Encephalitis in rickettsial diseases classified elsewhere***

Code first underlying disease (080-083.9)

DEF: Inflammation of the brain caused by rickettsial disease carried by louse, tick, or mite.

323.2 ***Encephalitis in protozoal diseases classified elsewhere***

Code first underlying disease, as:
- malaria (084.0-084.9)
- trypanosomiasis (086.0-086.9)

DEF: Inflammation of the brain caused by protozoal disease carried by mosquitoes and flies.

323.4 ***Other encephalitis due to infection classified elsewhere***

Code first underlying disease

EXCLUDES *encephalitis (in):*
- *meningococcal (036.1)*
- *syphilis:*
  - *NOS (094.81)*
  - *congenital (090.41)*
- *toxoplasmosis (130.0)*
- *tuberculosis (013.6)*
- *meningoencephalitis due to free-living ameba [Naegleria] (136.2)*

323.5 Encephalitis following immunization procedures

Encephalitis / Encephalomyelitis } postimmunization or postvaccinal

Use additional E code to identify vaccine

323.6 ***Postinfectious encephalitis***

▶Infectious acute disseminated encephalomyelitis (ADEM)◀

Code first underlying disease

EXCLUDES *encephalitis:*
- *postchickenpox (052.0)*
- *postmeasles (055.0)*

DEF: Infection, inflammation of brain several weeks following the outbreak of a systemic infection.

323.7 ***Toxic encephalitis***

Code first underlying cause, as:
- carbon tetrachloride (982.1)
- hydroxyquinoline derivatives (961.3)
- lead (984.0-984.9)
- mercury (985.0)
- thallium (985.8)

AHA: 2Q, '97, 8

323.8 Other causes of encephalitis

▶Noninfectious acute disseminated encephalomyelitis (ADEM)◀

323.9 Unspecified cause of encephalitis

✓4th **324 Intracranial and intraspinal abscess**

324.0 Intracranial abscess

Abscess (embolic):
- cerebellar
- cerebral

Abscess (embolic) of brain [any part]:
- epidural
- extradural
- otogenic
- subdural

EXCLUDES *tuberculous (013.3)*

324.1 Intraspinal abscess

Abscess (embolic) of spinal cord [any part]:
- epidural
- extradural
- subdural

EXCLUDES *tuberculous (013.5)*

324.9 Of unspecified site

Extradural or subdural abscess NOS

325 Phlebitis and thrombophlebitis of intracranial venous sinuses

Embolism / Endophlebitis / Phlebitis, septic or suppurative / Thrombophlebitis / Thrombosis } of cavernous, lateral, or other intracranial or unspecified intracranial venous sinus

EXCLUDES *that specified as:*
- *complicating pregnancy, childbirth, or the puerperium (671.5)*
- *of nonpyogenic origin (437.6)*

DEF: Inflammation and formation of blood clot in a vein within the brain or its lining.

326 Late effects of intracranial abscess or pyogenic infection

Note: This category is to be used to indicate conditions whose primary classification is to 320-325 [excluding 320.7, 321.0-321.8, 323.0-323.4, 323.6-323.7] as the cause of late effects, themselves classifiable elsewhere. The "late effects" include conditions specified as such, or as sequelae, which may occur at any time after the resolution of the causal condition.

Use additional code to identify condition, as:
- hydrocephalus (331.4)
- paralysis (342.0-342.9, 344.0-344.9)

● ✓4th **327 Organic sleep disorders**

● ✓5th **327.0 Organic disorders of initiating and maintaining sleep [Organic insomnia]**

EXCLUDES
- *insomnia NOS (780.52)*
- *insomnia not due to a substance or known physiological condition (307.41-307.42)*
- *insomnia with sleep apnea NOS (780.51)*

● **327.00 Organic insomnia, unspecified**

● **327.01 Insomnia due to medical condition classified elsewhere**

Code first underlying condition

EXCLUDES *insomnia due to mental disorder (327.02)*

● **327.02 Insomnia due to mental disorder**

Code first mental disorder

EXCLUDES
- *alcohol induced insomnia (291.82)*
- *drug induced insomnia (292.85)*

● **327.09 Other organic insomnia**

● ✓5th **327.1 Organic disorder of excessive somnolence [Organic hypersomnia]**

EXCLUDES
- *hypersomnia NOS (780.54)*
- *hypersomnia not due to a substance or known physiological condition (307.43-307.44)*
- *hypersomnia with sleep apnea NOS (780.53)*

● 327.10 **Organic hypersomnia, unspecified**

● 327.11 **Idiopathic hypersomnia with long sleep time**

● 327.12 **Idiopathic hypersomnia without long sleep time**

● 327.13 **Recurrent hypersomnia**
Kleine-Levin syndrome
Menstrual related hypersomnia

● 327.14 **Hypersomnia due to medical condition classified elsewhere**
Code first underlying condition
EXCLUDES *hypersomnia due to mental disorder (327.15)*

● 327.15 **Hypersomnia due to mental disorder**
Code first mental disorder
EXCLUDES *alcohol induced hypersomnia (291.82)*
drug induced hypersomnia (292.85)

● 327.19 **Other organic hypersomnia**

● ✓5th 327.2 **Organic sleep apnea**
EXCLUDES *Cheyne-Stokes breathing (786.04)*
hypersomnia with sleep apnea NOS (780.53)
insomnia with sleep apnea NOS (780.51)
sleep apnea in newborn (770.81-770.82)
sleep apnea NOS (780.57)

● 327.20 **Organic sleep apnea, unspecified**

● 327.21 **Primary central sleep apnea**

● 327.22 **High altitude periodic breathing**

● 327.23 **Obstructive sleep apnea (adult) (pediatric)**

● 327.24 **Idiopathic sleep related nonobstructive alveolar hypoventilation**
Sleep related hypoxia

● 327.25 **Congenital central alveolar hypoventilation syndrome**

● 327.26 **Sleep related hypoventilation/hypoxemia in conditions classifiable elsewhere**
Code first underlying condition

● 327.27 **Central sleep apnea in conditions classified elsewhere**
Code first underlying condition

● 327.29 **Other organic sleep apnea**

● ✓5th 327.3 **Circadian rhythm sleep disorder**
Organic disorder of sleep wake cycle
Organic disorder of sleep wake schedule
EXCLUDES *alcohol induced circadian rhythm sleep disorder (291.82)*
circadian rhythm sleep disorder of nonorganic origin (307.45)
disruption of 24 hour sleep wake cycle NOS (780.55)
drug induced circadian rhythm sleep disorder (292.85)

● 327.30 **Circadian rhythm sleep disorder, unspecified**

● 327.31 **Circadian rhythm sleep disorder, delayed sleep phase type**

● 327.32 **Circadian rhythm sleep disorder, advanced sleep phase type**

● 327.33 **Circadian rhythm sleep disorder, irregular sleep-wake type**

● 327.34 **Circadian rhythm sleep disorder, free-running type**

● 327.35 **Circadian rhythm sleep disorder, jet lag type**

● 327.36 **Circadian rhythm sleep disorder, shift work type**

● 327.37 **Circadian rhythm sleep disorder in conditions classified elsewhere**
Code first underlying condition

● 327.39 **Other circadian rhythm sleep disorder**

● ✓5th 327.4 **Organic parasomnia**
EXCLUDES *alcohol induced parasomnia (291.82)*
drug induced parasomnia (292.85)
parasomnia not due to a known physiological condition (307.47)

● 327.40 **Organic parasomnia, unspecified**

● 327.41 **Confusional arousals**

● 327.42 **REM sleep behavior disorder**

● 327.43 **Recurrent isolated sleep paralysis**

● 327.44 **Parasomnia in conditions classified elsewhere**
Code first underlying condition

● 327.49 **Other organic parasomnia**

● ✓5th 327.5 **Organic sleep related movement disorders**
EXCLUDES *restless leg syndrome (333.99)*
sleep related movement disorder NOS (780.58)

● 327.51 **Periodic limb movement disorder**
Periodic limb movement sleep disorder

● 327.52 **Sleep related leg cramps**

● 327.53 **Sleep related bruxism**

● 327.59 **Other organic sleep related movement disorders**

● 327.8 **Other organic sleep disorders**

HEREDITARY AND DEGENERATIVE DISEASES OF THE CENTRAL NERVOUS SYSTEM (330-337)

EXCLUDES *hepatolenticular degeneration (275.1)*
multiple sclerosis (340)
other demyelinating diseases of central nervous system (341.0-341.9)

✓4th 330 **Cerebral degenerations usually manifest in childhood**
Use additional code to identify associated mental retardation

330.0 **Leukodystrophy**
Krabbe's disease
Leukodystrophy
NOS
globoid cell
metachromatic
sudanophilic
Pelizaeus-Merzbacher disease
Sulfatide lipidosis

DEF: Hereditary disease of arylsulfatase or cerebroside sulfatase; characterized by a diffuse loss of myelin in CNS; infantile form causes blindness, motor disturbances, rigidity, mental deterioration and, occasionally, convulsions.

330.1 **Cerebral lipidoses**
Amaurotic (familial) idiocy
Disease:
Batten
Jansky-Bielschowsky
Kufs'
Disease:
Spielmeyer-Vogt
Tay-Sachs
Gangliosidosis

DEF: Genetic disorder causing abnormal lipid accumulation in the reticuloendothelial cells of the brain.

330.2 ***Cerebral degeneration in generalized lipidoses***
Code first underlying disease, as:
Fabry's disease (272.7)
Gaucher's disease (272.7)
Niemann-Pick disease (272.7)
sphingolipidosis (272.7)

330.3 ***Cerebral degeneration of childhood in other diseases classified elsewhere***
Code first underlying disease, as:
Hunter's disease (277.5)
mucopolysaccharidosis (277.5)

✓4th ✓5th Additional Digit Required | Unspecified Code | Other Specified Code | Manifestation Code | ►◄ Revised Text | ● New Code | ▲ Revised Code Title

330.8 **Other specified cerebral degenerations in childhood**
Alpers' disease or gray-matter degeneration
Infantile necrotizing encephalomyelopathy
Leigh's disease
Subacute necrotizing encephalopathy or encephalomyelopathy
AHA: N-D, '85, 5

330.9 **Unspecified cerebral degeneration in childhood**

✓4th **331 Other cerebral degenerations**

331.0 **Alzheimer's disease**
AHA: 4Q, '00, 41; 4Q, '99, 7; N-D, '84, 20
DEF: Diffuse atrophy of cerebral cortex; causing a progressive decline in intellectual and physical functions, including memory loss, personality changes and profound dementia.

✓5th 331.1 **Frontotemporal dementia**
Use additional code for associated behavioral disturbance (294.10-294.11)
AHA: 4Q, '03, 57
DEF: Rare, progressive degenerative brain disease, similar to Alzheimer's; cortical atrophy affects the frontal and temporal lobes.

331.11 **Pick's disease**
DEF: A less common form of progressive frontotemporal dementia with asymmetrical atrophy of the frontal and temporal regions of the cerebral cortex including abnormal rounded brain cells called Pick cells together with the presence of abnormal staining of protein (called tau) within the cells, called Pick bodies; symptoms include prominent apathy, deterioration of social skills, behavioral changes such as disinhibition and restlessness, echolalia, impairment of language, memory, and intellect, increased carelessness, poor personal hygiene, and decreased attention span.

331.19 **Other frontotemporal dementia**
Frontal dementia

331.2 **Senile degeneration of brain**
EXCLUDES *senility NOS (797)*

331.3 **Communicating hydrocephalus**
EXCLUDES *congenital hydrocephalus (741.0, 742.3)*
AHA: S-O, '85, 12
DEF: Subarachnoid hemorrhage and meningitis causing excess buildup of cerebrospinal fluid in cavities due to nonabsorption of fluid back through fluid pathways.

331.4 **Obstructive hydrocephalus**
Acquired hydrocephalus NOS
EXCLUDES *congenital hydrocephalus (741.0, 742.3)*
AHA: 4Q, '03, 106; 1Q, '99, 9
DEF: Obstruction of cerebrospinal fluid passage from brain into spinal canal.

331.7 ***Cerebral degeneration in diseases classified elsewhere***
Code first underlying disease, as:
alcoholism (303.0-303.9)
beriberi (265.0)
cerebrovascular disease (430-438)
congenital hydrocephalus (741.0, 742.3)
neoplastic disease (140.0-239.9)
myxedema (244.0-244.9)
vitamin B_{12} deficiency (266.2)
EXCLUDES *cerebral degeneration in:*
Jakob-Creutzfeldt disease (046.1)
progressive multifocal leukoencephalopathy (046.3)
subacute spongiform encephalopathy (046.1)

✓5th 331.8 **Other cerebral degeneration**

331.81 **Reye's syndrome** P
DEF: Rare childhood illness, often developed after a bout of viral upper respiratory infection; characterized by vomiting, elevated serum transaminase, changes in liver and other viscera; symptoms may be followed by an encephalopathic phase with brain swelling, disturbances of consciousness and seizures; can be fatal.

331.82 **Dementia with Lewy bodies**
Dementia with Parkinsonism
Lewy body dementia
Lewy body disease
Use additional code for associated behavioral disturbance (294.10-294.11)
AHA: 4Q, '03, 57
DEF: A cerebral dementia with neurophysiologic changes including increased hippocampal volume, hypoperfusion in the occipital lobes, and beta amyloid deposits with neurofibrillarity tangles, atrophy of cortex and brainstem, hallmark neuropsychologic characteristics are fluctuating cognition with pronounced variation in attention and alertness; recurrent hallucinations; and parkinsonism.

331.89 **Other**
Cerebral ataxia

331.9 **Cerebral degeneration, unspecified**

✓4th **332 Parkinson's disease**
EXCLUDES *dementia with Parkinsonism (331.82)*

332.0 **Paralysis agitans**
Parkinsonism or Parkinson's disease:
NOS
idiopathic
primary
AHA: M-A, '87, 7
DEF: Form of parkinsonism; progressive, occurs in senior years; characterized by masklike facial expression; condition affects ability to stand erect, walk smoothly; weakened muscles, also tremble and involuntarily movement.

332.1 **Secondary Parkinsonism**
▶Neuroleptic-induced Parkinsonism◀
Parkinsonism due to drugs
Use additional E code to identify drug, if drug-induced
EXCLUDES *Parkinsonism (in):*
Huntington's disease (333.4)
progressive supranuclear palsy (333.0)
Shy-Drager syndrome (333.0)
syphilitic (094.82)

✓4th **333 Other extrapyramidal disease and abnormal movement disorders**
INCLUDES other forms of extrapyramidal, basal ganglia, or striatopallidal disease
EXCLUDES *abnormal movements of head NOS (781.0)*
▶*sleep related movement disorders (327.51-327.59)*◀

333.0 **Other degenerative diseases of the basal ganglia**
Atrophy or degeneration:
olivopontocerebellar [Déjérine-Thomas syndrome]
pigmentary pallidal [Hallervorden-Spatz disease]
striatonigral
Parkinsonian syndrome associated with:
idiopathic orthostatic hypotension
symptomatic orthostatic hypotension
Progressive supranuclear ophthalmoplegia
Shy-Drager syndrome
AHA: 3Q, '96, 8

333.1 **Essential and other specified forms of tremor**
Benign essential tremor
Familial tremor
▶Medication-induced postural tremor◀
Use additional E code to identify drug, if drug-induced
EXCLUDES *tremor NOS (781.0)*

333.2 Myoclonus
Familial essential myoclonus
Progressive myoclonic epilepsy
Unverricht-Lundborg disease
Use additional E code to identify drug, if drug-induced
AHA: 3Q, '97, 4; M-A, '87, 12

DEF: Spontaneous movements or contractions of muscles.

333.3 Tics of organic origin
Use additional E code to identify drug, if drug-induced
EXCLUDES *Gilles de la Tourette's syndrome (307.23)*
habit spasm (307.22)
tic NOS (307.20)

333.4 Huntington's chorea
DEF: Genetic disease; characterized by chronic progressive mental deterioration; dementia and death within 15 years of onset.

333.5 Other choreas
Hemiballism(us)
Paroxysmal choreo-athetosis
Use additional E code to identify drug, if drug-induced
EXCLUDES *Sydenham's or rheumatic chorea (392.0-392.9)*

333.6 Idiopathic torsion dystonia
Dystonia:
deformans progressiva
musculorum deformans
(Schwalbe-) Ziehen-Oppenheim disease
DEF: Sustained muscular contractions, causing twisting and repetitive movements that result in abnormal postures of trunk and limbs; etiology unknown.

333.7 Symptomatic torsion dystonia
Athetoid cerebral palsy [Vogt's disease]
Double athetosis (syndrome)
▶Neuroleptic-induced acute dystonia◀
Use additional E code to identify drug, if drug-induced

✓5th **333.8 Fragments of torsion dystonia**
Use additional E code to identify drug, if drug-induced

333.81 Blepharospasm
DEF: Uncontrolled winking or blinking due to orbicularis oculi muscle spasm.

333.82 Orofacial dyskinesia
▶Neuroleptic-induced tardive dyskinesia◀
DEF: Uncontrolled movement of mouth or facial muscles.

333.83 Spasmodic torticollis
EXCLUDES *torticollis:*
NOS (723.5)
hysterical (300.11)
psychogenic (306.0)
DEF: Uncontrolled movement of head due to spasms of neck muscle.

333.84 Organic writers' cramp
EXCLUDES *pychogenic (300.89)*

333.89 Other

✓5th **333.9 Other and unspecified extrapyramidal diseases and abnormal movement disorders**

333.90 Unspecified extrapyramidal disease and abnormal movement disorder
▶Medication-induced movement disorders NOS
Use additional E code to identify drug, if drug-induced◀

333.91 Stiff-man syndrome

333.92 Neuroleptic malignant syndrome
Use additional E code to identify drug
AHA: 4Q, '94, 37

333.93 Benign shuddering attacks
AHA: 4Q, '94, 37

333.99 Other
▶Neuroleptic-induced acute akathisia◀
Restless legs
▶Use additional E code to identify drug, if drug-induced◀
AHA: 4Q, '04, 95; 2Q, '04, 12; 4Q, '94, 37

✓4th **334 Spinocerebellar disease**
EXCLUDES *olivopontocerebellar degeneration (333.0)*
peroneal muscular atrophy (356.1)

334.0 Friedreich's ataxia
DEF: Genetic recessive disease of children; sclerosis of dorsal, lateral spinal cord columns; characterized by ataxia, speech impairment, swaying and irregular movements, with muscle paralysis, especially of lower limbs.

334.1 Hereditary spastic paraplegia

334.2 Primary cerebellar degeneration
Cerebellar ataxia:
Marie's
Sanger-Brown
Dyssynergia cerebellaris myoclonica
Primary cerebellar degeneration:
NOS
hereditary
sporadic
AHA: M-A, '87, 9

334.3 Other cerebellar ataxia
Cerebellar ataxia NOS
Use additional E code to identify drug, if drug-induced

334.4 Cerebellar ataxia in diseases classified elsewhere
Code first underlying disease, as:
alcoholism (303.0-303.9)
myxedema (244.0-244.9)
neoplastic disease (140.0-239.9)

334.8 Other spinocerebellar diseases
Ataxia-telangiectasia [Louis-Bar syndrome]
Corticostriatal-spinal degeneration

334.9 Spinocerebellar disease, unspecified

✓4th **335 Anterior horn cell disease**

335.0 Werdnig-Hoffmann disease
Infantile spinal muscular atrophy
Progressive muscular atrophy of infancy
DEF: Spinal muscle atrophy manifested in prenatal period or shortly after birth; symptoms include hypotonia, atrophy of skeletal muscle; death occurs in infancy.

✓5th **335.1 Spinal muscular atrophy**

335.10 Spinal muscular atrophy, unspecified

335.11 Kugelberg-Welander disease
Spinal muscular atrophy:
familial
juvenile
DEF: Hereditary; juvenile muscle atrophy; appears during first two decades of life; due to lesions of anterior horns of spinal cord; includes wasting, diminution of lower body muscles and twitching.

335.19 Other
Adult spinal muscular atrophy

✓5th **335.2 Motor neuron disease**

335.20 Amyotrophic lateral sclerosis A
Motor neuron disease (bulbar) (mixed type)
AHA: 4Q, '95, 81

335.21 Progressive muscular atrophy
Duchenne-Aran muscular atrophy
Progressive muscular atrophy (pure)

335.22 Progressive bulbar palsy

335.23 Pseudobulbar palsy

335.24 Primary lateral sclerosis

335.29 Other

335.8 Other anterior horn cell diseases

335.9 Anterior horn cell disease, unspecified

✓4th **336 Other diseases of spinal cord**

336.0 Syringomyelia and syringobulbia
AHA: 1Q, '89, 10

336.1 Vascular myelopathies
Acute infarction of spinal cord (embolic) (nonembolic)
Arterial thrombosis of spinal cord
Edema of spinal cord
Hematomyelia
Subacute necrotic myelopathy

336.2 Subacute combined degeneration of spinal cord in diseases classified elsewhere
Code first underlying disease, as:
pernicious anemia (281.0)
other vitamin B_{12} deficiency anemia (281.1)
vitamin B_{12} deficiency (266.2)

336.3 Myelopathy in other diseases classified elsewhere
Code first underlying disease, as:
myelopathy in neoplastic disease (140.0-239.9)
EXCLUDES *myelopathy in:*
intervertebral disc disorder (722.70-722.73)
spondylosis (721.1, 721.41-721.42, 721.91)
AHA: 3Q, '99, 5

336.8 Other myelopathy
Myelopathy: drug-induced
Myelopathy: radiation-induced
Use additonal E code to identify cause

336.9 Unspecified disease of spinal cord
Cord compression NOS
Myelopathy NOS
EXCLUDES *myelitis (323.0-323.9)*
spinal (canal) stenosis (723.0, 724.00-724.09)

✓4th **337 Disorders of the autonomic nervous system**
INCLUDES disorders of peripheral autonomic, sympathetic, parasympathetic, or vegetative system
EXCLUDES *familial dysautonomia [Riley-Day syndrome] (742.8)*

337.0 Idiopathic peripheral autonomic neuropathy
Carotid sinus syncope or syndrome
Cervical sympathetic dystrophy or paralysis

337.1 Peripheral autonomic neuropathy in disorders classified elsewhere
Code first underlying disease, as:
amyloidosis (277.3)
diabetes (250.6)
AHA: 2Q, '93, 6; 3Q, '91, 9; N-D, '84, 9

✓5th **337.2 Reflex sympathetic dystrophy**
AHA: 4Q, '93, 24

DEF: Disturbance of the sympathetic nervous system evidenced by sweating, pain, pallor and edema following injury to nerves or blood vessels.

337.20 Reflex sympathetic dystrophy,unspecified
337.21 Reflex sympathetic dystrophy of the upper limb
337.22 Reflex sympathetic dystrophy of the lower limb
337.29 Reflex sympathetic dystrophy of other specified site

337.3 Autonomic dysreflexia
Use additional code to identify the cause, such as:
decubitus ulcer (707.00-707.09)
fecal impaction (560.39)
urinary tract infection (599.0)
AHA: 4Q, '98, 37

DEF: Noxious stimuli evokes paroxysmal hypertension, bradycardia, excess sweating, headache, pilomotor responses, facial flushing, and nasal congestion due to uncontrolled parasympathetic nerve response; usually occurs in patients with spinal cord injury above major sympathetic outflow tract (T_6).

337.9 Unspecified disorder of autonomic nervous system

OTHER DISORDERS OF THE CENTRAL NERVOUS SYSTEM (340-349)

340 Multiple sclerosis
Disseminated or multiple sclerosis:
NOS
brain stem
cord
generalized

✓4th **341 Other demyelinating diseases of central nervous system**

341.0 Neuromyelitis optica

341.1 Schilder's disease
Baló's concentric sclerosis
Encephalitis periaxialis:
concentrica [Baló's]
diffusa [Schilder's]

DEF: Chronic leukoencephalopathy of children and adolescents; symptoms include blindness, deafness, bilateral spasticity and progressive mental deterioration.

341.8 Other demyelinating diseases of central nervous system
Central demyelination of corpus callosum
Central pontine myelinosis
Marchiafava (-Bignami) disease
AHA: N-D, '87, 6

341.9 Demyelinating disease of central nervous system, unspecified

✓4th **342 Hemiplegia and hemiparesis**
Note: This category is to be used when hemiplegia (complete) (incomplete) is reported without further specification, or is stated to be old or long-standing but of unspecified cause. The category is also for use in multiple coding to identify these types of hemiplegia resulting from any cause.
EXCLUDES *congenital (343.1)*
hemiplegia due to late effect of cerebrovascular accident (438.20-438.22)
infantile NOS (343.4)

The following fifth-digits are for use with codes 342.0-342.9:
0 affecting unspecified side
1 affecting dominant side
2 affecting nondominant side

AHA: 4Q, '94, 38

✓5th **342.0 Flaccid hemiplegia**
✓5th **342.1 Spastic hemiplegia**
✓5th **342.8 Other specified hemiplegia**
✓5th **342.9 Hemiplegia, unspecified**
AHA: 4Q, '98, 87

✓4th **343 Infantile cerebral palsy**
INCLUDES cerebral:
palsy NOS
spastic infantile paralysis
congenital spastic paralysis (cerebral)
Little's disease
paralysis (spastic) due to birth injury:
intracranial
spinal
EXCLUDES *hereditary cerebral paralysis, such as:*
hereditary spastic paraplegia (334.1)
Vogt's disease (333.7)
spastic paralysis specified as noncongenital or noninfantile (344.0-344.9)

343.0 Diplegic
Congenital diplegia
Congenital paraplegia
DEF: Paralysis affecting both sides of the body simultaneously.

343.1 Hemiplegic
Congenital hemiplegia
EXCLUDES *infantile hemiplegia NOS (343.4)*

343.2 Quadriplegic
Tetraplegic

343.3 Monoplegic

N Newborn Age: 0 P Pediatric Age: 0-17 M Maternity Age: 12-55 A Adult Age: 15-124 MSP Medicare Secondary Payer

343.4 Infantile hemiplegia
Infantile hemiplegia (postnatal) NOS

343.8 Other specified infantile cerebral palsy

343.9 Infantile cerebral palsy, unspecified
Cerebral palsy NOS

✓4th **344 Other paralytic syndromes**

Note: This category is to be used when the listed conditions are reported without further specification or are stated to be old or long-standing but of unspecified cause. The category is also for use in multiple coding to identify these conditions resulting from any cause.

INCLUDES paralysis (complete) (incomplete), except as classifiable to 342 and 343

EXCLUDES *congenital or infantile cerebral palsy (343.0-343.9)*
hemiplegia (342.0-342.9)
congenital or infantile (343.1, 343.4)

✓5th **344.0 Quadriplegia and quadriparesis**

344.00 Quadriplegia unspecified
AHA: 4Q, '03, 103; 4Q, '98, 38

344.01 C_1-C_4 complete

344.02 C_1-C_4 incomplete

344.03 C_5-C_7 complete

344.04 C_5-C_7 incomplete

344.09 Other
AHA: 1Q, '01, 12; 4Q, '98, 39

344.1 Paraplegia
Paralysis of both lower limbs
Paraplegia (lower)
AHA: 4Q, '03, 110; M-A, '87, 10

344.2 Diplegia of upper limbs
Diplegia (upper)
Paralysis of both upper limbs

✓5th **344.3 Monoplegia of lower limb**
Paralysis of lower limb
EXCLUDES *monoplegia of lower limb due to late effect of cerebrovascular accident (438.40-438.42)*

344.30 Affecting unspecified side

344.31 Affecting dominant side

344.32 Affecting nondominant side

✓5th **344.4 Monoplegia of upper limb**
Paralysis of upper limb
EXCLUDES *monoplegia of upper limb due to late effect of cerebrovascular accident (438.30-438.32)*

344.40 Affecting unspecified side

344.41 Affecting dominant side

344.42 Affecting nondominant side

344.5 Unspecified monoplegia

✓5th **344.6 Cauda equina syndrome**
DEF: Dull pain and paresthesias in sacrum, perineum and bladder due to compression of spinal nerve roots; pain radiates down buttocks, back of thigh, calf of leg and into foot with prickling, burning sensations.

344.60 Without mention of neurogenic bladder

344.61 With neurogenic bladder
Acontractile bladder
Autonomic hyperreflexia of bladder
Cord bladder
Detrusor hyperreflexia
AHA: M-J, '87, 12; M-A, '87, 10

✓5th **344.8 Other specified paralytic syndromes**

344.81 Locked-in state
AHA: 4Q, '93, 24
DEF: State of consciousness where patients are paralyzed and unable to respond to environmental stimuli; patients have eye movements, and stimuli can enter the brain but patients cannot respond to stimuli.

344.89 Other specified paralytic syndrome
AHA: 2Q, '99, 4

344.9 Paralysis, unspecified

✓4th **345 Epilepsy**

EXCLUDES *progressive myoclonic epilepsy (333.2)*

The following fifth-digit subclassification is for use with categories 345.0, .1, .4–.9:
0 without mention of intractable epilepsy
1 with intractable epilepsy

AHA: 1Q, '93, 24; 2Q, '92, 8 4Q, '92, 23

DEF: Brain disorder characterized by electrical-like disturbances; may include occasional impairment or loss of consciousness, abnormal motor phenomena and psychic or sensory disturbances.

✓5th **345.0 Generalized nonconvulsive epilepsy**
Absences:
atonic
typical
Minor epilepsy
Petit mal
Pykno-epilepsy
Seizures:
akinetic
atonic
AHA: For code 345.00: 1Q, '04, 18

✓5th **345.1 Generalized convulsive epilepsy**
Epileptic seizures:
clonic
myoclonic
tonic
Epileptic seizures:
tonic-clonic
Grand mal
Major epilepsy
EXCLUDES *convulsions:*
NOS (780.3)
infantile (780.3)
newborn (779.0)
infantile spasms (345.6)
AHA: 3Q, '97, 4
DEF: Convulsive seizures with tension of limbs (tonic) or rhythmic contractions (clonic).

345.2 Petit mal status
Epileptic absence status
DEF: Minor myoclonic spasms and sudden momentary loss of consciousness in epilepsy.

345.3 Grand mal status
Status epilepticus NOS
EXCLUDES *epilepsia partialis continua (345.7)*
status:
psychomotor (345.7)
temporal lobe (345.7)
DEF: Sudden loss of consciousness followed by generalized convulsions in epilepsy.

✓5th **345.4 Partial epilepsy, with impairment of consciousness**
Epilepsy:
limbic system
partial:
secondarily generalized
with memory and ideational disturbances
psychomotor
psychosensory
temporal lobe
Epileptic automatism

✓5th **345.5 Partial epilepsy, without mention of impairment of consciousness**
Epilepsy:
Bravais-Jacksonian NOS
focal (motor) NOS
Jacksonian NOS
motor partial
partial NOS
Epilepsy:
sensory-induced
somatomotor
somatosensory
visceral
visual

✓5th **345.6 Infantile spasms**
Hypsarrhythmia
Lightning spasms
Salaam attacks
EXCLUDES *salaam tic (781.0)*
AHA: N-D, '84, 12

✓5th **345.7 Epilepsia partialis continua**
Kojevnikov's epilepsy
DEF: Continuous muscle contractions and relaxation; result of abnormal neural discharge.

§ ✓5th **345.8 Other forms of epilepsy**

Epilepsy: cursive [running]

Epilepsy: gelastic

§ ✓5th **345.9 Epilepsy, unspecified**

Epileptic convulsions, fits, or seizures NOS

EXCLUDES *convulsive seizure or fit NOS (780.3)*

AHA: N-D, '87, 12

✓4th **346 Migraine**

DEF: Benign vascular headache of extreme pain; commonly associated with irritability, nausea, vomiting and often photophobia; premonitory visual hallucination of a crescent in the visual field (scotoma).

The following fifth-digit subclassification is for use with category 346:

0 without mention of intractable migraine

1 with intractable migraine, so stated

✓5th **346.0 Classical migraine**

Migraine preceded or accompanied by transient focal neurological phenomena

Migraine with aura

✓5th **346.1 Common migraine**

Atypical migraine

Sick headache

✓5th **346.2 Variants of migraine**

Cluster headache

Histamine cephalgia

Horton's neuralgia

Migraine: abdominal, basilar

Migraine: lower half, retinal

Neuralgia: ciliary, migrainous

✓5th **346.8 Other forms of migraine**

Migraine: hemiplegic

Migraine: ophthalmoplegic

✓5th **346.9 Migraine, unspecified**

AHA: N-D, '85, 16

✓4th **347 Cataplexy and narcolepsy**

DEF: Cataplexy: sudden onset of muscle weakness with loss of tone and strength; caused by aggressive or spontaneous emotions.

DEF: Narcolepsy: brief, recurrent, uncontrollable episodes of sound sleep.

✓5th **347.0 Narcolepsy**

347.00 Without cataplexy

Narcolepsy NOS

347.01 With cataplexy

✓5th **347.1 Narcolepsy in conditions classified elsewhere**

Code first underlying condition

347.10 Without cataplexy

347.11 With cataplexy

✓4th **348 Other conditions of brain**

348.0 Cerebral cysts

Arachnoid cyst

Porencephalic cyst

Porencephaly, acquired

Pseudoporencephaly

EXCLUDES *porencephaly (congenital) (742.4)*

348.1 Anoxic brain damage

EXCLUDES *that occurring in:*
abortion (634-638 with .7, 639.8)
ectopic or molar pregnancy (639.8)
labor or delivery (668.2, 669.4)
that of newborn (767.0, 768.0-768.9, 772.1-772.2)

Use additional E code to identify cause

DEF: Brain injury due to lack of oxygen, other than birth trauma.

348.2 Benign intracranial hypertension

Pseudotumor cerebri

EXCLUDES *hypertensive encephalopathy (437.2)*

DEF: Elevated pressure in brain due to fluid retention in brain cavities.

✓5th **348.3 Encephalopathy, not elsewhere classified**

AHA: 4Q, '03, 58; 3Q, '97, 4

348.30 Encephalopathy, unspecified

348.31 Metabolic encephalopathy

Septic encephalopathy

§ Requres fifth-digit. See category 345 for codes and definitions.

Cranial Nerves

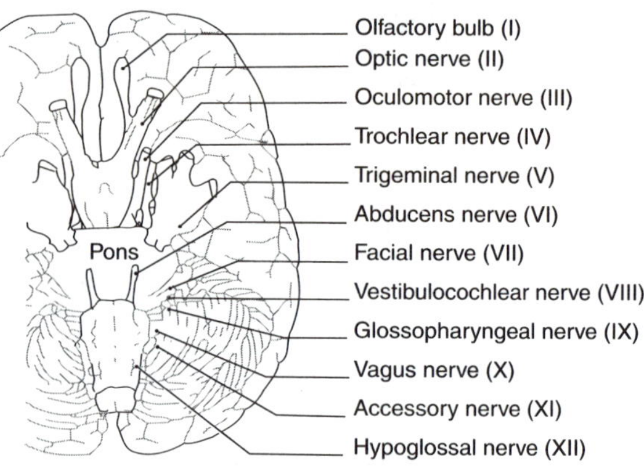

348.39 Other encephalopathy

EXCLUDES *encephalopathy:*
alcoholic (291.2)
hepatic (572.2)
hypertensive (437.2)
toxic (349.82)

348.4 Compression of brain

Compression } brain (stem)
Herniation }

Posterior fossa compression syndrome

AHA: 4Q, '94, 37

DEF: Elevated pressure in brain due to blood clot, tumor, fracture, abscess, other condition.

348.5 Cerebral edema

DEF: Elevated pressure in the brain due to fluid retention in brain tissues.

348.8 Other conditions of brain

Cerebral: calcification

Cerebral: fungus

AHA: S-O, '87, 9

348.9 Unspecified condition of brain

✓4th **349 Other and unspecified disorders of the nervous system**

349.0 Reaction to spinal or lumbar puncture

Headache following lumbar puncture

AHA: 2Q, '99, 9; 3Q, '90, 18

349.1 Nervous system complications from surgically implanted device

EXCLUDES *immediate postoperative complications (997.00-997.09)*
mechanical complications of nervous system device (996.2)

349.2 Disorders of meninges, not elsewhere classified

Adhesions, meningeal (cerebral) (spinal)

Cyst, spinal meninges

Meningocele, acquired

Pseudomeningocele, acquired

AHA: 2Q, '98, 18; 3Q, '94, 4

✓5th **349.8 Other specified disorders of nervous system**

349.81 Cerebrospinal fluid rhinorrhea

EXCLUDES *cerebrospinal fluid otorrhea (388.61)*

DEF: Cerebrospinal fluid discharging from the nose; caused by fracture of frontal bone with tearing of dura mater and arachnoid.

349.82 Toxic encephalopathy

Use additional E code, if desired, to identify cause

AHA 4Q, '93, 29

DEF: Brain tissue degeneration due to toxic substance.

349.89 Other

349.9 Unspecified disorders of nervous system

Disorder of nervous system (central) NOS

N Newborn Age: 0 P Pediatric Age: 0-17 M Maternity Age: 12-55 A Adult Age: 15-124 MSP Medicare Secondary Payer

DISORDERS OF THE PERIPHERAL NERVOUS SYSTEM (350-359)

EXCLUDES *diseases of:*
acoustic [8th] nerve (388.5)
oculomotor [3rd, 4th, 6th] nerves (378.0-378.9)
optic [2nd] nerve (377.0-377.9)
peripheral autonomic nerves (337.0-337.9)
neuralgia, neuritis, radiculitis } NOS or "rheumatic" (729.2)
peripheral neuritis in pregnancy (646.4)

✓4th 350 Trigeminal nerve disorders
INCLUDES disorders of 5th cranial nerve

350.1 Trigeminal neuralgia
Tic douloureux
Trifacial neuralgia
Trigeminal neuralgia NOS
EXCLUDES *postherpetic (053.12)*

350.2 Atypical face pain

350.8 Other specified trigeminal nerve disorders

350.9 Trigeminal nerve disorder, unspecified

✓4th 351 Facial nerve disorders
INCLUDES disorders of 7th cranial nerve
EXCLUDES *that in newborn (767.5)*

351.0 Bell's palsy
Facial palsy
DEF: Unilateral paralysis of face due to lesion on facial nerve; produces facial distortion.

Peripheral Nervous System

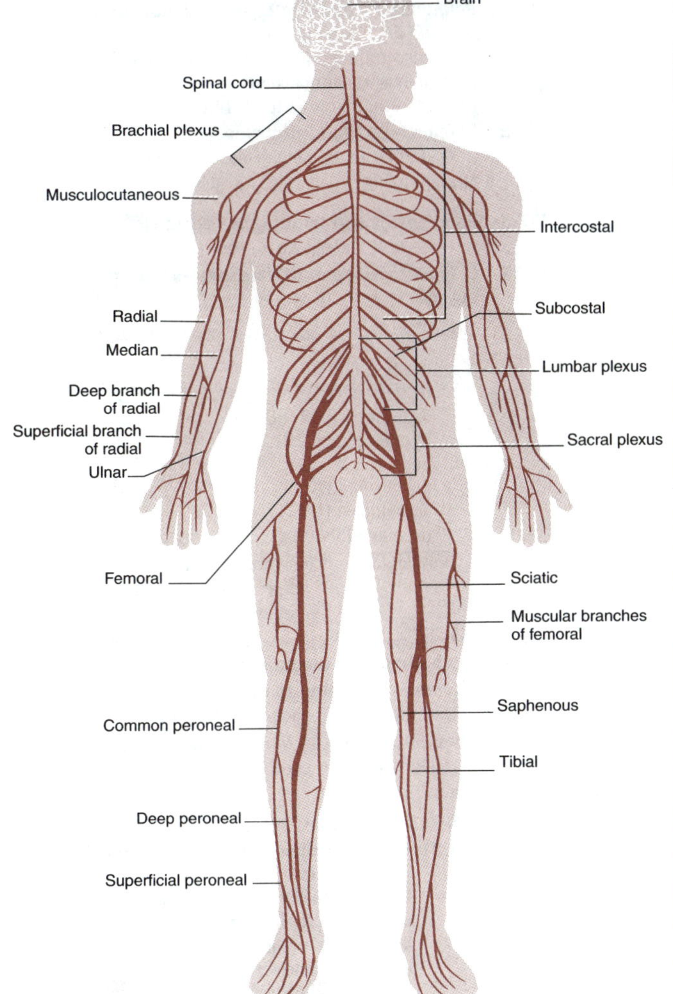

351.1 Geniculate ganglionitis
Geniculate ganglionitis NOS
EXCLUDES *herpetic (053.11)*
DEF: Inflammation of tissue at bend in facial nerve.

351.8 Other facial nerve disorders
Facial myokymia
Melkersson's syndrome
AHA: 3Q, '02, 13

351.9 Facial nerve disorder, unspecified

✓4th 352 Disorders of other cranial nerves

352.0 Disorders of olfactory [lst] nerve

352.1 Glossopharyngeal neuralgia
AHA: 2Q, '02, 8
DEF: Pain between throat and ear along petrosal and jugular ganglia.

352.2 Other disorders of glossopharyngeal [9th] nerve

352.3 Disorders of pneumogastric [10th] nerve
Disorders of vagal nerve
EXCLUDES *paralysis of vocal cords or larynx (478.30-478.34)*
DEF: Nerve disorder affecting ear, tongue, pharynx, larynx, esophagus, viscera and thorax.

352.4 Disorders of accessory [11th] nerve
DEF: Nerve disorder affecting palate, pharynx, larynx, thoracic viscera, sternocleidomastoid and trapezius muscles.

352.5 Disorders of hypoglossal [12th] nerve
DEF: Nerve disorder affecting tongue muscles.

352.6 Multiple cranial nerve palsies
Collet-Sicard syndrome
Polyneuritis cranialis

352.9 Unspecified disorder of cranial nerves

✓4th 353 Nerve root and plexus disorders
EXCLUDES *conditions due to:*
intervertebral disc disorders (722.0-722.9)
spondylosis (720.0-721.9)
vertebrogenic disorders (723.0-724.9)

353.0 Brachial plexus lesions
Cervical rib syndrome
Costoclavicular syndrome
Scalenus anticus syndrome
Thoracic outlet syndrome
EXCLUDES *brachial neuritis or radiculitis NOS (723.4)*
that in newborn (767.6)
DEF: Acquired disorder in tissue along nerves in shoulder; causes corresponding motor and sensory dysfunction.

353.1 Lumbosacral plexus lesions
DEF: Acquired disorder in tissue along nerves in lower back; causes corresponding motor and sensory dysfunction.

353.2 Cervical root lesions, not elsewhere classified

353.3 Thoracic root lesions, not elsewhere classified

353.4 Lumbosacral root lesions, not elsewhere classified

353.5 Neuralgic amyotrophy
Parsonage-Aldren-Turner syndrome

Trigeminal and Facial Nerve Branches

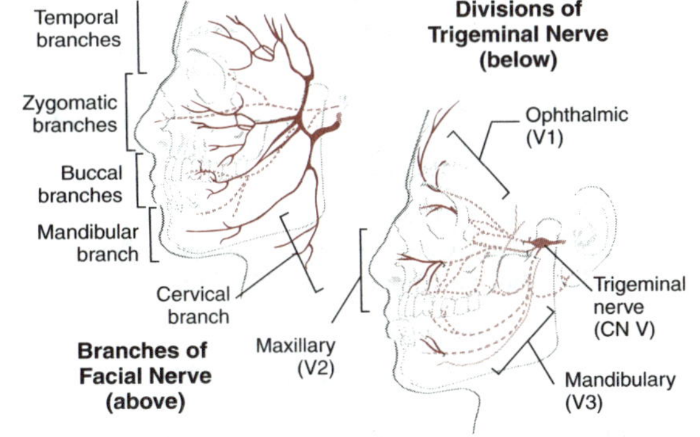

353.6 Phantom limb (syndrome)
DEF: Abnormal tingling or a burning sensation, transient aches, and intermittent or continuous pain perceived as originating in the absent limb.

353.8 Other nerve root and plexus disorders

353.9 Unspecified nerve root and plexus disorder

✓4th **354 Mononeuritis of upper limb and mononeuritis multiplex**
DEF: Inflammation of a single nerve; known as mononeuritis multiplex when several nerves in unrelated body areas are affected.

354.0 Carpal tunnel syndrome
Median nerve entrapment Partial thenar atrophy
DEF: Compression of median nerve by tendons; causes pain, tingling, numbness and burning sensation in hand.

354.1 Other lesion of median nerve
Median nerve neuritis

354.2 Lesion of ulnar nerve
Cubital tunnel syndrome
Tardy ulnar nerve palsy

354.3 Lesion of radial nerve
Acute radial nerve palsy
AHA: N-D, '87, 6

354.4 Causalgia of upper limb
EXCLUDES *causalgia:*
NOS (355.9)
lower limb (355.71)
DEF: Peripheral nerve damage, upper limb; usually due to injury; causes burning sensation and trophic skin changes.

354.5 Mononeuritis multiplex
Combinations of single conditions classifiable to 354 or 355

354.8 Other mononeuritis of upper limb

354.9 Mononeuritis of upper limb, unspecified

✓4th **355 Mononeuritis of lower limb**

355.0 Lesion of sciatic nerve
EXCLUDES *sciatica NOS (724.3)*
AHA: 2Q, '89, 12
DEF: Acquired disorder of sciatic nerve; causes motor and sensory dysfunction in back, buttock and leg.

355.1 Meralgia paresthetica
Lateral cutaneous femoral nerve of thigh compression or syndrome
DEF: Inguinal ligament entraps lateral femoral cutaneous nerve; causes tingling, pain and numbness along outer thigh.

355.2 Other lesion of femoral nerve

355.3 Lesion of lateral popliteal nerve
Lesion of common peroneal nerve

355.4 Lesion of medial popliteal nerve

355.5 Tarsal tunnel syndrome
DEF: Compressed, entrapped posterior tibial nerve; causes tingling, pain and numbness in sole of foot.

355.6 Lesion of plantar nerve
Morton's metatarsalgia, neuralgia, or neuroma

✓5th **355.7 Other mononeuritis of lower limb**

355.71 Causalgia of lower limb
EXCLUDES *causalgia:*
NOS (355.9)
upper limb (354.4)
DEF: Dysfunction of lower limb peripheral nerve, usually due to injury; causes burning pain and trophic skin changes.

355.79 Other mononeuritis of lower limb

355.8 Mononeuritis of lower limb, unspecified

355.9 Mononeuritis of unspecified site
Causalgia NOS
EXCLUDES *causalgia:*
lower limb (355.71)
upper limb (354.4)

✓4th **356 Hereditary and idiopathic peripheral neuropathy**

356.0 Hereditary peripheral neuropathy
Déjérine-Sottas disease

356.1 Peroneal muscular atrophy
Charcôt-Marie-Tooth disease
Neuropathic muscular atrophy
DEF: Genetic disorder, in muscles innervated by peroneal nerves; symptoms include muscle wasting in lower limbs and locomotor difficulties.

356.2 Hereditary sensory neuropathy
DEF: Inherited disorder in dorsal root ganglia, optic nerve, and cerebellum, causing sensory losses, shooting pains, and foot ulcers.

356.3 Refsum's disease
Heredopathia atactica polyneuritiformis
DEF: Genetic disorder of lipid metabolism; causes persistent, painful inflammation of nerves and retinitis pigmentosa.

356.4 Idiopathic progressive polyneuropathy

356.8 Other specified idiopathic peripheral neuropathy
Supranuclear paralysis

356.9 Unspecified

✓4th **357 Inflammatory and toxic neuropathy**

357.0 Acute infective polyneuritis
Guillain-Barré syndrome Postinfectious polyneuritis
AHA: 2Q, '98, 12
DEF: Guillain-Barré syndrome: acute demyelinatry polyneuropathy preceded by viral illness (i.e., herpes, cytomegalovirus [CMV], Epstein-Barr virus [EBV]) or a bacterial illness; areflexic motor paralysis with mild sensory disturbance and acellular rise in spinal fluid protein.

357.1 Polyneuropathy in collagen vascular disease
Code first underlying disease, as:
disseminated lupus erythematosus (710.0)
polyarteritis nodosa (446.0)
rheumatoid arthritis (714.0)

357.2 Polyneuropathy in diabetes
Code first underlying disease (250.6)
AHA: 4Q, '03, 105; 2Q, '92, 15; 3Q, '91, 9

357.3 Polyneuropathy in malignant disease
Code first underlying disease (140.0-208.9)

357.4 Polyneuropathy in other diseases classified elsewhere
Code first underlying disease, as:
amyloidosis (277.3)
beriberi (265.0)
deficiency of B vitamins (266.0-266.9)
diphtheria (032.0-032.9)
hypoglycemia (251.2)
pellagra (265.2)
porphyria (277.1)
sarcoidosis (135)
uremia ▶(585.9)◀
EXCLUDES *polyneuropathy in:*
herpes zoster (053.13)
mumps (072.72)
AHA: 2Q, '98, 15

357.5 Alcoholic polyneuropathy

357.6 Polyneuropathy due to drugs
Use additional E code to identify drug

357.7 Polyneuropathy due to other toxic agents
Use additional E code to identify toxic agent

✓5th **357.8 Other**
AHA: 4Q, '02, 47; 2Q, '98, 12

357.81 Chronic inflammatory demyelinating polyneuritis
DEF: Chronic inflammatory demyelinating polyneuritis: inflammation of peripheral nerves resulting in destruction of myelin sheath; associated with diabetes mellitus, dysproteinemias, renal failure and malnutrition; symptoms include tingling, numbness, burning pain, diminished tendon reflexes, weakness, and atrophy in lower extremities.

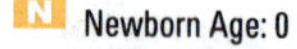
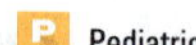

N Newborn Age: 0 P Pediatric Age: 0-17 M Maternity Age: 12-55 A Adult Age: 15-124 MSP Medicare Secondary Payer

357.82 **Critical illness polyneuropathy**
Acute motor neuropathy
AHA: 4Q, '03, 111
DEF: An acute axonal neuropathy, both sensory and motor, that is associated with Systemic Inflammatory Response Syndrome (SIRS).

357.89 **Other inflammatory and toxicneuropathy**

357.9 **Unspecified**

✓4th 358 **Myoneural disorders**

✓5th 358.0 **Myasthenia gravis**
AHA: 4Q, '03, 59
DEF: Autoimmune disorder of acetylcholine at neuromuscular junction; causing fatigue of voluntary muscles.

358.00 **Myasthenia gravis without (acute) exacerbation**
Myasthenia gravis NOS

358.01 **Myasthenia gravis with (acute) exacerbation**
Myasthenia gravis in crisis
AHA: ▶1Q, '05, 4:◀ 4Q, '04, 139

358.1 ***Myasthenic syndromes in diseases classified elsewhere***
Amyotrophy } from stated cause classified elsewhere
Eaton-Lambert syndrome }
Code first underlying disease, as:
botulism (005.1)
diabetes mellitus (250.6)
hypothyroidism (244.0-244.9)
malignant neoplasm (140.0-208.9)
pernicious anemia (281.0)
thyrotoxicosis (242.0-242.9)

358.2 **Toxic myoneural disorders**
Use additional E code to identify toxic agent

358.8 **Other specified myoneural disorders**

358.9 **Myoneural disorders, unspecified**
AHA: 2Q, '02, 16

✓4th 359 **Muscular dystrophies and other myopathies**
EXCLUDES *idiopathic polymyositis (710.4)*

359.0 **Congenital hereditary muscular dystrophy**
Benign congenital myopathy
Central core disease
Centronuclear myopathy
Myotubular myopathy
Nemaline body disease
EXCLUDES *arthrogryposis multiplex congenita (754.89)*
DEF: Genetic disorder; causing progressive or nonprogressive muscle weakness.

359.1 **Hereditary progressive muscular dystrophy**

Muscular dystrophy:	Muscular dystrophy:
NOS	Gower's
distal	Landouzy-Déjérine
Duchenne	limb-girdle
Erb's	ocular
fascioscapulohumeral	oculopharyngeal

DEF: Genetic degenerative, muscle disease; causes progressive weakness, wasting of muscle with no nerve involvement.

359.2 **Myotonic disorders**

Dystrophia myotonica	Paramyotonia congenita
Eulenburg's disease	Steinert's disease
Myotonia congenita	Thomsen's disease

DEF: Impaired movement due to spasmatic, rigid muscles.

359.3 **Familial periodic paralysis**
Hypokalemic familial periodic paralysis
DEF: Genetic disorder; characterized by rapidly progressive flaccid paralysis; attacks often occur after exercise or exposure to cold or dietary changes.

359.4 **Toxic myopathy**
Use additional E code to identify toxic agent
AHA: 1Q, '88, 5
DEF: Muscle disorder caused by toxic agent.

359.5 ***Myopathy in endocrine diseases classified elsewhere***
Code first underlying disease, as:
Addison's disease (255.4)
Cushing's syndrome (255.0)
hypopituitarism (253.2)
myxedema (244.0-244.9)
thyrotoxicosis (242.0-242.9)
DEF: Muscle disorder secondary to dysfunction in hormone secretion.

359.6 ***Symptomatic inflammatory myopathy in diseases classified elsewhere***
Code first underlying disease, as:
amyloidosis (277.3)
disseminated lupus erythematosus (710.0)
malignant neoplasm (140.0-208.9)
polyarteritis nodosa (446.0)
rheumatoid arthritis (714.0)
sarcoidosis (135)
scleroderma (710.1)
Sjögren's disease (710.2)

✓5th 359.8 **Other myopathies**
AHA: 4Q, '02, 47; 3Q, '90, 17

359.81 **Critical illness myopathy**
Acute necrotizing myopathy
Acute quadriplegic myopathy
Intensive care (ICU) myopathy
Myopathy of critical illness

359.89 **Other myopathies**

359.9 **Myopathy, unspecified**

DISORDERS OF THE EYE AND ADNEXA (360-379)

✓4th 360 **Disorders of the globe**
INCLUDES disorders affecting multiple structures of eye

✓5th 360.0 **Purulent endophthalmitis**

360.00 **Purulent endophthalmitis, unspecified**

360.01 **Acute endophthalmitis**

360.02 **Panophthalmitis**

360.03 **Chronic endophthalmitis**

360.04 **Vitreous abscess**

✓5th 360.1 **Other endophthalmitis**

360.11 **Sympathetic uveitis**
DEF: Inflammation of vascular layer of uninjured eye; follows injury to other eye.

360.12 **Panuveitis**
DEF: Inflammation of entire vascular layer of eye, including choroid, iris and ciliary body.

360.13 **Parasitic endophthalmitis NOS**
DEF: Parasitic infection causing inflammation of the entire eye.

360.14 **Ophthalmia nodosa**
DEF: Conjunctival inflammation caused by embedded hairs.

360.19 **Other**
Phacoanaphylactic endophthalmitis

✓5th 360.2 **Degenerative disorders of globe**
AHA: 3Q, '91, 3

360.20 **Degenerative disorder of globe, unspecified**

360.21 **Progressive high (degenerative) myopia**
Malignant myopia
DEF: Severe, progressive nearsightedness in adults, complicated by serious disease of the choroid; leads to retinal detachment and blindness.

360.23 **Siderosis**
DEF: Iron pigment deposits within tissue of eyeball; caused by high iron content of blood.

360.24 **Other metallosis**
Chalcosis
DEF: Metal deposits, other than iron, within eyeball tissues.

360.29 **Other**
EXCLUDES *xerophthalmia (264.7)*

✓5th 360.3 **Hypotony of eye**

360.30 **Hypotony, unspecified**
DEF: Low osmotic pressure causing lack of tone, tension and strength.

360.31 **Primary hypotony**

360.32 **Ocular fistula causing hypotony**
DEF: Low intraocular pressure due to leak through abnormal passage.

360.33 **Hypotony associated with other ocular disorders**

360.34 **Flat anterior chamber**
DEF: Low pressure behind cornea, causing compression.

✓5th 360.4 **Degenerated conditions of globe**

360.40 **Degenerated globe or eye, unspecified**

360.41 **Blind hypotensive eye**
Atrophy of globe
Phthisis bulbi
DEF: Vision loss due to extremely low intraocular pressure.

360.42 **Blind hypertensive eye**
Absolute glaucoma
DEF: Vision loss due to painful, high intraocular pressure.

360.43 **Hemophthalmos, except current injury**
EXCLUDES *traumatic (871.0-871.9, 921.0-921.9)*
DEF: Pool of blood within eyeball, not from current injury.

360.44 **Leucocoria**
DEF: Whitish mass or reflex in the pupil behind lens; also called cat's eye reflex; often indicative of retinoblastoma.

✓5th 360.5 **Retained (old) intraocular foreign body, magnetic**
EXCLUDES *current penetrating injury with magnetic foreign body (871.5)*
retained (old) foreign body of orbit (376.6)

Eye

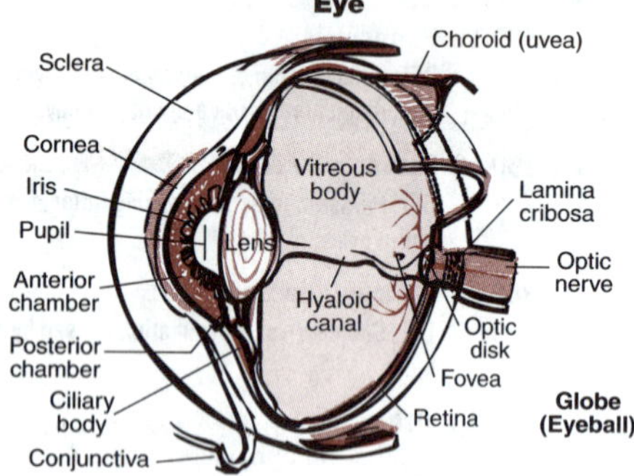

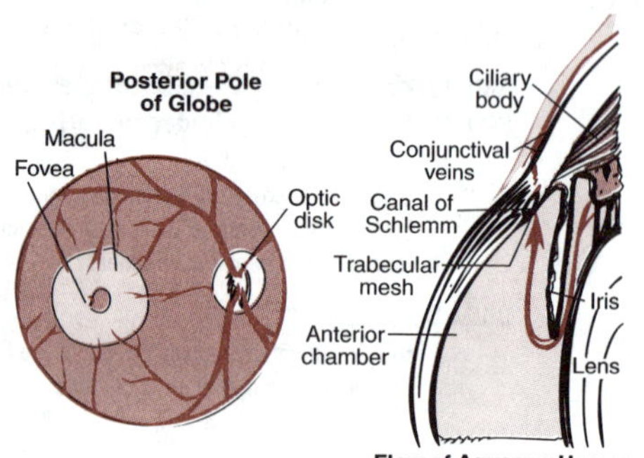

Adnexa

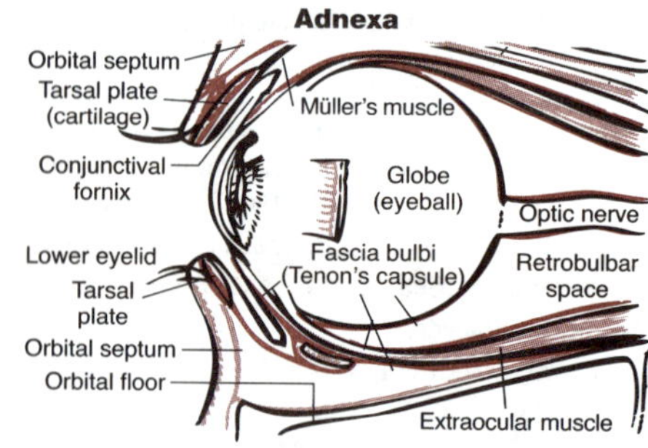

360.50 **Foreign body, magnetic, intraocular, unspecified**

360.51 **Foreign body, magnetic, in anterior chamber**

360.52 **Foreign body, magnetic, in iris or ciliary body**

360.53 **Foreign body, magnetic, in lens**

360.54 **Foreign body, magnetic, in vitreous**

360.55 **Foreign body, magnetic, in posterior wall**

360.59 **Foreign body, magnetic, in other or multiple sites**

✓5th 360.6 **Retained (old) intraocular foreign body, nonmagnetic**
Retained (old) foreign body:
NOS
nonmagnetic
EXCLUDES *current penetrating injury with (nonmagnetic) foreign body (871.6)*
retained (old) foreign body in orbit (376.6)

360.60 **Foreign body, intraocular, unspecified**

360.61 **Foreign body in anterior chamber**

360.62 **Foreign body in iris or ciliary body**

360.63 **Foreign body in lens**

360.64 **Foreign body in vitreous**

360.65 **Foreign body in posterior wall**

360.69 **Foreign body in other or multiple sites**

✓5th 360.8 **Other disorders of globe**

360.81 **Luxation of globe**
DEF: Displacement of eyeball.

360.89 **Other**

360.9 **Unspecified disorder of globe**

✓4th 361 **Retinal detachments and defects**
DEF: Light-sensitive layer at back of eye, separates from blood supply; disrupting vision.

✓5th 361.0 **Retinal detachment with retinal defect**
Rhegmatogenous retinal detachment
EXCLUDES *detachment of retinal pigment epithelium (362.42-362.43)*
retinal detachment (serous) (without defect) (361.2)

361.00 **Retinal detachment with retinal defect, unspecified**

361.01 **Recent detachment, partial, with single defect**

361.02 **Recent detachment, partial, with multiple defects**

361.03 **Recent detachment, partial, with giant tear**

361.04 **Recent detachment, partial, with retinal dialysis**
Dialysis (juvenile) of retina (with detachment)

361.05 **Recent detachment, total or subtotal**

361.06 **Old detachment, partial**
Delimited old retinal detachment

361.07 **Old detachment, total or subtotal**

✓5th **361.1 Retinoschisis and retinal cysts**

EXCLUDES *juvenile retinoschisis (362.73)*
microcystoid degeneration of retina (362.62)
parasitic cyst of retina (360.13)

361.10 Retinoschisis, unspecified

DEF: Separation of retina due to degenerative process of aging; should not be confused with acute retinal detachment.

361.11 Flat retinoschisis

DEF: Slow, progressive split of retinal sensory layers.

361.12 Bullous retinoschisis

DEF: Fluid retention between split retinal sensory layers.

361.13 Primary retinal cysts

361.14 Secondary retinal cysts

361.19 Other

Pseudocyst of retina

361.2 Serous retinal detachment

Retinal detachment without retinal defect

EXCLUDES *central serous retinopathy (362.41)*
retinal pigment epithelium detachment (362.42-362.43)

✓5th **361.3 Retinal defects without detachment**

EXCLUDES *chorioretinal scars after surgery for detachment (363.30-363.35)*
peripheral retinal degeneration without defect (362.60-362.66)

361.30 Retinal defect, unspecified

Retinal break(s) NOS

361.31 Round hole of retina without detachment

361.32 Horseshoe tear of retina without detachment

Operculum of retina without mention of detachment

361.33 Multiple defects of retina without detachment

✓5th **361.8 Other forms of retinal detachment**

361.81 Traction detachment of retina

Traction detachment with vitreoretinal organization

361.89 Other

AHA: 3Q, '99, 12

361.9 Unspecified retinal detachment

AHA: N-D, '87, 10

✓4th **362 Other retinal disorders**

EXCLUDES *chorioretinal scars (363.30-363.35)*
chorioretinitis (363.0-363.2)

✓5th **362.0 Diabetic retinopathy**

Code first diabetes (250.5)

AHA: 3Q, '91, 8

DEF: Retinal changes in diabetes of long duration; causes hemorrhages, microaneurysms, waxy deposits and proliferative noninflammatory degenerative disease of retina.

362.01 Background diabetic retinopathy

Diabetic retinal microaneurysms
Diabetic retinopathy NOS

362.02 Proliferative diabetic retinopathy

AHA: 3Q, '96, 5

● ***362.03 Nonproliferative diabetic retinopathy NOS***

● ***362.04 Mild nonproliferative diabetic retinopathy***

● ***362.05 Moderate nonproliferative diabetic retinopathy***

● ***362.06 Severe nonproliferative diabetic retinopathy***

● ***362.07 Diabetic macular edema***

Note: Code 362.07 must be used with a code for diabetic retinopathy (362.01-362.06)

Diabetic retinal edema

✓5th **362.1 Other background retinopathy and retinal vascular changes**

362.10 Background retinopathy, unspecified

362.11 Hypertensive retinopathy

AHA: 3Q, '90, 3

DEF: Retinal irregularities caused by systemic hypertension.

362.12 Exudative retinopathy

Coats' syndrome

AHA: 3Q, '99, 12

362.13 Changes in vascular appearance

Vascular sheathing of retina
Use additional code for any associated atherosclerosis (440.8)

362.14 Retinal microaneurysms NOS

DEF: Microscopic dilation of retinal vessels in nondiabetic.

362.15 Retinal telangiectasia

DEF: Dilation of blood vessels of the retina.

362.16 Retinal neovascularization NOS

Neovascularization:
- choroidal
- subretinal

DEF: New and abnormal vascular growth in the retina.

362.17 Other intraretinal microvascular abnormalities

Retinal varices

362.18 Retinal vasculitis

Eales' disease
Retinal:
- arteritis
- endarteritis
- perivasculitis
- phlebitis

DEF: Inflammation of retinal blood vessels.

✓5th **362.2 Other proliferative retinopathy**

362.21 Retrolental fibroplasia

DEF: Fibrous tissue in vitreous, from retina to lens, causing blindness; associated with premature infants requiring high amounts of oxygen.

362.29 Other nondiabetic proliferative retinopathy

AHA: 3Q, '96, 5

✓5th **362.3 Retinal vascular occlusion**

DEF: Obstructed blood flow to and from retina.

362.30 Retinal vascular occlusion, unspecified

362.31 Central retinal artery occlusion

362.32 Arterial branch occlusion

362.33 Partial arterial occlusion

Hollenhorst plaque
Retinal microembolism

362.34 Transient arterial occlusion

Amaurosis fugax

AHA: 1Q, '00, 16

362.35 Central retinal vein occlusion

AHA: 2Q, '93, 6

362.36 Venous tributary (branch) occlusion

362.37 Venous engorgement

Occlusion:
- incipient } of retinal vein
- partial } of retinal vein

✓5th **362.4 Separation of retinal layers**

EXCLUDES *retinal detachment (serous) (361.2)*
rhegmatogenous (361.00-361.07)

362.40 Retinal layer separation, unspecified

362.41 Central serous retinopathy

DEF: Serous-filled blister causing detachment of retina from pigment epithelium.

362.42 Serous detachment of retinal pigment epithelium
Exudative detachment of retinal pigment epithelium
DEF: Blister of fatty fluid causing detachment of retina from pigment epithelium.

362.43 Hemorrhagic detachment of retinal pigment epithelium
DEF: Blood-filled blister causing detachment of retina from pigment epithelium.

✓5th **362.5 Degeneration of macula and posterior pole**
EXCLUDES *degeneration of optic disc (377.21-377.24)*
hereditary retinal degeneration [dystrophy] (362.70-362.77)

362.50 Macular degeneration (senile), unspecified

362.51 Nonexudative senile macular degeneration
Senile macular degeneration:
atrophic
dry

362.52 Exudative senile macular degeneration
Kuhnt-Junius degeneration
Senile macular degeneration:
disciform
wet
DEF: Leakage in macular blood vessels with loss of visual acuity.

362.53 Cystoid macular degeneration
Cystoid macular edema
DEF: Retinal swelling and cyst formation in macula.

362.54 Macular cyst, hole, or pseudohole

362.55 Toxic maculopathy
Use additional E code to identify drug, if drug induced

362.56 Macular puckering
Preretinal fibrosis

362.57 Drusen (degenerative)
DEF: White, hyaline deposits on Bruch's membrane (lamina basalis choroideae).

✓5th **362.6 Peripheral retinal degenerations**
EXCLUDES *hereditary retinal degeneration [dystrophy] (362.70-362.77)*
retinal degeneration with retinal defect (361.00-361.07)

362.60 Peripheral retinal degeneration, unspecified

362.61 Paving stone degeneration
DEF: Degeneration of peripheral retina; causes thinning through which choroid is visible.

362.62 Microcystoid degeneration
Blessig's cysts Iwanoff's cysts

362.63 Lattice degeneration
Palisade degeneration of retina
DEF: Degeneration of retina; often bilateral, usually benign; characterized by lines intersecting at irregular intervals in peripheral retina; retinal thinning and retinal holes may occur.

362.64 Senile reticular degeneration
DEF: Net-like appearance of retina; sign of degeneration.

362.65 Secondary pigmentary degeneration
Pseudoretinitis pigmentosa

362.66 Secondary vitreoretinal degenerations

✓5th **362.7 Hereditary retinal dystrophies**
DEF: Genetically induced progressive changes in retina.

362.70 Hereditary retinal dystrophy, unspecified

362.71 Retinal dystrophy in systemic or cerebroretinal lipidoses
Code first underlying disease, as:
cerebroretinal lipidoses (330.1)
systemic lipidoses (272.7)

362.72 Retinal dystrophy in other systemic disorders and syndromes
Code first underlying disease, as:
Bassen-Kornzweig syndrome (272.5)
Refsum's disease (356.3)

362.73 Vitreoretinal dystrophies
Juvenile retinoschisis

362.74 Pigmentary retinal dystrophy
Retinal dystrophy, albipunctate
Retinitis pigmentosa

362.75 Other dystrophies primarily involving the sensory retina
Progressive cone(-rod) dystrophy
Stargardt's disease

362.76 Dystrophies primarily involving the retinal pigment epithelium
Fundus flavimaculatus
Vitelliform dystrophy

362.77 Dystrophies primarily involving Bruch's membrane
Dystrophy:
hyaline
pseudoinflammatory foveal
Hereditary drusen

✓5th **362.8 Other retinal disorders**
EXCLUDES *chorioretinal inflammations (363.0-363.2)*
chorioretinal scars (363.30-363.35)

362.81 Retinal hemorrhage
Hemorrhage:
preretinal
retinal (deep) (superficial)
subretinal
AHA: 4Q, '96, 43

362.82 Retinal exudates and deposits

362.83 Retinal edema
Retinal:
cotton wool spots
edema (localized) (macular) (peripheral)
DEF: Retinal swelling due to fluid accumulation.

362.84 Retinal ischemia
DEF: Reduced retinal blood supply.

362.85 Retinal nerve fiber bundle defects

362.89 Other retinal disorders

362.9 Unspecified retinal disorder

✓4th **363 Chorioretinal inflammations, scars, and other disorders of choroid**

✓5th **363.0 Focal chorioretinitis and focal retinochoroiditis**
EXCLUDES *focal chorioretinitis or retinochoroiditis in:*
histoplasmosis (115.02, 115.12, 115.92)
toxoplasmosis (130.2)
congenital infection (771.2)

363.00 Focal chorioretinitis, unspecified
Focal:
choroiditis or chorioretinitis NOS
retinitis or retinochoroiditis NOS

363.01 Focal choroiditis and chorioretinitis, juxtapapillary

363.03 Focal choroiditis and chorioretinitis of other posterior pole

363.04 Focal choroiditis and chorioretinitis, peripheral

363.05 Focal retinitis and retinochoroiditis, juxtapapillary
Neuroretinitis

363.06 Focal retinitis and retinochoroiditis, macular or paramacular

363.07 Focal retinitis and retinochoroiditis of other posterior pole

363.08 Focal retinitis and retinochoroiditis, peripheral

✓5th **363.1 Disseminated chorioretinitis and disseminated retinochoroiditis**

EXCLUDES *disseminated choroiditis or chorioretinitis in secondary syphilis (091.51)*
neurosyphilitic disseminated retinitis or retinochoroiditis (094.83)
retinal (peri)vasculitis (362.18)

363.10 Disseminated chorioretinitis, unspecified
Disseminated:
choroiditis or chorioretinitis NOS
retinitis or retinochoroiditis NOS

363.11 Disseminated choroiditis and chorioretinitis, posterior pole

363.12 Disseminated choroiditis and chorioretinitis, peripheral

363.13 Disseminated choroiditis and chorioretinitis, generalized
Code first any underlying disease, as:
tuberculosis (017.3)

363.14 Disseminated retinitis and retinochoroiditis, metastatic

363.15 Disseminated retinitis and retinochoroiditis, pigment epitheliopathy
Acute posterior multifocal placoid pigment epitheliopathy
DEF: Widespread inflammation of retina and choroid; characterized by pigmented epithelium involvement.

✓5th **363.2 Other and unspecified forms of chorioretinitis and retinochoroiditis**

EXCLUDES *panophthalmitis (360.02)*
sympathetic uveitis (360.11)
uveitis NOS (364.3)

363.20 Chorioretinitis, unspecified
Choroiditis NOS
Retinitis NOS
Uveitis, posterior NOS

363.21 Pars planitis
Posterior cyclitis
DEF: Inflammation of peripheral retina and ciliary body; characterized by bands of white cells.

363.22 Harada's disease
DEF: Retinal detachment and bilateral widespread exudative choroiditis; symptoms include headache, vomiting, increased lymphocytes in cerebrospinal fluid; and temporary or permanent deafness may occur.

✓5th **363.3 Chorioretinal scars**
Scar (postinflammatory) (postsurgical) (posttraumatic):
choroid
retina

363.30 Chorioretinal scar, unspecified

363.31 Solar retinopathy
DEF: Retinal scarring caused by solar radiation.

363.32 Other macular scars

363.33 Other scars of posterior pole

363.34 Peripheral scars

363.35 Disseminated scars

✓5th **363.4 Choroidal degenerations**

363.40 Choroidal degeneration, unspecified
Choroidal sclerosis NOS

363.41 Senile atrophy of choroid
DEF: Wasting away of choroid; due to aging.

363.42 Diffuse secondary atrophy of choroid
DEF: Wasting away of choroid in systemic disease.

363.43 Angioid streaks of choroid
DEF: Degeneration of choroid; characterized by dark brown steaks radiating from optic disk; occurs with pseudoxanthoma, elasticum or Paget's disease.

✓5th **363.5 Hereditary choroidal dystrophies**
Hereditary choroidal atrophy:
partial [choriocapillaris]
total [all vessels]

363.50 Hereditary choroidal dystrophy or atrophy, unspecified

363.51 Circumpapillary dystrophy of choroid, partial

363.52 Circumpapillary dystrophy of choroid, total
Helicoid dystrophy of choroid

363.53 Central dystrophy of choroid, partial
Dystrophy, choroidal:
central areolar
Dystrophy, choroidal:
circinate

363.54 Central choroidal atrophy, total
Dystrophy, choroidal:
central gyrate
Dystrophy, choroidal:
serpiginous

363.55 Choroideremia
DEF: Hereditary choroid degeneration, occurs in first decade; characterized by constricted visual field and ultimately blindness in males; less debilitating in females.

363.56 Other diffuse or generalized dystrophy, partial
Diffuse choroidal sclerosis

363.57 Other diffuse or generalized dystrophy, total
Generalized gyrate atrophy, choroid

✓5th **363.6 Choroidal hemorrhage and rupture**

363.61 Choroidal hemorrhage, unspecified

363.62 Expulsive choroidal hemorrhage

363.63 Choroidal rupture

✓5th **363.7 Choroidal detachment**

363.70 Choroidal detachment, unspecified

363.71 Serous choroidal detachment
DEF: Detachment of choroid from sclera; due to blister of serous fluid.

363.72 Hemorrhagic choroidal detachment
DEF: Detachment of choroid from sclera; due to blood-filled blister.

363.8 Other disorders of choroid

363.9 Unspecified disorder of choroid

✓4th **364 Disorders of iris and ciliary body**

✓5th **364.0 Acute and subacute iridocyclitis**
Anterior uveitis
Cyclitis
Iridocyclitis
Iritis
} acute, subacute

EXCLUDES *gonococcal (098.41)*
herpes simplex (054.44)
herpes zoster (053.22)

364.00 Acute and subacute iridocyclitis, unspecified

364.01 Primary iridocyclitis

364.02 Recurrent iridocyclitis

364.03 Secondary iridocyclitis, infectious

364.04 Secondary iridocyclitis, noninfectious
Aqueous:
cells
fibrin
Aqueous:
flare

364.05 Hypopyon
DEF: Accumulation of white blood cells between cornea and lens.

✓5th **364.1 Chronic iridocyclitis**

EXCLUDES *posterior cyclitis (363.21)*

364.10 Chronic iridocyclitis, unspecified

364.11 Chronic iridocyclitis in diseases classified elsewhere

Code first underlying disease, as:
sarcoidosis (135)
tuberculosis (017.3)

EXCLUDES *syphilitic iridocyclitis (091.52)*

DEF: Persistent inflammation of iris and ciliary body; due to underlying disease or condition.

✓5th **364.2 Certain types of iridocyclitis**

EXCLUDES *posterior cyclitis (363.21)*
sympathetic uveitis (360.11)

364.21 Fuchs' heterochromic cyclitis

DEF: Chronic cyclitis characterized by differences in the color of the two irises; the lighter iris appears in the inflamed eye.

364.22 Glaucomatocyclitic crises

DEF: One-sided form of secondary open angle glaucoma; recurrent, uncommon and of short duration; causes high intraocular pressure, rarely damage.

364.23 Lens-induced iridocyclitis

DEF: Inflammation of iris; due to immune reaction to proteins in lens following trauma or other lens abnormality.

364.24 Vogt-Koyanagi syndrome

DEF: Uveomeningitis with exudative iridocyclitis and choroiditis; causes depigmentation of hair and skin, detached retina; tinnitus and loss of hearing may occur.

364.3 Unspecified iridocyclitis

Uveitis NOS

✓5th **364.4 Vascular disorders of iris and ciliary body**

364.41 Hyphema

Hemorrhage of iris or ciliary body

DEF: Hemorrhage in anterior chamber; also called hyphemia or "blood shot" eyes.

364.42 Rubeosis iridis

Neovascularization of iris or ciliary body

DEF: Blood vessel and connective tissue formation on surface of iris; symptomatic of diabetic retinopathy, central retinal vein occlusion and retinal detachment.

✓5th **364.5 Degenerations of iris and ciliary body**

364.51 Essential or progressive iris atrophy

364.52 Iridoschisis

DEF: Splitting of iris into two layers.

364.53 Pigmentary iris degeneration

Acquired heterochromia, Pigment dispersion syndrome, Translucency } of iris

364.54 Degeneration of pupillary margin

Atrophy of sphincter, Ectropion of pigment epithelium } of iris

364.55 Miotic cysts of pupillary margin

DEF: Serous-filled sacs in pupillary margin of iris.

364.56 Degenerative changes of chamber angle

364.57 Degenerative changes of ciliary body

364.59 Other iris atrophy

Iris atrophy (generalized) (sector shaped)

✓5th **364.6 Cysts of iris, ciliary body, and anterior chamber**

EXCLUDES *miotic pupillary cyst (364.55)*
parasitic cyst (360.13)

364.60 Idiopathic cysts

DEF: Fluid-filled sacs in iris or ciliary body; unknown etiology.

364.61 Implantation cysts

Epithelial down-growth, anterior chamber
Implantation cysts (surgical) (traumatic)

364.62 Exudative cysts of iris or anterior chamber

364.63 Primary cyst of pars plana

DEF: Fluid-filled sacs of outermost ciliary ring.

364.64 Exudative cyst of pars plana

DEF: Protein, fatty-filled sacs of outermost ciliary ring; due to fluid lead from blood vessels.

✓5th **364.7 Adhesions and disruptions of iris and ciliary body**

EXCLUDES *flat anterior chamber (360.34)*

364.70 Adhesions of iris, unspecified

Synechiae (iris) NOS

364.71 Posterior synechiae

DEF: Adhesion binding iris to lens.

364.72 Anterior synechiae

DEF: Adhesion binding the iris to cornea.

364.73 Goniosynechiae

Peripheral anterior synechiae

DEF: Adhesion binding the iris to cornea at the angle of the anterior chamber.

364.74 Pupillary membranes

Iris bombé
Pupillary:
occlusion
Pupillary:
seclusion

DEF: Membrane traversing the pupil and blocking vision.

364.75 Pupillary abnormalities

Deformed pupil
Ectopic pupil
Rupture of sphincter, pupil

364.76 Iridodialysis

DEF: Separation of the iris from the ciliary body base; due to trauma or surgical accident.

364.77 Recession of chamber angle

DEF: Receding of anterior chamber angle of the eye; restricts vision.

364.8 Other disorders of iris and ciliary body

Prolapse of iris NOS

EXCLUDES *prolapse of iris in recent wound (871.1)*

364.9 Unspecified disorder of iris and ciliary body

✓4th **365 Glaucoma**

EXCLUDES *blind hypertensive eye [absolute glaucoma] (360.42)*
congenital glaucoma (743.20-743.22)

DEF: Rise in intraocular pressure which restricts blood flow; multiple causes.

✓5th **365.0 Borderline glaucoma [glaucoma suspect]**

AHA: 1Q, '90, 8

365.00 Preglaucoma, unspecified

365.01 Open angle with borderline findings

Open angle with:
borderline intraocular pressure
cupping of optic discs

DEF: Minor block of aqueous outflow from eye.

365.02 Anatomical narrow angle

365.03 Steroid responders

365.04 Ocular hypertension

DEF: High fluid pressure within eye; no apparent cause.

✓5th **365.1 Open-angle glaucoma**

365.10 Open-angle glaucoma, unspecified

Wide-angle glaucoma NOS

365.11 Primary open angle glaucoma

Chronic simple glaucoma

DEF: High intraocular pressure, despite free flow of aqueous.

365.12 Low tension glaucoma

365.13 **Pigmentary glaucoma**
DEF: High intraocular pressure; due to iris pigment granules blocking aqueous flow.

365.14 **Glaucoma of childhood**
Infantile or juvenile glaucoma

365.15 **Residual stage of open angle glaucoma**

✓5th 365.2 **Primary angle-closure glaucoma**

365.20 **Primary angle-closure glaucoma, unspecified**

365.21 **Intermittent angle-closure glaucoma**
Angle-closure glaucoma:
interval
subacute
DEF: Recurring attacks of high intraocular pressure; due to blocked aqueous flow.

365.22 **Acute angle-closure glaucoma**
DEF: Sudden, severe rise in intraocular pressure due to blockage in aqueous drainage.

365.23 **Chronic angle-closure glaucoma**
AHA: 2Q, '98, 16

365.24 **Residual stage of angle-closure glaucoma**

✓5th 365.3 **Corticosteroid-induced glaucoma**
DEF: Elevated intraocular pressure; due to long-term corticosteroid therapy.

365.31 **Glaucomatous stage**

365.32 **Residual stage**

✓5th 365.4 **Glaucoma associated with congenital anomalies, dystrophies, and systemic syndromes**

365.41 ***Glaucoma associated with chamber angle anomalies***
Code first associated disorder, as:
Axenfeld's anomaly (743.44)
Rieger's anomaly or syndrome (743.44)

365.42 ***Glaucoma associated with anomalies of iris***
Code first associated disorder, as:
aniridia (743.45)
essential iris atrophy (364.51)

365.43 ***Glaucoma associated with other anterior segment anomalies***
Code first associated disorder, as:
microcornea (743.41)

365.44 ***Glaucoma associated with systemic syndromes***
Code first associated disease, as
neurofibromatosis (237.7)
Sturge-Weber (-Dimitri) syndrome (759.6)

✓5th 365.5 **Glaucoma associated with disorders of the lens**

365.51 **Phacolytic glaucoma**
Use additional code for associated hypermature cataract (366.18)
DEF: Elevated intraocular pressure; due to lens protein blocking aqueous flow.

365.52 **Pseudoexfoliation glaucoma**
Use additional code for associated pseudoexfoliation of capsule (366.11)
DEF: Glaucoma characterized by small grayish particles deposited on the lens.

365.59 **Glaucoma associated with other lens disorders**
Use additional code for associated disorder, as:
dislocation of lens (379.33-379.34)
spherophakia (743.36)

✓5th 365.6 **Glaucoma associated with other ocular disorders**

365.60 **Glaucoma associated with unspecified ocular disorder**

365.61 **Glaucoma associated with pupillary block**
Use additional code for associated disorder, as:
seclusion of pupil [iris bombé] (364.74)
DEF: Acute, open-angle glaucoma caused by mature cataract; aqueous flow is blocked by lens material and macrophages.

365.62 **Glaucoma associated with ocular inflammations**
Use additional code for associated disorder, as:
glaucomatocyclitic crises (364.22)
iridocyclitis (364.0-364.3)

365.63 **Glaucoma associated with vascular disorders**
Use additional code for associated disorder, as:
central retinal vein occlusion (362.35)
hyphema (364.41)

365.64 **Glaucoma associated with tumors or cysts**
Use additional code for associated disorder, as:
benign neoplasm (224.0-224.9)
epithelial down-growth (364.61)
malignant neoplasm (190.0-190.9)

365.65 **Glaucoma associated with ocular trauma**
Use additional code for associated condition, as:
contusion of globe (921.3)
recession of chamber angle (364.77)

✓5th 365.8 **Other specified forms of glaucoma**

365.81 **Hypersecretion glaucoma**

365.82 **Glaucoma with increased episcleral venous pressure**

365.83 **Aqueous misdirection**
Malignant glaucoma
AHA: 4Q, '02, 48
DEF: A form of glaucoma that occurs when aqueous humor flows into the posterior chamber of the eye (vitreous) rather than through the normal recycling channels into the anterior chamber.

365.89 **Other specified glaucoma**
AHA: 2Q, '98, 16

365.9 **Unspecified glaucoma**
AHA: 3Q, '03, 14; 2Q, '01, 16

✓4th **366 Cataract**
EXCLUDES *congenital cataract (743.30-743.34)*
DEF: A variety of conditions that create a cloudy, or calcified lens that obstructs vision.

✓5th 366.0 **Infantile, juvenile, and presenile cataract**

366.00 **Nonsenile cataract, unspecified**

366.01 **Anterior subcapsular polar cataract**
DEF: Defect within the front, center lens surface.

Aqueous Misdirection Syndrome

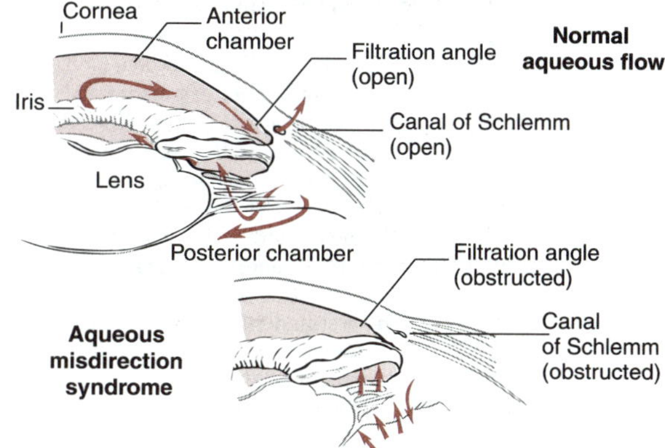

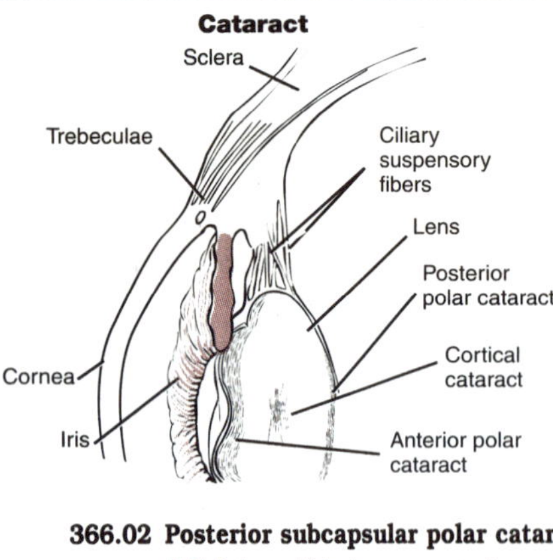

366.02 Posterior subcapsular polar cataract
DEF: Defect within the rear, center lens surface.

366.03 Cortical, lamellar, or zonular cataract
DEF: Opacities radiating from center to edge of lens; appear as thin, concentric layers of lens.

366.04 Nuclear cataract

366.09 Other and combined forms of nonsenile cataract

✓5th **366.1 Senile cataract**
AHA: 3Q, '91, 9; S-0, '85, 10

366.10 Senile cataract, unspecified A
AHA: 1Q, '03, 5

366.11 Pseudoexfoliation of lens capsule A

366.12 Incipient cataract A
Cataract: coronary, immature NOS
Cataract: punctate
Water clefts
DEF: Minor disorders of lens not affecting vision; due to aging.

366.13 Anterior subcapsular polar senile cataract A

366.14 Posterior subcapsular polar senile cataract A

366.15 Cortical senile cataract A

366.16 Nuclear sclerosis A
Cataracta brunescens
Nuclear cataract

366.17 Total or mature cataract A

366.18 Hypermature cataract A
Morgagni cataract

366.19 Other and combined forms of senile cataract A

✓5th **366.2 Traumatic cataract**

366.20 Traumatic cataract, unspecified

366.21 Localized traumatic opacities
Vossius' ring

366.22 Total traumatic cataract

366.23 Partially resolved traumatic cataract

✓5th **366.3 Cataract secondary to ocular disorders**

366.30 Cataracta complicata, unspecified

366.31 Glaucomatous flecks (subcapsular)
Code first underlying glaucoma (365.0-365.9)

366.32 Cataract in inflammatory disorders
Code first underlying condition, as:
chronic choroiditis (363.0-363.2)

366.33 Cataract with neovascularization
Code first underlying condition, as:
chronic iridocyclitis (364.10)

366.34 Cataract in degenerative disorders
Sunflower cataract
Code first underlying condition, as:
chalcosis (360.24)
degenerative myopia (360.21)
pigmentary retinal dystrophy (362.74)

✓5th **366.4 Cataract associated with other disorders**

366.41 Diabetic cataract
Code first diabetes (250.5)
AHA: 3Q, '91, 9; S-0, '85, 11

366.42 Tetanic cataract
Code first underlying disease, as:
calcinosis (275.4)
hypoparathyroidism (252.1)

366.43 Myotonic cataract
Code first underlying disorder (359.2)

366.44 Cataract associated with other syndromes
Code first underlying condition, as:
craniofacial dysostosis (756.0)
galactosemia (271.1)

366.45 Toxic cataract
Drug-induced cataract
Use additional E code to identify drug or other toxic substance

366.46 Cataract associated with radiation and other physical influences
Use additional E code to identify cause

✓5th **366.5 After-cataract**

366.50 After-cataract, unspecified
Secondary cataract NOS

366.51 Soemmering's ring
DEF: A donut-shaped lens remnant and a capsule behind the pupil as a result of cataract surgery or trauma.

366.52 Other after-cataract, not obscuring vision

366.53 After-cataract, obscuring vision

366.8 Other cataract
Calcification of lens

366.9 Unspecified cataract

✓4th **367 Disorders of refraction and accommodation**

367.0 Hypermetropia
Far-sightedness
Hyperopia
DEF: Refraction error, called also hyperopia, focal point is posterior to retina; abnormally short anteroposterior diameter or subnormal refractive power; causes farsightedness.

367.1 Myopia
Near-sightedness
DEF: Refraction error, focal point is anterior to retina; causes near-sightedness.

✓5th **367.2 Astigmatism**

367.20 Astigimatism, unspecified

367.21 Regular astigmatism

367.22 Irregular astigmatism

✓5th **367.3 Anisometropia and aniseikonia**

367.31 Anisometropia
DEF: Eyes with refractive powers that differ by at least one diopter.

367.32 Aniseikonia
DEF: Eyes with unequal retinal imaging; usually due to refractive error.

367.4 Presbyopia
DEF: Loss of crystalline lens elasticity; causes errors of accommodation; due to aging.

✓5th **367.5 Disorders of accommodation**

367.51 Paresis of accommodation
Cycloplegia
DEF: Partial paralysis of ciliary muscle; causing focus problems.

367.52 Total or complete internal ophthalmoplegia
DEF: Total paralysis of ciliary muscle; large pupil incapable of focus.

367.53 Spasm of accommodation
DEF: Abnormal contraction of ciliary muscle; causes focus problems.

Classification "legal"	Classification WHO	LEVELS OF VISUAL IMPAIRMENT — Visual acuity and/or visual field limitation (whichever is worse)	Additional descriptors which may be encountered
	(NEAR-) NORMAL VISION	RANGE OF NORMAL VISION 20/10 20/13 20/16 20/20 20/25 2.0 1.6 1.25 1.0 0.8	
		NEAR-NORMAL VISION 20/30 20/40 20/50 20/60 0.7 0.6 0.5 0.4 0.3	
	LOW VISION	MODERATE VISUAL IMPAIRMENT 20/70 20/80 20/100 20/125 20/160 0.25 0.20 0.16 0.12	Moderate low vision
LEGAL BLINDNESS (U.S.A.) both eyes		SEVERE VISUAL IMPAIRMENT 20/200 20/250 20/320 20/400 0.10 0.08 0.06 0.05 Visual field: 20 degrees or less	Severe low vision, "Legal" blindness
	BLINDNESS (WHO) one or both eyes	PROFOUND VISUAL IMPAIRMENT 20/500 20/630 20/800 20/1000 0.04 0.03 0.025 0.02 Count fingers at: less than 3m (10 ft.) Visual field: 10 degrees or less	Profound low vision, Moderate blindness
		NEAR-TOTAL VISUAL IMPAIRMENT Visual acuity: less than 0.02 (20/1000) Count fingers at: 1m (3 ft.) or less Hand movements: 5m (15 ft.) or less Light projection, light perception Visual field: 5 degrees or less	Severe blindness, Near-total blindness
		TOTAL VISUAL IMPAIRMENT No light perception (NLP)	Total blindness

Visual acuity refers to best achievable acuity with correction.
Non-listed Snellen fractions may be classified by converting to the nearest decimal equivalent, e.g. 10/200 = 0.05, 6/30 = 0.20.
CF (count fingers) without designation of distance, may be classified to profound impairment.
HM (hand motion) without designation of distance, may be classified to near-total impairment.
Visual field measurements refer to the largest field diameter for a 1/100 white test object.

✓5th **367.8 Other disorders of refraction and accommodation**

367.81 Transient refractive change

367.89 Other

Drug-induced } disorders of refraction
Toxic } & accommodation

367.9 Unspecified disorder of refraction and accommodation

✓4th **368 Visual disturbances**

EXCLUDES *electrophysiological disturbances (794.11-794.14)*

✓5th **368.0 Amblyopia ex anopsia**

DEF: Vision impaired due to disuse; esotropia often cause.

368.00 Amblyopia, unspecified

368.01 Strabismic amblyopia

Suppression amblyopia

368.02 Deprivation amblyopia

DEF: Decreased vision associated with suppressed retinal image of one eye.

368.03 Refractive amblyopia

✓5th **368.1 Subjective visual disturbances**

368.10 Subjective visual disturbance, unspecified

368.11 Sudden visual loss

368.12 Transient visual loss

Concentric fading
Scintillating scotoma

368.13 Visual discomfort

Asthenopia
Eye strain
Photophobia

368.14 Visual distortions of shape and size

Macropsia
Metamorphopsia
Micropsia

368.15 Other visual distortions and entoptic phenomena

Photopsia
Refractive:
 diplopia
Refractive:
 polyopia
Visual halos

368.16 Psychophysical visual disturbances

Visual:
 agnosia
 disorientation syndrome
Visual:
 hallucinations

368.2 Diplopia

Double vision

✓5th **368.3 Other disorders of binocular vision**

368.30 Binocular vision disorder, unspecified

368.31 Suppression of binocular vision

368.32 Simultaneous visual perception without fusion

368.33 Fusion with defective stereopsis

DEF: Faulty depth perception though normal ability to focus.

368.34 Abnormal retinal correspondence

✓5th **368.4 Visual field defects**

368.40 Visual field defect, unspecified

368.41 Scotoma involving central area

Scotoma:
 central
 centrocecal
Scotoma:
 paracentral

DEF: Vision loss (blind spot) in central five degrees of visual field.

368.42 Scotoma of blind spot area

Enlarged:
 angioscotoma
 blind spot
Paracecal scotoma

368.43 Sector or arcuate defects

Scotoma:
 arcuate
 Bjerrum
 Seidel

DEF: Arc-shaped blind spot caused by retinal nerve damage.

368.44 Other localized visual field defect

Scotoma:
 NOS
 ring
Visual field defect:
 nasal step
 peripheral

368.45 Generalized contraction or constriction

368.46 Homonymous bilateral field defects

Hemianopsia (altitudinal) (homonymous)
Quadrant anopia

DEF: Disorders found in the corresponding vertical halves of the visual fields of both eyes.

368.47 Heteronymous bilateral field defects

Hemianopsia:
 binasal
Hemianopsia:
 bitemporal

DEF: Disorders in the opposite halves of the visual fields of both eyes.

✓5th **368.5 Color vision deficiencies**

Color blindness

368.51 Protan defect

Protanomaly
Protanopia

DEF: Mild difficulty distinguishing green and red hues with shortened spectrum; sex-linked affecting one percent of males.

368.52 Deutan defect
Deuteranomaly Deuteranopia
DEF: Male-only disorder; difficulty in distinguishing green and red, no shortened spectrum.

368.53 Tritan defect
Tritanomaly Tritanopia
DEF: Difficulty in distinguishing blue and yellow; occurs often due to drugs, retinal detachment and central nervous system diseases.

368.54 Achromatopsia
Monochromatism (cone) (rod)
DEF: Complete color blindness; caused by disease, injury to retina, optic nerve or pathway.

368.55 Acquired color vision deficiencies

368.59 Other color vision deficiencies

✓5th **368.6 Night blindness**
Nyctalopia
DEF: Nyctalopia: disorder of vision in dim light or night blindness.

368.60 Night blindness, unspecified

368.61 Congenital night blindness
Hereditary night blindness
Oguchi's disease

368.62 Acquired night blindness
EXCLUDES *that due to vitamin A deficiency (264.5)*

368.63 Abnormal dark adaptation curve
Abnormal threshold } of cones or rods
Delayed adaptation } of cones or rods

368.69 Other night blindness

368.8 Other specified visual disturbances
Blurred vision NOS
AHA: 4Q, '02, 56

368.9 Unspecified visual disturbance
AHA: 1Q, '04, 15

✓4th **369 Blindness and low vision**

Note: Visual impairment refers to a functional limitation of the eye (e.g., limited visual acuity or visual field). It should be distinguished from visual disability, indicating a limitation of the abilities of the individual (e.g., limited reading skills, vocational skills), and from visual handicap, indicating a limitation of personal and socioeconomic independence (e.g., limited mobility, limited employability).

The levels of impairment defined in the table on page 95 are based on the recommendations of the WHO Study Group on Prevention of Blindness (Geneva, November 6–10, 1972; WHO Technical Report Series 518), and of the International Council of Ophthalmology (1976).

Note that definitions of blindness vary in different settings.

For international reporting WHO defines blindness as profound impairment. This definition can be applied to blindness of one eye (369.1, 369.6) and to blindness of the individual (369.0).

For determination of benefits in the U.S.A., the definition of legal blindness as severe impairment is often used. This definition applies to blindness of the individual only.

EXCLUDES *correctable impaired vision due to refractive errors (367.0-367.9)*

✓5th **369.0 Profound impairment, both eyes**

369.00 Impairment level not further specified
Blindness:
NOS according to WHO definition
both eyes

369.01 Better eye: total impairment; lesser eye: total impairment

369.02 Better eye: near-total impairment; lesser eye: not further specified

369.03 Better eye: near-total impairment; lesser eye: total impairment

369.04 Better eye: near-total impairment; lesser eye: near-total impairment

369.05 Better eye: profound impairment; lesser eye: not further specified

369.06 Better eye: profound impairment; lesser eye: total impairment

369.07 Better eye: profound impairment; lesser eye: near-total impairment

369.08 Better eye: profound impairment; lesser eye: profound impairment

✓5th **369.1 Moderate or severe impairment, better eye, profound impairment lesser eye**

369.10 Impairment level not further specified
Blindness, one eye, low vision other eye

369.11 Better eye: severe impairment; lesser eye: blind, not further specified

369.12 Better eye: severe impairment; lesser eye: total impairment

369.13 Better eye: severe impairment; lesser eye: near-total impairment

369.14 Better eye: severe impairment; lesser eye: profound impairment

369.15 Better eye: moderate impairment; lesser eye: blind, not further specified

369.16 Better eye: moderate impairment; lesser eye: total impairment

369.17 Better eye: moderate impairment; lesser eye: near-total impairment

369.18 Better eye: moderate impairment; lesser eye: profound impairment

✓5th **369.2 Moderate or severe impairment, both eyes**

369.20 Impairment level not further specified
Low vision, both eyes NOS

369.21 Better eye: severe impairment; lesser eye: not further specified

369.22 Better eye: severe impairment; lesser eye: severe impairment

369.23 Better eye: moderate impairment; lesser eye: not further specified

369.24 Better eye: moderate impairment; lesser eye: severe impairment

369.25 Better eye: moderate impairment; lesser eye: moderate impairment

369.3 Unqualified visual loss, both eyes
EXCLUDES *blindness NOS:*
legal [U.S.A. definition] (369.4)
WHO definition (369.00)

369.4 Legal blindness, as defined in U.S.A.
Blindness NOS according to U.S.A. definition
EXCLUDES *legal blindness with specification of impairment level (369.01-369.08, 369.11-369.14, 369.21-369.22)*

✓5th **369.6 Profound impairment, one eye**

369.60 Impairment level not further specified
Blindness, one eye

369.61 One eye: total impairment; other eye: not specified

369.62 One eye: total impairment; other eye: near-normal vision

369.63 One eye: total impairment; other eye: normal vision

369.64 One eye: near-total impairment; other eye: not specified

369.65 One eye: near-total impairment; other eye: near-normal vision

369.66 One eye: near-total impairment; other eye: normal vision

369.67 One eye: profound impairment; other eye: not specified

369.68 One eye: profound impairment; other eye: near-normal vision

369.69 One eye: profound impairment; other eye: normal vision

✓5th **369.7 Moderate or severe impairment, one eye**

369.70 Impairment level not further specified

Low vision, one eye

369.71 One eye: severe impairment; other eye: not specified

369.72 One eye: severe impairment; other eye: near-normal vision

369.73 One eye: severe impairment; other eye: normal vision

369.74 One eye: moderate impairment; other eye: not specified

369.75 One eye: moderate impairment; other eye: near-normal vision

369.76 One eye: moderate impairment; other eye: normal vision

369.8 Unqualified visual loss, one eye

369.9 Unspecified visual loss

AHA: 4Q, '02, 114; 3Q, '02, 20

✓4th **370 Keratitis**

✓5th **370.0 Corneal ulcer**

EXCLUDES *that due to vitamin A deficiency (264.3)*

370.00 Corneal ulcer, unspecified

370.01 Marginal corneal ulcer

370.02 Ring corneal ulcer

370.03 Central corneal ulcer

370.04 Hypopyon ulcer

Serpiginous ulcer

DEF: Corneal ulcer with an accumulation of pus in the eye's anterior chamber.

370.05 Mycotic corneal ulcer

DEF: Fungal infection causing corneal tissue loss.

370.06 Perforated corneal ulcer

DEF: Tissue loss through all layers of cornea.

370.07 Mooren's ulcer

DEF: Tissue loss, with chronic inflammation, at junction of cornea and sclera; seen in elderly.

✓5th **370.2 Superficial keratitis without conjunctivitis**

EXCLUDES *dendritic [herpes simplex] keratitis (054.42)*

370.20 Superficial keratitis, unspecified

370.21 Punctate keratitis

Thygeson's superficial punctate keratitis

DEF: Formation of cellular and fibrinous deposits (keratic precipitates) on posterior surface; deposits develop after injury or iridocyclitis.

370.22 Macular keratitis

Keratitis:	Keratitis:
areolar	stellate
nummular	striate

370.23 Filamentary keratitis

DEF: Keratitis characterized by twisted filaments of mucoid material on the cornea's surface.

370.24 Photokeratitis

Snow blindness
Welders' keratitis

AHA: 3Q, '96, 6

DEF: Painful, inflamed cornea; due to extended exposure to ultraviolet light.

✓5th **370.3 Certain types of keratoconjunctivitis**

370.31 Phlyctenular keratoconjunctivitis

Phlyctenulosis

Use additional code for any associated tuberculosis (017.3)

DEF: Miniature blister on conjunctiva or cornea; associated with tuberculosis and malnutrition disorders.

370.32 Limbar and corneal involvement in vernal conjunctivitis

Use additional code for vernal conjunctivitis (372.13)

DEF: Corneal itching and inflammation in conjunctivitis; often limited to lining of eyelids.

370.33 Keratoconjunctivitis sicca, not specified as Sjögren's

EXCLUDES *Sjögren's syndrome (710.2)*

DEF: Inflammation of conjunctiva and cornea; characterized by "horny" looking tissue and excess blood in these areas; decreased flow of lacrimal (tear) is a contributing factor.

370.34 Exposure keratoconjunctivitis

AHA: 3Q, '96, 6

DEF: Incomplete closure of eyelid causing dry, inflamed eye.

370.35 Neurotrophic keratoconjunctivitis

✓5th **370.4 Other and unspecified keratoconjunctivitis**

370.40 Keratoconjunctivitis, unspecified

Superficial keratitis with conjunctivitis NOS

370.44 Keratitis or keratoconjunctivitis in exanthema

Code first underlying condition (050.0-052.9)

EXCLUDES *herpes simplex (054.43)*
herpes zoster (053.21)
measles (055.71)

370.49 Other

EXCLUDES *epidemic keratoconjunctivitis (077.1)*

✓5th **370.5 Interstitial and deep keratitis**

370.50 Interstitial keratitis, unspecified

370.52 Diffuse interstitial keratitis

Cogan's syndrome

DEF: Inflammation of cornea; with deposits in middle corneal layers; may obscure vision.

370.54 Sclerosing keratitis

DEF: Chronic corneal inflammation leading to opaque scarring.

370.55 Corneal abscess

DEF: Pocket of pus and inflammation on the cornea.

370.59 Other

EXCLUDES *disciform herpes simplex keratitis (054.43)*
syphilitic keratitis (090.3)

✓5th **370.6 Corneal neovascularization**

370.60 Corneal neovascularization, unspecified

370.61 Localized vascularization of cornea

DEF: Limited infiltration of cornea by new blood vessels.

370.62 Pannus (corneal)

AHA: 3Q, '02, 20

DEF: Buildup of superficial vascularization and granulated tissue under epithelium of cornea.

370.63 Deep vascularization of cornea

DEF: Deep infiltration of cornea by new blood vessels.

370.64 Ghost vessels (corneal)

370.8 **Other forms of keratitis**
AHA: 3Q, '94, 5

370.9 **Unspecified keratitis**

✓4th 371 **Corneal opacity and other disorders of cornea**

✓5th 371.0 **Corneal scars and opacities**
EXCLUDES *that due to vitamin A deficiency (264.6)*

371.00 **Corneal opacity, unspecified**
Corneal scar NOS

371.01 **Minor opacity of cornea**
Corneal nebula

371.02 **Peripheral opacity of cornea**
Corneal macula not interfering with central vision

371.03 **Central opacity of cornea**
Corneal:
leucoma } interfering with central vision
macula }

371.04 **Adherent leucoma**
DEF: Dense, opaque corneal growth adhering to the iris; also spelled as leukoma.

371.05 ***Phthisical cornea***
Code first underlying tuberculosis (017.3)

✓5th 371.1 **Corneal pigmentations and deposits**

371.10 **Corneal deposit, unspecified**

371.11 **Anterior pigmentations**
Stähli's lines

371.12 **Stromal pigmentations**
Hematocornea

371.13 **Posterior pigmentations**
Krukenberg spindle

371.14 **Kayser-Fleischer ring**
DEF: Copper deposits forming ring at outer edge of cornea; seen in Wilson's disease and other liver disorders.

371.15 **Other deposits associated with metabolic disorders**

371.16 **Argentous deposits**
DEF: Silver deposits in cornea.

✓5th 371.2 **Corneal edema**

371.20 **Corneal edema, unspecified**

371.21 **Idiopathic corneal edema**
DEF: Corneal swelling and fluid retention of unknown cause.

371.22 **Secondary corneal edema**
DEF: Corneal swelling and fluid retention caused by an underlying disease, injury, or condition.

371.23 **Bullous keratopathy**
DEF: Corneal degeneration; characterized by recurring, rupturing epithelial "blisters;" ruptured blebs expose corneal nerves, cause great pain; occurs in glaucoma, iridocyclitis and Fuchs' epithelial dystrophy.

371.24 **Corneal edema due to wearing of contact lenses**

✓5th 371.3 **Changes of corneal membranes**

371.30 **Corneal membrane change, unspecified**

371.31 **Folds and rupture of Bowman's membrane**

371.32 **Folds in Descemet's membrane**

371.33 **Rupture in Descemet's membrane**

✓5th 371.4 **Corneal degenerations**

371.40 **Corneal degeneration, unspecified**

371.41 **Senile corneal changes**
Arcus senilis Hassall-Henle bodies

371.42 **Recurrent erosion of cornea**
EXCLUDES *Mooren's ulcer (370.07)*

371.43 **Band-shaped keratopathy**
DEF: Horizontal bands of superficial corneal calcium deposits.

371.44 **Other calcerous degenerations of cornea**

371.45 **Keratomalacia NOS**
EXCLUDES *that due to vitamin A deficiency (264.4)*
DEF: Destruction of the cornea by keratinization of the epithelium with ulceration and perforation of the cornea; seen in cases of vitamin A deficiency.

371.46 **Nodular degeneration of cornea**
Salzmann's nodular dystrophy

371.48 **Peripheral degenerations of cornea**
Marginal degeneration of cornea [Terrien's]

371.49 **Other**
Discrete colliquative keratopathy

✓5th 371.5 **Hereditary corneal dystrophies**
DEF: Genetic disorder; leads to opacities, edema or lesions of cornea.

371.50 **Corneal dystrophy, unspecified**

371.51 **Juvenile epithelial corneal dystrophy**

371.52 **Other anterior corneal dystrophies**
Corneal dystrophy:
microscopic cystic
ring-like

371.53 **Granular corneal dystrophy**

371.54 **Lattice corneal dystrophy**

371.55 **Macular corneal dystrophy**

371.56 **Other stromal corneal dystrophies**
Crystalline corneal dystrophy

371.57 **Endothelial corneal dystrophy**
Combined corneal dystrophy
Cornea guttata
Fuchs' endothelial dystrophy

371.58 **Other posterior corneal dystrophies**
Polymorphous corneal dystrophy

✓5th 371.6 **Keratoconus**
DEF: Bilateral bulging protrusion of anterior cornea; often due to noninflammatory thinning.

371.60 **Keratoconus, unspecified**

371.61 **Keratoconus, stable condition**

371.62 **Keratoconus, acute hydrops**

✓5th 371.7 **Other corneal deformities**

371.70 **Corneal deformity, unspecified**

371.71 **Corneal ectasia**
DEF: Bulging protrusion of thinned, scarred cornea.

371.72 **Descemetocele**
DEF: Protrusion of Descemet's membrane into cornea.

371.73 **Corneal staphyloma**
DEF: Protrusion of cornea into adjacent tissue.

✓5th 371.8 **Other corneal disorders**

371.81 **Corneal anesthesia and hypoesthesia**
DEF: Decreased or absent sensitivity of cornea.

371.82 **Corneal disorder due to contact lens**
EXCLUDES *corneal edema due to contact lens (371.24)*
DEF: Contact lens wear causing cornea disorder, excluding swelling.

371.89 **Other**
AHA: 3Q, '99, 12

371.9 **Unspecified corneal disorder**

372 Disorders of conjunctiva

EXCLUDES *keratoconjunctivitis (370.3-370.4)*

372.0 Acute conjunctivitis

372.00 Acute conjunctivitis, unspecified

372.01 Serous conjunctivitis, except viral

EXCLUDES *viral conjunctivitis NOS (077.9)*

372.02 Acute follicular conjunctivitis

Conjunctival folliculosis NOS

EXCLUDES *conjunctivitis:*
adenoviral (acute follicular) (077.3)
epidemic hemorrhagic (077.4)
inclusion (077.0)
Newcastle (077.8)
epidemic keratoconjunctivitis (077.1)
pharyngoconjunctival fever (077.2)

DEF: Severe conjunctival inflammation with dense infiltrations of lymphoid tissues of inner eyelids; may be traced to a viral or chlamydial etiology.

372.03 Other mucopurulent conjunctivitis

Catarrhal conjunctivitis

EXCLUDES *blennorrhea neonatorum (gonococcal) (098.40)*
neonatal conjunctivitis(771.6)
ophthalmia neonatorum NOS (771.6)

372.04 Pseudomembranous conjunctivitis

Membranous conjunctivitis

EXCLUDES *diphtheritic conjunctivitis (032.81)*

DEF: Severe inflammation of conjunctiva; false membrane develops on inner surface of eyelid; membrane can be removed without harming epithelium, due to bacterial infections, toxic and allergic factors, and viral infections.

372.05 Acute atopic conjunctivitis

DEF: Sudden, severe conjunctivitis due to allergens.

372.1 Chronic conjunctivitis

372.10 Chronic conjunctivitis, unspecified

372.11 Simple chronic conjunctivitis

372.12 Chronic follicular conjunctivitis

DEF: Persistent inflammation of conjunctiva; with infiltration of lymphoid tissue of inner eyelids.

372.13 Vernal conjunctivitis

AHA: 3Q, '96, 8

372.14 Other chronic allergic conjunctivitis

AHA: 3Q, '96, 8

372.15 Parasitic conjunctivitis

Code first underlying disease, as:
filariasis (125.0-125.9)
mucocutaneous leishmaniasis (085.5)

372.2 Blepharoconjunctivitis

372.20 Blepharoconjunctivitis, unspecified

372.21 Angular blepharoconjunctivitis

DEF: Inflammation at junction of upper and lower eyelids; may block lacrimal secretions.

372.22 Contact blepharoconjunctivitis

372.3 Other and unspecified conjunctivitis

372.30 Conjunctivitis, unspecified

372.31 Rosacea conjunctivitis

Code first underlying rosacea dermatitis (695.3)

372.33 Conjunctivitis in mucocutaneous disease

Code first underlying disease, as:
erythema multiforme (695.1)
Reiter's disease (099.3)

EXCLUDES *ocular pemphigoid (694.61)*

372.39 Other

372.4 Pterygium

EXCLUDES *pseudopterygium (372.52)*

DEF: Wedge-shaped, conjunctival thickening that advances from the inner corner of the eye toward the cornea.

372.40 Pterygium, unspecified

372.41 Peripheral pterygium, stationary

372.42 Peripheral pterygium, progressive

372.43 Central pterygium

372.44 Double pterygium

372.45 Recurrent pterygium

372.5 Conjunctival degenerations and deposits

372.50 Conjunctival degeneration, unspecified

372.51 Pinguecula

DEF: Proliferative spot on the bulbar conjunctiva located near the sclerocorneal junction, usually on the nasal side; it is seen in elderly people.

372.52 Pseudopterygium

DEF: Conjunctival scar joined to the cornea; it looks like a pterygium but is not attached to the tissue.

372.53 Conjunctival xerosis

EXCLUDES *conjunctival xerosis due to vitamin A deficiency (264.0, 264.1, 264.7)*

DEF: Dry conjunctiva due to vitamin A deficiency; related to Bitot's spots; may develop into xerophthalmia and keratomalacia.

372.54 Conjunctival concretions

DEF: Calculus or deposit on conjunctiva.

372.55 Conjunctival pigmentations

Conjunctival argyrosis

DEF: Color deposits in conjunctiva.

372.56 Conjunctival deposits

372.6 Conjunctival scars

372.61 Granuloma of conjunctiva

372.62 Localized adhesions and strands of conjunctiva

DEF: Abnormal fibrous connections in conjunctiva.

372.63 Symblepharon

Extensive adhesions of conjunctiva

DEF: Adhesion of the eyelids to the eyeball.

372.64 Scarring of conjunctiva

Contraction of eye socket (after enucleation)

372.7 Conjunctival vascular disorders and cysts

372.71 Hyperemia of conjunctiva

DEF: Conjunctival blood vessel congestion causing eye redness.

372.72 Conjunctival hemorrhage

Hyposphagma
Subconjunctival hemorrhage

372.73 Conjunctival edema

Chemosis of conjunctiva
Subconjunctival edema

DEF: Fluid retention and swelling in conjunctival tissue.

372.74 Vascular abnormalities of conjunctiva

Aneurysm(ata) of conjunctiva

372.75 Conjunctival cysts

DEF: Abnormal sacs of fluid in conjunctiva.

✓5th 372.8 **Other disorders of conjunctiva**

372.81 **Conjunctivochalasis**

AHA: 4Q, '00, 41

DEF: Bilateral condition of redundant conjunctival tissue between globe and lower eyelid margin; may cover lower punctum, interferring with normal tearing.

372.89 **Other disorders of conjunctiva**

372.9 **Unspecified disorder of conjunctiva**

✓4th 373 **Inflammation of eyelids**

✓5th 373.0 **Blepharitis**

EXCLUDES *blepharoconjunctivitis (372.20-372.22)*

373.00 **Blepharitis, unspecified**

373.01 **Ulcerative blepharitis**

373.02 **Squamous blepharitis**

✓5th 373.1 **Hordeolum and other deep inflammation of eyelid**

DEF: Purulent, localized, staphylococcal infection in sebaceous glands of eyelids.

373.11 **Hordeolum externum**

Hordeolum NOS
Stye

DEF: Infection of oil gland in eyelash follicles.

373.12 **Hordeolum internum**

Infection of meibomian gland

DEF: Infection of oil gland of eyelid margin.

373.13 **Abscess of eyelid**

Furuncle of eyelid

DEF: Inflamed pocket of pus on eyelid.

373.2 **Chalazion**

Meibomian (gland) cyst

EXCLUDES *infected meibomian gland (373.12)*

DEF: Chronic inflammation of the meibomian gland, causing an eyelid mass.

✓5th 373.3 **Noninfectious dermatoses of eyelid**

373.31 **Eczematous dermatitis of eyelid**

373.32 **Contact and allergic dermatitis of eyelid**

373.33 **Xeroderma of eyelid**

373.34 **Discoid lupus erythematosus of eyelid**

373.4 ***Infective dermatitis of eyelid of types resulting in deformity***

Code first underlying disease, as:
leprosy (030.0-030.9)
lupus vulgaris (tuberculous) (017.0)
yaws (102.0-102.9)

373.5 ***Other infective dermatitis of eyelid***

Code first underlying disease, as:
actinomycosis (039.3)
impetigo (684)
mycotic dermatitis (110.0-111.9)
vaccinia (051.0)
postvaccination (999.0)

EXCLUDES *herpes:*
simplex (054.41)
zoster (053.20)

373.6 ***Parasitic infestation of eyelid***

Code first underlying disease, as:
leishmaniasis (085.0-085.9)
loiasis (125.2)
onchocerciasis (125.3)
pediculosis (132.0)

373.8 **Other inflammations of eyelids**

373.9 **Unspecified inflammation of eyelid**

✓4th 374 **Other disorders of eyelids**

✓5th 374.0 **Entropion and trichiasis of eyelid**

DEF: Entropion: turning inward of eyelid edge toward eyeball.

DEF: Trichiasis: ingrowing eyelashes marked by irritation with possible distortion of sight.

Entropion and Ectropion

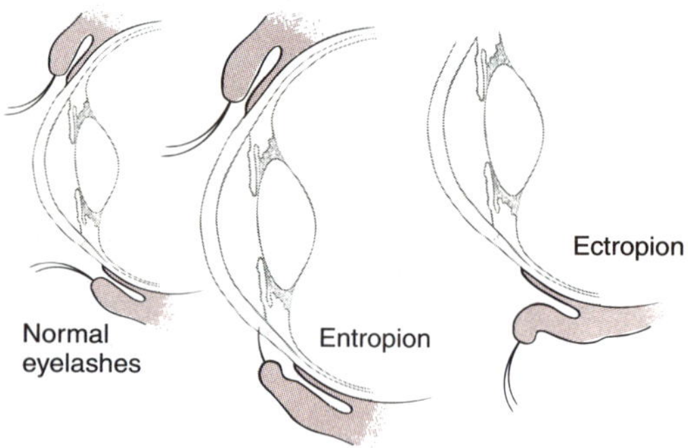

374.00 **Entropion, unspecified**

374.01 **Senile entropion** A

374.02 **Mechanical entropion**

374.03 **Spastic entropion**

374.04 **Cicatricial entropion**

374.05 **Trichiasis without entropion**

✓5th 374.1 **Ectropion**

DEF: Turning outward (eversion) of eyelid edge; exposes palpebral conjunctiva; dryness, irritation result.

374.10 **Ectropion, unspecified**

374.11 **Senile ectropion** A

374.12 **Mechanical ectropion**

374.13 **Spastic ectropion**

374.14 **Cicatricial ectropion**

✓5th 374.2 **Lagophthalmos**

DEF: Incomplete closure of eyes; causes dry eye and other complications.

374.20 **Lagophthalmos, unspecified**

374.21 **Paralytic lagophthalmos**

374.22 **Mechanical lagophthalmos**

374.23 **Cicatricial lagophthalmos**

✓5th 374.3 **Ptosis of eyelid**

374.30 **Ptosis of eyelid, unspecified**

AHA: 2Q, '96, 11

374.31 **Paralytic ptosis**

DEF: Drooping of upper eyelid due to nerve disorder.

374.32 **Myogenic ptosis**

DEF: Drooping of upper eyelid due to muscle disorder.

374.33 **Mechanical ptosis**

DEF: Outside force causes drooping of upper eyelid.

374.34 **Blepharochalasis**

Pseudoptosis

DEF: Loss of elasticity, thickened or indurated skin of eyelids associated with recurrent episodes of idiopathic edema causing intracellular tissue atrophy.

✓5th 374.4 **Other disorders affecting eyelid function**

EXCLUDES *blepharoclonus (333.81)*
blepharospasm (333.81)
facial nerve palsy (351.0)
third nerve palsy or paralysis (378.51-378.52)
tic (psychogenic) (307.20-307.23)
organic (333.3)

374.41 **Lid retraction or lag**

374.43 **Abnormal innervation syndrome**

Jaw-blinking
Paradoxical facial movements

374.44 **Sensory disorders**

N Newborn Age: 0 P Pediatric Age: 0-17 M Maternity Age: 12-55 A Adult Age: 15-124 MSP Medicare Secondary Payer

374.45 **Other sensorimotor disorders**
Deficient blink reflex

374.46 **Blepharophimosis**
Ankyloblepharon
DEF: Narrowing of palpebral fissure horizontally; caused by laterally displaced inner canthi; either acquired or congenital.

5th 374.5 **Degenerative disorders of eyelid and periocular area**

374.50 **Degenerative disorder of eyelid, unspecified**

374.51 ***Xanthelasma***
Xanthoma (planum) (tuberosum) of eyelid
Code first underlying condition (272.0-272.9)
DEF: Fatty tumors of eyelid linked to high fat content of blood.

374.52 **Hyperpigmentation of eyelid**
Chloasma Dyspigmentation
DEF: Excess pigment of eyelid.

374.53 **Hypopigmentation of eyelid**
Vitiligo of eyelid
DEF: Lack of color pigment of the eyelid.

374.54 **Hypertrichosis of eyelid**
DEF: Excess eyelash growth.

374.55 **Hypotrichosis of eyelid**
Madarosis of eyelid
DEF: Less than normal, or .absent, eyelashes.

374.56 **Other degenerative disorders of skin affecting eyelid**

5th 374.8 **Other disorders of eyelid**

374.81 **Hemorrhage of eyelid**
EXCLUDES *black eye (921.0)*

374.82 **Edema of eyelid**
Hyperemia of eyelid
DEF: Swelling and fluid retention in eyelid.

374.83 **Elephantiasis of eyelid**
DEF: Filarial disease causing dermatitis and enlarged eyelid.

374.84 **Cysts of eyelids**
Sebaceous cyst of eyelid

374.85 **Vascular anomalies of eyelid**

374.86 **Retained foreign body of eyelid**

374.87 **Dermatochalasis**
DEF: Acquired form of connective tissue disorder associated with decreased elastic tissue and abnormal elastin formation resulting in loss of elasticity of the skin of the eyelid, generally associated with aging.

374.89 **Other disorders of eyelid**

374.9 **Unspecified disorder of eyelid**

4th 375 **Disorders of lacrimal system**

5th 375.0 **Dacryoadenitis**

375.00 **Dacryoadenitis, unspecified**

375.01 **Acute dacryoadenitis**
DEF: Severe, sudden inflammation of lacrimal gland.

375.02 **Chronic dacryoadenitis**
DEF: Persistent inflammation of lacrimal gland.

375.03 **Chronic enlargement of lacrimal gland**

5th 375.1 **Other disorders of lacrimal gland**

375.11 **Dacryops**
DEF: Overproduction and constant flow of tears; may cause distended lacrimal duct.

375.12 **Other lacrimal cysts and cystic degeneration**

375.13 **Primary lacrimal atrophy**

375.14 **Secondary lacrimal atrophy**
DEF: Wasting away of lacrimal gland due to another disease.

375.15 **Tear film insufficiency, unspecified**
Dry eye syndrome
AHA: 3Q, '96, 6
DEF: Eye dryness and irritation due to insufficient tear production.

375.16 **Dislocation of lacrimal gland**

5th 375.2 **Epiphora**
DEF: Abnormal development of tears due to stricture of lacrimal passages.

375.20 **Epiphora, unspecified as to cause**

375.21 **Epiphora due to excess lacrimation**
DEF: Tear overflow due to overproduction.

375.22 **Epiphora due to insufficient drainage**
DEF: Tear overflow due to blocked drainage.

5th 375.3 **Acute and unspecified inflammation of lacrimal passages**
EXCLUDES *neonatal dacryocystitis (771.6)*

375.30 **Dacryocystitis, unspecified**

375.31 **Acute canaliculitis, lacrimal**

375.32 **Acute dacryocystitis**
Acute peridacryocystitis

375.33 **Phlegmonous dacryocystitis**
DEF: Infection of tear sac with pockets of pus.

5th 375.4 **Chronic inflammation of lacrimal passages**

375.41 **Chronic canaliculitis**

375.42 **Chronic dacryocystitis**

375.43 **Lacrimal mucocele**

5th 375.5 **Stenosis and insufficiency of lacrimal passages**

375.51 **Eversion of lacrimal punctum**
DEF: Abnormal turning outward of tear duct.

375.52 **Stenosis of lacrimal punctum**
DEF: Abnormal narrowing of tear duct.

375.53 **Stenosis of lacrimal canaliculi**

375.54 **Stenosis of lacrimal sac**
DEF: Abnormal narrowing of tear sac.

375.55 **Obstruction of nasolacrimal duct, neonatal**
EXCLUDES *congenital anomaly of nasolacrimal duct (743.65)*
DEF: Acquired, abnormal obstruction of lacrimal system, from eye to nose; in an infant.

375.56 **Stenosis of nasolacrimal duct, acquired**

375.57 **Dacryolith**
DEF: Concretion or stone in lacrimal system.

5th 375.6 **Other changes of lacrimal passages**

375.61 **Lacrimal fistula**
DEF: Abnormal communication from lacrimal system.

375.69 **Other**

5th 375.8 **Other disorders of lacrimal system**

375.81 **Granuloma of lacrimal passages**
DEF: Abnormal nodules within lacrimal system.

375.89 **Other**

375.9 **Unspecified disorder of lacrimal system**

4th 376 **Disorders of the orbit**

5th 376.0 **Acute inflammation of orbit**

376.00 **Acute inflammation of orbit, unspecified**

376.01 **Orbital cellulitis**
Abscess of orbit
DEF: Infection of tissue between orbital bone and eyeball.

376.02 **Orbital periostitis**
DEF: Inflammation of connective tissue covering orbital bone.

376.03 **Orbital osteomyelitis**
DEF: Inflammation of orbital bone.

376.04 **Tenonitis**

Lacrimal System

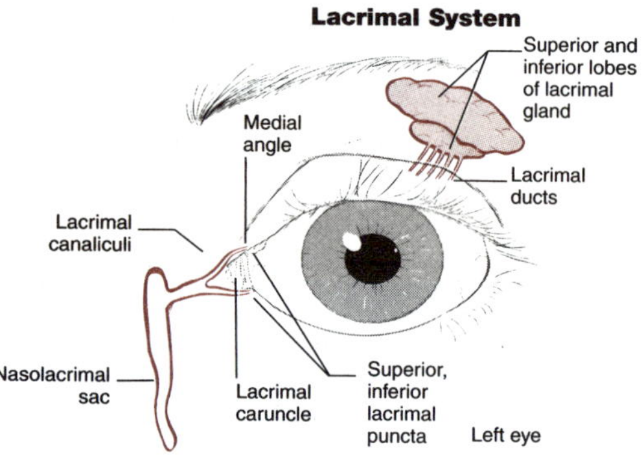

✓5th **376.1 Chronic inflammatory disorders of orbit**

376.10 Chronic inflammation of orbit, unspecified

376.11 Orbital granuloma

Pseudotumor (inflammatory) of orbit

DEF: Abnormal nodule between orbital bone and eyeball.

376.12 Orbital myositis

DEF: Painful inflammation of eye muscles.

376.13 Parasitic infestation of orbit

Code first underlying disease, as:

hydatid infestation of orbit (122.3, 122.6, 122.9)

myiasis of orbit (134.0)

✓5th **376.2 Endocrine exophthalmos**

Code first underlying thyroid disorder (242.0-242.9)

376.21 Thyrotoxic exophthalmos

DEF: Bulging eyes due to hyperthyroidism.

376.22 Exophthalmic ophthalmoplegia

DEF: Inability to rotate eye due to bulging eyes.

✓5th **376.3 Other exophthalmic conditions**

376.30 Exophthalmos, unspecified

DEF: Abnormal protrusion of eyeball.

376.31 Constant exophthalmos

DEF: Continuous, abnormal protrusion or bulging of eyeball.

376.32 Orbital hemorrhage

DEF: Bleeding behind the eyeball, causing forward bulge.

376.33 Orbital edema or congestion

DEF: Fluid retention behind eyeball, causing forward bulge.

376.34 Intermittent exophthalmos

376.35 Pulsating exophthalmos

DEF: Bulge or protrusion; associated with a carotid-cavernous fistula.

376.36 Lateral displacement of globe

DEF: Abnormal displacement of the eyeball away from nose, toward temple.

✓5th **376.4 Deformity of orbit**

376.40 Deformity of orbit, unspecified

376.41 Hypertelorism of orbit

DEF: Abnormal increase in interorbital distance; associated with congenital facial deformities; may be accompanied by mental deficiency.

376.42 Exostosis of orbit

DEF: Abnormal bony growth of orbit.

376.43 Local deformities due to bone disease

DEF: Acquired abnormalities of orbit; due to bone disease.

376.44 Orbital deformities associated with craniofacial deformities

376.45 Atrophy of orbit

DEF: Wasting away of bone tissue of orbit.

376.46 Enlargement of orbit

376.47 Deformity due to trauma or surgery

✓5th **376.5 Enophthalmos**

DEF: Recession of eyeball deep into eye socket.

376.50 Enophthalmos, unspecified as to cause

376.51 Enophthalmos due to atrophy of orbital tissue

376.52 Enophthalmos due to trauma or surgery

376.6 Retained (old) foreign body following penetrating wound of orbit

Retrobulbar foreign body

✓5th **376.8 Other orbital disorders**

376.81 Orbital cysts

Encephalocele of orbit

AHA: 3Q, '99, 13

376.82 Myopathy of extraocular muscles

DEF: Disease in the muscles that control eyeball movement.

376.89 Other

376.9 Unspecified disorder of orbit

✓4th **377 Disorders of optic nerve and visual pathways**

✓5th **377.0 Papilledema**

377.00 Papilledema, unspecified

377.01 Papilledema associated with increased intracranial pressure

377.02 Papilledema associated with decreased ocular pressure

377.03 Papilledema associated with retinal disorder

377.04 Foster-Kennedy syndrome

DEF: Retrobulbar optic neuritis, central scotoma and optic atrophy; caused by tumors in frontal lobe of brain that press downward.

✓5th **377.1 Optic atrophy**

377.10 Optic atrophy, unspecified

377.11 Primary optic atrophy

EXCLUDES *neurosyphilitic optic atrophy (094.84)*

377.12 Postinflammatory optic atrophy

DEF: Adverse effect of inflammation causing wasting away of eye.

377.13 Optic atrophy associated with retinal dystrophies

DEF: Progressive changes in retinal tissue due to metabolic disorder causing wasting away of eye.

377.14 Glaucomatous atrophy [cupping] of optic disc

377.15 Partial optic atrophy

Temporal pallor of optic disc

377.16 Hereditary optic atrophy

Optic atrophy:
- dominant hereditary
- Leber's

✓5th **377.2 Other disorders of optic disc**

377.21 Drusen of optic disc

377.22 Crater-like holes of optic disc

377.23 Coloboma of optic disc

DEF: Ocular malformation caused by the failure of fetal fissure of optic stalk to close.

377.24 Pseudopapilledema

✓5th **377.3 Optic neuritis**

EXCLUDES *meningococcal optic neuritis (036.81)*

377.30 Optic neuritis, unspecified

377.31 Optic papillitis

DEF: Swelling and inflammation of optic disc.

377.32 **Retrobulbar neuritis (acute)**
EXCLUDES *syphilitic retrobulbar neuritis (094.85)*
DEF: Inflammation of optic nerve immediately behind the eyeball.

377.33 **Nutritional optic neuropathy**
DEF: Malnutrition causing optic nerve disorder.

377.34 **Toxic optic neuropathy**
Toxic amblyopia
DEF: Toxic substance causing optic nerve disorder.

377.39 **Other**
EXCLUDES *ischemic optic neuropathy (377.41)*

5th 377.4 **Other disorders of optic nerve**
377.41 **Ischemic optic neuropathy**
DEF: Decreased blood flow affecting optic nerve.

377.42 **Hemorrhage in optic nerve sheaths**
DEF: Bleeding in meningeal lining of optic nerve.

377.49 **Other**
Compression of optic nerve

5th 377.5 **Disorders of optic chiasm**
377.51 **Associated with pituitary neoplasms and disorders**
DEF: Abnormal pituitary growth causing disruption in nerve chain from retina to brain.

377.52 **Associated with other neoplasms**
DEF: Abnormal growth, other than pituitary, causing disruption in nerve chain from retina to brain.

377.53 **Associated with vascular disorders**
DEF: Vascular disorder causing disruption in nerve chain from retina to brain.

377.54 **Associated with inflammatory disorders**
DEF: Inflammatory disease causing disruption in nerve chain from retina to brain.

5th 377.6 **Disorders of other visual pathways**
377.61 **Associated with neoplasms**
377.62 **Associated with vascular disorders**
377.63 **Associated with inflammatory disorders**

5th 377.7 **Disorders of visual cortex**
EXCLUDES *visual:*
agnosia (368.16)
hallucinations (368.16)
halos (368.15)
377.71 **Associated with neoplasms**
377.72 **Associated with vascular disorders**
377.73 **Associated with inflammatory disorders**
377.75 **Cortical blindness**
DEF: Blindness due to brain disorder, rather than eye disorder.

377.9 **Unspecified disorder of optic nerve and visual pathways**

4th 378 **Strabismus and other disorders of binocular eye movements**
EXCLUDES *nystagmus and other irregular eye movements (379.50-379.59)*
DEF: Misalignment of the eyes due to imbalance in extraocular muscles.

5th 378.0 **Esotropia**
Convergent concomitant strabismus
EXCLUDES *intermittent esotropia (378.20-378.22)*
DEF: Visual axis deviation created by one eye fixing upon an image and the other eye deviating inward.

378.00 **Esotropia, unspecified**
378.01 **Monocular esotropia**
378.02 **Monocular esotropia with A pattern**
378.03 **Monocular esotropia with V pattern**

Eye Musculature

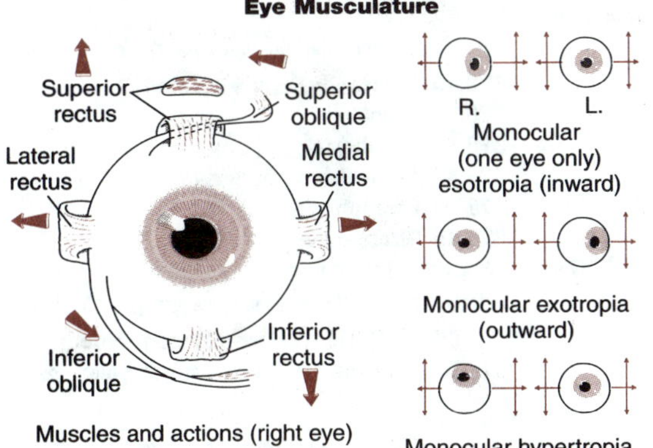

378.04 **Monocular esotropia with other noncomitancies**
Monocular esotropia with X or Y pattern
378.05 **Alternating esotropia**
378.06 **Alternating esotropia with A pattern**
378.07 **Alternating esotropia with V pattern**
378.08 **Alternating esotropia with other noncomitancies**
Alternating esotropia with X or Y pattern

5th 378.1 **Exotropia**
Divergent concomitant strabismus
EXCLUDES *intermittent exotropia (378.20, 378.23-378.24)*
DEF: Visual axis deviation created by one eye fixing upon an image and the other eye deviating outward.

378.10 **Exotropia, unspecified**
378.11 **Monocular exotropia**
378.12 **Monocular exotropia with A pattern**
378.13 **Monocular exotropia with V pattern**
378.14 **Monocular exotropia with other noncomitancies**
Monocular exotropia with X or Y pattern
378.15 **Alternating exotropia**
378.16 **Alternating exotropia with A pattern**
378.17 **Alternating exotropia with V pattern**
378.18 **Alternating exotropia with other noncomitancies**
Alternating exotropia with X or Y pattern

5th 378.2 **Intermittent heterotropia**
EXCLUDES *vertical heterotropia (intermittent) (378.31)*
DEF: Deviation of eyes seen only at intervals; it is also called strabismus.

378.20 **Intermittent heterotropia, unspecified**
Intermittent:
esotropia NOS
exotropia NOS
378.21 **Intermittent esotropia, monocular**
378.22 **Intermittent esotropia, alternating**
378.23 **Intermittent exotropia, monocular**
378.24 **Intermittent exotropia, alternating**

5th 378.3 **Other and unspecified heterotropia**
378.30 **Heterotropia, unspecified**
378.31 **Hypertropia**
Vertical heterotropia (constant) (intermittent)
378.32 **Hypotropia**
378.33 **Cyclotropia**
378.34 **Monofixation syndrome**
Microtropia
378.35 **Accommodative component in esotropia**

✓5th **378.4 Heterophoria**

DEF: Deviation occurring only when the other eye is covered.

378.40 Heterophoria, unspecified

378.41 Esophoria

378.42 Exophoria

378.43 Vertical heterophoria

378.44 Cyclophoria

378.45 Alternating hyperphoria

✓5th **378.5 Paralytic strabismus**

DEF: Deviation of the eye due to nerve paralysis affecting muscle.

378.50 Paralytic strabismus, unspecified

378.51 Third or oculomotor nerve palsy, partial

AHA: 3Q, '91, 9

378.52 Third or oculomotor nerve palsy, total

AHA: 2Q, '89, 12

378.53 Fourth or trochlear nerve palsy

AHA: 2Q, '01, 21

378.54 Sixth or abducens nerve palsy

AHA: 2Q, '89, 12

378.55 External ophthalmoplegia

378.56 Total ophthalmoplegia

✓5th **378.6 Mechanical strabismus**

DEF: Deviation of the eye due to an outside force on extraocular muscle.

378.60 Mechanical strabismus, unspecified

378.61 Brown's (tendon) sheath syndrome

DEF: Congenital or acquired shortening of the anterior sheath of the superior oblique muscle; the eye is unable to move upward and inward; it is usually unilateral.

378.62 Mechanical strabismus from other musculofascial disorders

378.63 Limited duction associated with other conditions

✓5th **378.7 Other specified strabismus**

378.71 Duane's syndrome

DEF: Congenital, affects one eye; due to abnormal fibrous bands attached to rectus muscle; inability to abduct affected eye with retraction of globe.

378.72 Progressive external ophthalmoplegia

DEF: Paralysis progressing from one eye muscle to another.

378.73 Strabismus in other neuromuscular disorders

✓5th **378.8 Other disorders of binocular eye movements**

EXCLUDES *nystagmus (379.50-379.56)*

378.81 Palsy of conjugate gaze

DEF: Muscle dysfunction impairing parallel movement of the eye.

378.82 Spasm of conjugate gaze

DEF: Muscle contractions impairing parallel movement of eye.

378.83 Convergence insufficiency or palsy

378.84 Convergence excess or spasm

378.85 Anomalies of divergence

378.86 Internuclear ophthalmoplegia

DEF: Eye movement anomaly due to brainstem lesion.

378.87 Other dissociated deviation of eye movements

Skew deviation

378.9 Unspecified disorder of eye movements

Ophthalmoplegia NOS Strabismus NOS

AHA: 2Q, '01, 21

✓4th **379 Other disorders of eye**

✓5th **379.0 Scleritis and episcleritis**

EXCLUDES *syphilitic episcleritis (095.0)*

379.00 Scleritis, unspecified

Episcleritis NOS

379.01 Episcleritis periodica fugax

DEF: Hyperemia (engorgement) of the sclera and overlying conjunctiva characterized by a sudden onset and short duration.

379.02 Nodular episcleritis

DEF: Inflammation of the outermost layer of the sclera, with formation of nodules.

379.03 Anterior scleritis

379.04 Scleromalacia perforans

DEF: Scleral thinning, softening and degeneration; seen with rheumatoid arthritis.

379.05 Scleritis with corneal involvement

Scleroperikeratitis

379.06 Brawny scleritis

DEF: Severe inflammation of the sclera; with thickened corneal margins.

379.07 Posterior scleritis

Sclerotenonitis

379.09 Other

Scleral abscess

✓5th **379.1 Other disorders of sclera**

EXCLUDES *blue sclera (743.47)*

379.11 Scleral ectasia

Scleral staphyloma NOS

DEF: Protrusion of the contents of the eyeball where the sclera has thinned.

379.12 Staphyloma posticum

DEF: Ring-shaped protrusion or bulging of sclera and uveal tissue at posterior pole of eye.

379.13 Equatorial staphyloma

DEF: Ring-shaped protrusion or bulging of sclera and uveal tissue midway between front and back of eye.

379.14 Anterior staphyloma, localized

379.15 Ring staphyloma

379.16 Other degenerative disorders of sclera

379.19 Other

✓5th **379.2 Disorders of vitreous body**

DEF: Disorder of clear gel that fills space between retina and lens.

379.21 Vitreous degeneration

Vitreous:
- cavitation
- detachment

Vitreous:
- liquefaction

379.22 Crystalline deposits in vitreous

Asteroid hyalitis

Synchysis scintillans

379.23 Vitreous hemorrhage

AHA: 3Q, '91, 15

379.24 Other vitreous opacities

Vitreous floaters

379.25 Vitreous membranes and strands

379.26 Vitreous prolapse

DEF: Slipping of vitreous from normal position.

379.29 Other disorders of vitreous

EXCLUDES *vitreous abscess (360.04)*

AHA: 1Q, '99, 11

✓5th **379.3 Aphakia and other disorders of lens**

EXCLUDES *after-cataract (366.50-366.53)*

379.31 Aphakia

EXCLUDES *cataract extraction status (V45.61)*

DEF: Absence of eye's crystalline lens.

379.32 Subluxation of lens

379.33 Anterior dislocation of lens

DEF: Lens displaced toward iris.

379.34 Posterior dislocation of lens

DEF: Lens displaced backward toward vitreous.

379.39 Other disorders of lens

5th **379.4 Anomalies of pupillary function**

379.40 Abnormal pupillary function, unspecified

379.41 Anisocoria

DEF: Unequal pupil diameter.

379.42 Miosis (persistent), not due to miotics

DEF: Abnormal contraction of pupil less than 2 millimeters.

379.43 Mydriasis (persistent), not due to mydriatics

DEF: Morbid dilation of pupil.

379.45 Argyll Robertson pupil, atypical

Argyll Robertson phenomenon or pupil, nonsyphilitic

EXCLUDES *Argyll Robertson pupil (syphilitic) (094.89)*

DEF: Failure of pupil to respond to light; affects both eyes; may be caused by diseases such as syphilis of the central nervous system or miosis.

379.46 Tonic pupillary reaction

Adie's pupil or syndrome

379.49 Other

Hippus
Pupillary paralysis

5th **379.5 Nystagmus and other irregular eye movements**

379.50 Nystagmus, unspecified

AHA: 4Q, '02, 68; 2Q, '01, 21

DEF: Involuntary, rapid, rhythmic movement of eyeball; vertical, horizontal, rotatory or mixed; cause may be congenital, acquired, physiological, neurological, myopathic, or due to ocular diseases.

379.51 Congenital nystagmus
379.52 Latent nystagmus
379.53 Visual deprivation nystagmus
379.54 Nystagmus associated with disorders of the vestibular system
379.55 Dissociated nystagmus
379.56 Other forms of nystagmus
379.57 Deficiencies of saccadic eye movements

Abnormal optokinetic response

DEF: Saccadic eye movements; small, rapid, involuntary movements by both eyes simultaneously, due to changing point of fixation on visualized object.

379.58 Deficiencies of smooth pursuit movements
379.59 Other irregularities of eye movements

Opsoclonus

379.8 Other specified disorders of eye and adnexa

5th **379.9 Unspecified disorder of eye and adnexa**

379.90 Disorder of eye, unspecified
379.91 Pain in or around eye
379.92 Swelling or mass of eye
379.93 Redness or discharge of eye
379.99 Other ill-defined disorders of eye

EXCLUDES *blurred vision NOS (368.8)*

DISEASES OF THE EAR AND MASTOID PROCESS (380-389)

4th **380 Disorders of external ear**

5th **380.0 Perichondritis and chondritis of pinna**

Chondritis of auricle
Perichondritis of auricle

380.00 Perichondritis of pinna, unspecified
380.01 Acute perichondritis of pinna
380.02 Chronic perichondritis of pinna

Ear and Mastoid Process

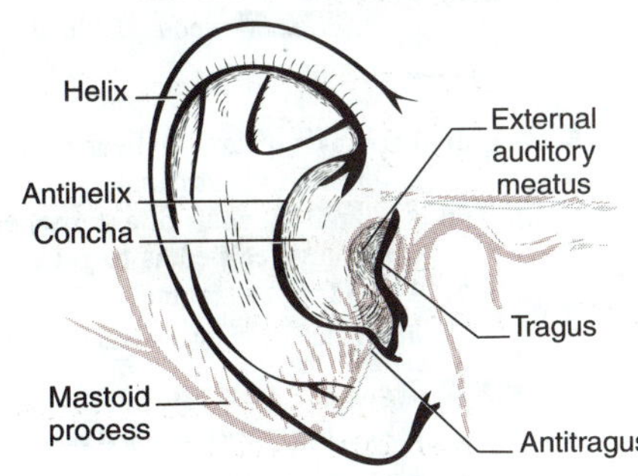

380.03 Chondritis of pinna

AHA: ▶4Q, '04, 76◀

DEF: ▶ Infection that has progressed into the cartilage; presents as indurated and edematous skin over the pinna; vascular compromise occurs with tissue necrosis and deformity.◀

5th **380.1 Infective otitis externa**

380.10 Infective otitis externa, unspecified

Otitis externa (acute):
NOS
circumscribed
diffuse
hemorrhagica
infective NOS

380.11 Acute infection of pinna

EXCLUDES *furuncular otitis externa (680.0)*

380.12 Acute swimmers' ear

Beach ear
Tank ear

DEF: Otitis externa due to swimming.

380.13 Other acute infections of external ear

Code first underlying disease, as:
erysipelas (035)
impetigo (684)
seborrheic dermatitis (690.10-690.18)

EXCLUDES *herpes simplex (054.73)*
herpes zoster (053.71)

380.14 Malignant otitis externa

DEF: Severe necrotic otitis externa; due to bacteria.

380.15 Chronic mycotic otitis externa

Code first underlying disease, as:
aspergillosis (117.3)
otomycosis NOS (111.9)

EXCLUDES *candidal otitis externa (112.82)*

380.16 Other chronic infective otitis externa

Chronic infective otitis externa NOS

5th **380.2 Other otitis externa**

380.21 Cholesteatoma of external ear

Keratosis obturans of external ear (canal)

EXCLUDES *cholesteatoma NOS (385.30-385.35)*
postmastoidectomy (383.32)

DEF: Cystlike mass filled with debris, including cholesterol; rare, congenital condition.

380.22 Other acute otitis externa

Acute otitis externa:
actinic
chemical
contact
eczematoid
reactive

380.23 Other chronic otitis externa

Chronic otitis externa NOS

5th **380.3 Noninfectious disorders of pinna**

380.30 Disorder of pinna, unspecified
380.31 Hematoma of auricle or pinna
380.32 Acquired deformities of auricle or pinna

EXCLUDES *cauliflower ear (738.7)*

AHA: 3Q, '03, 12

380.39 **Other**

EXCLUDES *gouty tophi of ear (274.81)*

380.4 **Impacted cerumen**
Wax in ear

✓5th 380.5 **Acquired stenosis of external ear canal**
Collapse of external ear canal

380.50 **Acquired stenosis of external ear canal, unspecified as to cause**

380.51 **Secondary to trauma**
DEF: Narrowing of external ear canal; due to trauma.

380.52 **Secondary to surgery**
DEF: Postsurgical narrowing of external ear canal.

380.53 **Secondary to inflammation**
DEF: Narrowing, external ear canal; due to chronic inflammation.

✓5th 380.8 **Other disorders of external ear**

380.81 **Exostosis of external ear canal**

380.89 **Other**

380.9 **Unspecified disorder of external ear**

✓4th 381 **Nonsuppurative otitis media and Eustachian tube disorders**

✓5th 381.0 **Acute nonsuppurative otitis media**
Acute tubotympanic catarrh
Otitis media, acute or subacute:
catarrhal
exudative
transudative
with effusion

EXCLUDES *otitic barotrauma (993.0)*

381.00 **Acute nonsuppurative otitis media, unspecified**

381.01 **Acute serous otitis media**
Acute or subacute secretory otitis media
DEF: Sudden, severe infection of middle ear.

381.02 **Acute mucoid otitis media**
Acute or subacute seromucinous otitis media
Blue drum syndrome
DEF: Sudden, severe infection of middle ear, with mucous.

381.03 **Acute sanguinous otitis media**
DEF: Sudden, severe infection of middle ear, with blood.

381.04 **Acute allergic serous otitis media**

381.05 **Acute allergic mucoid otitis media**

381.06 **Acute allergic sanguinous otitis media**

✓5th 381.1 **Chronic serous otitis media**
Chronic tubotympanic catarrh

381.10 **Chronic serous otitis media, simple or unspecified**
DEF: Persistent infection of middle ear, without pus.

381.19 **Other**
Serosanguinous chronic otitis media

✓5th 381.2 **Chronic mucoid otitis media**
Glue ear

EXCLUDES *adhesive middle ear disease (385.10-385.19)*

DEF: Chronic condition; characterized by viscous fluid in middle ear; due to obstructed Eustachian tube.

381.20 **Chronic mucoid otitis media, simple or unspecified**

381.29 **Other**
Mucosanguinous chronic otitis media

381.3 **Other and unspecified chronic nonsuppurative otitis media**
Otitis media, chronic:
allergic
exudative
secretory
seromucinous
transudative
with effusion

381.4 **Nonsuppurative otitis media, not specified as acute or chronic**
Otitis media:
allergic
catarrhal
exudative
mucoid
secretory
seromucinous
serous
transudative
with effusion

✓5th 381.5 **Eustachian salpingitis**

381.50 **Eustachian salpingitis, unspecified**

381.51 **Acute Eustachian salpingitis**
DEF: Sudden, severe inflammation of Eustachian tube.

381.52 **Chronic Eustachian salpingitis**
DEF: Persistent inflammation of Eustachian tube.

✓5th 381.6 **Obstruction of Eustachian tube**
Stenosis } of Eustachian tube
Stricture }

381.60 **Obstruction of Eustachian tube, unspecified**

381.61 **Osseous obstruction of Eustachian tube**
Obstruction of Eustachian tube from cholesteatoma, polyp, or other osseous lesion

381.62 **Intrinsic cartilagenous obstruction of Eustachian tube**
DEF: Blockage of Eustachian tube; due to cartilage overgrowth.

381.63 **Extrinsic cartilagenous obstruction of Eustachian tube**
Compression of Eustachian tube

381.7 **Patulous Eustachian tube**
DEF: Distended, oversized Eustachian tube.

✓5th 381.8 **Other disorders of Eustachian tube**

381.81 **Dysfunction of Eustachian tube**

381.89 **Other**

381.9 **Unspecified Eustachian tube disorder**

✓4th 382 **Suppurative and unspecified otitis media**

✓5th 382.0 **Acute suppurative otitis media**
Otitis media, acute:
necrotizing NOS
purulent

382.00 **Acute suppurative otitis media without spontaneous rupture of ear drum**
DEF: Sudden, severe inflammation of middle ear, with pus.

382.01 **Acute suppurative otitis media with spontaneous rupture of ear drum**
DEF: Sudden, severe inflammation of middle ear, with pressure tearing ear drum tissue.

382.02 ***Acute suppurative otitis media in diseases classified elsewhere***
Code first underlying disease, as:
influenza (487.8)
scarlet fever (034.1)

EXCLUDES *postmeasles otitis (055.2)*

382.1 **Chronic tubotympanic suppurative otitis media**
Benign chronic suppurative otitis media } (with anterior perforation of ear drum)
Chronic tubotympanic disease }
DEF: Inflammation of tympanic cavity and auditory tube; with pus formation.

382.2 **Chronic atticoantral suppurative otitis media**
Chronic atticoantral disease } (with posterior or superior marginal perforation of ear drum)
Persistent mucosal disease }
DEF: Inflammation of upper tympanic membrane and mastoid antrum; with pus formation.

382.3 Unspecified chronic suppurative otitis media
Chronic purulent otitis media
EXCLUDES *tuberculous otitis media (017.4)*

382.4 Unspecified suppurative otitis media
Purulent otitis media NOS

382.9 Unspecified otitis media
Otitis media: NOS, acute NOS
Otitis media: chronic NOS
AHA: N-D, '84, 16

✓4th **383 Mastoiditis and related conditions**

✓5th **383.0 Acute mastoiditis**
Abscess of mastoid
Empyema of mastoid

383.00 Acute mastoiditis without complications
DEF: Sudden, severe inflammation of mastoid air cells.

383.01 Subperiosteal abscess of mastoid
DEF: Pocket of pus within mastoid bone.

383.02 Acute mastoiditis with other complications
Gradenigo's syndrome

383.1 Chronic mastoiditis
Caries of mastoid
Fistula of mastoid
EXCLUDES *tuberculous mastoiditis (015.6)*
DEF: Persistent inflammation of mastoid air cells.

✓5th **383.2 Petrositis**
Coalescing osteitis, Inflammation, Osteomyelitis } of petrous bone

383.20 Petrositis, unspecified

383.21 Acute petrositis
DEF: Sudden, severe inflammation of dense bone behind ear.

383.22 Chronic petrositis
DEF: Persistent inflammation of dense bone behind ear.

✓5th **383.3 Complications following mastoidectomy**

383.30 Postmastoidectomy complication, unspecified

383.31 Mucosal cyst of postmastoidectomy cavity
DEF: Mucous-lined cyst cavity following removal of mastoid bone.

383.32 Recurrent cholesteatoma of postmastoidectomy cavity
DEF: Cystlike mass of cell debris in cavity following removal of mastoid bone.

383.33 Granulations of postmastoidectomy cavity
Chronic inflammation of postmastoidectomy cavity
DEF: Granular tissue in cavity following removal of mastoid bone.

✓5th **383.8 Other disorders of mastoid**

383.81 Postauricular fistula
DEF: Abnormal passage behind mastoid cavity.

383.89 Other

383.9 Unspecified mastoiditis

✓4th **384 Other disorders of tympanic membrane**

✓5th **384.0 Acute myringitis without mention of otitis media**

384.00 Acute myringitis, unspecified
Acute tympanitis NOS
DEF: Sudden, severe inflammation of ear drum.

384.01 Bullous myringitis
Myringitis bullosa hemorrhagica
DEF: Type of viral otitis media characterized by the appearance of serous or hemorrhagic blebs on the tympanic membrane.

384.09 Other

Middle and Inner Ear

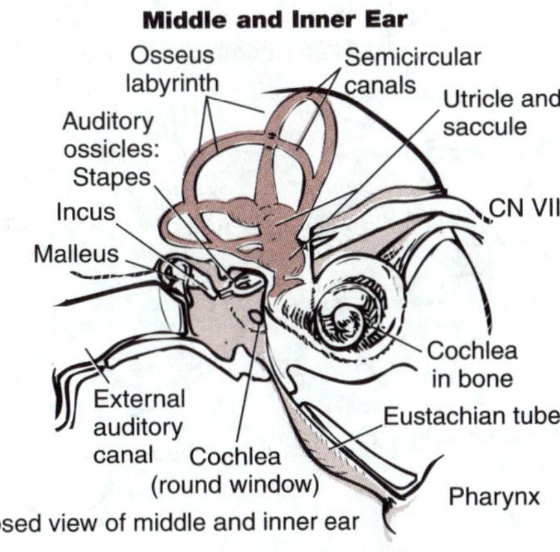

Exposed view of middle and inner ear

384.1 Chronic myringitis without mention of otitis media
Chronic tympanitis
DEF: Persistent inflammation of ear drum; with no evidence of middle ear infection.

✓5th **384.2 Perforation of tympanic membrane**
Perforation of ear drum: NOS, persistent posttraumatic
Perforation of ear drum: postinflammatory
EXCLUDES *otitis media with perforation of tympanic membrane (382.00-382.9)*
traumatic perforation [current injury] (872.61)

384.20 Perforation of tympanic membrane, unspecified

384.21 Central perforation of tympanic membrane

384.22 Attic perforation of tympanic membrane
Pars flaccida

384.23 Other marginal perforation of tympanic membrane

384.24 Multiple perforations of tympanic membrane

384.25 Total perforation of tympanic membrane

✓5th **384.8 Other specified disorders of tympanic membrane**

384.81 Atrophic flaccid tympanic membrane
Healed perforation of ear drum

384.82 Atrophic nonflaccid tympanic membrane

384.9 Unspecified disorder of tympanic membrane

✓4th **385 Other disorders of middle ear and mastoid**
EXCLUDES *mastoiditis (383.0-383.9)*

✓5th **385.0 Tympanosclerosis**

385.00 Tympanosclerosis, unspecified as to involvement

385.01 Tympanosclerosis involving tympanic membrane only
DEF: Tough, fibrous tissue impeding functions of ear drum.

385.02 Tympanosclerosis involving tympanic membrane and ear ossicles
DEF: Tough, fibrous tissue impeding functions of middle ear bones (stapes, malleus, incus).

385.03 Tympanosclerosis involving tympanic membrane, ear ossicles, and middle ear
DEF: Tough, fibrous tissue impeding functions of ear drum, middle ear bones and middle ear canal.

385.09 Tympanosclerosis involving other combination of structures

✓5th **385.1 Adhesive middle ear disease**
Adhesive otitis
Otitis media: chronic adhesive
Otitis media: fibrotic
EXCLUDES *glue ear (381.20-381.29)*
DEF: Adhesions of middle ear structures.

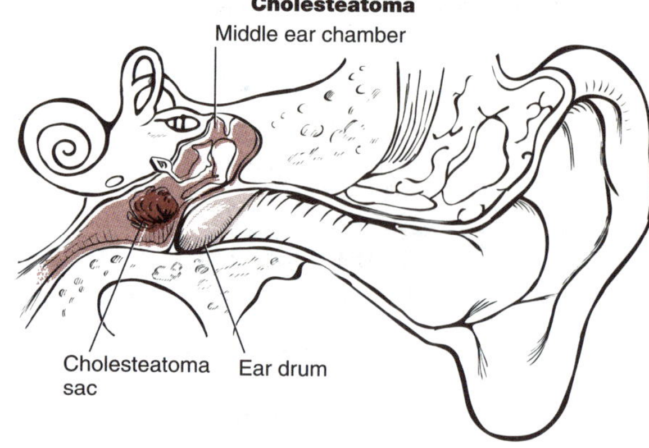

385.10 Adhesive middle ear disease, unspecified as to involvement
385.11 Adhesions of drum head to incus
385.12 Adhesions of drum head to stapes
385.13 Adhesions of drum head to promontorium
385.19 Other adhesions and combinations

✓5th **385.2 Other acquired abnormality of ear ossicles**
385.21 Impaired mobility of malleus
Ankylosis of malleus
385.22 Impaired mobility of other ear ossicles
Ankylosis of ear ossicles, except malleus
385.23 Discontinuity or dislocation of ear ossicles
DEF: Disruption in auditory chain; created by malleus, incus and stapes.
385.24 Partial loss or necrosis of ear ossicles
DEF: Tissue loss in malleus, incus and stapes.

✓5th **385.3 Cholesteatoma of middle ear and mastoid**
Cholesterosis, Epidermosis, Keratosis, Polyp } of (middle) ear
EXCLUDES *cholesteatoma:*
external ear canal (380.21)
recurrent of postmastoidectomy cavity (383.32)
DEF: Cystlike mass of middle ear and mastoid antrum filled with debris, including cholesterol.
385.30 Cholesteatoma, unspecified
385.31 Cholesteatoma of attic
385.32 Cholesteatoma of middle ear
385.33 Cholesteatoma of middle ear and mastoid
AHA: 3Q, '00, 10
DEF: Cystlike mass of cell debris in middle ear and mastoid air cells behind ear.
385.35 Diffuse cholesteatosis

✓5th **385.8 Other disorders of middle ear and mastoid**
385.82 Cholesterin granuloma
DEF: Granuloma formed of fibrotic tissue; contains cholesterol crystals surrounded by foreign-body cells; found in the middle ear and mastoid area.
385.83 Retained foreign body of middle ear
AHA: 3Q, '94, 7; N-D, '87, 9
385.89 Other

385.9 Unspecified disorder of middle ear and mastoid

✓4th **386 Vertiginous syndromes and other disorders of vestibular system**
EXCLUDES *vertigo NOS (780.4)*
AHA: M-A, '85, 12

✓5th **386.0 Ménière's disease**
Endolymphatic hydrops
Lermoyez's syndrome
Ménière's syndrome or vertigo
DEF: Distended membranous labyrinth of middle ear from endolymphatic hydrops; causes ischemia, failure of nerve function; hearing and balance dysfunction; symptoms include fluctuating deafness, ringing in ears and dizziness.
386.00 Ménière's disease, unspecified
Ménière's disease (active)
386.01 Active Ménière's disease, cochleovestibular
386.02 Active Ménière's disease, cochlear
386.03 Active Ménière's disease, vestibular
386.04 Inactive Ménière's disease
Ménière's disease in remission

✓5th **386.1 Other and unspecified peripheral vertigo**
EXCLUDES *epidemic vertigo (078.81)*
386.10 Peripheral vertigo, unspecified
386.11 Benign paroxysmal positional vertigo
Benign paroxysmal positional nystagmus
386.12 Vestibular neuronitis
Acute (and recurrent) peripheral vestibulopathy
DEF: Transient benign vertigo, unknown cause; characterized by response to caloric stimulation on one side, nystagmus with rhythmic movement of eyes; normal auditory function present; occurs in young adults.
386.19 Other
Aural vertigo
Otogenic vertigo

386.2 Vertigo of central origin
Central positional nystagmus
Malignant positional vertigo

✓5th **386.3 Labyrinthitis**
386.30 Labyrinthitis, unspecified
386.31 Serous labyrinthitis
Diffuse labyrinthitis
DEF: Inflammation of labyrinth; with fluid buildup.
386.32 Circumscribed labyrinthitis
Focal labyrinthitis
386.33 Suppurative labyrinthitis
Purulent labyrinthitis
DEF: Inflammation of labyrinth; with pus.
386.34 Toxic labyrinthitis
DEF: Inflammation of labyrinth; due to toxic reaction.
386.35 Viral labyrinthitis

✓5th **386.4 Labyrinthine fistula**
386.40 Labyrinthine fistula, unspecified
386.41 Round window fistula
386.42 Oval window fistula
386.43 Semicircular canal fistula
386.48 Labyrinthine fistula of combined sites

✓5th **386.5 Labyrinthine dysfunction**
386.50 Labyrinthine dysfunction, unspecified
386.51 Hyperactive labyrinth, unilateral
DEF: Oversensitivity of labyrinth to auditory signals; affecting one ear.
386.52 Hyperactive labyrinth, bilateral
DEF: Oversensitivity of labyrinth to auditory signals; affecting both ears.
386.53 Hypoactive labyrinth, unilateral
DEF: Reduced sensitivity of labyrinth to auditory signals; affecting one ear.
386.54 Hypoactive labyrinth, bilateral
DEF: Reduced sensitivity of labyrinth to auditory signals; affecting both ears.

386.55 Loss of labyrinthine reactivity, unilateral
DEF: Reduced reaction of labyrinth to auditory signals, affecting one ear.

386.56 Loss of labyrinthine reactivity, bilateral
DEF: Reduced reaction of labyrinth to auditory signals; affecting both ears.

386.58 Other forms and combinations

386.8 Other disorders of labyrinth

386.9 Unspecified vertiginous syndromes and labyrinthine disorders

✓4th **387 Otosclerosis**

INCLUDES otospongiosis

DEF: Synonym for otospongiosis, spongy bone formation in the labyrinth bones of the ear; it causes progressive hearing impairment.

387.0 Otosclerosis involving oval window, nonobliterative
DEF: Tough, fibrous tissue impeding functions of oval window.

387.1 Otosclerosis involving oval window, obliterative
DEF: Tough, fibrous tissue blocking oval window.

387.2 Cochlear otosclerosis
Otosclerosis involving: otic capsule
Otosclerosis involving: round window
DEF: Tough, fibrous tissue impeding functions of cochlea.

387.8 Other otosclerosis

387.9 Otosclerosis, unspecified

✓4th **388 Other disorders of ear**

✓5th **388.0 Degenerative and vascular disorders of ear**

388.00 Degenerative and vascular disorders, unspecified

388.01 Presbyacusis
DEF: Progressive, bilateral perceptive hearing loss caused by advancing age; it is also known as presbycusis.

388.02 Transient ischemic deafness
DEF: Restricted blood flow to auditory organs causing temporary hearing loss.

✓5th **388.1 Noise effects on inner ear**

388.10 Noise effects on inner ear, unspecified

388.11 Acoustic trauma (explosive) to ear
Otitic blast injury

388.12 Noise-induced hearing loss

388.2 Sudden hearing loss, unspecified

✓5th **388.3 Tinnitus**
DEF: Abnormal noises in ear; may be heard by others beside the affected individual; noises include ringing, clicking, roaring and buzzing.

388.30 Tinnitus, unspecified

388.31 Subjective tinnitus

388.32 Objective tinnitus

✓5th **388.4 Other abnormal auditory perception**

388.40 Abnormal auditory perception, unspecified

388.41 Diplacusis
DEF: Perception of a single auditory sound as two sounds at two different levels of intensity.

388.42 Hyperacusis
DEF: Exceptionally acute sense of hearing caused by such conditions as Bell's palsy; this term may also refer to painful sensitivity to sounds.

388.43 Impairment of auditory discrimination
DEF: Impaired ability to distinguish tone of sound.

388.44 Recruitment
DEF: Perception of abnormally increased loudness caused by a slight increase in sound intensity; it is a term used in audiology.

388.5 Disorders of acoustic nerve
Acoustic neuritis
Degeneration } of acoustic or eighth nerve
Disorder } of acoustic or eighth nerve

EXCLUDES *acoustic neuroma (225.1)*
syphilitic acoustic neuritis (094.86)

AHA: M-A, '87, 8

✓5th **388.6 Otorrhea**

388.60 Otorrhea, unspecified
Discharging ear NOS

388.61 Cerebrospinal fluid otorrhea
EXCLUDES *cerebrospinal fluid rhinorrhea (349.81)*
DEF: Spinal fluid leakage from ear.

388.69 Other
Otorrhagia

✓5th **388.7 Otalgia**

388.70 Otalgia, unspecified
Earache NOS

388.71 Otogenic pain

388.72 Referred pain

388.8 Other disorders of ear

388.9 Unspecified disorder of ear

✓4th **389 Hearing loss**

✓5th **389.0 Conductive hearing loss**
Conductive deafness
AHA: 4Q, '89, 5
DEF: Dysfunction in sound-conducting structures of external or middle ear causing hearing loss.

389.00 Conductive hearing loss, unspecified

389.01 Conductive hearing loss, external ear

389.02 Conductive hearing loss, tympanic membrane

389.03 Conductive hearing loss, middle ear

389.04 Conductive hearing loss, inner ear

389.08 Conductive hearing loss of combined types

✓5th **389.1 Sensorineural hearing loss**
Perceptive hearing loss or deafness

EXCLUDES *abnormal auditory perception (388.40-388.44)*
psychogenic deafness (306.7)

AHA: 4Q, '89, 5
DEF: Nerve conduction causing hearing loss.

389.10 Sensorineural hearing loss, unspecified
AHA: 1Q, '93, 29

389.11 Sensory hearing loss

389.12 Neural hearing loss

389.14 Central hearing loss

389.18 Sensorineural hearing loss of combined types

389.2 Mixed conductive and sensorineural hearing loss
Deafness or hearing loss of type classifiable to 389.0 with type classifiable to 389.1

389.7 Deaf mutism, not elsewhere classifiable
Deaf, nonspeaking

389.8 Other specified forms of hearing loss

389.9 Unspecified hearing loss
Deafness NOS
AHA: 1Q, '04, 15

7. DISEASES OF THE CIRCULATORY SYSTEM (390-459)

ACUTE RHEUMATIC FEVER (390-392)

DEF: Febrile disease occurs mainly in children or young adults following throat infection by group A streptococci; symptoms include fever, joint pain, lesions of heart, blood vessels and joint connective tissue, abdominal pain, skin changes, and chorea.

390 Rheumatic fever without mention of heart involvement
Arthritis, rheumatic, acute or subacute
Rheumatic fever (active) (acute)
Rheumatism, articular, acute or subacute
EXCLUDES *that with heart involvement (391.0-391.9)*

✓4th **391 Rheumatic fever with heart involvement**
EXCLUDES *chronic heart diseases of rheumatic origin (393.0-398.9) unless rheumatic fever is also present or there is evidence of recrudescence or activity of the rheumatic process*

391.0 Acute rheumatic pericarditis
Rheumatic:
fever (active) (acute) with pericarditis
pericarditis (acute)
Any condition classifiable to 390 with pericarditis
EXCLUDES *that not specified as rheumatic (420.0-420.9)*
DEF: Sudden, severe inflammation of heart lining due to rheumatic fever.

391.1 Acute rheumatic endocarditis
Rheumatic:
endocarditis, acute
fever (active) (acute) with endocarditis or valvulitis
valvulitis acute
Any condition classifiable to 390 with endocarditis or valvulitis
DEF: Sudden, severe inflammation of heart cavities due to rheumatic fever.

391.2 Acute rheumatic myocarditis
Rheumatic fever (active) (acute) with myocarditis
Any condition classifiable to 390 with myocarditis
DEF: Sudden, severe inflammation of heart muscles due to rheumatic fever.

391.8 Other acute rheumatic heart disease
Rheumatic:
fever (active) (acute) with other or multiple types of heart involvement
pancarditis, acute
Any condition classifiable to 390 with other or multiple types of heart involvement

391.9 Acute rheumatic heart disease, unspecified
Rheumatic:
carditis, acute
fever (active) (acute) with unspecified type of heart involvement
heart disease, active or acute
Any condition classifiable to 390 with unspecified type of heart involvement

✓4th **392 Rheumatic chorea**
INCLUDES Sydenham's chorea
EXCLUDES *chorea:*
NOS (333.5)
Huntington's (333.4)
DEF: Childhood disease linked with rheumatic fever and streptococcal infections; symptoms include spasmodic, involuntary movements of limbs or facial muscles, psychic symptoms, and irritability.

392.0 With heart involvement
Rheumatic chorea with heart involvement of any type classifiable to 391

392.9 Without mention of heart involvement

CHRONIC RHEUMATIC HEART DISEASE (393-398)

393 Chronic rheumatic pericarditis
Adherent pericardium, rheumatic
Chronic rheumatic:
mediastinopericarditis
myopericarditis
EXCLUDES *pericarditis NOS or not specified as rheumatic (423.0-423.9)*
DEF: Persistent inflammation of heart lining due to rheumatic heart disease.

✓4th **394 Diseases of mitral valve**
EXCLUDES *that with aortic valve involvement (396.0-396.9)*

394.0 Mitral stenosis
Mitral (valve):
obstruction (rheumatic)
stenosis NOS
DEF: Narrowing, of mitral valve between left atrium and left ventricle due to rheumatic heart disease.

394.1 Rheumatic mitral insufficiency
Rheumatic mitral:
incompetence
regurgitation
EXCLUDES *that not specified as rheumatic (424.0)*
DEF: Malfunction of mitral valve between left atrium and left ventricle due to rheumatic heart disease.

394.2 Mitral stenosis with insufficiency
Mitral stenosis with incompetence or regurgitation
DEF: A narrowing or stricture of the mitral valve situated between the left atrium and left ventricle. The stenosis interferes with blood flow from the atrium into the ventricle. If the valve does not completely close, it becomes insufficient (inadequate) and cannot prevent regurgitation (abnormal backward flow) into the atrium when the left ventricle contracts. This abnormal function is also called incompetence.

394.9 Other and unspecified mitral valve diseases
Mitral (valve):
disease (chronic)
failure

✓4th **395 Diseases of aortic valve**
EXCLUDES *that not specified as rheumatic (424.1)*
that with mitral valve involvement (396.0-396.9)

395.0 Rheumatic aortic stenosis
Rheumatic aortic (valve) obstruction
AHA: 4Q, '88, 8
DEF: Narrowing of the aortic valve; results in backflow into ventricle due to rheumatic heart disease.

395.1 Rheumatic aortic insufficiency
Rheumatic aortic:
incompetence
regurgitation
DEF: Malfunction of the aortic valve; results in backflow into left ventricle due to rheumatic heart disease.

395.2 Rheumatic aortic stenosis with insufficiency
Rheumatic aortic stenosis with incompetence or regurgitation
DEF: Malfunction and narrowing, of the aortic valve; results in backflow into left ventricle due to rheumatic heart disease.

395.9 Other and unspecified rheumatic aortic diseases
Rheumatic aortic (valve) disease

✓4th **396 Diseases of mitral and aortic valves**
INCLUDES involvement of both mitral and aortic valves, whether specified as rheumatic or not
AHA: N-D, '87, 8

396.0 Mitral valve stenosis and aortic valve stenosis
Atypical aortic (valve) stenosis
Mitral and aortic (valve) obstruction (rheumatic)

396.1 Mitral valve stenosis and aortic valve insufficiency

396.2 Mitral valve insufficiency and aortic valve stenosis
AHA: 2Q, '00, 16

396.3 Mitral valve insufficiency and aortic valve insufficiency

Mitral and aortic (valve): incompetence

Mitral and aortic (valve): regurgitation

396.8 Multiple involvement of mitral and aortic valves

Stenosis and insufficiency of mitral or aortic valve with stenosis or insufficiency, or both, of the other valve

396.9 Mitral and aortic valve diseases, unspecified

4th 397 Diseases of other endocardial structures

397.0 Diseases of tricuspid valve

Tricuspid (valve) (rheumatic):
- disease
- insufficiency
- obstruction
- regurgitation
- stenosis

AHA: 2Q, '00, 16

DEF: Malfunction of the valve between right atrium and right ventricle due to rheumatic heart disease.

397.1 Rheumatic diseases of pulmonary valve

EXCLUDES *that not specified as rheumatic (424.3)*

397.9 Rheumatic diseases of endocardium, valve unspecified

Rheumatic:
- endocarditis (chronic)
- valvulitis (chronic)

EXCLUDES *that not specified as rheumatic (424.90-424.99)*

4th 398 Other rheumatic heart disease

398.0 Rheumatic myocarditis

Rheumatic degeneration of myocardium

EXCLUDES *myocarditis not specified as rheumatic (429.0)*

DEF: Chronic inflammation of heart muscle due to rheumatic heart disease.

5th 398.9 Other and unspecified rheumatic heart diseases

398.90 Rheumatic heart disease, unspecified

Rheumatic: carditis

Rheumatic: heart disease NOS

EXCLUDES *carditis not specified as rheumatic (429.89)*
heart disease NOS not specified as rheumatic (429.9)

398.91 Rheumatic heart failure (congestive)

Rheumatic left ventricular failure

AHA: 1Q, '95, 6; 3Q, '88, 3

DEF: Decreased cardiac output, edema and hypertension due to rheumatic heart disease.

398.99 Other

Sections of Heart Muscle

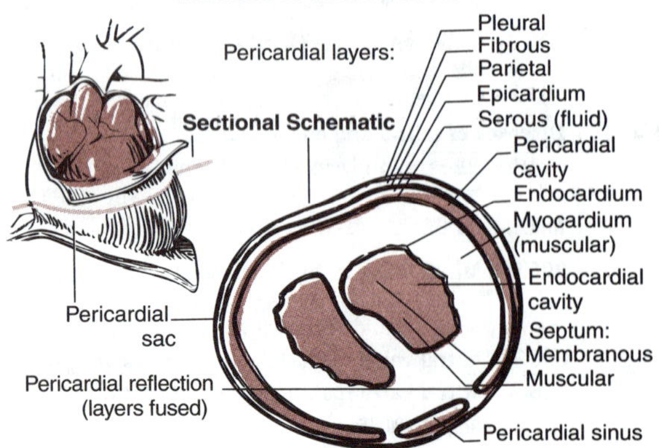

Acute Myocardial Infarction

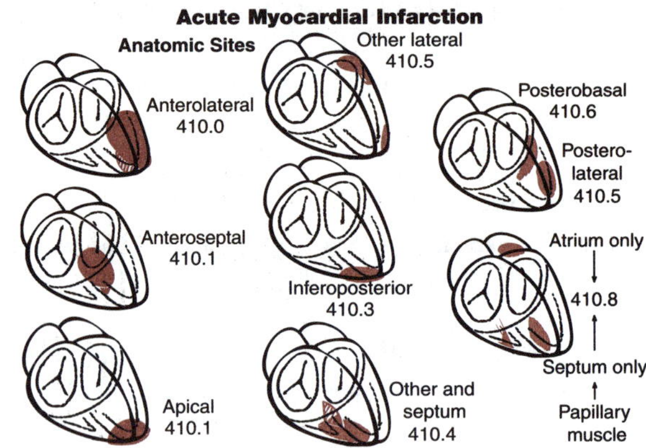

HYPERTENSIVE DISEASE (401-405)

EXCLUDES *that complicating pregnancy, childbirth, or the puerperium (642.0-642.9)*
that involving coronary vessels (410.00-414.9)

AHA: 3Q, '90, 3; 2Q, '89, 12; S-O, '87, 9; J-A, '84, 11

4th 401 Essential hypertension

INCLUDES high blood pressure
hyperpiesia
hyperpiesis
hypertension (arterial) (essential) (primary) (systemic)
hypertensive vascular:
- degeneration
- disease

EXCLUDES *elevated blood pressure without diagnosis of hypertension (796.2)*
pulmonary hypertension (416.0-416.9)
that involving vessels of:
- *brain (430-438)*
- *eye (362.11)*

AHA: 2Q, '92, 5

DEF: Hypertension that occurs without apparent organic cause; idiopathic.

401.0 Malignant

AHA: M-J, '85, 19

DEF: Severe high arterial blood pressure; results in necrosis in kidney, retina, etc.; hemorrhages occur and death commonly due to uremia or rupture of cerebral vessel.

401.1 Benign

DEF: Mildly elevated arterial blood pressure.

401.9 Unspecified

AHA: 4Q, '04, 78; 4Q, '03, 105, 108, 111; 3Q, '03, 14; 2Q, '03, 16; 4Q, '97, 37

4th 402 Hypertensive heart disease

INCLUDES hypertensive:
- cardiomegaly
- cardiopathy
- cardiovascular disease
- heart (disease) (failure)

any condition classifiable to 429.0-429.3, 429.8, 429.9 due to hypertension

Use additional code to specify type of heart failure ▶(428.0-428.43), if known◀

AHA: 4Q, '02, 49; 2Q, '93, 9; N-D, '84, 18

5th 402.0 Malignant

402.00 Without heart failure

402.01 With heart failure

5th 402.1 Benign

402.10 Without heart failure

402.11 With heart failure

5th 402.9 Unspecified

402.90 Without heart failure

402.91 With heart failure

AHA: 4Q, '02, 52; 1Q, '93, 19; 2Q, '89, 12

N Newborn Age: 0   P Pediatric Age: 0-17   M Maternity Age: 12-55   A Adult Age: 15-124   MSP Medicare Secondary Payer

▲ ✓4th **403 Hypertensive kidney disease**

INCLUDES arteriolar nephritis
arteriosclerosis of:
kidney
renal arterioles
arteriosclerotic nephritis (chronic) (interstitial)
hypertensive:
nephropathy
renal failure
uremia (chronic)
nephrosclerosis
renal sclerosis with hypertension
any condition classifiable to 585, 586, or 587 with any condition classifiable to 401

EXCLUDES *acute renal failure (584.5-584.9)*
renal disease stated as not due to hypertension
renovascular hypertension (405.0-405.9 with fifth-digit 1)

▶Use additional code to identify the stage of chronic kidney disease (585.1-585.6), if known◀

The following fifth-digit subclassification is for use with category 403:
▲ 0 **without chronic kidney disease**
▲ 1 **with chronic kidney disease**

AHA: 4Q, '92, 22; 2Q, '92, 5

▲ ✓5th **403.0 Malignant**
▲ ✓5th **403.1 Benign**
▲ ✓5th **403.9 Unspecified**
AHA: For code 403.91: 1Q, '04, 14; 1Q, '03, 20; 2Q, '01, 11; 3Q, '91, 8

▲ ✓4th **404 Hypertensive heart and kidney disease**

INCLUDES disease:
cardiorenal
cardiovascular renal
any condition classifiable to 402 with any condition classifiable to 403

Use additional code to specify type of heart failure ▶(428.0-428.43), if known◀

▶Use additional code to identify the stage of chronic kidney disease (585.1-585.6), if known◀

The following fifth-digit subclassification is for use with category 404:
▲ 0 **without heart failure or chronic kidney disease**
1 **with heart failure**
▲ 2 **with chronic kidney disease**
▲ 3 **with heart failure and chronic kidney disease**

AHA: 4Q, '02, 49; 3Q, '90, 3; J-A, '84, 14

▲ ✓5th **404.0 Malignant**
▲ ✓5th **404.1 Benign**
▲ ✓5th **404.9 Unspecified**

✓4th **405 Secondary hypertension**
AHA: 3Q, '90, 3; S-O, '87, 9, 11; J-A, '84, 14

DEF: High arterial blood pressure due to or with a variety of primary diseases, such as renal disorders, CNS disorders, endocrine, and vascular diseases.

✓5th **405.0 Malignant**
405.01 Renovascular
405.09 Other

✓5th **405.1 Benign**
405.11 Renovascular
405.19 Other

✓5th **405.9 Unspecified**
405.91 Renovascular
405.99 Other
AHA: 3Q, '00, 4

ISCHEMIC HEART DISEASE (410-414)

INCLUDES that with mention of hypertension

Use additional code to identify presence of hypertension (401.0-405.9)

AHA: 3Q, '91, 10; J-A, '84, 5

✓4th **410 Acute myocardial infarction**

INCLUDES cardiac infarction
coronary (artery):
embolism
occlusion
rupture
thrombosis
infarction of heart, myocardium, or ventricle
rupture of heart, myocardium, or ventricle
▶ST elevation (STEMI) and non-ST elevation (NSTEMI) myocardial infarction◀
any condition classifiable to 414.1-414.9 specified as acute or with a stated duration of 8 weeks or less

The following fifth-digit subclassification is for use with category 410:
0 **episode of care unspecified**
Use when the source document does not contain sufficient information for the assignment of fifth digit 1 or 2.
1 **initial episode of care**
Use fifth-digit 1 to designate the first episode of care (regardless of facility site) for a newly diagnosed myocardial infarction. The fifth-digit 1 is assigned regardless of the number of times a patient may be transferred during the initial episode of care.
2 **subsequent episode of care**
Use fifth-digit 2 to designate an episode of care following the initial episode when the patient is admitted for further observation, evaluation or treatment for a myocardial infarction that has received initial treatment, but is still less than 8 weeks old.

AHA: 3Q, '01, 21; 3Q, '98, 15; 4Q, '97, 37; 3Q, '95, 9; 4Q, '92, 24; 1Q, '92,10; 3Q, '91, 18; 1Q, '91, 14; 3Q, '89, 3

DEF: A sudden insufficiency of blood supply to an area of the heart muscle; usually due to a coronary artery occlusion.

✓5th **410.0 Of anterolateral wall**
▶ST elevation myocardial infarction (STEMI) of anterolateral wall◀

✓5th **410.1 Of other anterior wall**
Infarction:
anterior (wall) NOS } (with contiguous portion of intraventricular septum)
anteroapical
anteroseptal
▶ST elevation myocardial infarction (STEMI) of other anterior wall◀
AHA: For code 410.11: 3Q, '03, 10

✓5th **410.2 Of inferolateral wall**
▶ST elevation myocardial infarction (STEMI) of inferolateral wall◀

✓5th **410.3 Of inferoposterior wall**
▶ST elevation myocardial infarction (STEMI) of inferoposterior wall◀

§ 5th **410.4 Of other inferior wall**

Infarction:
diaphragmatic wall NOS } (with contiguous portion of intraventricular septum)
inferior (wall) NOS

▶ST elevation myocardial infarction (STEMI) of other inferior wall◀

AHA: 1Q, '00, 7, 26; 4Q, '99, 9; 3Q, '97, 10; **For code 410.41:** 2Q, '01, 8, 9

§ 5th **410.5 Of other lateral wall**

Infarction:
apical-lateral
basal-lateral
high lateral
posterolateral

▶ST elevation myocardial infarction (STEMI) of other lateral wall◀

§ 5th **410.6 True posterior wall infarction**

Infarction:
posterobasal
strictly posterior

▶ST elevation myocardial infarction (STEMI) of true posterior wall◀

§ 5th **410.7 Subendocardial infarction**

▶Non-ST elevation myocardial infarction (NSTEMI)◀
Nontransmural infarction

AHA: 1Q, '00, 7

§ 5th **410.8 Of other specified sites**

Infarction of:
atrium
papillary muscle
septum alone

▶ST elevation myocardial infarction (STEMI) of other specified sites◀

§ 5th **410.9 Unspecified site**

Acute myocardial infarction NOS
Coronary occlusion NOS
▶Myocardial infarction NOS◀

AHA: 1Q, '96, 17; 1Q, '92, 9; **For code 410.91:** 3Q,'02, 5

4th **411 Other acute and subacute forms of ischemic heart disease**

AHA: 4Q, '94, 55; 3Q, '91, 24

411.0 Postmyocardial infarction syndrome

Dressler's syndrome

DEF: Complication developing several days/weeks after myocardial infarction; symptoms include fever, leukocytosis, chest pain, evidence of pericarditis, pleurisy, and pneumonitis; tendency to recur.

411.1 Intermediate coronary syndrome

Impending infarction
Preinfarction angina
Preinfarction syndrome
Unstable angina

EXCLUDES *angina (pectoris) (413.9)*
decubitus (413.0)

AHA: 2Q, '04, 3; 1Q, '03, 12; 3Q, '01, 15; 2Q, '01, 7, 9; 4Q, '98, 86; 2Q, '96, 10; 3Q, '91, 24; 1Q, '91, 14; 3Q, '90, 6; 4Q, '89, 10

DEF: A condition representing an intermediate stage between angina of effort and acute myocardial infarction. It is often documented by the physician as "unstable angina."

5th **411.8 Other**

AHA: 3Q, '91, 18; 3Q, '89, 4

Arteries of the Heart

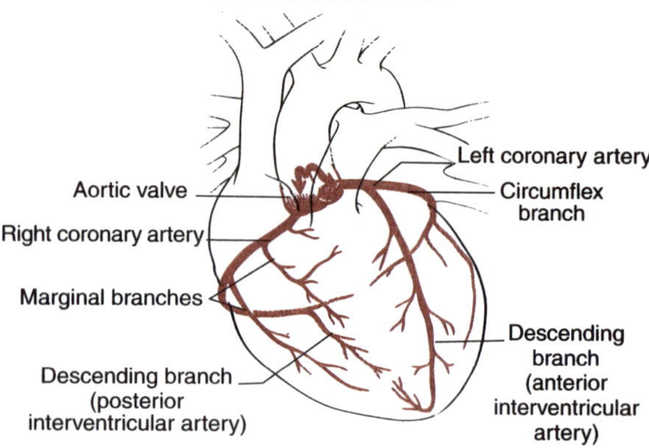

411.81 Acute coronary occlusion without myocardial infarction

Acute coronary (artery):
embolism
obstruction
occlusion
thrombosis
} without or not resulting in myocardial infarction

EXCLUDES *obstruction without infarction due to atherosclerosis (414.00-414.0*
occlusion without infarction due to atherosclerosis (414.00-414.07)

AHA: 3Q, '91, 24; 1Q, '91, 14

DEF: Interrupted blood flow to a portion of the heart; without tissue death.

411.89 Other

Coronary insufficiency (acute)
Subendocardial ischemia

AHA: 3Q, '01, 14; 1Q, '92, 9

412 Old myocardial infarction

Healed myocardial infarction
Past myocardial infarction diagnosed on ECG [EKG] or other special investigation, but currently presenting no symptoms

AHA: 2Q, '03, 10; 2Q, '01, 9; 3Q, '98, 15; 2Q, '91, 22; 3Q, '90, 7

4th **413 Angina pectoris**

DEF: Severe constricting pain in the chest, often radiating from the precordium to the left shoulder and down the arm, due to ischemia of the heart muscle; usually caused by coronary disease; pain is often precipitated by effort or excitement.

413.0 Angina decubitus

Nocturnal angina

DEF: Angina occurring only in the recumbent position.

413.1 Prinzmetal angina

Variant angina pectoris

DEF: Angina occurring when patient is recumbent; associated with ST-segment elevations.

413.9 Other and unspecified angina pectoris

Angina:
NOS
cardiac
of effort
Anginal syndrome
Status anginosus
Stenocardia
Syncope anginosa

EXCLUDES *preinfarction angina (411.1)*

AHA: 3Q, '02, 4; 3Q, '91, 16; 3Q, '90, 6

§ Requires fifth-digit. See category 410 for codes and definitions.

414 Other forms of chronic ischemic heart disease

EXCLUDES *arteriosclerotic cardiovascular disease [ASCVD] (429.2)*
cardiovascular:
arteriosclerosis or sclerosis (429.2)
degeneration or disease (429.2)

414.0 Coronary atherosclerosis

Arteriosclerotic heart disease [ASHD]
Atherosclerotic heart disease
Coronary (artery):
arteriosclerosis
arteritis or endarteritis
atheroma
sclerosis
stricture

EXCLUDES *embolism of graft (996.72)*
occlusion NOS of graft (996.72)
thrombus of graft (996.72)

AHA: 2Q, '97, 13; 2Q, '95, 17; 4Q, '94, 49; 2Q, '94, 13; 1Q, '94, 6; 3Q, '90, 7

DEF: A chronic condition marked by thickening and loss of elasticity of the coronary artery; caused by deposits of plaque containing cholesterol, lipoid material and lipophages.

414.00 Of unspecified type of vessel, native or graft A

AHA: 1Q, '04, 24; 2Q, '03, 16; 3Q, '01, 15; 4Q, '99, 4; 3Q, '97, 15; 4Q, '96, 31

414.01 Of native coronary artery A

AHA: ►2Q, '04, 3;◄ 4Q, '03, 108; 3Q, '03, 9, 14; 3Q, '02, 4-9; 3Q, '01, 15; 2Q, '01, 8, 9; 3Q, '97, 15; 2Q, '96, 10; 4Q, '96, 31

DEF: Plaque deposits in natural heart vessels.

414.02 Of autologous vein bypass graft A

DEF: Plaque deposit in grafted vein originating within patient.

414.03 Of nonautologous biological bypass graft A

DEF: Plaque deposits in grafted vessel originating outside patient.

414.04 Of artery bypass graft A

Internal mammary artery

AHA: 4Q, '96, 31

DEF: Plaque deposits in grafted artery originating within patient.

414.05 Of unspecified type of bypass graft A

Bypass graft NOS

AHA: 3Q, '97, 15; 4Q, '96, 31

414.06 Of native coronary artery of transplanted heart

AHA: 4Q, '03, 60

414.07 Of bypass graft (artery) (vein) of transplanted heart A

414.1 Aneurysm and dissection of heart

AHA: 4Q, '02, 54

414.10 Aneurysm of heart (wall)

Aneurysm (arteriovenous):
mural
ventricular

414.11 Aneurysm of coronary vessels

Aneurysm (arteriovenous) of coronary vessels

AHA: 3Q, '03, 10; 1Q, '99, 17

DEF: Dilatation of all three-vessel wall layers forming a sac filled with blood.

Anatomy

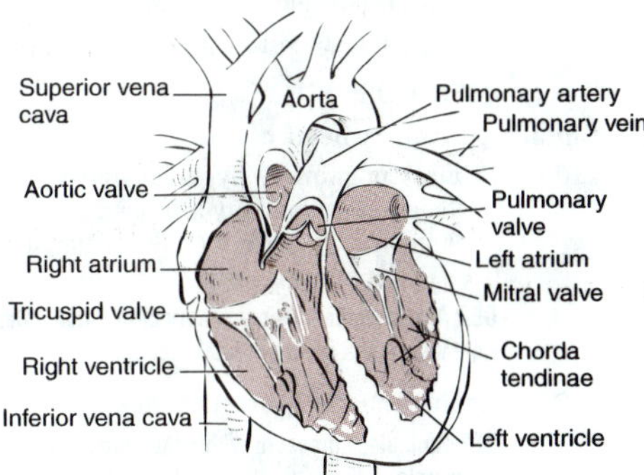

Blood Flow

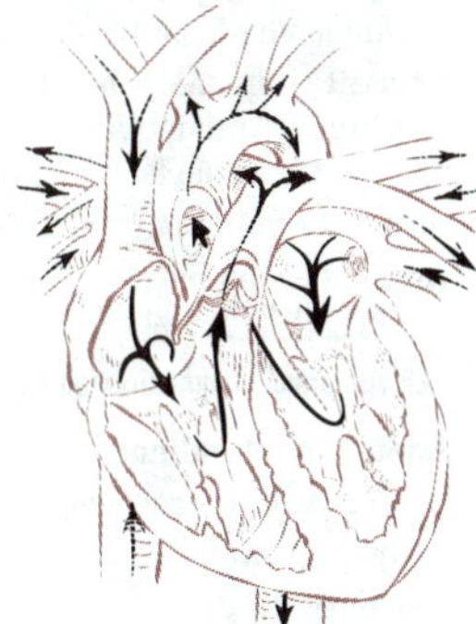

414.12 Dissection of coronary artery

DEF: A tear in the intimal arterial wall of a coronary artery resulting in the sudden intrusion of blood within the layers of the wall.

414.19 Other aneurysm of heart

Arteriovenous fistula, acquired, of heart

414.8 Other specified forms of chronic ischemic heart disease

Chronic coronary insufficiency
Ischemia, myocardial (chronic)
Any condition classifiable to 410 specified as chronic, or presenting with symptoms after 8 weeks from date of infarction

EXCLUDES *coronary insufficiency (acute) (411.89)*

AHA: 3Q, '01, 15; 1Q, '92, 10; 3Q, '90, 7, 15; 2Q, '90, 19

414.9 Chronic ischemic heart disease, unspecified

Ischemic heart disease NOS

DISEASES OF PULMONARY CIRCULATION (415-417)

415 Acute pulmonary heart disease

415.0 Acute cor pulmonale

EXCLUDES *cor pulmonale NOS (416.9)*

DEF: A heart-lung disease marked by dilation and failure of the right side of heart; due to pulmonary embolism; ventilatory function is impaired and pulmonary hypertension results within hours.

415.1 Pulmonary embolism and infarction

Pulmonary (artery) (vein):
apoplexy
embolism
infarction (hemorrhagic)
thrombosis

EXCLUDES *that complicating:*
abortion (634-638 with .6, 639.6)
ectopic or molar pregnancy (639.6)
pregnancy, childbirth, or the puerperium (673.0-673.8)

AHA: 4Q, '90, 25

DEF: Embolism: closure of the pulmonary artery or branch; due to thrombosis (blood clot).

DEF: Infarction: necrosis of lung tissue; due to obstructed arterial blood supply, most often by pulmonary embolism.

415.11 **Iatrogenic pulmonary embolism and infarction**
AHA: 4Q, '95, 58

415.19 **Other**

✓4th **416 Chronic pulmonary heart disease**

416.0 **Primary pulmonary hypertension**
Idiopathic pulmonary arteriosclerosis
Pulmonary hypertension (essential) (idiopathic) (primary)
DEF: A rare increase in pulmonary circulation, often resulting in right ventricular failure or fatal syncope.

416.1 **Kyphoscoliotic heart disease**
DEF: High blood pressure within the lungs as a result of curvature of the spine.

416.8 **Other chronic pulmonary heart diseases**
Pulmonary hypertension, secondary

416.9 **Chronic pulmonary heart disease, unspecified**
Chronic cardiopulmonary disease
Cor pulmonale (chronic) NOS

✓4th **417 Other diseases of pulmonary circulation**

417.0 **Arteriovenous fistula of pulmonary vessels**
EXCLUDES *congenital arteriovenous fistula (747.3)*
DEF: Abnormal communication between blood vessels within lung.

417.1 **Aneurysm of pulmonary artery**
EXCLUDES *congenital aneurysm (747.3)*

417.8 **Other specified diseases of pulmonary circulation**
Pulmonary:
arteritis
endarteritis
Rupture } of pulmonary vessel
Stricture } of pulmonary vessel

417.9 **Unspecified disease of pulmonary circulation**

OTHER FORMS OF HEART DISEASE (420-429)

✓4th **420 Acute pericarditis**
INCLUDES acute:
mediastinopericarditis
myopericarditis
pericardial effusion
pleuropericarditis
pneumopericarditis
EXCLUDES *acute rheumatic pericarditis (391.0)*
postmyocardial infarction syndrome [Dressler's] (411.0)
DEF: Inflammation of the pericardium (heart sac); pericardial friction rub results from this inflammation and is heard as a scratchy or leathery sound.

420.0 ***Acute pericarditis in diseases classified elsewhere***
Code first underlying disease, as:
actinomycosis (039.8)
amebiasis (006.8)
nocardiosis (039.8)
tuberculosis (017.9)
uremia ▶(585.9)◀
EXCLUDES *pericarditis (acute) (in):*
Coxsackie (virus) (074.21)
gonococcal (098.83)
histoplasmosis (115.0-115.9 with fifth-digit 3)
meningococcal infection (036.41)
syphilitic (093.81)

✓5th 420.9 **Other and unspecified acute pericarditis**

420.90 **Acute pericarditis, unspecified**
Pericarditis (acute):
NOS
infective NOS
sicca
AHA: 2Q, '89, 12

420.91 **Acute idiopathic pericarditis**
Pericarditis, acute:
benign
nonspecific
viral

420.99 **Other**
Pericarditis (acute):
pneumococcal
purulent
staphylococcal
streptococcal
suppurative
Pneumopyopericardium
Pyopericardium
EXCLUDES *pericarditis in diseases classified elsewhere (420.0)*

✓4th **421 Acute and subacute endocarditis**
DEF: Bacterial inflammation of the endocardium (intracardiac area); major symptoms include fever, fatigue, heart murmurs, splenomegaly, embolic episodes and areas of infarction.

421.0 **Acute and subacute bacterial endocarditis**
Endocarditis (acute) (chronic) (subacute):
bacterial
infective NOS
lenta
malignant
purulent
septic
ulcerative
vegetative
Infective aneurysm
Subacute bacterial endocarditis [SBE]
Use additional code to identify infectious organism [e.g., Streptococcus 041.0, Staphylococcus 041.1]
AHA: 1Q, '99, 12; 1Q, '91, 15

421.1 ***Acute and subacute infective endocarditis in diseases classified elsewhere***
Code first underlying disease, as:
blastomycosis (116.0)
Q fever (083.0)
typhoid (fever) (002.0)
EXCLUDES *endocarditis (in):*
Coxsackie (virus) (074.22)
gonococcal (098.84)
histoplasmosis (115.0-115.9 with fifth-digit 4)
meningococcal infection (036.42)
monilial (112.81)

421.9 **Acute endocarditis, unspecified**
Endocarditis } acute or subacute
Myoendocarditis } acute or subacute
Periendocarditis } acute or subacute
EXCLUDES *acute rheumatic endocarditis (391.1)*

✓4th **422 Acute myocarditis**
EXCLUDES *acute rheumatic myocarditis (391.2)*
DEF: Acute inflammation of the muscular walls of the heart (myocardium).

422.0 ***Acute myocarditis in diseases classified elsewhere***
Code first underlying disease, as:
myocarditis (acute):
influenzal (487.8)
tuberculous (017.9)
EXCLUDES *myocarditis (acute) (due to):*
aseptic, of newborn (074.23)
Coxsackie (virus) (074.23)
diphtheritic (032.82)
meningococcal infection (036.43)
syphilitic (093.82)
toxoplasmosis (130.3)

✓5th 422.9 **Other and unspecified acute myocarditis**

422.90 **Acute myocarditis, unspecified**
Acute or subacute (interstitial) myocarditis

422.91 Idiopathic myocarditis
Myocarditis (acute or subacute):
Fiedler's
giant cell
isolated (diffuse) (granulomatous)
nonspecific granulomatous

422.92 Septic myocarditis
Myocarditis, acute or subacute:
pneumococcal
staphylococcal
Use additional code to identify infectious organism [e.g., Staphylococcus 041.1]
EXCLUDES *myocarditis, acute or subacute:*
in bacterial diseases classified elsewhere (422.0)
streptococcal (391.2)

422.93 Toxic myocarditis
DEF: Inflammation of the heart muscle due to an adverse reaction to certain drugs or chemicals reaching the heart through the bloodstream.

422.99 Other

✓4th **423 Other diseases of pericardium**
EXCLUDES *that specified as rheumatic (393)*

423.0 Hemopericardium
DEF: Blood in the pericardial sac (pericardium).

423.1 Adhesive pericarditis
Adherent pericardium
Fibrosis of pericardium
Milk spots
Pericarditis:
adhesive
obliterative
Soldiers' patches
DEF: Two layers of serous pericardium adhere to each other by fibrous adhesions.

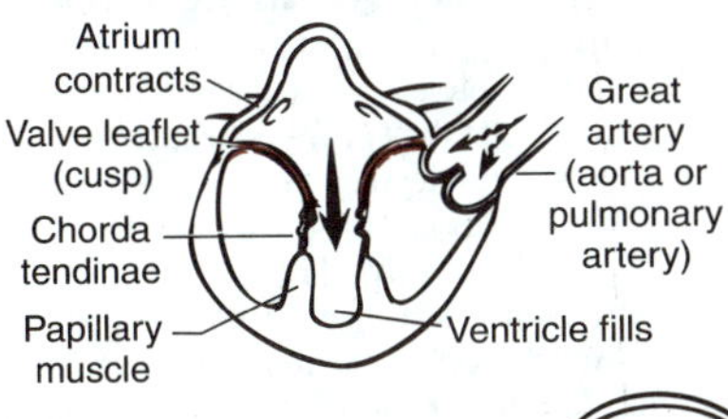

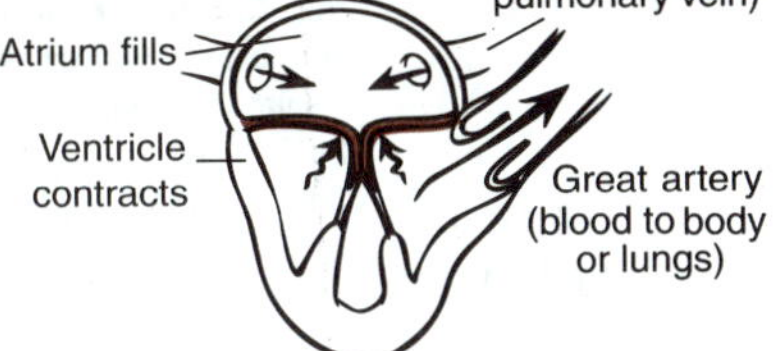

Heart Valve Disorders

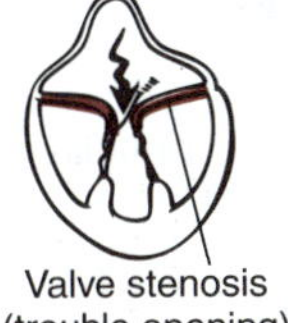

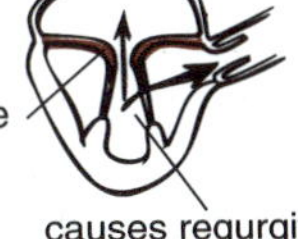

423.2 Constrictive pericarditis
Concato's disease
Pick's disease of heart (and liver)
DEF: Inflammation identified by a rigid, thickened and sometimes calcified pericardium; ventricles of the heart cannot be adequately filled and congestive heart failure may result.

423.8 Other specified diseases of pericardium
Calcification } of pericardium
Fistula }
AHA: 2Q, '89, 12

423.9 Unspecified disease of pericardium

✓4th **424 Other diseases of endocardium**
EXCLUDES *bacterial endocarditis (421.0-421.9)*
rheumatic endocarditis (391.1, 394.0-397.9)
syphilitic endocarditis (093.20-093.24)

424.0 Mitral valve disorders
Mitral (valve):
incompetence } NOS of specified cause, except rheumatic
insufficiency }
regurgitation }
EXCLUDES *mitral (valve):*
disease (394.9)
failure (394.9)
stenosis (394.0)
the listed conditions:
specified as rheumatic (394.1)
unspecified as to cause but with mention of:
diseases of aortic valve (396.0-396.9)
mitral stenosis or obstruction (394.2)
AHA: 2Q, '00, 16; 3Q, '98, 11; N-D, '87, 8; N-D, '84, 8

424.1 Aortic valve disorders
Aortic (valve):
incompetence } NOS of specified cause, except rheumatic
insufficiency }
regurgitation }
stenosis }
EXCLUDES *hypertrophic subaortic stenosis (425.1)*
that specified as rheumatic (395.0-395.9)
that of unspecified cause but with mention of diseases of mitral valve (396.0-396.9)
AHA: 4Q, '88, 8; N-D, '87, 8

Nerve Conduction of the Heart

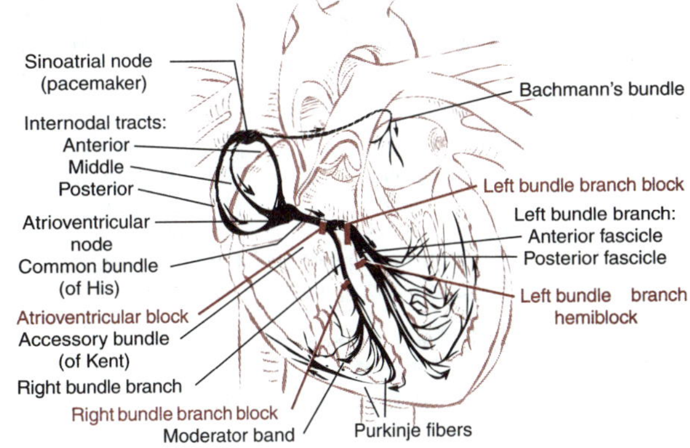

424.2 Tricuspid valve disorders, specified as nonrheumatic

Tricuspid valve:
- incompetence
- insufficiency
- regurgitation
- stenosis

} of specified cause, except rheumatic

EXCLUDES *rheumatic or of unspecified cause (397.0)*

424.3 Pulmonary valve disorders

Pulmonic:
- incompetence NOS
- insufficiency NOS
- regurgitation NOS
- stenosis NOS

EXCLUDES *that specified as rheumatic (397.1)*

✓5th **424.9 Endocarditis, valve unspecified**

424.90 Endocarditis, valve unspecified, unspecified cause

Endocarditis (chronic):
- NOS
- nonbacterial thrombotic

Valvular:
- incompetence
- insufficiency
- regurgitation
- stenosis

Valvulitis (chronic)

} of unspecified valve, unspecified cause

424.91 Endocarditis in diseases classified elsewhere

Code first underlying disease as:
- atypical verrucous endocarditis [Libman-Sacks] (710.0)
- disseminated lupus erythematosus (710.0)
- tuberculosis (017.9)

EXCLUDES *syphilitic (093.20-093.24)*

424.99 Other

Any condition classifiable to 424.90 with specified cause, except rheumatic

EXCLUDES *endocardial fibroelastosis (425.3)*
that specified as rheumatic (397.9)

✓4th **425 Cardiomyopathy**

INCLUDES myocardiopathy

AHA: J-A, '85, 15

425.0 Endomyocardial fibrosis

425.1 Hypertrophic obstructive cardiomyopathy

Hypertrophic subaortic stenosis (idiopathic)

DEF: Cardiomyopathy marked by left ventricle hypertrophy, enlarged septum; results in obstructed blood flow.

425.2 Obscure cardiomyopathy of Africa

Becker's disease

Idiopathic mural endomyocardial disease

425.3 Endocardial fibroelastosis

Elastomyofibrosis

DEF: A condition marked by left ventricle hypertrophy and conversion of the endocardium into a thick fibroelastic coat; capacity of the ventricle may be reduced, but is often increased.

425.4 Other primary cardiomyopathies

Cardiomyopathy:
- NOS
- congestive
- constrictive
- familial
- hypertrophic

Cardiomyopathy:
- idiopathic
- nonobstructive
- obstructive
- restrictive

Cardiovascular collagenosis

AHA: 1Q, '00, 22; 4Q, '97, 55; 2Q, '90, 19

425.5 Alcoholic cardiomyopathy

AHA: S-O, '85, 15

DEF: Heart disease as result of excess alcohol consumption.

425.7 Nutritional and metabolic cardiomyopathy

Code first underlying disease, as:
- amyloidosis (277.3)
- beriberi (265.0)
- cardiac glycogenosis (271.0)
- mucopolysaccharidosis (277.5)
- thyrotoxicosis (242.0-242.9)

EXCLUDES *gouty tophi of heart (274.82)*

425.8 Cardiomyopathy in other diseases classified elsewhere

Code first underlying disease, as:
- Friedreich's ataxia (334.0)
- myotonia atrophica (359.2)
- progressive muscular dystrophy (359.1)
- sarcoidosis (135)

EXCLUDES *cardiomyopathy in Chagas' disease (086.0)*

AHA: 2Q, '93, 9

425.9 Secondary cardiomyopathy, unspecified

✓4th **426 Conduction disorders**

DEF: Disruption or disturbance in the electrical impulses that regulate heartbeats.

426.0 Atrioventricular block, complete

Third degree atrioventricular block

✓5th **426.1 Atrioventricular block, other and unspecified**

426.10 Atrioventricular block, unspecified

Atrioventricular [AV] block (incomplete) (partial)

426.11 First degree atrioventricular block

Incomplete atrioventricular block, first degree

Prolonged P-R interval NOS

426.12 Mobitz (type) II atrioventricular block

Incomplete atrioventricular block:
- Mobitz (type) II
- second degree, Mobitz (type) II

DEF: Impaired conduction of excitatory impulse from cardiac atrium to ventricle through AV node.

426.13 Other second degree atrioventricular block

Incomplete atrioventricular block:
- Mobitz (type) I [Wenckebach's]
- second degree:
  - NOS
  - Mobitz (type) I
- with 2:1 atrioventricular response [block]

Wenckebach's phenomenon

DEF: Wenckebach's phenomenon: impulses generated at constant rate to sinus node, P-R interval lengthens; results in cycle of ventricular inadequacy and shortened P-R interval; second-degree A-V block commonly called "Mobitz type 1."

426.2 Left bundle branch hemiblock

Block:
- left anterior fascicular
- left posterior fascicular

426.3 Other left bundle branch block

Left bundle branch block:
- NOS
- anterior fascicular with posterior fascicular
- complete
- main stem

426.4 Right bundle branch block

AHA: 3Q, '00, 3

✓5th **426.5 Bundle branch block, other and unspecified**

426.50 Bundle branch block, unspecified

426.51 Right bundle branch block and left posterior fascicular block

426.52 Right bundle branch block and left anterior fascicular block

426.53 Other bilateral bundle branch block
Bifascicular block NOS
Bilateral bundle branch block NOS
Right bundle branch with left bundle branch block (incomplete) (main stem)

426.54 Trifascicular block

426.6 Other heart block
Intraventricular block:
NOS
diffuse
myofibrillar
Sinoatrial block
Sinoauricular block

426.7 Anomalous atrioventricular excitation
Atrioventricular conduction:
accelerated
accessory
pre-excitation
Ventricular pre-excitation
Wolff-Parkinson-White syndrome
DEF: Wolff-Parkinson-White: normal conduction pathway is bypassed; results in short P-R interval on EKG; tendency to supraventricular tachycardia.

✓5th **426.8 Other specified conduction disorders**

426.81 Lown-Ganong-Levine syndrome
Syndrome of short P-R interval, normal QRS complexes, and supraventricular tachycardias

● **426.82 Long QT syndrome**

426.89 Other
Dissociation:
atrioventricular [AV]
interference
isorhythmic
Nonparoxysmal AV nodal tachycardia

426.9 Conduction disorder, unspecified
Heart block NOS
Stokes-Adams syndrome

✓4th **427 Cardiac dysrhythmias**

EXCLUDES *that complicating:*
abortion (634-638 with .7, 639.8)
ectopic or molar pregnancy (639.8)
labor or delivery (668.1, 669.4)

AHA: J-A, '85, 15
DEF: Disruption or disturbance in the rhythm of heartbeats.

427.0 Paroxysmal supraventricular tachycardia
Paroxysmal tachycardia:
atrial [PAT]
atrioventricular [AV]
junctional
nodal
DEF: Rapid atrial rhythm.

427.1 Paroxysmal ventricular tachycardia
Ventricular tachycardia (paroxysmal)
AHA: 3Q, '95, 9; M-A, '86, 11
DEF: Rapid ventricular rhythm.

427.2 Paroxysmal tachycardia, unspecified
Bouveret-Hoffmann syndrome
Paroxysmal tachycardia:
NOS
essential

✓5th **427.3 Atrial fibrillation and flutter**

427.31 Atrial fibrillation
AHA: 4Q, '04, 78, 121; 3Q, '04, 7; 4Q, '03, 95, 105; 1Q, '03, 8; 2Q, '99, 17; 3Q, '95, 8
DEF: Irregular, rapid atrial contractions.

427.32 Atrial flutter
AHA: 4Q, '03, 94
DEF: Regular, rapid atrial contractions.

✓5th **427.4 Ventricular fibrillation and flutter**

427.41 Ventricular fibrillation
AHA: 3Q, '02, 5
DEF: Irregular, rapid ventricular contractions.

427.42 Ventricular flutter
DEF: Regular, rapid, ventricular contractions.

427.5 Cardiac arrest
Cardiorespiratory arrest
AHA: 3Q,'02, 5; 2Q, '00, 12; 3Q, '95, 8; 2Q, '88, 8

✓5th **427.6 Premature beats**

427.60 Premature beats, unspecified
Ectopic beats
Extrasystoles
Extrasystolic arrhythmia
Premature contractions or systoles NOS

427.61 Supraventricular premature beats
Atrial premature beats, contractions, or systoles

427.69 Other
Ventricular premature beats, contractions, or systoles
AHA: 4Q, '93, 42

✓5th **427.8 Other specified cardiac dysrhythmias**

427.81 Sinoatrial node dysfunction
Sinus bradycardia:
persistent
severe
Syndrome:
sick sinus
tachycardia-bradycardia

EXCLUDES *sinus bradycardia NOS (427.89)*

AHA: 3Q, '00, 8
DEF: Complex cardiac arrhythmia; appears as severe sinus bradycardia, sinus bradycardia with tachycardia, or sinus bradycardia with atrioventricular block.

427.89 Other
Rhythm disorder:
coronary sinus
ectopic
Rhythm disorder:
nodal
Wandering (atrial) pacemaker

EXCLUDES *carotid sinus syncope (337.0)*
neonatal bradycardia (779.81)
neonatal tachycardia (779.82)
reflex bradycardia (337.0)
tachycardia NOS (785.0)

427.9 Cardiac dysrhythmia, unspecified
Arrhythmia (cardiac) NOS
AHA: 2Q, '89, 10

✓4th **428 Heart failure**

Code, if applicable, heart failure due to hypertension first (402.0-402.9, with fifth-digit 1 or 404.0-404.9 with fifth-digit 1 or 3)

EXCLUDES *following cardiac surgery (429.4)*
rheumatic (398.91)
that complicating:
abortion (634-638 with .7, 639.8)
ectopic or molar pregnancy (639.8)
labor or delivery (668.1, 669.4)

AHA: 4Q, '02, 49; 3Q, '98, 5; 2Q, '90, 16; 2Q, '90, 19; 2Q, '89, 10; 3Q, '88, 3

428.0 Congestive heart failure, unspecified
Congestive heart disease
Right heart failure (secondary to left heart failure)

EXCLUDES *fluid overload NOS (276.6)*

AHA: ►1Q, '05, 5, 9;◄ 4Q, '04, 140; 3Q, '04, 7; 4Q, '03, 109; 1Q, '03, 9; 4Q, '02, 52; 2Q, '01, 13; 4Q, '00, 48; 2Q, '00, 16; 1Q, '00, 22; 4Q, '99, 4; 1Q, '99, 11; 4Q, '97, 55; 3Q, '97, 10; 3Q, '96, 9; 3Q, '91, 18; 3Q, '91, 19; 2Q, '89, 12

DEF: Mechanical inadequacy; caused by inability of heart to pump and circulate blood; results in fluid collection in lungs, hypertension, congestion and edema of tissue.

428.1 Left heart failure
Acute edema of lung } with heart disease NOS
Acute pulmonary edema } or heart failure
Cardiac asthma
Left ventricular failure
DEF: Mechanical inadequacy of left ventricle; causing fluid in lungs.

✓5th **428.2 Systolic heart failure**

EXCLUDES *combined systolic and diastolic heart failure (428.40-428.43)*

DEF: Heart failure due to a defect in expulsion of blood caused by an abnormality in systolic function, or ventricular contractile dysfunction.

428.20 Unspecified

428.21 Acute

428.22 Chronic

428.23 Acute on chronic

AHA: 1Q, '03, 9

✓5th **428.3 Diastolic heart failure**

EXCLUDES *combined systolic and diastolic heart failure (428.40-428.43)*

DEF: Heart failure due to resistance to ventricular filling caused by an abnormality in the diastolic function.

428.30 Unspecified

AHA: 4Q, '02, 52

428.31 Acute

428.32 Chronic

428.33 Acute on chronic

✓5th **428.4 Combined systolic and diastolic heart failure**

428.40 Unspecified

428.41 Acute

AHA: ▶4Q, '04, 140◀

428.42 Chronic

428.43 Acute on chronic

AHA: 4Q, '02, 52

428.9 Heart failure, unspecified

Cardiac failure NOS
Heart failure NOS
Myocardial failure NOS
Weak heart

AHA: 2Q, '89, 10; N-D, '85, 14

✓4th **429 Ill-defined descriptions and complications of heart disease**

429.0 Myocarditis, unspecified

Myocarditis:
- NOS
- chronic (interstitial)
- fibroid
- senile

} (with mention of arteriosclerosis)

Use additional code to identify presence of arteriosclerosis

EXCLUDES *acute or subacute (422.0-422.9)*
rheumatic (398.0)
acute (391.2)
that due to hypertension (402.0-402.9)

429.1 Myocardial degeneration

Degeneration of heart or myocardium:
- fatty
- mural
- muscular

Myocardial:
- degeneration
- disease

} (with mention of arteriosclerosis)

Use additional code to identify presence of arteriosclerosis

EXCLUDES *that due to hypertension (402.0-402.9)*

429.2 Cardiovascular disease, unspecified

Arteriosclerotic cardiovascular disease [ASCVD]
Cardiovascular arteriosclerosis
Cardiovascular:
- degeneration
- disease
- sclerosis

} (with mention of arteriosclerosis)

Use additional code to identify presence of arteriosclerosis

EXCLUDES *that due to hypertension (402.0-402.9)*

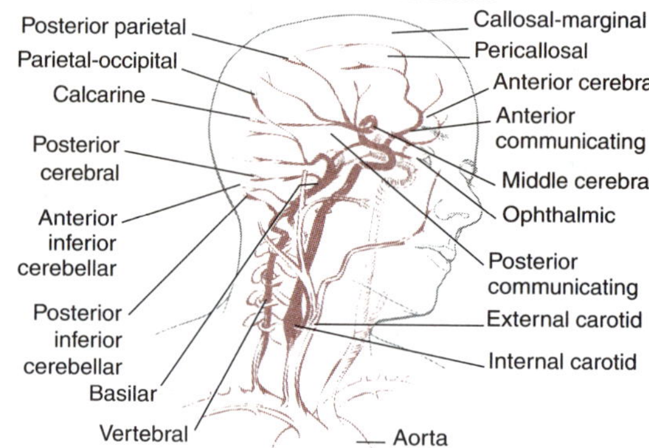

Echocardiography of Heart Failure

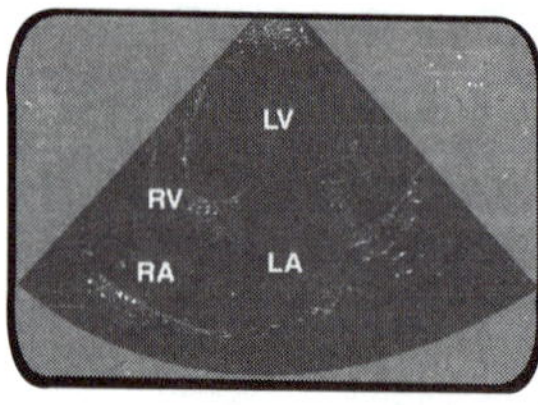

Four-chamber echocardiograms, two-dimensional views.
LV: Left ventricle
RV: Right ventricle
RA: Right atrium
LA: Left atrium

Systolic dysfunction with dilated LV

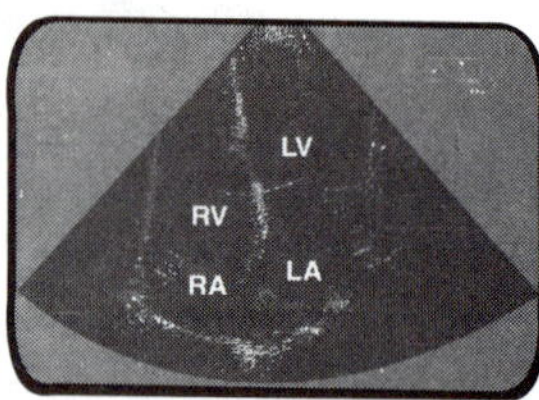

Diastolic dysfunction with LV hypertrophy

429.3 Cardiomegaly

Cardiac:
- dilatation
- hypertrophy

Ventricular dilatation

EXCLUDES *that due to hypertension (402.0-402.9)*

429.4 Functional disturbances following cardiac surgery

Cardiac insufficiency
Heart failure
} following cardiac surgery or due to prosthesis

Postcardiotomy syndrome
Postvalvulotomy syndrome

EXCLUDES *cardiac failure in the immediate postoperative period (997.1)*

AHA: 2Q, '02, 12; N-D, '85, 6

429.5 Rupture of chordae tendineae

DEF: Torn tissue, between heart valves and papillary muscles.

429.6 Rupture of papillary muscle

DEF: Torn muscle, between chordae tendineae and heart wall.

✓5th **429.7 Certain sequelae of myocardial infarction, not elsewhere classified**

Use additional code to identify the associated myocardial infarction:
- with onset of 8 weeks or less (410.00-410.92)
- with onset of more than 8 weeks (414.8)

EXCLUDES *congenital defects of heart (745, 746)*
coronary aneurysm (414.11)
disorders of papillary muscle (429.6, 429.81)
postmyocardial infarction syndrome (411.0)
rupture of chordae tendineae (429.5)

AHA: 3Q, '89, 5

429.71 Acquired cardiac septal defect A

EXCLUDES *acute septal infarction (410.00-410.92)*

DEF: Abnormal communication, between opposite heart chambers; due to defect of septum; not present at birth.

429.79 **Other** A

Mural thrombus (atrial) (ventricular), acquired, following myocardial infarction

AHA: 1Q, '92, 10

✓5th 429.8 **Other ill-defined heart diseases**

429.81 **Other disorders of papillary muscle**

Papillary muscle:	Papillary muscle:
atrophy	incompetence
degeneration	incoordination
dysfunction	scarring

429.82 **Hyperkinetic heart disease**

DEF: Condition of unknown origin in young adults; marked by increased cardiac output at rest, increased rate of ventricular ejection; may lead to heart failure.

429.89 **Other**

Carditis

EXCLUDES *that due to hypertension (402.0-402.9)*

AHA: 1Q, '92, 10

429.9 **Heart disease, unspecified**

Heart disease (organic) NOS Morbus cordis NOS

EXCLUDES *that due to hypertension (402.0-402.9)*

AHA: 1Q, '93, 19

CEREBROVASCULAR DISEASE (430-438)

INCLUDES with mention of hypertension (conditions classifiable to 401-405)

Use additional code to identify presence of hypertension

EXCLUDES *any condition classifiable to 430-434, 436, 437 occurring during pregnancy, childbirth, or the puerperium, or specified as puerperal (674.0)*

iatrogenic cerebrovascular infarction or hemorrhage (997.02)

AHA: 1Q, '93, 27; 3Q, '91, 10; 3Q, '90, 3; 2Q, '89, 8; M-A, '85, 6

430 **Subarachnoid hemorrhage**

Meningeal hemorrhage

Ruptured:
- berry aneurysm
- (congenital) cerebral aneurysm NOS

EXCLUDES *syphilitic ruptured cerebral aneurysm (094.87)*

AHA: ▶4Q, '04, 77◀

DEF: Bleeding in space between brain and lining.

431 **Intracerebral hemorrhage**

Hemorrhage (of):	Hemorrhage (of):
basilar	internal capsule
bulbar	intrapontine
cerebellar	pontine
cerebral	subcortical
cerebromeningeal	ventricular
cortical	Rupture of blood vessel in brain

DEF: Bleeding within the brain.

AHA: ▶4Q, '04, 77◀

Berry Aneurysm

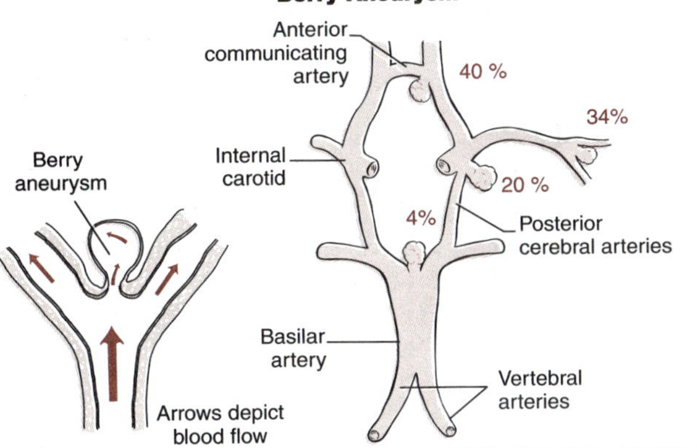

✓4th 432 **Other and unspecified intracranial hemorrhage**

AHA: ▶4Q, '04, 77◀

432.0 **Nontraumatic extradural hemorrhage**

Nontraumatic epidural hemorrhage

DEF: Bleeding, nontraumatic, between skull and brain lining.

432.1 **Subdural hemorrhage**

Subdural hematoma, nontraumatic

DEF: Bleeding, between outermost and other layers of brain lining.

432.9 **Unspecified intracranial hemorrhage**

Intracranial hemorrhage NOS

✓4th 433 **Occlusion and stenosis of precerebral arteries**

INCLUDES embolism, narrowing, obstruction, thrombosis } of basilar, carotid, and vertebral arteries

EXCLUDES *insufficiency NOS of precerebral arteries (435.0-435.9)*

The following fifth-digit subclassification is for use with category 433:
- **0 without mention of cerebral infarction**
- **1 with cerebral infarction**

AHA: 2Q, '95, 14; 3Q, '90, 16

DEF: Blockage, stricture, arteries branching into brain.

✓5th 433.0 **Basilar artery**

✓5th 433.1 **Carotid artery**

AHA: 1Q, '00, 16; For code 433.10: 1Q, '02, 7, 10

✓5th 433.2 **Vertebral artery**

✓5th 433.3 **Multiple and bilateral**

AHA: 2Q, '02, 19

✓5th 433.8 **Other specified precerebral artery**

✓5th 433.9 **Unspecified precerebral artery**

Precerebral artery NOS

✓4th 434 **Occlusion of cerebral arteries**

The following fifth-digit subclassification is for use with category 434:
- **0 without mention of cerebral infarction**
- **1 with cerebral infarction**

AHA: 2Q, '95, 14

✓5th 434.0 **Cerebral thrombosis**

Thrombosis of cerebral arteries

AHA: For code 434.01: ▶4Q, '04, 77◀

✓5th 434.1 **Cerebral embolism**

AHA: 3Q, '97, 11; For code 434.11: ▶4Q, '04, 77◀

✓5th 434.9 **Cerebral artery occlusion, unspecified**

AHA: 4Q, '98, 87; For code 434.91: ▶4Q, '04, 77-78◀

✓4th 435 **Transient cerebral ischemia**

INCLUDES cerebrovascular insufficiency (acute) with transient focal neurological signs and symptoms

insufficiency of basilar, carotid, and vertebral arteries

spasm of cerebral arteries

EXCLUDES *acute cerebrovascular insufficiency NOS (437.1)*

that due to any condition classifiable to 433 (433.0-433.9)

DEF: Temporary restriction of blood flow, to arteries branching into brain.

435.0 **Basilar artery syndrome**

435.1 **Vertebral artery syndrome**

435.2 **Subclavian steal syndrome**

DEF: Cerebrovascular insufficiency, due to occluded subclavian artery; symptoms include pain in mastoid and posterior head regions, flaccid paralysis of arm and diminished or absent radial pulse on affected side.

435.3 **Vertebrobasilar artery syndrome**

AHA: 4Q, '95, 60

DEF: Transient ischemic attack; due to brainstem dysfunction; symptoms include confusion, vertigo, binocular blindness, diplopia, unilateral or bilateral weakness and paresthesis of extremities.

Circulatory System

429.79–435.3

Map of Major Arteries

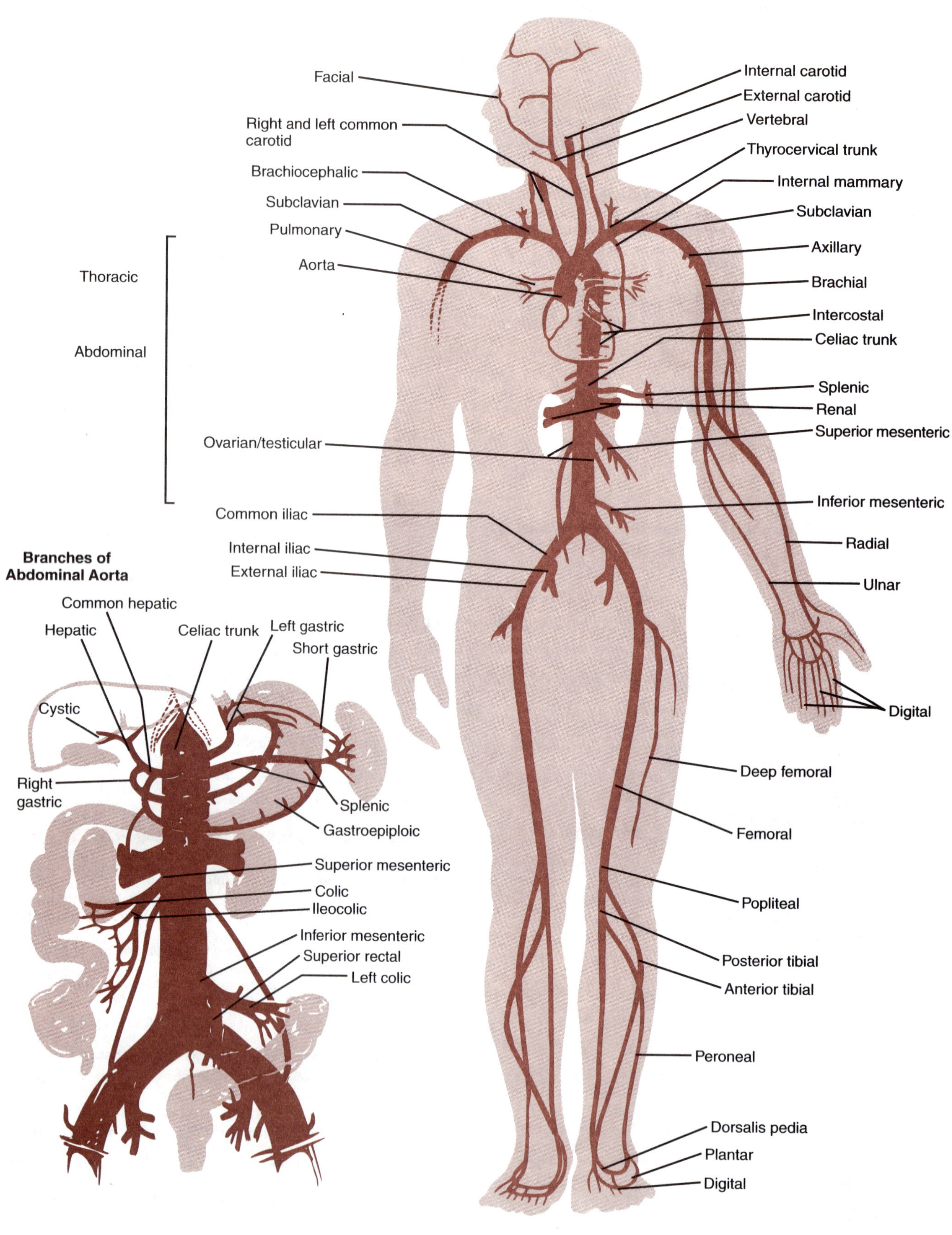

435.8 Other specified transient cerebral ischemias

435.9 Unspecified transient cerebral ischemia
Impending cerebrovascular accident
Intermittent cerebral ischemia
Transient ischemic attack [TIA]
AHA: N-D, '85, 12

436 Acute, but ill-defined, cerebrovascular disease
Apoplexy, apoplectic:
NOS
attack
cerebral
Apoplexy, apoplectic:
seizure
Cerebral seizure

EXCLUDES *any condition classifiable to categories 430-435*
cerebrovascular accident (434.91)
CVA (ischemic) (434.91)
embolic (434.11)
hemorrhagic (430, 431, 432.0-432.9)
thrombotic (434.01)
postoperative cerebrovascular accident (997.02)
stroke (ischemic) (434.91)
embolic (434.11)
hemorrhagic (430, 431, 432.0-432.9)
thrombotic (434.01)

AHA: ▶4Q, '04, 77;◀ 4Q, '99, 3

✓4th **437 Other and ill-defined cerebrovascular disease**

437.0 Cerebral atherosclerosis A
Atheroma of cerebral arteries
Cerebral arteriosclerosis

437.1 Other generalized ischemic cerebrovascular disease
Acute cerebrovascular insufficiency NOS
Cerebral ischemia (chronic)

437.2 Hypertensive encephalopathy
AHA: J-A, '84, 14
DEF: Cerebral manifestations (such as visual disturbances and headache) due to high blood pressure.

437.3 Cerebral aneurysm, nonruptured
Internal carotid artery, intracranial portion
Internal carotid artery NOS
EXCLUDES *congenital cerebral aneurysm, nonruptured (747.81)*
internal carotid artery, extracranial portion (442.81)

437.4 Cerebral arteritis
AHA: 4Q, '99, 21
DEF: Inflammation of a cerebral artery or arteries.

437.5 Moyamoya disease
DEF: Cerebrovascular ischemia; vessels occlude and rupture causing tiny hemorrhages at base of brain; predominantly affects Japanese.

437.6 Nonpyogenic thrombosis of intracranial venous sinus
EXCLUDES *pyogenic (325)*

437.7 Transient global amnesia
AHA: 4Q, '92, 20
DEF: Episode of short-term memory loss, not often recurrent; pathogenesis unknown; with no signs or symptoms of neurological disorder.

437.8 Other

437.9 Unspecified
Cerebrovascular disease or lesion NOS

✓4th **438 Late effects of cerebrovascular disease**
Note: This category is to be used to indicate conditions in 430-437 as the cause of late effects. The "late effects" include conditions specified as such, as sequelae, which may occur at any time after the onset of the causal condition.
AHA: 4Q, '99, 4, 6, 7; 4Q, '98, 39, 88; 4Q, '97, 35, 37; 4Q, '92, 21;N-D,'86, 12; M-A, '86, 7

438.0 Cognitive deficits

✓5th **438.1 Speech and language deficits**

438.10 Speech and language deficit, unspecified

438.11 Aphasia
AHA: 4Q, '03, 105; 4Q, '97, 36
DEF: Impairment or absence of the ability to communicate by speech, writing or signs or to comprehend the spoken or written language due to disease or injury to the brain. Total aphasia is the loss of function of both sensory and motor areas of the brain.

438.12 Dysphasia
AHA: 4Q, '99, 3, 9
DEF: Impaired speech; marked by inability to sequence language.

438.19 Other speech and language deficits

✓5th **438.2 Hemiplegia/hemiparesis**
DEF: Paralysis of one side of the body.

438.20 Hemiplegia affecting unspecified side
AHA: 4Q, '03, 105; 4Q, '99, 3, 9

438.21 Hemiplegia affecting dominant side

438.22 Hemiplegia affecting nondominant side
AHA: 4Q, '03, 105; 1Q, '02, 16

✓5th **438.3 Monoplegia of upper limb**
DEF: Paralysis of one limb or one muscle group.

438.30 Monoplegia of upper limb affecting unspecified side

438.31 Monoplegia of upper limb affecting dominant side

438.32 Monoplegia of upper limb affecting nondominant side

✓5th **438.4 Monoplegia of lower limb**

438.40 Monoplegia of lower limb affecting unspecified side

438.41 Monoplegia of lower limb affecting dominant side

438.42 Monoplegia of lower limb affecting nondominant side

✓5th **438.5 Other paralytic syndrome**
Use additional code to identify type of paralytic syndrome, such as:
locked-in state (344.81)
quadriplegia (344.00-344.09)
EXCLUDES *late effects of cerebrovascular accident with:*
hemiplegia/hemiparesis (438.20-438.22)
monoplegia of lower limb (438.40-438.42)
monoplegia of upper limb (438.30-438.32)

438.50 Other paralytic syndrome affecting unspecified side

438.51 Other paralytic syndrome affecting dominant side

438.52 Other paralytic syndrome affecting nondominant side

438.53 Other paralytic syndrome, bilateral
AHA: 4Q, '98, 39

438.6 Alterations of sensations
Use additional code to identify the altered sensation

438.7 Disturbances of vision
Use additional code to identify the visual disturbance
AHA: 4Q, '02, 56

✓5th **438.8 Other late effects of cerebrovascular disease**

438.81 Apraxia
DEF: Inability to activate learned movements; no known sensory or motor impairment.

438.82 Dysphagia
DEF: Inability or difficulty in swallowing.

438.83 Facial weakness
Facial droop

438.84 Ataxia
AHA: 4Q, '02, 56

438.85 Vertigo

438.89 Other late effects of cerebrovascular disease
Use additional code to identify the late effect
AHA: ▶1Q, '05, 13;◀ 4Q, '98, 39

438.9 Unspecified late effects of cerebrovascular disease

DISEASES OF ARTERIES, ARTERIOLES, AND CAPILLARIES (440-448)

✓4th **440 Atherosclerosis**

INCLUDES
arteriolosclerosis
arteriosclerosis (obliterans) (senile)
arteriosclerotic vascular disease
atheroma
degeneration:
arterial
arteriovascular
vascular
endarteritis deformans or obliterans
senile:
arteritis
endarteritis

EXCLUDES
atheroembolism (445.01-445.89)
atherosclerosis of bypass graft of the extremities (440.30-440.32)

DEF: Stricture and reduced elasticity of an artery; due to plaque deposits.

440.0 Of aorta A
AHA: 2Q, '93, 7; 2Q, '93, 8; 4Q, '88, 8

440.1 Of renal artery A
EXCLUDES *atherosclerosis of renal arterioles (403.00-403.91)*

✓5th **440.2 Of native arteries of the extremities**
EXCLUDES *atherosclerosis of bypass graft of the extremities (440.30-440.32)*
AHA: 4Q, '94, 49; 4Q, '93, 27; 4Q, '92, 25; 3Q, '90, 15; M-A, '87, 6

440.20 Atherosclerosis of the extremities, unspecified A

440.21 Atherosclerosis of the extremities with intermittent claudication A
DEF: Atherosclerosis; marked by pain, tension and weakness after walking; no symptoms while at rest.

440.22 Atherosclerosis of the extremities with rest pain A
INCLUDES any condition classifiable to 440.21
DEF: Atherosclerosis, marked by pain, tension and weakness while at rest.

Thoracic, Abdominal and Aortic Aneurysm

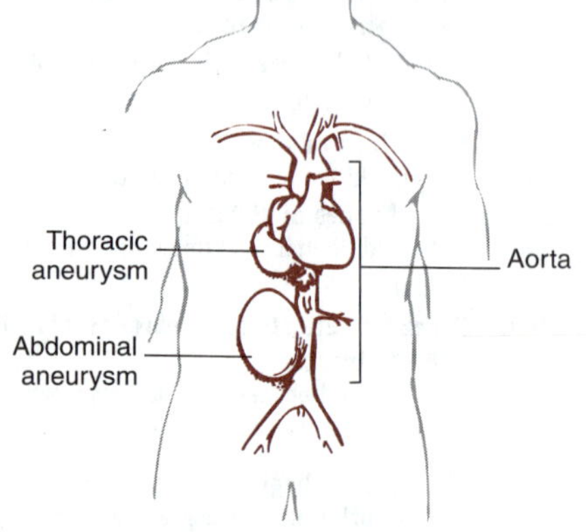

Arterial Diseases and Disorders

Intimal proliferation

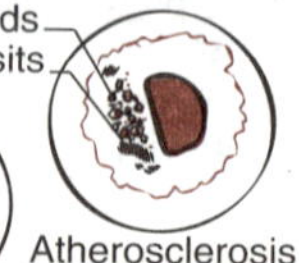

Atherosclerosis narrowing lumen

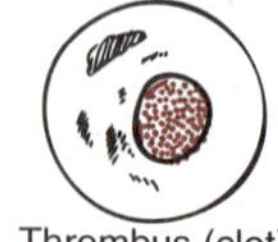
Thrombus (clot) forming in lumen

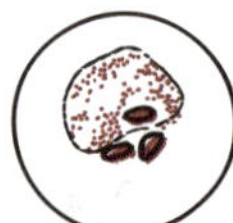
Organization of thrombus and recanalization

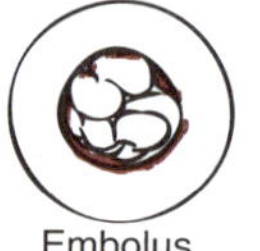
Embolus (from elsewhere) occluding lumen

Aneurysm bypasses lumen or... ...bulges from arterial wall

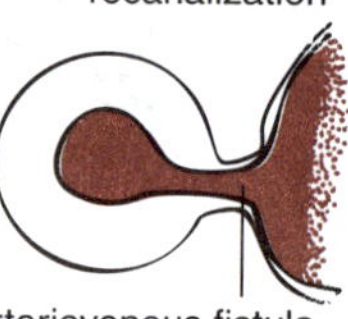
Arteriovenous fistula

440.23 Atherosclerosis of the extremities with ulceration A
Use additional code for any associated ulceration (707.10-707.9)
INCLUDES any condition classifiable to 440.21 and 440.22
AHA: 4Q, '00, 44

440.24 Atherosclerosis of the extremities with gangrene
INCLUDES any condition classifiable to 440.21, 440.22, and 440.23 with ischemic gangrene 785.4
EXCLUDES *gas gangrene (040.0)*
AHA: 4Q, '03, 109; 3Q. '03, 14; 4Q, '95, 54; 1Q, '95, 11

440.29 Other A

✓5th **440.3 Of bypass graft of extremities**
EXCLUDES *atherosclerosis of native arteries of the extremities (440.21-440.24)*
embolism [occlusion NOS] [thrombus] of graft (996.74)
AHA: 4Q, '94, 49

440.30 Of unspecified graft A
440.31 Of autologous vein bypass graft A
440.32 Of nonautologous biological bypass graft A

440.8 Of other specified arteries A
EXCLUDES
basilar (433.0)
carotid (433.1)
cerebral (437.0)
coronary (414.00-414.07)
mesenteric (557.1)
precerebral (433.0-433.9)
pulmonary (416.0)
vertebral (433.2)

440.9 Generalized and unspecified atherosclerosis A
Arteriosclerotic vascular disease NOS
EXCLUDES *arteriosclerotic cardiovascular disease [ASCVD] (429.2)*

✓4th **441 Aortic aneurysm and dissection**
EXCLUDES *syphilitic aortic aneurysm (093.0)*
traumatic aortic aneurysm (901.0, 902.0)

✓5th **441.0 Dissection of aorta**
AHA: 4Q, '89, 10
DEF: Dissection or splitting of wall of the aorta; due to blood entering through intimal tear or interstitial hemorrhage.

441.00 Unspecified site
441.01 Thoracic
441.02 Abdominal
441.03 Thoracoabdominal

441.1 Thoracic aneurysm, ruptured

441.2 Thoracic aneurysm without mention of rupture

AHA: 3Q, '92, 10

441.3 Abdominal aneurysm, ruptured

441.4 Abdominal aneurysm without mention of rupture

AHA: 4Q, '00, 64; 1Q, '99, 15, 16, 17; 3Q, '92, 10

441.5 Aortic aneurysm of unspecified site, ruptured

Rupture of aorta NOS

441.6 Thoracoabdominal aneurysm, ruptured

441.7 Thoracoabdominal aneurysm, without mention of rupture

441.9 Aortic aneurysm of unspecified site without mention of rupture

Aneurysm } of aorta
Dilatation } of aorta
Hyaline necrosis } of aorta

✓4th 442 Other aneurysm

INCLUDES aneurysm (ruptured) (cirsoid) (false) (varicose)
aneurysmal varix

EXCLUDES *arteriovenous aneurysm or fistula:*
acquired (447.0)
congenital (747.60-747.69)
traumatic (900.0-904.9)

DEF: Dissection or splitting of arterial wall; due to blood entering through intimal tear or interstitial hemorrhage.

442.0 Of artery of upper extremity

442.1 Of renal artery

442.2 Of iliac artery

AHA: 1Q, '99, 16, 17

442.3 Of artery of lower extremity

Aneurysm:
femoral } artery
popliteal } artery

AHA: 3Q, '02, 24-26; 1Q, '99, 16

✓5th 442.8 Of other specified artery

442.81 Artery of neck

Aneurysm of carotid artery (common) (external) (internal, extracranial portion)

EXCLUDES *internal carotid artery, intracranial portion (437.3)*

442.82 Subclavian artery

442.83 Splenic artery

442.84 Other visceral artery

Aneurysm:
celiac } artery
gastroduodenal } artery
gastroepiploic } artery
hepatic } artery
pancreaticoduodenal } artery
superior mesenteric } artery

442.89 Other

Aneurysm:
mediastinal } artery
spinal } artery

EXCLUDES *cerebral (nonruptured) (437.3)*
congenital (747.81)
ruptured (430)
coronary (414.11)
heart (414.10)
pulmonary (417.1)

442.9 Of unspecified site

✓4th 443 Other peripheral vascular disease

443.0 Raynaud's syndrome

Raynaud's:
disease
phenomenon (secondary)

Use additional code to identify gangrene (785.4)

DEF: Constriction of the arteries, due to cold or stress; bilateral ischemic attacks of fingers, toes, nose or ears; symptoms include pallor, paresthesia and pain; more common in females.

443.1 Thromboangiitis obliterans [Buerger's disease]

Presenile gangrene

DEF: Inflammatory disease of extremity blood vessels, mainly the lower; occurs primarily in young men and leads to tissue ischemia and gangrene.

✓5th 443.2 Other arterial dissection

EXCLUDES *dissection of aorta (441.00-441.03)*
dissection of coronary arteries (414.12)

AHA: 4Q, '02, 54

443.21 Dissection of carotid artery

443.22 Dissection of iliac artery

443.23 Dissection of renal artery

443.24 Dissection of vertebral artery

443.29 Dissection of other artery

✓5th 443.8 Other specified peripheral vascular diseases

443.81 Peripheral angiopathy in diseases classified elsewhere

Code first underlying disease, as:
diabetes mellitus (250.7)

AHA: 1Q, '04, 14; 3Q, '91, 10

● **443.82 Erythromelalgia**

443.89 Other

Acrocyanosis
Acroparesthesia:
simple [Schultze's type]
vasomotor [Nothnagel's type]
Erythrocyanosis

EXCLUDES *chilblains (991.5)*
frostbite (991.0-991.3)
immersion foot (991.4)

443.9 Peripheral vascular disease, unspecified

Intermittent claudication NOS
Peripheral:
angiopathy NOS
vascular disease NOS
Spasm of artery

EXCLUDES *atherosclerosis of the arteries of the extremities (440.20-440.22)*
spasm of cerebral artery (435.0-435.9)

AHA: 4Q, '92, 25; 3Q, '91, 10

✓4th 444 Arterial embolism and thrombosis

INCLUDES infarction:
embolic
thrombotic
occlusion

EXCLUDES *atheroembolism (445.01-445.89)*
that complicating:
abortion (634-638 with .6, 639.6)
ectopic or molar pregnancy (639.6)
pregnancy, childbirth, or the pueperium (673.0-673.8)

AHA: 2Q, '92, 11; 4Q, '90, 27

444.0 Of abdominal aorta

Aortic bifurcation syndrome
Aortoiliac obstruction
Leriche's syndrome
Saddle embolus

AHA: 2Q, '93, 7; 4Q, '90, 27

444.1 Of thoracic aorta

Embolism or thrombosis of aorta (thoracic)

Map of Major Veins

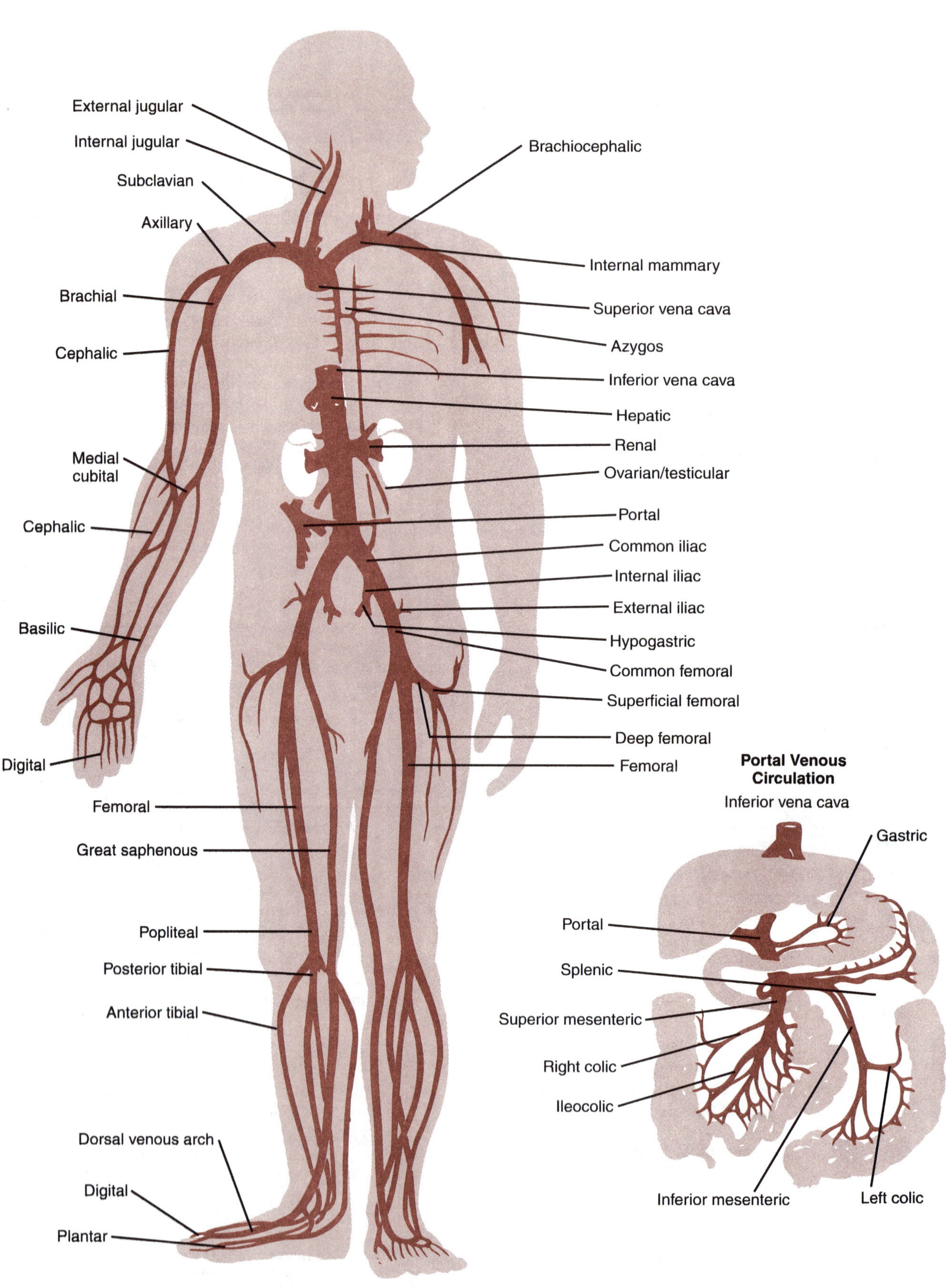

✓5th **444.2 Of arteries of the extremities**
AHA: M-A, '87, 6

444.21 Upper extremity

444.22 Lower extremity
Arterial embolism or thrombosis:
femoral
peripheral NOS
popliteal
EXCLUDES *iliofemoral (444.81)*
AHA: 3Q, '03, 10; 1Q, '03, 17; 3Q, '90, 16

✓5th **444.8 Of other specified artery**

444.81 Iliac artery
AHA: 1Q, '03, 16

444.89 Other
EXCLUDES *basilar (433.0)*
carotid (433.1)
cerebral (434.0-434.9)
coronary (410.00-410.92)
mesenteric (557.0)
ophthalmic (362.30-362.34)
precerebral (433.0-433.9)
pulmonary (415.19)
renal (593.81)
retinal (362.30-362.34)
vertebral (433.2)

444.9 Of unspecified artery

✓4th **445 Atheroembolism**
INCLUDES atherothrombotic microembolism
cholesterol embolism
AHA: 4Q, '02, 57

✓5th **445.0 Of extremities**

445.01 Upper extremity

445.02 Lower extremity

✓5th **445.8 Of other sites**

445.81 Kidney
Use additional code for any associated kidney failure (584, 585)

445.89 Other site

✓4th **446 Polyarteritis nodosa and allied conditions**

446.0 Polyarteritis nodosa
Disseminated necrotizing periarteritis
Necrotizing angiitis
Panarteritis (nodosa)
Periarteritis (nodosa)

DEF: Inflammation of small and mid-size arteries; symptoms related to involved arteries in kidneys, muscles, gastrointestinal tract and heart; results in tissue death.

446.1 Acute febrile mucocutaneous lymph node syndrome [MCLS]
Kawasaki disease

DEF: Acute febrile disease of children; marked by erythema of conjunctiva and mucous membranes of upper respiratory tract, skin eruptions and edema.

✓5th **446.2 Hypersensitivity angiitis**
EXCLUDES *antiglomerular basement membrane disease without pulmonary hemorrhage (583.89)*

446.20 Hypersensitivity angiitis, unspecified

446.21 Goodpasture's syndrome
Antiglomerular basement membrane antibody-mediated nephritis with pulmonary hemorrhage
Use additional code to identify renal disease (583.81)

DEF: Glomerulonephritis associated with hematuria, progresses rapidly; results in death from renal failure.

446.29 Other specified hypersensitivity angiitis
AHA: 1Q, '95, 3

446.3 Lethal midline granuloma
Malignant granuloma of face

DEF: Granulomatous lesion; in nose or paranasal sinuses; often fatal; occurs chiefly in males.
AHA: 3Q, '00, 11

446.4 Wegener's granulomatosis
Necrotizing respiratory granulomatosis
Wegener's syndrome

DEF: A disease occurring mainly in men; marked by necrotizing granulomas and ulceration of the upper respiratory tract; underlying condition is a vasculitis affecting small vessels and is possibly due to an immune disorder.
AHA: 3Q, '00, 11

446.5 Giant cell arteritis
Cranial arteritis
Horton's disease
Temporal arteritis

DEF: Inflammation of arteries; due to giant cells affecting carotid artery branches, resulting in occlusion; symptoms include fever, headache and neurological problems; occurs in elderly.

446.6 Thrombotic microangiopathy
Moschcowitz's syndrome
Thrombotic thrombocytopenic purpura

DEF: Blockage of small blood vessels; due to hyaline deposits; symptoms include purpura, CNS disorders; results in protracted disease or rapid death.

446.7 Takayasu's disease
Aortic arch arteritis
Pulseless disease

DEF: Progressive obliterative arteritis of brachiocephalic trunk, left subclavian, and left common carotid arteries above aortic arch; results in ischemia in brain, heart and arm; pulses impalpable in head, neck and arms; more common in young adult females.

✓4th **447 Other disorders of arteries and arterioles**

447.0 Arteriovenous fistula, acquired
Arteriovenous aneurysm, acquired
EXCLUDES *cerebrovascular (437.3)*
coronary (414.19)
pulmonary (417.0)
surgically created arteriovenous shunt or fistula:
complication (996.1, 996.61-996.62)
status or presence (V45.1)
traumatic (900.0-904.9)

DEF: Communication between an artery and vein caused by error in healing.

447.1 Stricture of artery
AHA: 2Q, '93, 8; M-A, '87, 6

447.2 Rupture of artery
Erosion
Fistula, except arteriovenous } of artery
Ulcer
EXCLUDES *traumatic rupture of artery (900.0-904.9)*

447.3 Hyperplasia of renal artery
Fibromuscular hyperplasia of renal artery

DEF: Overgrowth of cells in muscular lining of renal artery.

447.4 Celiac artery compression syndrome
Celiac axis syndrome
Marable's syndrome

447.5 Necrosis of artery

447.6 Arteritis, unspecified
Aortitis NOS
Endarteritis NOS
EXCLUDES *arteritis, endarteritis:*
aortic arch (446.7)
cerebral (437.4)
coronary (414.00-414.07)
deformans (440.0-440.9)
obliterans (440.0-440.9)
pulmonary (417.8)
senile (440.0-440.9)
polyarteritis NOS (446.0)
syphilitic aortitis (093.1)
AHA: 1Q, '95, 3

447.8 Other specified disorders of arteries and arterioles
Fibromuscular hyperplasia of arteries, except renal

447.9 Unspecified disorders of arteries and arterioles

✓4th **448 Disease of capillaries**

448.0 Hereditary hemorrhagic telangiectasia
Rendu-Osler-Weber disease
DEF: Genetic disease with onset after puberty; results in multiple telangiectases, dilated venules on skin and mucous membranes; recurrent bleeding may occur.

448.1 Nevus, non-neoplastic
Nevus:
araneus
senile
spider
stellar
EXCLUDES *neoplastic (216.0-216.9)*
port wine (757.32)
strawberry (757.32)
DEF: Enlarged or malformed blood vessels of skin; results in reddish swelling, skin patch, or birthmark.

448.9 Other and unspecified capillary diseases
Capillary:
hemorrhage
hyperpermeability
thrombosis
EXCLUDES *capillary fragility (hereditary) (287.8)*

DISEASES OF VEINS AND LYMPHATICS, AND OTHER DISEASES OF CIRCULATORY SYSTEM (451-459)

✓4th **451 Phlebitis and thrombophlebitis**
INCLUDES endophlebitis
inflammation, vein
periphlebitis
suppurative phlebitis
Use additional E code to identify drug, if drug-induced
EXCLUDES *that complicating:*
abortion (634-638 with .7, 639.8)
ectopic or molar pregnancy (639.8)
pregnancy, childbirth, or the puerperium (671.0-671.9)
that due to or following:
implant or catheter device (996.61-996.62)
infusion, perfusion, or transfusion (999.2)
AHA: 1Q, '92, 16
DEF: Inflammation of a vein (phlebitis) with formation of a thrombus (thrombophlebitis).

451.0 Of superficial vessels of lower extremities
AHA: 3Q, '91, 16
Saphenous vein (greater) (lesser)

✓5th **451.1 Of deep vessels of lower extremities**
AHA: 3Q, '91, 16

451.11 Femoral vein (deep) (superficial)

451.19 Other
Femoropopliteal vein
Popliteal vein
Tibial vein

451.2 Of lower extremities, unspecified
AHA: ▶4Q, '04, 80◀

✓5th **451.8 Of other sites**
EXCLUDES *intracranial venous sinus (325)*
nonpyogenic (437.6)
portal (vein) (572.1)

451.81 Iliac vein

451.82 Of superficial veins of upper extremities
Antecubital vein
Basilic vein
Cephalic vein

451.83 Of deep veins of upper extremities
Brachial vein
Radial vein
Ulnar vein

451.84 Of upper extremities, unspecified

451.89 Other
Axillary vein
Jugular vein
Subclavian vein
Thrombophlebitis of breast (Mondor's disease)

451.9 Of unspecified site

452 Portal vein thrombosis
Portal (vein) obstruction
EXCLUDES *hepatic vein thrombosis (453.0)*
phlebitis of portal vein (572.1)
DEF: Formation of a blood clot in main vein of liver.

✓4th **453 Other venous embolism and thrombosis**
EXCLUDES *that complicating:*
abortion (634-638 with .7, 639.8)
ectopic or molar pregnancy (639.8)
pregnancy, childbirth, or the puerperium (671.0-671.9)
that with inflammation, phlebitis, and thrombophlebitis (451.0-451.9)
AHA: 1Q, '92, 16

453.0 Budd-Chiari syndrome
Hepatic vein thrombosis
DEF: Thrombosis or other obstruction of hepatic vein; symptoms include enlarged liver, extensive collateral vessels, intractable ascites and severe portal hypertension.

453.1 Thrombophlebitis migrans
DEF: Slow, advancing thrombophlebitis; appearing first in one vein then another.

453.2 Of vena cava

453.3 Of renal vein

✓5th **453.4 Venous embolism and thrombosis of deep vessels of lower extremity**

453.40 Venous embolism and thrombosis of unspecified deep vessels of lower extremity
Deep vein thrombosis NOS
DVT NOS

453.41 Venous embolism and thrombosis of deep vessels of proximal lower extremity
Femoral
Iliac
Popliteal
Thigh
Upper leg NOS
AHA: ▶4Q, '04, 79◀

453.42 Venous embolism and thrombosis of deep vessels of distal lower extremity
Calf
Lower leg NOS
Peroneal
Tibial

453.8 Of other specified veins
EXCLUDES *cerebral (434.0-434.9)*
coronary (410.00-410.92)
intracranial venous sinus (325)
nonpyogenic (437.6)
mesenteric (557.0)
portal (452)
precerebral (433.0-433.9)
pulmonary (415.19)
AHA: 3Q, '91, 16; M-A, '87, 6

453.9 Of unspecified site
Embolism of vein
Thrombosis (vein)

✓4th **454 Varicose veins of lower extremities**
EXCLUDES *that complicating pregnancy, childbirth, or the puerperium (671.0)*
AHA: 2Q, '91, 20
DEF: Dilated leg veins; due to incompetent vein valves that allow reversed blood flow and cause tissue erosion or weakness of wall; may be painful.

454.0 With ulcer A
Varicose ulcer (lower extremity, any part)
Varicose veins with ulcer of lower extremity [any part] or of unspecified site
Any condition classifiable to 454.9 with ulcer or specified as ulcerated
AHA: 4Q, '99, 18

454.1 With inflammation A
Stasis dermatitis
Varicose veins with inflammation of lower extremity [any part] or of unspecified site
Any condition classifiable to 454.9 with inflammation or specified as inflamed

454.2 With ulcer and inflammation A
Varicose veins with ulcer and inflammation of lower extremity [any part] or of unspecified site
Any condition classifiable to 454.9 with ulcer and inflammation

454.8 With other complications
Edema
Pain
Swelling
AHA: 4Q, '02, 58

454.9 Asymptomatic varicose veins A
Phlebectasia, Varicose veins, Varix } of lower extremity [any part] or of unspecified site
Varicose veins NOS
AHA: 4Q, '02, 58

✓4th 455 Hemorrhoids

INCLUDES hemorrhoids (anus) (rectum)
piles
varicose veins, anus or rectum

EXCLUDES *that complicating pregnancy, childbirth, or the puerperium (671.8)*

DEF: Varicose condition of external hemorrhoidal veins causing painful swellings at the anus.

455.0 Internal hemorrhoids without mention of complication

455.1 Internal thrombosed hemorrhoids

455.2 Internal hemorrhoids with other complication
Internal hemorrhoids:
bleeding
prolapsed
strangulated
ulcerated
AHA: 1Q, '03, 8

455.3 External hemorrhoids without mention of complication

455.4 External thrombosed hemorrhoids

455.5 External hemorrhoids with other complication
External hemorrhoids:
bleeding
prolapsed
strangulated
ulcerated
AHA: 1Q, '03, 8

455.6 Unspecified hemorrhoids without mention of complication
Hemorrhoids NOS

455.7 Unspecified thrombosed hemorrhoids
Thrombosed hemorrhoids, unspecified whether internal or external

455.8 Unspecified hemorrhoids with other complication
Hemorrhoids, unspecified whether internal or external:
bleeding
prolapsed
strangulated
ulcerated

455.9 Residual hemorrhoidal skin tags
Skin tags, anus or rectum

✓4th 456 Varicose veins of other sites

456.0 Esophageal varices with bleeding
DEF: Distended, tortuous, veins of lower esophagus, usually due to portal hypertension.

456.1 Esophageal varices without mention of bleeding

✓5th **456.2 Esophageal varices in diseases classified elsewhere**
Code first underlying disease, as:
cirrhosis of liver (571.0-571.9)
portal hypertension (572.3)

456.20 With bleeding
AHA: N-D, '85, 14

456.21 Without mention of bleeding
AHA: 2Q, '02, 4

456.3 Sublingual varices
DEF: Distended, tortuous veins beneath tongue.

456.4 Scrotal varices ♂
Varicocele

456.5 Pelvic varices
Varices of broad ligament

456.6 Vulval varices ♀
Varices of perineum
EXCLUDES *that complicating pregnancy, childbirth, or the puerperium (671.1)*

456.8 Varices of other sites
Varicose veins of nasal septum (with ulcer)
EXCLUDES *placental varices (656.7)*
retinal varices (362.17)
varicose ulcer of unspecified site (454.0)
varicose veins of unspecified site (454.9)
AHA: 2Q, '02, 4

✓4th 457 Noninfectious disorders of lymphatic channels

457.0 Postmastectomy lymphedema syndrome A
Elephantiasis, Obliteration of lymphatic vessel } due to mastectomy

DEF: Reduced lymphatic circulation following mastectomy; symptoms include swelling of the arm on the operative side.

AHA: 2Q, '02, 12

457.1 Other lymphedema
Elephantiasis (nonfilarial) NOS
Lymphangiectasis
Lymphedema:
acquired (chronic)
praecox
secondary
Obliteration, lymphatic vessel
EXCLUDES *elephantiasis (nonfilarial):*
congenital (757.0)
eyelid (374.83)
vulva (624.8)
AHA: ►3Q, '04, 5◄

DEF: Fluid retention due to reduced lymphatic circulation; due to other than mastectomy.

457.2 Lymphangitis
Lymphangitis:
NOS
chronic
subacute
EXCLUDES *acute lymphangitis (682.0-682.9)*

457.8 Other noninfectious disorders of lymphatic channels
Chylocele (nonfilarial)
Chylous:
ascites
cyst
Lymph node or vessel:
fistula
infarction
rupture
EXCLUDES *chylocele:*
filarial (125.0-125.9)
tunica vaginalis (nonfilarial) (608.84)
AHA: 1Q, '04, 5; 3Q, '03, 17

457.9 Unspecified noninfectious disorder of lymphatic channels

✓4th ✓5th Additional Digit Required 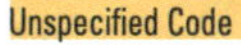 Unspecified Code | Other Specified Code | Manifestation Code | ►◄ Revised Text | ● New Code | ▲ Revised Code Title

Circulatory System
454.1–457.9

✓4th **458 Hypotension**

INCLUDES hypopiesis

EXCLUDES *cardiovascular collapse (785.50)*
maternal hypotension syndrome (669.2)
shock (785.50-785.59)
Shy-Drager syndrome (333.0)

458.0 Orthostatic hypotension
Hypotension: orthostatic (chronic)
Hypotension: postural
AHA: 3Q, '00, 8; 3Q, '91, 9
DEF: Low blood pressure; occurs when standing.

458.1 Chronic hypotension
Permanent idiopathic hypotension
DEF: Persistent low blood pressure.

✓5th **458.2 Iatrogenic hypotension**
AHA: 4Q, '03, 60; 3Q, '02, 12; 4Q, '95, 57
DEF: Abnormally low blood pressure; due to medical treatment.

458.21 Hypotension of hemodialysis
Intra-dialytic hypotension
AHA: 4Q, '03, 61

458.29 Other iatrogenic hypotension
Postoperative hypotension

458.8 Other specified hypotension
AHA: 4Q, '97, 37

458.9 Hypotension, unspecified
Hypotension (arterial) NOS

✓4th **459 Other disorders of circulatory system**

459.0 Hemorrhage, unspecified
Rupture of blood vessel NOS
Spontaneous hemorrhage NEC

EXCLUDES *hemorrhage:*
gastrointestinal NOS (578.9)
in newborn NOS (772.9)
secondary or recurrent following trauma (958.2)
traumatic rupture of blood vessel (900.0-904.9)

AHA: 4Q, '90, 26

✓5th **459.1 Postphlebitic syndrome**
Chronic venous hypertension due to deep vein thrombosis

EXCLUDES *chronic venous hypertension without deep vein thrombosis (459.30-459.39)*

AHA: 4Q, '02, 58; 2Q, '91, 20
DEF: Various conditions following deep vein thrombosis; including edema, pain, stasis dermatitis, cellulitis, varicose veins and ulceration of the lower leg.

459.10 Postphlebitic syndrome without complications
Asymptomatic postphlebitic syndrome
Postphlebitic syndrome NOS

459.11 Postphlebitic syndrome with ulcer

459.12 Postphlebitic syndrome with inflammation

459.13 Postphlebitic syndrome with ulcer and inflammation

459.19 Postphlebitic syndrome with other complication

459.2 Compression of vein
Stricture of vein
Vena cava syndrome (inferior) (superior)

✓5th **459.3 Chronic venous hypertension (idiopathic)**
Stasis edema

EXCLUDES *chronic venous hypertension due to deep vein thrombosis (459.10-459.19)*
varicose veins (454.0-454.9)

AHA: 4Q, '02, 59

459.30 Chronic venous hypertension without complications
Asymptomatic chronic venous hypertension
Chronic venous hypertension NOS

459.31 Chronic venous hypertension with ulcer
AHA: 4Q, '02, 43

459.32 Chronic venous hypertension with inflammation

459.33 Chronic venous hypertension with ulcer and inflammation

459.39 Chronic venous hypertension with other complication

✓5th **459.8 Other specified disorders of circulatory system**

459.81 Venous (peripheral) insufficiency, unspecified
Chronic venous insufficiency NOS
Use additional code for any associated ulceration (707.10-707.9)
AHA: ▶3Q, '04, 5;◀ 2Q, '91, 20; M-A, '87, 6
DEF: Insufficient drainage, venous blood, any part of body, results in edema or dermatosis.

459.89 Other
Collateral circulation (venous), any site
Phlebosclerosis
Venofibrosis

459.9 Unspecified circulatory system disorder

8. DISEASES OF THE RESPIRATORY SYSTEM (460-519)

Use additional code to identify infectious organism

ACUTE RESPIRATORY INFECTIONS (460-466)

EXCLUDES *pneumonia and influenza (480.0-487.8)*

460 Acute nasopharyngitis [common cold]

Coryza (acute)
Nasal catarrh, acute
Nasopharyngitis:
  NOS
  acute
Nasopharyngitis:
  infective NOS
Rhinitis:
  acute
  infective

EXCLUDES *nasopharyngitis, chronic (472.2)*
pharyngitis:
  acute or unspecified (462)
  chronic (472.1)
rhinitis:
  allergic (477.0-477.9)
  chronic or unspecified (472.0)
sore throat:
  acute or unspecified (462)
  chronic (472.1)

AHA: 1Q, '88, 12

DEF: Acute inflammation of mucous membranes; extends from nares to pharynx.

✓4th **461 Acute sinusitis**

INCLUDES abscess, empyema, infection, inflammation, suppuration } acute, of sinus (accessory) (nasal)

EXCLUDES *chronic or unspecified sinusitis (473.0-473.9)*

461.0 Maxillary
Acute antritis

461.1 Frontal

461.2 Ethmoidal

461.3 Sphenoidal

461.8 Other acute sinusitis
Acute pansinusitis

461.9 Acute sinusitis, unspecified
Acute sinusitis NOS

462 Acute pharyngitis

Acute sore throat NOS
Pharyngitis (acute):
  NOS
  gangrenous
  infective
  phlegmonous
  pneumococcal
Pharyngitis (acute):
  staphylococcal
  suppurative
  ulcerative
Sore throat (viral) NOS
Viral pharyngitis

EXCLUDES *abscess:*
  peritonsillar [quinsy] (475)
  pharyngeal NOS (478.29)
  retropharyngeal (478.24)
chronic pharyngitis (472.1)
infectious mononucleosis (075)
that specified as (due to):
  Coxsackie (virus) (074.0)
  gonococcus (098.6)
  herpes simplex (054.79)
  influenza (487.1)
  septic (034.0)
  streptococcal (034.0)

AHA: 4Q, '99, 26; S-O, '85, 8

463 Acute tonsillitis

Tonsillitis (acute):
  NOS
  follicular
  gangrenous
  infective
  pneumococcal
Tonsillitis (acute):
  septic
  staphylococcal
  suppurative
  ulcerative
  viral

EXCLUDES *chronic tonsillitis (474.0)*
hypertrophy of tonsils (474.1)
peritonsillar abscess [quinsy] (475)
sore throat:
  acute or NOS (462)
  septic (034.0)
streptococcal tonsillitis (034.0)

AHA: N-D, '84, 16

✓4th **464 Acute laryngitis and tracheitis**

EXCLUDES *that associated with influenza (487.1)*
that due to Streptococcus (034.0)

✓5th **464.0 Acute laryngitis**
Laryngitis (acute):
  NOS
  edematous
  Hemophilus influenzae [H. influenzae]
  pneumococcal
  septic
  suppurative
  ulcerative

EXCLUDES *chronic laryngitis (476.0-476.1)*
influenzal laryngitis (487.1)

AHA: 4Q, '01, 42

464.00 Without mention of obstruction

464.01 With obstruction

✓5th **464.1 Acute tracheitis**
Tracheitis (acute):
  NOS
  catarrhal
Tracheitis (acute):
  viral

EXCLUDES *chronic tracheitis (491.8)*

464.10 Without mention of obstruction

464.11 With obstruction

✓5th **464.2 Acute laryngotracheitis**
Laryngotracheitis (acute)
Tracheitis (acute) with laryngitis (acute)

EXCLUDES *chronic laryngotracheitis (476.1)*

464.20 Without mention of obstruction

464.21 With obstruction

✓5th **464.3 Acute epiglottitis**
Viral epiglottitis

EXCLUDES *epiglottitis, chronic (476.1)*

464.30 Without mention of obstruction

464.31 With obstruction

464.4 Croup
Croup syndrome

DEF: Acute laryngeal obstruction due to allergy, foreign body or infection; symptoms include barking cough, hoarseness and harsh, persistent high-pitched respiratory sound.

✓5th **464.5 Supraglottitis, unspecified**

AHA: 4Q, '01, 42

DEF: A rapidly advancing generalized upper respiratory infection of the lingual tonsillar area, epiglottic folds, false vocal cords, and the epiglottis; seen most commonly in children, but can affect people of any age.

464.50 Without mention of obstruction
AHA: 4Q, '01, 43

464.51 With obstruction

Respiratory System

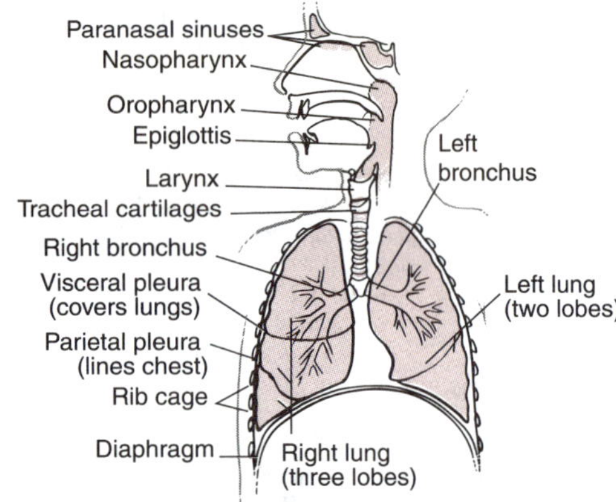

465 Acute upper respiratory infections of multiple or unspecified sites

EXCLUDES *upper respiratory infection due to:*
influenza (487.1)
Streptococcus (034.0)

465.0 Acute laryngopharyngitis

DEF: Acute infection of the vocal cords and pharynx.

465.8 Other multiple sites

Multiple URI

465.9 Unspecified site

Acute URI NOS
Upper respiratory infection (acute)

466 Acute bronchitis and bronchiolitis

INCLUDES that with:
bronchospasm
obstruction

466.0 Acute bronchitis

Bronchitis, acute or subacute:
fibrinous
membranous
pneumococcal
purulent
septic

Bronchitis, acute or subacute:
viral
with tracheitis
Croupous bronchitis
Tracheobronchitis, acute

EXCLUDES *acute bronchitis with chronic obstructive pulmonary disease (491.22)*

AHA: 4Q, '04, 137; 1Q, '04, 3; 4Q, '02, 46; 4Q, '96, 28; 4Q, '91, 24; 1Q, '88, 12

DEF: Acute inflammation of main branches of bronchial tree due to infectious or irritant agents; symptoms include cough with a varied production of sputum, fever, substernal soreness, and lung rales.

466.1 Acute bronchiolitis

Bronchiolitis (acute)
Capillary pneumonia

DEF: Acute inflammation of finer subdivisions of bronchial tree due to infectious or irritant agents; symptoms include cough with a varied production of sputum, fever, substernal soreness, and lung rales.

466.11 Acute bronchiolitis due to respiratory syncytial virus (RSV)

AHA: ▶1Q, '05, 10;◀ 4Q, '96, 27

466.19 Acute bronchiolitis due to other infectious organisms

Use additional code to identify organism

Upper Respiratory System

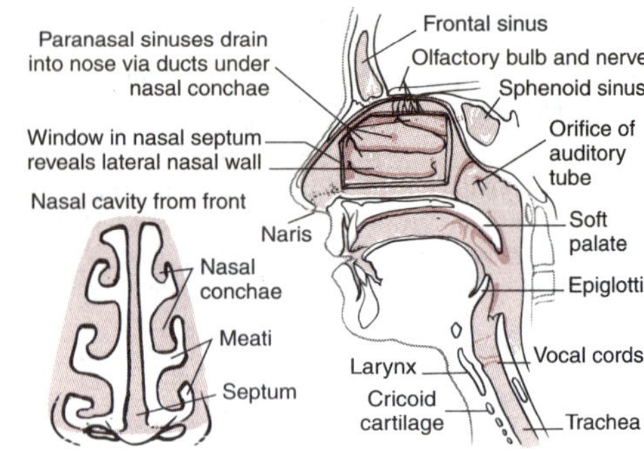

OTHER DISEASES OF THE UPPER RESPIRATORY TRACT (470-478)

470 Deviated nasal septum

Deflected septum (nasal) (acquired)

EXCLUDES *congenital (754.0)*

471 Nasal polyps

EXCLUDES *adenomatous polyps (212.0)*

471.0 Polyp of nasal cavity

Polyp:
choanal
nasopharyngeal

471.1 Polypoid sinus degeneration

Woakes' syndrome or ethmoiditis

471.8 Other polyp of sinus

Polyp of sinus:
accessory
ethmoidal

Polyp of sinus:
maxillary
sphenoidal

471.9 Unspecified nasal polyp

Nasal polyp NOS

472 Chronic pharyngitis and nasopharyngitis

472.0 Chronic rhinitis

Ozena
Rhinitis:
NOS
atrophic
granulomatous

Rhinitis:
hypertrophic
obstructive
purulent
ulcerative

EXCLUDES *allergic rhinitis (477.0-477.9)*

DEF: Persistent inflammation of mucous membranes of nose.

472.1 Chronic pharyngitis

Chronic sore throat
Pharyngitis:
atrophic

Pharyngitis:
granular (chronic)
hypertrophic

472.2 Chronic nasopharyngitis

EXCLUDES *acute or unspecified nasopharyngitis (460)*

DEF: Persistent inflammation of mucous membranes extending from nares to pharynx.

Paranasal Sinuses

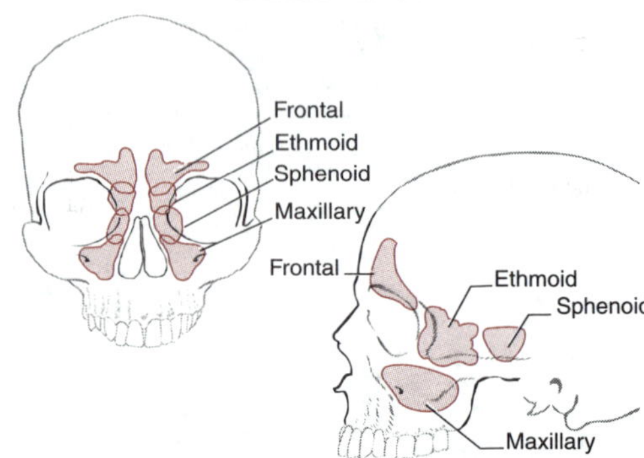

4th 473 Chronic sinusitis

INCLUDES abscess, empyema, infection, suppuration } (chronic) of sinus (accessory) (nasal)

EXCLUDES *acute sinusitis (461.0-461.9)*

473.0 Maxillary
Antritis (chronic)

473.1 Frontal

473.2 Ethmoidal
EXCLUDES *Woakes' ethmoiditis (471.1)*

473.3 Sphenoidal

473.8 Other chronic sinusitis
Pansinusitis (chronic)

473.9 Unspecified sinusitis (chronic)
Sinusitis (chronic) NOS

4th 474 Chronic disease of tonsils and adenoids

5th 474.0 Chronic tonsillitis and adenoiditis
EXCLUDES *acute or unspecified tonsillitis (463)*
AHA: 4Q, '97, 38

474.00 Chronic tonsillitis
474.01 Chronic adenoiditis
474.02 Chronic tonsillitis and adenoiditis

5th 474.1 Hypertrophy of tonsils and adenoids
Enlargement, Hyperplasia, Hypertrophy } of tonsils or adenoids
EXCLUDES *that with:*
adenoiditis (474.01)
adenoiditis and tonsillitis (474.02)
tonsillitis (474.00)

474.10 Tonsils with adenoids
474.11 Tonsils alone
474.12 Adenoids alone

474.2 Adenoid vegetations
DEF: Fungus-like growth of lymph tissue between the nares and pharynx.

474.8 Other chronic disease of tonsils and adenoids
Amygdalolith
Calculus, tonsil
Cicatrix of tonsil (and adenoid)
Tonsillar tag
Ulcer, tonsil

474.9 Unspecified chronic disease of tonsils and adenoids
Disease (chronic) of tonsils (and adenoids)

475 Peritonsillar abscess
Abscess of tonsil
Peritonsillar cellulitis
Quinsy
EXCLUDES *tonsillitis:*
acute or NOS (463)
chronic (474.0)

4th 476 Chronic laryngitis and laryngotracheitis

476.0 Chronic laryngitis
Laryngitis:
catarrhal
hypertrophic
Laryngitis:
sicca

476.1 Chronic laryngotracheitis
Laryngitis, chronic, with tracheitis (chronic)
Tracheitis, chronic, with laryngitis
EXCLUDES *chronic tracheitis (491.8)*
laryngitis and tracheitis, acute or unspecified (464.00-464.51)

4th 477 Allergic rhinitis

INCLUDES allergic rhinitis (nonseasonal) (seasonal)
hay fever
spasmodic rhinorrhea

EXCLUDES *allergic rhinitis with asthma (bronchial) (493.0)*

DEF: True immunoglobulin E (IgE)-mediated allergic reaction of nasal mucosa; seasonal (typical hay fever) or perennial (year-round allergens: dust, food, dander).

477.0 Due to pollen
Pollinosis

477.1 Due to food
AHA: 4Q, '00, 42

477.2 Due to animal (cat) (dog) hair and dander

477.8 Due to other allergen

477.9 Cause unspecified
AHA: 2Q, '97, 9

4th 478 Other diseases of upper respiratory tract

478.0 Hypertrophy of nasal turbinates
DEF: Overgrowth, enlargement of shell-shaped bones, in nasal cavity.

478.1 Other diseases of nasal cavity and sinuses
Abscess, Necrosis, Ulcer } of nose (septum)
Cyst or mucocele of sinus (nasal)
Rhinolith
EXCLUDES *varicose ulcer of nasal septum (456.8)*

5th 478.2 Other diseases of pharynx, not elsewhere classified

478.20 Unspecified disease of pharynx
478.21 Cellulitis of pharynx or nasopharynx
478.22 Parapharyngeal abscess
478.24 Retropharyngeal abscess
DEF: Purulent infection, behind pharynx and front of precerebral fascia.

478.25 Edema of pharynx or nasopharynx
478.26 Cyst of pharynx or nasopharynx
478.29 Other
Abscess of pharynx or nasopharynx
EXCLUDES *ulcerative pharyngitis (462)*

5th 478.3 Paralysis of vocal cords or larynx
DEF: Loss of motor ability of vocal cords or larynx; due to nerve or muscle damage.

478.30 Paralysis, unspecified
Laryngoplegia
Paralysis of glottis

478.31 Unilateral, partial
478.32 Unilateral, complete
478.33 Bilateral, partial
478.34 Bilateral, complete

478.4 Polyp of vocal cord or larynx
EXCLUDES *adenomatous polyps (212.1)*

478.5 Other diseases of vocal cords
Abscess, Cellulitis, Granuloma, Leukoplakia } of vocal cords
Chorditis (fibrinous) (nodosa) (tuberosa)
Singers' nodes

478.6 Edema of larynx
Edema (of):
glottis
subglottic
Edema (of):
supraglottic

5th 478.7 Other diseases of larynx, not elsewhere classified

478.70 Unspecified disease of larynx
478.71 Cellulitis and perichondritis of larynx
DEF: Inflammation of deep soft tissues or lining of bone of the larynx.

4th 5th Additional Digit Required | Unspecified Code | Other Specified Code | Manifestation Code | ▶◀ Revised Text | ● New Code | ▲ Revised Code Title

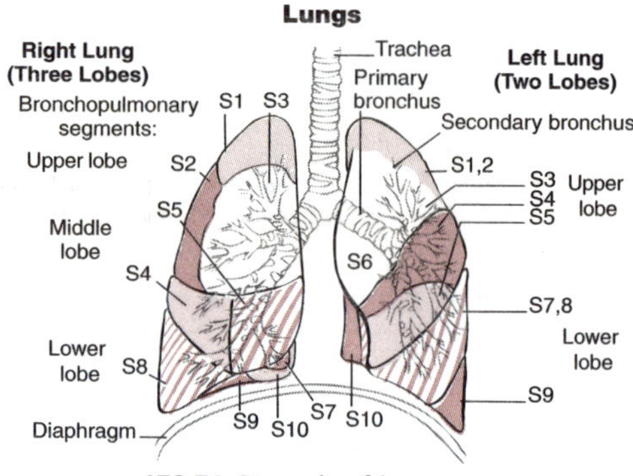

478.74 Stenosis of larynx

478.75 Laryngeal spasm

Laryngismus (stridulus)

DEF: Involuntary muscle contraction of the larynx.

478.79 Other

Abscess, Necrosis, Obstruction, Pachyderma, Ulcer } of larynx

EXCLUDES *ulcerative laryngitis (464.00-464.01)*

AHA: 3Q, '91, 20

478.8 Upper respiratory tract hypersensitivity reaction, site unspecified

EXCLUDES *hypersensitivity reaction of lower respiratory tract, as:*
extrinsic allergic alveolitis (495.0-495.9)
pneumoconiosis (500-505)

478.9 Other and unspecified diseases of upper respiratory tract

Abscess, Cicatrix } of trachea

PNEUMONIA AND INFLUENZA (480-487)

EXCLUDES *pneumonia:*
allergic or eosinophilic (518.3)
aspiration:
NOS (507.0)
newborn ▶(770.18)◀
solids and liquids (507.0-507.8)
congenital (770.0)
lipoid (507.1)
passive (514)
rheumatic (390)

✓4th **480 Viral pneumonia**

480.0 Pneumonia due to adenovirus

480.1 Pneumonia due to respiratory syncytial virus

AHA: 4Q, '96, 28; 1Q, '88, 12

480.2 Pneumonia due to parainfluenza virus

480.3 Pneumonia due to SARS-associated coronavirus

AHA: 4Q, '03, 46-47

DEF: A severe adult respiratory syndrome caused by the coronavirus, specified as inflammation of the lungs with consolidation.

480.8 Pneumonia due to other virus not elsewhere classified

EXCLUDES *congenital rubella pneumonitis (771.0)*
influenza with pneumonia, any form (487.0)
pneumonia complicating viral diseases classified elsewhere (484.1-484.8)

480.9 Viral pneumonia, unspecified

AHA: 3Q, '98, 5

481 Pneumococcal pneumonia [Streptococcus pneumoniae pneumonia]

Lobar pneumonia, organism unspecified

AHA: 2Q, '98, 7; 4Q, '92, 19; 1Q, '92, 18; 1Q, '91, 13; 1Q, '88, 13; M-A, '85, 6

✓4th **482 Other bacterial pneumonia**

AHA: 4Q, '93, 39

482.0 Pneumonia due to Klebsiella pneumoniae

482.1 Pneumonia due to Pseudomonas

482.2 Pneumonia due to Hemophilus influenzae [H. influenzae]

✓5th **482.3 Pneumonia due to Streptococcus**

EXCLUDES *Streptococcus pneumoniae (481)*

AHA: 1Q, '88, 13

482.30 Streptococcus, unspecified

482.31 Group A

482.32 Group B

482.39 Other Streptococcus

✓5th **482.4 Pneumonia due to Staphylococcus**

AHA: 3Q, '91, 16

482.40 Pneumonia due to Staphylococcus, unspecified

482.41 Pneumonia due to Staphylococcus aureus

482.49 Other Staphylococcus pneumonia

✓5th **482.8 Pneumonia due to other specified bacteria**

EXCLUDES *pneumonia, complicating infectious disease classified elsewhere (484.1-484.8)*

AHA: 3Q, '88, 11

482.81 Anaerobes

Bacteroides (melaninogenicus)
Gram-negative anaerobes

482.82 Escherichia coli [E. coli]

482.83 Other gram-negative bacteria

Gram-negative pneumonia NOS
Proteus
Serratia marcescens

EXCLUDES *gram-negative anaerobes (482.81)*
Legionnaires' disease (482.84)

AHA: 2Q, '98, 5; 3Q, '94, 9

482.84 Legionnaires' disease

AHA: 4Q, '97, 38

DEF: Severe and often fatal infection by *Legionella pneumophilia;* symptoms include high fever, gastrointestinal pain, headache, myalgia, dry cough, and pneumonia; transmitted airborne via air conditioning systems, humidifiers, water faucets, shower heads; not person-to-person contact.

482.89 Other specified bacteria

AHA: 2Q, '97, 6

482.9 Bacterial pneumonia unspecified

AHA: 2Q, '98, 6; 2Q, '97, 6; 1Q, '94, 17

✓4th **483 Pneumonia due to other specified organism**

AHA: N-D, '87, 5

483.0 Mycoplasma pneumoniae

Eaton's agent
Pleuropneumonia-like organism [PPLO]

483.1 Chlamydia

AHA: 4Q, '96, 31

483.8 Other specified organism

✓4th **484 Pneumonia in infectious diseases classified elsewhere**

EXCLUDES *influenza with pneumonia, any form (487.0)*

484.1 *Pneumonia in cytomegalic inclusion disease*
Code first underlying disease, as (078.5)

484.3 *Pneumonia in whooping cough*
Code first underlying disease, as (033.0-033.9)

484.5 *Pneumonia in anthrax*
Code first underlying disease (022.1)

484.6 *Pneumonia in aspergillosis*
Code first underlying disease (117.3)
AHA: 4Q, '97, 40

484.7 *Pneumonia in other systemic mycoses*
Code first underlying disease
EXCLUDES *pneumonia in:*
candidiasis (112.4)
coccidioidomycosis (114.0)
histoplasmosis (115.0-115.9 with fifth-digit 5)

484.8 *Pneumonia in other infectious diseases classified elsewhere*
Code first underlying disease, as:
Q fever (083.0)
typhoid fever (002.0)
EXCLUDES *pneumonia in:*
actinomycosis (039.1)
measles (055.1)
nocardiosis (039.1)
ornithosis (073.0)
Pneumocystis carinii (136.3)
salmonellosis (003.22)
toxoplasmosis (130.4)
tuberculosis (011.6)
tularemia (021.2)
varicella (052.1)

485 Bronchopneumonia, organism unspecified
Bronchopneumonia:
hemorrhagic
terminal
Pneumonia:
lobular
segmental
Pleurobronchopneumonia
EXCLUDES *bronchiolitis (acute) (466.11-466.19)*
chronic (491.8)
lipoid pneumonia (507.1)

486 Pneumonia, organism unspecified
EXCLUDES *hypostatic or passive pneumonia (514)*
influenza with pneumonia, any form (487.0)
inhalation or aspiration pneumonia due to foreign materials (507.0-507.8)
pneumonitis due to fumes and vapors (506.0)
AHA: 4Q, '99, 6; 3Q, '99, 9; 3Q, '98, 7; 2Q, '98, 4, 5; 1Q, '98, 8; 3Q, '97, 9; 3Q, '94, 10; 3Q, '88, 11

Bronchioli and Alveoli

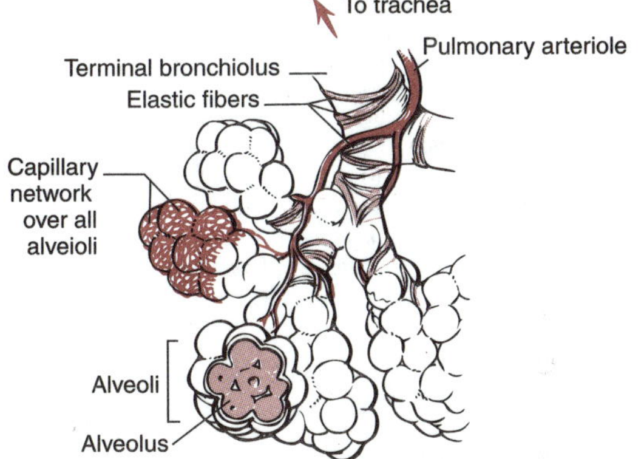

✓4th **487 Influenza**

EXCLUDES *Hemophilus influenzae [H. influenzae]:*
infection NOS (041.5)
laryngitis (464.00-464.01)
meningitis (320.0)

487.0 With pneumonia
Influenza with pneumonia, any form
Influenzal:
bronchopneumonia
pneumonia
▶Use additional code to identify the type of pneumonia (480.0-480.9, 481, 482.0-482.9, 483.0-483.8, 485)◀

487.1 With other respiratory manifestations
Influenza NOS
Influenzal:
laryngitis
pharyngitis
respiratory infection (upper) (acute)
AHA: 4Q, '99, 26

487.8 With other manifestations
Encephalopathy due to influenza
Influenza with involvement of gastrointestinal tract
EXCLUDES *"intestinal flu" [viral gastroenteritis] (008.8)*

CHRONIC OBSTRUCTIVE PULMONARY DISEASE AND ALLIED CONDITIONS (490-496)

AHA: 3Q, '88, 5

490 Bronchitis, not specified as acute or chronic
Bronchitis NOS:
catarrhal
with tracheitis NOS
Tracheobronchitis NOS
EXCLUDES *bronchitis:*
allergic NOS (493.9)
asthmatic NOS (493.9)
due to fumes and vapors (506.0)

✓4th **491 Chronic bronchitis**

EXCLUDES *chronic obstructive asthma (493.2)*

491.0 Simple chronic bronchitis
Catarrhal bronchitis, chronic
Smokers' cough

491.1 Mucopurulent chronic bronchitis
Bronchitis (chronic) (recurrent):
fetid
mucopurulent
purulent
AHA: 3Q, '88, 12

DEF: Chronic bronchial infection characterized by both mucus and pus secretions in the bronchial tree; recurs after asymptomatic periods; signs are coughing, expectoration and secondary changes in the lung.

✓5th **491.2 Obstructive chronic bronchitis**
Bronchitis:
emphysematous
obstructive (chronic) (diffuse)
Bronchitis with:
chronic airway obstruction
emphysema
EXCLUDES *asthmatic bronchitis (acute) NOS (493.9)*
chronic obstructive asthma (493.2)
AHA: 3Q, '97, 9; 4Q, '91, 25; 2Q, '91, 21

491.20 Without exacerbation
Emphysema with chronic bronchitis
AHA: 3Q, '97, 9

Interrelationship Between Chronic Airway Obstruction, Chronic Bronchitis and Emphysema

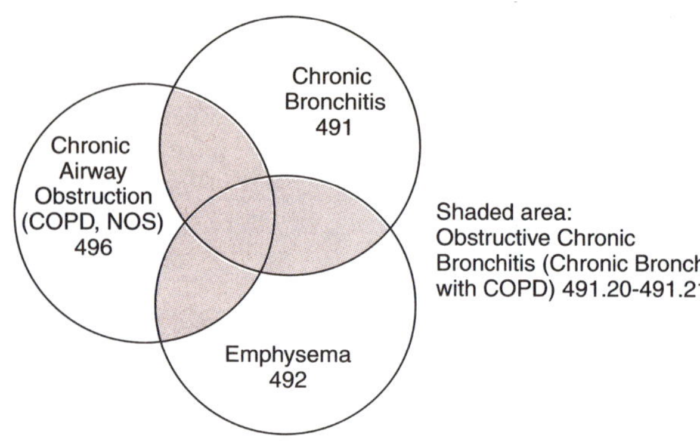

491.21 With (acute) exacerbation
Acute exacerbation of chronic obstructive pulmonary disease [COPD]
Decompensated chronic obstructive pulmonary disease [COPD]
Decompensated chronic obstructive pulmonary disease [COPD] with exacerbation
EXCLUDES *chronic obstructive asthma with acute exacerbation (493.22)*
AHA: 1Q, '04, 3; 3Q, '02, 18, 19; 4Q, '01, 43; 2Q, '96, 10

491.22 With acute bronchitis
AHA: 4Q, '04, 82

491.8 Other chronic bronchitis
Chronic:
tracheitis
tracheobronchitis

491.9 Unspecified chronic bronchitis

✓4th **492 Emphysema**
AHA: 2Q, '91, 21

492.0 Emphysematous bleb
Giant bullous emphysema
Ruptured emphysematous bleb
Tension pneumatocele
Vanishing lung
AHA: 2Q, '93, 3

DEF: Formation of vesicle or bulla in emphysematous lung, more than one millimeter; contains serum or blood.

492.8 Other emphysema
Emphysema (lung or pulmonary):
NOS
centriacinar
centrilobular
obstructive
panacinar
panlobular
unilateral
vesicular
MacLeod's syndrome
Swyer-James syndrome
Unilateral hyperlucent lung
EXCLUDES *emphysema:*
with chronic bronchitis (491.20-491.22)
compensatory (518.2)
due to fumes and vapors (506.4)
interstitial (518.1)
newborn (770.2)
mediastinal (518.1)
surgical (subcutaneous) (998.81)
traumatic (958.7)
AHA: ▶1Q, '05, 4;◀ 4Q, '93, 41; J-A, '84, 17

✓4th **493 Asthma**
EXCLUDES *wheezing NOS (786.07)*

The following fifth-digit subclassification is for use with codes 493.0-493.2, 493.9:
0 unspecified
1 with status asthmaticus
2 with (acute) exacerbation

AHA: 4Q, '04, 137; 4Q, '03, 62; 4Q, '01, 43; 4Q, '00, 42; 1Q, '91, 13; 3Q, '88, 9; J-A, '85, 8; N-D, '84, 17

DEF: Status asthmaticus: Severe, intractable episode of asthma unresponsive to normal therapeutic measures.

✓5th **493.0 Extrinsic asthma**
Asthma:
allergic with stated cause
atopic
childhood
Asthma:
hay
platinum
Hay fever with asthma
EXCLUDES *asthma:*
allergic NOS (493.9)
detergent (507.8)
miners' (500)
wood (495.8)

DEF: Transient stricture of airway diameters of bronchi; due to environmental factor; also called allergic (bronchial) asthma.

✓5th **493.1 Intrinsic asthma**
Late-onset asthma
AHA: 3Q, '88, 9; M-A, '85, 7

DEF: Transient stricture, of airway diameters of bronchi; due to pathophysiological disturbances.

✓5th **493.2 Chronic obstructive asthma**
Asthma with chronic obstructive pulmonary disease [COPD]
Chronic asthmatic bronchitis
EXCLUDES *acute bronchitis (466.0)*
chronic obstructive bronchitis (491.20-491.22)
AHA: 4Q, '03, 108; 2Q, '91, 21; 2Q, '90, 20

DEF: Persistent narrowing of airway diameters in the bronchial tree, restricting airflow and causing constant labored breathing.

✓5th **493.8 Other forms of asthma**
AHA: 4Q, '03, 62

493.81 Exercise induced bronchospasm
493.82 Cough variant asthma

✓5th **493.9 Asthma, unspecified**
Asthma (bronchial) (allergic NOS)
Bronchitis:
allergic
asthmatic
AHA: 4Q, '97, 40; **For code 493.90:** 4Q, '04, 137; 4Q, '03, 108; 4Q, '99, 25; 1Q, '97, 7; **For code 493.91:** ▶1Q, '05, 5;◀ **For code 493.92:** 1Q, '03, 9

✓4th **494 Bronchiectasis**
Bronchiectasis (fusiform) (postinfectious) (recurrent)
Bronchiolectasis
EXCLUDES *congenital (748.61)*
tuberculous bronchiectasis (current disease) (011.5)
AHA: 4Q, '00, 42

DEF: Dilation of bronchi; due to infection or chronic conditions; causes decreased lung capacity and recurrent infections of lungs.

494.0 Bronchiectasis without acute exacerbation
494.1 Bronchiectasis with acute exacerbation

✓4th **495 Extrinsic allergic alveolitis**

INCLUDES allergic alveolitis and pneumonitis due to inhaled organic dust particles of fungal, thermophilic actinomycete, or other origin

DEF: Pneumonitis due to particles inhaled into lung, often at workplace; symptoms include cough, chills, fever, increased heart and respiratory rates; develops within hours of exposure.

495.0 Farmers' lung

495.1 Bagassosis

495.2 Bird-fanciers' lung
Budgerigar-fanciers' disease or lung
Pigeon-fanciers' disease or lung

495.3 Suberosis
Cork-handlers' disease or lung

495.4 Malt workers' lung
Alveolitis due to Aspergillus clavatus

495.5 Mushroom workers' lung

495.6 Maple bark-strippers' lung
Alveolitis due to Cryptostroma corticale

495.7 "Ventilation" pneumonitis
Allergic alveolitis due to fungal, thermophilic actinomycete, and other organisms growing in ventilation [air conditioning] systems

495.8 Other specified allergic alveolitis and pneumonitis
Cheese-washers' lung
Coffee workers' lung
Fish-meal workers' lung
Furriers' lung
Grain-handlers' disease or lung
Pituitary snuff-takers' disease
Sequoiosis or red-cedar asthma
Wood asthma

495.9 Unspecified allergic alveolitis and pneumonitis
Alveolitis, allergic (extrinsic)
Hypersensitivity pneumonitis

496 Chronic airway obstruction, not elsewhere classified

Note: This code is not to be used with any code from categories 491-493

Chronic:
nonspecific lung disease
obstructive lung disease
obstructive pulmonary disease [COPD] NOS

EXCLUDES *chronic obstructive lung disease [COPD] specified (as) (with):*
allergic alveolitis (495.0-495.9)
asthma (493.20-493.22)
bronchiectasis (494.0-494.1)
bronchitis (491.20-491.22)
with emphysema (491.20-491.22)
emphysema (492.0-492.8)

AHA: 4Q, '03, 109; 2Q, '00, 15; 2Q, '92, 16; 2Q, '91, 21; 3Q, '88, 56

PNEUMOCONIOSES AND OTHER LUNG DISEASES DUE TO EXTERNAL AGENTS (500-508)

DEF: Permanent deposits of particulate matter, within lungs; due to occupational or environmental exposure; results in chronic induration and fibrosis. (See specific listings in 500-508 code range)

500 Coal workers' pneumoconiosis A
Anthracosilicosis
Anthracosis
Black lung disease
Coal workers' lung
Miner's asthma

501 Asbestosis A

502 Pneumoconiosis due to other silica or silicates
Pneumoconiosis due to talc
Silicotic fibrosis (massive) of lung
Silicosis (simple) (complicated)

503 Pneumoconiosis due to other inorganic dust
Aluminosis (of lung)
Bauxite fibrosis (of lung)
Berylliosis
Graphite fibrosis (of lung)
Siderosis
Stannosis

504 Pneumonopathy due to inhalation of other dust
Byssinosis
Cannabinosis
Flax-dressers' disease

EXCLUDES *allergic alveolitis (495.0-495.9)*
asbestosis (501)
bagassosis (495.1)
farmers' lung (495.0)

505 Pneumoconiosis, unspecified

✓4th **506 Respiratory conditions due to chemical fumes and vapors**
Use additional E code to identify cause

506.0 Bronchitis and pneumonitis due to fumes and vapors
Chemical bronchitis (acute)

506.1 Acute pulmonary edema due to fumes and vapors
Chemical pulmonary edema (acute)

EXCLUDES *acute pulmonary edema NOS (518.4)*
chronic or unspecified pulmonary edema (514)

AHA: 3Q, '88, 4

506.2 Upper respiratory inflammation due to fumes and vapors

506.3 Other acute and subacute respiratory conditions due to fumes and vapors

506.4 Chronic respiratory conditions due to fumes and vapors
Emphysema (diffuse) (chronic) } due to inhalation of chemical fumes and vapors
Obliterative bronchiolitis (chronic) (subacute) } due to inhalation of chemical fumes and vapors
Pulmonary fibrosis (chronic) } due to inhalation of chemical fumes and vapors

506.9 Unspecified respiratory conditions due to fumes and vapors
Silo-fillers' disease

✓4th **507 Pneumonitis due to solids and liquids**

EXCLUDES *fetal aspiration pneumonitis* ▶*(770.18)*◀

AHA: 3Q, '91, 16

507.0 Due to inhalation of food or vomitus
Aspiration pneumonia (due to):
NOS
food (regurgitated)
gastric secretions
milk
saliva
vomitus

AHA: 1Q, '89, 10

507.1 Due to inhalation of oils and essences
Lipoid pneumonia (exogenous)

EXCLUDES *endogenous lipoid pneumonia (516.8)*

507.8 Due to other solids and liquids
Detergent asthma

✓4th **508 Respiratory conditions due to other and unspecified external agents**
Use additional E code to identify cause

508.0 Acute pulmonary manifestations due to radiation
Radiation pneumonitis

AHA: 2Q, '88, 4

508.1 Chronic and other pulmonary manifestations due to radiation
Fibrosis of lung following radiation

508.8 Respiratory conditions due to other specified external agents

508.9 Respiratory conditions due to unspecified external agent

OTHER DISEASES OF RESPIRATORY SYSTEM (510-519)

✓4th **510 Empyema**
Use additional code to identify infectious organism (041.0-041.9)

EXCLUDES *abscess of lung (513.0)*

DEF: Purulent infection, within pleural space.

510.0 With fistula

Fistula:
- bronchocutaneous
- bronchopleural
- hepatopleural

Fistula:
- mediastinal
- pleural
- thoracic

Any condition classifiable to 510.9 with fistula

DEF: Purulent infection of respiratory cavity; with communication from cavity to another structure.

510.9 Without mention of fistula

Abscess:
- pleura
- thorax

Empyema (chest) (lung) (pleura)
Fibrinopurulent pleurisy
Pleurisy:
- purulent

Pleurisy:
- septic
- seropurulent
- suppurative

Pyopneumothorax
Pyothorax

AHA: 3Q, '94, 6

✓4th **511 Pleurisy**

EXCLUDES *malignant pleural effusion (197.2)*
pleurisy with mention of tuberculosis, current disease (012.0)

DEF: Inflammation of serous membrane of lungs and lining of thoracic cavity; causes exudation in cavity or membrane surface.

511.0 Without mention of effusion or current tuberculosis

Adhesion, lung or pleura
Calcification of pleura
Pleurisy (acute) (sterile):
- diaphragmatic
- fibrinous
- interlobar

Pleurisy:
- NOS
- pneumococcal
- staphylococcal
- streptococcal

Thickening of pleura

AHA: 3Q, '94, 5

511.1 With effusion, with mention of a bacterial cause other than tuberculosis

Pleurisy with effusion (exudative) (serous):
- pneumococcal
- staphylococcal
- streptococcal
- other specified nontuberculous bacterial cause

511.8 Other specified forms of effusion, except tuberculous

Encysted pleurisy
Hemopneumothorax
Hemothorax
Hydropneumothorax
Hydrothorax

EXCLUDES *traumatic (860.2-860.5, 862.29, 862.39)*

AHA: 1Q, '97, 10

511.9 Unspecified pleural effusion

Pleural effusion NOS
Pleurisy:
- exudative
- serofibrinous

Pleurisy:
- serous
- with effusion NOS

AHA: 2Q, '03, 7; 3Q, '91, 19; 4Q, '89, 11

✓4th **512 Pneumothorax**

DEF: Collapsed lung; due to gas or air in pleural space.

512.0 Spontaneous tension pneumothorax

AHA: 3Q, '94, 5

DEF: Leaking air from lung into lining causing collapse.

512.1 Iatrogenic pneumothorax

Postoperative pneumothorax

AHA: 4Q, '94, 40

DEF: Air trapped in the lining of the lung following surgery.

512.8 Other spontaneous pneumothorax

Pneumothorax:
- NOS
- acute

Pneumothorax:
- chronic

EXCLUDES *pneumothorax:*
- *congenital (770.2)*
- *traumatic (860.0-860.1, 860.4-860.5)*
- *tuberculous, current disease (011.7)*

AHA: 2Q, '93, 3

✓4th **513 Abscess of lung and mediastinum**

513.0 Abscess of lung

Abscess (multiple) of lung
Gangrenous or necrotic pneumonia
Pulmonary gangrene or necrosis

AHA: 2Q, '98, 7

513.1 Abscess of mediastinum

514 Pulmonary congestion and hypostasis

Hypostatic:
- bronchopneumonia
- pneumonia

Passive pneumonia
Pulmonary congestion (chronic) (passive)

Pulmonary edema:
- NOS
- chronic

EXCLUDES *acute pulmonary edema:*
- *NOS (518.4)*
- *with mention of heart disease or failure (428.1)*

AHA: 2Q, '98, 6; 3Q, '88, 5

DEF: Excessive retention of interstitial fluid in the lungs and pulmonary vessels; due to poor circulation.

515 Postinflammatory pulmonary fibrosis

Cirrhosis of lung
Fibrosis of lung (atrophic) (confluent) (massive) (perialveolar) (peribronchial)
Induration of lung
} chronic or unspecified

DEF: Fibrosis and scarring of the lungs due to inflammatory reaction.

✓4th **516 Other alveolar and parietoalveolar pneumonopathy**

516.0 Pulmonary alveolar proteinosis

DEF: Reduced ventilation; due to proteinaceous deposits on alveoli; symptoms include dyspnea, cough, chest pain, weakness, weight loss, and hemoptysis.

516.1 Idiopathic pulmonary hemosiderosis

Essential brown induration of lung
Code first underlying disease (275.0)

DEF: Fibrosis of alveolar walls; marked by abnormal amounts hemosiderin in lungs; primarily affects children; symptoms include anemia, fluid in lungs, and blood in sputum; etiology unknown.

516.2 Pulmonary alveolar microlithiasis

DEF: Small calculi in pulmonary alveoli resembling sand-like particles on x-ray.

516.3 Idiopathic fibrosing alveolitis

Alveolar capillary block
Diffuse (idiopathic) (interstitial) pulmonary fibrosis
Hamman-Rich syndrome

516.8 Other specified alveolar and parietoalveolar pneumonopathies

Endogenous lipoid pneumonia
Interstitial pneumonia (desquamative) (lymphoid)

EXCLUDES *lipoid pneumonia, exogenous or unspecified (507.1)*

AHA: 1Q, '92, 12

516.9 Unspecified alveolar and parietoalveolar pneumonopathy

✓4th 517 Lung involvement in conditions classified elsewhere

EXCLUDES *rheumatoid lung (714.81)*

517.1 *Rheumatic pneumonia*
Code first underlying disease (390)

517.2 *Lung involvement in systemic sclerosis*
Code first underlying disease (710.1)

517.3 *Acute chest syndrome*
Code first sickle-cell disease in crisis (282.42, 282.62, 282.64, 282.69)

AHA: 4Q, '03, 51, 56

517.8 *Lung involvement in other diseases classified elsewhere*
Code first underlying disease, as:
amyloidosis (277.3)
polymyositis (710.4)
sarcoidosis (135)
Sjögren's disease (710.2)
systemic lupus erythematosus (710.0)

EXCLUDES *syphilis (095.1)*

AHA: 2Q, '03, 7

✓4th 518 Other diseases of lung

518.0 Pulmonary collapse
Atelectasis
Collapse of lung
Middle lobe syndrome

EXCLUDES *atelectasis:*
congenital (partial) (770.5)
primary (770.4)
tuberculous, current disease (011.8)

AHA: 4Q, '90, 25

518.1 Interstitial emphysema
Mediastinal emphysema

EXCLUDES *surgical (subcutaneous) emphysema (998.81)*
that in fetus or newborn (770.2)
traumatic emphysema (958.7)

DEF: Escaped air from the alveoli trapped in the interstices of the lung; trauma or cough may cause the disease.

518.2 Compensatory emphysema

DEF: Distention of all or part of the lung caused by disease processes or surgical intervention that decreased volume in another part of the lung; overcompensation reaction to the loss of capacity in another part of the lung.

518.3 Pulmonary eosinophilia
Eosinophilic asthma
Löffler's syndrome
Pneumonia:
allergic
Pneumonia:
eosinophilic
Tropical eosinophilia

DEF: Infiltration, into pulmonary parenchyma of eosinophilia; results in cough, fever, and dyspnea.

518.4 Acute edema of lung, unspecified
Acute pulmonary edema NOS
Pulmonary edema, postoperative

EXCLUDES *pulmonary edema:*
acute, with mention of heart disease or failure (428.1)
chronic or unspecified (514)
due to external agents (506.0-508.9)

DEF: Severe, sudden fluid retention within lung tissues.

518.5 Pulmonary insufficiency following trauma and surgery
Adult respiratory distress syndrome
Pulmonary insufficiency following:
shock
surgery
trauma
Shock lung

EXCLUDES *adult respiratory distress syndrome associated with other conditions (518.82)*
pneumonia:
aspiration (507.0)
hypostatic (514)
respiratory failure in other conditions (518.81, 518.83-518.84)

AHA: 4Q, '04, 139; 3Q, '88, 3; 3Q, '88, 7; S-O, '87, 1

518.6 Allergic bronchopulmonary aspergillosis

AHA: 4Q, '97, 39

DEF: Noninvasive hypersensitive reaction; due to allergic reaction to *Aspergillus fumigatus* (mold).

✓5th 518.8 Other diseases of lung

518.81 Acute respiratory failure
Respiratory failure NOS

EXCLUDES *acute and chronic respiratory failure (518.84)*
acute respiratory distress (518.82)
chronic respiratory failure (518.83)
respiratory arrest (799.1)
respiratory failure, newborn (770.84)

AHA: ►1Q, '05, 3-8;◄ 4Q, '04, 139; 1Q, '03, 15; 4Q, '98, 41; 3Q, '91, 14; 2Q, '91, 3; 4Q, '90, 25; 2Q, '90, 20; 3Q, '88, 7; 3Q, '88, 10; S-O, '87, 1

518.82 Other pulmonary insufficiency, not elsewhere classified
Acute respiratory distress
Acute respiratory insufficiency
Adult respiratory distress syndrome NEC

EXCLUDES *adult respiratory distress syndrome associated with trauma and surgery (518.5)*
pulmonary insufficiency following trauma and surgery (518.5)
respiratory distress:
NOS (786.09)
newborn (770.89)
syndrome, newborn (769)
shock lung (518.5)

AHA: 4Q, '03, 105; 2Q, '91, 21; 3Q, '88, 7

518.83 Chronic respiratory failure

AHA: 4Q, '03, 103, 111

518.84 Acute and chronic respiratory failure
Acute on chronic respiratory failure

518.89 Other diseases of lung, not elsewhere classified
Broncholithiasis
Calcification of lung
Lung disease NOS
Pulmolithiasis

AHA: 3Q, '90, 18; 4Q, '88, 6

DEF: Broncholithiasis: calculi in lumen of transbronchial tree.

DEF: Pulmolithiasis: calculi in lung.

✓4th **519 Other diseases of respiratory system**

✓5th **519.0 Tracheostomy complications**

519.00 Tracheostomy complication, unspecified

519.01 Infection of tracheostomy

Use additional code to identify type of infection, such as:
- abscess or cellulitis of neck (682.1)
- septicemia (038.0-038.9)

Use additional code to identify organism (041.00-041.9)

AHA: 4Q, '98, 41

519.02 Mechanical complication of tracheostomy

Tracheal stenosis due to tracheostomy

519.09 Other tracheostomy complications

Hemorrhage due to tracheostomy
Tracheoesophageal fistula due to tracheostomy

519.1 Other diseases of trachea and bronchus, not elsewhere classified

Calcification, Stenosis, Ulcer } of bronchus or trachea

AHA: 3Q, '02, 18; 3Q, '88, 6

519.2 Mediastinitis

DEF: Inflammation of tissue between organs behind sternum.

519.3 Other diseases of mediastinum, not elsewhere classified

Fibrosis, Hernia, Retraction } of mediastinum

519.4 Disorders of diaphragm

Diaphragmitis
Paralysis of diaphragm
Relaxation of diaphragm

EXCLUDES *congenital defect of diaphragm (756.6)*
diaphragmatic hernia (551-553 with .3)
congenital (756.6)

519.8 Other diseases of respiratory system, not elsewhere classified

AHA: 4Q, '89, 12

519.9 Unspecified disease of respiratory system

Respiratory disease (chronic) NOS

9. DISEASES OF THE DIGESTIVE SYSTEM (520-579)

DISEASES OF ORAL CAVITY, SALIVARY GLANDS, AND JAWS (520-529)

✓4th **520 Disorders of tooth development and eruption**

520.0 Anodontia
Absence of teeth (complete) (congenital) (partial)
Hypodontia
Oligodontia
EXCLUDES *acquired absence of teeth (525.10-525.19)*

520.1 Supernumerary teeth
Distomolar
Fourth molar
Mesiodens
Paramolar
Supplemental teeth
EXCLUDES *supernumerary roots (520.2)*

520.2 Abnormalities of size and form
Concrescence }
Fusion } of teeth
Gemination }

Dens evaginatus
Dens in dente
Dens invaginatus
Enamel pearls
Macrodontia
Microdontia
Peg-shaped [conical] teeth
Supernumerary roots
Taurodontism
Tuberculum paramolare
EXCLUDES *that due to congenital syphilis (090.5)*
tuberculum Carabelli, which is regarded as a normal variation

520.3 Mottled teeth
Dental fluorosis
Mottling of enamel
Nonfluoride enamel opacities

Digestive System

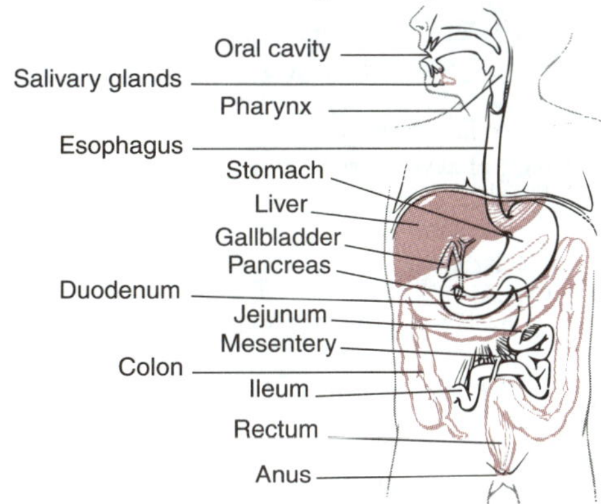

The Oral Cavity

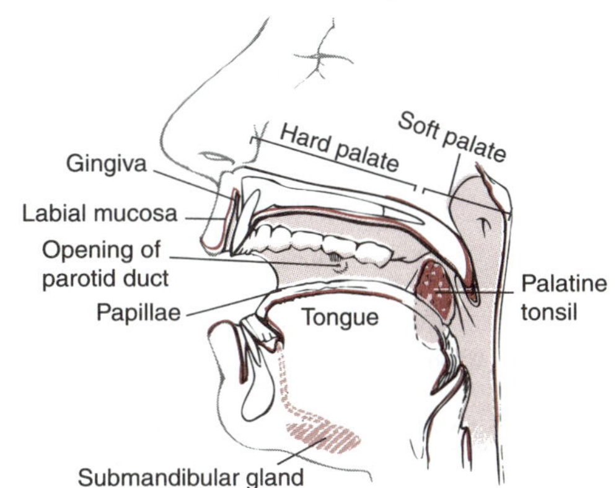

Teeth

Labial frenulum
Mucosa
Vestibule
Gingiva
Upper lip
Hard palate
Soft palate
Uvula
Tongue
Maxillary view

Enamel
Dentine
Gingiva (gum)
Root canal
Cementum
Section of molar

Uvula
Tongue
Gingiva
Lower lip
Mucosa
Frenulum
Vestibule
Mandibulary view

Enamel
Pulp cavity
Dentin
Alveolar bone
Mandible
Section of incisor

520.4 Disturbances of tooth formation
Aplasia and hypoplasia of cementum
Dilaceration of tooth
Enamel hypoplasia (neonatal) (postnatal) (prenatal)
Horner's teeth
Hypocalcification of teeth
Regional odontodysplasia
Turner's tooth
EXCLUDES *Hutchinson's teeth and mulberry molars in congenital syphilis (090.5)*
mottled teeth (520.3)

520.5 Hereditary disturbances in tooth structure, not elsewhere classified
Amelogenesis }
Dentinogenesis } imperfecta
Odontogenesis }

Dentinal dysplasia
Shell teeth

520.6 Disturbances in tooth eruption
Teeth:
- embedded
- impacted
- natal
- neonatal
- primary [deciduous]:
  - persistent
  - shedding, premature

Tooth eruption:
- late
- obstructed
- premature

EXCLUDES *exfoliation of teeth (attributable to disease of surrounding tissues) (525.0-525.19)*

520.7 Teething syndrome

520.8 Other specified disorders of tooth development and eruption
Color changes during tooth formation
Pre-eruptive color changes
EXCLUDES *posteruptive color changes (521.7)*

520.9 Unspecified disorder of tooth development and eruption

4th 521 Diseases of hard tissues of teeth

5th 521.0 Dental caries
AHA: 4Q, '01, 44

521.00 Dental caries, unspecified

521.01 Dental caries limited to enamel
Initial caries
White spot lesion

521.02 Dental caries extending into dentine

521.03 Dental caries extending into pulp

521.04 Arrested dental caries

521.05 Odontoclasia
Infantile melanodontia
Melanodontoclasia
EXCLUDES *internal and external resorption of teeth (521.40-521.49)*
DEF: A pathological dental condition described as stained areas, loss of tooth substance, and hypoplasia linked to nutritional deficiencies during tooth development and to cariogenic oral conditions; synonyms are melanodontoclasia and infantile melanodontia.

521.06 Dental caries pit and fissure

521.07 Dental caries of smooth surface

521.08 Dental caries of root surface

521.09 Other dental caries
AHA: 3Q, '02, 14

5th 521.1 Excessive attrition (approximal wear) (occlusal wear)

521.10 Excessive attrition, unspecified

521.11 Excessive attrition, limited to enamel

521.12 Excessive attrition, extending into dentine

521.13 Excessive attrition, extending into pulp

521.14 Excessive attrition, localized

521.15 Excessive attrition, generalized

5th 521.2 Abrasion
Abrasion:
- dentifrice
- habitual
- occupational
- ritual
- traditional

} of teeth

Wedge defect NOS

521.20 Abrasion, unspecified

521.21 Abrasion, limited to enamel

521.22 Abrasion, extending into dentine

521.23 Abrasion, extending into pulp

521.24 Abrasion, localized

521.25 Abrasion, generalized

5th 521.3 Erosion
Erosion of teeth:
- NOS
- due to:
  - medicine
  - persistent vomiting

Erosion of teeth:
- idiopathic
- occupational

521.30 Erosion, unspecified

521.31 Erosion, limited to enamel

521.32 Erosion, extending into dentine

521.33 Erosion, extending into pulp

521.34 Erosion, localized

521.35 Erosion, generalized

5th 521.4 Pathological resorption
DEF: Loss of dentin and cementum due to disease process.

521.40 Pathological resorption, unspecified

521.41 Pathological resorption, internal

521.42 Pathological resorption, external

521.49 Other pathological resorption
Internal granuloma of pulp

521.5 Hypercementosis
Cementation hyperplasia
DEF: Excess deposits of cementum, on tooth root.

521.6 Ankylosis of teeth
DEF: Adhesion of tooth to surrounding bone.

521.7 Intrinsic posteruptive color changes
Staining [discoloration] of teeth:
- NOS
- due to:
  - drugs
  - metals
  - pulpal bleeding

EXCLUDES *accretions [deposits] on teeth (523.6)*
extrinsic color changes (523.6)
pre-eruptive color changes (520.8)

521.8 Other specified diseases of hard tissues of teeth
Irradiated enamel
Sensitive dentin

521.9 Unspecified disease of hard tissues of teeth

4th 522 Diseases of pulp and periapical tissues

522.0 Pulpitis
Pulpal:
- abscess
- polyp

Pulpitis:
- acute

Pulpitis:
- chronic (hyperplastic) (ulcerative)
- suppurative

522.1 Necrosis of the pulp
Pulp gangrene
DEF: Death of pulp tissue.

522.2 Pulp degeneration
Denticles
Pulp calcifications
Pulp stones

522.3 Abnormal hard tissue formation in pulp
Secondary or irregular dentin

522.4 Acute apical periodontitis of pulpal origin
DEF: Severe inflammation of periodontal ligament due to pulpal inflammation or necrosis.

522.5 Periapical abscess without sinus
Abscess:
- dental

Abscess:
- dentoalveolar

EXCLUDES *periapical abscess with sinus (522.7)*

522.6 Chronic apical periodontitis
Apical or periapical granuloma
Apical periodontitis NOS

522.7 Periapical abscess with sinus
Fistula:
- alveolar process

Fistula:
- dental

522.8 Radicular cyst
Cyst:
- apical (periodontal)
- periapical

Cyst:
- radiculodental
- residual radicular

EXCLUDES *lateral developmental or lateral periodontal cyst (526.0)*
DEF: Cyst in tissue around tooth apex due to chronic infection of granuloma around root.

522.9 Other and unspecified diseases of pulp and periapical tissues

4th 523 Gingival and periodontal diseases

523.0 Acute gingivitis
EXCLUDES *acute necrotizing ulcerative gingivitis (101)*
herpetic gingivostomatitis (054.2)

523.1 Chronic gingivitis
Gingivitis (chronic):
- NOS
- desquamative
- hyperplastic

Gingivitis (chronic):
- simple marginal
- ulcerative

Gingivostomatitis
EXCLUDES *herpetic gingivostomatitis (054.2)*

5th 523.2 Gingival recession
Gingival recession (postinfective) (postoperative)

523.20 Gingival recession, unspecified

523.21 Gingival recession, minimal

523.22 Gingival recession, moderate

523.23 Gingival recession, severe

523.24 Gingival recession, localized

523.25 Gingival recession, generalized

523.3 Acute periodontitis

Acute:
- pericementitis
- pericoronitis

Paradontal abscess
Periodontal abscess

EXCLUDES *acute apical periodontitis (522.4)*
periapical abscess (522.5, 522.7)

DEF: Severe inflammation, of tissues supporting teeth.

523.4 Chronic periodontitis

Alveolar pyorrhea
Chronic pericoronitis
Pericementitis (chronic)
Periodontitis:
- NOS
- complex
- simplex

EXCLUDES *chronic apical periodontitis (522.6)*

523.5 Periodontosis

523.6 Accretions on teeth

Dental calculus:
- subgingival
- supragingival

Deposits on teeth:
- betel
- materia alba
- soft
- tartar
- tobacco

Extrinsic discoloration of teeth

EXCLUDES *intrinsic discoloration of teeth (521.7)*

DEF: Foreign material on tooth surface, usually plaque or calculus.

523.8 Other specified periodontal diseases

Giant cell:
- epulis
- peripheral granuloma

Gingival:
- cysts
- enlargement NOS
- fibromatosis

Gingival polyp
Periodontal lesions due to traumatic occlusion
Peripheral giant cell granuloma

EXCLUDES *leukoplakia of gingiva (528.6)*

523.9 Unspecified gingival and periodontal disease

AHA: 3Q,'02, 14

✓4th **524 Dentofacial anomalies, including malocclusion**

✓5th **524.0 Major anomalies of jaw size**

EXCLUDES *hemifacial atrophy or hypertrophy (754.0)*
unilateral condylar hyperplasia or hypoplasia of mandible (526.89)

524.00 Unspecified anomaly

DEF: Unspecified deformity of jaw size.

524.01 Maxillary hyperplasia

DEF: Overgrowth or overdevelopment of upper jaw bone.

524.02 Mandibular hyperplasia

DEF: Overgrowth or overdevelopment of lower jaw bone.

524.03 Maxillary hypoplasia

DEF: Incomplete or underdeveloped, upper jaw bone.

524.04 Mandibular hypoplasia

DEF: Incomplete or underdeveloped, lower jaw bone.

524.05 Macrogenia

DEF: Enlarged, jaw, especially chin; affects bone, soft tissue, or both.

524.06 Microgenia

DEF: Underdeveloped mandible, characterized by an extremely small chin.

524.07 Excessive tuberosity of jaw

524.09 Other specified anomaly

✓5th **524.1 Anomalies of relationship of jaw to cranial base**

524.10 Unspecified anomaly

Prognathism
Retrognathism

DEF: Prognathism: protrusion of lower jaw.

DEF: Retrognathism: jaw is located posteriorly to a normally positioned jaw; backward position of mandible.

524.11 Maxillary asymmetry

DEF: Absence of symmetry of maxilla.

524.12 Other jaw asymmetry

524.19 Other specified anomaly

✓5th **524.2 Anomalies of dental arch relationship**

EXCLUDES *hemifacial atrophy or hypertrophy (754.0)*
soft tissue impingement (524.81-524.82)
unilateral condylar hyperplasia or hypoplasia of mandible (526.89)

524.20 Unspecified anomaly of dental arch relationship

524.21 Angle's class I

Neutro-occlusion

524.22 Angle's class II

Disto-occlusion Division I
Disto-occlusion Division II

524.23 Angle's class III

Mesio-occlusion

524.24 Open anterior occlusal relationship

524.25 Open posterior occlusal relationship

524.26 Excessive horizontal overlap

524.27 Reverse articulation

Anterior articulation
Posterior articulation

524.28 Anomalies of interarch distance

Excessive interarch distance
Inadequate interarch distance

524.29 Other anomalies of dental arch relationship

✓5th **524.3 Anomalies of tooth position of fully erupted teeth**

EXCLUDES *impacted or embedded teeth with abnormal position of such teeth or adjacent teeth (520.6)*

524.30 Unspecified anomaly of tooth position

Diastema of teeth NOS
Displacement of teeth NOS
Transposition of teeth NOS

524.31 Crowding of teeth

524.32 Excessive spacing of teeth

524.33 Horizontal displacement of teeth

Tipping of teeth

524.34 Vertical displacement of teeth

Infraeruption of teeth
Supraeruption of teeth

524.35 Rotation of teeth

524.36 Insufficient interocclusal distance of teeth (ridge)

524.37 Excessive interocclusal distance of teeth

Loss of occlusal vertical dimension

524.39 Other anomalies of tooth position

▶Angle's Classification of Malocclusion◀

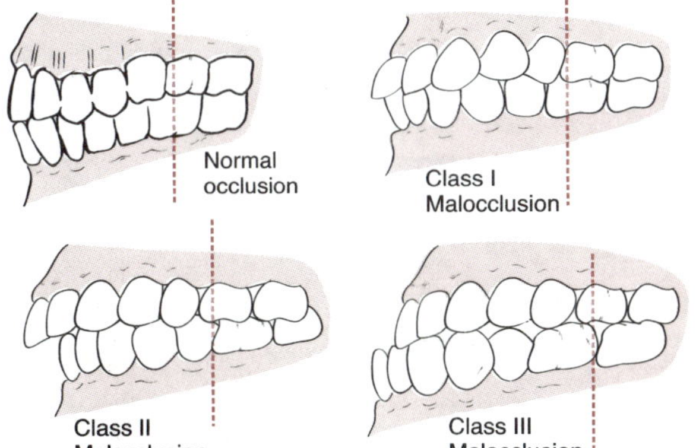

✓4th ✓5th Additional Digit Required — Unspecified Code — Other Specified Code — Manifestation Code — ▶◀ Revised Text — ● New Code — ▲ Revised Code Title

524.4 Malocclusion, unspecified
DEF: Malposition of top and bottom teeth; interferes with chewing.

✓5th **524.5 Dentofacial functional abnormalities**

524.50 Dentofacial functional abnormality, unspecified

524.51 Abnormal jaw closure

524.52 Limited mandibular range of motion

524.53 Deviation in opening and closing of the mandible

524.54 Insufficient anterior guidance

524.55 Centric occlusion maximum intercuspation discrepancy

524.56 Non-working side interference

524.57 Lack of posterior occlusal support

524.59 Other dentofacial functional abnormalities
Abnormal swallowing
Mouth breathing
Sleep postures
Tongue, lip, or finger habits

✓5th **524.6 Temporomandibular joint disorders**
EXCLUDES *current temporomandibular joint:*
dislocation (830.0-830.1)
strain (848.1)

524.60 Temporomandibular joint disorders, unspecified
Temporomandibular joint-pain-dysfunction syndrome [TMJ]

524.61 Adhesions and ankylosis (bony or fibrous)
DEF: Stiffening or union of temporomandibular joint due to bony or fibrous union across joint.

524.62 Arthralgia of temporomandibular joint
DEF: Pain in temporomandibular joint; not inflammatory in nature.

524.63 Articular disc disorder (reducing or non-reducing)

524.64 Temporomandibular joint sounds on opening and/or closing the jaw

524.69 Other specified temporomandibular joint disorders

✓5th **524.7 Dental alveolar anomalies**

524.70 Unspecified alveolar anomaly

524.71 Alveolar maxillary hyperplasia
DEF: Excessive tissue formation in the dental alveoli of upper jaw.

524.72 Alveolar mandibular hyperplasia
DEF: Excessive tissue formation in the dental alveoli of lower jaw.

524.73 Alveolar maxillary hypoplasia
DEF: Incomplete or underdeveloped, alveolar tissue of upper jaw.

524.74 Alveolar mandibular hypoplasia
DEF: Incomplete or underdeveloped, alveolar tissue of lower jaw.

524.75 Vertical displacement of alveolus and teeth
Extrusion of alveolus and teeth

524.76 Occlusal plane deviation

524.79 Other specified alveolar anomaly

✓5th **524.8 Other specified dentofacial anomalies**

524.81 Anterior soft tissue impingement

524.82 Posterior soft tissue impingement

524.89 Other specified dentofacial anomalies

524.9 Unspecified dentofacial anomalies

✓4th **525 Other diseases and conditions of the teeth and supporting structures**

525.0 Exfoliation of teeth due to systemic causes
DEF: Deterioration of teeth and surrounding structures due to systemic disease.

✓5th **525.1 Loss of teeth due to trauma, extraction, or periodontal disease**
▶Code first class of edentulism (525.40-525.44, 525.50-525.54)◀
AHA: 4Q, '01, 44

525.10 Acquired absence of teeth, unspecified
Tooth extraction status, NOS

525.11 Loss of teeth due to trauma

525.12 Loss of teeth due to periodontal disease

525.13 Loss of teeth due to caries

525.19 Other loss of teeth

✓5th **525.2 Atrophy of edentulous alveolar ridge**

525.20 Unspecified atrophy of edentulous alveolar ridge
Atrophy of the mandible NOS
Atrophy of the maxilla NOS

525.21 Minimal atrophy of the mandible

525.22 Moderate atrophy of the mandible

525.23 Severe atrophy of the mandible

525.24 Minimal atrophy of the maxilla

525.25 Moderate atrophy of the maxilla

525.26 Severe atrophy of the maxilla

525.3 Retained dental root

● ✓5th **525.4 Complete edentulism**
Use additional code to identify cause of edentulism (525.10-525.19)

● **525.40 Complete edentulism, unspecified**
Edentulism NOS

● **525.41 Complete edentulism, class I**

● **525.42 Complete edentulism, class II**

● **525.43 Complete edentulism, class III**

● **525.44 Complete edentulism, class IV**

● ✓5th **525.5 Partial edentulism**
Use additional code to identify cause of edentulism (525.10-525.19)

● **525.50 Partial edentulism, unspecified**

● **525.51 Partial edentulism, class I**

● **525.52 Partial edentulism, class II**

● **525.53 Partial edentulism, class III**

● **525.54 Partial edentulism, class IV**

525.8 Other specified disorders of the teeth and supporting structures
Enlargement of alveolar ridge NOS
Irregular alveolar process

525.9 Unspecified disorder of the teeth and supporting structures

✓4th **526 Diseases of the jaws**

526.0 Developmental odontogenic cysts
Cyst:
dentigerous
eruption
follicular
lateral developmental
Cyst:
lateral periodontal
primordial
Keratocyst
EXCLUDES *radicular cyst (522.8)*

526.1 Fissural cysts of jaw
Cyst:
globulomaxillary
incisor canal
median anterior maxillary
Cyst:
median palatal
nasopalatine
palatine of papilla
EXCLUDES *cysts of oral soft tissues (528.4)*

526.2 Other cysts of jaws
Cyst of jaw:
NOS
aneurysmal
Cyst of jaw:
hemorrhagic
traumatic

526.3 Central giant cell (reparative) granuloma
EXCLUDES *peripheral giant cell granuloma (523.8)*

N Newborn Age: 0 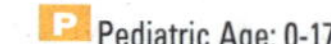 P Pediatric Age: 0-17 M Maternity Age: 12-55 A Adult Age: 15-124 MSP Medicare Secondary Payer

526.4 Inflammatory conditions

Abscess, Osteitis, Osteomyelitis (neonatal), Periostitis } of jaw (acute) (chronic) (suppurative)

Sequestrum of jaw bone

EXCLUDES *alveolar osteitis (526.5)*

526.5 Alveolitis of jaw

Alveolar osteitis
Dry socket

DEF: Inflammation, of alveoli or tooth socket.

✓5th **526.8 Other specified diseases of the jaws**

526.81 Exostosis of jaw

Torus mandibularis
Torus palatinus

DEF: Spur or bony outgrowth on the jaw.

526.89 Other

Cherubism, Fibrous dysplasia, Latent bone cyst, Osteoradionecrosis } of jaw(s)

Unilateral condylar hyperplasia or hypoplasia of mandible

526.9 Unspecified disease of the jaws

✓4th **527 Diseases of the salivary glands**

527.0 Atrophy

DEF: Wasting away, necrosis of salivary gland tissue.

527.1 Hypertrophy

DEF: Overgrowth or overdeveloped salivary gland tissue.

527.2 Sialoadenitis

Parotitis:
- NOS
- allergic
- toxic

Sialoangitis
Sialodochitis

EXCLUDES *epidemic or infectious parotitis (072.0-072.9)*
uveoparotid fever (135)

DEF: Inflammation of salivary gland.

527.3 Abscess

527.4 Fistula

EXCLUDES *congenital fistula of salivary gland (750.24)*

527.5 Sialolithiasis

Calculus, Stone } of salivary gland or duct

Sialodocholithiasis

527.6 Mucocele

Mucous:
- extravasation cyst of salivary gland
- retention cyst of salivary gland

Ranula

DEF: Dilated salivary gland cavity filled with mucous.

527.7 Disturbance of salivary secretion

Hyposecretion
Ptyalism
Sialorrhea
Xerostomia

527.8 Other specified diseases of the salivary glands

Benign lymphoepithelial lesion of salivary gland
Sialectasia
Sialosis
Stenosis, Stricture } of salivary duct

527.9 Unspecified disease of the salivary glands

✓4th **528 Diseases of the oral soft tissues, excluding lesions specific for gingiva and tongue**

528.0 Stomatitis

Stomatitis:
- NOS
- ulcerative

Vesicular stomatitis

EXCLUDES *stomatitis:*
- *acute necrotizing ulcerative (101)*
- *aphthous (528.2)*
- *gangrenous (528.1)*
- *herpetic (054.2)*
- *Vincent's (101)*

AHA: 2Q, '99, 9

DEF: Inflammation of oral mucosa; labial and buccal mucosa, tongue, plate, floor of the mouth, and gingivae.

528.1 Cancrum oris

Gangrenous stomatitis
Noma

DEF: A severely gangrenous lesion of mouth due to fusospirochetal infection; destroys buccal, labial and facial tissues; can be fatal; found primarily in debilitated and malnourished children.

528.2 Oral aphthae

Aphthous stomatitis
Canker sore
Periadenitis mucosa necrotica recurrens
Recurrent aphthous ulcer
Stomatitis herpetiformis

EXCLUDES *herpetic stomatitis (054.2)*

DEF: Small oval or round ulcers of the mouth marked by a grayish exudate and a red halo effect.

528.3 Cellulitis and abscess

Cellulitis of mouth (floor)
Ludwig's angina
Oral fistula

EXCLUDES *abscess of tongue (529.0)*
cellulitis or abscess of lip (528.5)
fistula (of):
- *dental (522.7)*
- *lip (528.5)*

gingivitis (523.0-523.1)

528.4 Cysts

Dermoid cyst, Epidermoid cyst, Epstein's pearl, Lymphoepithelial cyst, Nasoalveolar cyst, Nasolabial cyst } of mouth

EXCLUDES *cyst:*
- *gingiva (523.8)*
- *tongue (529.8)*

528.5 Diseases of lips

Abscess, Cellulitis, Fistula, Hypertrophy } of lip(s)

Cheilitis:
- NOS
- angular

Cheilodynia
Cheilosis

EXCLUDES *actinic cheilitis (692.79)*
congenital fistula of lip (750.25)
leukoplakia of lips (528.6)

AHA: S-O, '86, 10

528.6 Leukoplakia of oral mucosa, including tongue

Leukokeratosis of oral mucosa
Leukoplakia of:
- gingiva

Leukoplakia of:
- lips
- tongue

EXCLUDES *carcinoma in situ (230.0, 232.0)*
leukokeratosis nicotina palati (528.79)

DEF: Thickened white patches of epithelium on mucous membranes of mouth.

Digestive System 526.4–528.6

✓5th **528.7 Other disturbances of oral epithelium, including tongue**

EXCLUDES *carcinoma in situ (230.0, 232.0)*
leukokeratosis NOS (702)

528.71 Minimal keratinized residual ridge mucosa

528.72 Excessive keratinized residual ridge mucosa

528.79 Other disturbances of oral epithelium, including tongue
Erythroplakia of mouth or tongue
Focal epithelial hyperplasia of mouth or tongue
Leukoedema of mouth or tongue
Leukokeratosis nicotina palate

528.8 Oral submucosal fibrosis, including of tongue

528.9 Other and unspecified diseases of the oral soft tissues
Cheek and lip biting
Denture sore mouth
Denture stomatitis
Melanoplakia
Papillary hyperplasia of palate
Eosinophilic granuloma, Irritative hyperplasia, Pyogenic granuloma, Ulcer (traumatic) } of oral mucosa

✓4th **529 Diseases and other conditions of the tongue**

529.0 Glossitis
Abscess, Ulceration (traumatic) } of tongue

EXCLUDES *glossitis:*
benign migratory (529.1)
Hunter's (529.4)
median rhomboid (529.2)
Moeller's (529.4)

529.1 Geographic tongue
Benign migratory glossitis
Glossitis areata exfoliativa
DEF: Chronic glossitis; marked by filiform papillae atrophy and inflammation; no known etiology.

529.2 Median rhomboid glossitis
DEF: A noninflammatory, congenital disease characterized by rhomboid-like lesions at the middle third of the tongue's dorsal surface.

529.3 Hypertrophy of tongue papillae
Black hairy tongue
Coated tongue
Hypertrophy of foliate papillae
Lingua villosa nigra

529.4 Atrophy of tongue papillae
Bald tongue
Glazed tongue
Glossitis:
Hunter's
Glossitis:
Moeller's
Glossodynia exfoliativa
Smooth atrophic tongue

529.5 Plicated tongue
Fissured, Furrowed, Scrotal } tongue

EXCLUDES *fissure of tongue, congenital (750.13)*

DEF: Cracks, fissures or furrows, on dorsal surface of tongue.

529.6 Glossodynia
Glossopyrosis
Painful tongue

EXCLUDES *glossodynia exfoliativa (529.4)*

529.8 Other specified conditions of the tongue
Atrophy, Crenated, Enlargement, Hypertrophy } (of) tongue
Glossocele
Glossoptosis

EXCLUDES *erythroplasia of tongue (528.79)*
leukoplakia of tongue (528.6)
macroglossia (congenital) (750.15)
microglossia (congenital) (750.16)
oral submucosal fibrosis (528.8)

529.9 Unspecified condition of the tongue

DISEASES OF ESOPHAGUS, STOMACH, AND DUODENUM (530-537)

✓4th **530 Diseases of esophagus**

EXCLUDES *esophageal varices (456.0-456.2)*

530.0 Achalasia and cardiospasm
Achalasia (of cardia)
Megaesophagus
Aperistalsis of esophagus

EXCLUDES *congenital cardiospasm (750.7)*

DEF: Failure of smooth muscle fibers to relax, at gastrointestinal junctures; such as esophagogastric sphincter when swallowing.

✓5th **530.1 Esophagitis**
Abscess of esophagus
Esophagitis:
NOS
chemical
Esophagitis:
peptic
postoperative
regurgitant
Use additional E code to identify cause, if induced by chemical

EXCLUDES *tuberculous esophagitis (017.8)*

AHA: 4Q, '93, 27; 1Q, '92, 17; 3Q, '91, 20

530.10 Esophagitis, unspecified

530.11 Reflux esophagitis
AHA: 4Q, '95, 82
DEF: Inflammation of lower esophagus; due to regurgitated gastric acid from malfunctioning lower esophageal sphincter; causes heartburn and substernal pain.

530.12 Acute esophagitis
AHA: 4Q, '01, 45
DEF: An acute inflammation of the mucous lining or submucosal coat of the esophagus.

530.19 Other esophagitis
AHA: 3Q, '01, 10

✓5th **530.2 Ulcer of esophagus**
Ulcer of esophagus
fungal
peptic
Ulcer of esophagus due to ingestion of:
aspirin
chemicals
medicines
Use additional E code to identify cause, if induced by chemical or drug

AHA: 4Q, '03, 63

530.20 Ulcer of esophagus without bleeding
Ulcer of esophagus NOS

530.21 Ulcer of esophagus with bleeding
EXCLUDES *bleeding esophageal varices (456.0, 456.20)*

530.3 Stricture and stenosis of esophagus
Compression of esophagus
Obstruction of esophagus

EXCLUDES *congenital stricture of esophagus (750.3)*

AHA: 2Q, '01, 4; 2Q, '97, 3; 1Q, '88, 13

530.4 Perforation of esophagus
Rupture of esophagus

EXCLUDES *traumatic perforation of esophagus (862.22, 862.32, 874.4-874.5)*

Esophagus

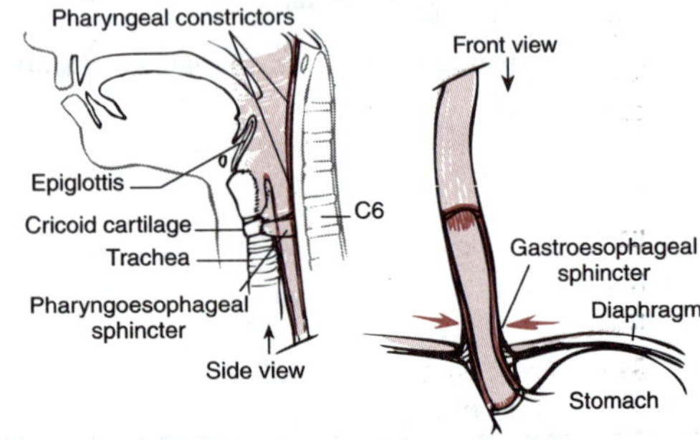

530.5 Dyskinesia of esophagus
Corkscrew esophagus
Curling esophagus
Esophagospasm
Spasm of esophagus
EXCLUDES *cardiospasm (530.0)*
AHA: 1Q, '88, 13; N-D, '84, 19
DEF: Difficulty performing voluntary esophageal movements.

530.6 Diverticulum of esophagus, acquired
Diverticulum, acquired:
epiphrenic
pharyngoesophageal
pulsion
subdiaphragmatic
traction
Zenker's (hypopharyngeal)
Esophageal pouch, acquired
Esophagocele, acquired
EXCLUDES *congenital diverticulum of esophagus (750.4)*
AHA: J-F, '85, 3

530.7 Gastroesophageal laceration-hemorrhage syndrome
Mallory-Weiss syndrome
DEF: Laceration of distal esophagus and proximal stomach due to vomiting, hiccups or other sustained activity.

✓5th **530.8 Other specified disorders of esophagus**

530.81 Esophageal reflux
Gastroesophageal reflux
EXCLUDES *reflux esophagitis (530.11)*
AHA: 2Q, '01, 4; 1Q, '95, 7; 4Q, '92, 27
DEF: Regurgitation of the gastric contents into esophagus and possibly pharynx; where aspiration may occur between the vocal cords and down into the trachea.

530.82 Esophageal hemorrhage
EXCLUDES *hemorrhage due to esophageal varices (456.0-456.2)*
AHA: ▶1Q, '05, 17◀

530.83 Esophageal leukoplakia

530.84 Tracheoesophageal fistula
EXCLUDES *congenital tracheoesophageal fistula (750.3)*

530.85 Barrett's esophagus
AHA: 4Q, '03, 63
DEF: A metaplastic disorder in which specialized columnar epithelial cells replace the normal squamous epithelial cells; an acquired condition secondary to chronic gastroesophageal reflux damage to the mucosa; associated with increased risk of developing adenocarcinoma.

530.86 Infection of esophagostomy
Use additional code to specify infection

530.87 Mechanical complication of esophagostomy
Malfunction of esophagostomy

530.89 Other
EXCLUDES *Paterson-Kelly syndrome (280.8)*

530.9 Unspecified disorder of esophagus

✓4th **531 Gastric ulcer**
INCLUDES ulcer (peptic):
prepyloric
pylorus
stomach
Use additional E code to identify drug, if drug-induced
EXCLUDES *peptic ulcer NOS (533.0-533.9)*

The following fifth-digit subclassification is for use with category 531:
0 without mention of obstruction
1 with obstruction

AHA: 1Q, '91, 15; 4Q, '90, 27
DEF: Destruction of tissue in lumen of stomach due to action of gastric acid and pepsin on gastric mucosa decreasing resistance to ulcers.

✓5th **531.0 Acute with hemorrhage**
AHA: N-D, '84, 15

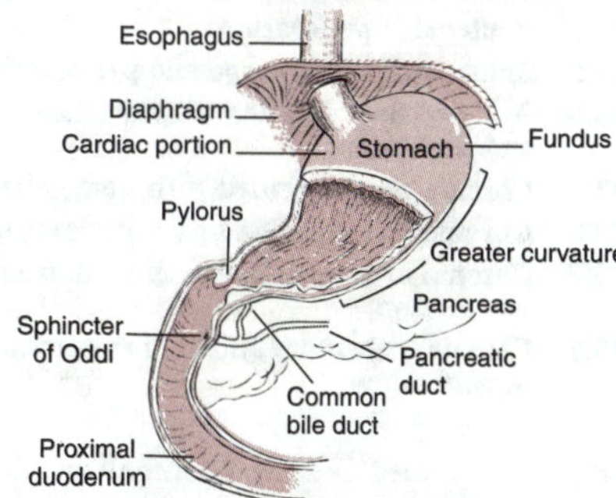

✓5th **531.1 Acute with perforation**
✓5th **531.2 Acute with hemorrhage and perforation**
✓5th **531.3 Acute without mention of hemorrhage or perforation**
✓5th **531.4 Chronic or unspecified with hemorrhage**
AHA: 4Q, '90, 22
✓5th **531.5 Chronic or unspecified with perforation**
✓5th **531.6 Chronic or unspecified with hemorrhage and perforation**
✓5th **531.7 Chronic without mention of hemorrhage or perforation**
✓5th **531.9 Unspecified as acute or chronic, without mention of hemorrhage or perforation**

✓4th **532 Duodenal ulcer**
INCLUDES erosion (acute) of duodenum
ulcer (peptic):
duodenum
postpyloric
Use additional E code to identify drug, if drug-induced
EXCLUDES *peptic ulcer NOS (533.0-533.9)*

The following fifth-digit subclassification is for use with category 532:
0 without mention of obstruction
1 with obstruction

AHA: 4Q, '90, 27, 1Q, '91, 15
DEF: Ulcers in duodenum due to action of gastric acid and pepsin on mucosa decreasing resistance to ulcers.

✓5th **532.0 Acute with hemorrhage**
AHA: 4Q, '90, 22
✓5th **532.1 Acute with perforation**
✓5th **532.2 Acute with hemorrhage and perforation**
✓5th **532.3 Acute without mention of hemorrhage or perforation**
✓5th **532.4 Chronic or unspecified with hemorrhage**
✓5th **532.5 Chronic or unspecified with perforation**
✓5th **532.6 Chronic or unspecified with hemorrhage and perforation**
✓5th **532.7 Chronic without mention of hemorrhage or perforation**
✓5th **532.9 Unspecified as acute or chronic, without mention of hemorrhage or perforation**

✓4th **533 Peptic ulcer, site unspecified**
INCLUDES gastroduodenal ulcer NOS
peptic ulcer NOS
stress ulcer NOS
Use additional E code to identify drug, if drug-induced
EXCLUDES *peptic ulcer:*
duodenal (532.0-532.9)
gastric (531.0-531.9)

The following fifth-digit subclassification is for use with category 533:
0 without mention of obstruction
1 with obstruction

AHA: 1Q, '91, 15; 4Q, '90, 27

§ ✓5th **533.0 Acute with hemorrhage**

§ ✓5th **533.1 Acute with perforation**

§ ✓5th **533.2 Acute with hemorrhage and perforation**

§ ✓5th **533.3 Acute without mention of hemorrhage and perforation**

§ ✓5th **533.4 Chronic or unspecified with hemorrhage**

§ ✓5th **533.5 Chronic or unspecified with perforation**

§ ✓5th **533.6 Chronic or unspecified with hemorrhage and perforation**

§ ✓5th **533.7 Chronic without mention of hemorrhage or perforation**
AHA: 2Q, '89, 16

§ ✓5th **533.9 Unspecified as acute or chronic, without mention of hemorrhage or perforation**

✓4th **534 Gastrojejunal ulcer**

INCLUDES ulcer (peptic) or erosion:
anastomotic
gastrocolic
gastrointestinal
gastrojejunal
jejunal
marginal
stomal

EXCLUDES *primary ulcer of small intestine (569.82)*

The following fifth-digit subclassification is for use with category 534:
0 without mention of obstruction
1 with obstruction

AHA: 1Q, '91, 15; 4Q, '90, 27

✓5th **534.0 Acute with hemorrhage**

✓5th **534.1 Acute with perforation**

✓5th **534.2 Acute with hemorrhage and perforation**

✓5th **534.3 Acute without mention of hemorrhage or perforation**

✓5th **534.4 Chronic or unspecified with hemorrhage**

✓5th **534.5 Chronic or unspecified with perforation**

✓5th **534.6 Chronic or unspecified with hemorrhage and perforation**

✓5th **534.7 Chronic without mention of hemorrhage or perforation**

✓5th **534.9 Unspecified as acute or chronic, without mention of hemorrhage or perforation**

✓4th **535 Gastritis and duodenitis**

The following fifth-digit subclassification is for use with category 535:
0 without mention of hemorrhage
1 with hemorrhage

AHA: 2Q, '92, 9; 4Q, '91, 25

✓5th **535.0 Acute gastritis**
AHA: 2Q, '92, 8; N-D, '86, 9

✓5th **535.1 Atrophic gastritis**
Gastritis:
atrophic-hyperplastic
Gastritis:
chronic (atrophic)
AHA: 1Q, '94, 18
DEF: Inflammation of stomach, with mucous membrane atrophy and peptic gland destruction.

✓5th **535.2 Gastric mucosal hypertrophy**
Hypertrophic gastritis

✓5th **535.3 Alcoholic gastritis**

✓5th **535.4 Other specified gastritis**
Gastritis:
allergic
bile induced
irritant
Gastritis:
superficial
toxic
AHA: 4Q, '90, 27

✓5th **535.5 Unspecified gastritis and gastroduodenitis**
AHA: For code 535.50: 4Q, '99, 25

✓5th **535.6 Duodenitis**
DEF: Inflammation of intestine, between pylorus and jejunum.

✓4th **536 Disorders of function of stomach**

EXCLUDES *functional disorders of stomach specified as psychogenic (306.4)*

536.0 Achlorhydria
DEF: Absence of gastric acid due to gastric mucosa atrophy; unresponsive to histamines; also known as gastric anacidity.

536.1 Acute dilatation of stomach
Acute distention of stomach

536.2 Persistent vomiting
Habit vomiting
Persistent vomiting [not of pregnancy]
Uncontrollable vomiting

EXCLUDES *excessive vomiting in pregnancy (643.0-643.9)*
vomiting NOS (787.0)

536.3 Gastroparesis
Gastroparalysis
AHA: ►2Q, '04, 7;◄ 2Q, '01, 4; 4Q, '94, 42
DEF: Slight degree of paralysis within muscular coat of stomach.

✓5th **536.4 Gastrostomy complications**
AHA: 4Q, '98, 42

536.40 Gastrostomy complication, unspecified

536.41 Infection of gastrostomy
Use additional code to specify type of infection, such as:
abscess or cellulitis of abdomen (682.2)
septicemia (038.0-038.9)
Use additional code to identify organism (041.00-041.9)
AHA: 4Q, '98, 42

536.42 Mechanical complication of gastrostomy

536.49 Other gastrostomy complications
AHA: 4Q, '98, 42

536.8 Dyspepsia and other specified disorders of function of stomach
Achylia gastrica
Hourglass contraction of stomach
Hyperacidity
Hyperchlorhydria
Hypochlorhydria
Indigestion

EXCLUDES *achlorhydria (536.0)*
heartburn (787.1)

AHA: 2Q, '93, 6; 2Q, '89, 16; N-D, '84, 9

536.9 Unspecified functional disorder of stomach
Functional gastrointestinal:
disorder
disturbance
irritation

✓4th **537 Other disorders of stomach and duodenum**

537.0 Acquired hypertrophic pyloric stenosis
Constriction
Obstruction
Stricture
} of pylorus, acquired or adult

EXCLUDES *congenital or infantile pyloric stenosis (750.5)*

AHA: 2Q, '01, 4; J-F, '85, 14

Duodenum

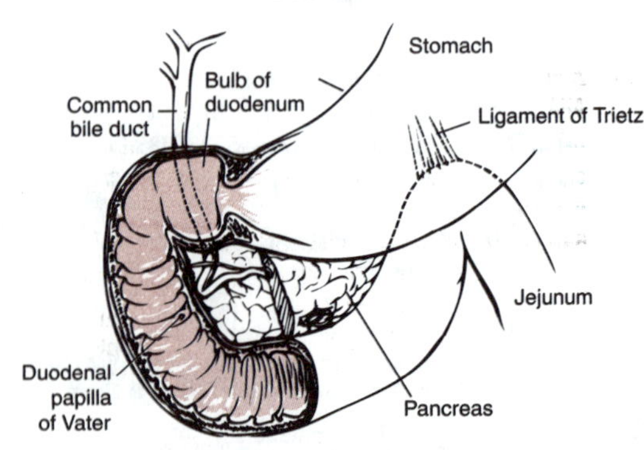

§ Requires fifth-digit. See category 533 for codes and definitions.

537.1 Gastric diverticulum

EXCLUDES *congenital diverticulum of stomach (750.7)*

AHA: J-F, '85, 4

DEF: Herniated sac or pouch, within stomach or duodenum.

537.2 Chronic duodenal ileus

DEF: Persistent obstruction between pylorus and jejunum.

537.3 Other obstruction of duodenum

Cicatrix, Stenosis, Stricture, Volvulus } of duodenum

EXCLUDES *congenital obstruction of duodenum (751.1)*

537.4 Fistula of stomach or duodenum

Gastrocolic fistula
Gastrojejunocolic fistula

537.5 Gastroptosis

DEF: Downward displacement of stomach.

537.6 Hourglass stricture or stenosis of stomach

Cascade stomach

EXCLUDES *congenital hourglass stomach (750.7)*
hourglass contraction of stomach (536.8)

5th **537.8 Other specified disorders of stomach and duodenum**

AHA: 4Q, '91, 25

537.81 Pylorospasm

EXCLUDES *congenital pylorospasm (750.5)*

DEF: Spasm of the pyloric sphincter.

537.82 Angiodysplasia of stomach and duodenum (without mention of hemorrhage)

AHA: 3Q, '96, 10; 4Q, '90, 4

537.83 Angiodysplasia of stomach and duodenum with hemorrhage

DEF: Bleeding of stomach and duodenum due to vascular abnormalities.

537.84 Dieulafoy lesion (hemorrhagic) of stomach and duodenum

AHA: 4Q, '02, 60

DEF: An abnormally large and convoluted submucosal artery protruding through a defect in the mucosa in the stomach or intestines that can erode the epithelium causing hemorrhaging; also called Dieulafoy's vascular malformation.

537.89 Other

Gastric or duodenal:
- prolapse
- rupture

Intestinal metaplasia of gastric mucosa
Passive congestion of stomach

EXCLUDES *diverticula of duodenum (562.00-562.01)*
gastrointestinal hemorrhage (578.0-578.9)

AHA: N-D, '84, 7

537.9 Unspecified disorder of stomach and duodenum

APPENDICITIS (540-543)

4th **540 Acute appendicitis**

AHA: N-D, '84, 19

DEF: Inflammation of vermiform appendix due to fecal obstruction, neoplasm or foreign body of appendiceal lumen; causes infection, edema and infarction of appendiceal wall; may result in mural necrosis, and perforation.

540.0 With generalized peritonitis

Appendicitis (acute): fulminating, gangrenous, obstructive; Cecitis (acute) } with: perforation, peritonitis (generalized), rupture

Rupture of appendix

EXCLUDES *acute appendicitis with peritoneal abscess (540.1)*

Appendix

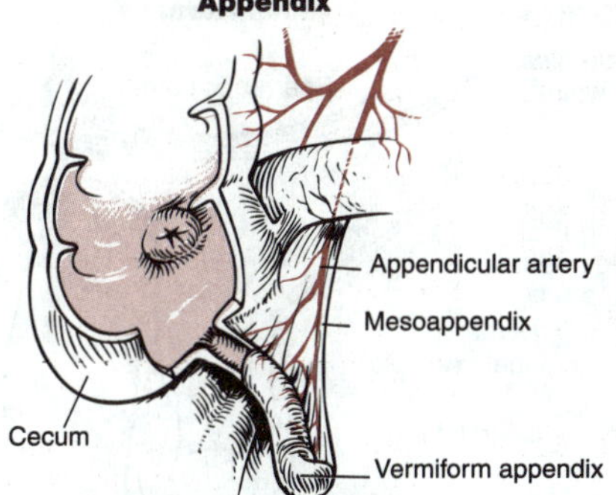

540.1 With peritoneal abscess

With generalized peritonitis
Abscess of appendix

AHA: N-D, '84, 19

540.9 Without mention of peritonitis

Acute: appendicitis: fulminating, gangrenous, inflamed, obstructive; cecitis } without mention of perforation, peritonitis, or rupture

AHA: 1Q, '01, 15; 4Q, '97, 52

541 Appendicitis, unqualified

AHA: 2Q, '90, 26

542 Other appendicitis

Appendicitis:
- chronic
- recurrent

Appendicitis:
- relapsing
- subacute

EXCLUDES *hyperplasia (lymphoid) of appendix (543.0)*

AHA: 1Q, '01, 15

4th **543 Other diseases of appendix**

543.0 Hyperplasia of appendix (lymphoid)

DEF: Proliferation of cells in appendix tissue.

543.9 Other and unspecified diseases of appendix

Appendicular or appendiceal:
- colic
- concretion
- fistula

Diverticulum, Fecalith, Intussusception, Mucocele, Stercolith } of appendix

HERNIA OF ABDOMINAL CAVITY (550-553)

INCLUDES hernia:
- acquired
- congenital, except diaphragmatic or hiatal

4th **550 Inguinal hernia**

INCLUDES bubonocele
inguinal hernia (direct) (double) (indirect) (oblique) (sliding)
scrotal hernia

The following fifth-digit subclassification is for use with category 550:

0 unilateral or unspecified (not specified as recurrent)
Unilateral NOS
1 unilateral or unspecified, recurrent
2 bilateral (not specified as recurrent)
Bilateral NOS
3 bilateral, recurrent

AHA: N-D, '85, 12

DEF: Hernia: protrusion of an abdominal organ or tissue through inguinal canal.

DEF: Indirect inguinal hernia: (external or oblique) leaves abdomen through deep inguinal ring, passes through inguinal canal lateral to the inferior epigastric artery.

DEF: Direct inguinal hernia: (internal) emerges between inferior epigastric artery and rectus muscle edge.

Inguinal Hernia

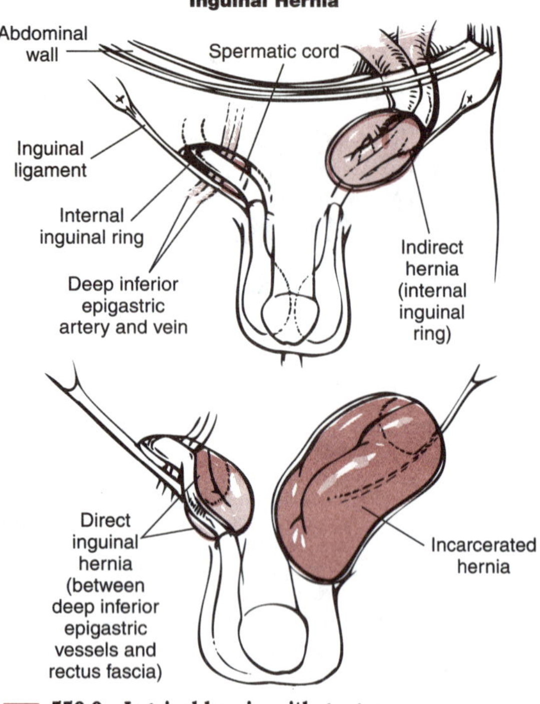

§ ✓5th **550.0 Inguinal hernia, with gangrene**
Inguinal hernia with gangrene (and obstruction)

§ ✓5th **550.1 Inguinal hernia, with obstruction, without mention of gangrene**
Inguinal hernia with mention of incarceration, irreducibility, or strangulation

§ ✓5th **550.9 Inguinal hernia, without mention of obstruction or gangrene**
Inguinal hernia NOS
AHA: For code 550.91: 3Q, '03, 10; 1Q, '03, 4

✓4th **551 Other hernia of abdominal cavity, with gangrene**
INCLUDES that with gangrene (and obstruction)

✓5th **551.0 Femoral hernia with gangrene**

551.00 Unilateral or unspecified (not specified as recurrent)
Femoral hernia NOS with gangrene

551.01 Unilateral or unspecified, recurrent

551.02 Bilateral (not specified as recurrent)

551.03 Bilateral, recurrent

551.1 Umbilical hernia with gangrene
Parumbilical hernia specified as gangrenous

✓5th **551.2 Ventral hernia with gangrene**

551.20 Ventral, unspecified, with gangrene

Femoral Hernia

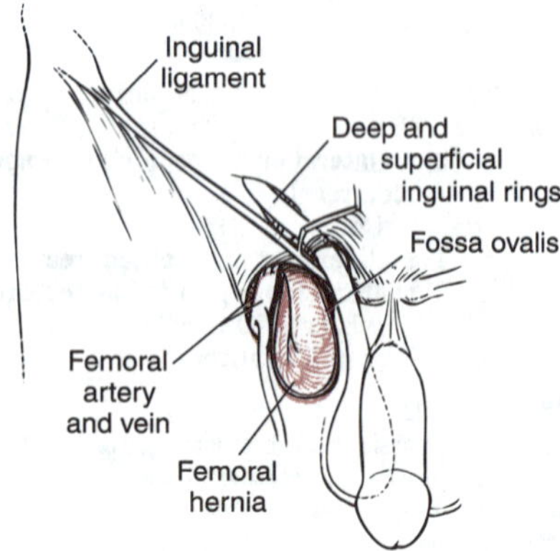

§ Requires fifth-digit. See category 550 for codes and definitions.

Hernias of Abdominal Cavity

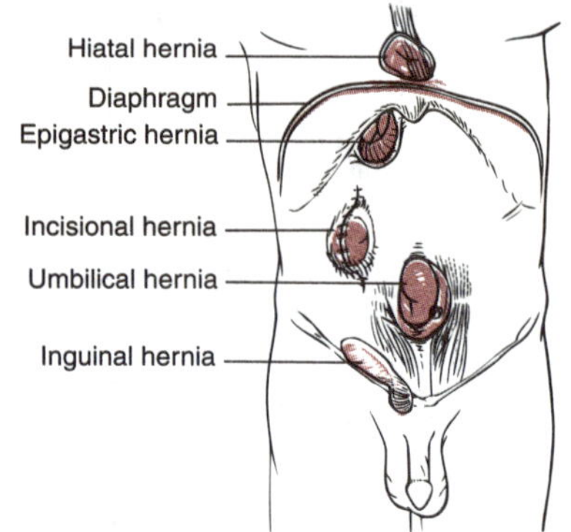

551.21 Incisional, with gangrene
Hernia:
postoperative } specified as gangrenous
recurrent, ventral } specified as gangrenous

551.29 Other
Epigastric hernia specified as gangrenous

551.3 Diaphragmatic hernia with gangrene
Hernia:
hiatal (esophageal) (sliding) } specified as gangrenous
paraesophageal } specified as gangrenous
Thoracic stomach } specified as gangrenous

EXCLUDES *congenital diaphragmatic hernia (756.6)*

551.8 Hernia of other specified sites, with gangrene
Any condition classifiable to 553.8 if specified as gangrenous

551.9 Hernia of unspecified site, with gangrene
Any condition classifiable to 553.9 if specified as gangrenous

✓4th **552 Other hernia of abdominal cavity, with obstruction, but without mention of gangrene**
EXCLUDES *that with mention of gangrene (551.0-551.9)*

✓5th **552.0 Femoral hernia with obstruction**
Femoral hernia specified as incarcerated, irreducible, strangulated, or causing obstruction

552.00 Unilateral or unspecified (not specified as recurrent)

552.01 Unilateral or unspecified, recurrent

552.02 Bilateral (not specified as recurrent)

552.03 Bilateral, recurrent

552.1 Umbilical hernia with obstruction
Parumbilical hernia specified as incarcerated, irreducible, strangulated, or causing obstruction

✓5th **552.2 Ventral hernia with obstruction**
Ventral hernia specified as incarcerated, irreducible, strangulated, or causing obstruction

552.20 Ventral, unspecified, with obstruction

Diaphragmatic Hernia

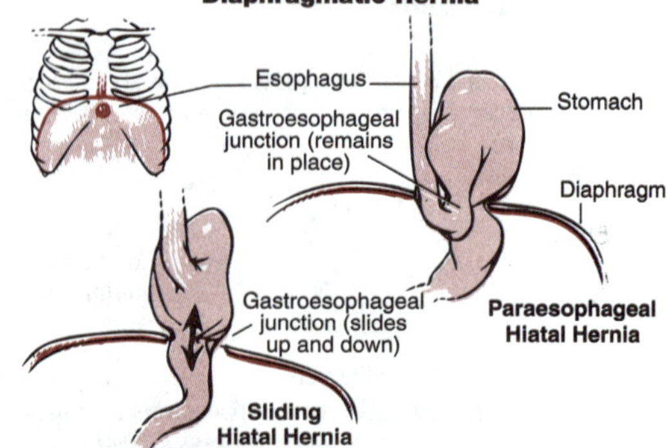

552.21 Incisional, with obstruction
Hernia:
postoperative, recurrent, ventral } specified as incarcerated, irreducible, strangulated, or causing obstruction
AHA: 3Q, '03, 11

552.29 Other
Epigastric hernia specified as incarcerated, irreducible, strangulated, or causing obstruction

552.3 Diaphragmatic hernia with obstruction
Hernia:
hiatal (esophageal) (sliding), paraesophageal, Thoracic stomach } specified as incarcerated, irreducible, strangulated, or causing obstruction
EXCLUDES *congenital diaphragmatic hernia (756.6)*

552.8 Hernia of other specified sites, with obstruction
Any condition classifiable to 553.8 if specified as incarcerated, irreducible, strangulated, or causing obstruction
EXCLUDES ▶ *hernia due to adhesion with obstruction (560.81)*◀
AHA: 1Q, '04, 10

552.9 Hernia of unspecified site, with obstruction
Any condition classifiable to 553.9 if specified as incarcerated, irreducible, strangulated, or causing obstruction

✓4th **553 Other hernia of abdominal cavity without mention of obstruction or gangrene**
EXCLUDES *the listed conditions with mention of:*
gangrene (and obstruction) (551.0-551.9)
obstruction (552.0-552.9)

✓5th **553.0 Femoral hernia**
553.00 Unilateral or unspecified (not specified as recurrent)
Femoral hernia NOS
553.01 Unilateral or unspecified, recurrent
553.02 Bilateral (not specified as recurrent)
553.03 Bilateral, recurrent

553.1 Umbilical hernia
Parumbilical hernia

✓5th **553.2 Ventral hernia**
553.20 Ventral, unspecified
AHA: 3Q, '03, 6
553.21 Incisional
Hernia: postoperative
Hernia: recurrent, ventral
AHA: 3Q, '03, 6
553.29 Other
Hernia: epigastric
Hernia: spigelian

553.3 Diaphragmatic hernia
Hernia:
hiatal (esophageal) (sliding)
paraesophageal
Thoracic stomach
EXCLUDES *congenital:*
diaphragmatic hernia (756.6)
hiatal hernia (750.6)
esophagocele (530.6)
AHA: 2Q, '01, 6; 1Q, '00, 6

553.8 Hernia of other specified sites
Hernia:
ischiatic
ischiorectal
lumbar
obturator
pudendal
Hernia:
retroperitoneal
sciatic
Other abdominal hernia of specified site
EXCLUDES *vaginal enterocele (618.6)*

553.9 Hernia of unspecified site
Enterocele
Epiplocele
Hernia:
NOS
interstitial
Hernia:
intestinal
intra-abdominal
Rupture (nontraumatic)
Sarcoepiplocele

NONINFECTIOUS ENTERITIS AND COLITIS (555-558)

✓4th **555 Regional enteritis**
INCLUDES Crohn's disease
Granulomatous enteritis
EXCLUDES *ulcerative colitis (556)*
DEF: Inflammation of intestine; classified to site.

555.0 Small intestine
Ileitis:
regional
segmental
terminal
Regional enteritis or Crohn's disease of:
duodenum
ileum
jejunum

555.1 Large intestine
Colitis:
granulmatous
regional
transmural
Regional enteritis or Crohn's disease of:
colon
large bowel
rectum
AHA: 3Q, '99, 8

555.2 Small intestine with large intestine
Regional ileocolitis
AHA: 1Q, '03, 18

555.9 Unspecified site
Crohn's disease NOS
Regional enteritis NOS
AHA: 3Q, '99, 8; 4Q, '97, 42; 2Q, '97, 3

✓4th **556 Ulcerative colitis**
AHA: 3Q, '99, 8
DEF: Chronic inflammation of mucosal lining of intestinal tract; may be single area or entire colon.

556.0 Ulcerative (chronic) enterocolitis
556.1 Ulcerative (chronic) ileocolitis
556.2 Ulcerative (chronic) proctitis
556.3 Ulcerative (chronic) proctosigmoiditis
556.4 Pseudopolyposis of colon
556.5 Left-sided ulcerative (chronic) colitis
556.6 Universal ulcerative (chronic) colitis
Pancolitis
556.8 Other ulcerative colitis
556.9 Ulcerative colitis, unspecified
Ulcerative enteritis NOS
AHA: 1Q, '03, 10

✓4th **557 Vascular insufficiency of intestine**
EXCLUDES *necrotizing enterocolitis of the newborn (777.5)*
DEF: Inadequacy of intestinal vessels.

Large Intestine

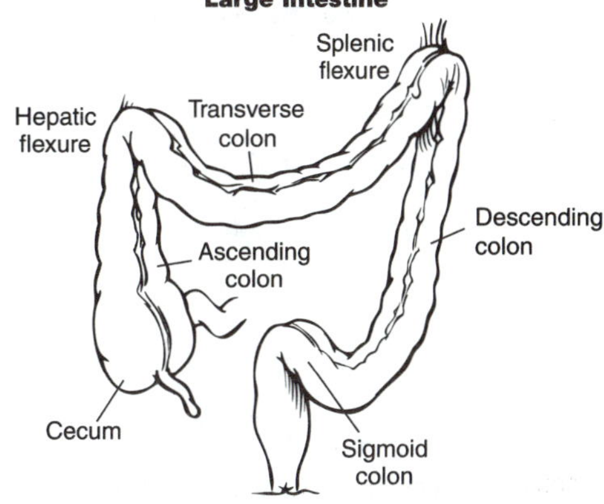

557.0 Acute vascular insufficiency of intestine
Acute:
hemorrhagic enterocolitis
ischemic colitis, enteritis, or enterocolitis
massive necrosis of intestine
Bowel infarction
Embolism of mesenteric artery
Fulminant enterocolitis
Hemorrhagic necrosis of intestine
Infarction of appendices epiploicae
Intestinal gangrene
Intestinal infarction (acute) (agnogenic) (hemorrhagic) (nonocclusive)
Mesenteric infarction (embolic) (thrombotic)
Necrosis of intestine
Terminal hemorrhagic enteropathy
Thrombosis of mesenteric artery
AHA: 4Q, '01, 53

557.1 Chronic vascular insufficiency of intestine
Angina, abdominal
Chronic ischemic colitis, enteritis, or enterocolitis
Ischemic stricture of intestine
Mesenteric:
angina
artery syndrome (superior)
vascular insufficiency
AHA: 3Q, '96, 9; 4Q, '90, 4; N-D, '86, 11; N-D, '84, 7

557.9 Unspecified vascular insufficiency of intestine
Alimentary pain due to vascular insufficiency
Ischemic colitis, enteritis, or enterocolitis NOS

✓4th **558 Other and unspecified noninfectious gastroenteritis and colitis**
EXCLUDES *infectious:*
colitis, enteritis, or gastroenteritis (009.0-009.1)
diarrhea (009.2-009.3)

558.1 Gastroenteritis and colitis due to radiation
Radiation enterocolitis

558.2 Toxic gastroenteritis and colitis
Use additional E code, if desired, to identify cause

558.3 Allergic gastroenteritis and colitis
Use additional code to identify type of food allergy (V15.01-V15.05)
AHA: 1Q, '03, 12; 4Q, '00, 42

DEF: True immunoglobulin E (IgE)-mediated allergic reaction of the lining of the stomach, intestines, or colon to food proteins; causes nausea, vomiting, diarrhea, and abdominal cramping.

558.9 Other and unspecified noninfectious gastroenteritis and colitis
Colitis, Enteritis, Gastroenteritis, Ileitis, Jejunitis, Sigmoiditis — NOS, dietetic, or noninfectious
AHA: 3Q, '99, 4, 6; N-D, '87, 7

Volvulus, Diverticulitis

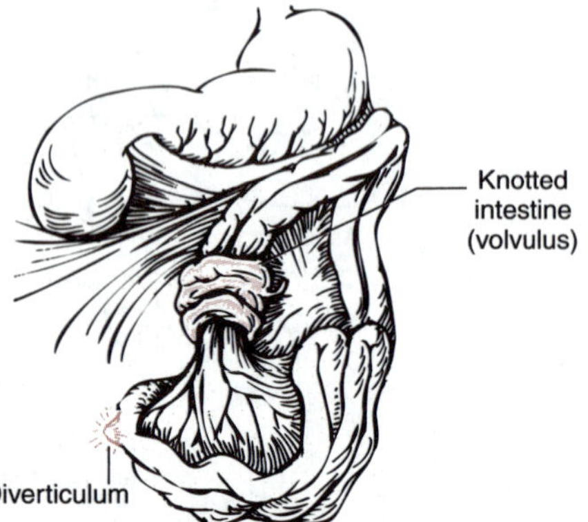

OTHER DISEASES OF INTESTINES AND PERITONEUM (560-569)

✓4th **560 Intestinal obstruction without mention of hernia**
EXCLUDES *duodenum (537.2-537.3)*
inguinal hernia with obstruction (550.1)
intestinal obstruction complicating hernia (552.0-552.9)
mesenteric:
embolism (557.0)
infarction (557.0)
thrombosis (557.0)
neonatal intestinal obstruction (277.01, 777.1-777.2, 777.4)

560.0 Intussusception
Intussusception (colon) (intestine) (rectum)
Invagination of intestine or colon
EXCLUDES *intussusception of appendix (543.9)*
AHA: 4Q, '98, 82

DEF: Prolapse of a bowel section into adjacent section; occurs primarily in children; symptoms include paroxysmal pain, vomiting, presence of lower abdominal tumor and blood, and mucous passage from rectum.

560.1 Paralytic ileus
Adynamic ileus
Ileus (of intestine) (of bowel) (of colon)
Paralysis of intestine or colon
EXCLUDES *gallstone ileus (560.31)*
AHA: J-F, '87, 13

DEF: Obstruction of ileus due to inhibited bowel motility.

560.2 Volvulus
Knotting, Strangulation, Torsion, Twist — of intestine, bowel, or colon

DEF: Entanglement of bowel; causes obstruction; may compromise bowel circulation.

✓5th **560.3 Impaction of intestine**

560.30 Impaction of intestine, unspecified
Impaction of colon

560.31 Gallstone ileus
Obstruction of intestine by gallstone

560.39 Other
Concretion of intestine
Enterolith
Fecal impaction
AHA: 4Q, '98, 38

✓5th **560.8 Other specified intestinal obstruction**

560.81 Intestinal or peritoneal adhesions with obstruction (postoperative) (postinfection)
EXCLUDES *adhesions without obstruction (568.0)*
AHA: 4Q, '95, 55; 3Q, '95, 6; N-D, '87, 9

DEF: Obstruction of peritoneum or intestine due to abnormal union of tissues.

560.89 Other
Acute pseudo-obstruction of intestine
Mural thickening causing obstruction
EXCLUDES *ischemic stricture of intestine (557.1)*
AHA: 2Q, '97, 3; 1Q, '88, 6

560.9 Unspecified intestinal obstruction
Enterostenosis
Obstruction, Occlusion, Stenosis, Stricture — of intestine or colon
EXCLUDES *congenital stricture or stenosis of intestine (751.1-751.2)*

N Newborn Age: 0 P Pediatric Age: 0-17 M Maternity Age: 12-55 A Adult Age: 15-124 MSP Medicare Secondary Payer

✓4th **562 Diverticula of intestine**

Use additional code to identify any associated:
peritonitis (567.0-567.9)

EXCLUDES *congenital diverticulum of colon (751.5)*
diverticulum of appendix (543.9)
Meckel's diverticulum (751.0)

AHA: 4Q, '91, 25; J-F, '85, 1

✓5th **562.0 Small intestine**

562.00 Diverticulosis of small intestine (without mention of hemorrhage)

Diverticulosis:
duodenum, ileum, jejunum } without mention of diverticulitis

DEF: Saclike herniations of mucous lining of small intestine\

562.01 Diverticulitis of small intestine (without mention of hemorrhage)

Diverticulitis (with diverticulosis):
duodenum
ileum
jejunum
small intestine

DEF: Inflamed saclike herniations of mucous lining of small intestine.

562.02 Diverticulosis of small intestine with hemorrhage

562.03 Diverticulitis of small intestine with hemorrhage

✓5th **562.1 Colon**

562.10 Diverticulosis of colon (without mention of hemorrhage)

Diverticulosis:
NOS
intestine (large)
Diverticular disease (colon)
} without mention of diverticulitis

AHA: 3Q, '02, 15; 4Q, '90, 21; J-F, '85, 5

DEF: Saclike herniations of mucous lining of large intestine

562.11 Diverticulitis of colon (without mention of hemorrhage)

Diverticulitis (with diverticulosis):
NOS
colon
intestine (large)

AHA: 1Q, '96, 14; J-F, '85, 5

DEF: Inflamed saclike herniations of mucosal lining of large intestine.

562.12 Diverticulosis of colon with hemorrhage

562.13 Diverticulitis of colon with hemorrhage

✓4th **564 Functional digestive disorders, not elsewhere classified**

EXCLUDES *functional disorders of stomach (536.0-536.9)*
those specified as psychogenic (306.4)

Anal Fistula and Abscess

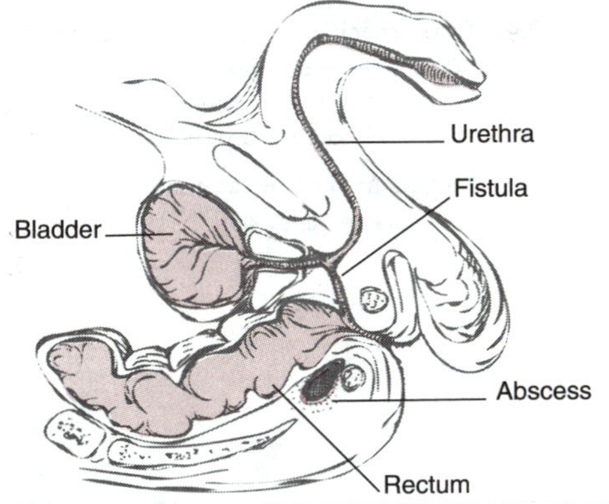

✓5th **564.0 Constipation**

AHA: 4Q, '01, 45

564.00 Constipation, unspecified

564.01 Slow transit constipation

DEF: Delay in the transit of fecal material through the colon secondary to smooth muscle dysfunction or decreased peristaltic contractions along the colon: also called colonic inertia or delayed transit.

564.02 Outlet dysfunction constipation

DEF: Failure to relax the paradoxical contractions of the striated pelvic floor muscles during the attempted defecation.

564.09 Other constipation

564.1 Irritable bowel syndrome

Irritable colon
Spastic colon

AHA: 1Q, '88, 6

DEF: Functional gastrointestinal disorder (FGID); symptoms following meals include diarrhea, constipation, abdominal pain; other symptoms include bloating, gas, distended abdomen, nausea, vomiting, appetite loss, emotional distress, and depression.

564.2 Postgastric surgery syndromes

Dumping syndrome
Jejunal syndrome
Postgastrectomy syndrome
Postvagotomy syndrome

EXCLUDES *malnutrition following gastrointestinal surgery (579.3)*
postgastrojejunostomy ulcer (534.0-534.9)

AHA: 1Q, '95, 11

564.3 Vomiting following gastrointestinal surgery

Vomiting (bilious) following gastrointestinal surgery

564.4 Other postoperative functional disorders

Diarrhea following gastrointestinal surgery

EXCLUDES *colostomy and enterostomy complications (569.60-569.69)*

564.5 Functional diarrhea

EXCLUDES *diarrhea:*
NOS (787.91)
psychogenic (306.4)

DEF: Diarrhea with no detectable organic cause.

564.6 Anal spasm

Proctalgia fugax

564.7 Megacolon, other than Hirschsprung's

Dilatation of colon

EXCLUDES *megacolon:*
congenital [Hirschsprung's] (751.3)
toxic (556)

DEF: Enlarged colon; congenital or acquired; can occur acutely or become chronic.

✓5th **564.8 Other specified functional disorders of intestine**

EXCLUDES *malabsorption (579.0-579.9)*

AHA: 1Q, '88, 6

Rectum and Anus

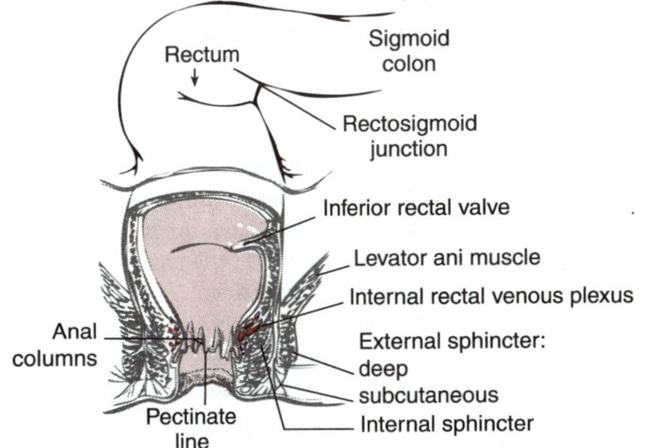

564.81 Neurogenic bowel
AHA: 1Q, '01, 12; 4Q, '98, 45
DEF: Disorder of bowel due to spinal cord lesion above conus medullaris; symptoms include precipitous micturition, nocturia, catheter intolerance, headache, sweating, nasal obstruction and spastic contractions.

564.89 Other functional disorders of intestine
Atony of colon
DEF: Absence of normal bowel tone or strength.

564.9 Unspecified functional disorder of intestine

565 Anal fissure and fistula

565.0 Anal fissure
Tear of anus, nontraumatic
EXCLUDES *traumatic (863.89, 863.99)*
DEF: Ulceration of cleft at anal mucosa; causes pain, itching, bleeding, infection, and sphincter spasm; may occur with hemorrhoids.

565.1 Anal fistula
Fistula:
anorectal
rectal
rectum to skin
EXCLUDES *fistula of rectum to internal organs—see Alphabetic Index*
ischiorectal fistula (566)
rectovaginal fistula (619.1)
DEF: Abnormal opening on cutaneous surface near anus; may lack connection with rectum.

566 Abscess of anal and rectal regions
Abscess:
ischiorectal
perianal
perirectal
Cellulitis:
anal
perirectal
rectal
Ischiorectal fistula

▲ **567 Peritonitis and retroperitoneal infections**
EXCLUDES *peritonitis:*
benign paroxysmal (277.3)
pelvic, female (614.5, 614.7)
periodic familial (277.3)
puerperal (670)
with or following:
abortion (634-638 with .0, 639.0)
appendicitis (540.0-540.1)
ectopic or molar pregnancy (639.0)
DEF: Inflammation of the peritoneal cavity.

567.0 Peritonitis in infectious diseases classified elsewhere
Code first underlying disease
EXCLUDES *peritonitis:*
gonococcal (098.86)
syphilitic (095.2)
tuberculous (014.0)

567.1 Pneumococcal peritonitis

567.2 Other suppurative peritonitis
AHA: 2Q, '01, 11, 12; 3Q, '99, 9; 2Q, '98, 19

● **567.21 Peritonitis (acute) generalized**
Pelvic peritonitis, male

● **567.22 Peritoneal abscess**
Abscess (of):
abdominopelvic
mesenteric
omentum
peritoneum
retrocecal
subdiaphragmatic
subhepatic
subphrenic

● **567.23 Spontaneous bacterial peritonitis**

● **567.29 Other suppurative peritonitis**
Subphrenic peritonitis

● **567.3 Retroperitoneal infections**

● **567.31 Psoas muscle abscess**

● **567.38 Other retroperitoneal abscess**

● **567.39 Other retroperitoneal infections**

567.8 Other specified peritonitis

● **567.81 Choleperitonitis**
Peritonitis due to bile

● **567.82 Sclerosing mesenteritis**
Fat necrosis of peritoneum
(Idiopathic) sclerosing mesenteric fibrosis
Mesenteric lipodystrophy
Mesenteric panniculitis
Retractile mesenteritis

● **567.89 Other specified peritonitis**
Chronic proliferative peritonitis
Mesenteric saponification
Peritonitis due to urine

567.9 Unspecified peritonitis
Peritonitis:
NOS
of unspecified cause
AHA: 1Q, '04, 10

568 Other disorders of peritoneum

568.0 Peritoneal adhesions (postoperative) (postinfection)
Adhesions (of):
abdominal (wall)
diaphragm
intestine
male pelvis
mesenteric
omentum
stomach
Adhesive bands
EXCLUDES *adhesions:*
pelvic, female (614.6)
with obstruction:
duodenum (537.3)
intestine (560.81)
AHA: 3Q, '03, 7, 11; 4Q, '95, 55; 3Q, '95, 7; S-O, '85, 11
DEF: Abnormal union of tissues in peritoneum.

568.8 Other specified disorders of peritoneum

568.81 Hemoperitoneum (nontraumatic)

568.82 Peritoneal effusion (chronic)
EXCLUDES *ascites NOS (789.5)*
DEF: Persistent leakage of fluid within peritoneal cavity.

568.89 Other
Peritoneal:
cyst
granuloma

568.9 Unspecified disorder of peritoneum

569 Other disorders of intestine

569.0 Anal and rectal polyp
Anal and rectal polyp NOS
EXCLUDES *adenomatous anal and rectal polyp (211.4)*

569.1 Rectal prolapse
Procidentia:
anus (sphincter)
rectum (sphincter)
Proctoptosis
Prolapse:
anal canal
rectal mucosa
EXCLUDES *prolapsed hemorrhoids (455.2, 455.5)*

569.2 Stenosis of rectum and anus
Stricture of anus (sphincter)

569.3 Hemorrhage of rectum and anus
EXCLUDES *gastrointestinal bleeding NOS (578.9)*
melena (578.1)

569.4 Other specified disorders of rectum and anus

569.41 Ulcer of anus and rectum
Solitary ulcer / Stercoral ulcer } of anus (sphincter) or rectum (sphincter)

569.42 Anal or rectal pain
AHA: 1Q, '03, 8; 1Q, '96, 13

N Newborn Age: 0 P Pediatric Age: 0-17 M Maternity Age: 12-55 A Adult Age: 15-124 MSP Medicare Secondary Payer

569.49 Other
Granuloma } of rectum (sphincter)
Rupture
Hypertrophy of anal papillae
Proctitis NOS
EXCLUDES *fistula of rectum to:*
internal organs—see Alphabetic Index
skin (565.1)
hemorrhoids (455.0-455.9)
incontinence of sphincter ani (787.6)

569.5 Abscess of intestine
EXCLUDES *appendiceal abscess (540.1)*

✓5th **569.6 Colostomy and enterostomy complications**
AHA: 4Q, '95, 58
DEF: Complication in a surgically created opening, from intestine to surface skin.

569.60 Colostomy and enterostomy complication, unspecified

569.61 Infection of colostomy or enterostomy
Use additional code to identify organism (041.00-041.9)
Use additional code to specify type of infection, such as:
abscess or cellulitis of abdomen (682.2)
septicemia (038.0-038.9)

569.62 Mechanical complication of colostomy and enterostomy
Malfunction of colostomy and enterostomy
AHA: 1Q, '03, 10; 4Q, '98, 44

569.69 Other complication
Fistula
Hernia
Prolapse
AHA: 3Q, '98, 16

✓5th **569.8 Other specified disorders of intestine**
AHA: 4Q, '91, 25

569.81 Fistula of intestine, excluding rectum and anus
Fistula:
abdominal wall
enterocolic
enteroenteric
ileorectal
EXCLUDES *fistula of intestine to internal organs—see Alphabetic Index*
persistent postoperative fistula (998.6)
AHA: 3Q, '99, 8

569.82 Ulceration of intestine
Primary ulcer of intestine
Ulceration of colon
EXCLUDES *that with perforation (569.83)*

569.83 Perforation of intestine

569.84 Angiodysplasia of intestine (without mention of hemorrhage)
AHA: 3Q, '96, 10; 4Q, '90, 4; 4Q, '90, 21
DEF: Small vascular abnormalities of the intestinal tract without bleeding problems.

569.85 Angiodysplasia of intestine with hemorrhage
AHA: 3Q, '96, 9
DEF: Small vascular abnormalities of the intestinal tract with bleeding problems.

569.86 Dieulafoy lesion (hemorrhagic) of intestine
AHA: 4Q, '02, 60-61

569.89 Other
Enteroptosis
Granuloma } of intestine
Prolapse
Pericolitis
Perisigmoiditis
Visceroptosis
EXCLUDES *gangrene of intestine, mesentery, or omentum (557.0)*
hemorrhage of intestine NOS (578.9)
obstruction of intestine (560.0-560.9)
AHA: 3Q, '96, 9

569.9 Unspecified disorder of intestine

OTHER DISEASES OF DIGESTIVE SYSTEM (570-579)

570 Acute and subacute necrosis of liver
Acute hepatic failure
Acute or subacute hepatitis, not specified as infective
Necrosis of liver (acute) (diffuse) (massive) (subacute)
Parenchymatous degeneration of liver
Yellow atrophy (liver) (acute) (subacute)
EXCLUDES *icterus gravis of newborn (773.0-773.2)*
serum hepatitis (070.2-070.3)
that with:
abortion (634-638 with .7, 639.8)
ectopic or molar pregnancy (639.8)
pregnancy, childbirth, or the puerperium (646.7)
viral hepatitis (070.0-070.9)
AHA: 1Q, '00, 22

✓4th **571 Chronic liver disease and cirrhosis**

571.0 Alcoholic fatty liver A

571.1 Acute alcoholic hepatitis A
Acute alcoholic liver disease
AHA: 2Q, '02, 4

571.2 Alcoholic cirrhosis of liver A
Florid cirrhosis
Laennec's cirrhosis (alcoholic)
AHA: 2Q, '02, 4; 1Q, '02, 3; N-D, '85, 14
DEF: Fibrosis and dysfunction, of liver; due to alcoholic liver disease.

571.3 Alcoholic liver damage, unspecified A

✓5th **571.4 Chronic hepatitis**
EXCLUDES *viral hepatitis (acute) (chronic) (070.0-070.9)*

571.40 Chronic hepatitis, unspecified

571.41 Chronic persistent hepatitis

571.49 Other
Chronic hepatitis:
active
aggressive
Recurrent hepatitis
AHA: 3Q, '99, 19; N-D, '85, 14

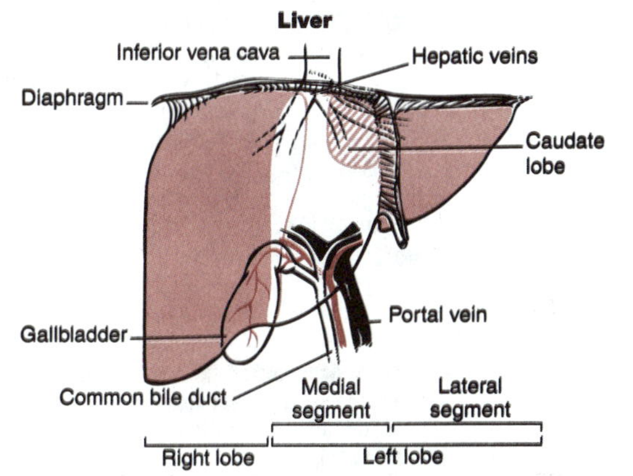

571.5 Cirrhosis of liver without mention of alcohol

Cirrhosis of liver:
- NOS
- cryptogenic
- macronodular
- micronodular
- posthepatitic

Cirrhosis of liver:
- postnecrotic

Healed yellow atrophy (liver)
Portal cirrhosis

DEF: Fibrosis and dysfunction of liver; not alcohol related.

571.6 Biliary cirrhosis

Chronic nonsuppurative destructive cholangitis
Cirrhosis:
- cholangitic
- cholestatic

571.8 Other chronic nonalcoholic liver disease

Chronic yellow atrophy (liver)
Fatty liver, without mention of alcohol
AHA: 2Q, '96, 12

571.9 Unspecified chronic liver disease without mention of alcohol

4th **572 Liver abscess and sequelae of chronic liver disease**

572.0 Abscess of liver

EXCLUDES *amebic liver abscess (006.3)*

572.1 Portal pyemia

Phlebitis of portal vein
Portal thrombophlebitis
Pylephlebitis
Pylethrombophlebitis

DEF: Inflammation of portal vein or branches; may be due to intestinal disease; symptoms include fever, chills, jaundice, sweating, and abscess in various body parts.

572.2 Hepatic coma

Hepatic encephalopathy
Hepatocerebral intoxication
Portal-systemic encephalopathy
AHA: 1Q, '02, 3; 3Q, '95, 14

572.3 Portal hypertension

DEF: Abnormally high blood pressure in the portal vein.

572.4 Hepatorenal syndrome

EXCLUDES *that following delivery (674.8)*

AHA: 3Q, '93, 15

DEF: Hepatic and renal failure characterized by cirrhosis with ascites or obstructive jaundice, oliguria, and low sodium concentration.

572.8 Other sequelae of chronic liver disease

4th **573 Other disorders of liver**

EXCLUDES *amyloid or lardaceous degeneration of liver (277.3)*
congenital cystic disease of liver (751.62)
glycogen infiltration of liver (271.0)
hepatomegaly NOS (789.1)
portal vein obstruction (452)

573.0 Chronic passive congestion of liver

DEF: Blood accumulation in liver tissue.

573.1 Hepatitis in viral diseases classified elsewhere

Code first underlying disease as:
- Coxsackie virus disease (074.8)
- cytomegalic inclusion virus disease (078.5)
- infectious mononucleosis (075)

EXCLUDES *hepatitis (in):*
- *mumps (072.71)*
- *viral (070.0-070.9)*
- *yellow fever (060.0-060.9)*

573.2 Hepatitis in other infectious diseases classified elsewhere

Code first underlying disease, as:
- malaria (084.9)

EXCLUDES *hepatitis in:*
- *late syphilis (095.3)*
- *secondary syphilis (091.62)*
- *toxoplasmosis (130.5)*

573.3 Hepatitis, unspecified

Toxic (noninfectious) hepatitis
Use additional E code to identify cause
AHA: 3Q, '98, 3, 4; 4Q, '90, 26

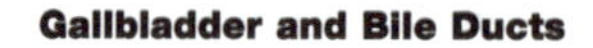

Gallbladder and Bile Ducts

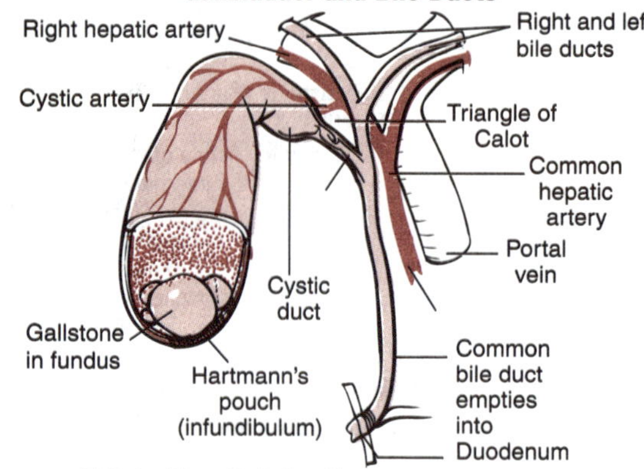

573.4 Hepatic infarction

573.8 Other specified disorders of liver

Hepatoptosis

573.9 Unspecified disorder of liver

4th **574 Cholelithiasis**

The following fifth-digit subclassification is for use with category 574:
- **0 without mention of obstruction**
- **1 with obstruction**

5th **574.0 Calculus of gallbladder with acute cholecystitis**

Biliary calculus, Calculus of cystic duct, Cholelithiasis } with acute cholecystitis

Any condition classifiable to 574.2 with acute cholecystitis
AHA: 4Q, '96, 32

5th **574.1 Calculus of gallbladder with other cholecystitis**

Biliary calculus, Calculus of cystic duct, Cholelithiasis } with cholecystitis

Cholecystitis with cholelithiasis NOS
Any condition classifiable to 574.2 with cholecystitis (chronic)
AHA: 3Q, '99, 9; 4Q, '96, 32, 69; 2Q, '96, 13; For code 574.10: 1Q, '03, 5

5th **574.2 Calculus of gallbladder without mention of cholecystitis**

Biliary:
- calculus NOS
- colic NOS

Calculus of cystic duct
Cholelithiasis NOS
Colic (recurrent) of gallbladder
Gallstone (impacted)
AHA: For code 574.20: 1Q, '88, 14

5th **574.3 Calculus of bile duct with acute cholecystitis**

Calculus of bile duct [any], Choledocholithiasis } with acute cholecystitis

Any condition classifiable to 574.5 with acute cholecystitis

5th **574.4 Calculus of bile duct with other cholecystitis**

Calculus of bile duct [any], Choledocholithiasis } with cholecystitis (chronic)

Any condition classifiable to 574.5 with cholecystitis (chronic)

5th **574.5 Calculus of bile duct without mention of cholecystitis**

Calculus of:
- bile duct [any]
- common duct
- hepatic duct

Choledocholithiasis
Hepatic:
- colic (recurrent)
- lithiasis

AHA: 3Q, '94, 11

✓5th **574.6 Calculus of gallbladder and bile duct with acute cholecystitis**

Any condition classifiable to 574.0 and 574.3

AHA: 4Q, '96, 32

✓5th **574.7 Calculus of gallbladder and bile duct with other cholecystitis**

Any condition classifiable to 574.1 and 574.4

AHA: 4Q, '96, 32

✓5th **574.8 Calculus of gallbladder and bile duct with acute and chronic cholecystitis**

Any condition classifiable to 574.6 and 574.7

AHA: 4Q, '96, 32

✓5th **574.9 Calculus of gallbladder and bile duct without cholecystitis**

Any condition classifiable to 574.2 and 574.5

AHA: 4Q, '96, 32

✓4th **575 Other disorders of gallbladder**

575.0 Acute cholecystitis

Abscess of gallbladder
Angiocholecystitis
Cholecystitis:
emphysematous (acute)
gangrenous
suppurative
Empyema of gallbladder
Gangrene of gallbladder
} without mention of calculus

EXCLUDES *that with:*
acute and chronic cholecystitis (575.12)
choledocholithiasis (574.3)
choledocholithiasis and cholelithiasis (574.6)
cholelithiasis (574.0)

AHA: 3Q, '91, 17

✓5th **575.1 Other cholecystitis**

Cholecystitis:
NOS
chronic
} without mention of calculus

EXCLUDES *that with:*
choledocholithiasis (574.4)
choledocholithiasis and cholelithiasis (574.8)
cholelithiasis (574.1)

AHA: 4Q, '96, 32

575.10 Cholecystitis, unspecified

Cholecystitis NOS

575.11 Chronic cholecystitis

575.12 Acute and chronic cholecystitis

AHA: 4Q, '97, 52; 4Q, '96, 32

575.2 Obstruction of gallbladder

Occlusion
Stenosis
Stricture
} of cystic duct or gallbladder without mention of calculus

EXCLUDES *that with calculus (574.0-574.2 with fifth-digit 1)*

575.3 Hydrops of gallbladder

Mucocele of gallbladder

AHA: 2Q, '89, 13

DEF: Serous fluid accumulation in bladder.

575.4 Perforation of gallbladder

Rupture of cystic duct or gallbladder

575.5 Fistula of gallbladder

Fistula:
cholecystoduodenal
cholecystoenteric

575.6 Cholesterolosis of gallbladder

Strawberry gallbladder

AHA: 4Q, '90, 17

DEF: Cholesterol deposits in gallbladder tissue.

575.8 Other specified disorders of gallbladder

Adhesions
Atrophy
Cyst
Hypertrophy
Nonfunctioning
Ulcer
} (of) cystic duct or gallbladder

Biliary dyskinesia

EXCLUDES *Hartmann's pouch of intestine (V44.3)*
nonvisualization of gallbladder (793.3)

AHA: 4Q, '90, 26; 2Q, '89, 13

575.9 Unspecified disorder of gallbladder

✓4th **576 Other disorders of biliary tract**

EXCLUDES *that involving the:*
cystic duct (575.0-575.9)
gallbladder (575.0-575.9)

576.0 Postcholecystectomy syndrome

AHA: 1Q, '88, 10

DEF: Jaundice or abdominal pain following cholecystectomy.

576.1 Cholangitis

Cholangitis:
NOS
acute
ascending
chronic
primary

Cholangitis:
recurrent
sclerosing
secondary
stenosing
suppurative

AHA: 2Q, '99, 13

576.2 Obstruction of bile duct

Occlusion
Stenosis
Stricture
} of bile duct, except cystic duct, without mention of calculus

EXCLUDES *congenital (751.61)*
that with calculus (574.3-574.5 with fifth-digit 1)

AHA: 3Q, '03, 17-18; 1Q, '01, 8; 2Q, '99, 13

576.3 Perforation of bile duct

Rupture of bile duct, except cystic duct

576.4 Fistula of bile duct

Choledochoduodenal fistula

576.5 Spasm of sphincter of Oddi

576.8 Other specified disorders of biliary tract

Adhesions
Atrophy
Cyst
Hypertrophy
Stasis
Ulcer
} of bile duct [any]

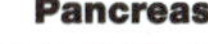

EXCLUDES *congenital choledochal cyst (751.69)*

AHA: 3Q, '03, 17; 2Q, '99, 14

576.9 Unspecified disorder of biliary tract

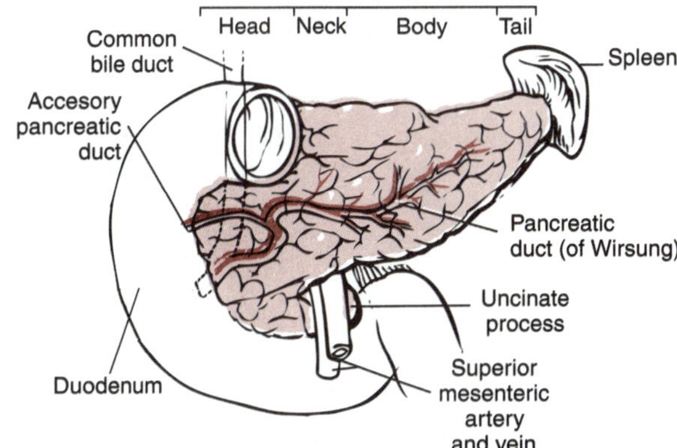

4th 577 Diseases of pancreas

577.0 Acute pancreatitis

Abscess of pancreas
Necrosis of pancreas:
acute
infective
Pancreatitis:
NOS
Pancreatitis:
acute (recurrent)
apoplectic
hemorrhagic
subacute
suppurative

EXCLUDES *mumps pancreatitis (072.3)*

AHA: 3Q, '99, 9; 2Q, '98, 19; 2Q, '96, 13; 2Q, '89, 9

577.1 Chronic pancreatitis

Chronic pancreatitis:
NOS
infectious
interstitial
Pancreatitis:
painless
recurrent
relapsing

AHA: 1Q, '01, 8; 2Q, '96, 13; 3Q, '94, 11

577.2 Cyst and pseudocyst of pancreas

577.8 Other specified diseases of pancreas

Atrophy, Calculus, Cirrhosis, Fibrosis } of pancreas

Pancreatic:
infantilism
necrosis:
NOS
aseptic
Pancreatic:
necrosis:
fat
Pancreatolithiasis

EXCLUDES *fibrocystic disease of pancreas (277.00-277.09)*
islet cell tumor of pancreas (211.7)
pancreatic steatorrhea (579.4)

AHA: 1Q, '01, 8

577.9 Unspecified disease of pancreas

4th 578 Gastrointestinal hemorrhage

EXCLUDES *that with mention of:*
angiodysplasia of stomach and duodenum (537.83)
angiodysplasia of intestine (569.85)
diverticulitis, intestine:
large (562.13)
small (562.03)
diverticulosis, intestine:
large (562.12)
small (562.02)
gastritis and duodenitis (535.0-535.6)
ulcer:
duodenal, gastric, gastrojejuunal or peptic (531.00-534.91)

AHA: 2Q, '92, 9; 4Q, '90, 20

578.0 Hematemesis

Vomiting of blood

AHA: 2Q, '02, 4

578.1 Blood in stool

Melena

EXCLUDES *melena of the newborn (772.4, 777.3)*
occult blood (792.1)

AHA: 2Q, '92, 8

578.9 Hemorrhage of gastrointestinal tract, unspecified

Gastric hemorrhage
Intestinal hemorrhage

AHA: N-D, '86, 9

4th 579 Intestinal malabsorption

579.0 Celiac disease

Celiac:
crisis
infantilism
rickets
Gee (-Herter) disease
Gluten enteropathy
Idiopathic steatorrhea
Nontropical sprue

DEF: Malabsorption syndrome due to gluten consumption; symptoms include fetid, bulky, frothy, oily stools; distended abdomen, gas, weight loss, asthenia, electrolyte depletion and vitamin B, D and K deficiency.

579.1 Tropical sprue

Sprue:
NOS
tropical
Tropical steatorrhea

DEF: Diarrhea, occurs in tropics; may be due to enteric infection and malnutrition.

579.2 Blind loop syndrome

Postoperative blind loop syndrome

DEF: Obstruction or impaired passage in small intestine due to alterations, from strictures or surgery; causes stasis, abnormal bacterial flora, diarrhea, weight loss, multiple vitamin deficiency, and megaloblastic anemia.

579.3 Other and unspecified postsurgical nonabsorption

Hypoglycemia, Malnutrition } following gastrointestinal surgery

AHA: 4Q, '03, 104

579.4 Pancreatic steatorrhea

DEF: Excess fat in feces due to absence of pancreatic juice in intestine.

579.8 Other specified intestinal malabsorption

Enteropathy:
exudative
protein-losing
Steatorrhea (chronic)

AHA: 1Q, '88, 6

579.9 Unspecified intestinal malabsorption

Malabsorption syndrome NOS

AHA: ►4Q, '04, 59◄

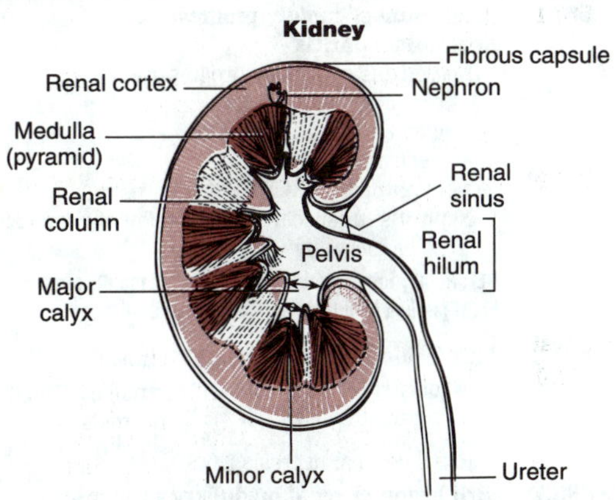

10. DISEASES OF THE GENITOURINARY SYSTEM (580-629)

NEPHRITIS, NEPHROTIC SYNDROME, AND NEPHROSIS (580-589)

EXCLUDES *hypertensive renal disease (403.00-403.91)*

✓4th **580 Acute glomerulonephritis**

INCLUDES acute nephritis

DEF: Acute, severe inflammation in tuft of capillaries that filter the kidneys.

580.0 With lesion of proliferative glomerulonephritis
Acute (diffuse) proliferative glomerulonephritis
Acute poststreptococcal glomerulonephritis

580.4 With lesion of rapidly progressive glomerulonephritis
Acute nephritis with lesion of necrotizing glomerulitis

DEF: Acute glomerulonephritis; progresses to ESRD with diffuse epithelial proliferation.

✓5th **580.8 With other specified pathological lesion in kidney**

580.81 Acute glomerulonephritis in diseases classified elsewhere
Code first underlying disease, as:
infectious hepatitis (070.0-070.9)
mumps (072.79)
subacute bacterial endocarditis (421.0)
typhoid fever (002.0)

580.89 Other
Glomerulonephritis, acute, with lesion of:
exudative nephritis
interstitial (diffuse) (focal) nephritis

580.9 Acute glomerulonephritis with unspecified pathological lesion in kidney
Glomerulonephritis: NOS, hemorrhagic; Nephritis; Nephropathy — specified as acute

Nephron
Proximal convoluted tubule
Distal convoluted tubule
Renal corpuscle: Bowman's capsule
Glomerulus
Afferent arteriole
Collecting duct
Cortex
Medulla
Interlobar artery and vein
Loop of Henle
To minor calyx
Renal papilla

✓4th **581 Nephrotic syndrome**

DEF: Disease process marked by symptoms such as; extensive edema, notable proteinuria, hypoalbuminemia, and susceptibility to intercurrent infections.

581.0 With lesion of proliferative glomerulonephritis

581.1 With lesion of membranous glomerulonephritis
Epimembranous nephritis
Idiopathic membranous glomerular disease
Nephrotic syndrome with lesion of:
focal glomerulosclerosis
sclerosing membranous glomerulonephritis
segmental hyalinosis

581.2 With lesion of membranoproliferative glomerulonephritis
Nephrotic syndrome with lesion (of):
endothelial; hypocomplementemic persistent; lobular; mesangiocapillary; mixed membranous and proliferative — glomerulonephritis

DEF: Glomerulonephritis combined with clinical features of nephrotic syndrome; characterized by uneven thickening of glomerular capillary walls and mesangial cell increase; slowly progresses to ESRD.

581.3 With lesion of minimal change glomerulonephritis
Foot process disease
Lipoid nephrosis
Minimal change:
glomerular disease
glomerulitis
nephrotic syndrome

✓5th **581.8 With other specified pathological lesion in kidney**

581.81 Nephrotic syndrome in diseases classified elsewhere
Code first underlying disease, as:
amyloidosis (277.3)
diabetes mellitus (250.4)
malaria (084.9)
polyarteritis (446.0)
systemic lupus erythematosus (710.0)

EXCLUDES *nephrosis in epidemic hemorrhagic fever (078.6)*

AHA: 3Q, '91, 8,12; S-O, '85, 3

581.89 Other
Glomerulonephritis with edema and lesion of:
exudative nephritis
interstitial (diffuse) (focal) nephritis

581.9 Nephrotic syndrome with unspecified pathological lesion in kidney
Glomerulonephritis with edema NOS
Nephritis:
nephrotic NOS
with edema NOS
Nephrosis NOS
Renal disease with edema NOS

✓4th **582 Chronic glomerulonephritis**

INCLUDES chronic nephritis

DEF: Slow progressive type of nephritis characterized by inflammation of the capillary loops in the glomeruli of the kidney, which leads to renal failure.

582.0 With lesion of proliferative glomerulonephritis
Chronic (diffuse) proliferative glomerulonephritis

582.1 With lesion of membranous glomerulonephritis
Chronic glomerulonephritis:
membranous
sclerosing
Focal glomerulosclerosis
Segmental hyalinosis

AHA: S-O, '84, 16

✓4th ✓5th Additional Digit Required | Unspecified Code | Other Specified Code | Manifestation Code | ►◄ Revised Text | ● New Code | ▲ Revised Code Title

582.2 With lesion of membranoproliferative glomerulonephritis

Chronic glomerulonephritis:
- endothelial
- hypocomplementemic persistent
- lobular
- membranoproliferative
- mesangiocapillary
- mixed membranous and proliferative

DEF: Chronic glomerulonephritis with mesangial cell proliferation.

582.4 With lesion of rapidly progressive glomerulonephritis

Chronic nephritis with lesion of necrotizing glomerulitis

DEF: Chronic glomerulonephritisrapidly progresses to ESRD; marked by diffuse epithelial proliferation.

✓5th **582.8 With other specified pathological lesion in kidney**

582.81 Chronic glomerulonephritis in diseases classified elsewhere

Code first underlying disease, as:
- amyloidosis (277.3)
- systemic lupus erythematosus (710.0)

582.89 Other

Chronic glomerulonephritis with lesion of:
- exudative nephritis
- interstitial (diffuse) (focal) nephritis

582.9 Chronic glomerulonephritis with unspecified pathological lesion in kidney

Glomerulonephritis:
- NOS
- hemorrhagic

Nephritis
Nephropathy
} specified as chronic

AHA: 2Q, '01, 12

✓4th **583 Nephritis and nephropathy, not specified as acute or chronic**

INCLUDES "renal disease" so stated, not specified as acute or chronic but with stated pathology or cause

583.0 With lesion of proliferative glomerulonephritis

Proliferative:
- glomerulonephritis (diffuse) NOS

Proliferative
- nephritis NOS
- nephropathy NOS

583.1 With lesion of membranous glomerulonephritis

Membranous:
- glomerulonephritis NOS
- nephritis NOS

Membranous nephropathy:
- NOS

DEF: Kidney inflammation or dysfunction with deposits on glomerular capillary basement membranes.

583.2 With lesion of membranoproliferative glomerulonephritis

Membranoproliferative:
- glomerulonephritis NOS
- nephritis NOS
- nephropathy NOS

Nephritis NOS, with lesion of:
- hypocomplementemic persistent
- lobular
- mesangiocapillary
- mixed membranous and proliferative

} glomerulonephritis

DEF: Kidney inflammation or dysfunction with mesangial cell proliferation.

583.4 With lesion of rapidly progressive glomerulonephritis

Necrotizing or rapidly progressive:
- glomerulitis NOS
- glomerulonephritis NOS
- nephritis NOS
- nephropathy NOS

Nephritis, unspecified, with lesion of necrotizing glomerulitis

DEF: Kidney inflammation or dysfunction; rapidly progresses to ESRD marked by diffuse epithelial proliferation.

583.6 With lesion of renal cortical necrosis

Nephritis NOS
Nephropathy NOS
} with (renal) cortical necrosis

Renal cortical necrosis NOS

583.7 With lesion of renal medullary necrosis

Nephritis NOS
Nephropathy NOS
} with (renal) medullary [papillary] necrosis

✓5th **583.8 With other specified pathological lesion in kidney**

583.81 Nephritis and nephropathy, not specified as acute or chronic, in diseases classified elsewhere

Code first underlying disease, as:
- amyloidosis (277.3)
- diabetes mellitus (250.4)
- gonococcal infection (098.19)
- Goodpasture's syndrome (446.21)
- systemic lupus erythematosus (710.0)
- tuberculosis (016.0)

EXCLUDES *gouty nephropathy (274.10)*
syphilitic nephritis (095.4)

AHA: 2Q, '03, 7; 3Q, '91, 8; S-O, '85, 3

583.89 Other

Glomerulitis
Glomerulonephritis
Nephritis
Nephropathy
Renal disease
} with lesion of:
- exudative nephritis
- interstitial nephritis

583.9 With unspecified pathological lesion in kidney

Glomerulitis NOS
Glomerulonephritis NOS
Nephritis NOS
Nephropathy NOS

EXCLUDES *nephropathy complicating pregnancy, labor, or the puerperium (642.0-642.9, 646.2)*
renal disease NOS with no stated cause (593.9)

✓4th **584 Acute renal failure**

EXCLUDES *following labor and delivery (669.3)*
posttraumatic (958.5)
that complicating:
- *abortion (634-638 with .3, 639.3)*
- *ectopic or molar pregnancy (639.3)*

AHA: 1Q, '93, 18; 2Q, '92, 5; 4Q, '92, 22

DEF: State resulting from increasing urea and related substances from the blood (azotemia), often with urine output of less than 500 ml per day.

584.5 With lesion of tubular necrosis

Lower nephron nephrosis
Renal failure with (acute) tubular necrosis
Tubular necrosis:
- NOS
- acute

DEF: Acute decline in kidney efficiency with destruction of tubules.

584.6 With lesion of renal cortical necrosis

DEF: Acute decline in kidney efficiency with destruction of renal tissues that filter blood.

584.7 With lesion of renal medullary [papillary] necrosis
Necrotizing renal papillitis
DEF: Acute decline in kidney efficiency with destruction of renal tissues that collect urine.

584.8 With other specified pathological lesion in kidney
AHA: N-D, '85, 1

584.9 Acute renal failure, unspecified
AHA: 2Q, '03, 7; 1Q, 03, 22; 3Q, '02, 21, 28; 2Q, '01, 14; 1Q, '00, 22; 3Q, '96, 9; 4Q, '88, 1

▲ ✓4th **585 Chronic kidney disease (CKD)**
Chronic uremia
▶Use additional code to identify kidney transplant status, if applicable (V42.0)◀
Use additional code to identify manifestation as:
uremic:
neuropathy (357.4)
pericarditis (420.0)
EXCLUDES *that with any condition classifiable to 401 (403.0-403.9 with fifth-digit 1)*
AHA: 1Q, '04, 5; 4Q, '03, 61, 111; 2Q, '03, 7; 2Q, '01, 12, 13; 1Q, '01, 3; 4Q, '98, 55; 3Q, '98, 6, 7; 2Q, '98, 20; 3Q, '96, 9; 1Q, '93, 18; 3Q, '91, 8; 4Q, '89, 1; N-D, '85, 15; S-O, '84, 3

● **585.1 Chronic kidney disease, Stage I**
● **585.2 Chronic kidney disease, Stage II (mild)**
● **585.3 Chronic kidney disease, Stage III (moderate)**
● **585.4 Chronic kidney disease, Stage IV (severe)**
● **585.5 Chronic kidney disease, Stage V**
● **585.6 End stage renal disease**
● **585.9 Chronic kidney disease, unspecified**
Chronic renal disease
Chronic renal failure NOS
Chronic renal insufficiency

586 Renal failure, unspecified
Uremia NOS
EXCLUDES *following labor and delivery (669.3)*
posttraumatic renal failure (958.5)
that complicating:
abortion (634-638 with .3, 639.3)
ectopic or molar pregnancy (639.3)
uremia:
extrarenal (788.9)
prerenal (788.9)
with any condition classifiable to 401 (403.0-403.9 with fifth-digit 1)
AHA: 3Q, '98, 6; 1Q, '93, 18
DEF: Renal failure: kidney functions cease; malfunction may be due to inability to excrete metabolized substances or retain level of electrolytes.
DEF: Uremia: excess urea, creatinine and other nitrogenous products of protein and amino acid metabolism in blood due to reduced excretory function in bilateral kidney disease; also called azotemia.

587 Renal sclerosis, unspecified
Atrophy of kidney
Contracted kidney
Renal:
cirrhosis
fibrosis
EXCLUDES *nephrosclerosis (arteriolar) (arteriosclerotic) (403.00-403.92)*
with hypertension (403.00-403.91)

✓4th **588 Disorders resulting from impaired renal function**

588.0 Renal osteodystrophy
Azotemic osteodystrophy
Phosphate-losing tubular disorders
Renal:
dwarfism
infantilism
rickets
DEF: Bone disorder that results in various bone diseases such as osteomalacia, osteoporosis or osteosclerosis; caused by impaired renal function, an abnormal level of phosphorus in the blood and impaired stimulation of the parathyroid.

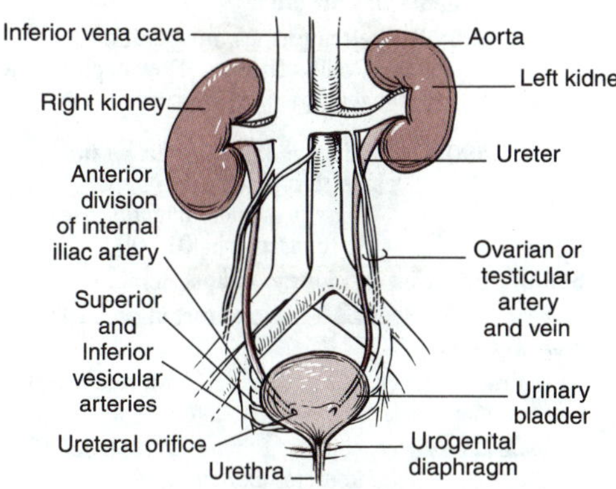
Genitourinary System

588.1 Nephrogenic diabetes insipidus
EXCLUDES *diabetes insipidus NOS (253.5)*
DEF: Type of diabetes due to renal tubules inability to reabsorb water; not responsive to vasopressin; may develop into chronic renal insufficiency.

✓5th **588.8 Other specified disorders resulting from impaired renal function**
EXCLUDES *secondary hypertension (405.0-405.9)*

588.81 Secondary hyperparathyroidism (of renal origin)
Secondary hyperparathyroidism NOS
AHA: 4Q, '04, 58-59
DEF: Parathyroid dysfunction caused by chronic renal failure; phosphate clearance is impaired, phosphate is released from bone, vitamin D is not produced, intestinal calcium absorption is low, and blood levels of calcium are lowered causing excessive production of parathyroid hormone.

588.89 Other specified disorders resulting from impaired renal function
Hypokalemic nephropathy

588.9 Unspecified disorder resulting from impaired renal function

✓4th **589 Small kidney of unknown cause**
589.0 Unilateral small kidney
589.1 Bilateral small kidneys
589.9 Small kidney, unspecified

OTHER DISEASES OF URINARY SYSTEM (590-599)

✓4th **590 Infections of kidney**
Use additional code to identify organism, such as Escherichia coli [E. coli] (041.4)

✓5th **590.0 Chronic pyelonephritis**
Chronic pyelitis
Chronic pyonephrosis
Code, if applicable, any causal condition first
590.00 Without lesion of renal medullary necrosis
590.01 With lesion of renal medullary necrosis

✓5th **590.1 Acute pyelonephritis**
Acute pyelitis
Acute pyonephrosis
590.10 Without lesion of renal medullary necrosis
590.11 With lesion of renal medullary necrosis

590.2 Renal and perinephric abscess
Abscess:
kidney
nephritic
Abscess:
perirenal
Carbuncle of kidney

590.3 Pyeloureteritis cystica
Infection of renal pelvis and ureter
Ureteritis cystica
DEF: Inflammation and formation of submucosal cysts in the kidney, pelvis, and ureter.

✓5th **590.8 Other pyelonephritis or pyonephrosis, not specified as acute or chronic**

590.80 Pyelonephritis, unspecified
Pyelitis NOS
Pyelonephritis NOS
AHA: 1Q, '98, 10; 4Q, '97, 40

590.81 Pyelitis or pyelonephritis in diseases classified elsewhere
Code first underlying disease, as:
tuberculosis (016.0)

590.9 Infection of kidney, unspecified
EXCLUDES *urinary tract infection NOS (599.0)*

591 Hydronephrosis
Hydrocalycosis
Hydronephrosis
Hydroureteronephrosis
EXCLUDES *congenital hydronephrosis (753.29)*
hydroureter (593.5)
AHA: 2Q, '98, 9
DEF: Distention of kidney and pelvis, with urine build-up due to ureteral obstruction; pyonephrosis may result.

✓4th **592 Calculus of kidney and ureter**
EXCLUDES *nephrocalcinosis (275.4)*

592.0 Calculus of kidney
Nephrolithiasis NOS
Renal calculus or stone
Staghorn calculus
Stone in kidney
EXCLUDES *uric acid nephrolithiasis (274.11)*
AHA: 1Q, '00, 4

592.1 Calculus of ureter
Ureteric stone
Ureterolithiasis
AHA: 2Q, '98, 9; 1Q, '98, 10; 1Q, '91, 11

592.9 Urinary calculus, unspecified
AHA: 1Q, '98, 10; 4Q, '97, 40

✓4th **593 Other disorders of kidney and ureter**

593.0 Nephroptosis
Floating kidney
Mobile kidney

593.1 Hypertrophy of kidney

593.2 Cyst of kidney, acquired
Cyst (multiple) (solitary) of kidney, not congenital
Peripelvic (lymphatic) cyst
EXCLUDES *calyceal or pyelogenic cyst of kidney (591)*
congenital cyst of kidney (753.1)
polycystic (disease of) kidney (753.1)
AHA: 4Q, '90, 3
DEF: Abnormal, fluid-filled sac in the kidney, not present at birth.

593.3 Stricture or kinking of ureter
Angulation } of ureter (post-operative)
Constriction }
Stricture of pelviureteric junction
AHA: 2Q, '98, 9
DEF: Stricture or knot in tube connecting kidney to bladder.

593.4 Other ureteric obstruction
Idiopathic retroperitoneal fibrosis
Occlusion NOS of ureter
EXCLUDES *that due to calculus (592.1)*
AHA: 2Q, '97, 4

593.5 Hydroureter
EXCLUDES *congenital hydroureter (753.22)*
hydroureteronephrosis (591)

593.6 Postural proteinuria
Benign postural proteinuria
Orthostatic proteinuria
EXCLUDES *proteinuria NOS (791.0)*
DEF: Excessive amounts of serum protein in the urine caused by the body position, e.g., orthostatic and lordotic.

✓5th **593.7 Vesicoureteral reflux**
AHA: 4Q, '94, 42
DEF: Backflow of urine, from bladder into ureter due to obstructed bladder neck.

593.70 Unspecified or without reflux nephropathy
593.71 With reflux nephropathy, unilateral
593.72 With reflux nephropathy, bilateral
593.73 With reflux nephropathy NOS

✓5th **593.8 Other specified disorders of kidney and ureter**

593.81 Vascular disorders of kidney
Renal (artery):
embolism
hemorrhage
thrombosis
Renal infarction

593.82 Ureteral fistula
Intestinoureteral fistula
EXCLUDES *fistula between ureter and female genital tract (619.0)*
DEF: Abnormal communication, between tube connecting kidney to bladder and another structure.

593.89 Other
Adhesions, kidney or ureter
Periureteritis
Polyp of ureter
Pyelectasia
Ureterocele
EXCLUDES *tuberculosis of ureter (016.2)*
ureteritis cystica (590.3)

593.9 Unspecified disorder of kidney and ureter
▶Acute renal disease
Acute renal insufficiency
Renal disease NOS◀
Salt-losing nephritis or syndrome
EXCLUDES ▶ *chronic renal insufficiency (585.9)*◀
cystic kidney disease (753.1)
nephropathy, so stated (583.0-583.9)
renal disease:
arising in pregnancy or the puerperium (642.1-642.2, 642.4-642.7, 646.2)
not specified as acute or chronic, but with stated pathology or cause (583.0-583.9)
AHA: 1Q, '93, 17

✓4th **594 Calculus of lower urinary tract**

594.0 Calculus in diverticulum of bladder
DEF: Stone or mineral deposit in abnormal sac on the bladder wall.

594.1 Other calculus in bladder
Urinary bladder stone
EXCLUDES *staghorn calculus (592.0)*
DEF: Stone or mineral deposit in bladder.

594.2 Calculus in urethra
DEF: Stone or mineral deposit in tube that empties urine from bladder.

594.8 Other lower urinary tract calculus
AHA: J-F, '85, 16

594.9 Calculus of lower urinary tract, unspecified
EXCLUDES *calculus of urinary tract NOS (592.9)*

✓4th **595 Cystitis**
EXCLUDES *prostatocystitis (601.3)*
Use additional code to identify organism, such as Escherichia coli [E. coli] (041.4)

595.0 Acute cystitis
EXCLUDES *trigonitis (595.3)*
AHA: 2Q, '99, 15
DEF: Acute inflammation of bladder.

595.1 Chronic interstitial cystitis
Hunner's ulcer
Submucous cystitis
Panmural fibrosis of bladder
DEF: Inflamed lesion affecting bladder wall; symptoms include urinary frequency, pain on bladder filling, nocturia, and distended bladder.

595.2 Other chronic cystitis
Chronic cystitis NOS
Subacute cystitis
EXCLUDES *trigonitis (595.3)*
DEF: Persistent inflammation of bladder.

595.3 Trigonitis
Follicular cystitis
Urethrotrigonitis
Trigonitis (acute) (chronic)
DEF: Inflammation of the triangular area of the bladder called the trigonum vesicae.

595.4 Cystitis in diseases classified elsewhere
Code first underlying disease, as:
actinomycosis (039.8)
amebiasis (006.8)
bilharziasis (120.0-120.9)
Echinococcus infestation (122.3, 122.6)
EXCLUDES *cystitis:*
diphtheritic (032.84)
gonococcal (098.11, 098.31)
monilial (112.2)
trichomonal (131.09)
tuberculous (016.1)

✓5th **595.8 Other specified types of cystitis**

595.81 Cystitis cystica
DEF: Inflammation of the bladder characterized by formation of multiple cysts.

595.82 Irradiation cystitis
Use additional E code to identify cause
DEF: Inflammation of the bladder due to effects of radiation.

595.89 Other
Abscess of bladder
Cystitis:
bullous
Cystitis:
emphysematous
glandularis

595.9 Cystitis, unspecified

✓4th **596 Other disorders of bladder**
Use additional code to identify urinary incontinence (625.6, 788.30-788.39)
AHA: M-A, '87, 10

596.0 Bladder neck obstruction
Contracture (acquired) } of bladder neck or vesicourethral orifice
Obstruction (acquired) } of bladder neck or vesicourethral orifice
Stenosis (acquired) } of bladder neck or vesicourethral orifice
EXCLUDES *congenital (753.6)*
AHA: 3Q '02, 28; 2Q, '01, 14; N-D, '86, 10
DEF: Bladder outlet and vesicourethral obstruction; occurs more often in males as a consequence of benign prostatic hypertrophy or prostatic cancer; may also occur in either sex due to strictures, following radiation, cystoscopy, catheterization, injury, infection, blood clots, bladder cancer, impaction or disease compressing bladder neck.

596.1 Intestinovesical fistula
Fistula:
enterovesical
vesicocolic
Fistula:
vesicoenteric
vesicorectal
DEF: Abnormal communication, between intestine and bladder.

596.2 Vesical fistula, not elsewhere classified
Fistula:
bladder NOS
urethrovesical
Fistula:
vesicocutaneous
vesicoperineal
EXCLUDES *fistula between bladder and female genital tract (619.0)*
DEF: Abnormal communication between bladder and another structure.

596.3 Diverticulum of bladder
Diverticulitis } of bladder
Diverticulum (acquired) (false) } of bladder
EXCLUDES *that with calculus in diverticulum of bladder (594.0)*
DEF: Abnormal pouch in bladder wall.

596.4 Atony of bladder
High compliance bladder
Hypotonicity } of bladder
Inertia } of bladder
EXCLUDES *neurogenic bladder (596.54)*
DEF: Distended, bladder with loss of expulsive force; linked to CNS disease.

✓5th **596.5 Other functional disorders of bladder**
EXCLUDES *cauda equina syndrome with neurogenic bladder (344.61)*

596.51 Hypertonicity of bladder
Hyperactivity
Overactive bladder
DEF: Abnormal tension of muscular wall of bladder; may appear after surgery of voluntary nerve.

596.52 Low bladder compliance
DEF: Low bladder capacity; causes increased pressure and frequent urination.

596.53 Paralysis of bladder
DEF: Impaired bladder motor function due to nerve or muscle damage.

596.54 Neurogenic bladder NOS
AHA: 1Q, '01, 12
DEF: Unspecified dysfunctional bladder due to lesion of central, peripheral nervous system; may result in incontinence, residual urine retention, urinary infection, stones and renal failure.

596.55 Detrusor sphincter dyssynergia
DEF: Instability of the urinary bladder sphincter muscle associated with urinary incontinence.

596.59 Other functional disorder of bladder
Detrusor instability
DEF: Detrusor instability: instability of bladder; marked by uninhibited contractions often leading to incontinence.

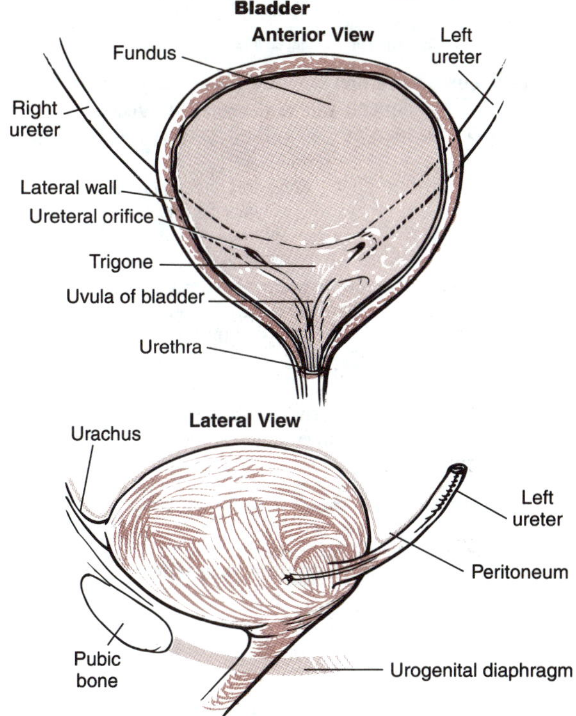

596.6 Rupture of bladder, nontraumatic

596.7 Hemorrhage into bladder wall

Hyperemia of bladder

EXCLUDES *acute hemorrhagic cystitis (595.0)*

596.8 Other specified disorders of bladder

Bladder: calcified, contracted, hemorrhage, hypertrophy

EXCLUDES *cystocele, female (618.01-618.02, 618.09, 618.2-618.4)*
hernia or prolapse of bladder, female (618.01-618.02, 618.09, 618.2-618.4)

AHA: J-F, '85, 8

596.9 Unspecified disorder of bladder

AHA: J-F, '85, 8

4th 597 Urethritis, not sexually transmitted, and urethral syndrome

EXCLUDES *nonspecific urethritis, so stated (099.4)*

597.0 Urethral abscess

Abscess:
- periurethral
- urethral (gland)

Abscess of:
- bulbourethral gland

Abscess of:
- Cowper's gland
- Littré's gland

Periurethral cellulitis

EXCLUDES *urethral caruncle (599.3)*

DEF: Pocket of pus in tube that empties urine from the bladder.

5th 597.8 Other urethritis

597.80 Urethritis, unspecified

597.81 Urethral syndrome NOS

597.89 Other

Adenitis, Skene's glands
Cowperitis
Meatitis, urethral
Ulcer, urethra (meatus)
Verumontanitis

EXCLUDES *trichomonal (131.02)*

4th 598 Urethral stricture

Use additional code to identify urinary incontinence (625.6, 788.30-788.39)

INCLUDES pinhole meatus
stricture of urinary meatus

EXCLUDES *congenital stricture of urethra and urinary meatus (753.6)*

DEF: Narrowing of tube that empties urine from bladder.

5th 598.0 Urethral stricture due to infection

598.00 Due to unspecified infection

598.01 Due to infective diseases classified elsewhere

Code first underlying disease, as:
gonococcal infection (098.2)
schistosomiasis (120.0-120.9)
syphilis (095.8)

598.1 Traumatic urethral stricture

Stricture of urethra: late effect of injury

Stricture of urethra: postobstetric

EXCLUDES *postoperative following surgery on genitourinary tract (598.2)*

598.2 Postoperative urethral stricture

Postcatheterization stricture of urethra

AHA: 3Q, '97, 6

598.8 Other specified causes of urethral stricture

AHA: N-D, '84, 9

598.9 Urethral stricture, unspecified

4th 599 Other disorders of urethra and urinary tract

599.0 Urinary tract infection, site not specified

EXCLUDES *candidiasis of urinary tract (112.2)*
urinary tract infection of newborn (771.82)

Use additional code to identify organism, such as Escherichia coli [E. coli] (041.4)

AHA: 2Q, '04, 13; 4Q, '03, 79; 4Q, '99, 6; 2Q, '99, 15;1Q, '98, 5; 2Q, '96, 7; 4Q, '96, 33; 2Q, '95, 7; 1Q, '92, 13

599.1 Urethral fistula

Fistula:
- urethroperineal
- urethrorectal

Urinary fistula NOS

EXCLUDES *fistula:*
urethroscrotal (608.89)
urethrovaginal (619.0)
urethrovesicovaginal (619.0)

AHA: 3Q, '97, 6

599.2 Urethral diverticulum

DEF: Abnormal pouch in urethral wall.

599.3 Urethral caruncle

Polyp of urethra

599.4 Urethral false passage

DEF: Abnormal opening in urethra due to surgery, trauma or disease.

599.5 Prolapsed urethral mucosa

Prolapse of urethra
Urethrocele

EXCLUDES *urethrocele, female (618.03, 618.09, 618.2-618.4)*

▲ **5th 599.6 Urinary obstruction**

Use additional code to identify urinary incontinence (625.6, 788.30-788.39)

EXCLUDES *obstructive nephropathy NOS (593.89)*
►urinary obstruction due to hyperplasia of prostate (600.0-600.9 with fifth-digit 1)◄

● **599.60 Urinary obstruction, unspecified**

Obstructive uropathy NOS
Urinary (tract) obstruction NOS

● **599.69 Urinary obstruction, not elsewhere classified**

599.7 Hematuria

Hematuria (benign) (essential)

EXCLUDES *hemoglobinuria (791.2)*

AHA: 1Q, '00, 5; 3Q, '95, 8

DEF: Blood in urine.

5th 599.8 Other specified disorders of urethra and urinary tract

Use additional code to identify urinary incontinence (625.6, 788.30-788.39)

EXCLUDES *symptoms and other conditions classifiable to 788.0-788.2, 788.4-788.9, 791.0-791.9*

599.81 Urethral hypermobility

DEF: Hyperactive urethra.

599.82 Intrinsic (urethral) spincter deficiency [ISD]

AHA: 2Q, '96, 15

DEF: Malfunctioning urethral sphincter.

599.83 Urethral instability

DEF: Inconsistent functioning of urethra.

599.84 Other specified disorders of urethra

Rupture of urethra (nontraumatic)
Urethral:
- cyst
- granuloma

DEF: Rupture of urethra; due to herniation or breaking down of tissue; not due to trauma.
DEF: Urethral cyst: abnormal sac in urethra; usually fluid filled.
DEF: Granuloma: inflammatory cells forming small nodules in urethra.

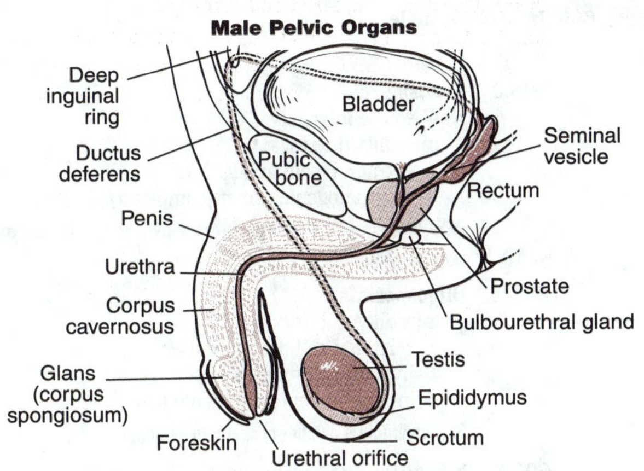

599.89 **Other specified disorders of urinary tract**

599.9 **Unspecified disorder of urethra and urinary tract**

DISEASES OF MALE GENITAL ORGANS (600-608)

✓4th **600 Hyperplasia of prostate**

Use additional code to identify urinary incontinence (788.30-788.39)

AHA: 4Q, '00, 43; 3Q, '94, 12; 3Q, '92, 7; N-D, '86, 10

DEF: Fibrostromal proliferation in periurethral glands, causes blood in urine; etiology unknown.

✓5th **600.0 Hypertrophy (benign) of prostate**

Benign prostatic hypertrophy
Enlargement of prostate
Smooth enlarged prostate
Soft enlarged prostate

AHA: 4Q, '03, 63; 1Q, '03, 6; 3Q '02, 28; 2Q, '01, 14

600.00 Hypertrophy (benign) of prostate without urinary obstruction A ♂

Hypertrophy (benign) of prostate NOS

600.01 Hypertrophy (benign) of prostate with urinary obstruction A ♂

Hypertrophy (benign) of prostate with urinary retention

AHA: 4Q, '03, 64

✓5th **600.1 Nodular prostate**

Hard, firm prostate
Multinodular prostate

EXCLUDES *malignant neoplasm of prostate (185)*

AHA: 4Q, '03, 63

DEF: Hard, firm nodule in prostate.

600.10 Nodular prostate without urinary obstruction A ♂

Nodular prostate NOS

600.11 Nodular prostate with urinary obstruction A ♂

Nodular prostate with urinary retention

✓5th **600.2 Benign localized hyperplasia of prostate**

Adenofibromatous hypertrophy of prostate
Adenoma of prostate
Fibroadenoma of prostate
Fibroma of prostate
Myoma of prostate
Polyp of prostate

EXCLUDES *benign neoplasms of prostate (222.2)*
hypertrophy of prostate (600.00-600.01)
malignant neoplasm of prostate (185)

AHA: 4Q, '03, 63

DEF: Benign localized hyperplasia is a clearly defined epithelial tumor. Other terms used for this condition are adenofibromatous hypertrophy of prostate, adenoma of prostate, fibroadenoma of prostate, fibroma of prostate, myoma of prostate, and polyp of prostate.

600.20 Benign localized hyperplasia of prostate without urinary obstruction A ♂

Benign localized hyperplasia of prostate NOS

600.21 Benign localized hyperplasia of prostate with urinary obstruction A ♂

Benign localized hyperplasia of prostate with urinary retention

600.3 Cyst of prostate A ♂

DEF: Sacs of fluid, which differentiate this from either nodular or adenomatous tumors.

✓5th **600.9 Hyperplasia of prostate, unspecified**

Median bar
Prostatic obstruction NOS

AHA: 4Q, '03, 63

600.90 Hyperplasia of prostate, unspecified, without urinary obstruction A ♂

Hyperplasia of prostate NOS

600.91 Hyperplasia of prostate, unspecified, with urinary obstruction A ♂

Hyperplasia of prostate, unspecified, with urinary retention

✓4th **601 Inflammatory diseases of prostate**

Use additional code to identify organism, such as Staphylococcus (041.1), or Streptococcus (041.0)

601.0 Acute prostatitis A ♂

601.1 Chronic prostatitis A ♂

601.2 Abscess of prostate A ♂

601.3 Prostatocystitis A ♂

601.4 ***Prostatitis in diseases classified elsewhere*** A ♂

Code first underlying disease, as:
actinomycosis (039.8)
blastomycosis (116.0)
syphilis (095.8)
tuberculosis (016.5)

EXCLUDES *prostatitis:*
gonococcal (098.12, 098.32)
monilial (112.2)
trichomonal (131.03)

601.8 Other specified inflammatory diseases of prostate A ♂

Prostatitis:
cavitary
diverticular
granulomatous

601.9 Prostatitis, unspecified A ♂

Prostatitis NOS

Common Inguinal Canal Anomalies

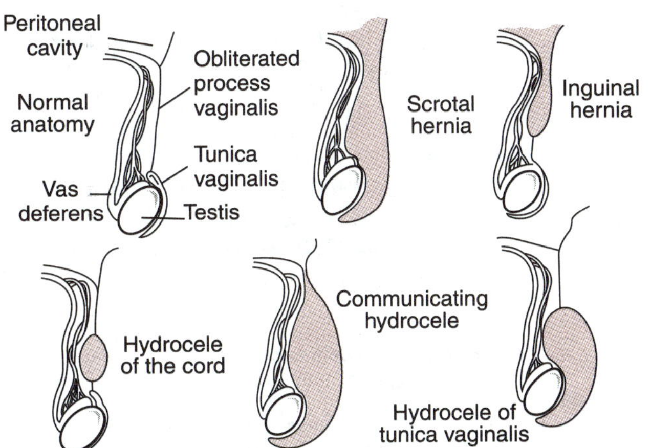

✓4th **602 Other disorders of prostate**

602.0 Calculus of prostate A ♂
Prostatic stone
DEF: Stone or mineral deposit in prostate.

602.1 Congestion or hemorrhage of prostate A ♂
DEF: Bleeding or fluid collection in prostate.

602.2 Atrophy of prostate A ♂

602.3 Dysplasia of prostate ♂
Prostatic intraepithelial neoplasia I (PIN I)
Prostatic intraepithelial neoplasia II (PIN II)
EXCLUDES *prostatic intraepithelial neoplasia III (PIN III) (233.4)*
AHA: 4Q, '01, 46
DEF: Abnormality of shape and size of the intraepithelial tissues of the prostate; pre-malignant condition characterized by stalks and absence of a basilar cell layer; synonyms are intraductal dysplasia, large acinar atypical hyperplasia, atypical primary hyperplasia, hyperplasia with malignant changes, marked atypia, or duct-acinar dysplasia.

602.8 Other specified disorders of prostate A ♂
Fistula, Infarction, Stricture } of prostate
Periprostatic adhesions

602.9 Unspecified disorder of prostate A ♂

✓4th **603 Hydrocele**
INCLUDES hydrocele of spermatic cord, testis, or tunica vaginalis
EXCLUDES *congenital (778.6)*
DEF: Circumscribed collection of fluid in tunica vaginalis, spermatic cord or testis.

603.0 Encysted hydrocele

603.1 Infected hydrocele
Use additional code to identify organism

603.8 Other specified types of hydrocele

603.9 Hydrocele, unspecified

✓4th **604 Orchitis and epididymitis**
Use additional code to identify organism, such as Escherichia coli [E. coli] (041.4), Staphylococcus (041.1), or Streptococcus (041.0)

604.0 Orchitis, epididymitis, and epididymo-orchitis, with abscess ♂
Abscess of epididymis or testis

✓5th **604.9 Other orchitis, epididymitis, and epididymo-orchitis, without mention of abscess**

604.90 Orchitis and epididymitis, unspecified ♂

604.91 Orchitis and epididymitis in diseases classified elsewhere ♂
Code first underlying disease, as:
diphtheria (032.89)
filariasis (125.0-125.9)
syphilis (095.8)
EXCLUDES *orchitis:*
gonococcal (098.13, 098.33)
mumps (072.0)
tuberculous (016.5)
tuberculous epididymitis (016.4)

604.99 Other ♂

605 Redundant prepuce and phimosis ♂
Adherent prepuce
Paraphimosis
Phimosis (congenital)
Tight foreskin
DEF: Constriction of preputial orifice causing inability of the prepuce to be drawn back over the glans; it may be congenital or caused by infection.

✓4th **606 Infertility, male**
AHA: 2Q, '96, 9

606.0 Azoospermia A ♂
Absolute infertility
Infertility due to:
germinal (cell) aplasia
spermatogenic arrest (complete)
DEF: Absence of spermatozoa in the semen or inability to produce spermatozoa.

606.1 Oligospermia A ♂
Infertility due to:
germinal cell desquamation
hypospermatogenesis
incomplete spermatogenic arrest
DEF: Insufficient number of sperm in semen.

606.8 Infertility due to extratesticular causes A ♂
Infertility due to:
drug therapy
infection
obstruction of efferent ducts
radiation
systemic disease

606.9 Male infertility, unspecified A ♂

✓4th **607 Disorders of penis**
EXCLUDES *phimosis (605)*

607.0 Leukoplakia of penis ♂
Kraurosis of penis
EXCLUDES *carcinoma in situ of penis (233.5)*
erythroplasia of Queyrat (233.5)
DEF: White, thickened patches on glans penis.

607.1 Balanoposthitis ♂
Balanitis
Use additional code to identify organism
DEF: Inflammation of glans penis and prepuce.

607.2 Other inflammatory disorders of penis ♂
Abscess, Boil, Carbuncle, Cellulitis } of corpus cavernosum or penis
Cavernitis (penis)
Use additional code to identify organism
EXCLUDES *herpetic infection (054.13)*

607.3 Priapism ♂
Painful erection
DEF: Prolonged penile erection without sexual stimulation.

✓5th **607.8 Other specified disorders of penis**

607.81 Balanitis xerotica obliterans ♂
Induratio penis plastica
DEF: Inflammation of the glans penis, caused by stricture of the opening of the prepuce.

607.82 Vascular disorders of penis ♂
Embolism, Hematoma (nontraumatic), Hemorrhage, Thrombosis } of corpus cavernosum or penis

607.83 Edema of penis ♂
DEF: Fluid retention within penile tissues.

607.84 Impotence of organic origin A ♂
EXCLUDES ▶ *nonorganic (302.72)*◀
AHA: 3Q, '91, 11
DEF: Physiological cause interfering with erection.

607.85 Peyronie's disease ♂
AHA: 4Q, '03, 64
DEF: A severe curvature of the erect penis due to fibrosis of the cavernous sheaths.

Torsion of Testis

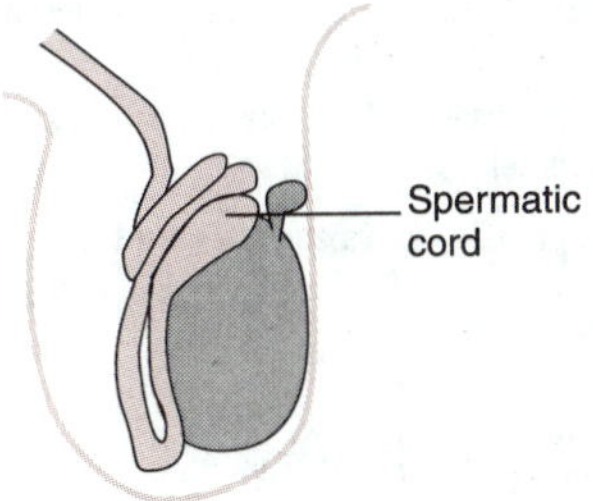

Torsion of testis

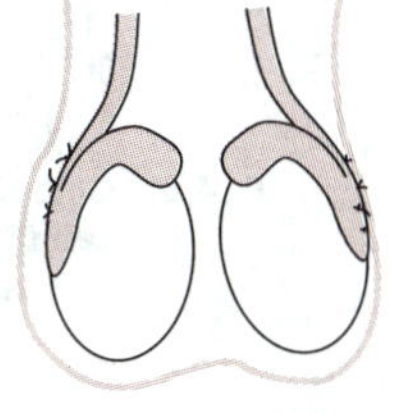
Testes after correction showing bilateral fixation

607.89 Other ♂
Atrophy, Fibrosis, Hypertrophy, Ulcer (chronic) } of corpus cavernosum or penis

607.9 Unspecified disorder of penis ♂

✓4th **608 Other disorders of male genital organs**

608.0 Seminal vesiculitis ♂
Abscess, Cellulitis } of seminal vesicle
Vesiculitis (seminal)
Use additional code to identify organism
EXCLUDES *gonococcal infection (098.14, 098.34)*
DEF: Inflammation of seminal vesicle.

608.1 Spermatocele ♂
DEF: Cystic enlargement of the epididymis or the testis; the cysts contain spermatozoa.

608.2 Torsion of testis ♂
Torsion of:
epididymis
spermatic cord
Torsion of:
testicle
DEF: Twisted or rotated testis; may compromise blood flow.

608.3 Atrophy of testis ♂

608.4 Other inflammatory disorders of male genital organs ♂
Abscess, Boil, Carbuncle, Cellulitis } of scrotum, spermatic cord, testis [except abscess], tunica vaginalis, or vas deferens
Vasitis
Use additional code to identify organism
EXCLUDES *abscess of testis (604.0)*

✓5th **608.8 Other specified disorders of male genital organs**

608.81 Disorders of male genital organs in diseases classified elsewhere ♂
Code first underlying disease, as:
filariasis (125.0-125.9)
tuberculosis (016.5)

608.82 Hematospermia ♂
AHA: 4Q, '01, 46
DEF: Presence of blood in the ejaculate; relatively common, affecting men of any age after puberty; cause is often difficult to determine since the semen originates in several organs, often the result of a viral bacterial infection and inflammation.

608.83 Vascular disorders ♂
Hematoma (non-traumatic), Hemorrhage, Thrombosis } of seminal vesicle, spermatic cord, testis, scrotum, tunica vaginalis, or vas deferens
Hematocele NOS, male
AHA: 4Q, '03, 110

608.84 Chylocele of tunica vaginalis ♂
DEF: Chylous effusion into tunica vaginalis; due to infusion of lymphatic fluids.

608.85 Stricture ♂
Stricture of:
spermatic cord
tunica vaginalis
Stricture of:
vas deferens

608.86 Edema ♂

608.87 Retrograde ejaculation ♂
AHA: 4Q, '01, 46
DEF: Condition where the semen travels to the bladder rather than out through the urethra due to damaged nerves causing the bladder neck to remain open during ejaculation.

608.89 Other ♂
Atrophy, Fibrosis, Hypertrophy, Ulcer } of seminal vesicle, spermatic cord, testis, scrotum, tunica vaginalis, or vas deferens
EXCLUDES *atrophy of testis (608.3)*

608.9 Unspecified disorder of male genital organs ♂

DISORDERS OF BREAST (610-611)

✓4th **610 Benign mammary dysplasias**

610.0 Solitary cyst of breast
Cyst (solitary) of breast

610.1 Diffuse cystic mastopathy A
Chronic cystic mastitis
Cystic breast
Fibrocystic disease of breast
DEF: Extensive formation of nodular cysts in breast tissue; symptoms include tenderness, change in size and hyperplasia of ductal epithelium.

610.2 Fibroadenosis of breast
Fibroadenosis of breast:
NOS
chronic
cystic
Fibroadenosis of breast:
diffuse
periodic
segmental
DEF: Non-neoplastic nodular condition of breast.

610.3 Fibrosclerosis of breast
DEF: Fibrous tissue in breast.

610.4 Mammary duct ectasia
Comedomastitis
Duct ectasia
Mastitis:
periductal
plasma cell
DEF: Atrophy of duct epithelium; causes distended collecting ducts of mammary gland; drying up of breast secretion, intraductal inflammation and periductal and interstitial chronic inflammatory reaction.

610.8 Other specified benign mammary dysplasias
Mazoplasia
Sebaceous cyst of breast

610.9 Benign mammary dysplasia, unspecified

✓4th **611 Other disorders of breast**
EXCLUDES *that associated with lactation or the puerperium (675.0-676.9)*

611.0 Inflammatory disease of breast
Abscess (acute) (chronic) (nonpuerperal) of:
areola
breast
Mammillary fistula
Mastitis (acute) (subacute) (nonpuerperal):
NOS
infective
retromammary
submammary
EXCLUDES *carbuncle of breast (680.2)*
chronic cystic mastitis (610.1)
neonatal infective mastitis (771.5)
thrombophlebitis of breast [Mondor's disease] (451.89)

611.1 Hypertrophy of breast
Gynecomastia
Hypertrophy of breast:
NOS
massive pubertal

611.2 Fissure of nipple

611.3 Fat necrosis of breast
Fat necrosis (segmental) of breast

DEF: Splitting of neutral fats in adipose tissue cells as a result of trauma; a firm circumscribed mass is then formed in the breast.

611.4 Atrophy of breast

611.5 Galactocele

DEF: Milk-filled cyst in breast; due to blocked duct.

611.6 Galactorrhea not associated with childbirth

DEF: Flow of milk not associated with childbirth or pregnancy.

✓5th **611.7 Signs and symptoms in breast**

611.71 Mastodynia
Pain in breast

611.72 Lump or mass in breast
AHA: 2Q, '03, 4-5

611.79 Other
Induration of breast
Inversion of nipple
Nipple discharge
Retraction of nipple

611.8 Other specified disorders of breast
Hematoma (nontraumatic) } of breast
Infarction } of breast
Occlusion of breast duct
Subinvolution of breast (postlactational) (postpartum)

611.9 Unspecified breast disorder

INFLAMMATORY DISEASE OF FEMALE PELVIC ORGANS (614-616)

Use additional code to identify organism, such as Staphylococcus (041.1), or Streptococcus (041.0)

EXCLUDES *that associated with pregnancy, abortion, childbirth, or the puerperium (630-676.9)*

✓4th **614 Inflammatory disease of ovary, fallopian tube, pelvic cellular tissue, and peritoneum**

EXCLUDES *endometritis (615.0-615.9)*
major infection following delivery (670)
that complicating:
abortion (634-638 with .0, 639.0)
ectopic or molar pregnancy (639.0)
pregnancy or labor (646.6)

614.0 Acute salpingitis and oophoritis ♀
Any condition classifiable to 614.2, specified as acute or subacute

DEF: Acute inflammation, of ovary and fallopian tube.

614.1 Chronic salpingitis and oophoritis ♀
Hydrosalpinx
Salpingitis:
follicularis
isthmica nodosa
Any condition classifiable to 614.2, specified as chronic

DEF: Persistent inflammation of ovary and fallopian tube.

614.2 Salpingitis and oophoritis not specified as acute, subacute, or chronic ♀
Abscess (of):
fallopian tube
ovary
tubo-ovarian
Oophoritis
Perioophoritis
Pyosalpinx
Perisalpingitis
Salpingitis
Salpingo-oophoritis
Tubo-ovarian inflammatory disease

EXCLUDES *gonococcal infection (chronic) (098.37)*
acute (098.17)
tuberculous (016.6)

AHA: 2Q, '91, 5

614.3 Acute parametritis and pelvic cellulitis ♀
Acute inflammatory pelvic disease
Any condition classifiable to 614.4, specified as acute

DEF: Parametritis: inflammation of the parametrium; pelvic cellulitis is a synonym for parametritis.

614.4 Chronic or unspecified parametritis and pelvic cellulitis ♀
Abscess (of):
broad ligament } chronic or NOS
parametrium } chronic or NOS
pelvis, female } chronic or NOS
pouch of Douglas } chronic or NOS
Chronic inflammatory pelvic disease
Pelvic cellulitis, female

EXCLUDES *tuberculous (016.7)*

614.5 Acute or unspecified pelvic peritonitis, female ♀

614.6 Pelvic peritoneal adhesions, female (postoperative) (postinfection) ♀
Adhesions:
peritubal
tubo-ovarian
Use additional code to identify any associated infertility (628.2)

AHA: 3Q, '03, 6; 1Q, '03, 4; 3Q, '95, 7; 3Q, '94, 12

DEF: Fibrous scarring abnormally joining structures within abdomen.

614.7 Other chronic pelvic peritonitis, female ♀

EXCLUDES *tuberculous (016.7)*

614.8 Other specified inflammatory disease of female pelvic organs and tissues ♀

614.9 Unspecified inflammatory disease of female pelvic organs and tissues ♀
Pelvic infection or inflammation, female NOS
Pelvic inflammatory disease [PID]

✓4th **615 Inflammatory diseases of uterus, except cervix**

EXCLUDES *following delivery (670)*
hyperplastic endometritis (621.30-621.33)
that complicating:
abortion (634-638 with .0, 639.0)
ectopic or molar pregnancy (639.0)
pregnancy or labor (646.6)

615.0 Acute ♀
Any condition classifiable to 615.9, specified as acute or subacute

615.1 Chronic ♀
Any condition classifiable to 615.9, specified as chronic

615.9 Unspecified inflammatory disease of uterus ♀
Endometritis
Endomyometritis
Metritis
Myometritis
Perimetritis
Pyometra
Uterine abscess

Female Genitourinary System

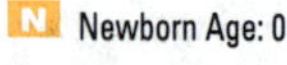 Newborn Age: 0
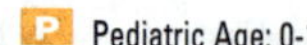 Pediatric Age: 0-17
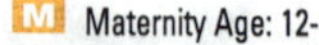 Maternity Age: 12-55
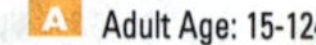 Adult Age: 15-124
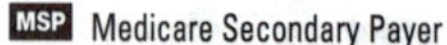 Medicare Secondary Payer

Common Sites of Endometriosis

Common sites of endometriosis, in descending order of frequency:
(1) ovary
(2) cul de sac
(3) utersacral ligaments
(4) broad ligaments
(5) fallopian tube
(6) uterovesical fold
(7) round ligament
(8) vermiform appedix
(9) vagina
(10) rectovaginal septum

✓4th **616 Inflammatory disease of cervix, vagina, and vulva**

EXCLUDES *that complicating:*
abortion (634-638 with .0, 639.0)
ectopic or molar pregnancy (639.0)
pregnancy, childbirth, or the puerperium (646.6)

616.0 Cervicitis and endocervicitis ♀

Cervicitis } with or without mention of
Endocervicitis } erosion or ectropion

Nabothian (gland) cyst or follicle

EXCLUDES *erosion or ectropion without mention of cervicitis (622.0)*

✓5th **616.1 Vaginitis and vulvovaginitis**

DEF: Inflammation or infection of vagina or external female genitalia.

616.10 Vaginitis and vulvovaginitis, unspecified ♀

Vaginitis:
NOS
postirradiation
Vulvitis NOS
Vulvovaginitis NOS
Use additional code to identify organism, such as Escherichia coli [E. coli] (041.4), Staphylococcus (041.1), or Streptococcus (041.0)

EXCLUDES *noninfective leukorrhea (623.5)*
postmenopausal or senile vaginitis (627.3)

616.11 Vaginitis and vulvovaginitis in diseases classified elsewhere ♀

Code first underlying disease, as:
pinworm vaginitis (127.4)

EXCLUDES *herpetic vulvovaginitis (054.11)*
monilial vulvotaginitis (112.1)
trichomonal vaginitis or vulvovaginitis (131.01)

616.2 Cyst of Bartholin's gland ♀

Bartholin's duct cyst

DEF: Fluid-filled sac within gland of vaginal orifice.

616.3 Abscess of Bartholin's gland ♀

Vulvovaginal gland abscess

616.4 Other abscess of vulva ♀

Abscess }
Carbuncle } of vulva
Furuncle }

✓5th **616.5 Ulceration of vulva**

616.50 Ulceration of vulva, unspecified ♀

Ulcer NOS of vulva

616.51 Ulceration of vulva in diseases classified elsewhere ♀

Code first underlying disease, as:
Behçet's syndrome (136.1)
tuberculosis (016.7)

EXCLUDES *vulvar ulcer (in):*
gonococcal (098.0)
herpes simplex (054.12)
syphilitic (091.0)

616.8 Other specified inflammatory diseases of cervix, vagina, and vulva ♀

Caruncle, vagina or labium
Ulcer, vagina

EXCLUDES *noninflammatory disorders of:*
cervix (622.0-622.9)
vagina (623.0-623.9)
vulva (624.0-624.9)

616.9 Unspecified inflammatory disease of cervix, vagina, and vulva ♀

OTHER DISORDERS OF FEMALE GENITAL TRACT (617-629)

✓4th **617 Endometriosis**

617.0 Endometriosis of uterus ♀

Adenomyosis
Endometriosis:
cervix
internal
myometrium

EXCLUDES *stromal endometriosis (236.0)*

AHA: 3Q, '92, 7

DEF: Aberrant uterine mucosal tissue; creating products of menses and inflamed uterine tissues.

617.1 Endometriosis of ovary ♀

Chocolate cyst of ovary
Endometrial cystoma of ovary

DEF: Aberrant uterine tissue; creating products of menses and inflamed ovarian tissues.

617.2 Endometriosis of fallopian tube ♀

DEF: Aberrant uterine tissue; creating products of menses and inflamed tissues of fallopian tubes.

617.3 Endometriosis of pelvic peritoneum ♀

Endometriosis:
broad ligament
cul-de-sac (Douglas')
parametrium
round ligament

DEF: Aberrant uterine tissue; creating products of menses and inflamed peritoneum tissues.

617.4 Endometriosis of rectovaginal septum and vagina ♀

DEF: Aberrant uterine tissue; creating products of menses and inflamed tissues in and behind vagina.

617.5 Endometriosis of intestine ♀

Endometriosis:
appendix
colon
rectum

DEF: Aberrant uterine tissue; creating products of menses and inflamed intestinal tissues.

Types of Vaginal Hernias

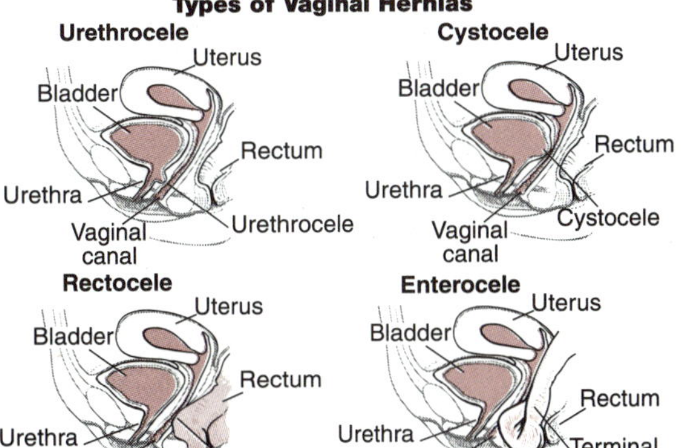

▶Vaginal Midline Cystocele◀

Normal vaginal support

Uterus
Pubocervical fascia
Bladder
Rectum
Urethra
Rectovaginal fascia
Uterus
Vaginal epithelium
Bladder
Urethra
Defect of pubocervical fascia

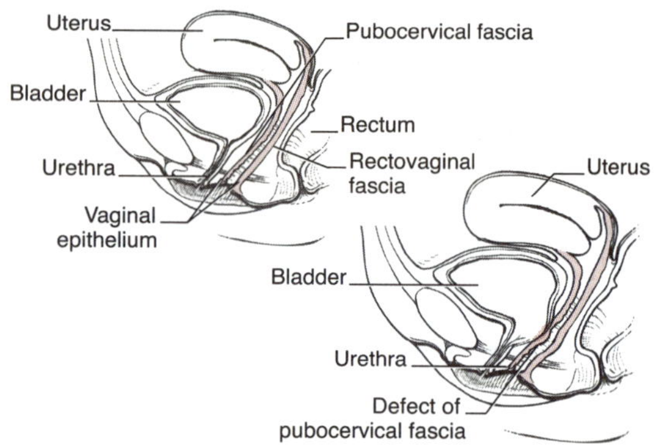

617.6 Endometriosis in scar of skin ♀

617.8 Endometriosis of other specified sites ♀

Endometriosis:
- bladder
- lung

Endometriosis:
- umbilicus
- vulva

617.9 Endometriosis, site unspecified ♀

✓4th **618 Genital prolapse**

Use additional code to identify urinary incontinence (625.6, 788.31, 788.33-788.39)

EXCLUDES *that complicating pregnancy, labor, or delivery (654.4)*

✓5th **618.0 Prolapse of vaginal walls without mention of uterine prolapse**

EXCLUDES *that with uterine prolapse (618.2-618.4)*
enterocele (618.6)
vaginal vault prolapse following hysterectomy (618.5)

618.00 Unspecified prolapse of vaginal walls ♀

Vaginal prolapse NOS

618.01 Cystocele, midline ♀

Cystocele NOS

DEF: ▶Defect in the pubocervical fascia, the supportive layer of the bladder, causing bladder drop and herniated into the vagina along the midline.◀

618.02 Cystocele, lateral ♀

Paravaginal

DEF: ▶Loss of support of the lateral attachment of the vagina at the arcus tendinous results in bladder drop; bladder herniates into the vagina laterally; also called paravaginal defect.◀

618.03 Urethrocele ♀

618.04 Rectocele ♀

Proctocele

618.05 Perineocele ♀

618.09 Other prolapse of vaginal walls without mention of uterine prolapse ♀

Cystourethrocele

▶Vaginal Lateral Cystocele◀

Normal vaginal support

Symphysis pubis
Cooper's ligament
Arcus tendineus
Bladder
Pubocervical fascia
Arcus tendineus defect

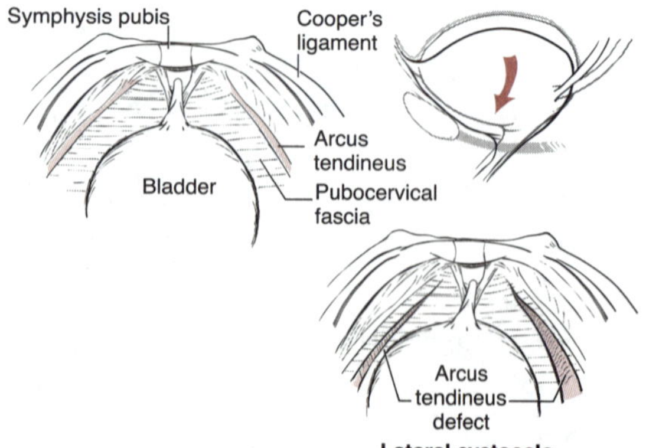

Lateral cystocele

618.1 Uterine prolapse without mention of vaginal wall prolapse ♀

Descensus uteri
Uterine prolapse:
- NOS
- complete

Uterine prolapse:
- first degree
- second degree
- third degree

EXCLUDES *that with mention of cystocele, urethrocele, or rectocele (618.2-618.4)*

618.2 Uterovaginal prolapse, incomplete ♀

DEF: Downward displacement of uterus downward into vagina.

618.3 Uterovaginal prolapse, complete ♀

DEF: Downward displacement of uterus exposed within external genitalia.

618.4 Uterovaginal prolapse, unspecified ♀

618.5 Prolapse of vaginal vault after hysterectomy ♀

618.6 Vaginal enterocele, congenital or acquired ♀

Pelvic enterocele, congenital or acquired

DEF: Vaginal vault hernia formed by the loop of the small intestine protruding into the rectal vaginal pouch; can also accompany uterine prolapse or follow hysterectomy.

618.7 Old laceration of muscles of pelvic floor ♀

✓5th **618.8 Other specified genital prolapse**

618.81 Incompetence or weakening of pubocervical tissue ♀

618.82 Incompetence or weakening of rectovaginal tissue ♀

618.83 Pelvic muscle wasting ♀

Disuse atrophy of pelvic muscles and anal sphincter

618.89 Other specified genital prolapse ♀

Incompetence or weakening of pelvic fundus
Relaxation of vaginal outlet or pelvis

618.9 Unspecified genital prolapse ♀

✓4th **619 Fistula involving female genital tract**

EXCLUDES *vesicorectal and intestinovesical fistula (596.1)*

619.0 Urinary-genital tract fistula, female ♀

Fistula:
- cervicovesical
- ureterovaginal
- urethrovaginal
- urethrovesicovaginal

Fistula:
- uteroureteric
- uterovesical
- vesicocervicovaginal
- vesicovaginal

619.1 Digestive-genital tract fistula, female ♀

Fistula:
- intestinouterine
- intestinovaginal
- rectovaginal

Fistula:
- rectovulval
- sigmoidovaginal
- uterorectal

619.2 Genital tract-skin fistula, female ♀

Fistula:
- uterus to abdominal wall
- vaginoperineal

619.8 Other specified fistulas involving female genital tract ♀

Fistula:
- cervix
- cul-de-sac (Douglas')

Fistula:
- uterus
- vagina

DEF: Abnormal communication between female reproductive tract and skin.

619.9 Unspecified fistula involving female genital tract ♀

✓4th **620 Noninflammatory disorders of ovary, fallopian tube, and broad ligament**

EXCLUDES *hydrosalpinx (614.1)*

620.0 Follicular cyst of ovary ♀

Cyst of graafian follicle

DEF: Fluid-filled, encapsulated cyst due to occluded follicle duct that secretes hormones into ovaries.

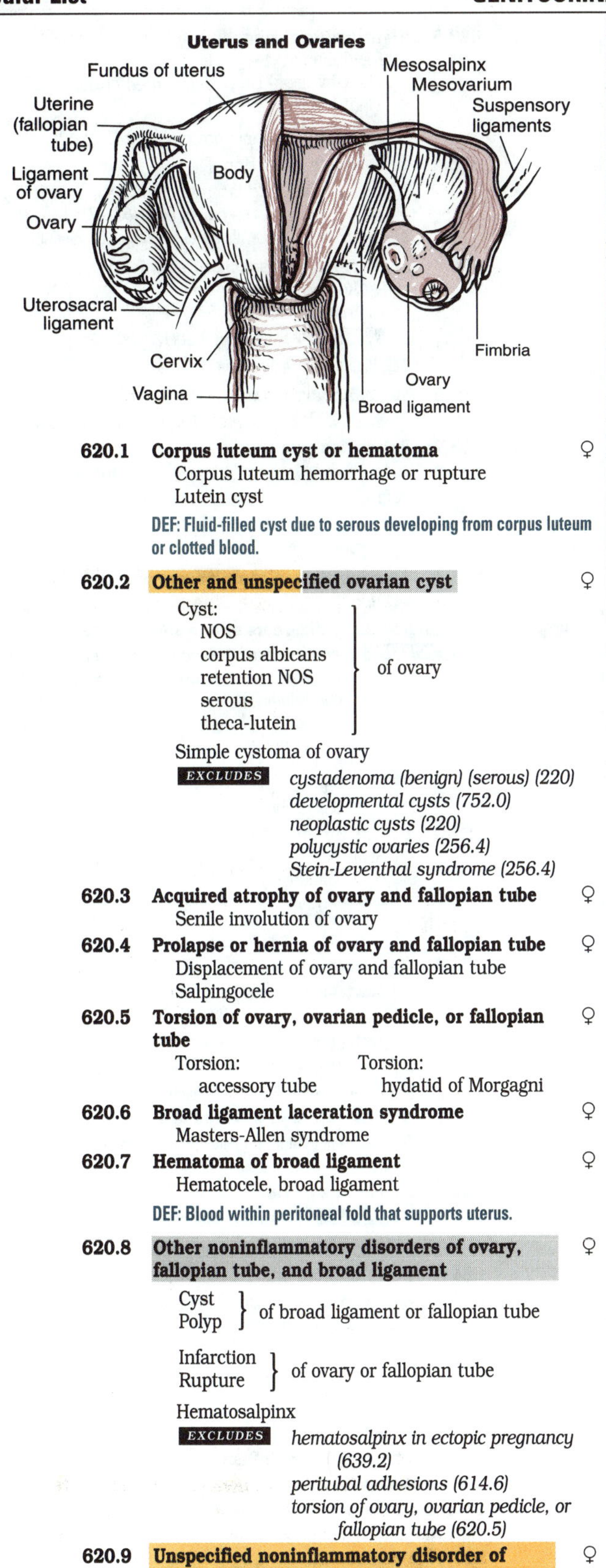

620.1 Corpus luteum cyst or hematoma ♀
Corpus luteum hemorrhage or rupture
Lutein cyst
DEF: Fluid-filled cyst due to serous developing from corpus luteum or clotted blood.

620.2 Other and unspecified ovarian cyst ♀
Cyst:
- NOS
- corpus albicans
- retention NOS
- serous
- theca-lutein

} of ovary

Simple cystoma of ovary
EXCLUDES *cystadenoma (benign) (serous) (220)*
developmental cysts (752.0)
neoplastic cysts (220)
polycystic ovaries (256.4)
Stein-Leventhal syndrome (256.4)

620.3 Acquired atrophy of ovary and fallopian tube ♀
Senile involution of ovary

620.4 Prolapse or hernia of ovary and fallopian tube ♀
Displacement of ovary and fallopian tube
Salpingocele

620.5 Torsion of ovary, ovarian pedicle, or fallopian tube ♀
Torsion: accessory tube
Torsion: hydatid of Morgagni

620.6 Broad ligament laceration syndrome ♀
Masters-Allen syndrome

620.7 Hematoma of broad ligament ♀
Hematocele, broad ligament
DEF: Blood within peritoneal fold that supports uterus.

620.8 Other noninflammatory disorders of ovary, fallopian tube, and broad ligament ♀
Cyst, Polyp } of broad ligament or fallopian tube
Infarction, Rupture } of ovary or fallopian tube
Hematosalpinx
EXCLUDES *hematosalpinx in ectopic pregnancy (639.2)*
peritubal adhesions (614.6)
torsion of ovary, ovarian pedicle, or fallopian tube (620.5)

620.9 Unspecified noninflammatory disorder of ovary, fallopian tube, and broad ligament ♀

✓4th **621 Disorders of uterus, not elsewhere classified**

621.0 Polyp of corpus uteri ♀
Polyp: endometrium
Polyp: uterus NOS
EXCLUDES *cervical polyp NOS (622.7)*

621.1 Chronic subinvolution of uterus ♀
EXCLUDES *puerperal (674.8)*
AHA: 1Q, '91, 11
DEF: Abnormal size of uterus after delivery; the uterus does not return to its normal size after the birth of a child.

621.2 Hypertrophy of uterus ♀
Bulky or enlarged uterus
EXCLUDES *puerperal (674.8)*

✓5th **621.3 Endometrial hyperplasia**
Hyperplasia (adenomatous) (cystic) (glandular) of endometrium
DEF: Abnormal cystic overgrowth of endometrial tissue.

621.30 Endometrial hyperplasia, unspecified ♀
Endometrial hyperplasia NOS

621.31 Simple endometrial hyperplasia without atypia ♀

621.32 Complex endometrial hyperplasia without atypia ♀

621.33 Endometrial hyperplasia with atypia ♀

621.4 Hematometra ♀
Hemometra
EXCLUDES *that in congenital anomaly (752.2-752.3)*
DEF: Accumulated blood in uterus.

621.5 Intrauterine synechiae ♀
Adhesions of uterus
Band(s) of uterus

621.6 Malposition of uterus ♀
Anteversion, Retroflexion, Retroversion } of uterus
EXCLUDES *malposition complicating pregnancy, labor, or delivery (654.3-654.4)*
prolapse of uterus (618.1-618.4)

621.7 Chronic inversion of uterus ♀
EXCLUDES *current obstetrical trauma (665.2)*
prolapse of uterus (618.1-618.4)

621.8 Other specified disorders of uterus, not elsewhere classified ♀
Atrophy, acquired
Cyst
Fibrosis NOS
Old laceration (postpartum)
Ulcer
} of uterus
EXCLUDES *bilharzial fibrosis (120.0-120.9)*
endometriosis (617.0)
fistulas (619.0-619.8)
inflammatory diseases (615.0-615.9)

621.9 Unspecified disorder of uterus ♀

✓4th **622 Noninflammatory disorders of cervix**
EXCLUDES *abnormality of cervix complicating pregnancy, labor, or delivery (654.5-654.6)*
fistula (619.0-619.8)

622.0 Erosion and ectropion of cervix ♀
Eversion, Ulcer } of cervix
EXCLUDES *that in chronic cervicitis (616.0)*
DEF: Ulceration or turning outward of uterine cervix.

✓5th **622.1 Dysplasia of cervix (uteri)**
EXCLUDES *abnormal results from cervical cytologic examination without histologic confirmation (795.00-795.09)*
carcinoma in situ of cervix (233.1)
cervical intraepithelial neoplasia III [CIN III] (233.1)
AHA: 1Q, '91, 11
DEF: Abnormal cell structures in portal between uterus and vagina.

622.10 Dysplasia of cervix, unspecified ♀
Anaplasia of cervix
Cervical atypism
Cervical dysplasia NOS

622.11 Mild dysplasia of cervix ♀
Cervical intraepithelial neoplasia I [CIN I]

622.12 Moderate dysplasia of cervix ♀
Cervical intraepithelial neoplasia II [CIN II]
EXCLUDES *carcinoma in situ of cervix (233.1)*
cervical intraepithelial neoplasia III [CIN III] (233.1)
severe dysplasia (233.1)

622.2 Leukoplakia of cervix (uteri) ♀
DEF: Abnormal cell structures in portal between uterus and vagina.
EXCLUDES *carcinoma in situ of cervix (233.1)*
DEF: Thickened, white patches on portal between uterus and vagina.

622.3 Old laceration of cervix ♀
Adhesions / Band(s) / Cicatrix (postpartum) } of cervix
EXCLUDES *current obstetrical trauma (665.3)*
DEF: Scarring or other evidence of old wound on cervix.

622.4 Stricture and stenosis of cervix ♀
Atresia (acquired) / Contracture / Occlusion } of cervix
Pinpoint os uteri
EXCLUDES *congenital (752.49)*
that complicating labor (654.6)

622.5 Incompetence of cervix ♀
EXCLUDES *complicating pregnancy (654.5)*
that affecting fetus or newborn (761.0)
DEF: Inadequate functioning of cervix; marked by abnormal widening during pregnancy; causing miscarriage.

622.6 Hypertrophic elongation of cervix ♀
DEF: Overgrowth of cervix tissues extending down into vagina.

622.7 Mucous polyp of cervix ♀
Polyp NOS of cervix
EXCLUDES *adenomatous polyp of cervix (219.0)*

622.8 Other specified noninflammatory disorders of cervix ♀
Atrophy (senile) / Cyst / Fibrosis / Hemorrhage } of cervix
EXCLUDES *endometriosis (617.0)*
fistula (619.0-619.8)
inflammatory diseases (616.0)

622.9 Unspecified noninflammatory disorder of cervix ♀

✓4th **623 Noninflammatory disorders of vagina**
EXCLUDES *abnormality of vagina complicating pregnancy, labor, or delivery (654.7)*
congenital absence of vagina (752.49)
congenital diaphragm or bands (752.49)
fistulas involving vagina (619.0-619.8)

623.0 Dysplasia of vagina ♀
EXCLUDES *carcinoma in situ of vagina (233.3)*

623.1 Leukoplakia of vagina ♀
DEF: Thickened white patches on vaginal canal.

623.2 Stricture or atresia of vagina ♀
Adhesions (postoperative) (postradiation) of vagina
Occlusion of vagina
Stenosis, vagina
Use additional E code to identify any external cause
EXCLUDES *congenital atresia or stricture (752.49)*

623.3 Tight hymenal ring ♀
Rigid hymen / Tight hymenal ring / Tight introitus } acquired or congenital
EXCLUDES *imperforate hymen (752.42)*

623.4 Old vaginal laceration ♀
EXCLUDES *old laceration involving muscles of pelvic floor (618.7)*
DEF: Scarring or other evidence of old wound on vagina.

623.5 Leukorrhea, not specified as infective ♀
Leukorrhea NOS of vagina
Vaginal discharge NOS
EXCLUDES *trichomonal (131.00)*
DEF: Viscid whitish discharge, from vagina.

623.6 Vaginal hematoma ♀
EXCLUDES *current obstetrical trauma (665.7)*

623.7 Polyp of vagina ♀

623.8 Other specified noninflammatory disorders of vagina ♀
Cyst / Hemorrhage } of vagina

623.9 Unspecified noninflammatory disorder of vagina ♀

✓4th **624 Noninflammatory disorders of vulva and perineum**
EXCLUDES *abnormality of vulva and perineum complicating pregnancy, labor, or delivery (654.8)*
condyloma acuminatum (078.1)
fistulas involving:
perineum — see Alphabetic Index
vulva (619.0-619.8)
vulval varices (456.6)
vulvar involvement in skin conditions (690-709.9)

624.0 Dystrophy of vulva ♀
Kraurosis / Leukoplakia } of vulva
EXCLUDES *carcinoma in situ of vulva (233.3)*

624.1 Atrophy of vulva ♀

624.2 Hypertrophy of clitoris ♀
EXCLUDES *that in endocrine disorders (255.2, 256.1)*

624.3 Hypertrophy of labia ♀
Hypertrophy of vulva NOS
DEF: Overgrowth of fleshy folds on either side of vagina.

624.4 Old laceration or scarring of vulva ♀
DEF: Scarring or other evidence of old wound on external female genitalia.

624.5 Hematoma of vulva ♀
EXCLUDES *that complicating delivery (664.5)*
DEF: Blood in tissue of external genitalia.

624.6 Polyp of labia and vulva ♀

624.8 Other specified noninflammatory disorders of vulva and perineum ♀
Cyst / Edema / Stricture } of vulva
AHA: 1Q, '03, 13; 1Q, '95, 8

624.9 Unspecified noninflammatory disorder of vulva and perineum ♀

✓4th **625 Pain and other symptoms associated with female genital organs**

625.0 Dyspareunia ♀
EXCLUDES *psychogenic dyspareunia (302.76)*
DEF: Difficult or painful sexual intercourse.

625.1 Vaginismus ♀
Colpospasm
Vulvismus
EXCLUDES *psychogenic vaginismus (306.51)*
DEF: Vaginal spasms; due to involuntary contraction of musculature; prevents intercourse.

625.2 Mittelschmerz ♀
Intermenstrual pain Ovulation pain
DEF: Pain occurring between menstrual periods.

625.3 Dysmenorrhea ♀
Painful menstruation
EXCLUDES *psychogenic dysmenorrhea (306.52)*
AHA: 2Q, '94, 12

625.4 Premenstrual tension syndromes ♀
Menstrual:
migraine
molimen
Premenstrual dysphoric disorder
Premenstrual syndrome
Premenstrual tension NOS
AHA: 4Q, '03, 116

625.5 Pelvic congestion syndrome ♀
Congestion-fibrosis syndrome Taylor's syndrome
DEF: Excessive accumulated of blood in vessels of pelvis; may occur after orgasm; causes abnormal menstruation, lower back pain and vaginal discharge.

625.6 Stress incontinence, female ♀
EXCLUDES *mixed incontinence (788.33)*
stress incontinence, male (788.32)
DEF: Involuntary leakage of urine due to insufficient sphincter control; occurs upon sneezing, laughing, coughing, sudden movement or lifting.

625.8 Other specified symptoms associated with female genital organs ♀
AHA: N-D, '85, 16

625.9 Unspecified symptom associated with female genital organs ♀

✓4th **626 Disorders of menstruation and other abnormal bleeding from female genital tract**
EXCLUDES *menopausal and premenopausal bleeding (627.0)*
pain and other symptoms associated with menstrual cycle (625.2-625.4)
postmenopausal bleeding (627.1)

626.0 Absence of menstruation ♀
Amenorrhea (primary) (secondary)

626.1 Scanty or infrequent menstruation ♀
Hypomenorrhea Oligomenorrhea

626.2 Excessive or frequent menstruation ♀
Heavy periods Menorrhagia
Menometrorrhagia Plymenorrhea
EXCLUDES *premenopausal(627.0)*
that in puberty (626.3)

626.3 Puberty bleeding ♀
Excessive bleeding associated with onset of menstrual periods
Pubertal menorrhagia

626.4 Irregular menstrual cycle ♀
Irregular:
bleeding NOS
menstruation
Irregular:
periods

626.5 Ovulation bleeding ♀
Regular intermenstrual bleeding

626.6 Metrorrhagia ♀
Bleeding unrelated to menstrual cycle
Irregular intermenstrual bleeding

626.7 Postcoital bleeding ♀
DEF: Bleeding from vagina after sexual intercourse.

626.8 Other ♀
Dysfunctional or functional uterine hemorrhage NOS
Menstruation:
retained
suppression of

626.9 Unspecified ♀

✓4th **627 Menopausal and postmenopausal disorders**
EXCLUDES *asymptomatic age-related (natural) postmenopausal status (V49.81)*

627.0 Premenopausal menorrhagia ♀
Excessive bleeding associated with onset of menopause
Menorrhagia:
climacteric
menopausal
preclimacteric

627.1 Postmenopausal bleeding ♀

627.2 Symptomatic menopausal or female climacteric states ♀
Symptoms, such as flushing, sleeplessness, headache, lack of concentration, associated with the menopause

627.3 Postmenopausal atrophic vaginitis ♀
Senile (atrophic) vaginitis

627.4 Symptomatic states associated with artificial menopause ♀
Postartificial menopause syndromes
Any condition classifiable to 627.1, 627.2, or 627.3 which follows induced menopause
DEF: Conditions arising after hysterectomy.

627.8 Other specified menopausal and postmenopausal disorders ♀
EXCLUDES *premature menopause NOS (256.31)*

627.9 Unspecified menopausal and postmenopausal disorder ♀

✓4th **628 Infertility, female**
INCLUDES primary and secondary sterility
AHA: 2Q, '96, 9; 1Q, '95, 7
DEF: Infertility: inability to conceive for at least one year with regular intercourse.
DEF: Primary infertility: occurring in patients who have never conceived.
DEF: Secondary infertility; occurring in patients who have previously conceived.

628.0 Associated with anovulation ♀
Anovulatory cycle
Use additional code for any associated Stein-Leventhal syndrome (256.4)

628.1 Of pituitary-hypothalamic origin ♀
Code first underlying cause, as:
adiposogenital dystrophy (253.8)
anterior pituitary disorder (253.0-253.4)

628.2 Of tubal origin ♀
Infertility associated with congenital anomaly of tube
Tubal:
block
occlusion
stenosis
Use additional code for any associated peritubal adhesions (614.6)

628.3 Of uterine origin ♀
Infertility associated with congenital anomaly of uterus
Nonimplantation
Use additional code for any associated tuberculous endometritis (016.7)

628.4 Of cervical or vaginal origin ♀
Infertility associated with:
anomaly of cervical mucus
congenital structural anomaly
dysmucorrhea

628.8 Of other specified origin ♀

628.9 Of unspecified origin ♀

✓4th **629 Other disorders of female genital organs**

629.0 Hematocele, female, not elsewhere classified ♀

EXCLUDES *hematocele or hematoma:*
broad ligament (620.7)
fallopian tube (620.8)
that associated with ectopic pregnancy (633.00-633.91)
uterus (621.4)
vagina (623.6)
vulva (624.5)

629.1 Hydrocele, canal of Nuck ♀

Cyst of canal of Nuck (acquired)

EXCLUDES *congenital (752.41)*

✓5th **629.2 Female genital mutilation status**

Female circumcision status

AHA: ▶4Q, '04, 88◀

629.20 Female genital mutilation status, unspecified ♀

Female genital mutilation status NOS

629.21 Female genital mutilation Type I status ♀

Clitorectomy status

DEF: ▶Female genital mutilation involving clitorectomy, with part or all of the clitoris removed.◀

629.22 Female genital mutilation Type II status ♀

Clitorectomy with excision of labia minora status

AHA: ▶4Q, '04, 90◀

DEF: ▶Female genital mutilation involving clitoris and the labia minora amputation.◀

629.23 Female genital mutilation Type III status ♀

Infibulation status

AHA: ▶4Q, '04, 90◀

DEF: ▶Female genital mutilation involving removal, most or all of the labia minora excised, labia majora incised which is then made into a hood of skin over the urethral and vaginal opening.◀

629.8 Other specified disorders of female genital organs ♀

629.9 Unspecified disorder of female genital organs ♀

Habitual aborter without current pregnancy

11. COMPLICATIONS OF PREGNANCY, CHILDBIRTH AND THE PUERPERIUM (630-677)

ECTOPIC AND MOLAR PREGNANCY (630-633)

Use additional code from category 639 to identify any complications

630 Hydatidiform mole M ♀

Trophoblastic disease NOS
Vesicularmole

EXCLUDES *chorioadenoma (destruens) (236.1)*
chorionepithelioma (181)
malignant hydatidiform mole (236.1)

DEF: Abnormal product of pregnancy; marked by mass of cysts resembling bunch of grapes due to chorionic villi proliferation, and dissolution; must be surgically removed.

631 Other abnormal product of conception M ♀

Blighted ovum
Mole:
NOS
carneous
Mole:
fleshy
stone

632 Missed abortion M ♀

Early fetal death before completion of 22 weeks' gestation with retention of dead fetus
Retained products of conception, not following spontaneous or induced abortion or delivery

EXCLUDES *failed induced abortion (638.0-638.9)*
fetal death (intrauterine) (late) (656.4)
missed delivery (656.4)
that with abnormal product of conception (630, 631)

AHA: 1Q, '01, 5

✓4th **633 Ectopic pregnancy**

INCLUDES ruptured ectopic pregnancy

AHA: 4Q, '02, 61

DEF: Fertilized egg develops outside uterus.

✓5th **633.0 Abdominal pregnancy**

Intraperitoneal pregnancy

633.00 Abdominal pregnancy without intrauterine pregnancy M ♀

633.01 Abdominal pregnancy with intrauterine pregnancy M ♀

✓5th **633.1 Tubal pregnancy**

Fallopian pregnancy
Rupture of (fallopian) tube due to pregnancy
Tubal abortion

AHA: 2Q, '90, 27

633.10 Tubal pregnancy without intrauterine pregnancy M ♀

633.11 Tubal pregnancy with intrauterine pregnancy M ♀

✓5th **633.2 Ovarian pregnancy**

633.20 Ovarian pregnancy without intrauterine pregnancy M ♀

633.21 Ovarian pregnancy with intrauterine pregnancy M ♀

✓5th **633.8 Other ectopic pregnancy**

Pregnancy:
cervical
combined
cornual
Pregnancy:
intraligamentous
mesometric
mural

633.80 Other ectopic pregnancy without intrauterine pregnancy M ♀

633.81 Other ectopic pregnancy with intrauterine pregnancy M ♀

✓5th **633.9 Unspecified ectopic pregnancy**

633.90 Unspecified ectopic pregnancy without intrauterine pregnancy M ♀

633.91 Unspecified ectopic pregnancy with intrauterine pregnancy M ♀

Ectopic Pregnancy Sites

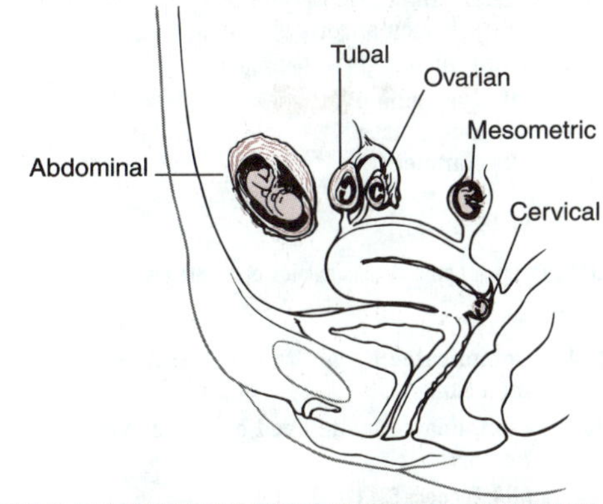

OTHER PREGNANCY WITH ABORTIVE OUTCOME (634-639)

The following fourth-digit subdivisions are for use with categories 634-638:

.0 Complicated by genital tract and pelvic infection

Endometritis
Salpingo-oophoritis
Sepsis NOS
Septicemia NOS
Any condition classifiable to 639.0, with condition classifiable to 634-638

EXCLUDES *urinary tract infection (634-638 with .7)*

.1 Complicated by delayed or excessive hemorrhage

Afibrinogenemia
Defibrination syndrome
Intravascular hemolysis
Any condition classifiable to 639.1, with condition classifiable to 634-638

.2 Complicated by damage to pelvic organs and tissues

Laceration, perforation, or tear of:
bladder
uterus
Any condition classifiable to 639.2, with condition classifiable to 634-638

.3 Complicated by renal failure

Oliguria
Uremia
Any condition classifiable to 639.3, with condition classifiable to 634-638

.4 Complicated by metabolic disorder

Electrolyte imbalance with conditions classifiable to 634-638

.5 Complicated by shock

Circulatory collapse
Shock (postoperative) (septic)
Any condition classifiable to 639.5, with condition classifiable to 634-638

.6 Complicated by embolism

Embolism:
NOS
amniotic fluid
pulmonary
Any condition classifiable to 639.6, with condition classifiable to 634-638

.7 With other specified complications

Cardiac arrest or failure
Urinary tract infection
Any condition classifiable to 639.8, with condition classifiable to 634-638

.8 With unspecified complication

.9 Without mention of complication

§ ✓4th **634 Spontaneous abortion**

INCLUDES miscarriage
spontaneous abortion

Requires fifth-digit to identify stage:
- **0 unspecified**
- **1 incomplete**
- **2 complete**

AHA: 2Q, '91, 16

DEF: Spontaneous premature expulsion of the products of conception from the uterus.

- ✓5th **634.0 Complicated by genital tract and pelvic infection** M♀
- ✓5th **634.1 Complicated by delayed or excessive hemorrhage** M♀
  AHA: For code 634.11: 1Q, '03, 6
- ✓5th **634.2 Complicated by damage to pelvic organs or tissues** M♀
- ✓5th **634.3 Complicated by renal failure** M♀
- ✓5th **634.4 Complicated by metabolic disorder** M♀
- ✓5th **634.5 Complicated by shock** M♀
- ✓5th **634.6 Complicated by embolism** M♀
- ✓5th **634.7 With other specified complications** M♀
- ✓5th **634.8 With unspecified complication** M♀
- ✓5th **634.9 Without mention of complication** M♀

§ ✓4th **635 Legally induced abortion**

INCLUDES abortion or termination of pregnancy:
elective
legal
therapeutic

EXCLUDES *menstrual extraction or regulation (V25.3)*

Requires fifth-digit to identify stage:
- **0 unspecified**
- **1 incomplete**
- **2 complete**

AHA: 2Q, '94, 14

DEF: Intentional expulsion of products of conception from uterus performed by medical professionals inside boundaries of law.

- ✓5th **635.0 Complicated by genital tract and pelvic infection** M♀
- ✓5th **635.1 Complicated by delayed or excessive hemorrhage** M♀
- ✓5th **635.2 Complicated by damage to pelvic organs or tissues** M♀
- ✓5th **635.3 Complicated by renal failure** M♀
- ✓5th **635.4 Complicated by metabolic disorder** M♀
- ✓5th **635.5 Complicated by shock** M♀
- ✓5th **635.6 Complicated by embolism** M♀
- ✓5th **635.7 With other specified complications** M♀
- ✓5th **635.8 With unspecified complication** M♀
- ✓5th **635.9 Without mention of complication** M♀

§ ✓4th **636 Illegally induced abortion**

INCLUDES abortion:
criminal
illegal
abortion:
self-induced

Requires fifth-digit to identify stage:
- **0 unspecified**
- **1 incomplete**
- **2 complete**

DEF: Intentional expulsion of products of conception from uterus; outside boundaries of law.

- ✓5th **636.0 Complicated by genital tract and pelvic infection** M♀
- ✓5th **636.1 Complicated by delayed or excessive hemorrhage** M♀
- ✓5th **636.2 Complicated by damage to pelvic organs or tissues** M♀
- ✓5th **636.3 Complicated by renal failure** M♀
- ✓5th **636.4 Complicated by metabolic disorder** M♀
- ✓5th **636.5 Complicated by shock** M♀
- ✓5th **636.6 Complicated by embolism** M♀
- ✓5th **636.7 With other specified complications** M♀
- ✓5th **636.8 With unspecified complication** M♀
- ✓5th **636.9 Without mention of complication** M♀

§ ✓4th **637 Unspecified abortion**

INCLUDES abortion NOS
retained products of conception following abortion, not classifiable elsewhere

Requires fifth-digit to identify stage:
- **0 unspecified**
- **1 incomplete**
- **2 complete**

- ✓5th **637.0 Complicated by genital tract and pelvic infection** M♀
- ✓5th **637.1 Complicated by delayed or excessive hemorrhage** M♀
- ✓5th **637.2 Complicated by damage to pelvic organs or tissues** M♀
- ✓5th **637.3 Complicated by renal failure** M♀
- ✓5th **637.4 Complicated by metabolic disorder** M♀
- ✓5th **637.5 Complicated by shock** M♀
- ✓5th **637.6 Complicated by embolism** M♀
- ✓5th **637.7 With other specified complications** M♀
- ✓5th **637.8 With unspecified complication** M♀
- ✓5th **637.9 Without mention of complication** M♀

§ ✓4th **638 Failed attempted abortion**

INCLUDES failure of attempted induction of (legal) abortion

EXCLUDES *incomplete abortion (634.0-637.9)*

DEF: Continued pregnancy despite an attempted legal abortion.

- **638.0 Complicated by genital tract and pelvic infection** M♀
- **638.1 Complicated by delayed or excessive hemorrhage** M♀
- **638.2 Complicated by damage to pelvic organs or tissues** M♀
- **638.3 Complicated by renal failure** M♀
- **638.4 Complicated by metabolic disorder** M♀
- **638.5 Complicated by shock** M♀
- **638.6 Complicated by embolism** M♀
- **638.7 With other specified complications** M♀
- **638.8 With unspecified complication** M♀
- **638.9 Without mention of complication** M♀

✓4th **639 Complications following abortion and ectopic and molar pregnancies**

Note: This category is provided for use when it is required to classify separately the complications classifiable to the fourth-digit level in categories 634-638; for example:

a) when the complication itself was responsible for an episode of medical care, the abortion, ectopic or molar pregnancy itself having been dealt with at a previous episode

b) when these conditions are immediate complications of ectopic or molar pregnancies classifiable to 630-633 where they cannot be identified at fourth-digit level.

§ See beginning of section 634–639 for fourth-digit definitions.

639.0 Genital tract and pelvic infection M ♀

Endometritis, Parametritis, Pelvic peritonitis, Salpingitis, Salpingo-oophoritis, Sepsis NOS, Septicemia NOS — following conditions classifiable to 630-638

EXCLUDES *urinary tract infection (639.8)*

639.1 Delayed or excessive hemorrhage M ♀

Afibrinogenemia, Defibrination syndrome, Intravascular hemolysis — following conditions classifiable to 630-638

639.2 Damage to pelvic organs and tissues M ♀

Laceration, perforation, or tear of: bladder, bowel, broad ligament, cervix, periurethral tissue, uterus, vagina — following conditions classifiable to 630-638

639.3 Renal failure M ♀

Oliguria; Renal: failure (acute), shutdown, tubular necrosis; Uremia — following conditions classifiable to 630-638

639.4 Metabolic disorders M ♀

Electrolyte imbalance following conditions classifiable to 630-638

639.5 Shock M ♀

Circulatory collapse, Shock (postoperative) (septic) — following conditions classifiable to 630-638

639.6 Embolism M ♀

Embolism: NOS, air, amniotic fluid, blood-clot, fat, pulmonary, pyemic, septic, soap — following conditions classifiable to 630-638

639.8 Other specified complications following abortion or ectopic and molar pregnancy M ♀

Acute yellow atrophy or necrosis of liver, Cardiac arrest or failure, Cerebral anoxia, Urinary tract infection — following conditions classifiable to 630-638

639.9 Unspecified complication following abortion or ectopic and molar pregnancy M ♀

Complication(s) not further specified following conditions classifiable to 630-638

COMPLICATIONS MAINLY RELATED TO PREGNANCY (640-648)

INCLUDES the listed conditions even if they arose or were present during labor, delivery, or the puerperium

The following fifth-digit subclassification is for use with categories 640-648 to denote the current episode of care. Valid fifth-digits are in [brackets] under each code.

0 unspecified as to episode of care or not applicable

1 delivered, with or without mention of antepartum condition
- Antepartum condition with delivery
- Delivery NOS (with mention of antepartum complication during current episode of care)
- Intrapartum obstetric condition (with mention of antepartum complication during current episode of care)
- Pregnancy, delivered (with mention of antepartum complication during current episode of care)

2 delivered, with mention of postpartum complication
- Delivery with mention of puerperal complication during current episode of care

3 antepartum condition or complication
- Antepartum obstetric condition, not delivered during the current episode of care

4 postpartum condition or complication
- Postpartum or puerperal obstetric condition or complication following delivery that occurred:
  - during previous episode of care
  - outside hospital, with subsequent admission for observation or care

AHA: 2Q, '90, 11

✓4th **640 Hemorrhage in early pregnancy**

INCLUDES hemorrhage before completion of 22 weeks' gestation

✓5th **640.0 Threatened abortion** M ♀
[0,1,3]
DEF: Bloody discharge during pregnancy; cervix may be dilated and pregnancy is threatened, but the pregnancy is not terminated.

✓5th **640.8 Other specified hemorrhage in early pregnancy** M ♀
[0,1,3]

✓5th **640.9 Unspecified hemorrhage in early pregnancy** M ♀
[0,1,3]

✓4th **641 Antepartum hemorrhage, abruptio placentae, and placenta previa**

✓5th **641.0 Placenta previa without hemorrhage** M ♀
[0,1,3]

Low implantation of placenta; Placenta previa noted: during pregnancy, before labor (and delivered by cesarean delivery) — without hemorrhage

DEF: Placenta implanted in lower segment of uterus; commonly causes hemorrhage in the last trimester of pregnancy.

✓5th **641.1 Hemorrhage from placenta previa** M ♀
[0,1,3]

Low-lying placenta; Placenta previa: incomplete, marginal, partial, total — NOS or with hemorrhage (intrapartum)

EXCLUDES *hemorrhage from vasa previa (663.5)*

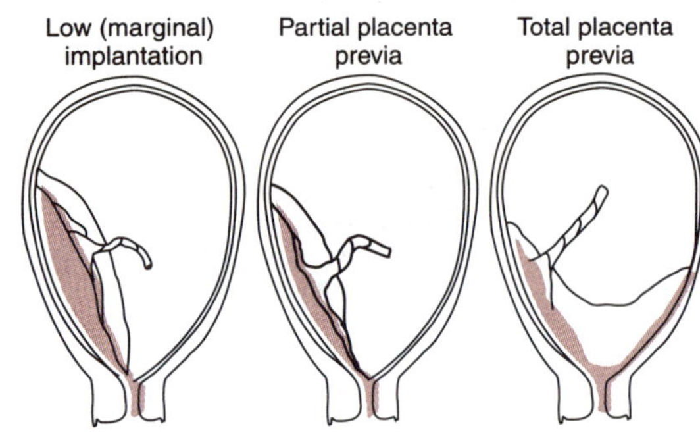

§ ✓5th **641.2 Premature separation of placenta** M♀
[0,1,3]
Ablatio placentae
Abruptio placentae
Accidental antepartum hemorrhage
Couvelaire uterus
Detachment of placenta (premature)
Premature separation of normally implanted placenta

DEF: Abruptio placentae: premature detachment of the placenta, characterized by shock, oliguria and decreased fibrinogen.

§ ✓5th **641.3 Antepartum hemorrhage associated with coagulation defects** M♀
[0,1,3]
Antepartum or intrapartum hemorrhage associated with:
afibrinogenemia
hyperfibrinolysis
hypofibrinogenemia

DEF: Uterine hemorrhage prior to delivery.

§ ✓5th **641.8 Other antepartum hemorrhage** M♀
[0,1,3]
Antepartum or intrapartum hemorrhage associated with:
trauma
uterine leiomyoma

§ ✓5th **641.9 Unspecified antepartum hemorrhage** M♀
[0,1,3]
Hemorrhage:
antepartum NOS
intrapartum NOS
Hemorrhage:
of pregnancy NOS

✓4th **642 Hypertension complicating pregnancy, childbirth, and the puerperium**

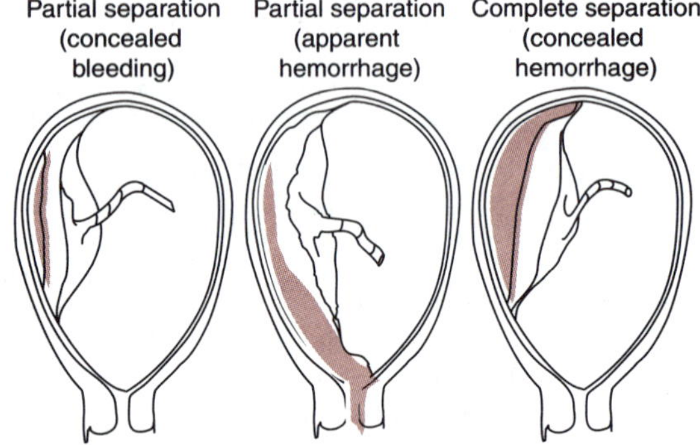

§ ✓5th **642.0 Benign essential hypertension complicating pregnancy, childbirth, and the puerperium** M♀
[0-4]
Hypertension:
benign essential
chronic NOS
essential
pre-existing NOS
} specified as complicating, or as a reason for obstetric care during pregnancy, childbirth or the puerperium

§ ✓5th **642.1 Hypertension secondary to renal disease, complicating pregnancy, childbirth, and the puerperium** M♀
[0-4]
Hypertension secondary to renal disease, specified as complicating, or as a reason for obstetric care during pregnancy, childbirth or the puerperium

§ ✓5th **642.2 Other pre-existing hypertension complicating pregnancy, childbirth, and the puerperium** M♀
[0-4]
Hypertensive:
heart and renal disease
heart disease
renal disease
Malignant hypertension
} specified as complicating, or as a reason for obstetric care during pregnancy, childbirth or the puerperium

§ ✓5th **642.3 Transient hypertension of pregnancy** M♀
[0-4]
Gestational hypertension
Transient hypertension, so described, in pregnancy, childbirth or the puerperium

AHA: 3Q, '90, 4

§ ✓5th **642.4 Mild or unspecified pre-eclampsia** M♀
[0-4]
Hypertension in pregnancy, childbirth or the puerperium, not specified as pre-existing, with either albuminuria or edema, or both; mild or unspecified
Pre-eclampsia:
NOS
mild
Toxemia (pre-eclamptic):
NOS
mild

EXCLUDES *albuminuria in pregnancy, without mention of hypertension (646.2)*
edema in pregnancy, without mention of hypertension (646.1)

§ ✓5th **642.5 Severe pre-eclampsia** M♀
[0-4]
Hypertension in pregnancy, childbirth or the puerperium, not specified as pre-existing, with either albuminuria or edema, or both; specified as severe
Pre-eclampsia, severe
Toxemia (pre-eclamptic), severe

AHA: N-D, '85, 3

§ ✓5th **642.6 Eclampsia** M♀
[0-4]
Toxemia:
eclamptic
Toxemia:
with convulsions

§ ✓5th **642.7 Pre-eclampsia or eclampsia superimposed on pre-existing hypertension** M♀
[0-4]
Conditions classifiable to 642.4-642.6, with conditions classifiable to 642.0-642.2

§ ✓5th **642.9 Unspecified hypertension complicating pregnancy, childbirth, or the puerperium** M♀
[0-4]
Hypertension NOS, without mention of albuminuria or edema, complicating pregnancy, childbirth or the puerperium

✓4th **643 Excessive vomiting in pregnancy**

INCLUDES hyperemesis
vomiting:
persistent
vicious
} arising during pregnancy

hyperemesis gravidarum

§ Requires fifth digit. Valid digits are in [brackets] under each code. See beginning of section 640–648 for codes and definitions.

§ ✓5th **643.0 Mild hyperemesis gravidarum** M♀
[0,1,3] Hyperemesis gravidarum, mild or unspecified, starting before the end of the 22nd week of gestation
DEF: Detrimental vomiting and nausea.

§ ✓5th **643.1 Hyperemesis gravidarum with metabolic disturbance** M♀
[0,1,3] Hyperemesis gravidarum, starting before the end of the 22nd week of gestation, with metabolic disturbance, such as:
carbohydrate depletion
dehydration
electrolyte imbalance

§ ✓5th **643.2 Late vomiting of pregnancy** M♀
[0,1,3] Excessive vomiting starting after 22 completed weeks of gestation

§ ✓5th **643.8 Other vomiting complicating pregnancy** M♀
[0,1,3] Vomiting due to organic disease or other cause, specified as complicating pregnancy, or as a reason for obstetric care during pregnancy
Use additional code to specify cause

§ ✓5th **643.9 Unspecified vomiting of pregnancy** M♀
[0,1,3] Vomiting as a reason for care during pregnancy, length of gestation unspecified

✓4th **644 Early or threatened labor**

§ ✓5th **644.0 Threatened premature labor** M♀
[0,3] Premature labor after 22 weeks, but before 37 completed weeks of gestation without delivery
EXCLUDES *that occurring before 22 completed weeks of gestation (640.0)*

§ ✓5th **644.1 Other threatened labor** M♀
[0,3] False labor:
NOS } without delivery
after 37 completed weeks of gestation } without delivery
Threatened labor NOS } without delivery

§ ✓5th **644.2 Early onset of delivery** M♀
[0,1] Onset (spontaneous) of delivery } before 37 completed weeks of gestation
Premature labor with onset of delivery } before 37 completed weeks of gestation
AHA: 2Q, '91, 16

✓4th **645 Late pregnancy**
AHA: 4Q. '00, 43; 4Q, '91, 26

§ ✓5th **645.1 Post term pregnancy** M♀
[0,1,3] Pregnancy over 40 completed weeks to 42 completed weeks gestation

§ ✓5th **645.2 Prolonged pregnancy** M♀
[0,1,3] Pregnancy which has advanced beyond 42 completed weeks of gestation

✓4th **646 Other complications of pregnancy, not elsewhere classified**
Use additional code(s) to further specify complication
AHA: 4Q, '95, 59

§ ✓5th **646.0 Papyraceous fetus** M♀
[0,1,3] DEF: Fetus retained in the uterus beyond natural term, exhibits parchment-like skin.

§ ✓5th **646.1 Edema or excessive weight gain in pregnancy, without mention of hypertension** M♀
[0-4] Gestational edema
Maternal obesity syndrome
EXCLUDES *that with mention of hypertension (642.0-642.)*

§ ✓5th **646.2 Unspecified renal disease in pregnancy, without mention of hypertension** M♀
[0-4] Albuminuria } in pregnancy or the puerperium, without mention of hypertension
Nephropathy NOS } in pregnancy or the puerperium, without mention of hypertension
Renal disease NOS } in pregnancy or the puerperium, without mention of hypertension
Uremia } in pregnancy or the puerperium, without mention of hypertension
Gestational proteinuria
EXCLUDES *that with mention of hypertension (642.0-642.9)*

§ ✓5th **646.3 Habitual aborter** M♀
[0,1,3] EXCLUDES *with current abortion (634.0-634.9)*
without current pregnancy (629.9)
DEF: Three or more consecutive spontaneous abortions.

§ ✓5th **646.4 Peripheral neuritis in pregnancy** M♀
[0-4]

§ ✓5th **646.5 Asymptomatic bacteriuria in pregnancy** M♀
[0-4]

§ ✓5th **646.6 Infections of genitourinary tract in pregnancy** M♀
[0-4] Conditions classifiable to 590, 595, 597, 599.0, 616 complicating pregnancy, childbirth or the puerperium
Conditions classifiable to (614.0-614.5, 614.7-614.9, 615) complicating pregnancy or labor
EXCLUDES *major puerperal infection (670)*
AHA: For code 646.63: ▶4Q, '04, 90◀

§ ✓5th **646.7 Liver disorders in pregnancy** M♀
[0,1,3] Acute yellow atrophy of liver (obstetric) (true) } of pregnancy
Icterus gravis } of pregnancy
Necrosis of liver } of pregnancy
EXCLUDES *hepatorenal syndrome following delivery (674.8)*
viral hepatitis (647.6)

§ ✓5th **646.8 Other specified complications of pregnancy** M♀
[0-4] Fatigue during pregnancy
Herpes gestationis
Insufficient weight gain of pregnancy
Uterine size-date discrepancy
AHA: 3Q, '98, 16, J-F, '85, 15

§ ✓5th **646.9 Unspecified complication of pregnancy** M♀
[0,1,3]

✓4th **647 Infectious and parasitic conditions in the mother classifiable elsewhere, but complicating pregnancy, childbirth, or the puerperium**
INCLUDES the listed conditions when complicating the pregnant state, aggravated by the pregnancy, or when a main reason for obstetric care
EXCLUDES *those conditions in the mother known or suspected to have affected the fetus (655.0-655.9)*
Use additional code(s) to further specify complication

§ ✓5th **647.0 Syphilis** M♀
[0-4] Conditions classifiable to 090-097

§ ✓5th **647.1 Gonorrhea** M♀
[0-4] Conditions classifiable to 098

§ ✓5th **647.2 Other venereal diseases** M♀
[0-4] Conditions classifiable to 099

§ ✓5th **647.3 Tuberculosis** M♀
[0-4] Conditions classifiable to 010-018

§ ✓5th **647.4 Malaria** M♀
[0-4] Conditions classifiable to 084

§ ✓5th **647.5 Rubella** M♀
[0-4] Conditions classifiable to 056

§ Requires fifth digit. Valid digits are in [brackets] under each code. See beginning of section 640–648 for codes and definitions.

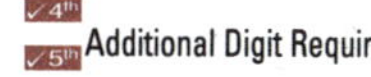
Additional Digit Required   Unspecified Code   Other Specified Code   Manifestation Code   ▶◀ Revised Text   ● New Code   ▲ Revised Code Title

§ ✓5th **647.6 Other viral diseases** M ♀
[0-4]
Conditions classifiable to 042 and 050-079, except 056
AHA: J-F, '85, 15

§ ✓5th **647.8 Other specified infectious and parasitic diseases** M ♀
[0-4]

§ ✓5th **647.9 Unspecified infection or infestation** M ♀
[0-4]

✓4th **648 Other current conditions in the mother classifiable elsewhere, but complicating pregnancy, childbirth, or the puerperium**

INCLUDES the listed conditions when complicating the pregnant state, aggravated by the pregnancy, or when a main reason for obstetric care

EXCLUDES *those conditions in the mother known or suspected to have affected the fetus (655.0-665.9)*

Use additional code(s) to identify the condition

§ ✓5th **648.0 Diabetes mellitus** M ♀
[0-4]
Conditions classifiable to 250
EXCLUDES *gestational diabetes (648.8)*
AHA: 3Q, '91, 5, 11

§ ✓5th **648.1 Thyroid dysfunction** M ♀
[0-4]
Conditions classifiable to 240-246

§ ✓5th **648.2 Anemia** M ♀
[0-4]
Conditions classifiable to 280-285
AHA: For Code 648.22: 1Q, '02, 14

§ ✓5th **648.3 Drug dependence** M ♀
[0-4]
Conditions classifiable to 304
AHA: 2Q, '98, 13; 4Q, '88, 8

§ ✓5th **648.4 Mental disorders** M ♀
[0-4]
Conditions classifiable to 290-303, 305-316, 317-319
AHA: 2Q, '98, 13; 4Q, '95, 63

§ ✓5th **648.5 Congenital cardiovascular disorders** M ♀
[0-4]
Conditions classifiable to 745-747

§ ✓5th **648.6 Other cardiovascular diseases** M ♀
[0-4]
Conditions classifiable to 390-398, 410-429
EXCLUDES *cerebrovascular disorders in the puerperium (674.0)*
peripartum cardiomyopathy (674.5)
venous complications (671.0-671.9)
AHA: 3Q, '98, 11

§ ✓5th **648.7 Bone and joint disorders of back, pelvis, and lower limbs** M ♀
[0-4]
Conditions classifiable to 720-724, and those classifiable to 711-719 or 725-738, specified as affecting the lower limbs

§ ✓5th **648.8 Abnormal glucose tolerance** M ♀
[0-4]
Conditions classifiable to ▶790.21-790.29◀
Gestational diabetes
▶Use additional code, if applicable, for associated long-term (current) insulin use (V58.67)◀
AHA: 3Q, '91, 5; **For code 648.83:** 4Q, '04, 56

DEF: Glucose intolerance arising in pregnancy, resolving at end of pregnancy.

§ ✓5th **648.9 Other current conditions classifiable elsewhere** M ♀
[0-4]
Conditions classifiable to 440-459
Nutritional deficiencies [conditions classifiable to 260-269]
AHA: 4Q, '04, 88; N-D, '87, 10; **For code 648.91:** 1Q, '02, 14; **For code 648.93:** 4Q, '04, 90

NORMAL DELIVERY, AND OTHER INDICATIONS FOR CARE IN PREGNANCY, LABOR, AND DELIVERY (650-659)

The following fifth-digit subclassification is for use with categories 651-659 to denote the current episode of care. Valid fifth-digits are in [brackets] under each code.

0 unspecified as to episode of care or not applicable
1 delivered, with or without mention of antepartum condition
2 delivered, with mention of postpartum complication
3 antepartum condition or complication
4 postpartum condition or complication

650 Normal delivery M ♀
Delivery requiring minimal or no assistance, with or without episiotomy, without fetal manipulation [e.g., rotation version] or instrumentation [forceps] of spontaneous, cephalic, vaginal, full-term, single, live-born infant. This code is for use as a single diagnosis code and is not to be used with any other code in the range 630-676.
EXCLUDES *breech delivery (assisted) (spontaneous) NOS (652.2)*
delivery by vacuum extractor, forceps, cesarean section, or breech extraction, without specified complication (669.5-669.7)
Use additional code to indicate outcome of delivery (V27.0)
AHA: 2Q, '02, 10; 3Q, '01, 12; 3Q, '00, 5; 4Q, '95, 28, 59

✓4th **651 Multiple gestation**

§ ✓5th **651.0 Twin pregnancy** M ♀
[0,1,3]

§ ✓5th **651.1 Triplet pregnancy** M ♀
[0,1,3]

§ ✓5th **651.2 Quadruplet pregnancy** M ♀
[0,1,3]

§ ✓5th **651.3 Twin pregnancy with fetal loss and retention of one fetus** M ♀
[0,1,3]
Vanishing twin syndrome (651.33)

§ ✓5th **651.4 Triplet pregnancy with fetal loss and retention of one or more fetus(es)** M ♀
[0,1,3]

§ ✓5th **651.5 Quadruplet pregnancy with fetal loss and retention of one or more fetus(es)** M ♀
[0,1,3]

§ ✓5th **651.6 Other multiple pregnancy with fetal loss and retention of one or more fetus(es)** M ♀
[0,1,3]

● § ✓5th **651.7 Multiple gestation following (elective) fetal reduction** M ♀
[0,1,3]
Fetal reduction of multiple fetuses reduced to single fetus

§ ✓5th **651.8 Other specified multiple gestation** M ♀
[0,1,3]

§ ✓5th **651.9 Unspecified multiple gestation** M ♀
[0,1,3]

✓4th **652 Malposition and malpresentation of fetus**
Code first any associated obstructed labor (660.0)

§ ✓5th **652.0 Unstable lie** M ♀
[0,1,3]
DEF: Changing fetal position.

§ ✓5th **652.1 Breech or other malpresentation successfully converted to cephalic presentation** M ♀
[0,1,3]
Cephalic version NOS

§ ✓5th **652.2 Breech presentation without mention of version** M ♀
[0,1,3]
Breech delivery (assisted) (spontaneous) NOS
Buttocks presentation
Complete breech
Frank breech
EXCLUDES *footling presentation (652.8)*
incomplete breech (652.8)
DEF: Fetal presentation of buttocks or feet at birth canal.

§ Requires fifth digit. Valid digits are in [brackets] under each code. See beginning of section 640–648 for codes and definitions.

N Newborn Age: 0 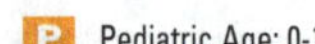 P Pediatric Age: 0-17 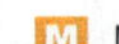 M Maternity Age: 12-55 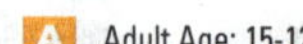 A Adult Age: 15-124 MSP Medicare Secondary Payer

Malposition and Malpresentation

Breech
Shoulder (arm prolapse)
Mother's pelvis
Face (mentum)
Compound (extremity together with head)
Oblique

§ 5th **652.3 Transverse or oblique presentation** M♀
[0,1,3] Oblique lie Transverse lie
EXCLUDES *transverse arrest of fetal head (660.3)*
DEF: Delivery of fetus, shoulder first.

§ 5th **652.4 Face or brow presentation** M♀
[0,1,3] Mentum presentation

§ 5th **652.5 High head at term** M♀
[0,1,3] Failure of head to enter pelvic brim

§ 5th **652.6 Multiple gestation with malpresentation of one fetus or more** M♀
[0,1,3]

§ 5th **652.7 Prolapsed arm** M♀
[0,1,3]

§ 5th **652.8 Other specified malposition or malpresentation** M♀
[0,1,3] Compound presentation

§ 5th **652.9 Unspecified malposition or malpresentation** M♀
[0,1,3]

4th **653 Disproportion**
Code first any associated obstructed labor (660.1)

§ 5th **653.0 Major abnormality of bony pelvis, not further specified** M♀
[0,1,3] Pelvic deformity NOS

§ 5th **653.1 Generally contracted pelvis** M♀
[0,1,3] Contracted pelvis NOS

§ 5th **653.2 Inlet contraction of pelvis** M♀
[0,1,3] Inlet contraction (pelvis)

§ 5th **653.3 Outlet contraction of pelvis** M♀
[0,1,3] Outlet contraction (pelvis)

§ 5th **653.4 Fetopelvic disproportion** M♀
[0,1,3] Cephalopelvic disproportion NOS
Disproportion of mixed maternal and fetal origin, with normally formed fetus

§ 5th **653.5 Unusually large fetus causing disproportion** M♀
[0,1,3] Disproportion of fetal origin with normally formed fetus
Fetal disproportion NOS
EXCLUDES *that when the reason for medical care was concern for the fetus (656.6)*

§ 5th **653.6 Hydrocephalic fetus causing disproportion** M♀
[0,1,3] EXCLUDES *that when the reason for medical care was concern for the fetus (655.0)*

§ 5th **653.7 Other fetal abnormality causing disproportion** M♀
[0,1,3] Conjoined twins
Fetal:
ascites
hydrops
Fetal:
myelomeningocele
sacral teratoma
tumor

Cephalopelvic Disproportion

Pubic symphysis
Cephalopelvic disproportion due to: Contraction of pelvic inlet, or large fetus, or hydrocephalus
Ischial tuberosity
Contraction of pelvic outlet (from below)
Pubic symphysis
Pelvic inlet from above

§ 5th **653.8 Disproportion of other origin** M♀
[0,1,3] EXCLUDES *shoulder (girdle) dystocia (660.4)*

§ 5th **653.9 Unspecified disproportion** M♀
[0,1,3]

4th **654 Abnormality of organs and soft tissues of pelvis**
INCLUDES the listed conditions during pregnancy, childbirth or the puerperium
Code first any associated obstructed labor (660.2)

§ 5th **654.0 Congenital abnormalities of uterus** M♀
[0-4] Double uterus Uterus bicornis

§ 5th **654.1 Tumors of body of uterus** M♀
[0-4] Uterine fibroids

§ 5th **654.2 Previous cesarean delivery** M♀
[0,1,3] Uterine scar from previous cesarean delivery
AHA: 1Q, '92, 8

§ 5th **654.3 Retroverted and incarcerated gravid uterus** M♀
[0-4] DEF: Retroverted: tilted back uterus; no change in angle of longitudinal axis.
DEF: Incarcerated: immobile, fixed uterus.

§ 5th **654.4 Other abnormalities in shape or position of gravid uterus and of neighboring structures** M♀
[0-4] Cystocele Prolapse of gravid uterus
Pelvic floor repair Rectocele
Pendulous abdomen Rigid pelvic floor

§ 5th **654.5 Cervical incompetence** M♀
[0-4] Presence of Shirodkar suture with or without mention of cervical incompetence
DEF: Abnormal cervix; tendency to dilate in second trimester; causes premature fetal expulsion.
DEF: Shirodkar suture: purse-string suture used to artificially close incompetent cervix.

§ 5th **654.6 Other congenital or acquired abnormality of cervix** M♀
[0-4] Cicatricial cervix Rigid cervix (uteri)
Polyp of cervix Stenosis or stricture of cervix
Previous surgery to cervix Tumor of cervix

§ 5th **654.7 Congenital or acquired abnormality of vagina** M♀
[0-4] Previous surgery to vagina Stricture of vagina
Septate vagina Tumor of vagina
Stenosis of vagina (acquired) (congenital)

§ 5th **654.8 Congenital or acquired abnormality of vulva** M♀
[0-4] Fibrosis of perineum Rigid perineum
Persistent hymen Tumor of vulva
Previous surgery to perineum or vulva
EXCLUDES *varicose veins of vulva (671.1)*
AHA: 1Q, '03, 14

§ 5th **654.9 Other and unspecified** M♀
[0-4] Uterine scar NEC

§ Requires fifth digit. Valid digits are in [brackets] under each code. See beginning of section 640–648 for codes and definitions.

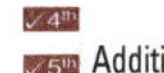 Additional Digit Required 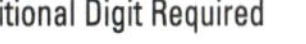 Unspecified Code 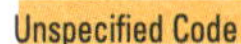 Other Specified Code Manifestation Code ▶◀ Revised Text ● New Code ▲ Revised Code Title

✓4th **655 Known or suspected fetal abnormality affecting management of mother**

INCLUDES the listed conditions in the fetus as a reason for observation or obstetrical care of the mother, or for termination of pregnancy

AHA: 3Q, '90, 4

§✓5th **655.0 Central nervous system malformation in fetus** M ♀
[0,1,3]
Fetal or suspected fetal:
- anencephaly
- hydrocephalus
- spina bifida (with myelomeningocele)

§✓5th **655.1 Chromosomal abnormality in fetus** M ♀
[0,1,3]

§✓5th **655.2 Hereditary disease in family possibly affecting fetus** M ♀
[0,1,3]

§✓5th **655.3 Suspected damage to fetus from viral disease in the mother** M ♀
[0,1,3]
Suspected damage to fetus from maternal rubella

§✓5th **655.4 Suspected damage to fetus from other disease in the mother** M ♀
[0,1,3]
Suspected damage to fetus from maternal:
- alcohol addiction
- listeriosis
- toxoplasmosis

§✓5th **655.5 Suspected damage to fetus from drugs** M ♀
[0,1,3]

§✓5th **655.6 Suspected damage to fetus from radiation** M ♀
[0,1,3]

§✓5th **655.7 Decreased fetal movements** M ♀
[0,1,3]
AHA: 4Q, '97, 41

§✓5th **655.8 Other known or suspected fetal abnormality, not elsewhere classified** M ♀
[0,1,3]
Suspected damage to fetus from:
- environmental toxins
- intrauterine contraceptive device

§✓5th **655.9 Unspecified** M ♀
[0,1,3]

✓4th **656 Other fetal and placental problems affecting management of mother**

§✓5th **656.0 Fetal-maternal hemorrhage** M ♀
[0,1,3]
Leakage (microscopic) of fetal blood into maternal circulation

§✓5th **656.1 Rhesus isoimmunization** M ♀
[0,1,3]
Anti-D [Rh] antibodies
Rh incompatibility

DEF: Antibodies developing against Rh factor; mother with Rh negative develops antibodies against Rh positive fetus.

§✓5th **656.2 Isoimmunization from other and unspecified blood-group incompatibility** M ♀
[0,1,3]
ABO isoimmunization

§✓5th **656.3 Fetal distress** M ♀
[0,1,3]
Fetal metabolic acidemia

EXCLUDES *abnormal fetal acid-base balance (656.8)*
abnormality in fetal heart rate or rhythm (659.7)
fetal bradycardia (659.7)
fetal tachycardia (659.7)
meconium in liquor (656.8)

AHA: N-D, '86, 4

DEF: Life-threatening disorder; fetal anoxia, hemolytic disease and other miscellaneous diseases cause fetal distress.

§✓5th **656.4 Intrauterine death** M ♀
[0,1,3]
Fetal death:
- NOS
- after completion of 22 weeks' gestation
- late

Missed delivery

EXCLUDES *missed abortion (632)*

§✓5th **656.5 Poor fetal growth** M ♀
[0,1,3]
"Light-for-dates"
"Small-for-dates"
"Placental insufficiency"

§✓5th **656.6 Excessive fetal growth** M ♀
[0,1,3]
"Large-for-dates"

§✓5th **656.7 Other placental conditions** M ♀
[0,1,3]
Abnormal placenta
Placental infarct

EXCLUDES *placental polyp (674.4)*
placentitis (658.4)

§✓5th **656.8 Other specified fetal and placental problems** M ♀
[0,1,3]
Abnormal acid-base balance
Intrauterine acidosis
Lithopedian
Meconium in liquor

DEF: Lithopedion: Calcified fetus; not expelled by mother.

§✓5th **656.9 Unspecified fetal and placental problem** M ♀
[0,1,3]

✓4th **657 Polyhydramnios** M ♀
[0,1,3]
§✓5th Use 0 as fourth-digit for this category
Hydramnios

AHA: 4Q, '91, 26

DEF: Excess amniotic fluid.

✓4th **658 Other problems associated with amniotic cavity and membranes**

EXCLUDES *amniotic fluid embolism (673.1)*

§✓5th **658.0 Oligohydramnios** M ♀
[0,1,3]
Oligohydramnios without mention of rupture of membranes

DEF: Deficient amount of amniotic fluid.

§✓5th **658.1 Premature rupture of membranes** M ♀
[0,1,3]
Rupture of amniotic sac less than 24 hours prior to the onset of labor

AHA: For code 658.13: 1Q, '01, 5; 4Q, '98, 77

§✓5th **658.2 Delayed delivery after spontaneous or unspecified rupture of membranes** M ♀
[0,1,3]
Prolonged rupture of membranes NOS
Rupture of amniotic sac 24 hours or more prior to the onset of labor

§✓5th **658.3 Delayed delivery after artificial rupture of membranes** M ♀
[0,1,3]

§✓5th **658.4 Infection of amniotic cavity** M ♀
[0,1,3]
Amnionitis
Chorioamnionitis
Membranitis
Placentitis

§✓5th **658.8 Other** M ♀
[0,1,3]
Amnion nodosum
Amniotic cyst

§✓5th **658.9 Unspecified** M ♀
[0,1,3]

✓4th **659 Other indications for care or intervention related to labor and delivery, not elsewhere classified**

§✓5th **659.0 Failed mechanical induction** M ♀
[0,1,3]
Failure of induction of labor by surgical or other instrumental methods

§✓5th **659.1 Failed medical or unspecified induction** M ♀
[0,1,3]
Failed induction NOS
Failure of induction of labor by medical methods, such as oxytocic drugs

§ Requires fifth digit. Valid digits are in [brackets] under each code. See beginning of section 640–648 for codes and definitions.

N Newborn Age: 0 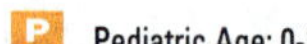 P Pediatric Age: 0-17 M Maternity Age: 12-55 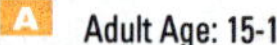 A Adult Age: 15-124 MSP Medicare Secondary Payer

§ 5th **659.2 Maternal pyrexia during labor, unspecified** M ♀
[0,1,3]
DEF: Fever during labor.

§ 5th **659.3 Generalized infection during labor** M ♀
[0,1,3]
Septicemia during labor

§ 5th **659.4 Grand multiparity** M ♀
[0,1,3]
EXCLUDES *supervision only, in pregnancy (V23.3)*
without current pregnancy (V61.5)
DEF: Having borne six or more children previously.

§ 5th **659.5 Elderly primigravida** M ♀
[0,1,3]
First pregnancy in a woman who will be 35 years of age or older at expected date of delivery
EXCLUDES *supervision only, in pregnancy (V23.81)*
AHA: 3Q, '01, 12

§ 5th **659.6 Elderly multigravida** M ♀
[0,1,3]
Second or more pregnancy in a woman who will be 35 years of age or older at expected date of delivery
EXCLUDES *elderly primigravida 659.5*
supervision only, in pregnancy (V23.82)
AHA: 3Q, '01, 12

§ 5th **659.7 Abnormality in fetal heart rate or rhythm** M ♀
[0,1,3]
Depressed fetal heart tones
Fetal:
bradycardia
tachycardia
Fetal heart rate decelerations
Non-reassuring fetal heart rate or rhythm
AHA: 4Q, '98, 48

§ 5th **659.8 Other specified indications for care or intervention related to labor and delivery** M ♀
[0,1,3]
Pregnancy in a female less than 16 years old at expected date of delivery
Very young maternal age
AHA: 3Q, '01, 12

§ 5th **659.9 Unspecified indication for care or intervention related to labor and delivery** M ♀
[0,1,3]

COMPLICATIONS OCCURRING MAINLY IN THE COURSE OF LABOR AND DELIVERY (660-669)

The following fifth-digit subclassification is for use with categories 660-669 to denote the current episode of care. Valid fifth-digits are in [brackets] under each code.

0 unspecified as to episode of care or not applicable
1 delivered, with or without mention of antepartum condition
2 delivered, with mention of postpartum complication
3 antepartum condition or complication
4 postpartum condition or complication

4th **660 Obstructed labor**
AHA: 3Q, '95, 10

§ 5th **660.0 Obstruction caused by malposition of fetus at onset of labor** M ♀
[0,1,3]
Any condition classifiable to 652, causing obstruction during labor
Use additional code from 652.0-652.9 to identify condition

§ 5th **660.1 Obstruction by bony pelvis** M ♀
[0,1,3]
Any condition classifiable to 653, causing obstruction during labor
Use additional code from 653.0-653.9 to identify condition

§ 5th **660.2 Obstruction by abnormal pelvic soft tissues** M ♀
[0,1,3]
Prolapse of anterior lip of cervix
Any condition classifiable to 654, causing obstruction during labor
Use additional code from 654.0-654.9 to identify condition

§ 5th **660.3 Deep transverse arrest and persistent occipitoposterior position** M ♀
[0,1,3]

§ 5th **660.4 Shoulder (girdle) dystocia** M ♀
[0,1,3]
Impacted shoulders
DEF: Obstructed labor due to impacted fetal shoulders.

§ 5th **660.5 Locked twins** M ♀
[0,1,3]

§ 5th **660.6 Failed trial of labor, unspecified** M ♀
[0,1,3]
Failed trial of labor, without mention of condition or suspected condition

§ 5th **660.7 Failed forceps or vacuum extractor, unspecified** M ♀
[0,1,3]
Application of ventouse or forceps, without mention of condition

§ 5th **660.8 Other causes of obstructed labor** M ♀
[0,1,3]
▶Use additional code to identify condition◀
AHA: 4Q, '04, 88

§ 5th **660.9 Unspecified obstructed labor** M ♀
[0,1,3]
Dystocia:
NOS
fetal NOS
Dystocia:
maternal NOS

4th **661 Abnormality of forces of labor**

§ 5th **661.0 Primary uterine inertia** M ♀
[0,1,3]
Failure of cervical dilation
Hypotonic uterine dysfunction, primary
Prolonged latent phase of labor
DEF: Lack of efficient contractions during labor causing prolonged labor.

§ 5th **661.1 Secondary uterine inertia** M ♀
[0,1,3]
Arrested active phase of labor
Hypotonic uterine dysfunction, secondary

§ 5th **661.2 Other and unspecified uterine inertia** M ♀
[0,1,3]
Desultory labor
Irregular labor
Poor contractions
Slow slope active phase of labor

§ 5th **661.3 Precipitate labor** M ♀
[0,1,3]
DEF: Rapid labor and delivery.

§ 5th **661.4 Hypertonic, incoordinate, or prolonged uterine contractions** M ♀
[0,1,3]
Cervical spasm
Contraction ring (dystocia)
Dyscoordinate labor
Hourglass contraction of uterus
Hypertonic uterine dysfunction
Incoordinate uterine action
Retraction ring (Bandl's) (pathological)
Tetanic contractions
Uterine dystocia NOS
Uterine spasm

§ 5th **661.9 Unspecified abnormality of labor** M ♀
[0,1,3]

4th **662 Long labor**

§ 5th **662.0 Prolonged first stage** M ♀
[0,1,3]

§ 5th **662.1 Prolonged labor, unspecified** M ♀
[0,1,3]

§ 5th **662.2 Prolonged second stage** M ♀
[0,1,3]

§ 5th **662.3 Delayed delivery of second twin, triplet, etc.** M ♀
[0,1,3]

§ Requires fifth digit. Valid digits are in [brackets] under each code. See beginning of section 640–648 for codes and definitions.

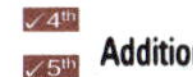
Additional Digit Required | Unspecified Code | Other Specified Code | Manifestation Code | ▶◀ Revised Text | ● New Code | ▲ Revised Code Title

✓4th **663 Umbilical cord complications**

§ ✓5th **663.0 Prolapse of cord** M♀
[0,1,3]
Presentation of cord
DEF: Abnormal presentation of fetus; marked by protruding umbilical cord during labor; can cause fetal death.

§ ✓5th **663.1 Cord around neck, with compression** M♀
[0,1,3]
Cord tightly around neck

§ ✓5th **663.2 Other and unspecified cord entanglement, with compression** M♀
[0,1,3]
Entanglement of cords of twins in mono-amniotic sac
Knot in cord (with compression)

§ ✓5th **663.3 Other and unspecified cord entanglement, without mention of compression** M♀
[0,1,3]
AHA: For code 663.31: 2Q, '03, 9

§ ✓5th **663.4 Short cord** M♀
[0,1,3]

§ ✓5th **663.5 Vasa previa** M♀
[0,1,3]
DEF: Abnormal presentation of fetus marked by blood vessels of umbilical cord in front of fetal head.

§ ✓5th **663.6 Vascular lesions of cord** M♀
[0,1,3]
Bruising of cord
Hematoma of cord
Thrombosis of vessels of cord

§ ✓5th **663.8 Other umbilical cord complications** M♀
[0,1,3]
Velamentous insertion of umbilical cord

§ ✓5th **663.9 Unspecified umbilical cord complication** M♀
[0,1,3]

✓4th **664 Trauma to perineum and vulva during delivery**
INCLUDES damage from instruments
that from extension of episiotomy
AHA: 1Q, '92, 11; N-D, '84, 10

§ ✓5th **664.0 First-degree perineal laceration** M♀
[0,1,4]
Perineal laceration, rupture, or tear involving:
fourchette
hymen
labia
skin
vagina
vulva

§ ✓5th **664.1 Second-degree perineal laceration** M♀
[0,1,4]
Perineal laceration, rupture, or tear (following episiotomy) involving:
pelvic floor
perineal muscles
vaginal muscles
EXCLUDES *that involving anal sphincter (664.2)*

Perineal Lacerations

§ ✓5th **664.2 Third-degree perineal laceration** M♀
[0,1,4]
Perineal laceration, rupture, or tear (following episiotomy) involving:
anal sphincter
rectovaginal septum
sphincter NOS
EXCLUDES *that with anal or rectal mucosal laceration (664.3)*

§ ✓5th **664.3 Fourth-degree perineal laceration** M♀
[0,1,4]
Perineal laceration, rupture, or tear as classifiable to 664.2 and involving also:
anal mucosa
rectal mucosa

§ ✓5th **664.4 Unspecified perineal laceration** M♀
[0,1,4]
Central laceration
AHA: 1Q, '92, 8

§ ✓5th **664.5 Vulval and perineal hematoma** M♀
[0,1,4]
AHA: N-D, '84, 10

§ ✓5th **664.8 Other specified trauma to perineum and vulva** M♀
[0,1,4]

§ ✓5th **664.9 Unspecified trauma to perineum and vulva** M♀
[0,1,4]

✓4th **665 Other obstetrical trauma**
INCLUDES damage from instruments

§ ✓5th **665.0 Rupture of uterus before onset of labor** M♀
[0,1,3]

§ ✓5th **665.1 Rupture of uterus during labor** M♀
[0,1]
Rupture of uterus NOS

§ ✓5th **665.2 Inversion of uterus** M♀
[0,2,4]

§ ✓5th **665.3 Laceration of cervix** M♀
[0,1,4]

§ ✓5th **665.4 High vaginal laceration** M♀
[0,1,4]
Laceration of vaginal wall or sulcus without mention of perineal laceration

§ ✓5th **665.5 Other injury to pelvic organs** M♀
[0,1,4]
Injury to:
bladder
urethra
AHA: M-A, '87, 10

§ ✓5th **665.6 Damage to pelvic joints and ligaments** M♀
[0,1,4]
Avulsion of inner symphyseal cartilage
Damage to coccyx
Separation of symphysis (pubis)
AHA: N-D, '84, 12

§ ✓5th **665.7 Pelvic hematoma** M♀
[0,1,2,4]
Hematoma of vagina

§ ✓5th **665.8 Other specified obstetrical trauma** M♀
[0-4]

§ ✓5th **665.9 Unspecified obstetrical trauma** M♀
[0-4]

✓4th **666 Postpartum hemorrhage**
AHA: 1Q, '88, 14

§ ✓5th **666.0 Third-stage hemorrhage** M♀
[0,2,4]
Hemorrhage associated with retained, trapped, or adherent placenta
Retained placenta NOS

§ ✓5th **666.1 Other immediate postpartum hemorrhage** M♀
[0,2,4]
Atony of uterus
Hemorrhage within the first 24 hours following delivery of placenta
Postpartum hemorrhage (atonic) NOS

§ Requires fifth digit. Valid digits are in [brackets] under each code. See beginning of section 640–648 for codes and definitions.

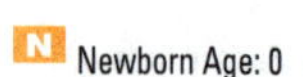 Newborn Age: 0
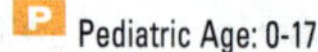 Pediatric Age: 0-17
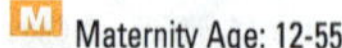 Maternity Age: 12-55
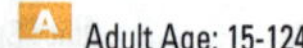 Adult Age: 15-124
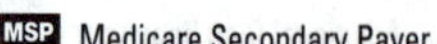 Medicare Secondary Payer

§ ✓5th **666.2 Delayed and secondary postpartum hemorrhage** M ♀
[0,2,4]
Hemorrhage:
after the first 24 hours following delivery
associated with retained portions of placenta or membranes
Postpartum hemorrhage specified as delayed or secondary
Retained products of conception NOS, following delivery

§ ✓5th **666.3 Postpartum coagulation defects** M ♀
[0,2,4]
Postpartum: afibrinogenemia
Postpartum: fibrinolysis

✓4th **667 Retained placenta or membranes, without hemorrhage**
Requires fifth-digit; valid digits are in [brackets] under each code. See beginning of section 660-669 for definitions.
AHA: 1Q, '88, 14

DEF: Postpartum condition resulting from failure to expel placental membrane tissues due to failed contractions of uterine wall.

§ ✓5th **667.0 Retained placenta without hemorrhage** M ♀
[0,2,4]
Placenta accreta
Retained placenta:
NOS
total
} without hemorrhage

§ ✓5th **667.1 Retained portions of placenta or membranes, without hemorrhage** M ♀
[0,2,4]
Retained products of conception following delivery, without hemorrhage

✓4th **668 Complications of the administration of anesthetic or other sedation in labor and delivery**
INCLUDES complications arising from the administration of a general or local anesthetic, analgesic, or other sedation in labor and delivery
EXCLUDES *reaction to spinal or lumbar puncture (349.0)*
spinal headache (349.0)
Use additional code(s) to further specify complication

§ ✓5th **668.0 Pulmonary complications** M ♀
[0-4]
Inhalation [aspiration] of stomach contents or secretions
Mendelson's syndrome
Pressure collapse of lung
} following anesthesia or other sedation in labor or delivery

§ ✓5th **668.1 Cardiac complications** M ♀
[0-4]
Cardiac arrest or failure following anesthesia or other sedation in labor and delivery

§ ✓5th **668.2 Central nervous system complications** M ♀
[0-4]
Cerebral anoxia following anesthesia or other sedation in labor and delivery

§ ✓5th **668.8 Other complications of anesthesia or other sedation in labor and delivery** M ♀
[0-4]
AHA: 2Q, '99, 9

§ ✓5th **668.9 Unspecified complication of anesthesia and other sedation** M ♀
[0-4]

✓4th **669 Other complications of labor and delivery, not elsewhere classified**

§ ✓5th **669.0 Maternal distress** M ♀
[0-4]
Metabolic disturbance in labor and delivery

§ ✓5th **669.1 Shock during or following labor and delivery** M ♀
[0-4]
Obstetric shock

§ ✓5th **669.2 Maternal hypotension syndrome** M ♀
[0-4]
DEF: Low arterial blood pressure, in mother, during labor and delivery.

§ ✓5th **669.3 Acute renal failure following labor and delivery** M ♀
[0,2,4]

§ ✓5th **669.4 Other complications of obstetrical surgery and procedures** M ♀
[0-4]
Cardiac:
arrest
failure
Cerebral anoxia
} following cesarean or other obstetrical surgery or procedure, including delivery NOS
EXCLUDES *complications of obstetrical surgical wounds (674.1-674.3)*

§ ✓5th **669.5 Forceps or vacuum extractor delivery without mention of indication** M ♀
[0,1]
Delivery by ventouse, without mention of indication

§ ✓5th **669.6 Breech extraction, without mention of indication** M ♀
[0,1]
EXCLUDES *breech delivery NOS (652.2)*

§ ✓5th **669.7 Cesarean delivery, without mention of indication** M ♀
[0,1]
AHA: For code 669.71: 1Q, '01, 11

§ ✓5th **669.8 Other complications of labor and delivery** M ♀
[0-4]

§ ✓5th **669.9 Unspecified complication of labor and delivery** M ♀
[0-4]

COMPLICATIONS OF THE PUERPERIUM (670-677)

Note: Categories 671 and 673-676 include the listed conditions even if they occur during pregnancy or childbirth.

The following fifth-digit subclassification is for use with categories 670-676 to denote the current episode of care. Valid fifth-digits are in [brackets] under each code.
- **0 unspecified as to episode of care or not applicable**
- **1 delivered, with or without mention of antepartum condition**
- **2 delivered, with mention of postpartum complication**
- **3 antepartum condition or complication**
- **4 postpartum condition or complication**

✓4th **670 Major puerperal infection** M ♀
[0,2,4]
§ ✓5th Use 0 as fourth-digit for this category
Puerperal:
endometritis
fever (septic)
pelvic:
cellulitis
sepsis
peritonitis
pyemia
salpingitis
septicemia
EXCLUDES *infection following abortion (639.0)*
minor genital tract infection following delivery (646.6)
puerperal pyrexia NOS (672)
puerperal fever NOS (672)
puerperal pyrexia of unknown origin (672)
urinary tract infection following delivery (646.6)
AHA: 4Q, '91, 26; 2Q, '91, 7

DEF: Infection and inflammation, following childbirth.

✓4th **671 Venous complications in pregnancy and the puerperium**

§ ✓5th **671.0 Varicose veins of legs** M ♀
[0-4]
Varicose veins NOS
DEF: Distended, tortuous veins on legs associated with pregnancy.

§ Requires fifth digit. Valid digits are in [brackets] under each code. See beginning of section 640–648 for codes and definitions.

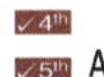
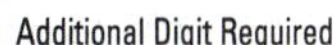
Additional Digit Required | Unspecified Code | Other Specified Code | Manifestation Code | ►◄ Revised Text | ● New Code | ▲ Revised Code Title

§ ✓5th **671.1 Varicose veins of vulva and perineum** M ♀
[0-4]
DEF: Distended, tortuous veins on external female genitalia associated with pregnancy.

§ ✓5th **671.2 Superficial thrombophlebitis** M ♀
[0-4]
Thrombophlebitis (superficial)

§ ✓5th **671.3 Deep phlebothrombosis, antepartum** M ♀
[0,1,3]
Deep-vein thrombosis, antepartum

§ ✓5th **671.4 Deep phlebothrombosis, postpartum** M ♀
[0,2,4]
Deep-vein thrombosis, postpartum
Pelvic thrombophlebitis, postpartum
Phlegmasia alba dolens (puerperal)

§ ✓5th **671.5 Other phlebitis and thrombosis** M ♀
[0-4]
Cerebral venous thrombosis
Thrombosis of intracranial venous sinus

§ ✓5th **671.8 Other venous complications** M ♀
[0-4]
Hemorrhoids

§ ✓5th **671.9 Unspecified venous complication** M ♀
[0-4]
Phlebitis NOS
Thrombosis NOS

✓4th **672 Pyrexia of unknown origin during the puerperium** M ♀
[0,2,4]
§ ✓5th Use 0 as fourth-digit for this category
Postpartum fever NOS
Puerperal fever NOS
Puerperal pyrexia NOS
AHA: 4Q, '91, 26

DEF: Fever of unknown origin experienced by the mother after childbirth.

✓4th **673 Obstetrical pulmonary embolism**
Requires fifth-digit; valid digits are in [brackets] under each code. See beginning of section 670-676 for definitions.
INCLUDES pulmonary emboli in pregnancy, childbirth or the puerperium, or specified as puerperal
EXCLUDES *embolism following abortion (639.6)*

§ ✓5th **673.0 Obstetrical air embolism** M ♀
[0-4]
DEF: Sudden blocking of pulmonary artery with air or nitrogen bubbles during puerperium..

§ ✓5th **673.1 Amniotic fluid embolism** M ♀
[0-4]
DEF: Sudden onset of pulmonary artery blockage from amniotic fluid entering the mother's circulation near the end of pregnancy due to strong uterine contractions.

§ ✓5th **673.2 Obstetrical blood-clot embolism** M ♀
[0-4]
Puerperal pulmonary embolism NOS
AHA: For code 673.24: ►1Q, '05, 6◄

DEF: Blood clot blocking artery in the lung; associated with pregnancy.

§ ✓5th **673.3 Obstetrical pyemic and septic embolism** M ♀
[0-4]

§ ✓5th **673.8 Other pulmonary embolism** M ♀
[0-4]
Fat embolism

✓4th **674 Other and unspecified complications of the puerperium, not elsewhere classified**

§ ✓5th **674.0 Cerebrovascular disorders in the puerperium** M ♀
[0-4]
Any condition classifiable to 430-434, 436-437 occurring during pregnancy, childbirth or the puerperium, or specified as puerperal
EXCLUDES *intracranial venous sinus thrombosis (671.5)*

§ ✓5th **674.1 Disruption of cesarean wound** M ♀
[0,2,4]
Dehiscence or disruption of uterine wound
EXCLUDES *uterine rupture before onset of labor (665.0)*
uterine rupture during labor (665.1)

§ ✓5th **674.2 Disruption of perineal wound** M ♀
[0,2,4]
Breakdown of perineum
Disruption of wound of:
episiotomy
Disruption of wound of:
perineal laceration
Secondary perineal tear
AHA: For code 674.24: 1Q, '97, 9

§ ✓5th **674.3 Other complications of obstetrical surgical wounds** M ♀
[0,2,4]
Hematoma
Hemorrhage
Infection
} of cesarean section or perineal wound
EXCLUDES *damage from instruments in delivery (664.0-665.9)*
AHA: 2Q, '91, 7

§ ✓5th **674.4 Placental polyp** M ♀
[0,2,4]

§ ✓5th **674.5 Peripartum cardiomyopathy** M ♀
[0-4]
Postpartum cardiomyopathy
AHA: 4Q, '03, 65

DEF: Any structural or functional abnormality of the ventricular myocardium, non-inflammatory disease of obscure or unknown etiology with onset during the postpartum period.

§ ✓5th **674.8 Other** M ♀
[0,2,4]
Hepatorenal syndrome, following delivery
Postpartum:
subinvolution of uterus
uterine hypertrophy
AHA: 3Q, '98, 16

§ ✓5th **674.9 Unspecified** M ♀
[0,2,4]
Sudden death of unknown cause during the puerperium

✓4th **675 Infections of the breast and nipple associated with childbirth**
INCLUDES the listed conditions during pregnancy, childbirth or the puerperium

§ ✓5th **675.0 Infections of nipple** M ♀
[0-4]
Abscess of nipple

§ ✓5th **675.1 Abscess of breast** M ♀
[0-4]
Abscess:
mammary
subareolar
submammary
Mastitis:
purulent
retromammary
submammary

§ ✓5th **675.2 Nonpurulent mastitis** M ♀
[0-4]
Lymphangitis of breast
Mastitis:
NOS
Mastitis:
interstitial
parenchymatous

§ ✓5th **675.8 Other specified infections of the breast and nipple** M ♀
[0-4]

Lactation Process: Ejection Reflex Arc

§ Requires fifth digit. Valid digits are in [brackets] under each code. See beginning of section 640-648 for codes and definitions.

§ 5th **675.9 Unspecified infection of the breast and nipple** M ♀
[0-4]

4th **676 Other disorders of the breast associated with childbirth and disorders of lactation**

INCLUDES the listed conditions during pregnancy, the puerperium, or lactation

§ 5th **676.0 Retracted nipple** M ♀
[0-4]

§ 5th **676.1 Cracked nipple** M ♀
[0-4]
Fissure of nipple

§ 5th **676.2 Engorgement of breasts** M ♀
[0-4]
DEF: Abnormal accumulation of milk in ducts of breast.

§ 5th **676.3 Other and unspecified disorder of breast** M ♀
[0-4]

§ 5th **676.4 Failure of lactation** M ♀
[0-4]
Agalactia
DEF: Abrupt ceasing of milk secretion by breast.

§ 5th **676.5 Suppressed lactation** M ♀
[0-4]

§ 5th **676.6 Galactorrhea** M ♀
[0-4]
EXCLUDES *galactorrhea not associated with childbirth (611.6)*
DEF: Excessive or persistent milk secretion by breast; may be in absence of nursing.

§ 5th **676.8 Other disorders of lactation** M ♀
[0-4]
Galactocele
DEF: Galactocele: obstructed mammary gland, creating retention cyst, results in milk-filled cysts enlarging mammary gland.

§ 5th **676.9 Unspecified disorder of lactation** M ♀
[0-4]

677 Late effect of complication of pregnancy, childbirth, and the puerperium ♀

Note: This category is to be used to indicate conditions in 632-648.9 and 651-676.9 as the cause of the late effect, themselves classifiable elsewhere. The "late effects" include conditions specified as such, or as sequelae, which may occur at any time after puerperium.

Code first any sequelae

AHA: 1Q, '97, 9; 4Q, '94, 42

§ Requires fifth digit. Valid digits are in [brackets] under each code. See beginning of section 640-648 for codes and definitions.

12. DISEASES OF THE SKIN AND SUBCUTANEOUS TISSUE (680-709)

INFECTIONS OF SKIN AND SUBCUTANEOUS TISSUE (680-686)

EXCLUDES *certain infections of skin classified under "Infectious and Parasitic Diseases," such as:*
erysipelas (035)
erysipeloid of Rosenbach (027.1)
herpes:
simplex (054.0-054.9)
zoster (053.0-053.9)
molluscum contagiosum (078.0)
viral warts (078.1)

✓4th **680 Carbuncle and furuncle**
INCLUDES boil
furunculosis
DEF: Carbuncle: necrotic boils in skin and subcutaneous tissue of neck or back mainly due to staphylococcal infection.
DEF: Furuncle: circumscribed inflammation of corium and subcutaneous tissue due to staphylococcal infection.

680.0 Face
Ear [any part] — Nose (septum)
Face [any part, except eye] — Temple (region)
EXCLUDES *eyelid (373.13)*
lacrimal apparatus (375.31)
orbit (376.01)

680.1 Neck

680.2 Trunk
Abdominal wall — Flank
Back [any part, except buttocks] — Groin
Breast — Pectoral region
Chest wall — Perineum
Umbilicus
EXCLUDES *buttocks (680.5)*
external genital organs:
female (616.4)
male (607.2, 608.4)

680.3 Upper arm and forearm
Arm [any part, except hand] — Axilla
Shoulder

680.4 Hand
Finger [any] — Wrist
Thumb

680.5 Buttock
Anus — Gluteal region

680.6 Leg, except foot
Ankle — Knee
Hip — Thigh

680.7 Foot
Heel — Toe

680.8 Other specified sites
Head [any part, except face]
Scalp
EXCLUDES *external genital organs:*
female (616.4)
male (607.2, 608.4)

680.9 Unspecified site
Boil NOS — Furuncle NOS
Carbuncle NOS

✓4th **681 Cellulitis and abscess of finger and toe**
INCLUDES that with lymphangitis
Use additional code to identify organism, such as Staphylococcus (041.1)
AHA: 2Q, '91, 5; J-F, '87, 12
DEF: Acute suppurative inflammation and edema in subcutaneous tissue or muscle of finger or toe.

✓5th **681.0 Finger**
681.00 Cellulitis and abscess, unspecified
681.01 Felon
Pulp abscess — Whitlow
EXCLUDES *herpetic whitlow (054.6)*
DEF: Painful abscess of fingertips caused by infection in the closed space of terminal phalanx.
681.02 Onychia and paronychia of finger
Panaritium } of finger
Perionychia }
DEF: Onychia: inflammation of nail matrix; causes nail loss.
DEF: Paronychia: inflammation of tissue folds around nail.

✓5th **681.1 Toe**
681.10 Cellulitis and abscess, unspecified
AHA: ►1Q, '05, 14◄
681.11 Onychia and paronychia of toe
Panaritium } of toe
Perionychia }

681.9 Cellulitis and abscess of unspecified digit
Infection of nail NOS

✓4th **682 Other cellulitis and abscess**
INCLUDES abscess (acute) } (with lymphangitis) except of finger or toe
cellulitis (diffuse) }
lymphangitis, acute }
Use additional code to identify organism, such as Staphylococcus (041.1)
EXCLUDES *lymphangitis (chronic) (subacute) (457.2)*
AHA: 2Q, '91, 5; J-F, '87, 12; S-O, '85, 10
DEF: Cellulitis: Acute suppurative inflammation of deep subcutaneous tissue and sometimes muscle due to infection of wound, burn or other lesion.

682.0 Face
Cheek, external — Nose, external
Chin — Submandibular
Forehead — Temple (region)
EXCLUDES *ear [any part] (380.10-380.16)*
eyelid (373.13)
lacrimal apparatus (375.31)
lip (528.5)
mouth (528.3)
nose (internal) (478.1)
orbit (376.01)

682.1 Neck

682.2 Trunk
Abdominal wall — Groin
Back [any part, except buttock] — Pectoral region
Chest wall — Perineum
Flank — Umbilicus, except newborn
EXCLUDES *anal and rectal regions (566)*
breast:
NOS (611.0)
puerperal (675.1)
external genital organs:
female (616.3-616.4)
male (604.0, 607.2, 608.4)
umbilicus, newborn (771.4)
AHA: 4Q, '98, 42

Skin and Subcutaneous Layer

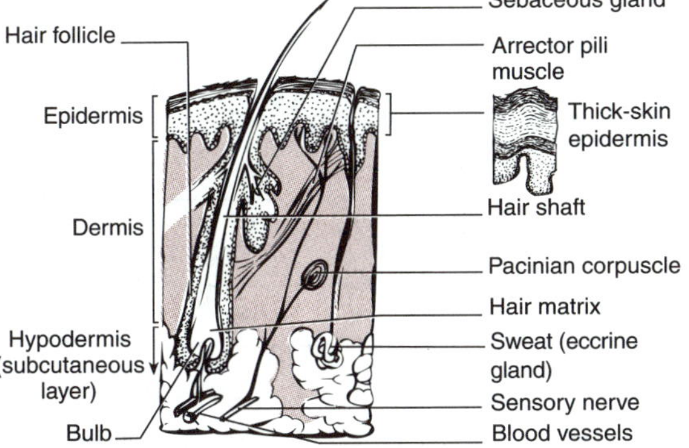

Skin and Subcutaneous Tissue

680–682.2

682.3 Upper arm and forearm
Arm [any part, except hand]
Axilla
Shoulder
EXCLUDES *hand (682.4)*
AHA: 2Q, '03, 7

682.4 Hand, except fingers and thumb
Wrist
EXCLUDES *finger and thumb (681.00-681.02)*

682.5 Buttock
Gluteal region
EXCLUDES *anal and rectal regions (566)*

682.6 Leg, except foot
Ankle
Hip
Knee
Thigh
AHA: ▶3Q, '04, 5;◀ 4Q, '03, 108

682.7 Foot, except toes
Heel
EXCLUDES *toe (681.10-681.11)*

682.8 Other specified sites
Head [except face]
Scalp
EXCLUDES *face (682.0)*

682.9 Unspecified site
Abscess NOS
Cellulitis NOS
Lymphangitis, acute NOS
EXCLUDES *lymphangitis NOS (457.2)*

683 Acute lymphadenitis
Abscess (acute) } lymph gland or node, except mesenteric
Adenitis, acute } lymph gland or node, except mesenteric
Lymphadenitis, acute } lymph gland or node, except mesenteric

Use additional code to identify organism, such as Staphylococcus (041.1)
EXCLUDES *enlarged glands NOS (785.6)*
lymphadenitis:
chronic or subacute, except mesenteric (289.1)
mesenteric (acute) (chronic) (subacute) (289.2)
unspecified (289.3)

DEF: Acute inflammation of lymph nodes due to primary infection located elsewhere in the body.

684 Impetigo
Impetiginization of other dermatoses
Impetigo (contagiosa) [any site] [any organism]:
bullous
circinate
neonatorum
simplex
Pemphigus neonatorum
EXCLUDES *impetigo herpetiformis (694.3)*

DEF: Infectious skin disease commonly occurring in children; caused by group A streptococci or *Staphylococcus aureus*; skin lesions usually appear on the face and consist of subcorneal vesicles and bullae that burst and form yellow crusts.

✓4th **685 Pilonidal cyst**
INCLUDES fistula } coccygeal or pilonidal
sinus } coccygeal or pilonidal

DEF: Hair-containing cyst or sinus in the tissues of the sacrococcygeal area; often drains through opening at the postanal dimple.

685.0 With abscess

685.1 Without mention of abscess

✓4th **686 Other local infections of skin and subcutaneous tissue**
Use additional code to identify any infectious organism (041.0-041.8)

✓5th **686.0 Pyoderma**
Dermatitis:
purulent
septic
suppurative

DEF: Nonspecific purulent skin disease related most to furuncles, pustules, or possibly carbuncles.

Lymphatic System of Head and Neck

Afferent vessels (in)
Blood vessels
Hilum
Efferent vessel (out)
Schematic of lymph node

Superficial parotid
Jugulodigastric
Submental
Occipital
Submandibular
Jugulomyohyoid
Anterior cervical
Lymphatic drainage of the head, neck, and face

686.00 Pyoderma, unspecified

686.01 Pyoderma gangrenosum
AHA: 4Q, '97, 42

DEF: Persistent debilitating skin disease, characterized by irregular, boggy, blue-red ulcerations, with central healing and undermined edges.

686.09 Other pyoderma

686.1 Pyogenic granuloma
Granuloma:
septic
suppurative
telangiectaticum
EXCLUDES *pyogenic granuloma of oral mucosa (528.9)*

DEF: Solitary polypoid capillary hemangioma often associated with local irritation, trauma, and superimposed inflammation; located on the skin and gingival or oral mucosa.

686.8 Other specified local infections of skin and subcutaneous tissue
Bacterid (pustular)
Dermatitis vegetans
Ecthyma
Perlèche
EXCLUDES *dermatitis infectiosa eczematoides (690.8)*
panniculitis (729.30-729.39)

686.9 Unspecified local infection of skin and subcutaneous tissue
Fistula of skin NOS
Skin infection NOS
EXCLUDES *fistula to skin from internal organs — see Alphabetic Index*

OTHER INFLAMMATORY CONDITIONS OF SKIN AND SUBCUTANEOUS TISSUE (690-698)

EXCLUDES *panniculitis (729.30-729.39)*

✓4th **690 Erythematosquamous dermatosis**
EXCLUDES *eczematous dermatitis of eyelid (373.31)*
parakeratosis variegata (696.2)
psoriasis (696.0-696.1)
seborrheic keratosis (702.11-702.19)

DEF: Dry material desquamated from the scalp, associated with disease.

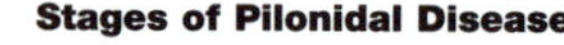

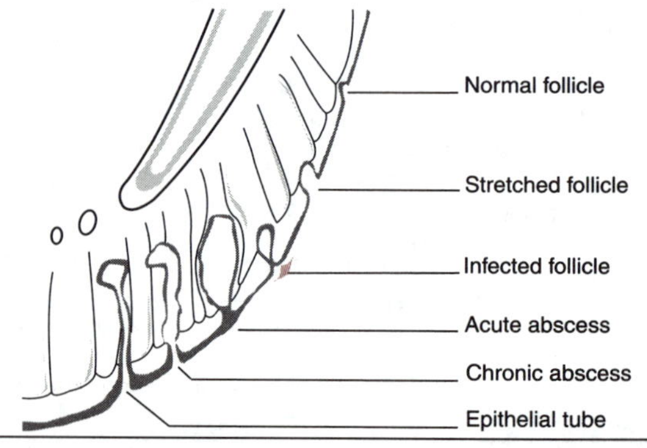

✓5th **690.1 Seborrheic dermatitis**
AHA: 4Q, '95, 58

690.10 Seborrheic dermatitis, unspecified
Seborrheic dermatitis NOS

690.11 Seborrhea capitis P
Cradle cap

690.12 Seborrheic infantile dermatitis P

690.18 Other seborrheic dermatitis

690.8 Other erythematosquamous dermatosis

✓4th **691 Atopic dermatitis and related conditions**
DEF: Atopic dermatitis: chronic, pruritic, inflammatory skin disorder found on the face and antecubital and popliteal fossae; noted in persons with a hereditary predisposition to pruritus, and often accompanied by allergic rhinitis, hay fever, asthma, and extreme itching; also called allergic dermatitis, allergic or atopic eczema, or disseminated neurodermatitis.

691.0 Diaper or napkin rash
Ammonia dermatitis
Diaper or napkin:
  dermatitis
  erythema
Diaper or napkin:
  rash
Psoriasiform napkin eruption

691.8 Other atopic dermatitis and related conditions
Atopic dermatitis
Besnier's prurigo
Eczema:
  atopic
  flexural
  intrinsic (allergic)
Neurodermatitis:
  atopic
  diffuse (of Brocq)

✓4th **692 Contact dermatitis and other eczema**
INCLUDES dermatitis:
  NOS
  contact
  occupational
  venenata
eczema (acute) (chronic):
  NOS
  allergic
  erythematous
  occupational

EXCLUDES *allergy NOS (995.3)*
contact dermatitis of eyelids (373.32)
dermatitis due to substances taken internally (693.0-693.9)
eczema of external ear (380.22)
perioral dermatitis (695.3)
urticarial reactions (708.0-708.9, 995.1)

DEF: Contact dermatitis: acute or chronic dermatitis caused by initial irritant effect of a substance, or by prior sensitization to a substance coming once again in contact with skin.

692.0 Due to detergents

692.1 Due to oils and greases

692.2 Due to solvents
Dermatitis due to solvents of:
  chlorocompound
  cyclohexane
  ester
  glycol
  hydrocarbon
  ketone
} group

692.3 Due to drugs and medicines in contact with skin
Dermatitis (allergic) (contact) due to:
  arnica
  fungicides
  iodine
  keratolytics
  mercurials
Dermatitis (allergic) (contact) due to:
  neomycin
  pediculocides
  phenols
  scabicides
  any drug applied to skin
Dermatitis medicamentosa due to drug applied to skin
Use additional E code to identify drug

EXCLUDES *allergy NOS due to drugs (995.2)*
dermatitis due to ingested drugs (693.0)
dermatitis medicamentosa NOS (693.0)

692.4 Due to other chemical products
Dermatitis due to:
  acids
  adhesive plaster
  alkalis
  caustics
  dichromate
Dermatitis due to:
  insecticide
  nylon
  plastic
  rubber
AHA: 2Q, '89, 16

692.5 Due to food in contact with skin
Dermatitis, contact, due to:
  cereals
  fish
  flour
Dermatitis, contact, due to:
  fruit
  meat
  milk

EXCLUDES *dermatitis due to:*
dyes (692.89)
ingested foods (693.1)
preservatives (692.89)

692.6 Due to plants [except food]
Dermatitis due to:
  lacquer tree [Rhus verniciflua]
  poison:
    ivy [Rhus toxicodendron]
    oak [Rhus diversiloba]
    sumac [Rhus venenata]
    vine [Rhus radicans]
  primrose [Primula]
  ragweed [Senecio jacobae]
  other plants in contact with the skin

EXCLUDES *allergy NOS due to pollen (477.0)*
nettle rash (708.8)

✓5th **692.7 Due to solar radiation**
EXCLUDES *sunburn due to other ultraviolet radiation exposure (692.82)*

692.70 Unspecified dermatitis due to sun

692.71 Sunburn
First degree sunburn
Sunburn NOS
AHA: 4Q, '01, 47

692.72 Acute dermatitis due to solar radiation
Acute solar skin damage NOS
Berlogue dermatitis
Photoallergic response
Phototoxic response
Polymorphus light eruption

EXCLUDES *sunburn (692.71, 692.76-692.77)*

Use additional E code to identify drug, if drug induced

DEF: Berloque dermatitis: phytophotodermatitis due to sun exposure after use of a product containing bergamot oil; causes red patches, which may turn brown.

DEF: Photoallergic response: dermatitis due to hypersensitivity to the sun; causes papulovesicular, eczematous or exudative eruptions.

DEF: Phototoxic response: chemically induced sensitivity to sun causes burn-like reaction, occasionally vesiculation and subsequent hyperpigmentation.

DEF: Polymorphous light eruption: inflammatory skin eruptions due to sunlight exposure; eruptions differ in size and shape.

DEF: Acute solar skin damage (NOS): rapid, unspecified injury to skin from sun.

692.73 Actinic reticuloid and actinic granuloma
DEF: Actinic reticuloid: dermatosis aggravated by light, causes chronic eczema-like eruption on exposed skin which extends to other unexposed surfaces; occurs in the eldery.

DEF: Actinic granuloma: inflammatory response of skin to sun causing small nodule of microphages.

692.74 Other chronic dermatitis due to solar radiation
Solar elastosis
Chronic solar skin damage NOS
EXCLUDES *actinic [solar] keratosis (702.0)*
DEF: Solar elastosis: premature aging of skin of light-skinned people; causes inelasticity, thinning or thickening, wrinkling, dryness, scaling and hyperpigmentation.
DEF: Chronic solar skin damage (NOS): chronic skin impairment due to exposure to the sun, not otherwise specified.

692.75 Disseminated superficial actinic porokeratosis (DSAP)
AHA: 4Q, '00, 43
DEF: Autosomal dominant skin condition occurring in skin that has been overexposed to the sun. Primarily affects women over the age of 16; characterized by numerous superficial annular, keratotic, brownish-red spots or thickenings with depressed centers and sharp, ridged borders. High risk that condition will evolve into squamous cell carcinoma.

692.76 Sunburn of second degree
AHA: 4Q, '01, 47

692.77 Sunburn of third degree
AHA: 4Q, '01, 47

692.79 Other dermatitis due to solar radiation
Hydroa aestivale
Photodermatitis } (due to sun)
Photosensitiveness } (due to sun)
Solar skin damage NOS

✓5th **692.8 Due to other specified agents**

692.81 Dermatitis due to cosmetics

692.82 Dermatitis due to other radiation
Infrared rays
Light
Radiation NOS
Tanning bed
Ultraviolet rays
X-rays
EXCLUDES *solar radiation (692.70-692.79)*
AHA: 4Q, '01, 47; 3Q, '00, 5

692.83 Dermatitis due to metals
Jewelry

692.84 Due to animal (cat) (dog) dander
Due to animal (cat) (dog) hair

692.89 Other
Dermatitis due to:
cold weather
dyes
hot weather
preservatives
EXCLUDES *allergy (NOS) (rhinitis) due to animal hair or dander (477.2)*
allergy to dust (477.8)
sunburn (692.71, 692.76-692.77)

692.9 Unspecified cause
Dermatitis:
NOS
contact NOS
venenata NOS
Eczema NOS

✓4th **693 Dermatitis due to substances taken internally**
EXCLUDES *adverse effect NOS of drugs and medicines (995.2)*
allergy NOS (995.3)
contact dermatitis (692.0-692.9)
urticarial reactions (708.0-708.9, 995.1)
DEF: Inflammation of skin due to ingested substance.

693.0 Due to drugs and medicines
Dermatitis medicamentosa NOS
Use additional E code to identify drug
EXCLUDES *that due to drugs in contact with skin (692.3)*

693.1 Due to food

693.8 Due to other specified substances taken internally

693.9 Due to unspecified substance taken internally
EXCLUDES *dermatitis NOS (692.9)*

✓4th **694 Bullous dermatoses**

694.0 Dermatitis herpetiformis
Dermatosis herpetiformis
Hydroa herpetiformis
Duhring's disease
EXCLUDES *herpes gestationis (646.8)*
dermatitis herpetiformis:
juvenile (694.2)
senile (694.5)
DEF: Chronic, relapsing multisystem disease manifested most in the cutaneous system; seen as an extremely pruritic eruption of various combinations of lesions that frequently heal leaving hyperpigmentation or hypopigmentation and occasionally scarring; usually associated with an asymptomatic gluten-sensitive enteropathy, and immunogenic factors are believed to play a role in its origin.

694.1 Subcorneal pustular dermatosis
Sneddon-Wilkinson disease or syndrome
DEF: Chronic relapses of sterile pustular blebs beneath the horny skin layer of the trunk and skin folds; resembles dermatitis herpetiformis.

694.2 Juvenile dermatitis herpetiformis
Juvenile pemphigoid

694.3 Impetigo herpetiformis
DEF: Rare dermatosis associated with pregnancy; marked by itching pustules in third trimester, hypocalcemia, tetany, fever and lethargy; may result in maternal or fetal death.

694.4 Pemphigus
Pemphigus:
NOS
erythematosus
foliaceus
malignant
vegetans
vulgaris
EXCLUDES *pemphigus neonatorum (684)*
DEF: Chronic, relapsing, sometimes fatal skin diseases; causes vesicles, bullae; autoantibodies against intracellular connections cause acantholysis.

694.5 Pemphigoid
Benign pemphigus NOS
Bullous pemphigoid
Herpes circinatus bullosus
Senile dermatitis herpetiformis

✓5th **694.6 Benign mucous membrane pemphigoid**
Cicatricial pemphigoid
Mucosynechial atrophic bullous dermatitis

694.60 Without mention of ocular involvement

694.61 With ocular involvement
Ocular pemphigus

694.8 Other specified bullous dermatoses
EXCLUDES *herpes gestationis (646.8)*

694.9 Unspecified bullous dermatoses

✓4th **695 Erythematous conditions**

695.0 Toxic erythema
Erythema venenatum

695.1 Erythema multiforme
Erythema iris
Herpes iris
Lyell's syndrome
Scalded skin syndrome
Stevens-Johnson syndrome
Toxic epidermal necrolysis
DEF: Symptom complex with a varied skin eruption pattern of macular, bullous, papular, nodose, or vesicular lesions on the neck, face, and legs; gastritis and rheumatic pains are also noticeable, first-seen symptoms; complex is secondary to a number of factors, including infections, ingestants, physical agents, malignancy and pregnancy.

695.2 Erythema nodosum
EXCLUDES *tuberculous erythema nodosum (017.1)*
DEF: Panniculitis (an inflammatory reaction of the subcutaneous fat) of women, usually seen as a hypersensitivity reaction to various infections, drugs, sarcoidosis, and specific enteropathies; the acute stage is often associated with other symptoms, including fever, malaise, and arthralgia; the lesions are pink to blue in color, appear in crops as tender nodules and are found on the front of the legs below the knees.

695.3 Rosacea
Acne:
erythematosa
rosacea
Perioral dermatitis
Rhinophyma
DEF: Chronic skin disease, usually of the face, characterized by persistent erythema and sometimes by telangiectasis with acute episodes of edema, engorgement papules, and pustules.

695.4 Lupus erythematosus
Lupus:
erythematodes (discoid)
erythematosus (discoid), not disseminated
EXCLUDES *lupus (vulgaris) NOS (017.0)*
systemic [disseminated] lupus erythematosus (710.0)
DEF: Group of connective tissue disorders occurring as various cutaneous diseases of unknown origin; it primarily affects women between the ages of 20 and 40.

✓5th **695.8 Other specified erythematous conditions**
695.81 Ritter's disease
Dermatitis exfoliativa neonatorum
DEF: Infectious skin disease of infants and young children marked by eruptions ranging from a localized bullous type to widespread development of easily ruptured fine vesicles and bullae; results in exfoliation of large planes of skin and leaves raw areas; also called staphylococcal scalded skin syndrome.

695.89 Other
Erythema intertrigo
Intertrigo
Pityriasis rubra (Hebra)
EXCLUDES *mycotic intertrigo (111.0-111.9)*
AHA:: S-O, '86, 10

695.9 Unspecified erythematous condition
Erythema NOS
Erythroderma (secondary)

✓4th **696 Psoriasis and similar disorders**

696.0 Psoriatic arthropathy
DEF: Psoriasis associated with inflammatory arthritis; often involves interphalangeal joints.

696.1 Other psoriasis
Acrodermatitis continua
Dermatitis repens
Psoriasis:
NOS
any type, except arthropathic
EXCLUDES *psoriatic arthropathy (696.0)*

696.2 Parapsoriasis
Parakeratosis variegata
Parapsoriasis lichenoides chronica
Pityriasis lichenoides et varioliformis
DEF: Erythrodermas similar to lichen, planus and psoriasis; symptoms include redness and itching; resistant to treatment.

696.3 Pityriasis rosea
Pityriasis circinata (et maculata)
DEF: Common, self-limited rash of unknown etiology marked by a solitary erythematous, salmon or fawn-colored herald plaque on the trunk, arms or thighs; followed by development of papular or macular lesions that tend to peel and form a scaly collarette.

696.4 Pityriasis rubra pilaris
Devergie's disease
Lichen ruber acuminatus
EXCLUDES *pityriasis rubra (Hebra) (695.89)*
DEF: Inflammatory disease of hair follicles; marked by firm, red lesions topped by horny plugs; may form patches; occurs on fingers elbows, knees.

696.5 Other and unspecified pityriasis
Pityriasis:
NOS
alba
streptogenes
EXCLUDES *pityriasis:*
simplex (690.18)
versicolor (111.0)

696.8 Other

✓4th **697 Lichen**
EXCLUDES *lichen:*
obtusus corneus (698.3)
pilaris (congenital) (757.39)
ruber acuminatus (696.4)
sclerosus et atrophicus (701.0)
scrofulosus (017.0)
simplex chronicus (698.3)
spinulosus (congenital) (757.39)
urticatus (698.2)

697.0 Lichen planus
Lichen:
planopilaris
ruber planus
DEF: Inflammatory, pruritic skin disease; marked by angular, flat-top, violet-colored papules; may be acute and widespread or chronic and localized.

697.1 Lichen nitidus
Pinkus' disease
DEF: Chronic, inflammatory, usually asymptomatic skin disorder, characterized by numerous glistening, flat-topped, discrete, smooth, skin-colored micropapules most often on penis, lower abdomen, inner thighs, wrists, forearms, breasts and buttocks.

697.8 Other lichen, not elsewhere classified
Lichen:
ruber moniliforme
striata

697.9 Lichen, unspecified

✓4th **698 Pruritus and related conditions**
EXCLUDES *pruritus specified as psychogenic (306.3)*
DEF: Pruritus: Intense, persistent itching due to irritation of sensory nerve endings from organic or psychogenic causes.

698.0 Pruritus ani
Perianal itch

698.1 Pruritus of genital organs

698.2 Prurigo
Lichen urticatus
Prurigo:
NOS
Hebra's
mitis
simplex
Urticaria papulosa (Hebra)
EXCLUDES *prurigo nodularis (698.3)*

698.3 Lichenification and lichen simplex chronicus
Hyde's disease
Neurodermatitis (circumscripta) (local)
Prurigo nodularis
EXCLUDES *neurodermatitis, diffuse (of Brocq) (691.8)*
DEF: Lichenification: thickening of skin due to prolonged rubbing or scratching.
DEF: Lichen simplex chronicus: eczematous dermatitis, of face, neck, extremities, scrotum, vulva, and perianal region due to repeated itching, rubbing and scratching; spontaneous or evolves with other dermatoses.

698.4 Dermatitis factitia [artefacta]
Dermatitis ficta
Neurotic excoriation
Use additional code to identify any associated mental disorder
DEF: Various types of self-inflicted skin lesions characterized in appearance as an erythema to a gangrene.

698.8 Other specified pruritic conditions
Pruritus:
hiemalis
senilis
Winter itch

698.9 Unspecified pruritic disorder
Itch NOS
Pruritus NOS

OTHER DISEASES OF SKIN AND SUBCUTANEOUS TISSUE (700-709)

EXCLUDES *conditions confined to eyelids (373.0-374.9)*
congenital conditions of skin, hair, and nails (757.0-757.9)

700 Corns and callosities
Callus
Clavus

DEF: Corns: conical or horny thickening of skin on toes, due to friction, pressure from shoes and hosiery; pain and inflammation may develop.

DEF: Callosities: localized overgrowth (hyperplasia) of the horny epidermal layer due to pressure or friction.

4th **701 Other hypertrophic and atrophic conditions of skin**

EXCLUDES *dermatomyositis (710.3)*
hereditary edema of legs (757.0)
scleroderma (generalized) (710.1)

701.0 Circumscribed scleroderma
Addison's keloid
Dermatosclerosis, localized
Lichen sclerosus et atrophicus
Morphea
Scleroderma, circumscribed or localized

DEF: Thickened, hardened, skin and subcutaneous tissue; may involve musculoskeletal system.

701.1 Keratoderma, acquired
Acquired:
ichthyosis
keratoderma palmaris et plantaris
Elastosis perforans serpiginosa
Hyperkeratosis:
NOS
follicularis in cutem penetrans
palmoplantaris climacterica
Keratoderma:
climactericum
tylodes, progressive
Keratosis (blennorrhagica)

EXCLUDES *Darier's disease [keratosis follicularis] (congenital) (757.39)*
keratosis:
arsenical (692.4)
gonococcal (098.81)

AHA: 4Q, '94, 48

701.2 Acquired acanthosis nigricans
Keratosis nigricans

DEF: Diffuse velvety hyperplasia of the spinous skin layer of the axilla and other body folds marked by gray, brown, or black pigmentation; in adult form it is often associated with an internal carcinoma (malignant acanthosis nigricans) in a benign, nevoid form it is relatively generalized; benign juvenile form with obesity is sometimes caused by an endocrine disturbance.

701.3 Striae atrophicae
Atrophic spots of skin
Atrophoderma maculatum
Atrophy blanche (of Milian)
Degenerative colloid atrophy
Senile degenerative atrophy
Striae distensae

DEF: Bands of atrophic, depressed, wrinkled skin associated with stretching of skin from pregnancy, obesity, or rapid growth during puberty.

701.4 Keloid scar
Cheloid
Hypertrophic scar
Keloid

DEF: Overgrowth of scar tissue due to excess amounts of collagen during connective tissue repair; occurs mainly on upper trunk, face.

701.5 Other abnormal granulation tissue
Excessive granulation

701.8 Other specified hypertrophic and atrophic conditions of skin
Acrodermatitis atrophicans chronica
Atrophia cutis senilis
Atrophoderma neuriticum
Confluent and reticulate papillomatosis
Cutis laxa senilis
Elastosis senilis
Folliculitis ulerythematosa reticulata
Gougerot-Carteaud syndrome or disease

701.9 Unspecified hypertrophic and atrophic conditions of skin
Atrophoderma

4th **702 Other dermatoses**

EXCLUDES *carcinoma in situ (232.0-232.9)*

702.0 Actinic keratosis
AHA: 1Q, '92, 18

DEF: Wart-like growth, red or skin-colored; may form a cutaneous horn.

5th **702.1 Seborrheic keratosis**

DEF: Common, benign, lightly pigmented, warty growth composed of basaloid cells.

702.11 Inflamed seborrheic keratosis
AHA: 4Q, '94, 48

702.19 Other seborrheic keratosis
Seborrheic keratosis NOS

702.8 Other specified dermatoses

4th **703 Diseases of nail**

EXCLUDES *congenital anomalies (757.5)*
onychia and paronychia (681.02, 681.11)

703.0 Ingrowing nail
Ingrowing nail with infection
Unguis incarnatus

EXCLUDES *infection, nail NOS (681.9)*

703.8 Other specified diseases of nail
Dystrophia unguium
Hypertrophy of nail
Koilonychia
Leukonychia (punctata) (striata)
Onychauxis
Onychogryposis
Onycholysis

703.9 Unspecified disease of nail

4th **704 Diseases of hair and hair follicles**

EXCLUDES *congenital anomalies (757.4)*

5th **704.0 Alopecia**

EXCLUDES *madarosis (374.55)*
syphilitic alopecia (091.82)

DEF: Lack of hair, especially on scalp; often called baldness; may be partial or total; occurs at any age.

704.00 Alopecia, unspecified
Baldness
Loss of hair

704.01 Alopecia areata
Ophiasis

DEF: Alopecia areata: usually reversible, inflammatory, patchy hair loss found in beard or scalp.
DEF: Ophiasis: alopecia areata of children; marked by band around temporal and occipital scalp margins.

704.02 Telogen effluvium

DEF: Shedding of hair from premature telogen development in follicles due to stress, including shock, childbirth, surgery, drugs or weight loss.

704.09 Other
Folliculitis decalvans
Hypotrichosis:
NOS
postinfectional NOS
Pseudopelade

704.1 Hirsutism
Hypertrichosis:
NOS
lanuginosa, acquired
Polytrichia

EXCLUDES *hypertrichosis of eyelid (374.54)*

DEF: Excess hair growth; often in unexpected places and amounts.

704.2 Abnormalities of the hair
Atrophic hair
Clastothrix
Fragilitas crinium
Trichiasis:
NOS
cicatrical
Trichorrhexis (nodosa)
EXCLUDES *trichiasis of eyelid (374.05)*

704.3 Variations in hair color
Canities (premature)
Grayness, hair (premature)
Heterochromia of hair
Poliosis:
NOS
circumscripta, acquired

704.8 Other specified diseases of hair and hair follicles
Folliculitis:
NOS
abscedens et suffodiens
pustular
Perifolliculitis:
NOS
capitis abscedens et suffodiens
scalp
Sycosis:
NOS
barbae [not parasitic]
lupoid
vulgaris

704.9 Unspecified disease of hair and hair follicles

✓4th **705 Disorders of sweat glands**

705.0 Anhidrosis
Hypohidrosis
Oligohidrosis
DEF: Lack or deficiency of ability to sweat.

705.1 Prickly heat
Heat rash
Miliaria rubra (tropicalis)
Sudamina

✓5th **705.2 Focal hyperhidrosis**
EXCLUDES *generalized (secondary) hyperhidrosis (780.8)*

705.21 Primary focal hyperhidrosis
Focal hyperhidrosis NOS
Hyperhidrosis NOS
Hyperhidrosis of:
axilla
face
palms
soles
AHA: 4Q, '04, 91
DEF: A rare condition that is a disorder of the sweat glands resulting in excessive production of sweat; occurs in the absence of any underlying or causative condition and is almost always focal, confined to one or more specific areas of the body.

705.22 Secondary focal hyperhidrosis
Frey's syndrome
AHA: 4Q, '04, 91
DEF: Secondary focal hyperhidrosis: a symptom of an underlying disease process resulting in excessive sweating beyond what the body requires to maintain thermal control, confined to one or more specific areas of the body.
DEF: Frey's syndrome: an auriculotemporal syndrome due to lesion on the parotid gland; characteristic redness and excessive sweating on the cheek in connection with eating.

✓5th **705.8 Other specified disorders of sweat glands**

705.81 Dyshidrosis
Cheiropompholyx
Pompholyx
DEF: Vesicular eruption, on hands, feet causing itching and burning.

705.82 Fox-Fordyce disease
DEF: Chronic, usually pruritic disease chiefly of women evidenced by small follicular papular eruptions, especially in the axillary and pubic areas; develops from the closure and rupture of the affected apocrine glands' intraepidermal portion of the ducts.

705.83 Hidradenitis
Hidradenitis suppurativa
DEF: Inflamed sweat glands.

705.89 Other
Bromhidrosis
Chromhidrosis
Granulosis rubra nasi
Urhidrosis
EXCLUDES *generalized hyperhidrosis (780.8)*
hidrocystoma (216.0-216.9)
DEF: Bromhidrosis: foul-smelling axillary sweat due to decomposed bacteria.
DEF: Chromhidrosis: secretion of colored sweat.
DEF: Granulosis rubra nasi: ideopathic condition of children; causes redness, sweating around nose, face and chin; tends to end by puberty.
DEF: Urhidrosis: urinous substance, such as uric acid, in sweat; occurs in uremia.

705.9 Unspecified disorder of sweat glands
Disorder of sweat glands NOS

✓4th **706 Diseases of sebaceous glands**

706.0 Acne varioliformis
Acne:
frontalis
Acne:
necrotica
DEF: Rare form of acne characterized by persistent brown papulopustules usually on the brow and temporoparietal part of the scalp.

706.1 Other acne
Acne:
NOS
conglobata
cystic
pustular
Acne:
vulgaris
Blackhead
Comedo
EXCLUDES *acne rosacea (695.3)*

706.2 Sebaceous cyst
Atheroma, skin
Keratin cyst
Wen
DEF: Benign epidermal cyst, contains sebum and keratin; presents as firm, circumscribed nodule.

706.3 Seborrhea
EXCLUDES *seborrhea:*
capitis (690.11)
sicca (690.18)
seborrheic:
dermatitis (690.10)
keratosis (702.11-702.19)
DEF: Seborrheic dermatitis marked by excessive secretion of sebum; the sebum forms an oily coating, crusts, or scales on the skin; it is also called hypersteatosis.

706.8 Other specified diseases of sebaceous glands
Asteatosis (cutis)
Xerosis cutis

706.9 Unspecified disease of sebaceous glands

✓4th **707 Chronic ulcer of skin**
INCLUDES non-infected sinus of skin
non-healing ulcer
EXCLUDES *specific infections classified under "Infectious and Parasitic Diseases" (001.0-136.9)*
varicose ulcer (454.0, 454.2)
AHA: 4Q, '04, 92

✓5th **707.0 Decubitus ulcer**
Bed sore
Decubitus ulcer [any site]
Plaster ulcer
Pressure ulcer
AHA: 1Q, '04, 14; 4Q, '03, 110; 4Q, '99, 20; 1Q, '96, 15; 3Q, '90, 15; N-D, '87, 9

707.00 Unspecified site
707.01 Elbow
707.02 Upper back
Shoulder blades
707.03 Lower back
Sacrum
AHA: ▶1Q, '05, 16◀
707.04 Hip

✓4th ✓5th Additional Digit Required | Unspecified Code | Other Specified Code | Manifestation Code | ▶◀ Revised Text | ● New Code | ▲ Revised Code Title

707.05 Buttock

707.06 Ankle

707.07 Heel

AHA: ▶1Q, '05, 16◀

707.09 Other site

Head

✓5th **707.1 Ulcer of lower limbs, except decubitus**

Ulcer, chronic: neurogenic, trophic } of lower limb

Code, if applicable, any casual condition first:
- atherosclerosis of the extremities with ulceration (440.23)
- chronic venous hypertension with ulcer (459.31)
- chronic venous hypertension with ulcer and inflammation (459.33)
- diabetes mellitus (250.80-250.83)
- postphlebitic syndrome with ulcer (459.11)
- postphlebitic syndrome with ulcer and inflammation (459.13)

AHA: 4Q, '00, 44; 4Q, '99, 15

707.10 Ulcer of lower limb, unspecified

AHA: 3Q, '04, 5; 4Q, '02, 43

707.11 Ulcer of thigh

707.12 Ulcer of calf

707.13 Ulcer of ankle

707.14 Ulcer of heel and midfoot

Plantar surface of midfoot

707.15 Ulcer of other part of foot

Toes

707.19 Ulcer of other part of lower limb

707.8 Chronic ulcer of other specified sites

Ulcer, chronic: neurogenic, trophic } of other specified sites

707.9 Chronic ulcer of unspecified site

Chronic ulcer NOS; Tropical ulcer NOS; Trophic ulcer NOS; Ulcer of skin NOS

✓4th **708 Urticaria**

EXCLUDES *edema:*
- *angioneurotic (995.1)*
- *Quincke's (995.1)*

hereditary angioedema (277.6)

urticaria:
- *giant (995.1)*
- *papulosa (Hebra) (698.2)*
- *pigmentosa (juvenile) (congenital) (757.33)*

DEF: Skin disorder marked by raised edematous patches of skin or mucous membrane with intense itching; also called hives.

708.0 Allergic urticaria

708.1 Idiopathic urticaria

708.2 Urticaria due to cold and heat

Thermal urticaria

708.3 Dermatographic urticaria

Dermatographia; Factitial urticaria

708.4 Vibratory urticaria

708.5 Cholinergic urticaria

708.8 Other specified urticaria

Nettle rash

Urticaria:
- chronic
- recurrent periodic

708.9 Urticaria, unspecified

Hives NOS

✓4th **709 Other disorders of skin and subcutaneous tissue**

✓5th **709.0 Dyschromia**

EXCLUDES *albinism (270.2)*
pigmented nevus (216.0-216.9)
that of eyelid (374.52-374.53)

DEF: Pigment disorder of skin or hair.

709.00 Dyschromia, unspecified

709.01 Vitiligo

DEF: Persistent, progressive development of nonpigmented white patches on otherwise normal skin.

709.09 Other

709.1 Vascular disorders of skin

Angioma serpiginosum

Purpura (primary)annularis telangiectodes

709.2 Scar conditions and fibrosis of skin

Adherent scar (skin); Fibrosis, skin NOS; Cicatrix; Scar NOS; Disfigurement (due to scar)

EXCLUDES *keloid scar (701.4)*

AHA: N-D, '84, 19

709.3 Degenerative skin disorders

Calcinosis:
- circumscripta
- cutis

Colloid milium

Degeneration, skin; Deposits, skin; Senile dermatosis NOS; Subcutaneous calcification

709.4 Foreign body granuloma of skin and subcutaneous tissue

EXCLUDES *residual foreign body without granuloma of skin and subcutaneous tissue (729.6)*
that of muscle (728.82)

709.8 Other specified disorders of skin

Epithelial hyperplasia; Vesicular eruption; Menstrual dermatosis

AHA: N-D, '87, 6

DEF: Epithelial hyperplasia: increased number of epitheleal cells.

DEF: Vesicular eruption: liquid-filled structures appearing through skin.

709.9 Unspecified disorder of skin and subcutaneous tissue

Dermatosis NOS

Four Stages of Decubitus Ulcers

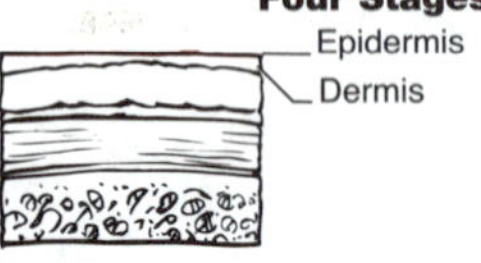
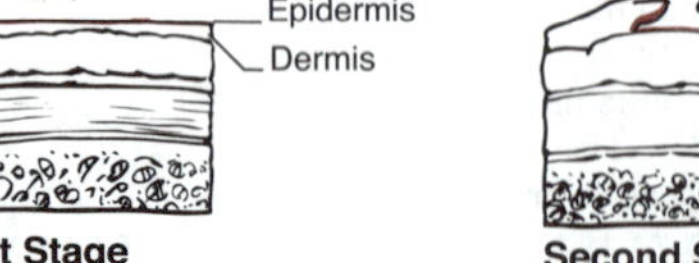

First Stage
Nonblanchable erythema

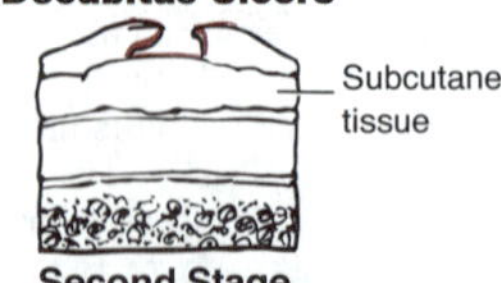

Second Stage
Partial thickness skin loss involving epidermis, dermis, or both

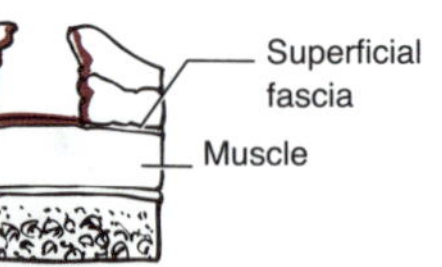

Third Stage
Full thickness skin loss extending through subcutaneous tissue

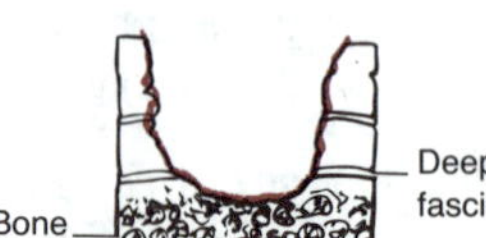

Fourth Stage
Full thickness skin loss extending to muscle and bone

Cutaneous Lesions

Surface Lesions

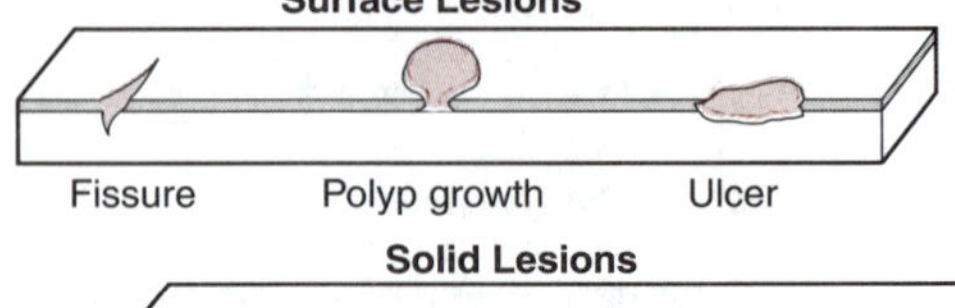

Solid Lesions

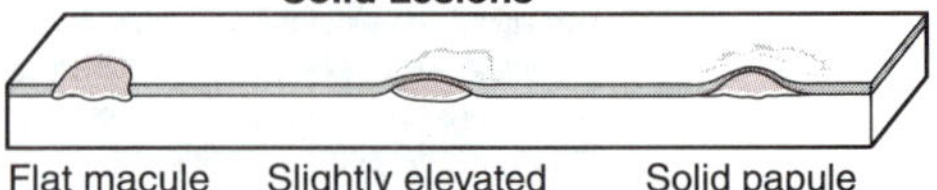

Sac Lesions

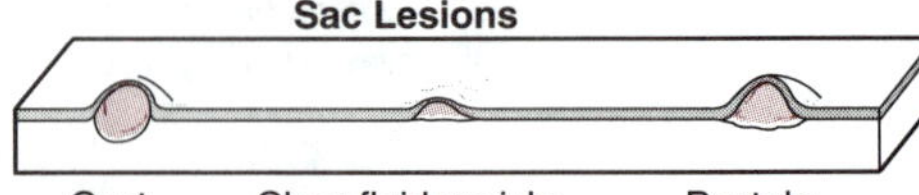

13. DISEASES OF THE MUSCULOSKELETAL SYSTEM AND CONNECTIVE TISSUE (710-739)

The following fifth-digit subclassification is for use with categories 711-712, 715-716, 718-719, and 730:

0 site unspecified

1 shoulder region
- Acromioclavicular joint(s)
- Clavicle
- Glenohumeral joint(s)
- Scapula
- Sternoclavicular joint(s)

2 upper arm
- Elbow joint
- Humerus

3 forearm
- Radius
- Ulna
- Wrist joint

4 hand
- Carpus
- Metacarpus
- Phalanges [fingers]

5 pelvic region and thigh
- Buttock
- Femur
- Hip (joint)

6 lower leg
- Fibula
- Knee joint
- Patella
- Tibia

7 ankle and foot
- Ankle joint
- Digits [toes]
- Metatarsus
- Phalanges, foot
- Tarsus
- Other joints in foot

8 other specified sites
- Head
- Neck
- Ribs
- Skull
- Trunk
- Vertebral column

9 multiple sites

ARTHROPATHIES AND RELATED DISORDERS (710-719)

EXCLUDES *disorders of spine (720.0-724.9)*

✓4th **710 Diffuse diseases of connective tissue**

INCLUDES all collagen diseases whose effects are not mainly confined to a single system

EXCLUDES *those affecting mainly the cardiovascular system, i.e., polyarteritis nodosa and allied conditions (446.0-446.7)*

710.0 Systemic lupus erythematosus

Disseminated lupus erythematosus
Libman-Sacks disease
Use additional code to identify manifestation, as:
- endocarditis (424.91)
- nephritis (583.81)
  - chronic (582.81)
- nephrotic syndrome (581.81)

EXCLUDES *lupus erythematosus (discoid) NOS (695.4)*

AHA: 2Q, '03, 7-8; 2Q, '97, 8

DEF: A chronic multisystemic inflammatory disease affecting connective tissue; marked by anemia, leukopenia, muscle and joint pains, fever, rash of a butterfly pattern around cheeks and forehead area; of unknown etiology.

710.1 Systemic sclerosis

Acrosclerosis
CRST syndrome
Progressive systemic sclerosis
Scleroderma

EXCLUDES *circumscribed scleroderma (701.0)*

Use additional code to identify manifestation, as:
- lung involvement (517.2)
- myopathy (359.6)

AHA: 1Q, '88, 6

DEF: Systemic disease, involving excess fibrotic collagen build-up; symptoms include thickened skin; fibrotic degenerative changes in various organs; and vascular abnomalities; condition occurs more often in females.

Joint Structures

710.2 Sicca syndrome

Keratoconjunctivitis sicca
Sjögren's disease

DEF: Autoimmune disease; associated with keratoconjunctivitis, laryngopharyngitis, rhinitis, dry mouth, enlarged parotid gland, and chronic polyarthritis.

710.3 Dermatomyositis

Poikilodermatomyositis
Polymyositis with skin involvement

DEF: Polymyositis associated with flat-top purple papules on knuckles; marked by upper eyelid rash, edema of eyelids and orbit area, red rash on forehead, neck, shoulders, trunk and arms; symptoms include fever, weight loss aching muscles; visceral cancer (in individuals older than 40).

710.4 Polymyositis

DEF: Chronic, progressive, inflammatory skeletal muscle disease; causes weakness of limb girdles, neck, pharynx; may precede or follow scleroderma, Sjogren's disease, systemic lupus erythematosus, arthritis, or malignancy.

710.5 Eosinophilia myalgia syndrome

Toxic oil syndrome
Use additional E code to identify drug, if drug induced

AHA: 4Q, '92, 21

DEF: Eosinophilia myalgia syndrome (EMS): inflammatory, multisystem fibrosis; associated with ingesting elemetary L-tryptophan; symptoms include myalgia, weak limbs and bulbar muscles, distal sensory loss, areflexia, arthralgia, cough, fever, fatigue, skin rashes, myopathy, and eosinophil counts greater than 1000/microliter.

DEF: Toxic oil syndrome: syndrome similar to EMS due to ingesting contaminated cooking oil.

710.8 Other specified diffuse diseases of connective tissue

Multifocal fibrosclerosis (idiopathic) NEC
Systemic fibrosclerosing syndrome

AHA: M-A, '87, 12

710.9 Unspecified diffuse connective tissue disease

Collagen disease NOS

✓4th 711 Arthropathy associated with infections

INCLUDES arthritis, arthropathy, polyarthritis, polyarthropathy } associated with conditions classifiable below

EXCLUDES *rheumatic fever (390)*

The following fifth-digit subclassification is for use with category 711; valid digits are in [brackets] under each code. See list at beginning of chapter for definitions.

- **0 site unspecified**
- **1 shoulder region**
- **2 upper arm**
- **3 forearm**
- **4 hand**
- **5 pelvic region and thigh**
- **6 lower leg**
- **7 ankle and foot**
- **8 other specified sites**
- **9 multiple sites**

AHA: 1Q, '92, 17

§ ✓5th **711.0 Pyogenic arthritis**
[0-9]
Arthritis or polyarthritis (due to):
coliform [Escherichia coli]
Hemophilus influenzae [H. influenzae]
pneumococcal
Pseudomonas
staphylococcal
streptococcal
Pyarthrosis
Use additional code to identify infectious organism (041.0-041.8)

AHA: 1Q, '92, 16; 1Q, '91, 15

DEF: Infectious arthritis caused by various bacteria; marked by inflamed synovial membranes, and purulent effusion in joints.

§ ✓5th ***711.1 Arthropathy associated with Reiter's disease and nonspecific urethritis***
[0-9]
Code first underlying disease as:
nonspecific urethritis (099.4)
Reiter's disease (099.3)

DEF: Reiter's disease: joint disease marked by diarrhea, urethritis, conjunctivitis, keratosis and arthritis; of unknown etiology; affects young males.

DEF: Urethritis: inflamed urethra.

§ ✓5th ***711.2 Arthropathy in Behçet's syndrome***
[0-9]
Code first underlying disease (136.1)

DEF: Behçet's syndrome: chronic inflammatory disorder, of unknown etiology; affects small blood vessels; causes ulcers of oral and pharyngeal mucous membranes and genitalia, skin lesions, retinal vasculitis, optic atrophy and severe uveitis.

§ ✓5th ***711.3 Postdysenteric arthropathy***
[0-9]
Code first underlying disease as:
dysentery (009.0)
enteritis, infectious (008.0-009.3)
paratyphoid fever (002.1-002.9)
typhoid fever (002.0)

EXCLUDES *salmonella arthritis (003.23)*

§ ✓5th ***711.4 Arthropathy associated with other bacterial diseases***
[0-9]
Code first underlying disease as:
diseases classifiable to 010-040, 090-099, except as in 711.1, 711.3, and 713.5
leprosy (030.0-030.9)
tuberculosis (015.0-015.9)

EXCLUDES *gonococcal arthritis (098.50)*
meningococcal arthritis (036.82)

§ ✓5th ***711.5 Arthropathy associated with other viral diseases***
[0-9]
Code first underlying disease as:
diseases classifiable to 045-049, 050-079, 480, 487
O'nyong nyong (066.3)

EXCLUDES *that due to rubella (056.71)*

§ ✓5th ***711.6 Arthropathy associated with mycoses***
[0-9]
Code first underlying disease (110.0-118)

§ ✓5th ***711.7 Arthropathy associated with helminthiasis***
[0-9]
Code first underlying disease as:
filariasis (125.0-125.9)

§ ✓5th ***711.8 Arthropathy associated with other infectious and parasitic diseases***
[0-9]
Code first underlying disease as:
diseases classifiable to 080-088, 100-104, 130-136

EXCLUDES *arthropathy associated with sarcoidosis (713.7)*

AHA: 4Q, '91, 15; 3Q, '90, 14

§ ✓5th **711.9 Unspecified infective arthritis**
[0-9]
Infective arthritis or polyarthritis (acute) (chronic) (subacute) NOS

✓4th 712 Crystal arthropathies

INCLUDES crystal-induced arthritis andsynovitis

EXCLUDES *gouty arthropathy (274.0)*

DEF: Joint disease due to urate crystal deposit in joints or synovial membranes.

The following fifth-digit subclassification is for use with category 712; valid digits are in [brackets] under each code. See list at beginning of chapter for definitions.

- **0 site unspecified**
- **1 shoulder region**
- **2 upper arm**
- **3 forearm**
- **4 hand**
- **5 pelvic region and thigh**
- **6 lower leg**
- **7 ankle and foot**
- **8 other specified sites**
- **9 multiple sites**

§ ✓5th ***712.1 Chondrocalcinosis due to dicalcium phosphate crystals***
[0-9]
Chondrocalcinosis due to dicalcium phosphate crystals (with other crystals)
Code first underlying disease (275.4)

§ ✓5th ***712.2 Chondrocalcinosis due to pyrophosphate crystals***
[0-9]
Code first underlying disease (275.4)

§ ✓5th ***712.3 Chondrocalcinosis, unspecified***
[0-9]
Code first underlying disease (275.4)

§ ✓5th **712.8 Other specified crystal arthropathies**
[0-9]

§ ✓5th **712.9 Unspecified crystal arthropathy**
[0-9]

✓4th 713 Arthropathy associated with other disorders classified elsewhere

INCLUDES arthritis, arthropathy, polyarthritis, polyarthropathy } associated with conditions classifiable below

§ Requires fifth digit. Valid digits are in [brackets] under each code. See beginning of section 710–739 for codes and definitions.

713.0 ***Arthropathy associated with other endocrine and metabolic disorders***

Code first underlying disease as:
- acromegaly (253.0)
- hemochromatosis (275.0)
- hyperparathyroidism (252.00-252.08)
- hypogammaglobulinemia (279.00-279.09)
- hypothyroidism (243-244.9)
- lipoid metabolism disorder (272.0-272.9)
- ochronosis (270.2)

EXCLUDES *arthropathy associated with:*
amyloidosis (713.7)
crystal deposition disorders, except gout (712.1-712.9)
diabetic neuropathy (713.5)
gouty arthropathy (274.0)

713.1 ***Arthropathy associated with gastrointestinal conditions other than infections***

Code first underlying disease as:
- regional enteritis (555.0-555.9)
- ulcerative colitis (556)

713.2 ***Arthropathy associated with hematological disorders***

Code first underlying disease as:
- hemoglobinopathy (282.4-282.7)
- hemophilia (286.0-286.2)
- leukemia (204.0-208.9)
- malignant reticulosis (202.3)
- multiple myelomatosis (203.0)

EXCLUDES *arthropathy associated with Henoch-Schönlein purpura (713.6)*

713.3 ***Arthropathy associated with dermatological disorders***

Code first underlying disease as:
- erythema multiforme (695.1)
- erythema nodosum (695.2)

EXCLUDES *psoriatic arthropathy (696.0)*

713.4 ***Arthropathy associated with respiratory disorders***

Code first underlying disease as:
- diseases classifiable to 490-519

EXCLUDES *arthropathy associated with respiratory infections (711.0, 711.4-711.8)*

713.5 ***Arthropathy associated with neurological disorders***

Charcôt's arthropathy } associated with diseases classifiable elsewhere
Neuropathic arthritis }

Code first underlying disease as:
neuropathic joint disease [Charcôt's joints]:
- NOS (094.0)
- diabetic (250.6)
- syringomyelic (336.0)
- tabetic [syphilitic] (094.0)

713.6 ***Arthropathy associated with hypersensitivity reaction***

Code first underlying disease as:
- Henoch (-Schönlein) purpura (287.0)
- serum sickness (999.5)

EXCLUDES *allergic arthritis NOS (716.2)*

713.7 ***Other general diseases with articular involvement***

Code first underlying disease as:
- amyloidosis (277.3)
- familial Mediterranean fever (277.3)
- sarcoidosis (135)

AHA: 2Q, '97, 12

713.8 ***Arthropathy associated with other conditions classifiable elsewhere***

Code first underlying disease as:
conditions classifiable elsewhere except as in 711.1-711.8, 712, and 713.0-713.7

✓4th **714 Rheumatoid arthritis and other inflammatory polyarthropathies**

EXCLUDES *rheumatic fever (390)*
rheumatoid arthritis of spine NOS (720.0)

AHA: 2Q, '95, 3

714.0 Rheumatoid arthritis

Arthritis or polyarthritis:
- atrophic
- rheumatic (chronic)

Use additional code to identify manifestation, as:
- myopathy (359.6)
- polyneuropathy (357.1)

EXCLUDES *juvenile rheumatoid arthritis NOS (714.30)*

AHA: 1Q, '90, 5

DEF: Chronic systemic disease principally of joints, manifested by inflammatory changes in articular structures and synovial membranes, atrophy, and loss in bone density.

714.1 Felty's syndrome

Rheumatoid arthritis with splenoadenomegaly and leukopenia

DEF: Syndrome marked by rheumatoid arthritis, splenomegaly, leukopenia, pigmented spots on lower extremity skin, anemia, and thrombocytopenia.

714.2 Other rheumatoid arthritis with visceral or systemic involvement

Rheumatoid carditis

✓5th **714.3 Juvenile chronic polyarthritis**

DEF: Rheumatoid arthritis of more than one joint; lasts longer than six weeks in age 17 or younger; symptoms include fever, erythematous rash, weight loss, lymphadenopathy, hepatosplenomegaly and pericarditis.

714.30 Polyarticular juvenile rheumatoid arthritis, chronic or unspecified

Juvenile rheumatoid arthritis NOS
Still's disease

714.31 Polyarticular juvenile rheumatoid arthritis, acute

714.32 Pauciarticular juvenile rheumatoid arthritis

714.33 Monoarticular juvenile rheumatoid arthritis

714.4 Chronic postrheumatic arthropathy

Chronic rheumatoid nodular fibrositis
Jaccoud's syndrome

DEF: Persistent joint disorder; follows previous rheumatic infection.

✓5th **714.8 Other specified inflammatory polyarthropathies**

714.81 Rheumatoid lung

Caplan's syndrome
Diffuse interstitial rheumatoid disease of lung
Fibrosing alveolitis, rheumatoid

DEF: Lung disorders associated with rheumatoid arthritis.

714.89 Other

714.9 Unspecified inflammatory polyarthropathy

Inflammatory polyarthropathy or polyarthritis NOS

EXCLUDES *polyarthropathy NOS (716.5)*

✓4th 715 Osteoarthrosis and allied disorders

Note: Localized, in the subcategories below, includes bilateral involvement of the same site.

INCLUDES arthritis or polyarthritis:
degenerative
hypertrophic
degenerative joint disease
osteoarthritis

EXCLUDES *Marie-Strümpell spondylitis (720.0)*
osteoarthrosis [osteoarthritis] of spine (721.0-721.9)

The following fifth-digit subclassification is for use with category 715; valid digits are in [brackets] under each code. See list at beginning of chapter for definitions.

- **0 site unspecified**
- **1 shoulder region**
- **2 upper arm**
- **3 forearm**
- **4 hand**
- **5 pelvic region and thigh**
- **6 lower leg**
- **7 ankle and foot**
- **8 other specified sites**
- **9 multiple sites**

§ ✓5th **715.0 Osteoarthrosis, generalized**
[0,4,9]
Degenerative joint disease, involving multiple joints
Primary generalized hypertrophic osteoarthrosis
DEF: Chronic noninflammatory arthritis; marked by degenerated articular cartilage and enlarged bone; symptoms include pain and stiffness with activity; occurs among elderly.

§ ✓5th **715.1 Osteoarthrosis, localized, primary**
[0-8]
Localized osteoarthropathy, idiopathic

§ ✓5th **715.2 Osteoarthrosis, localized, secondary**
[0-8]
Coxae malum senilis

§ ✓5th **715.3 Osteoarthrosis, localized, not specified whether primary or secondary**
[0-8]
Otto's pelvis
AHA: For code 715.35: ►3Q, '04, 12; 2Q, '04, 15;◄ For code 715.36: 4Q, '03, 118; 2Q, '95, 5

§ ✓5th **715.8 Osteoarthrosis involving, or with mention of more than one site, but not specified as generalized**
[0,9]

§ ✓5th **715.9 Osteoarthrosis, unspecified whether generalized or localized**
[0-8]
AHA: For code 715.90: 2Q, '97, 12

✓4th 716 Other and unspecified arthropathies

EXCLUDES *cricoarytenoid arthropathy (478.79)*

The following fifth-digit subclassification is for use with category 716; valid digits are in [brackets] under each code. See list at beginning of chapter for definitions.

- **0 site unspecified**
- **1 shoulder region**
- **2 upper arm**
- **3 forearm**
- **4 hand**
- **5 pelvic region and thigh**
- **6 lower leg**
- **7 ankle and foot**
- **8 other specified sites**
- **9 multiple sites**

AHA: 2Q, '95, 3

§ ✓5th **716.0 Kaschin-Beck disease**
[0-9]
Endemic polyarthritis
DEF: Chronic degenerative disease of spine and peripheral joints; occurs in eastern Siberian, northern Chinese, and Korean youth; may a mycotoxicosis caused by eating cereals infected with fungus.

§ ✓5th **716.1 Traumatic arthropathy**
[0-9]
AHA: For Code 716.11: 1Q, '02, 9

§ ✓5th **716.2 Allergic arthritis**
[0-9]
EXCLUDES *arthritis associated with Henoch-Schönlein purpura or serum sickness (713.6)*

§ ✓5th **716.3 Climacteric arthritis** ♀
[0-9]
Menopausal arthritis
DEF: Ovarian hormone deficiency; causes pain in small joints, shoulders, elbows or knees; affects females at menopause; also called arthropathia ovaripriva.

§ ✓5th **716.4 Transient arthropathy**
[0-9]
EXCLUDES *palindromic rheumatism (719.3)*

§ ✓5th **716.5 Unspecified polyarthropathy or polyarthritis**
[0-9]

§ ✓5th **716.6 Unspecified monoarthritis**
[0-8]
Coxitis

§ ✓5th **716.8 Other specified arthropathy**
[0-9]

§ ✓5th **716.9 Arthropathy, unspecified**
[0-9]
Arthritis } (acute) (chronic) (subacute)
Arthropathy }
Articular rheumatism (chronic)
Inflammation of joint NOS

✓4th 717 Internal derangement of knee

INCLUDES degeneration } of articular cartilage or meniscus of knee
rupture, old }
tear, old }

EXCLUDES *acute derangement of knee (836.0-836.6)*
ankylosis (718.5)
contracture (718.4)
current injury (836.0-836.6)
deformity (736.4-736.6)
recurrent dislocation (718.3)

717.0 Old bucket handle tear of medial meniscus
Old bucket handle tear of unspecified cartilage

717.1 Derangement of anterior horn of medial meniscus

717.2 Derangement of posterior horn of medial meniscus

717.3 Other and unspecified derangement of medial meniscus
Degeneration of internal semilunar cartilage

Disruption and Tears of Meniscus

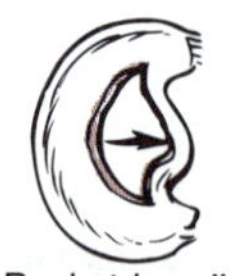
Bucket-handle

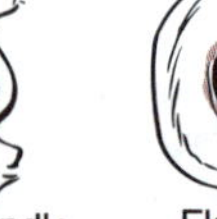
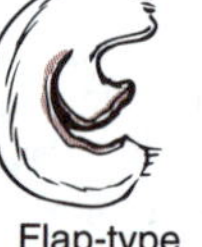
Flap-type

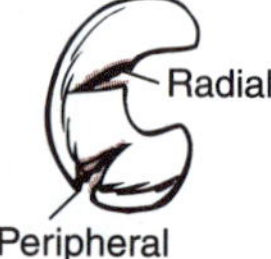

Peripheral

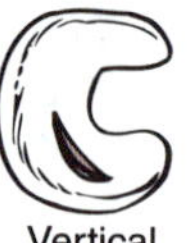
Horizontal cleavage

Vertical

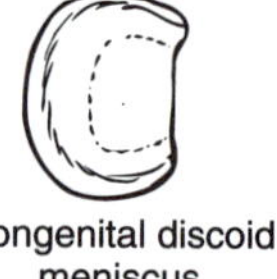
Congenital discoid meniscus

§ Requires fifth digit. Valid digits are in [brackets] under each code. See beginning of section 710–739 for codes and definitions.

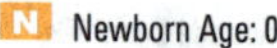 Newborn Age: 0 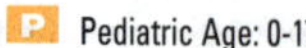 Pediatric Age: 0-17 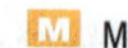 Maternity Age: 12-55 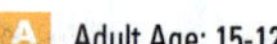 Adult Age: 15-124 MSP Medicare Secondary Payer

Internal Derangements of Knee

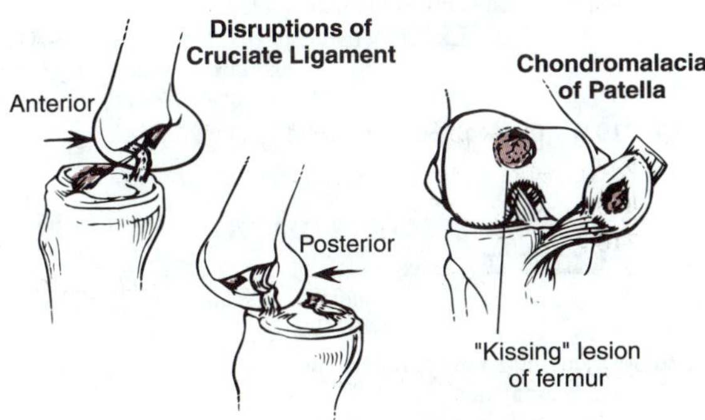

✓5th **717.4 Derangement of lateral meniscus**

717.40 Derangement of lateral meniscus, unspecified

717.41 Bucket handle tear of lateral meniscus

717.42 Derangement of anterior horn of lateral meniscus

717.43 Derangement of posterior horn of lateral meniscus

717.49 Other

717.5 Derangement of meniscus, not elsewhere classified

Congenital discoid meniscus
Cyst of semilunar cartilage
Derangement of semilunar cartilage NOS

717.6 Loose body in knee

Joint mice, knee
Rice bodies, knee (joint)

DEF: The presence in the joint synovial area of a small, frequently calcified, loose body created from synovial membrane, organized fibrin fragments of articular cartilage or arthritis osteophytes.

717.7 Chondromalacia of patella

Chondromalacia patellae
Degeneration [softening] of articular cartilage of patella

AHA: M-A, '85, 14; N-D, '84, 9

DEF: Softened patella cartilage.

✓5th **717.8 Other internal derangement of knee**

717.81 Old disruption of lateral collateral ligament

717.82 Old disruption of medial collateral ligament

717.83 Old disruption of anterior cruciate ligament

717.84 Old disruption of posterior cruciate ligament

717.85 Old disruption of other ligaments of knee

Capsular ligament of knee

717.89 Other

Old disruption of ligaments of knee NOS

717.9 Unspecified internal derangement of knee

Derangement NOS of knee

✓4th **718 Other derangement of joint**

EXCLUDES *current injury (830.0-848.9)*
jaw (524.60-524.69)

The following fifth-digit subclassification is for use with category 718; valid digits are in [brackets] under each code. See list at beginning of chapter for definitions.

0 site unspecified
1 shoulder region
2 upper arm
3 forearm
4 hand
5 pelvic region and thigh
6 lower leg
7 ankle and foot
8 other specified sites
9 multiple sites

§ ✓5th **718.0 Articular cartilage disorder**

[0-5,7-9]

Meniscus:
disorder
rupture, old

Meniscus:
tear, old

Old rupture of ligament(s) of joint NOS

EXCLUDES *articular cartilage disorder:*
in ochronosis (270.2)
knee (717.0-717.9)
chondrocalcinosis (275.4)
metastatic calcification (275.4)

§ ✓5th **718.1 Loose body in joint**

[0-5,7-9]

Joint mice

EXCLUDES *knee (717.6)*

AHA: For code **718.17**: 2Q, '01, 15

DEF: Calcified loose bodies in synovial fluid; due to arthritic osteophytes.

§ ✓5th **718.2 Pathological dislocation**

[0-9]

Dislocation or displacement of joint, not recurrent and not current injury
Spontaneous dislocation (joint)

§ ✓5th **718.3 Recurrent dislocation of joint**

[0-9]

AHA: N-D, '87, 7

§ ✓5th **718.4 Contracture of joint**

[0-9]

AHA: 4Q, '98, 40

§ ✓5th **718.5 Ankylosis of joint**

[0-9]

Ankylosis of joint (fibrous) (osseous)

EXCLUDES *spine (724.9)*
stiffness of joint without mention of ankylosis (719.5)

DEF: Immobility and solidification, of joint; due to disease, injury or surgical procedure.

§ ✓5th **718.6 Unspecified intrapelvic protrusion of acetabulum**

[0,5]

Protrusio acetabuli, unspecified

DEF: Sinking of the floor of acetabulum; causing femoral head to protrude, limits hip movement; of unknown etiology.

§ ✓5th **718.7 Developmental dislocation of joint**

[0-9]

EXCLUDES *congenital dislocation of joint (754.0-755.8)*
traumatic dislocation of joint (830-839)

AHA: 4Q, '01, 48

§ ✓5th **718.8 Other joint derangement, not elsewhere classified**

[0-9]

Flail joint (paralytic)
Instability of joint

EXCLUDES *deformities classifiable to 736 (736.0-736.9)*

AHA: For code **718.81**: 2Q, '00, 14

§ Requires fifth digit. Valid digits are in [brackets] under each code. See beginning of section 710–739 for codes and definitions.

Joint Derangements and Disorders

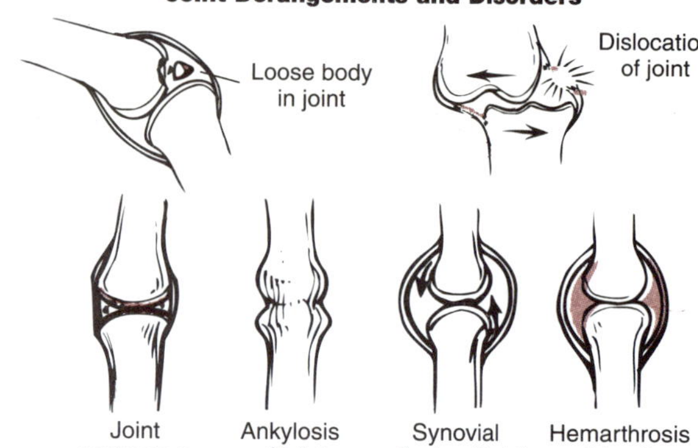

§ ✓5th **718.9 Unspecified derangement of joint**
[0-5,7-9] EXCLUDES *knee (717.9)*

✓4th **719 Other and unspecified disorders of joint**
EXCLUDES *jaw (524.60-524.69)*

The following fifth-digit subclassification is for use with codes 719.0-719.6, 719.8-719.9; valid digits are in [brackets] under each code. See list at beginning of chapter for definitions.

- **0 site unspecified**
- **1 shoulder region**
- **2 upper arm**
- **3 forearm**
- **4 hand**
- **5 pelvic region and thigh**
- **6 lower leg**
- **7 ankle and foot**
- **8 other specified sites**
- **9 multiple sites**

§ ✓5th **719.0 Effusion of joint**
[0-9]
Hydrarthrosis
Swelling of joint, with or without pain
EXCLUDES *intermittent hydrarthrosis (719.3)*

§ ✓5th **719.1 Hemarthrosis**
[0-9] EXCLUDES *current injury (840.0-848.9)*

§ ✓5th **719.2 Villonodular synovitis**
[0-9] DEF: Overgrowth of synovial tissue, especially at knee joint; due to macrophage infiltration of giant cells in synovial villi and fibrous nodules.

§ ✓5th **719.3 Palindromic rheumatism**
[0-9]
Hench-Rosenberg syndrome
Intermittent hydrarthrosis
DEF: Recurrent episodes of afebrile arthritis and periarthritis marked by their complete disappearance after a few days or hours; causes swelling, redness, and disability usually affecting only one joint; no known cause; affects adults of either sex.

§ ✓5th **719.4 Pain in joint**
[0-9]
Arthralgia
AHA: For code 719.46: 1Q, '01, 3

§ ✓5th **719.5 Stiffness of joint, not elsewhere classified**
[0-9]

§ ✓5th **719.6 Other symptoms referable to joint**
[0-9]
Joint crepitus
Snapping hip
AHA: 1Q, '94, 15

719.7 Difficulty in walking
EXCLUDES *abnormality of gait (781.2)*
AHA: ►2Q, '04, 15;◄ 4Q, '03, 66

§ ✓5th **719.8 Other specified disorders of joint**
[0-9]
Calcification of joint
Fistula of joint
EXCLUDES *temporomandibular joint-pain-dysfunction syndrome [Costen's syndrome] (524.60)*

§ ✓5th **719.9 Unspecified disorder of joint**
[0-9]

DORSOPATHIES (720-724)

EXCLUDES *curvature of spine (737.0-737.9)*
osteochondrosis of spine (juvenile) (732.0)
adult (732.8)

✓4th **720 Ankylosing spondylitis and other inflammatory spondylopathies**

720.0 Ankylosing spondylitis
Rheumatoid arthritis of spine NOS
Spondylitis:
Marie-Strümpell
rheumatoid
DEF: Rheumatoid arthritis of spine and sacroiliac joints; fusion and deformity in spine follows; affects mainly males; cause unknown.

720.1 Spinal enthesopathy
Disorder of peripheral ligamentous or muscular attachments of spine
Romanus lesion
DEF: Tendinous or muscular vertebral bone attachment abnormality.

720.2 Sacroiliitis, not elsewhere classified
Inflammation of sacroiliac joint NOS
DEF: Pain due to inflammation in joint, at juncture of sacrum and hip.

✓5th **720.8 Other inflammatory spondylopathies**

720.81 Inflammatory spondylopathies in diseases classified elsewhere
Code first underlying disease as:
tuberculosis (015.0)

720.89 Other

720.9 Unspecified inflammatory spondylopathy
Spondylitis NOS

✓4th **721 Spondylosis and allied disorders**
AHA: 2Q, '89, 14
DEF: Degenerative changes in spinal joint.

721.0 Cervical spondylosis without myelopathy
Cervical or cervicodorsal:
arthritis
osteoarthritis
Cervical or cervicodorsal:
spondylarthritis

721.1 Cervical spondylosis with myelopathy
Anterior spinal artery compression syndrome
Spondylogenic compression of cervical spinal cord
Vertebral artery compression syndrome

Normal Anatomy of Vertebral Disc

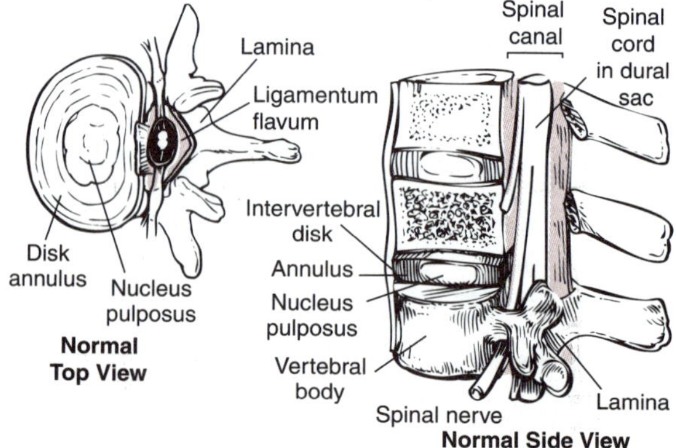

§ Requires fifth digit. Valid digits are in [brackets] under each code. See beginning of section 710–739 for codes and definitions.

721.2 Thoracic spondylosis without myelopathy
Thoracic:
arthritis
osteoarthritis
spondylarthritis

721.3 Lumbosacral spondylosis without myelopathy
Lumbar or lumbosacral:
arthritis
osteoarthritis
spondylarthritis
AHA: 4Q, '02, 107

✓5th **721.4 Thoracic or lumbar spondylosis with myelopathy**
721.41 Thoracic region
Spondylogenic compression of thoracic spinal cord
721.42 Lumbar region
Spondylogenic compression of lumbar spinal cord

721.5 Kissing spine
Baastrup's syndrome
DEF: Compression of spinous processes of adjacent vertebrae; due to mutual contact.

721.6 Ankylosing vertebral hyperostosis

721.7 Traumatic spondylopathy
Kümmell's disease or spondylitis

721.8 Other allied disorders of spine

✓5th **721.9 Spondylosis of unspecified site**
721.90 Without mention of myelopathy
Spinal:
arthritis (deformans) (degenerative) (hypertrophic)
osteoarthritis NOS
Spondylarthrosis NOS
721.91 With myelopathy
Spondylogenic compression of spinal cord NOS

✓4th **722 Intervertebral disc disorders**
AHA: 1Q, '88, 10

722.0 Displacement of cervical intervertebral disc without myelopathy
Neuritis (brachial) or radiculitis due to displacement or rupture of cervical intervertebral disc
Any condition classifiable to 722.2 of the cervical or cervicothoracic intervertebral disc

✓5th **722.1 Displacement of thoracic or lumbar intervertebral disc without myelopathy**
722.10 Lumbar intervertebral disc without myelopathy
Lumbago or sciatica due to displacement of intervertebral disc
Neuritis or radiculitis due to displacement or rupture of lumbar intervertebral disc
Any condition classifiable to 722.2 of the lumbar or lumbosacral intervertebral disc
AHA: 3Q, '03, 12; 1Q, '03, 7; 4Q, '02, 107
722.11 Thoracic intervertebral disc without myelopathy
Any condition classifiable to 722.2 of thoracic intervertebral disc

722.2 Displacement of intervertebral disc, site unspecified, without myelopathy
Discogenic syndrome NOS
Herniation of nucleus pulposus NOS
Intervertebral disc NOS:
extrusion
prolapse
protrusion
rupture
Neuritis or radiculitis due to displacement or rupture of intervertebral disc

✓5th **722.3 Schmorl's nodes**
DEF: Irregular bone defect in the margin of the vertebral body; causes herniation into end plate of vertebral body.
722.30 Unspecified region
722.31 Thoracic region
722.32 Lumbar region
722.39 Other

722.4 Degeneration of cervical intervertebral disc
Degeneration of cervicothoracic intervertebral disc

✓5th **722.5 Degeneration of thoracic or lumbar intervertebral disc**
722.51 Thoracic or thoracolumbar intervertebral disc
722.52 Lumbar or lumbosacral intervertebral disc
AHA: ▶4Q, '04, 133◀

722.6 Degeneration of intervertebral disc, site unspecified
Degenerative disc disease NOS
Narrowing of intervertebral disc or space NOS

✓5th **722.7 Intervertebral disc disorder with myelopathy**
722.70 Unspecified region
722.71 Cervical region
722.72 Thoracic region
722.73 Lumbar region

✓5th **722.8 Postlaminectomy syndrome**
AHA: J-F, '87, 7
DEF: Spinal disorder due to spinal laminectomy surgery.
722.80 Unspecified region
722.81 Cervical region
722.82 Thoracic region
722.83 Lumbar region
AHA: 2Q, '97, 15

✓5th **722.9 Other and unspecified disc disorder**
Calcification of intervertebral cartilage or disc
Discitis

Derangement of Vertebral Disc

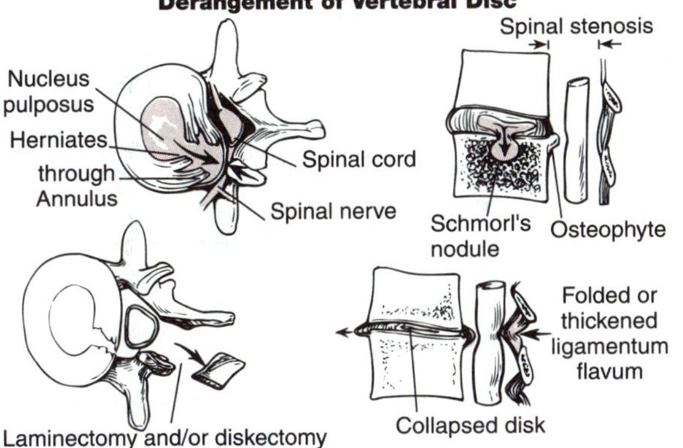

Spinal Stenosis in Cervical Region

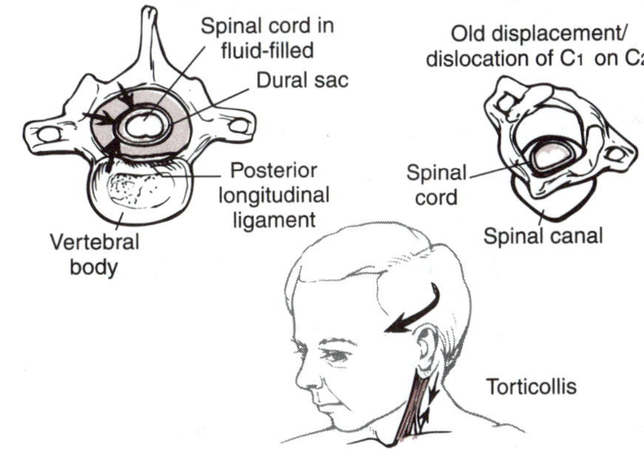

722.90 **Unspecified region**
AHA: N-D, '84, 19

722.91 **Cervical region**

722.92 **Thoracic region**

722.93 **Lumbar region**

✓4th **723 Other disorders of cervical region**

EXCLUDES *conditions due to:*
intervertebral disc disorders (722.0-722.9)
spondylosis (721.0-721.9)

AHA: 3Q, '94, 14; 2Q, '89, 14

723.0 Spinal stenosis in cervical region
AHA: 4Q, '03, 101

723.1 Cervicalgia
Pain in neck
DEF: Pain in cervical spine or neck region.

723.2 Cervicocranial syndrome
Barré-Liéou syndrome
Posterior cervical sympathetic syndrome
DEF: Neurologic disorder of upper cervical spine and nerve roots.

723.3 Cervicobrachial syndrome (diffuse)
AHA: N-D, '85, 12

DEF: Complex of symptoms due to scalenus anterior muscle compressing the brachial plexus; pain radiates from shoulder to arm or back of neck.

723.4 Brachial neuritis or radiculitis NOS
Cervical radiculitis
Radicular syndrome of upper limbs

723.5 Torticollis, unspecified
Contracture of neck

EXCLUDES *congenital (754.1)*
due to birth injury (767.8)
hysterical (300.11)
ocular torticollis (781.93)
psychogenic (306.0)
spasmodic (333.83)
traumatic, current (847.0)

AHA: 2Q, '01, 21; 1Q, '95, 7

DEF: Abnormally positioned neck relative to head; due to cervical muscle or fascia contractions; also called wryneck.

723.6 Panniculitis specified as affecting neck
DEF: Inflammation of the panniculus adiposus (subcutaneous fat) in the neck.

723.7 Ossification of posterior longitudinal ligament in cervical region

723.8 Other syndromes affecting cervical region
Cervical syndrome NEC
Klippel's disease
Occipital neuralgia
AHA: 1Q, '00, 7

723.9 Unspecified musculoskeletal disorders and symptoms referable to neck
Cervical (region) disorder NOS

✓4th **724 Other and unspecified disorders of back**

EXCLUDES *collapsed vertebra (code to cause, e.g., osteoporosis, 733.00-733.09)*
conditions due to:
intervertebral disc disorders (722.0-722.9)
spondylosis (721.0-721.9)

AHA: 2Q, '89, 14

✓5th **724.0 Spinal stenosis, other than cervical**

724.00 **Spinal stenosis, unspecified region**

724.01 **Thoracic region**

724.02 **Lumbar region**
AHA: 4Q, '99, 13

724.09 **Other**

724.1 Pain in thoracic spine

724.2 Lumbago
Low back pain
Low back syndrome
Lumbalgia
AHA: N-D, '85, 12

724.3 Sciatica
Neuralgia or neuritis of sciatic nerve

EXCLUDES *specified lesion of sciatic nerve (355.0)*

AHA: 2Q, '89, 12

724.4 Thoracic or lumbosacral neuritis or radiculitis, unspecified
Radicular syndrome of lower limbs
AHA: 2Q, '99, 3

724.5 Backache, unspecified
Vertebrogenic (pain) syndrome NOS

724.6 Disorders of sacrum
Ankylosis } lumbosacral or sacroiliac (joint)
Instability }

✓5th **724.7 Disorders of coccyx**

724.70 **Unspecified disorder of coccyx**

724.71 **Hypermobility of coccyx**

724.79 **Other**
Coccygodynia

724.8 Other symptoms referable to back
Ossification of posterior longitudinal ligament NOS
Panniculitis specified as sacral or affecting back

724.9 Other unspecified back disorders
Ankylosis of spine NOS
Compression of spinal nerve root NEC
Spinal disorder NOS

EXCLUDES *sacroiliitis (720.2)*

RHEUMATISM, EXCLUDING THE BACK (725-729)

INCLUDES disorders of muscles and tendons and their attachments, and of other soft tissues

725 Polymyalgia rheumatica
DEF: Joint and muscle pain, pelvis, and shoulder girdle stiffness, high sedimentation rate and temporal arteritis; occurs in elderly.

✓4th **726 Peripheral enthesopathies and allied syndromes**

Note: Enthesopathies are disorders of peripheral ligamentous or muscular attachments.

EXCLUDES *spinal enthesopathy (720.1)*

726.0 Adhesive capsulitis of shoulder

✓5th **726.1 Rotator cuff syndrome of shoulder and allied disorders**

726.10 **Disorders of bursae and tendons in shoulder region, unspecified**
Rotator cuff syndrome NOS
Supraspinatus syndrome NOS
AHA: 2Q, '01, 11

726.11 **Calcifying tendinitis of shoulder**

726.12 **Bicipital tenosynovitis**

726.19 **Other specified disorders**

EXCLUDES *complete rupture of rotator cuff, nontraumatic (727.61)*

726.2 Other affections of shoulder region, not elsewhere classified
Periarthritis of shoulder
Scapulohumeral fibrositis

✓5th **726.3 Enthesopathy of elbow region**

726.30 **Enthesopathy of elbow, unspecified**

726.31 **Medial epicondylitis**

726.32 **Lateral epicondylitis**
Epicondylitis NOS
Golfers' elbow
Tennis elbow

726.33 **Olecranon bursitis**
Bursitis of elbow

726.39 **Other**

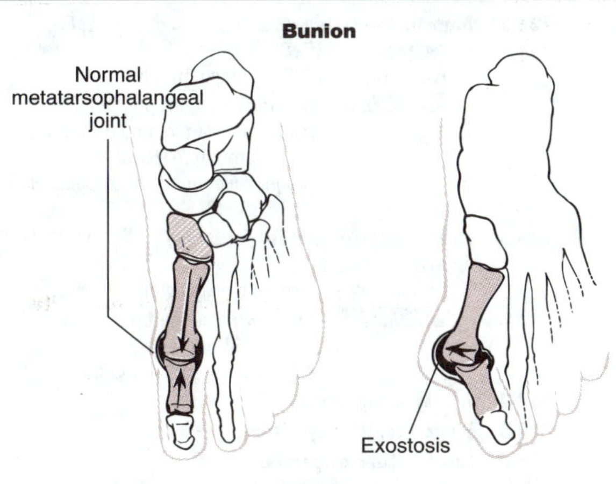

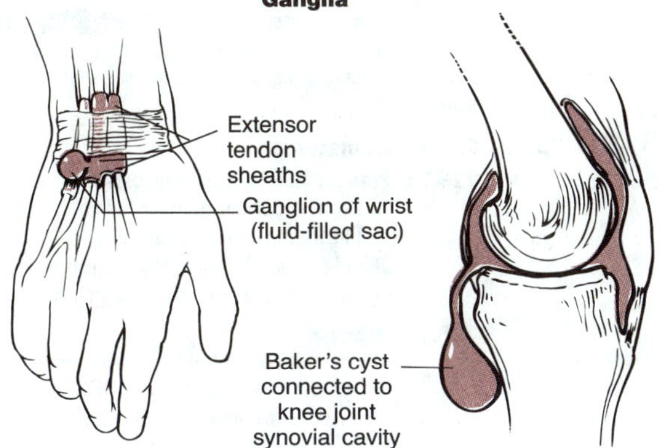

726.4 Enthesopathy of wrist and carpus
Bursitis of hand or wrist
Periarthritis of wrist

726.5 Enthesopathy of hip region
Bursitis of hip
Gluteal tendinitis
Iliac crest spur
Psoas tendinitis
Trochanteric tendinitis

✓5th **726.6 Enthesopathy of knee**

726.60 Enthesopathy of knee, unspecified
Bursitis of knee NOS

726.61 Pes anserinus tendinitis or bursitis
DEF: Inflamed tendons of sartorius, gracilis and semitendinosus muscles of medial aspect of knee.

726.62 Tibial collateral ligament bursitis
Pellegrini-Stieda syndrome

726.63 Fibular collateral ligament bursitis

726.64 Patellar tendinitis

726.65 Prepatellar bursitis

726.69 Other
Bursitis:
infrapatellar
subpatellar

✓5th **726.7 Enthesopathy of ankle and tarsus**

726.70 Enthesopathy of ankle and tarsus, unspecified
Metatarsalgia NOS
EXCLUDES *Morton's metatarsalgia (355.6)*

726.71 Achilles bursitis or tendinitis

726.72 Tibialis tendinitis
Tibialis (anterior) (posterior) tendinitis

726.73 Calcaneal spur
DEF: Overgrowth of calcaneous bone; causes pain on walking; due to chronic avulsion injury of plantar fascia from calcaneus.

726.79 Other
Peroneal tendinitis

726.8 Other peripheral enthesopathies

✓5th **726.9 Unspecified enthesopathy**

726.90 Enthesopathy of unspecified site
Capsulitis NOS
Periarthritis NOS
Tendinitis NOS

726.91 Exostosis of unspecified site
Bone spur NOS
AHA: 2Q, '01, 15

✓4th **727 Other disorders of synovium, tendon, and bursa**

✓5th **727.0 Synovitis and tenosynovitis**

727.00 Synovitis and tenosynovitis, unspecified
Synovitis NOS
Tenosynovitis NOS

727.01 Synovitis and tenosynovitis in diseases classified elsewhere
Code first underlying disease as:
tuberculosis (015.0-015.9)
EXCLUDES *crystal-induced (275.4)*
gonococcal (098.51)
gouty (274.0)
syphilitic (095.7)

727.02 Giant cell tumor of tendon sheath

727.03 Trigger finger (acquired)
DEF: Stenosing tenosynovitis or nodule in flexor tendon; cessation of flexion or extension movement in finger, followed by snapping into place.

727.04 Radial styloid tenosynovitis
de Quervain's disease

727.05 Other tenosynovitis of hand and wrist

727.06 Tenosynovitis of foot and ankle

727.09 Other

727.1 Bunion
DEF: Enlarged first metatarsal head due to inflamed bursa; results in laterally displaced great toe.

727.2 Specific bursitides often of occupational origin
Beat:
elbow
hand
knee
Miners':
elbow
knee
Chronic crepitant synovitis of wrist

727.3 Other bursitis
Bursitis NOS
EXCLUDES *bursitis:*
gonococcal (098.52)
subacromial (726.19)
subcoracoid (726.19)
subdeltoid (726.19)
syphilitic (095.7)
"frozen shoulder" (726.0)

✓5th **727.4 Ganglion and cyst of synovium, tendon, and bursa**

727.40 Synovial cyst, unspecified
EXCLUDES *that of popliteal space (727.51)*
AHA: 2Q, '97, 6

727.41 Ganglion of joint

727.42 Ganglion of tendon sheath

727.43 Ganglion, unspecified

727.49 Other
Cyst of bursa

✓5th **727.5 Rupture of synovium**

727.50 Rupture of synovium, unspecified

727.51 Synovial cyst of popliteal space
Baker's cyst (knee)

727.59 Other

✓5th **727.6 Rupture of tendon, nontraumatic**

727.60 Nontraumatic rupture of unspecified tendon

Musculoskeletal System and Connective Tissue 726.4–727.60

✓4th ✓5th Additional Digit Required | Unspecified Code | Other Specified Code | Manifestation Code | ▶◀ Revised Text | ● New Code | ▲ Revised Code Title

727.61 Complete rupture of rotator cuff
727.62 Tendons of biceps (long head)
727.63 Extensor tendons of hand and wrist
727.64 Flexor tendons of hand and wrist
727.65 Quadriceps tendon
727.66 Patellar tendon
727.67 Achilles tendon
727.68 Other tendons of foot and ankle
727.69 Other

✓5th **727.8 Other disorders of synovium, tendon, and bursa**

727.81 Contracture of tendon (sheath)
Short Achilles tendon (acquired)

727.82 Calcium deposits in tendon and bursa
Calcification of tendon NOS
Calcific tendinitis NOS
EXCLUDES *peripheral ligamentous or muscular attachments (726.0-726.9)*

727.83 Plica syndrome
Plica knee
AHA: 4Q, '00, 44
DEF: A fold in the synovial tissue that begins to form before birth, creating a septum between two pockets of synovial tissue; two most common plicae are the medial patellar plica and the suprapatellar plica. Plica syndrome, or plica knee, refers to symptomatic plica. Experienced by females more commonly than males.

727.89 Other
Abscess of bursa or tendon
EXCLUDES *xanthomatosis localized to tendons (272.7)*
AHA: 2Q, '89, 15

727.9 Unspecified disorder of synovium, tendon, and bursa

✓4th **728 Disorders of muscle, ligament, and fascia**
EXCLUDES *enthesopathies (726.0-726.9)*
muscular dystrophies (359.0-359.1)
myoneural disorders (358.00-358.9)
myopathies (359.2-359.9)
old disruption of ligaments of knee (717.81-717.89)

728.0 Infective myositis
Myositis:
purulent
suppurative
EXCLUDES *myositis:*
epidemic (074.1)
interstitial (728.81)
syphilitic (095.6)
tropical (040.81)
DEF: Inflamed connective septal tissue of muscle.

✓5th **728.1 Muscular calcification and ossification**

728.10 Calcification and ossification, unspecified
Massive calcification (paraplegic)

728.11 Progressive myositis ossificans
DEF: Progressive myositic disease; marked by bony tissue formed by voluntary muscle; occurs among very young.

728.12 Traumatic myositis ossificans
Myositis ossificans (circumscripta)

728.13 Postoperative heterotopic calcification
DEF: Abnormal formation of calcium deposits in muscular tissue after surgery, marked by a corresponding loss of muscle tone and tension.

728.19 Other
Polymyositis ossificans

728.2 Muscular wasting and disuse atrophy, not elsewhere classified
Amyotrophia NOS   Myofibrosis
EXCLUDES *neuralgic amyotrophy (353.5)*
pelvic muscle wasting and disuse atrophy (618.83)
progressive muscular atrophy (335.0-335.9)

728.3 Other specific muscle disorders
Arthrogryposis
Immobility syndrome (paraplegic)
EXCLUDES *arthrogryposis multiplex congenita (754.89)*
stiff-man syndrome (333.91)

728.4 Laxity of ligament

728.5 Hypermobility syndrome

728.6 Contracture of palmar fascia A
Dupuytren's contracture
DEF: Dupuytren's contracture: flexion deformity of finger, due to shortened, thickened fibrosing of palmar fascia; cause unknown; associated with long-standing epilepsy; occurs more often in males.

✓5th **728.7 Other fibromatoses**

728.71 Plantar fascial fibromatosis
Contracture of plantar fascia
Plantar fasciitis (traumatic)
DEF: Plantar fascia fibromatosis; causes nodular swelling and pain; not associated with contractures.

728.79 Other
Garrod's or knuckle pads
Nodular fasciitis
Pseudosarcomatous fibromatosis (proliferative) (subcutaneous)
DEF: Knuckle pads: pea-size nodules on dorsal surface of interphalangeal joints; new growth of fibrous tissue with thickened dermis and epidermis.

✓5th **728.8 Other disorders of muscle, ligament, and fascia**

728.81 Interstitial myositis
DEF: Inflammation of septal connective parts of muscle tissue.

728.82 Foreign body granuloma of muscle
Talc granuloma of muscle

728.83 Rupture of muscle, nontraumatic

728.84 Diastasis of muscle
Diastasis recti (abdomen)
EXCLUDES *diastasis recti complicating pregnancy, labor, and delivery (665.8)*
DEF: Muscle separation, such as recti abdominis after repeated pregnancies.

728.85 Spasm of muscle

728.86 Necrotizing fasciitis
Use additional code to identify:
infectious organism (041.00-041.89)
gangrene (785.4), if applicable
AHA: 4Q, '95, 54
DEF: Fulminating infection begins with extensive cellulitis, spreads to superficial and deep fascia; causes thrombosis of subcutaneous vessels, and gangrene of underlying tissue.

▲ **728.87 Muscle weakness (generalized)**
EXCLUDES *generalized weakness (780.79)*
AHA: ►1Q, '05, 13;◄ 4Q, '03, 66

728.88 Rhabdomyolysis
AHA: 4Q, '03, 66
DEF: A disintegration or destruction of muscle; an acute disease characterized by the excretion of myoglobin into the urine.

N Newborn Age: 0   P Pediatric Age: 0-17   M Maternity Age: 12-55   A Adult Age: 15-124   MSP Medicare Secondary Payer

728.89 Other
Eosinophilic fasciitis
Use additional E code to identify drug, if drug induced
AHA: 3Q, '02, 28; 2Q, '01, 14, 15
DEF: Eosinophilic fasciitis: inflammation of fascia of extremities associated with eosinophilia, edema, and swelling; occurs alone or as part of myalgia syndrome.

728.9 Unspecified disorder of muscle, ligament, and fascia
AHA: 4Q, '88, 11

✓4th **729 Other disorders of soft tissues**
EXCLUDES *acroparesthesia (443.89)*
carpal tunnel syndrome (354.0)
disorders of the back (720.0-724.9)
entrapment syndromes (354.0-355.9)
palindromic rheumatism (719.3)
periarthritis (726.0-726.9)
psychogenic rheumatism (306.0)

729.0 Rheumatism, unspecified and fibrositis
DEF: General term describes diseases of muscle, tendon, nerve, joint, or bone; symptoms include pain and stiffness.

729.1 Myalgia and myositis, unspecified
Fibromyositis NOS
DEF: Myalgia: muscle pain.
DEF: Myositis: inflamed voluntary muscle.
DEF: Fibromyositis: inflamed fibromuscular tissue.

729.2 Neuralgia, neuritis, and radiculitis, unspecified
EXCLUDES *brachial radiculitis (723.4)*
cervical radiculitis (723.4)
lumbosacral radiculitis (724.4)
mononeuritis (354.0-355.9)
radiculitis due to intervertebral disc involvement (722.0-722.2, 722.7)
sciatica (724.3)
DEF: Neuralgia: paroxysmal pain along nerve symptoms include brief pain and tenderness at point nerve exits.
DEF: Neuritis: inflamed nerve, symptoms include paresthesia, paralysis and loss of reflexes at nerve site.
DEF: Radiculitis: inflamed nerve root.

✓5th **729.3 Panniculitis, unspecified**
DEF: Inflammatory reaction of subcutaneous fat; causes nodules; often develops in abdominal region.

729.30 Panniculitis, unspecified site
Weber-Christian disease
DEF: Febrile, nodular, nonsuppurative, relapsing inflammation of subcutaneous fat.

729.31 Hypertrophy of fat pad, knee
Hypertrophy of infrapatellar fat pad

729.39 Other site
EXCLUDES *panniculitis specified as (affecting):*
back (724.8)
neck (723.6)
sacral (724.8)

729.4 Fasciitis, unspecified
EXCLUDES *necrotizing fasciitis (728.86)*
nodular fasciitis (728.79)
AHA: 2Q, '94, 13

729.5 Pain in limb

729.6 Residual foreign body in soft tissue
EXCLUDES *foreign body granuloma:*
muscle (728.82)
skin and subcutaneous tissue (709.4)

✓5th **729.8 Other musculoskeletal symptoms referable to limbs**

729.81 Swelling of limb
AHA: 4Q, '88, 6

729.82 Cramp

729.89 Other
EXCLUDES *abnormality of gait (781.2)*
tetany (781.7)
transient paralysis of limb (781.4)
AHA: 4Q, '88, 12

729.9 Other and unspecified disorders of soft tissue
Polyalgia

OSTEOPATHIES, CHONDROPATHIES, AND ACQUIRED MUSCULOSKELETAL DEFORMITIES (730-739)

✓4th **730 Osteomyelitis, periostitis, and other infections involving bone**
EXCLUDES *jaw (526.4-526.5)*
petrous bone (383.2)
Use additional code to identify organism, such as Staphylococcus (041.1)

The following fifth-digit subclassification is for use with category 730; valid digits are in [brackets] under each code. See list at beginning of chapter for definitions.
- **0 site unspecified**
- **1 shoulder region**
- **2 upper arm**
- **3 forearm**
- **4 hand**
- **5 pelvic region and thigh**
- **6 lower leg**
- **7 ankle and foot**
- **8 other specified sites**
- **9 multiple sites**

AHA: 4Q, '97, 43
DEF: Osteomyelitis: bacterial inflammation of bone tissue and marrow.
DEF: Periostitis: inflammation of specialized connective tissue; causes swelling of bone and aching pain.

§✓5th **730.0 Acute osteomyelitis**
[0-9]
Abscess of any bone except accessory sinus, jaw, or mastoid
Acute or subacute osteomyelitis, with or without mention of periostitis
AHA: For code 730.06: 1Q, '02, 4; For code 730.07: 1Q, '04, 14

§✓5th **730.1 Chronic osteomyelitis**
[0-9]
Brodie's abscess
Chronic or old osteomyelitis, with or without mention of periostitis
Sequestrum of bone
Sclerosing osteomyelitis of Garré
EXCLUDES *aseptic necrosis of bone (733.40-733.49)*
AHA: For code 730.17: 3Q, '00, 4

§✓5th **730.2 Unspecified osteomyelitis**
[0-9]
Osteitis or osteomyelitis NOS, with or without mention of periostitis

§✓5th **730.3 Periostitis without mention of osteomyelitis**
[0-9]
Abscess of periosteum } without mention of osteomyelitis
Periostosis } without mention of osteomyelitis
EXCLUDES *that in secondary syphilis (091.61)*

§ Requires fifth digit. Valid digits are in [brackets] under each code. See beginning of section 710–739 for codes and definitions.

✓4th ✓5th Additional Digit Required | Unspecified Code | Other Specified Code | Manifestation Code | ►◄ Revised Text | ● New Code | ▲ Revised Code Title

§ ✓5th **730.7** ***Osteopathy resulting from poliomyelitis***
[0-9]
Code first underlying disease (045.0-045.9)

§ ✓5th **730.8** ***Other infections involving bone in diseases classified elsewhere***
[0-9]
Code first underlying disease as:
tuberculosis (015.0-015.9)
typhoid fever (002.0)
EXCLUDES *syphilis of bone NOS (095.5)*
AHA: 2Q, '97, 16; 3Q, '91, 10

§ ✓5th **730.9** **Unspecified infection of bone**
[0-9]

✓4th **731 Osteitis deformans and osteopathies associated with other disorders classified elsewhere**
DEF: Osteitis deformans: Bone disease marked by episodes of increased bone loss, excessive repair attempts follow; causes weakened, deformed bones with increased mass, bowed long bones, deformed flat bones, pain and pathological fractures; may be fatal if associated with congestive heart failure, giant cell tumors or bone sarcoma; also called Paget's disease.

731.0 Osteitis deformans without mention of bone tumor
Paget's disease of bone

731.1 Osteitis deformans in diseases classified elsewhere
Code first underlying disease as:
malignant neoplasm of bone (170.0-170.9)

731.2 Hypertrophic pulmonary osteoarthropathy
Bamberger-Marie disease
DEF: Clubbing, of fingers and toes; related to enlarged ends of long bones; due to chronic lung and heart disease.

731.8 Other bone involvement in diseases classified elsewhere
Code first underlying disease as:
diabetes mellitus (250.8)
Use additional code to specify bone condition, such as:
acute osteomyelitis (730.00-730.09)
AHA: 1Q, '04, 14; 4Q, '97, 43; 2Q, '97, 16

✓4th **732 Osteochondropathies**
DEF: Conditions related to both bone and cartilage, or conditions in which cartilage is converted to bone (enchondral ossification).

732.0 Juvenile osteochondrosis of spine
Juvenile osteochondrosis (of):
marginal or vertebral epiphysis (of Scheuermann)
spine NOS
Vertebral epiphysitis
EXCLUDES *adolescent postural kyphosis (737.0)*

732.1 Juvenile osteochondrosis of hip and pelvis
Coxa plana
Ischiopubic synchondrosis (of van Neck)
Osteochondrosis (juvenile) of:
acetabulum
head of femur (of Legg-Calvé-Perthes)
iliac crest (of Buchanan)
symphysis pubis (of Pierson)
Pseudocoxalgia

732.2 Nontraumatic slipped upper femoral epiphysis
Slipped upper femoral epiphysis NOS

732.3 Juvenile osteochondrosis of upper extremity
Osteochondrosis (juvenile) of:
capitulum of humerus (of Panner)
carpal lunate (of Kienbock)
hand NOS
head of humerus (of Haas)
heads of metacarpals (of Mauclaire)
lower ulna (of Burns)
radial head (of Brailsford)
upper extremity NOS

732.4 Juvenile osteochondrosis of lower extremity, excluding foot
Osteochondrosis (juvenile) of:
lower extremity NOS
primary patellar center (of Köhler)
proximal tibia (of Blount)
secondary patellar center (of Sinding-Larsen)
tibial tubercle (of Osgood-Schlatter)
Tibia vara

732.5 Juvenile osteochondrosis of foot
Calcaneal apophysitis
Epiphysitis, os calcis
Osteochondrosis (juvenile) of:
astragalus (of Diaz)
calcaneum (of Sever)
foot NOS
metatarsal:
second (of Freiberg)
fifth (of Iselin)
os tibiale externum (of Haglund)
tarsal navicular (of Köhler)

732.6 Other juvenile osteochondrosis
Apophysitis, Epiphysitis, Osteochondritis, Osteochondrosis } specified as juvenile, of other site, or site NOS

732.7 Osteochondritis dissecans

732.8 Other specified forms of osteochondropathy
Adult osteochondrosis of spine

732.9 Unspecified osteochondropathy
Apophysitis, Epiphysitis, Osteochondritis, Osteochondrosis } NOS; not specified as adult or juvenile, of unspecified site

✓4th **733 Other disorders of bone and cartilage**
EXCLUDES *bone spur (726.91)*
cartilage of, or loose body in, joint (717.0-717.9, 718.0-718.9)
giant cell granuloma of jaw (526.3)
osteitis fibrosa cystica generalisata (252.01)
osteomalacia (268.2)
polyostotic fibrous dysplasia of bone (756.54)
prognathism, retrognathism (524.1)
xanthomatosis localized to bone (272.7)

✓5th **733.0 Osteoporosis**
DEF: Bone mass reduction that ultimately results in fractures after minimal trauma; dorsal kyphosis or loss of height often occur.

733.00 Osteoporosis, unspecified
Wedging of vertebra NOS
AHA: 3Q, '01, 19; 2Q, '98, 12

733.01 Senile osteoporosis
Postmenopausal osteoporosis

733.02 Idiopathic osteoporosis

733.03 Disuse osteoporosis

733.09 Other
Drug-induced osteoporosis
Use additional E code to identify drug
AHA: 4Q, '03, 108

✓5th **733.1 Pathologic fracture**
Spontaneous fracture
EXCLUDES *stress fracture (733.93-733.95)*
traumatic fracture (800-829)
AHA: 4Q, '93, 25; N-D, '86, 10; N-D, '85, 16
DEF: Fracture due to bone structure weakening by pathological processes (e.g., osteoporosis, neoplasms and osteomalacia).

733.10 Pathologic fracture, unspecified site

733.11 Pathologic fracture of humerus

§ Requires fifth digit. Valid digits are in [brackets] under each code. See beginning of section 710–739 for codes and definitions.

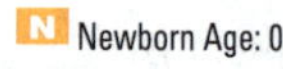
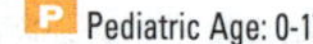

Acquired Deformities of Toe

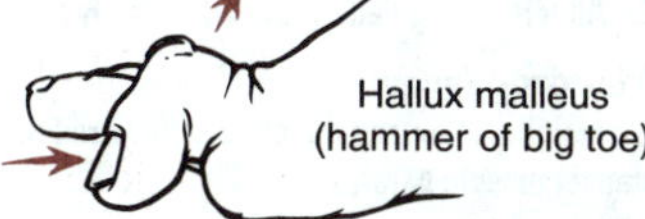
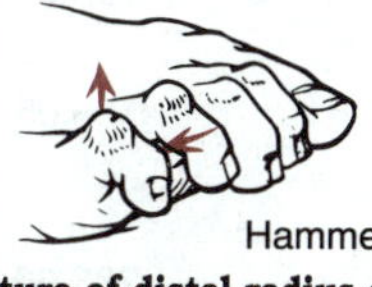

733.12 Pathologic fracture of distal radius and ulna
Wrist NOS

733.13 Pathologic fracture of vertebrae
Collapse of vertebra NOS
AHA: 3Q, '99, 5

733.14 Pathologic fracture of neck of femur
Femur NOS Hip NOS
AHA: 1Q, '01, 1; 1Q, '96, 16

733.15 Pathologic fracture of other specified part of femur
AHA: 2Q, '98, 12

733.16 Pathologic fracture of tibia or fibula
Ankle NOS

733.19 Pathologic fracture of other specified site

✓5th **733.2 Cyst of bone**

733.20 Cyst of bone (localized), unspecified

733.21 Solitary bone cyst
Unicameral bone cyst

733.22 Aneurysmal bone cyst
DEF: Solitary bone lesion, bulges into periosteum; marked by calcified rim.

733.29 Other
Fibrous dysplasia (monostotic)
EXCLUDES *cyst of jaw (526.0-526.2, 526.89)*
osteitis fibrosa cystica (252.01)
polyostotic fibrousdyplasia of bone (756.54)

733.3 Hyperostosis of skull
Hyperostosis interna frontalis
Leontiasis ossium
DEF: Abnormal bone growth on inner aspect of cranial bones.

✓5th **733.4 Aseptic necrosis of bone**
EXCLUDES *osteochondropathies (732.0-732.9)*
DEF: Infarction of bone tissue due to a nonfectious etiology, such as a fracture, ischemic disorder or administration of immunosuppressive drugs; leads to degenerative joint disease or nonunion of fractures.

733.40 Aseptic necrosis of bone, site unspecified

733.41 Head of humerus

733.42 Head and neck of femur
Femur NOS
EXCLUDES *Legg-Calvé-Perthes disease (732.1)*

733.43 Medial femoral condyle

733.44 Talus

733.49 Other

Acquired Deformities of Forearm

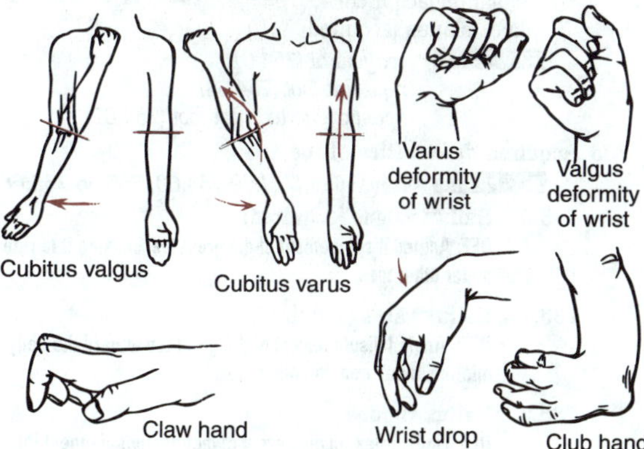

733.5 Osteitis condensans
Piriform sclerosis of ilium
DEF: Idiopathic condition marked by low back pain; associated with oval or triangular sclerotic, opaque bone next to sacroiliac joints in the ileum.

733.6 Tietze's disease
Costochondral junction syndrome
Costochondritis
DEF: Painful, idiopathic, nonsuppurative, swollen costal cartilage sometimes confused with cardiac symptoms because the anterior chest pain resembles that of coronary artery disease.

733.7 Algoneurodystrophy
Disuse atrophy of bone
Sudeck's atrophy
DEF: Painful, idiopathic.

✓5th **733.8 Malunion and nonunion of fracture**
AHA: 2Q, '94, 5

733.81 Malunion of fracture

733.82 Nonunion of fracture
Pseudoarthrosis (bone)

✓5th **733.9 Other and unspecified disorders of bone and cartilage**

733.90 Disorder of bone and cartilage, unspecified

733.91 Arrest of bone development or growth
Epiphyseal arrest

733.92 Chondromalacia
Chondromalacia:
NOS
localized, except patella
systemic
tibial plateau
EXCLUDES *chondromalacia of patella (717.7)*
DEF: Articular cartilage softening.

733.93 Stress fracture of tibia or fibula
Stress reaction of tibia or fibula
AHA: 4Q, '01, 48

733.94 Stress fracture of the metatarsals
Stress reaction of metatarsals
AHA: 4Q, '01, 48

733.95 Stress fracture of other bone
Stress reaction of other bone
AHA: 4Q, '01, 48

733.99 Other
Diaphysitis
Hypertrophy of bone
Relapsing polychondritis
AHA: J-F, '87, 14

734 Flat foot

Pes planus (acquired)

Talipes planus (acquired)

EXCLUDES *congenital (754.61)*
rigid flat foot (754.61)
spastic (everted) flat foot (754.61)

✓4th **735 Acquired deformities of toe**

EXCLUDES *congenital (754.60-754.69, 755.65-755.66)*

735.0 Hallux valgus (acquired)

DEF: Angled displacement of the great toe, causing it to ride over or under other toes.

735.1 Hallux varus (acquired)

DEF: Angled displacement of the great toe toward the body midline, away from the other toes.

735.2 Hallux rigidus

DEF: Limited flexion movement at metatarsophalangeal joint of great toe; due to degenerative joint disease.

735.3 Hallux malleus

DEF: Extended proximal phalanx, flexed distal phalanges, of great toe; foot resembles claw or hammer.

735.4 Other hammer toe (acquired)

735.5 Claw toe (acquired)

DEF: Hyperextended proximal phalanges, flexed middle and distal phalanges.

735.8 Other acquired deformities of toe

735.9 Unspecified acquired deformity of toe

✓4th **736 Other acquired deformities of limbs**

EXCLUDES *congenital (754.3-755.9)*

✓5th **736.0 Acquired deformities of forearm, excluding fingers**

736.00 Unspecified deformity

Deformity of elbow, forearm, hand, or wrist (acquired) NOS

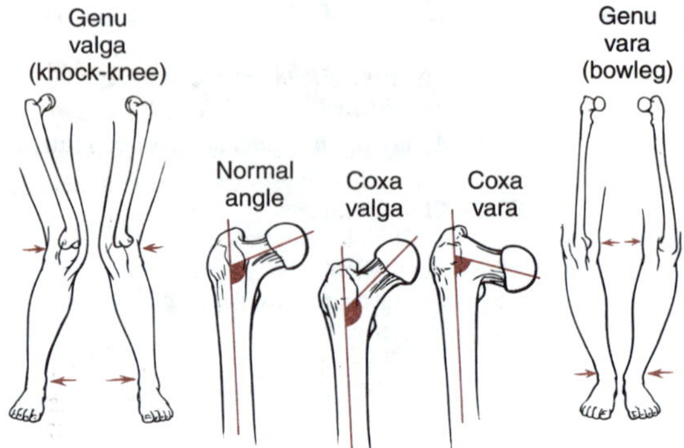

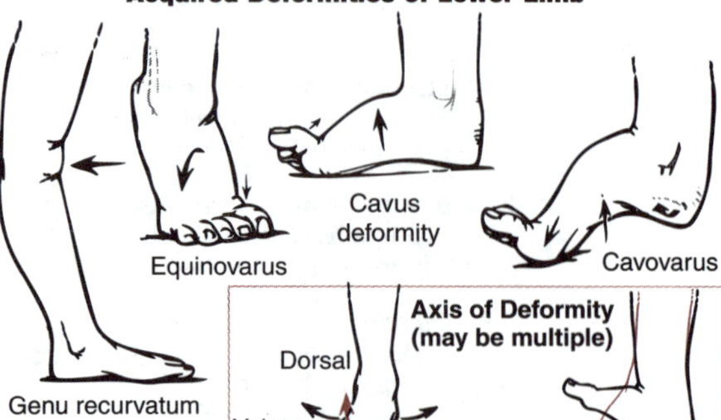

736.01 Cubitus valgus (acquired)

DEF: Deviation of the elbow away from the body midline upon extension; it occurs when the palm is turning outward.

736.02 Cubitus varus (acquired)

DEF: Elbow joint displacement angled laterally; when the forearm is extended, it is deviated toward the midline of the body; also called "gun stock" deformity.

736.03 Valgus deformity of wrist (acquired)

DEF: Abnormal angulation away from the body midline.

736.04 Varus deformity of wrist (acquired)

DEF: Abnormal angulation toward the body midline.

736.05 Wrist drop (acquired)

DEF: Inability to extend the hand at the wrist due to extensor muscle paralysis.

736.06 Claw hand (acquired)

DEF: Flexion and atrophy of the hand and fingers; found in ulnar nerve lesions, syringomyelia, and leprosy.

736.07 Club hand, acquired

DEF: Twisting of the hand out of shape or position; caused by the congenital absence of the ulna or radius.

736.09 Other

736.1 Mallet finger

DEF: Permanently flexed distal phalanx.

✓5th **736.2 Other acquired deformities of finger**

736.20 Unspecified deformity

Deformity of finger (acquired) NOS

736.21 Boutonniere deformity

DEF: A deformity of the finger caused by flexion of the proximal interphalangeal joint and hyperextension of the distal joint; also called buttonhole deformity.

736.22 Swan-neck deformity

DEF: Flexed distal and hyperextended proximal interphalangeal joint.

736.29 Other

EXCLUDES *trigger finger (727.03)*

AHA: 2Q, '89, 13

✓5th **736.3 Acquired deformities of hip**

736.30 Unspecified deformity

Deformity of hip (acquired) NOS

736.31 Coxa valga (acquired)

DEF: Increase of at least 140 degrees in the angle formed by the axis of the head and the neck of the femur, and the axis of its shaft.

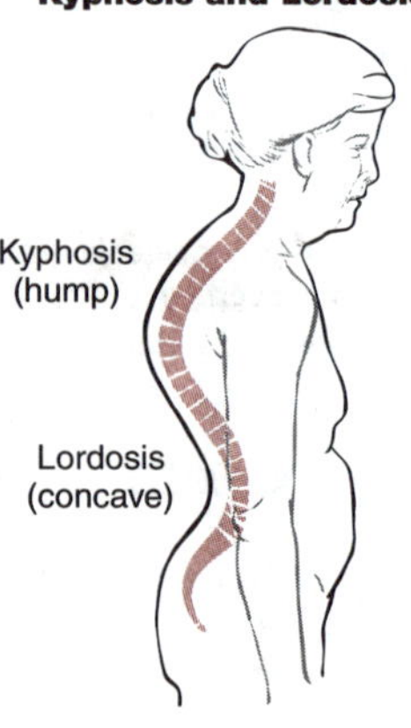

Scoliosis and Kyphoscoliosis

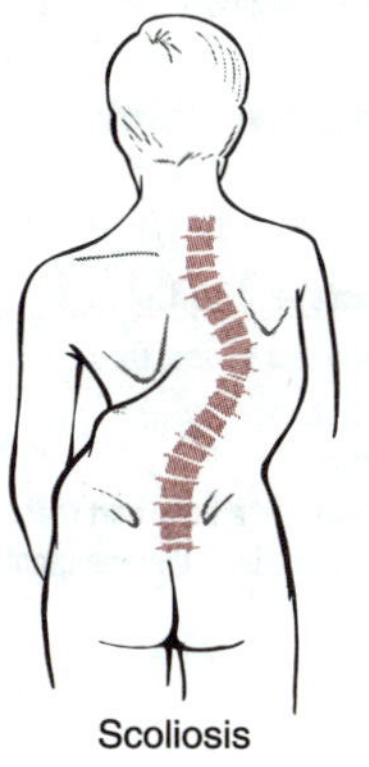
Scoliosis

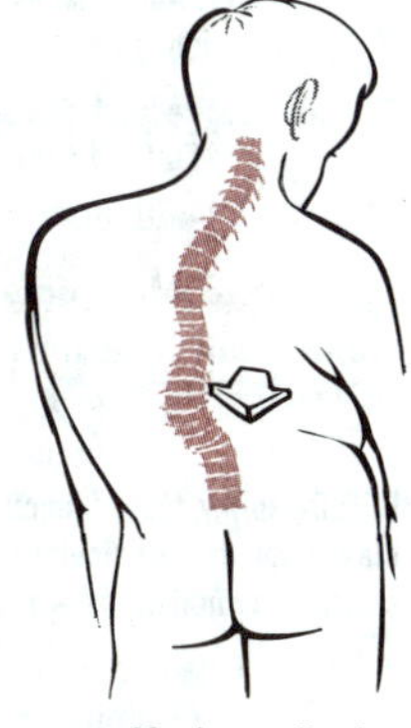
Kyphoscoliosis

736.32 Coxa vara (acquired)
DEF: The bending downward of the neck of the femur: causing difficulty in movement; a right angle or less may be formed by the axis of the head and neck of the femur, and the axis of its shaft.

736.39 Other
AHA: 2Q, '91, 18

✓5th **736.4 Genu valgum or varum (acquired)**

736.41 Genu valgum (acquired)
DEF: Abnormally close together and an abnormally large space between the ankles; also called "knock-knees."

736.42 Genu varum (acquired)
DEF: Abnormally separated knees and the inward bowing of the legs; it is also called "bowlegs."

736.5 Genu recurvatum (acquired)
DEF: Hyperextended knees; also called "backknee."

736.6 Other acquired deformities of knee
Deformity of knee (acquired) NOS

✓5th **736.7 Other acquired deformities of ankle and foot**
EXCLUDES *deformities of toe (acquired) (735.0-735.9)*
pes planus (acquired) (734)

736.70 Unspecified deformity of ankle and foot, acquired

736.71 Acquired equinovarus deformity
Clubfoot, acquired
EXCLUDES *clubfoot not specified as acquired (754.5-754.7)*

736.72 Equinus deformity of foot, acquired
DEF: A plantar flexion deformity that forces people to walk on their toes.

736.73 Cavus deformity of foot
EXCLUDES *that with claw foot (736.74)*
DEF: Abnormally high longitudinal arch of the foot.

736.74 Claw foot, acquired
DEF: High foot arch with hyperextended toes at metatarsophalangeal joint and flexed toes at distal joints; also called "main en griffe."

736.75 Cavovarus deformity of foot, acquired
DEF: Inward turning of the heel from the midline of the leg and an abnormally high longitudinal arch.

736.76 Other calcaneus deformity

736.79 Other
Acquired:
pes } not elsewhere classified
talipes }

✓5th **736.8 Acquired deformities of other parts of limbs**

736.81 Unequal leg length (acquired)

736.89 Other
Deformity (acquired):
arm or leg, not elsewhere classified
shoulder

736.9 Acquired deformity of limb, site unspecified

✓4th **737 Curvature of spine**
EXCLUDES *congenital (754.2)*

737.0 Adolescent postural kyphosis
EXCLUDES *osteochondrosis of spine (juvenile) (732.0)*
adult (732.8)

✓5th **737.1 Kyphosis (acquired)**

737.10 Kyphosis (acquired) (postural)

737.11 Kyphosis due to radiation

737.12 Kyphosis, postlaminectomy
AHA: J-F, '87, 7

737.19 Other
EXCLUDES *that associated with conditions classifiable elsewhere (737.41)*

✓5th **737.2 Lordosis (acquired)**
DEF: Swayback appearance created by an abnormally increased spinal curvature; it is also referred to as "hollow back" or "saddle back."

737.20 Lordosis (acquired) (postural)

737.21 Lordosis, postlaminectomy

737.22 Other postsurgical lordosis

737.29 Other
EXCLUDES *that associated with conditions classifiable elsewhere (737.42)*

✓5th **737.3 Kyphoscoliosis and scoliosis**
DEF: Kyphoscoliosis: backward and lateral curvature of the spinal column; it is found in vertebral osteochondrosis.

DEF: Scoliosis: an abnormal deviation of the spine to the left or right of the midline

737.30 Scoliosis [and kyphoscoliosis], idiopathic
AHA: 3Q, '03, 19

737.31 Resolving infantile idiopathic scoliosis

737.32 Progressive infantile idiopathic scoliosis
AHA: 3Q, '02, 12

737.33 Scoliosis due to radiation

737.34 Thoracogenic scoliosis

737.39 Other
EXCLUDES *that associated with conditions classifiable elsewhere (737.43)*
that in kyphoscoliotic heart disease (416.1)

AHA: 2Q, '02, 16

✓5th **737.4 Curvature of spine associated with other conditions**
Code first associated condition as:
Charcôt-Marie-Tooth disease (356.1)
mucopolysaccharidosis (277.5)
neurofibromatosis (237.7)
osteitis deformans (731.0)
osteitis fibrosa cystica (252.01)
osteoporosis (733.00-733.09)
poliomyelitis (138)
tuberculosis [Pott's curvature] (015.0)

737.40 Curvature of spine, unspecified

737.41 Kyphosis

737.42 Lordosis

737.43 Scoliosis

737.8 Other curvatures of spine

737.9 Unspecified curvature of spine
Curvature of spine (acquired) (idiopathic) NOS
Hunchback, acquired
EXCLUDES *deformity of spine NOS (738.5)*

✓4th **738 Other acquired deformity**
EXCLUDES *congenital (754.0-756.9, 758.0-759.9)*
dentofacial anomalies (524.0-524.9)

738.0 Acquired deformity of nose
Deformity of nose (acquired)
Overdevelopment of nasal bones
EXCLUDES *deflected or deviated nasal septum (470)*

✓5th **738.1 Other acquired deformity of head**

738.10 Unspecified deformity

738.11 Zygomatic hyperplasia
DEF: Abnormal enlargement of the zygoma (processus zygomaticus temporalis).

738.12 Zygomatic hypoplasia
DEF: Underdevelopment of the zygoma (processus zygomaticus temporalis).

738.19 Other specified deformity
AHA: 2Q, '03, 13

738.2 Acquired deformity of neck

738.3 Acquired deformity of chest and rib
Deformity:
chest (acquired)
rib (acquired)
Pectus:
carinatum, acquired
excavatum, acquired

738.4 Acquired spondylolisthesis
Degenerative spondylolisthesis
Spondylolysis, acquired
EXCLUDES *congenital (756.12)*
DEF: Vertebra displaced forward over another; due to bilateral defect in vertebral arch, eroded articular surface of posterior facts and elongated pedicle between fifth lumbar vertebra and sacrum.

738.5 Other acquired deformity of back or spine
Deformity of spine NOS
EXCLUDES *curvature of spine (737.0-737.9)*

738.6 Acquired deformity of pelvis
Pelvic obliquity
EXCLUDES *intrapelvic protrusion of acetabulum (718.6)*
that in relation to labor and delivery (653.0-653.4, 653.8-653.9)
DEF: Pelvic obliquity: slanting or inclination of the pelvis at an angle between 55 and 60 degrees between the plane of the pelvis and the horizontal plane.

738.7 Cauliflower ear
DEF: Abnormal external ear; due to injury, subsequent perichondritis.

738.8 Acquired deformity of other specified site
Deformity of clavicle
AHA: 2Q, '01, 15

738.9 Acquired deformity of unspecified site

✓4th **739 Nonallopathic lesions, not elsewhere classified**
INCLUDES segmental dysfunction
somatic dysfunction
DEF: Disability, loss of function or abnormality of a body part that is neither classifiable to a particular system nor brought about therapeutically to counteract another disease.

739.0 Head region
Occipitocervical region

739.1 Cervical region
Cervicothoracic region

739.2 Thoracic region
Thoracolumbar region

739.3 Lumbar region
Lumbosacral region

739.4 Sacral region
Sacrococcygeal region Sacroiliac region

739.5 Pelvic region
Hip region
Pubic region

739.6 Lower extremities

739.7 Upper extremities
Acromioclavicular region
Sternoclavicular region

739.8 Rib cage
Costochondral region Sternochondral region
Costovertebral region

739.9 Abdomen and other
AHA: 2Q, '89, 14

14. CONGENITAL ANOMALIES (740-759)

✓4th **740 Anencephalus and similar anomalies**

740.0 Anencephalus

Acrania
Amyelencephalus
Hemicephaly
Hemianencephaly

DEF: Fetus without cerebrum, cerebellum and flat bones of skull.

740.1 Craniorachischisis

DEF: Congenital slit in cranium and vertebral column.

740.2 Iniencephaly

DEF: Spinal cord passes through enlarged occipital bone (foramen magnum); absent vertebral bone layer and spinal processes; resulting in both reduction in number and proper fusion of the vertebrae.

✓4th **741 Spina bifida**

EXCLUDES *spina bifida occulta (756.17)*

The following fifth-digit subclassification is for use with category 741:

0 unspecified region
1 cervical region
2 dorsal [thoracic] region
3 lumbar region

AHA: 3Q, '94, 7

DEF: Lack of closure of spinal cord's bony encasement; marked by cord protrusion into lumbosacral area; evident by elevated alpha-fetoprotein of amniotic fluid.

✓5th **741.0 With hydrocephalus**

Arnold-Chiari syndrome, type II
Any condition classifiable to 741.9 with any condition classifiable to 742.3
Chiari malformation, type II

AHA: 4Q, '97, 51; 4Q, '94, 37; S-O, '87, 10

✓5th **741.9 Without mention of hydrocephalus**

Hydromeningocele (spinal)
Hydromyelocele
Meningocele (spinal)
Meningomyelocele
Myelocele
Myelocystocele
Rachischisis
Spina bifida (aperta)
Syringomyelocele

✓4th **742 Other congenital anomalies of nervous system**

EXCLUDES ▶*congenital central alveolar hypoventilation syndrome (327.25)*◀

742.0 Encephalocele

Encephalocystocele
Encephalomyelocele
Hydroencephalocele
Hydromeningocele, cranial
Meningocele, cerebral
Meningoencephalocele

AHA: 4Q, '94, 37

DEF: Brain tissue protrudes through skull defect.

742.1 Microcephalus

Hydromicrocephaly
Micrencephaly

DEF: Extremely small head or brain.

Spina Bifida

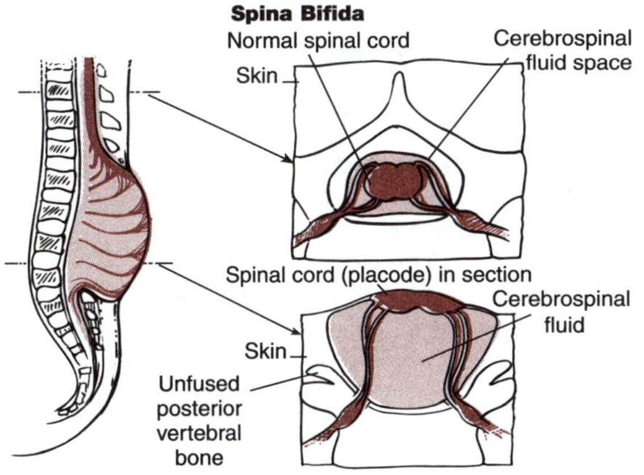

742.2 Reduction deformities of brain

Absence, Agenesis, Aplasia, Hypoplasia } of part of brain

Agyria
Arhinencephaly
Holoprosencephaly
Microgyria

AHA: 3Q, '03, 15; 4Q, '94, 37

742.3 Congenital hydrocephalus

Aqueduct of Sylvius:
- anomaly
- obstruction, congenital
- stenosis

Atresia of foramina of Magendie and Luschka
Hydrocephalus in newborn

EXCLUDES *hydrocephalus:*
acquired (331.3-331.4)
due to congenital toxoplasmosis (771.2)
with any condition classifiable to 741.9 (741.0)

DEF: Fluid accumulation within the skull; involves subarachnoid (external) or ventricular (internal) brain spaces.

742.4 Other specified anomalies of brain

Congenital cerebral cyst
Macroencephaly
Macrogyria
Megalencephaly
Multiple anomalies of brain NOS
Porencephaly
Ulegyria

AHA: 1Q, '99, 9; 3Q, '92, 12

✓5th **742.5 Other specified anomalies of spinal cord**

742.51 Diastematomyelia

DEF: Congenital anomaly often associated with spina bifida; the spinal cord is separated into halves by bony tissue resembling a "spike" (spicule), each half surrounded by a dural sac.

742.53 Hydromyelia

Hydrorhachis

DEF: Dilated central spinal cord canal; characterized by increased fluid accumulation.

Normal Ventricles and Hydrocephalus

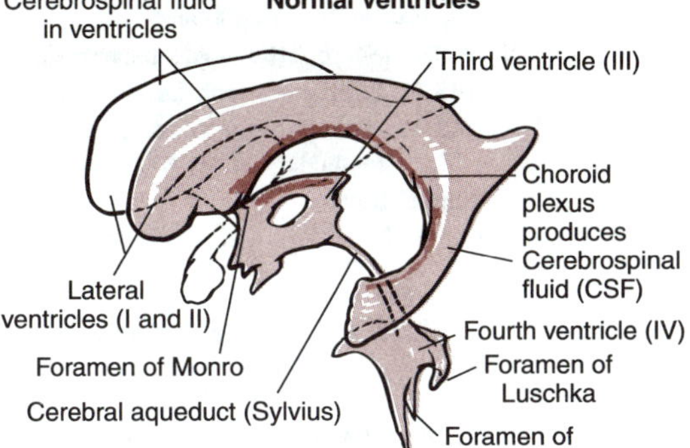

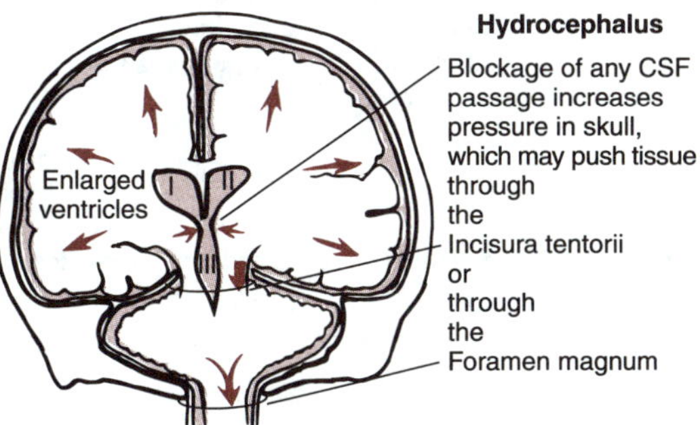

742.59 Other
Amyelia
Atelomyelia
Congenital anomaly of spinal meninges
Defective development of cauda equina
Hypoplasia of spinal cord
Myelatelia
Myelodysplasia
AHA: 2Q, '91, 14; 1Q, '89, 10

742.8 Other specified anomalies of nervous system
Agenesis of nerve
Displacement of brachial plexus
Familial dysautonomia
Jaw-winking syndrome
Marcus-Gunn syndrome
Riley-Day syndrome
EXCLUDES *neurofibromatosis (237.7)*

742.9 Unspecified anomaly of brain, spinal cord, and nervous system
Anomaly } of: brain
Congenital: } of: nervous system
disease } of: spinal cord
lesion
Deformity

✓4th 743 Congenital anomalies of eye

✓5th 743.0 Anophthalmos
DEF: Complete absence of the eyes or the presence of vestigial eyes.

743.00 Clinical anophthalmos, unspecified
Agenesis } of eye
Congenital absence } of eye
Anophthalmos NOS

743.03 Cystic eyeball, congenital

743.06 Cryptophthalmos
DEF: Eyelids continue over eyeball, results in apparent absence of eyelids.

✓5th 743.1 Microphthalmos
Dysplasia } of eye
Hypoplasia } of eye
Rudimentary eye
DEF: Abnormally small eyeballs, may be opacities of cornea and lens, scarring of choroid and retina.

743.10 Microphthalmos, unspecified

743.11 Simple microphthalmos

743.12 Microphthalmos associated with other anomalies of eye and adnexa

✓5th 743.2 Buphthalmos
Glaucoma:
congenital
newborn
Hydrophthalmos
EXCLUDES *glaucoma of childhood (365.14)*
traumatic glaucoma due to birth injury (767.8)
DEF: Distended, enlarged fibrous coats of eye; due to intraocular pressure of congenital glaucoma.

743.20 Buphthalmos, unspecified

743.21 Simple buphthalmos

743.22 Buphthalmos associated with other ocular anomalies
Keratoglobus, congenital } associated with buphthalmos
Megalocornea } associated with buphthalmos

✓5th 743.3 Congenital cataract and lens anomalies
EXCLUDES *infantile cataract (366.00-366.09)*
DEF: Opaque eye lens.

743.30 Congenital cataract, unspecified

743.31 Capsular and subcapsular cataract

743.32 Cortical and zonular cataract

743.33 Nuclear cataract

743.34 Total and subtotal cataract, congenital

743.35 Congenital aphakia
Congenital absence of lens

743.36 Anomalies of lens shape
Microphakia
Spherophakia

743.37 Congenital ectopic lens

743.39 Other

✓5th 743.4 Coloboma and other anomalies of anterior segment
DEF: Coloboma: ocular tissue defect associated with defect of ocular fetal intraocular fissure; may cause small pit on optic disk, major defects of iris, ciliary body, choroid, and retina.

743.41 Anomalies of corneal size and shape
Microcornea
EXCLUDES *that associated with buphthalmos (743.22)*

743.42 Corneal opacities, interfering with vision, congenital

743.43 Other corneal opacities, congenital

743.44 Specified anomalies of anterior chamber, chamber angle, and related structures
Anomaly:
Axenfeld's
Peters'
Anomaly:
Rieger's

743.45 Aniridia
AHA: 3Q, '02, 20
DEF: Incompletely formed or absent iris; affects both eyes; dominant trait; also called congenital hyperplasia of iris.

743.46 Other specified anomalies of iris and ciliary body
Anisocoria, congenital
Atresia of pupil
Coloboma of iris
Corectopia

743.47 Specified anomalies of sclera

743.48 Multiple and combined anomalies of anterior segment

743.49 Other

✓5th 743.5 Congenital anomalies of posterior segment

743.51 Vitreous anomalies
Congenital vitreous opacity

743.52 Fundus coloboma
DEF: Absent retinal and choroidal tissue; occurs in lower fundus; a bright white ectatic zone of exposed sclera extends into and changes the optic disk.

743.53 Chorioretinal degeneration, congenital

743.54 Congenital folds and cysts of posterior segment

743.55 Congenital macular changes

743.56 Other retinal changes, congenital
AHA: 3Q, '99, 12

743.57 Specified anomalies of optic disc
Coloboma of optic disc (congenital)

743.58 Vascular anomalies
Congenital retinal aneurysm

743.59 Other

✓5th 743.6 Congenital anomalies of eyelids, lacrimal system, and orbit

743.61 Congenital ptosis
DEF: Drooping of eyelid.

743.62 Congenital deformities of eyelids
Ablepharon
Absence of eyelid
Accessory eyelid
Congenital:
ectropion
entropion
AHA: 1Q, '00, 22

743.63 **Other specified congenital anomalies of eyelid**
Absence, agenesis, of cilia

743.64 **Specified congenital anomalies of lacrimal gland**

743.65 **Specified congenital anomalies of lacrimal passages**
Absence, agenesis of:
lacrimal apparatus
punctum lacrimale
Accessory lacrimal canal

743.66 **Specified congenital anomalies of orbit**

743.69 **Other**
Accessory eye muscles

743.8 **Other specified anomalies of eye**
EXCLUDES *congenital nystagmus (379.51)*
ocular albinism (270.2)
retinitis pigmentosa (362.74)

743.9 **Unspecified anomaly of eye**
Congenital:
anomaly NOS } of eye [any part]
deformity NOS

✓4th **744 Congenital anomalies of ear, face, and neck**
EXCLUDES *anomaly of:*
cervical spine (754.2, 756.10-756.19)
larynx (748.2-748.3)
nose (748.0-748.1)
parathyroid gland (759.2)
thyroid gland (759.2)
cleft lip (749.10-749.25)

✓5th 744.0 **Anomalies of ear causing impairment of hearing**
EXCLUDES *congenital deafness without mention of cause (389.0-389.9)*

744.00 **Unspecified anomaly of ear with impairment of hearing**

744.01 **Absence of external ear**
Absence of:
auditory canal (external)
auricle (ear) (with stenosis or atresia of auditory canal)

744.02 **Other anomalies of external ear with impairment of hearing**
Atresia or stricture of auditory canal (external)

744.03 **Anomaly of middle ear, except ossicles**
Atresia or stricture of osseous meatus (ear)

744.04 **Anomalies of ear ossicles**
Fusion of ear ossicles

744.05 **Anomalies of inner ear**
Congenital anomaly of:
membranous labyrinth
organ of Corti

744.09 **Other**
Absence of ear, congenital

744.1 **Accessory auricle**
Accessory tragus
Polyotia
Preauricular appendage
Supernumerary:
ear
lobule
DEF: Redundant tissue or structures of ear.

✓5th 744.2 **Other specified anomalies of ear**
EXCLUDES *that with impairment of hearing (744.00-744.09)*

744.21 **Absence of ear lobe, congenital**

744.22 **Macrotia**
DEF: Abnormally large pinna of ear.

744.23 **Microtia**
DEF: Hypoplasia of pinna; associated with absent or closed auditory canal.

744.24 **Specified anomalies of Eustachian tube**
Absence of Eustachian tube

744.29 **Other**
Bat ear
Darwin's tubercle
Pointed ear
Prominence of auricle
Ridge ear
EXCLUDES *preauricular sinus (744.46)*

744.3 **Unspecified anomaly of ear**
Congenital:
anomaly NOS } of ear, not elsewhere classified
deformity NOS

✓5th 744.4 **Branchial cleft cyst or fistula; preauricular sinus**

744.41 **Branchial cleft sinus or fistula**
Branchial:
sinus (external) (internal)
vestige
DEF: Cyst due to failed closure of embryonic branchial cleft.

744.42 **Branchial cleft cyst**

744.43 **Cervical auricle**

744.46 **Preauricular sinus or fistula**

744.47 **Preauricular cyst**

744.49 **Other**
Fistula (of):
auricle, congenital
cervicoaural

744.5 **Webbing of neck**
Pterygium colli
DEF: Thick, triangular skinfold, stretches from lateral side of neck across shoulder; associated with Turner's and Noonan's syndromes.

✓5th 744.8 **Other specified anomalies of face and neck**

744.81 **Macrocheilia**
Hypertrophy of lip, congenital
DEF: Abnormally large lips.

744.82 **Microcheilia**
DEF: Abnormally small lips.

744.83 **Macrostomia**
DEF: Bilateral or unilateral anomaly, of mouth due to malformed maxillary and mandibular processes; results in mouth extending toward ear.

744.84 **Microstomia**
DEF: Abnormally small mouth.

744.89 **Other**
EXCLUDES *congenital fistula of lip (750.25)*
musculoskeletal anomalies (754.0-754.1, 756.0)

744.9 **Unspecified anomalies of face and neck**
Congenital:
anomaly NOS } of face [any part] or neck [any part]
deformity NOS

✓4th **745 Bulbus cordis anomalies and anomalies of cardiac septal closure**

745.0 **Common truncus**
Absent septum } between aorta and pulmonary artery
Communication (abnormal)
Aortic septal defect
Common aortopulmonary trunk
Persistent truncus arteriosus

Heart Defects

Atrial septal defect
Aortic stenosis
Ventricular septal defect
Patent ductus arteriosus
Pulmonary stenosis
Transposition of the great vessels
Tetralogy of Fallot

✓5th **745.1 Transposition of great vessels**

745.10 Complete transposition of great vessels
Transposition of great vessels:
NOS
classical

745.11 Double outlet right ventricle
Dextratransposition of aorta
Incomplete transposition of great vessels
Origin of both great vessels from right ventricle
Taussig-Bing syndrome or defect

745.12 Corrected transposition of great vessels

745.19 Other

745.2 Tetralogy of Fallot
Fallot's pentalogy
Ventricular septal defect with pulmonary stenosis or atresia, dextraposition of aorta, and hypertrophy of right ventricle

EXCLUDES *Fallot's triad (746.09)*

DEF: Obstructed cardiac outflow causes pulmonary stenosis, interventricular septal defect and right ventricular hypertrophy.

745.3 Common ventricle
Cor triloculare biatriatum
Single ventricle

745.4 Ventricular septal defect
Eisenmenger's defect or complex
Gerbo dedefect
Interventricular septal defect
Left ventricular-right atrial communication
Roger's disease

EXCLUDES *common atrioventricular canal type (745.69)*
single ventricle (745.3)

745.5 Ostium secundum type atrial septal defect
Defect:
atrium secundum
fossa ovalis
Patent or persistent:
foramen ovale
ostium secundum
Lutembacher's syndrome

DEF: Opening in atrial septum due to failure of the septum secundum and the endocardial cushions to fuse; there is a rim of septum surrounding the defect.

✓5th **745.6 Endocardial cushion defects**

DEF: Atrial and/or ventricular septal defects causing abnormal fusion of cushions in atrioventricular canal.

745.60 Endocardial cushion defect, unspecified type

DEF: Septal defect due to imperfect fusion of endocardial cushions.

745.61 Ostium primum defect
Persistent ostium primum

DEF: Opening in low, posterior septum primum; causes cleft in basal portion of atrial septum; associated with cleft mitral valve.

745.69 Other
Absence of atrial septum
Atrioventricular canal type ventricular septal defect
Common atrioventricular canal
Common atrium

745.7 Cor biloculare
Absence of atrial and ventricular septa

DEF: Atrial and ventricular septal defect; marked by heart with two cardiac chambers (one atrium, one ventricle), and one atrioventricular valve.

745.8 Other

745.9 Unspecified defect of septal closure
Septal defect NOS

✓4th **746 Other congenital anomalies of heart**

EXCLUDES *endocardial fibroelastosis (425.3)*

✓5th **746.0 Anomalies of pulmonary valve**

EXCLUDES *infundibular or subvalvular pulmonic stenosis (746.83)*
tetralogy of Fallot (745.2)

746.00 Pulmonary valve anomaly, unspecified

746.01 Atresia, congenital
Congenital absence of pulmonary valve

746.02 Stenosis, congenital

DEF: Stenosis of opening between pulmonary artery and right ventricle; causes obstructed blood outflow from right ventricle.

746.09 Other
Congenital insufficiency of pulmonary valve
Fallot's triad or trilogy

746.1 Tricuspid atresia and stenosis, congenital
Absence of tricuspid valve

746.2 Ebstein's anomaly

DEF: Malformation of the tricuspid valve characterized by septal and posterior leaflets attaching to the wall of the right ventricle; causing the right ventricle to fuse with the atrium producing a large right atrium and a small ventricle; causes a malfunction of the right ventricle with accompanying complications such as heart failure and abnormal cardiac rhythm.

746.3 Congenital stenosis of aortic valve
Congenital aortic stenosis

EXCLUDES *congenital:*
subaortic stenosis (746.81)
supravalvular aortic stenosis (747.22)

AHA: 4Q, '88, 8

DEF: Stenosis of orifice of aortic valve; obstructs blood outflow from left ventricle.

746.4 Congenital insufficiency of aortic valve
Bicuspid aortic valve
Congenital aortic insufficiency

DEF: Impaired functioning of aortic valve due to incomplete closure; causes backflow (regurgitation) of blood from aorta to left ventricle.

746.5 Congenital mitral stenosis
Fused commissure } of mitral valve
Parachute deformity } of mitral valve
Supernumerary cusps } of mitral valve

DEF: Stenosis of left atrioventricular orifice.

746.6 Congenital mitral insufficiency

DEF: Impaired functioning of mitral valve due to incomplete closure; causes backflow of blood from left ventricle to left atrium.

746.7 Hypoplastic left heart syndrome
Atresia, or marked hypoplasia, of aortic orifice or valve, with hypoplasia of ascending aorta and defective development of left ventricle (with mitral valve atresia)

✓5th **746.8 Other specified anomalies of heart**

746.81 Subaortic stenosis

DEF: Stenosis, of left ventricular outflow tract due to fibrous tissue ring or septal hypertrophy below aortic valve.

746.82 Cor triatriatum

DEF: Transverse septum divides left atrium due to failed resorption of embryonic common pulmonary vein; results in three atrial chambers.

746.83 Infundibular pulmonic stenosis

Subvalvular pulmonic stenosis

DEF: Stenosis of right ventricle outflow tract within infundibulum due to fibrous diaphragm below valve or long, narrow fibromuscular channel.

746.84 Obstructive anomalies of heart, not elsewhere classified

Uhl's disease

746.85 Coronary artery anomaly

Anomalous origin or communication of coronary artery
Arteriovenous malformation of coronary artery
Coronary artery:
- absence
- arising from aorta or pulmonary trunk
- single

AHA: N-D, '85, 3

746.86 Congenital heart block

Complete or incomplete atrioventricular [AV] block

DEF: Impaired conduction of electrical impulses; due to maldeveloped junctional tissue.

746.87 Malposition of heart and cardiac apex

Abdominal heart
Dextrocardia
Ectopia cordis
Levocardia (isolated)
Mesocardia

EXCLUDES *dextrocardia with complete transposition of viscera (759.3)*

746.89 Other

Atresia } of cardiac vein
Hypoplasia } of cardiac vein

Congenital:
- cardiomegaly
- diverticulum, left ventricle
- pericardial defect

AHA: 3Q, '00, 3; 1Q, '99, 11; J-F, '85, 3

746.9 Unspecified anomaly of heart

Congenital:
- anomaly of heart NOS
- heart disease NOS

✓4th **747 Other congenital anomalies of circulatory system**

747.0 Patent ductus arteriosus

Patent ductus Botalli
Persistent ductus arteriosus

DEF: Open lumen in ductus arteriosus causes arterial blood recirculation in lungs; inhibits blood supply to aorta; symptoms such as shortness of breath more noticeable upon activity.

✓5th **747.1 Coarctation of aorta**

DEF: Localized deformity of aortic media seen as a severe constriction of the vessel lumen; major symptom is high blood pressure in the arms and low pressure in the legs; a CVA, rupture of the aorta, bacterial endocarditis or congestive heart failure can follow if left untreated.

747.10 Coarctation of aorta (preductal) (postductal)

Hypoplasia of aortic arch

AHA: 1Q, '99, 11; 4Q, '88, 8

747.11 Interruption of aortic arch

✓5th **747.2 Other anomalies of aorta**

747.20 Anomaly of aorta, unspecified

747.21 Anomalies of aortic arch

Anomalous origin, right subclavian artery
Dextraposition of aorta
Double aortic arch
Kommerell's diverticulum
Overriding aorta
Persistent:
- convolutions, aortic arch
- right aortic arch

Vascular ring

EXCLUDES *hypoplasia of aortic arch (747.10)*

AHA: 1Q, '03, 15

747.22 Atresia and stenosis of aorta

Absence } of aorta
Aplasia } of aorta
Hypoplasia } of aorta
Stricture } of aorta

Supra (valvular)-aortic stenosis

EXCLUDES *congenital aortic (valvular) stenosis or stricture, so stated (746.3)*
hypoplasia of aorta in hypoplastic left heart syndrome (746.7)

747.29 Other

Aneurysm of sinus of Valsalva
Congenital:
- aneurysm } of aorta
- dilation } of aorta

747.3 Anomalies of pulmonary artery

Agenesis } of pulmonary artery
Anomaly } of pulmonary artery
Atresia } of pulmonary artery
Coarctation } of pulmonary artery
Hypoplasia } of pulmonary artery
Stenosis } of pulmonary artery

Pulmonary arteriovenous aneurysm

AHA: 1Q, '94, 15; 4Q, '88, 8

✓5th **747.4 Anomalies of great veins**

747.40 Anomaly of great veins, unspecified

Anomaly NOS of:
- pulmonary veins
- vena cava

747.41 Total anomalous pulmonary venous connection

Total anomalous pulmonary venous return [TAPVR]:
- subdiaphragmatic
- supradiaphragmatic

747.42 Partial anomalous pulmonary venous connection

Partial anomalous pulmonary venous return

747.49 Other anomalies of great veins

Absence } of vena cava (inferior) (superior)
Congenital stenosis } of vena cava (inferior) (superior)

Persistent:
- left posterior cardinal vein
- left superior vena cava

Scimitar syndrome
Transposition of pulmonary veins NOS

747.5 Absence or hypoplasia of umbilical artery

Single umbilical artery

✓5th **747.6 Other anomalies of peripheral vascular system**

Absence / Anomaly / Atresia } of artery or vein, not elsewhere classified

Arteriovenous aneurysm (peripheral)
Arteriovenous malformation of the peripheral vascular system
Congenital:
aneurysm (peripheral)
Congenital:
phlebectasia
stricture, artery
varix
Multiple renal arteries

EXCLUDES *anomalies of:*
cerebral vessels (747.81)
pulmonary artery (747.3)
congenital retinal aneurysm (743.58)
hemangioma (228.00-228.09)
lymphangioma (228.1)

747.60 Anomaly of the peripheral vascular system, unspecified site

747.61 Gastrointestinal vessel anomaly
AHA: 3Q '96, 10

747.62 Renal vessel anomaly

747.63 Upper limb vessel anomaly

747.64 Lower limb vessel anomaly

747.69 Anomalies of other specified sites of peripheral vascular system

✓5th **747.8 Other specified anomalies of circulatory system**

747.81 Anomalies of cerebrovascular system
Arteriovenous malformation of brain
Cerebral arteriovenous aneurysm, congenital
Congenital anomalies of cerebral vessels
EXCLUDES *ruptured cerebral (arteriovenous) aneurysm (430)*

747.82 Spinal vessel anomaly
Arteriovenous malformation of spinal vessel
AHA: 3Q, '95, 5

747.83 Persistent fetal circulation N
Persistent pulmonary hypertension
Primary pulmonary hypertension of newborn
AHA: 4Q, '02, 62

DEF: A return to fetal-type circulation due to constriction of pulmonary arterioles and opening of the ductus arteriosus and foramen ovale, right-to-left shunting occurs, oxygenation of the blood does not occur, and the lungs remain constricted after birth; PFC is seen in term or post-term infants causes include asphyxiation, meconium aspiration syndrome, acidosis, sepsis, and developmental immaturity.

747.89 Other
Aneurysm, congenital, specified site not elsewhere classified
EXCLUDES *congenital aneurysm:*
coronary (746.85)
peripheral (747.6)
pulmonary (747.3)
retinal (743.58)
AHA: 4Q, '02, 63

747.9 Unspecified anomaly of circulatory system

✓4th **748 Congenital anomalies of respiratory system**
EXCLUDES ▶ *congenital central alveolar hypoventilation syndrome (327.25)*◀
congenital defect of diaphragm (756.6)

748.0 Choanal atresia
Atresia / Congenital stenosis } of nares (anterior) (posterior)

DEF: Occluded posterior nares (choana), bony or membranous due to failure of embryonic bucconasal membrane to rupture.

Persistent Fetal Circulation

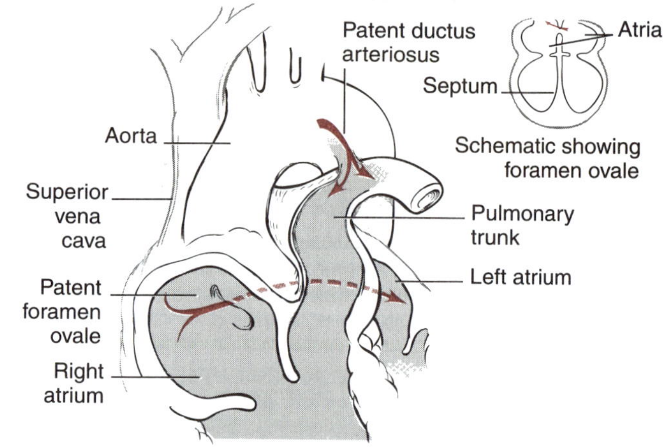

748.1 Other anomalies of nose
Absent nose
Accessory nose
Cleft nose
Congenital:
deformity of nose
Congenital:
notching of tip of nose
perforation of wall of nasal sinus
Deformity of wall of nasal sinus
EXCLUDES *congenital deviation of nasal septum (754.0)*

748.2 Web of larynx
Web of larynx:
NOS
glottic
subglottic

DEF: Malformed larynx; marked by thin, translucent, or thick, fibrotic spread between vocal folds; affects speech.

748.3 Other anomalies of larynx, trachea, and bronchus
Absence or agenesis of:
bronchus
larynx
trachea
Anomaly(of):
cricoid cartilage
epiglottis
thyroid cartilage
tracheal cartilage
Atresia (of):
epiglottis
glottis
larynx
trachea
Cleft thyroid, cartilage, congenital
Congenital:
dilation, trachea
stenosis:
larynx
trachea
tracheocele
Diverticulum:
bronchus
trachea
Fissure of epiglottis
Laryngocele
Posterior cleft of cricoid cartilage (congenital)
Rudimentary tracheal bronchus
Stridor, laryngeal, congenital
AHA: 1Q, '99, 14

748.4 Congenital cystic lung
Disease, lung:
cystic, congenital
polycystic, congenital
Honeycomb lung, congenital
EXCLUDES *acquired or unspecified cystic lung (518.89)*

DEF: Enlarged air spaces of lung parenchyma.

748.5 Agenesis, hypoplasia, and dysplasia of lung
Absence of lung (fissures) (lobe)
Aplasia of lung
Hypoplasia of lung (lobe)
Sequestration of lung

✓5th **748.6 Other anomalies of lung**

748.60 Anomaly of lung, unspecified

748.61 Congenital bronchiectasis

748.69 Other
Accessory lung (lobe)
Azygos lobe (fissure), lung

N Newborn Age: 0 · P Pediatric Age: 0-17 · M Maternity Age: 12-55 · A Adult Age: 15-124 · MSP Medicare Secondary Payer

Cleft Lip and Palate

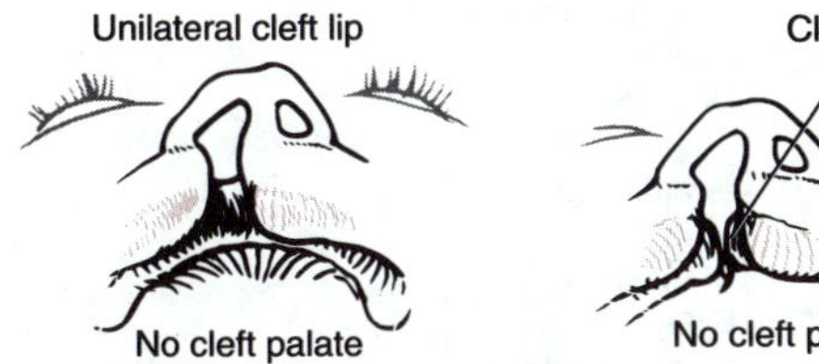

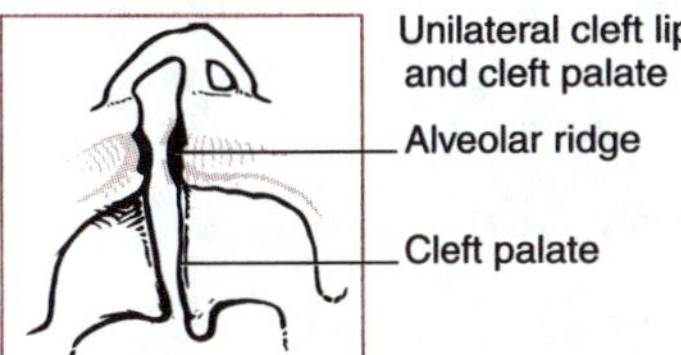

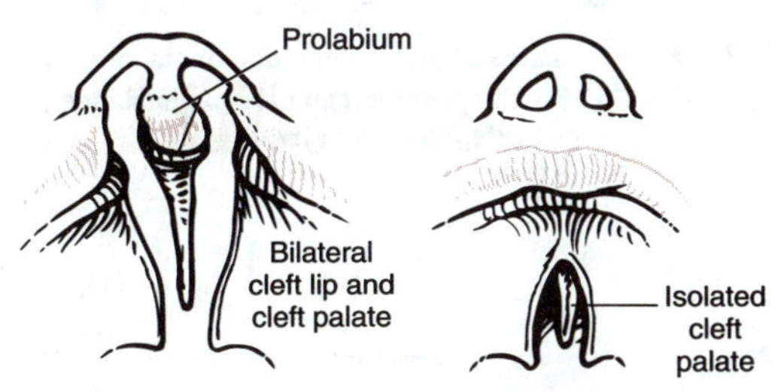

748.8 Other specified anomalies of respiratory system
Abnormal communication between pericardial and pleural sacs
Anomaly, pleural folds
Atresia of nasopharynx
Congenital cyst of mediastinum

748.9 Unspecified anomaly of respiratory system
Anomaly of respiratory system NOS

✓4th **749 Cleft palate and cleft lip**

✓5th **749.0 Cleft palate**
- **749.00 Cleft palate, unspecified**
- **749.01 Unilateral, complete**
- **749.02 Unilateral, incomplete**
  Cleft uvula
- **749.03 Bilateral, complete**
- **749.04 Bilateral, incomplete**

✓5th **749.1 Cleft lip**
Cheiloschisis
Congenital fissure of lip
Harelip
Labium leporinum
- **749.10 Cleft lip, unspecified**
- **749.11 Unilateral, complete**
- **749.12 Unilateral, incomplete**
- **749.13 Bilateral, complete**
- **749.14 Bilateral, incomplete**

✓5th **749.2 Cleft palate with cleft lip**
Cheilopalatoschisis
- **749.20 Cleft palate with cleft lip, unspecified**
- **749.21 Unilateral, complete**
- **749.22 Unilateral, incomplete**
- **749.23 Bilateral, complete**
  AHA: 1Q, '96, 14
- **749.24 Bilateral, incomplete**
- **749.25 Other combinations**

✓4th **750 Other congenital anomalies of upper alimentary tract**
EXCLUDES *dentofacial anomalies (524.0-524.9)*

750.0 Tongue tie
Ankyloglossia
DEF: Restricted tongue movement due to lingual frenum extending toward tip of tongue. Tongue may be fused to mouth floor affecting speech.

✓5th **750.1 Other anomalies of tongue**
- **750.10 Anomaly of tongue, unspecified**
- **750.11 Aglossia**
  DEF: Absence of tongue.
- **750.12 Congenital adhesions of tongue**
- **750.13 Fissure of tongue**
  Bifid tongue
  Double tongue
- **750.15 Macroglossia**
  Congenital hypertrophy of tongue
- **750.16 Microglossia**
  Hypoplasia of tongue
- **750.19 Other**

✓5th **750.2 Other specified anomalies of mouth and pharynx**
- **750.21 Absence of salivary gland**
- **750.22 Accessory salivary gland**
- **750.23 Atresia, salivary duct**
  Imperforate salivary duct
- **750.24 Congenital fistula of salivary gland**
- **750.25 Congenital fistula of lip**
  Congenital (mucus) lip pits
- **750.26 Other specified anomalies of mouth**
  Absence of uvula
- **750.27 Diverticulum of pharynx**
  Pharyngeal pouch
- **750.29 Other specified anomalies of pharynx**
  Imperforate pharynx

750.3 Tracheoesophageal fistula, esophageal atresia and stenosis
Absent esophagus
Atresia of esophagus
Congenital:
- esophageal ring
- stenosis of esophagus
- stricture of esophagus

Congenital fistula:
- esophagobronchial
- esophagotracheal

Imperforate esophagus
Webbed esophagus

750.4 Other specified anomalies of esophagus
Dilatation, congenital
Displacement, congenital
Diverticulum
Duplication
Giant
} (of) esophagus

Esophageal pouch
EXCLUDES *congenital hiatus hernia (750.6)*
AHA: J-F, '85, 3

750.5 Congenital hypertrophic pyloric stenosis
Congenital or infantile:
constriction
hypertrophy
spasm
stenosis
stricture
} of pylorus

DEF: Obstructed pylorus due to overgrowth of pyloric muscle.

750.6 Congenital hiatus hernia
Displacement of cardia through esophageal hiatus
EXCLUDES *congenital diaphragmatic hernia (756.6)*

750.7 Other specified anomalies of stomach
Congenital:
- cardiospasm
- hourglass stomach

Displacement of stomach
Diverticulum of stomach, congenital
Duplication of stomach
Megalogastria
Microgastria
Transposition of stomach

750.8 Other specified anomalies of upper alimentary tract

750.9 Unspecified anomaly of upper alimentary tract
Congenital:
anomaly NOS } of upper alimentary tract [any part, except tongue]
deformity NOS } of upper alimentary tract [any part, except tongue]

4th 751 Other congenital anomalies of digestive system

751.0 Meckel's diverticulum
Meckel's diverticulum (displaced) (hypertrophic)
Persistent:
omphalomesenteric duct
vitelline duct
AHA: 1Q, '04, 10

DEF: Malformed sacs or appendages of ileum of small intestine; can cause strangulation, volvulus and intussusception.

751.1 Atresia and stenosis of small intestine P
Atresia of:
duodenum
ileum
intestine NOS
Congenital:
absence } of small intestine or intestine NOS
obstruction } of small intestine or intestine NOS
stenosis } of small intestine or intestine NOS
stricture } of small intestine or intestine NOS
Imperforate jejunum

751.2 Atresia and stenosis of large intestine, rectum, and anal canal P
Absence:
anus (congenital)
appendix, congenital
large intestine, congenital
rectum
Atresia of:
anus
colon
rectum
Congenital or infantile:
obstruction of large intestine
occlusion of anus
stricture of anus
Imperforate:
anus
rectum
Stricture of rectum, congenital
AHA: 2Q, '98, 16

751.3 Hirschsprung's disease and other congenital functional disorders of colon
Aganglionosis
Congenital dilation of colon
Congenital megacolon
Macrocolon

DEF: Hirschsprung's disease: enlarged or dilated colon (megacolon), with absence of ganglion cells in the narrowed wall distally; causes inability to defecate.

751.4 Anomalies of intestinal fixation
Congenital adhesions:
omental, anomalous
peritoneal
Jackson's membrane
Malrotation of colon
Rotation of cecum or colon:
failure of
incomplete
insufficient
Universal mesentery

751.5 Other anomalies of intestine
Congenital diverticulum, colon
Dolichocolon
Duplication of:
anus
appendix
cecum
intestine
Ectopic anus
Megaloappendix
Megaloduodenum
Microcolon
Persistent cloaca
Transposition of:
appendix
colon
intestine
AHA: 3Q, '02, 11; 3Q, '01, 8

5th 751.6 Anomalies of gallbladder, bile ducts, and liver

751.60 Unspecified anomaly of gallbladder, bile ducts, and liver

751.61 Biliary atresia P
Congenital:
absence } of bile duct (common) or passage
hypoplasia } of bile duct (common) or passage
obstruction } of bile duct (common) or passage
stricture } of bile duct (common) or passage
AHA: S-O, '87, 8

751.62 Congenital cystic disease of liver
Congenital polycystic disease of liver
Fibrocystic disease of liver

751.69 Other anomalies of gallbladder, bile ducts, and liver
Absence of:
gallbladder, congenital
liver (lobe)
Accessory:
hepatic ducts
liver
Congenital:
choledochal cyst
hepatomegaly
Duplication of:
biliary duct
cystic duct
gallbladder
liver
Floating:
gallbladder
liver
Intrahepatic gallbladder
AHA: S-O, '87, 8

751.7 Anomalies of pancreas
Absence } (of) pancreas
Accessory } (of) pancreas
Agenesis } (of) pancreas
Annular } (of) pancreas
Hypoplasia } (of) pancreas
Ectopic pancreatic tissue
Pancreatic heterotopia
EXCLUDES *diabetes mellitus:*
congenital (250.0-250.9)
neonatal (775.1)
fibrocystic disease of pancreas (277.00-277.09)

751.8 Other specified anomalies of digestive system
Absence (complete) (partial) of alimentary tract NOS
Duplication } of digestive organs NOS
Malposition, congenital } of digestive organs NOS
EXCLUDES *congenital diaphragmatic hernia (756.6)*
congenital hiatus hernia (750.6)

751.9 Unspecified anomaly of digestive system

Congenital:
- anomaly NOS } of digestive system NOS
- deformity NOS } of digestive system NOS

752 Congenital anomalies of genital organs

EXCLUDES *syndromes associated with anomalies in the number and form of chromosomes (758.0-758.9)*
testicular feminization syndrome ▶(259.5)◀

752.0 Anomalies of ovaries ♀

Absence, congenital } (of) ovary
Accessory } (of) ovary
Ectopic } (of) ovary
Streak } (of) ovary

752.1 Anomalies of fallopian tubes and broad ligaments

752.10 Unspecified anomaly of fallopian tubes and broad ligaments ♀

752.11 Embryonic cyst of fallopian tubes and broad ligaments ♀

Cyst:
- epoophoron
- fimbrial
- parovarian

AHA: S-O, '85, 13

752.19 Other ♀

Absence } (of) fallopian tube or broad ligament
Accessory } (of) fallopian tube or broad ligament
Atresia } (of) fallopian tube or broad ligament

752.2 Doubling of uterus ♀

Didelphic uterus
Doubling of uterus [any degree] (associated with doubling of cervix and vagina)

752.3 Other anomalies of uterus ♀

Absence, congenital } (of) uterus
Agenesis } (of) uterus
Aplasia } (of) uterus
Bicornuate } (of) uterus

Uterus unicornis
Uterus with only one functioning horn

752.4 Anomalies of cervix, vagina, and external female genitalia

752.40 Unspecified anomaly of cervix, vagina, and external female genitalia ♀

752.41 Embryonic cyst of cervix, vagina, and external female genitalia ♀

Cyst of:
- canal of Nuck, congenital
- ▶Gartner's duct◀
- vagina, embryonal
- vulva, congenital

DEF: Embryonic fluid-filled cysts, of cervix, vagina or external female genitalia.

752.42 Imperforate hymen ♀

DEF: Complete closure of membranous fold around external opening of vagina.

752.49 Other anomalies of cervix, vagina, and external female genitalia ♀

Absence } of cervix, clitoris, vagina, or vulva
Agenesis } of cervix, clitoris, vagina, or vulva

Congenital stenosis or stricture of:
- cervical canal
- vagina

EXCLUDES *double vagina associated with total duplication (752.2)*

752.5 Undescended and retractile testicle

AHA: 4Q, '96, 33

752.51 Undescended testis ♂

Cryptorchism
Ectopic testis

752.52 Retractile testis ♂

Hypospadias and Epispadias

Glans penis
Glandular hypospadias
Penile hypospadias
Penile raphe
Scrotal hypospadias
Scrotum
Scrotal raphe
Normal external urethral orifice
Glans penis
Foreskin (retracted)
Epispadias

Hypospadias (ventral view)

Epispadias (dorsal view)

752.6 Hypospadias and epispadias and other penile anomalies

AHA: 4Q, '96, 34, 35

752.61 Hypospadias ♂

AHA: 3Q, '97, 6

DEF: Abnormal opening of urethra on the ventral surface of the penis or perineum; also a rare defect of vagina.

AHA: 4Q, '03, 67-68

752.62 Epispadias ♂

Anaspadias

DEF: Epispadias: urethra opening on dorsal surface of penis; in females appears as a slit in the upper wall of urethra.

752.63 Congenital chordee ♂

DEF: Ventral bowing of penis due to fibrous band along corpus spongiosum; occurs with hypospadias.

752.64 Micropenis ♂

752.65 Hidden penis ♂

752.69 Other penile anomalies ♂

752.7 Indeterminate sex and pseudohermaphroditism

Gynandrism
Hermaphroditism
Ovotestis
Pseudohermaphroditism (male) (female)
Pure gonadal dysgenesis

EXCLUDES *pseudohermaphroditism:*
female, with adrenocortical disorder (255.2)
male, with gonadal disorder (257.8)
with specified chromosomal anomaly (758.0-758.9)
testicular feminization syndrome ▶(259.5)◀

DEF: Pseudohermaphroditism: presence of gonads of one sex and external genitalia of other sex.

752.8 Other specified anomalies of genital organs

EXCLUDES *congenital hydrocele (778.6)*
penile anomalies (752.61-752.69)
phimosis or paraphimosis (605)

752.81 Scrotal transposition ♂

AHA: 4Q, '03, 67-68

752.89 Other specified anomalies of genital organs

Absence of:
- prostate
- spermatic cord
- vas deferens

Anorchism
Aplasia (congenital) of:
- prostate
- round ligament
- testicle

Atresia of:
- ejaculatory duct
- vas deferens

Fusion of testes
Hypoplasia of testis
Monorchism
Polyorchism

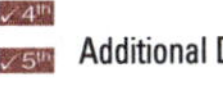

Additional Digit Required | Unspecified Code | Other Specified Code | Manifestation Code | ▶◀ Revised Text | ● New Code | ▲ Revised Code Title

752.9 Unspecified anomaly of genital organs
Congenital:
anomaly NOS } of genital organ, not
deformity NOS } elsewhere classified

✓4th **753 Congenital anomalies of urinary system**

753.0 Renal agenesis and dysgenesis
Atrophy of kidney:
congenital
infantile
Congenital absence of kidney(s)
Hypoplasia of kidney(s)

✓5th **753.1 Cystic kidney disease**
EXCLUDES *acquired cyst of kidney (593.2)*
AHA: 4Q, '90, 3

753.10 Cystic kidney disease, unspecified

753.11 Congenital single renal cyst

753.12 Polycystic kidney, unspecified type

753.13 Polycystic kidney, autosomal dominant
DEF: Slow progressive disease characterized by bilateral cysts causing increased kidney size and impaired function.

753.14 Polycystic kidney, autosomal recessive
DEF: Rare disease characterized by multiple cysts involving kidneys and liver, producing renal and hepatic failure in childhood or adolescence.

753.15 Renal dysplasia

753.16 Medullary cystic kidney
Nephronopthisis
DEF: Diffuse kidney disease results in uremia onset prior to age 20.

753.17 Medullary sponge kidney
DEF: Dilated collecting tubules; usually asymptomatic but calcinosis in tubules may cause renal insufficiency.

753.19 Other specified cystic kidney disease
Multicystic kidney

✓5th **753.2 Obstructive defects of renal pelvis and ureter**
AHA: 4Q, '96, 35

753.20 Unspecified obstructive defect of renal pelvis and ureter

753.21 Congenital obstruction of ureteropelvic junction
DEF: Stricture at junction of ureter and renal pelvis.

753.22 Congenital obstruction of ureterovesical junction
Adynamic ureter
Congenital hydroureter
DEF: Stricture at junction of ureter and bladder.

753.23 Congenital ureterocele

753.29 Other

753.3 Other specified anomalies of kidney
Accessory kidney
Congenital:
calculus of kidney
displaced kidney
Discoid kidney
Double kidney with double pelvis
Ectopic kidney
Fusion of kidneys
Giant kidney
Horseshoe kidney
Hyperplasia of kidney
Lobulation of kidney
Malrotation of kidney
Trifid kidney (pelvis)

753.4 Other specified anomalies of ureter
Absent ureter
Accessory ureter
Deviation of ureter
Displaced ureteric orifice
Double ureter
Ectopic ureter
Implantation, anomalous of ureter

753.5 Exstrophy of urinary bladder
Ectopia vesicae
Extroversion of bladder
DEF: Absence of lower abdominal and anterior bladder walls with posterior bladder wall protrusion.

753.6 Atresia and stenosis of urethra and bladder neck
Congenital obstruction:
bladder neck
urethra
Congenital stricture of:
urethra (valvular)
urinary meatus
vesicourethral orifice
Imperforate urinary meatus
Impervious urethra
Urethral valve formation

753.7 Anomalies of urachus
Cyst }
Fistula } (of) urachussinus
Patent }

Persistent umbilical sinus

753.8 Other specified anomalies of bladder and urethra
Absence, congenital of:
bladder
urethra
Accessory:
bladder
urethra
Congenital:
diverticulum of bladder
hernia of bladder
Congenital urethrorectal fistula
Congenital prolapse of:
bladder (mucosa)
urethra
Double:
urethra
urinary meatus

753.9 Unspecified anomaly of urinary system
Congenital:
anomaly NOS } of urinary system [any part,
deformity NOS } except urachus]

✓4th **754 Certain congenital musculoskeletal deformities**
INCLUDES nonteratogenic deformities which are considered to be due to intrauterine malposition and pressure

754.0 Of skull, face, and jaw
Asymmetry of face
Compression facies
Depressions in skull
Deviation of nasal septum, congenital
Dolichocephaly
Plagiocephaly
Potter's facies
Squashed or bent nose, congenital
EXCLUDES *dentofacial anomalies (524.0-524.9)*
syphilitic saddle nose (090.5)

754.1 Of sternocleidomastoid muscle
Congenital sternomastoid torticollis
Congenital wryneck
Contracture of sternocleidomastoid (muscle)
Sternomastoid tumor

754.2 Of spine
Congenital postural:
lordosis
scoliosis

✓5th **754.3 Congenital dislocation of hip**

754.30 Congenital dislocation of hip, unilateral
Congenital dislocation of hip NOS

754.31 Congenital dislocation of hip, bilateral

754.32 Congenital subluxation of hip, unilateral
Congenital flexion deformity, hip or thigh
Predislocation status of hip at birth
Preluxation of hip, congenital

754.33 Congenital subluxation of hip, bilateral

754.35 Congenital dislocation of one hip with subluxation of other hip

✓5th **754.4 Congenital genu recurvatum and bowing of long bones of leg**

754.40 Genu recurvatum
DEF: Backward curving of knee joint.

754.41 Congenital dislocation of knee (with genu recurvatum)
DEF: Elevated, outward rotation of heel; also called clubfoot.

754.42 Congenital bowing of femur

754.43 Congenital bowing of tibia and fibula

754.44 Congenital bowing of unspecified long bones of leg

✓5th **754.5 Varus deformities of feet**

EXCLUDES *acquired (736.71, 736.75, 736.79)*

754.50 Talipes varus

Congenital varus deformity of foot, unspecified

Pes varus

DEF: Inverted foot marked by outer sole resting on ground.

754.51 Talipes equinovarus

Equinovarus (congenital)

754.52 Metatarsus primus varus

DEF: Malformed first metatarsal bone, with bone angled toward body.

754.53 Metatarsus varus

754.59 Other

Talipes calcaneovarus

✓5th **754.6 Valgus deformities of feet**

EXCLUDES *valgus deformity of foot (acquired) (736.79)*

754.60 Talipes valgus

Congenital valgus deformity of foot, unspecified

754.61 Congenital pes planus

Congenital rocker bottom flat foot

Flat foot, congenital

EXCLUDES *pes planus (acquired) (734)*

754.62 Talipes calcaneovalgus

754.69 Other

Talipes:
- equinovalgus
- planovalgus

✓5th **754.7 Other deformities of feet**

EXCLUDES *acquired (736.70-736.79)*

754.70 Talipes, unspecified

Congenital deformity of foot NOS

754.71 Talipes cavus

Cavus foot (congenital)

754.79 Other

Asymmetric talipes

Talipes:
- calcaneus
- equinus

✓5th **754.8 Other specified nonteratogenic anomalies**

754.81 Pectus excavatum

Congenital funnel chest

754.82 Pectus carinatum

Congenital pigeon chest [breast]

754.89 Other

Club hand (congenital)

Congenital:
- deformity of chest wall
- dislocation of elbow

Generalized flexion contractures of lower limb joints, congenital

Spade-like hand (congenital)

✓4th **755 Other congenital anomalies of limbs**

EXCLUDES *those deformities classifiable to 754.0-754.8*

✓5th **755.0 Polydactyly**

755.00 Polydactyly, unspecified digits

Supernumerary digits

755.01 Of fingers

Accessory fingers

755.02 Of toes

Accessory toes

✓5th **755.1 Syndactyly**

Symphalangy

Webbing of digits

755.10 Of multiple and unspecified sites

755.11 Of fingers without fusion of bone

755.12 Of fingers with fusion of bone

755.13 Of toes without fusion of bone

755.14 Of toes with fusion of bone

✓5th **755.2 Reduction deformities of upper limb**

755.20 Unspecified reduction deformity of upper limb

Ectromelia NOS } of upper limb
Hemimelia NOS } of upper limb

Shortening of arm, congenital

755.21 Transverse deficiency of upper limb

Amelia of upper limb

Congenital absence of:
- fingers, all (complete or partial)
- forearm, including hand and fingers
- upper limb, complete

Congenital amputation of upper limb

Transverse hemimelia of upper limb

755.22 Longitudinal deficiency of upper limb, not elsewhere classified

Phocomelia NOS of upper limb

Rudimentary arm

755.23 Longitudinal deficiency, combined, involving humerus, radius, and ulna (complete or incomplete)

Congenital absence of arm and forearm (complete or incomplete) with or without metacarpal deficiency and/or phalangeal deficiency, incomplete

Phocomelia, complete, of upper limb

755.24 Longitudinal deficiency, humeral, complete or partial (with or without distal deficiencies, incomplete)

Congenital absence of humerus (with or without absence of some [but not all] distal elements)

Proximal phocomelia of upper limb

755.25 Longitudinal deficiency, radioulnar, complete or partial (with or without distal deficiencies, incomplete)

Congenital absence of radius and ulna (with or without absence of some [but not all] distal elements)

Distal phocomelia of upper limb

755.26 Longitudinal deficiency, radial, complete or partial (with or without distal deficiencies, incomplete)

Agenesis of radius

Congenital absence of radius (with or without absence of some [but not all] distal elements)

755.27 Longitudinal deficiency, ulnar, complete or partial (with or without distal deficiencies, incomplete)

Agenesis of ulna

Congenital absence of ulna (with or without absence of some [but not all] distal elements)

755.28 Longitudinal deficiency, carpals or metacarpals, complete or partial (with or without incomplete phalangeal deficiency)

755.29 Longitudinal deficiency, phalanges, complete or partial

Absence of finger, congenital

Aphalangia of upper limb, terminal, complete or partial

EXCLUDES *terminal deficiency of all five digits (755.21)*
transverse deficiency of phalanges (755.21)

✓5th **755.3 Reduction deformities of lower limb**

755.30 Unspecified reduction deformity of lower limb

Ectromelia NOS } of lower limb
Hemimelia NOS }

Shortening of leg, congenital

755.31 Transverse deficiency of lower limb

Amelia of lower limb
Congenital absence of:
- foot
- leg, including foot and toes
- lower limb, complete
- toes, all, complete

Transverse hemimelia of lower limb

755.32 Longitudinal deficiency of lower limb, not elsewhere classified

Phocomelia NOS of lower limb

755.33 Longitudinal deficiency, combined, involving femur, tibia, and fibula (complete or incomplete)

Congenital absence of thigh and (lower) leg (complete or incomplete) with or without metacarpal deficiency and/or phalangeal deficiency, incomplete
Phocomelia, complete, of lower limb

755.34 Longitudinal deficiency, femoral, complete or partial (with or without distal deficiencies, incomplete)

Congenital absence of femur (with or without absence of some [but not all] distal elements)
Proximal phocomelia of lower limb

755.35 Longitudinal deficiency, tibiofibular, complete or partial (with or without distal deficiencies, incomplete)

Congenital absence of tibia and fibula (with or without absence of some [but not all] distal elements)
Distal phocomelia of lower limb

755.36 Longitudinal deficiency, tibia, complete or partial (with or without distal deficiencies, incomplete)

Agenesis of tibia
Congenital absence of tibia (with or without absence of some [but not all] distal elements)

755.37 Longitudinal deficiency, fibular, complete or partial (with or without distal deficiencies, incomplete)

Agenesis of fibula
Congenital absence of fibula (with or without absence of some [but not all] distal elements)

755.38 Longitudinal deficiency, tarsals or metatarsals, complete or partial (with or without incomplete phalangeal deficiency)

755.39 Longitudinal deficiency, phalanges, complete or partial

Absence of toe, congenital
Aphalangia of lower limb, terminal, complete or partial

EXCLUDES *terminal deficiency of all five digits (755.31)*
transverse deficiency of phalanges (755.31)

755.4 Reduction deformities, unspecified limb

Absence, congenital (complete or partial) of limb NOS

Amelia } of unspecified limb
Ectromelia }
Hemimelia }
Phocomelia }

✓5th **755.5 Other anomalies of upper limb, including shoulder girdle**

755.50 Unspecified anomaly of upper limb

755.51 Congenital deformity of clavicle

755.52 Congenital elevation of scapula

Sprengel's deformity

755.53 Radioulnar synostosis

755.54 Madelung's deformity

DEF: Distal ulnar overgrowth or radial shortening; also called carpus curvus.

755.55 Acrocephalosyndactyly

Apert's syndrome

DEF: Premature cranial suture fusion (craniostenosis); marked by cone-shaped or pointed (acrocephaly) head and webbing of the fingers (syndactyly); it is very similar to craniofacial dysostosis.

755.56 Accessory carpal bones

755.57 Macrodactylia (fingers)

DEF: Abnormally large fingers, toes.

755.58 Cleft hand, congenital

Lobster-claw hand

DEF: Extended separation between fingers into metacarpus; also may refer to large fingers and absent middle fingers of hand.

755.59 Other

Cleidocranial dysostosis
Cubitus:
- valgus, congenital
- varus, congenital

EXCLUDES *club hand (congenital) (754.89)*
congenital dislocation of elbow (754.89)

✓5th **755.6 Other anomalies of lower limb, including pelvic girdle**

755.60 Unspecified anomaly of lower limb

755.61 Coxa valga, congenital

DEF: Abnormally wide angle between the neck and shaft of the femur.

755.62 Coxa vara, congenital

DEF: Diminished angle between neck and shaft of femur.

755.63 Other congenital deformity of hip (joint)

Congenital anteversion of femur (neck)

EXCLUDES *congenital dislocation of hip (754.30-754.35)*

AHA: 1Q, '94, 15; S-O, '84, 15

755.64 Congenital deformity of knee (joint)

Congenital:
- absence of patella
- genu valgum [knock-knee]
- genu varum [bowleg]

Rudimentary patella

755.65 Macrodactylia of toes

DEF: Abnormally large toes.

755.66 Other anomalies of toes

Congenital:
- hallux valgus
- hallux varus

Congenital:
- hammer toe

755.67 Anomalies of foot, not elsewhere classified

Astragaloscaphoid synostosis
Calcaneonavicular bar
Coalition of calcaneus
Talonavicular synostosis
Tarsal coalitions

755.69 Other

Congenital:
- angulation of tibia
- deformity (of):
  - ankle (joint)
  - sacroiliac (joint)
- fusion of sacroiliac joint

755.8 Other specified anomalies of unspecified limb

755.9 Unspecified anomaly of unspecified limb

Congenital:
- anomaly NOS } of unspecified limb
- deformity NOS } of unspecified limb

EXCLUDES *reduction deformity of unspecified limb (755.4)*

✓4th 756 Other congenital musculoskeletal anomalies

EXCLUDES *those deformities classifiable to 754.0-754.8*

756.0 Anomalies of skull and face bones

- Absence of skull bones
- Acrocephaly
- Congenital deformity of forehead
- Craniosynostosis
- Crouzon's disease
- Hyperteloris m
- Imperfect fusion of skull
- Oxycephaly
- Platybasia
- Premature closure of cranial sutures
- Tower skull
- Trigonocephaly

EXCLUDES *acrocephalosyndactyly [Apert's syndrome] (755.55)*
dentofacial anomalies (524.0-524.9)
skull defects associated with brain anomalies, such as:
anencephalus (740.0)
encephalocele (742.0)
hydrocephalus (742.3)
microcephalus (742.1)

AHA: 3Q, '98, 9; 3Q, '96, 15

✓5th 756.1 Anomalies of spine

756.10 Anomaly of spine, unspecified

756.11 Spondylolysis, lumbosacral region

Prespondylolisthesis (lumbosacral)

DEF: Bilateral or unilateral defect through the pars interarticularis of a vertebra causes spondylolisthesis.

756.12 Spondylolisthesis

DEF: Downward slipping of lumbar vertebra over next vertebra; usually related to pelvic deformity.

756.13 Absence of vertebra, congenital

756.14 Hemivertebra

DEF: Incomplete development of one side of a vertebra.

756.15 Fusion of spine [vertebra], congenital

756.16 Klippel-Feil syndrome

DEF: Short, wide neck; limits range of motion due to abnormal number of cervical vertebra or fused hemivertebrae.

756.17 Spina bifida occulta

EXCLUDES *spina bifida (aperta) (741.0-741.9)*

DEF: Spina bifida marked by a bony spinal canal defect without a protrusion of the cord or meninges; it is diagnosed by radiography and has no symptoms.

756.19 Other

Platyspondylia
Supernumerary vertebra

756.2 Cervical rib

Supernumerary rib in the cervical region

DEF: Costa cervicalis: extra rib attached to cervical vertebra.

756.3 Other anomalies of ribs and sternum

Congenital absence of:
- rib
- sternum

Congenital:
- fissure of sternum
- fusion of ribs

Sternum bifidum

EXCLUDES *nonteratogenic deformity of chest wall (754.81-754.89)*

756.4 Chondrodystrophy

- Achondroplasia
- Chondrodystrophia (fetalis)
- Dyschondroplasia
- Enchondromatosis
- Ollier's disease

EXCLUDES *lipochondrodystrophy [Hurler's syndrome] (277.5)*
Morquio's disease (277.5)

AHA: 2Q, '02, 16; S-O, '87, 10

DEF: Abnormal development of cartilage.

✓5th 756.5 Osteodystrophies

756.50 Osteodystrophy, unspecified

756.51 Osteogenesis imperfecta

Fragilitas ossium
Osteopsathyrosis

DEF: A collagen disorder commonly characterized by brittle, osteoporotic, easily fractured bones, hypermobility of joints, blue sclerae, and a tendency to hemorrhage.

756.52 Osteopetrosis

DEF: Abnormally dense bone, optic atrophy, hepatosplenomegaly, deafness; sclerosing depletes bone marrow and nerve foramina of skull; often fatal.

756.53 Osteopoikilosis

DEF: Multiple sclerotic foci on ends of long bones, stippling in round, flat bones; identified by x-ray.

756.54 Polyostotic fibrous dysplasia of bone

DEF: Fibrous tissue displaces bone results in segmented ragged-edge café-au-lait spots; occurs in girls of early puberty.

756.55 Chondroectodermal dysplasia

Ellis-van Creveld syndrome

DEF: Inadequate enchondral bone formation; impaired development of hair and teeth, polydactyly, and cardiac septum defects.

756.56 Multiple epiphyseal dysplasia

756.59 Other

Albright (-McCune)-Sternberg syndrome

756.6 Anomalies of diaphragm

- Absence of diaphragm
- Congenital hernia:
  - diaphragmatic
  - foramen of Morgagni
- Eventration of diaphragm

EXCLUDES *congenital hiatus hernia (750.6)*

✓5th 756.7 Anomalies of abdominal wall

756.70 Anomaly of abdominal wall, unspecified

756.71 Prune belly syndrome

Eagle-Barrett syndrome
Prolapse of bladder mucosa

AHA: 4Q, '97, 44

DEF: Prune belly syndrome: absence of lower rectus abdominis muscle and lower and medial oblique muscles; results in dilated bladder and ureters, dysplastic kidneys and hydronephrosis; more common in male infants with undescended testicles.

756.79 Other congenital anomalies of abdominal wall
Exomphalos
Omphalocele
Gastroschisis
EXCLUDES *umbilical hernia (551-553 with .1)*
DEF: Exomphalos: umbilical hernia prominent navel.
DEF: Gastroschisis: fissure of abdominal wall, results in protruding small or large intestine.
DEF: Omphalocele: hernia of umbilicus due to impaired abdominal wall; results in membrane-covered intestine protruding through peritoneum and amnion.

✓5th **756.8 Other specified anomalies of muscle, tendon, fascia, and connective tissue**

756.81 Absence of muscle and tendon
Absence of muscle (pectoral)

756.82 Accessory muscle

756.83 Ehlers-Danlos syndrome
DEF: Danlos syndrome: connective tissue disorder causes hyperextended skin and joints; results in fragile blood vessels with bleeding, poor wound healing and subcutaneous pseudotumors.

756.89 Other
Amyotrophia congenita
Congenital shortening of tendon
AHA: 3Q, '99, 16

756.9 Other and unspecified anomalies of musculoskeletal system
Congenital:
anomaly NOS } of musculoskeletal system, not elsewhere classified
deformity NOS } of musculoskeletal system, not elsewhere classified

✓4th **757 Congenital anomalies of the integument**
INCLUDES anomalies of skin, subcutaneous tissue, hair, nails, and breast
EXCLUDES *hemangioma (228.00-228.09)*
pigmented nevus (216.0-216.9)

757.0 Hereditary edema of legs
Congenital lymphedema
Hereditary trophedema
Milroy's disease

757.1 Ichthyosis congenita
Congenital ichthyosis
Harlequin fetus
Ichthyosiform erythroderma
DEF: Overproduction of skin cells causes scaling of skin; may result in stillborn fetus or death soon after birth.

757.2 Dermatoglyphic anomalies
Abnormal palmar creases
DEF: Abnormal skin-line patterns of fingers, palms, toes and soles; initial finding of possible chromosomal abnormalities.

✓5th **757.3 Other specified anomalies of skin**

757.31 Congenital ectodermal dysplasia
DEF: Tissues and structures originate in embryonic ectoderm; includes anhidrotic and hidrotic ectodermal dysplasia and EEC syndrome.

757.32 Vascular hamartomas
Birthmarks
Strawberry nevus
Port-wine stain
DEF: Benign tumor of blood vessels; due to malformed angioblastic tissues.

757.33 Congenital pigmentary anomalies of skin
Congenital poikiloderma
Urticaria pigmentosa
Xeroderma pigmentosum
EXCLUDES *albinism (270.2)*

757.39 Other
Accessory skin tags, congenital
Congenital scar
Epidermolysis bullosa
Keratoderma (congenital)
EXCLUDES *pilonidal cyst (685.0-685.1)*

757.4 Specified anomalies of hair
Congenital:
alopecia
atrichosis
beaded hair
Congenital:
hypertrichosis
monilethrix
Persistent lanugo

757.5 Specified anomalies of nails
Anonychia
Congenital:
clubnail
koilonychia
Congenital:
leukonychia
onychauxis
pachyonychia

757.6 Specified anomalies of breast
Absent } breast or nipple
Accessory } breast or nipple
Supernumerary } breast or nipple
Hypoplasia of breast
EXCLUDES *absence of pectoral muscle (756.81)*

757.8 Other specified anomalies of the integument

757.9 Unspecified anomaly of the integument
Congenital:
anomaly NOS } of integument
deformity NOS } of integument

✓4th **758 Chromosomal anomalies**
INCLUDES syndromes associated with anomalies in the number and form of chromosomes
Use additional codes for conditions associated with the chromosomal anomalies

758.0 Down's syndrome
Mongolism
Translocation Down's syndrome
Trisomy:
21 or 22
G

758.1 Patau's syndrome
Trisomy:
13
Trisomy:
D_1
DEF: Trisomy of 13th chromosome; characteristic failure to thrive, severe mental impairment, seizures, abnormal eyes, low-set ears and sloped forehead.

758.2 Edwards' syndrome
Trisomy:
18
Trisomy:
E_3
DEF: Trisomy of 18th chromosome; characteristic mental and physical impairments; mainly affects females.

✓5th **758.3 Autosomal deletion syndromes**

758.31 Cri-du-chat syndrome
Deletion 5p
DEF: Hereditary congenital syndrome caused by a microdeletion of short arm of chromosome 5; characterized by catlike cry in newborn, microencephaly, severe mental deficiency, and hypertelorism.

758.32 Velo-cardio-facial syndrome
Deletion 22q11.2
DEF: ►Microdeletion syndrome affecting multiple organs; characteristic cleft palate, heart defects, elongated face with almond-shaped eyes, wide nose, small ears, weak immune systems, weak musculature, hypothyroidism, short stature, and scoliosis; deletion at q11.2 on the long arm of the chromosome 22.◄

758.33 Other microdeletions
Miller-Dieker syndrome
Smith-Magenis syndrome
DEF: ►Miller-Dieker syndrome: deletion from the short arm of chromosome 17; characteristic mental retardation, speech and motor development delays, neurological complications, and multiple abnormalities affecting the kidneys, heart, gastrointestinal tract, and other organ; death in infancy or early childhood.◄
DEF: ►Smith-Magenis syndrome: deletion in a certain area of chromosome 17 that results in craniofacial changes, speech delay, hoarse voice, hearing loss in many, and behavioral problems, such as self-destructive head banging, wrist biting, and tearing at nails.◄

758.39 **Other autosomal deletions**

758.4 **Balanced autosomal translocation in normal individual**

758.5 **Other conditions due to autosomal anomalies**
Accessory autosomes NEC

758.6 **Gonadal dysgenesis**
Ovarian dysgenesis
XO syndrome
Turner's syndrome
EXCLUDES *pure gonadal dysgenesis (752.7)*
DEF: Impaired embryonic development of seminiferous tubes; results in small testes, azoospermia, infertility and enlarged mammary glands.

758.7 **Klinefelter's syndrome** ♂
XXY syndrome

✓5th 758.8 **Other conditions due to chromosome anomalies**

758.81 **Other conditions due to sex chromosome anomalies**

758.89 **Other**

758.9 **Conditions due to anomaly of unspecified chromosome**

✓4th 759 **Other and unspecified congenital anomalies**

759.0 **Anomalies of spleen**
Aberrant, Absent, Accessory } spleen
Congenital splenomegaly
Ectopic spleen
Lobulation of spleen

759.1 **Anomalies of adrenal gland**
Aberrant, Absent, Accessory } adrenal gland
EXCLUDES *adrenogenital disorders (255.2)*
congenital disorders of steroid metabolism (255.2)

759.2 **Anomalies of other endocrine glands**
Absent parathyroid gland
Accessory thyroid gland
Persistent thyroglossal or thyrolingual duct
Thyroglossal (duct) cyst
EXCLUDES *congenital:*
goiter (246.1)
hypothyroidism (243)

759.3 **Situs inversus**
Situs inversus or transversus:
abdominalis
thoracis
Transposition of viscera:
abdominal
thoracic
EXCLUDES *dextrocardia without mention of complete transposition (746.87)*
DEF: Laterally transposed thoracic and abdominal viscera.

759.4 **Conjoined twins**
Craniopagus
Dicephalus
Pygopagus
Thoracopagus
Xiphopagus

759.5 **Tuberous sclerosis**
Bourneville's disease
Epiloia
DEF: Hamartomas of brain, retina and viscera, impaired mental ability, seizures and adenoma sebaceum.

759.6 **Other hamartoses, not elsewhere classified**
Syndrome:
Peutz-Jeghers
Sturge-Weber (-Dimitri)
Syndrome:
von Hippel-Lindau
EXCLUDES *neurofibromatosis (237.7)*
AHA: 3Q, '92, 12
DEF: Peutz-Jeghers: hereditary syndrome characterized by hamartomas of small intestine.
DEF: Sturge-Weber: congenital syndrome characterized by unilateral port-wine stain over trigeminal nerve, underlying meninges and cerebral cortex.
DEF: von Hipple-Lindau: hereditary syndrome of congenital angiomatosis of the retina and cerebellum.

759.7 **Multiple congenital anomalies, so described**
Congenital:
anomaly, multiple NOS
deformity, multiple NOS

✓5th 759.8 **Other specified anomalies**
AHA: S-O, '87, 9; S-O, '85, 11

759.81 **Prader-Willi syndrome**

759.82 **Marfan syndrome**
AHA: 3Q, '93, 11

759.83 **Fragile X syndrome**
AHA: 4Q, '94, 41

759.89 **Other**
Congenital malformation syndromes affecting multiple systems, not elsewhere classified
Laurence-Moon-Biedl syndrome
AHA: ►2Q, '04, 12;◄ 1Q, '01, 3; 3Q, '99, 17, 18; 3Q, '98, 8

759.9 **Congenital anomaly, unspecified**

15. CERTAIN CONDITIONS ORIGINATING IN THE PERINATAL PERIOD (760-779)

INCLUDES ▶conditions which have their origin in the perinatal period, before birth through the first 28 days after birth, even though death or morbidity occurs later◀

Use additional code(s) to further specify condition

MATERNAL CAUSES OF PERINATAL MORBIDITY AND MORTALITY (760-763)

AHA: 2Q, '89, 14; 3Q, '90, 5

✓4th **760 Fetus or newborn affected by maternal conditions which may be unrelated to present pregnancy**

INCLUDES the listed maternal conditions only when specified as a cause of mortality or morbidity of the fetus or newborn

EXCLUDES *maternal endocrine and metabolic disorders affecting fetus or newborn (775.0-775.9)*

AHA: 1Q, '94, 8; 2Q, '92, 12; N-D, '84, 11

760.0 Maternal hypertensive disorders
Fetus or newborn affected by maternal conditions classifiable to 642

760.1 Maternal renal and urinary tract diseases
Fetus or newborn affected by maternal conditions classifiable to 580-599

760.2 Maternal infections
Fetus or newborn affected by maternal infectious disease classifiable to 001-136 and 487, but fetus or newborn not manifesting that disease

EXCLUDES *congenital infectious diseases (771.0-771.8)*
maternal genital tract and other localized infections (760.8)

760.3 Other chronic maternal circulatory and respiratory diseases
Fetus or newborn affected by chronic maternal conditions classifiable to 390-459, 490-519, 745-748

760.4 Maternal nutritional disorders
Fetus or newborn affected by:
maternal disorders classifiable to 260-269
maternal malnutrition NOS

EXCLUDES *fetal malnutrition (764.10-764.29)*

760.5 Maternal injury
Fetus or newborn affected by maternal conditions classifiable to 800-995

760.6 Surgical operation on mother

EXCLUDES *cesarean section for present delivery (763.4)*
damage to placenta from amniocentesis, cesarean section, or surgical induction (762.1)
previous surgery to uterus or pelvic organs (763.89)

✓5th **760.7 Noxious influences affecting fetus or newborn via placenta or breast milk**
Fetus or newborn affected by noxious substance transmitted via placenta or breast milk

EXCLUDES *anesthetic and analgesic drugs administered during labor and delivery (763.5)*
drug withdrawal syndrome in newborn (779.5)

AHA: 3Q, '91, 21

760.70 Unspecified noxious substance
Fetus or newborn affected by:
Drug NEC

760.71 Alcohol
Fetal alcohol syndrome

760.72 Narcotics

760.73 Hallucinogenic agents

760.74 Anti-infectives
Antibiotics
▶Antifungals◀

760.75 Cocaine
AHA: 3Q, '94, 6; 2Q, '92, 12; 4Q, '91, 26

760.76 Diethylstilbestrol [DES]
AHA: 4Q, '94, 45

● **760.77 Anticonvulsants**
Carbamazepine
Phenobarbital
Phenytoin
Valproic acid

● **760.78 Antimetabolic agents**
Methotrexate
Retinoic acid
Statins

760.79 Other
Fetus or newborn affected by:
immune sera, medicinal agents NEC, toxic substance NEC } transmitted via placenta or breast milk

760.8 Other specified maternal conditions affecting fetus or newborn
Maternal genital tract and other localized infection affecting fetus or newborn, but fetus or newborn not manifesting that disease

EXCLUDES *maternal urinary tract infection affecting fetus or newborn (760.1)*

760.9 Unspecified maternal condition affecting fetus or newborn

✓4th **761 Fetus or newborn affected by maternal complications of pregnancy**

INCLUDES the listed maternal conditions only when specified as a cause of mortality or morbidity of the fetus or newborn

761.0 Incompetent cervix
DEF: Inadequate functioning of uterine cervix.

761.1 Premature rupture of membranes

761.2 Oligohydramnios

EXCLUDES *that due to premature rupture of membranes (761.1)*

DEF: Deficient amniotic fluid.

761.3 Polyhydramnios
Hydramnios (acute) (chronic)
DEF: Excess amniotic fluid.

761.4 Ectopic pregnancy
Pregnancy:
abdominal
intraperitoneal
tubal

761.5 Multiple pregnancy
Triplet (pregnancy)
Twin (pregnancy)

761.6 Maternal death

761.7 Malpresentation before labor
Breech presentation, External version, Oblique lie, Transverse lie, Unstable lie } before labor

761.8 Other specified maternal complications of pregnancy affecting fetus or newborn
Spontaneous abortion, fetus

761.9 Unspecified maternal complication of pregnancy affecting fetus or newborn

4th 762 Fetus or newborn affected by complications of placenta, cord, and membranes

INCLUDES the listed maternal conditions only when specified as a cause of mortality or morbidity in the fetus or newborn

AHA: 1Q, '94, 8

762.0 Placenta previa N

DEF: Placenta developed in lower segment of uterus; causes hemorrhaging in last trimester.

762.1 Other forms of placental separation and hemorrhage N

Abruptio placentae
Antepartum hemorrhage
Damage to placenta from amniocentesis, cesarean section, or surgical induction
Maternal blood loss
Premature separation of placenta
Rupture of marginal sinus

762.2 Other and unspecified morphological and functional abnormalities of placenta N

Placental: dysfunction, infarction
Placental: insufficiency

762.3 Placental transfusion syndromes N

Placental and cord abnormality resulting in twin-to-twin or other transplacental transfusion
Use additional code to indicate resultant condition in fetus or newborn:
fetal blood loss (772.0)
polycythemia neonatorum (776.4)

762.4 Prolapsed cord N

Cord presentation

762.5 Other compression of umbilical cord N

Cord around neck
Entanglement of cord
Knot in cord
Torsion of cord

AHA: 2Q, '03, 9

762.6 Other and unspecified conditions of umbilical cord N

Short cord
Thrombosis, Varices, Velamentous insertion } of umbilical cord
Vasa previa

EXCLUDES *infection of umbilical cord (771.4)*
single umbilical artery (747.5)

762.7 Chorioamnionitis N

Amnionitis
Membranitis
Placentitis

DEF: Inflamed fetal membrane.

762.8 Other specified abnormalities of chorion and amnion N

762.9 Unspecified abnormality of chorion and amnion N

4th 763 Fetus or newborn affected by other complications of labor and delivery

INCLUDES the listed conditions only when specified as a cause of mortality or morbidity in the fetus or newborn

AHA: 1Q, '94, 8

763.0 Breech delivery and extraction N

763.1 Other malpresentation, malposition, and disproportion during labor and delivery N

Fetus or newborn affected by:
abnormality of bony pelvis
contracted pelvis
persistent occipitoposterior position
shoulder presentation
transverse lie
conditions classifiable to 652, 653, and 660

763.2 Forceps delivery N

Fetus or newborn affected by forceps extraction

763.3 Delivery by vacuum extractor N

763.4 Cesarean delivery N

EXCLUDES *placental separation or hemorrhage from cesarean section (762.1)*

763.5 Maternal anesthesia and analgesia N

Reactions and intoxications from maternal opiates and tranquilizers during labor and delivery

EXCLUDES *drug withdrawal syndrome in newborn (779.5)*

763.6 Precipitate delivery N

Rapid second stage

763.7 Abnormal uterine contractions N

Fetus or newborn affected by:
contraction ring
hypertonic labor
hypotonic uterine dysfunction
uterine inertia or dysfunction
conditions classifiable to 661, except 661.3

5th 763.8 Other specified complications of labor and delivery affecting fetus or newborn

AHA: 4Q, '98, 46

763.81 Abnormality in fetal heart rate or rhythm before the onset of labor N

763.82 Abnormality in fetal heart rate or rhythm during labor N

AHA: 4Q, '98, 46

763.83 Abnormality in fetal heart rate or rhythm, unspecified as to time of onset N

● **763.84 Meconium passage during delivery** N

EXCLUDES *meconium aspiration (770.11, 770.12)*
meconium staining (779.84)

763.89 Other specified complications of labor and delivery affecting fetus or newborn N

Fetus or newborn affected by:
abnormality of maternal soft tissues
destructive operation on live fetus to facilitate delivery
induction of labor (medical)
previous surgery to uterus or pelvic organs
other conditions classifiable to 650-669
other procedures used in labor and delivery

763.9 Unspecified complication of labor and delivery affecting fetus or newborn N

OTHER CONDITIONS ORIGINATING IN THE PERINATAL PERIOD (764-779)

The following fifth-digit subclassification is for use with category 764 and codes 765.0 and 765.1 to denote birthweight:

0 unspecified [weight]
1 less than 500 grams
2 500-749 grams
3 750-999 grams
4 1,000-1,249 grams
5 1,250-1,499 grams
6 1,500-1,749 grams
7 1,750-1,999 grams
8 2,000-2,499 grams
9 2,500 grams and over

4th 764 Slow fetal growth and fetal malnutrition

AHA: 3Q, '04, 4; 4Q, '02, 63; 1Q,'94, 8; 2Q, '91, 19; 2Q, '89, 15

5th 764.0 "Light-for-dates" without mention of fetal malnutrition N

Infants underweight for gestational age
"Small-for-dates"

5th **764.1 "Light-for-dates" with signs of fetal malnutrition** N
Infants "light-for-dates" classifiable to 764.0, who in addition show signs of fetal malnutrition, such as dry peeling skin and loss of subcutaneous tissue

5th **764.2 Fetal malnutrition without mention of "light-for-dates"** N
Infants, not underweight for gestational age, showing signs of fetal malnutrition, such as dry peeling skin and loss of subcutaneous tissue
Intrauterine malnutrition

5th **764.9 Fetal growth retardation, unspecified** N
Intrauterine growth retardation
AHA: For code 764.97: 1Q, '97, 6

4th **765 Disorders relating to short gestation and low birthweight**
INCLUDES the listed conditions, without further specification, as causes of mortality, morbidity, or additional care, in fetus or newborn
AHA: 1Q, '97, 6; 1Q, '94, 8; 2Q, '91, 19; 2Q, '89, 15

5th **765.0 Extreme immaturity** N
Note: Usually implies a birthweight of less than 1000 grams.
Use additional code for weeks of gestation (765.20-765.29)
AHA: ▶3Q, '04, 4;◀ 4Q, '02, 63; **For code 765.03:** 4Q, '01, 51

5th **765.1 Other preterm infants** N
Note: Usually implies a birthweight of 1000-2499 grams.
Prematurity NOS
Prematurity or small size, not classifiable to 765.0 or as "light-for-dates" in 764
Use additional code for weeks of gestation (765.20-765.29)
AHA: ▶3Q, '04, 4;◀ 4Q, '02, 63; **For code 765.10:** 1Q, '94, 14; **For code 765.17:** 1Q, '97, 6; **For code 765.18:** 4Q, '02, 64

5th **765.2 Weeks of gestation**
AHA: ▶3Q, '04, 4;◀ 4Q, '02, 63

765.20 Unspecified weeks of gestation N
765.21 Less than 24 completed weeks of gestation N
765.22 24 completed weeks of gestation N
765.23 25-26 completed weeks of gestation N
765.24 27-28 completed weeks of gestation N
765.25 29-30 completed weeks of gestation N
765.26 31-32 completed weeks of gestation N
765.27 33-34 completed weeks of gestation N
765.28 35-36 completed weeks of gestation N
AHA: 4Q, '02, 64
765.29 37 or more completed weeks of gestation N

4th **766 Disorders relating to long gestation and high birthweight**
INCLUDES the listed conditions, without further specification, as causes of mortality, morbidity, or additional care, in fetus or newborn

766.0 Exceptionally large baby N
Note: Usually implies a birthweight of 4500 grams or more.

766.1 Other "heavy-for-dates" infants N
Other fetus or infant "heavy-" or "large-for-dates" regardless of period of gestation

5th **766.2 Late infant, not "heavy-for-dates"**
AHA: 4Q, '03, 69

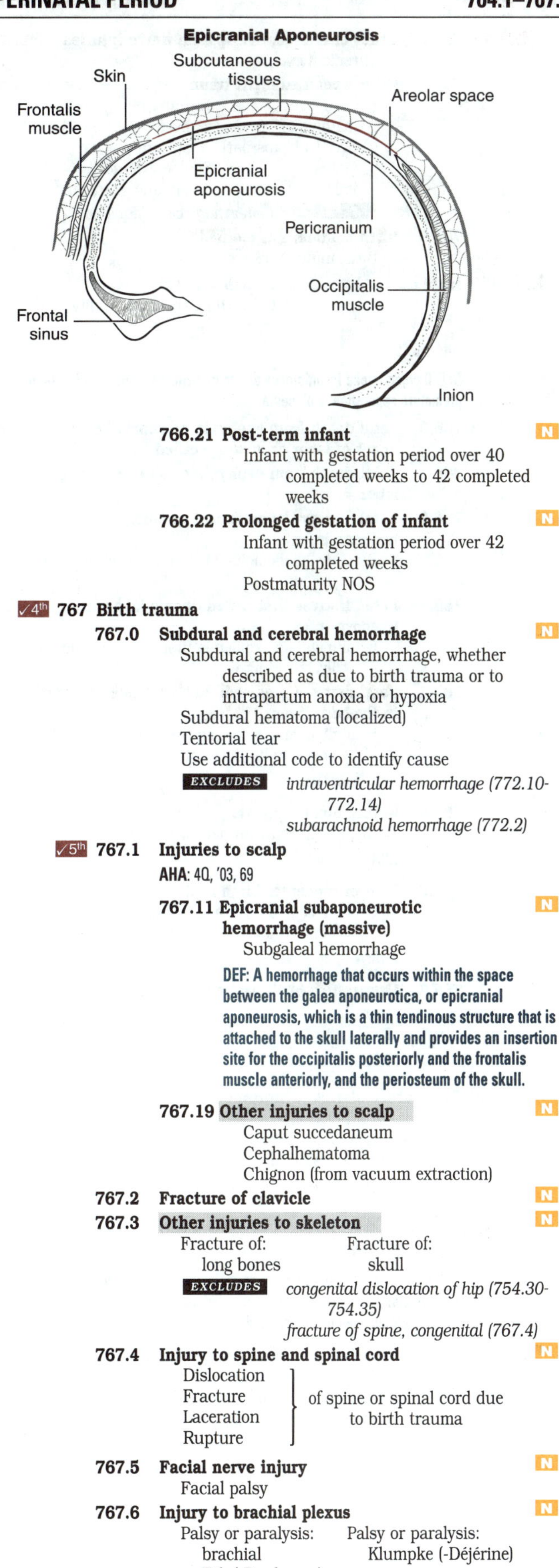

766.21 Post-term infant N
Infant with gestation period over 40 completed weeks to 42 completed weeks

766.22 Prolonged gestation of infant N
Infant with gestation period over 42 completed weeks
Postmaturity NOS

4th **767 Birth trauma**

767.0 Subdural and cerebral hemorrhage N
Subdural and cerebral hemorrhage, whether described as due to birth trauma or to intrapartum anoxia or hypoxia
Subdural hematoma (localized)
Tentorial tear
Use additional code to identify cause
EXCLUDES *intraventricular hemorrhage (772.10-772.14)*
subarachnoid hemorrhage (772.2)

5th **767.1 Injuries to scalp**
AHA: 4Q, '03, 69

767.11 Epicranial subaponeurotic hemorrhage (massive) N
Subgaleal hemorrhage
DEF: A hemorrhage that occurs within the space between the galea aponeurotica, or epicranial aponeurosis, which is a thin tendinous structure that is attached to the skull laterally and provides an insertion site for the occipitalis posteriorly and the frontalis muscle anteriorly, and the periosteum of the skull.

767.19 Other injuries to scalp N
Caput succedaneum
Cephalhematoma
Chignon (from vacuum extraction)

767.2 Fracture of clavicle N

767.3 Other injuries to skeleton N
Fracture of:
long bones
skull
EXCLUDES *congenital dislocation of hip (754.30-754.35)*
fracture of spine, congenital (767.4)

767.4 Injury to spine and spinal cord N
Dislocation, Fracture, Laceration, Rupture } of spine or spinal cord due to birth trauma

767.5 Facial nerve injury N
Facial palsy

767.6 Injury to brachial plexus N
Palsy or paralysis:
brachial
Erb (-Duchenne)
Klumpke (-Déjérine)

4th 5th Additional Digit Required | Unspecified Code | Other Specified Code | Manifestation Code | ▶◀ Revised Text | ● New Code | ▲ Revised Code Title

767.7 Other cranial and peripheral nerve injuries N
Phrenic nerve paralysis

767.8 Other specified birth trauma N
Eye damage
Hematoma of:
liver (subcapsular)
testes
vulva
Rupture of:
liver
spleen
Scalpel wound
Traumatic glaucoma
EXCLUDES *hemorrhage classifiable to 772.0-772.9*

767.9 Birth trauma, unspecified N
Birth injury NOS

✓4th **768 Intrauterine hypoxia and birth asphyxia**
Use only when associated with newborn morbidity classifiable elsewhere
AHA: 4Q, '92, 20

DEF: Oxygen intake insufficiency due to interrupted placental circulation or premature separation of placenta.

768.0 Fetal death from asphyxia or anoxia before onset of labor or at unspecified time N

768.1 Fetal death from asphyxia or anoxia during labor N

768.2 Fetal distress before onset of labor, in liveborn infant N
Fetal metabolic acidemia before onset of labor, in liveborn infant

768.3 Fetal distress first noted during labor, in liveborn infant N
Fetal metabolic acidemia first noted during labor, in liveborn infant

768.4 Fetal distress, unspecified as to time of onset, in liveborn infant N
Fetal metabolic acidemia unspecified as to time of onset, in liveborn infant
AHA: N-D, '86, 10

768.5 Severe birth asphyxia N
Birth asphyxia with neurologic involvement
AHA: N-D, '86, 3

768.6 Mild or moderate birth asphyxia N
Other specified birth asphyxia (without mention of neurologic involvement)
AHA: N-D, '86, 3

768.9 Unspecified birth asphyxia in liveborn infant N
Anoxia, Asphyxia, Hypoxia } NOS, in liveborn infant

769 Respiratory distress syndrome N
Cardiorespiratory distress syndrome of newborn
Hyaline membrane disease (pulmonary)
Idiopathic respiratory distress syndrome [IRDS or RDS] of newborn
Pulmonary hypoperfusion syndrome
EXCLUDES *transient tachypnea of newborn (770.6)*
AHA: 1Q, '89, 10; N-D, '86, 6

DEF: Severe chest contractions upon air intake and expiratory grunting; infant appears blue due to oxygen deficiency and has rapid respiratory rate; formerly called hyaline membrane disease.

✓4th **770 Other respiratory conditions of fetus and newborn**

770.0 Congenital pneumonia N
Infective pneumonia acquired prenatally
EXCLUDES *pneumonia from infection acquired after birth (480.0-486)*
AHA: ►1Q, '05, 10◄

▲ ✓5th **770.1 Fetal and newborn aspiration**
EXCLUDES ► *aspiration of postnatal stomach contents (770.85, 770.86)*
meconium passage during delivery (763.84)
meconium staining (779.84)◄

DEF: Meconium Aspiration: Aspiration of meconium by the newborn infant prior to delivery. Presence of meconium in the trachea or chest x-ray indicating patchy infiltrates in conjunction with chest hyperextension establishes this diagnosis.

● **770.10 Fetal and newborn aspiration, unspecified** N

● **770.11 Meconium aspiration without respiratory symptoms** N
Meconium aspiration NOS

● **770.12 Meconium aspiration with respiratory symptoms** N
Meconium aspiration pneumonia
Meconium aspiration pneumonitis
Meconium aspiration syndrome NOS
Use additional code to identify any secondary pulmonary hypertension (416.8), if applicable

● **770.13 Aspiration of clear amniotic fluid without respiratory symptoms** N
Aspiration of clear amniotic fluid NOS

● **770.14 Aspiration of clear amniotic fluid with respiratory symptoms** N
Aspiration of clear amniotic fluid with pneumonia
Aspiration of clear amniotic fluid with pneumonitis
Use additional code to identify any secondary pulmonary hypertension (416.8), if applicable

● **770.15 Aspiration of blood without respiratory symptoms** N
Aspiration of blood NOS

● **770.16 Aspiration of blood with respiratory symptoms** N
Aspiration of blood with pneumonia
Aspiration of blood with pneumonitis
Use additional code to identify any secondary pulmonary hypertension (416.8), if applicable

● **770.17 Other fetal and newborn aspiration without respiratory symptoms** N

● **770.18 Other fetal and newborn aspiration with respiratory symptoms** N
Other aspiration pneumonia
Other aspiration pneumonitis
Use additional code to identify any secondary pulmonary hypertension (416.8), if applicable

770.2 Interstitial emphysema and related conditions N
Pneumomediastinum, Pneumopericardium, Pneumothorax } originating in the perinatal period

770.3 Pulmonary hemorrhage N
Hemorrhage:
alveolar (lung), intra-alveolar (lung), massive pulmonary } originating in the perinatal period

770.4 Primary atelectasis N
Pulmonary immaturity NOS

DEF: Alveoli fail to expand causing insufficient air intake by newborn.

770.5 Other and unspecified atelectasis N
Atelectasis:
NOS
partial
secondary
Pulmonary collapse
} originating in the perinatal period

770.6 Transitory tachypnea of newborn N
Idiopathic tachypnea of newborn
Wet lung syndrome
EXCLUDES *respiratory distress syndrome (769)*
AHA: 4Q, '95, 4; 1Q, '94, 12; 3Q, '93, 7; 1Q, '89, 10; N-D, '86, 6
DEF: Quick, shallow breathing of newborn; short-term problem.

770.7 Chronic respiratory disease arising in the perinatal period
Bronchopulmonary dysplasia
Interstitial pulmonary fibrosis of prematurity
Wilson-Mikity syndrome
AHA: 2Q, '91, 19; N-D, '86, 11

✓5th **770.8 Other respiratory problems after birth**
AHA: 4Q, '02, 65; 2Q, '98, 10; 2Q, '96, 10

770.81 Primary apnea of newborn N
Apneic spells of newborn NOS
Essential apnea of newborn
Sleep apnea of newborn
DEF: Cessation of breathing when a neonate makes no respiratory effort for 15 seconds, resulting in cyanosis and bradycardia.

770.82 Other apnea of newborn N
Obstructive apnea of newborn

770.83 Cyanotic attacks of newborn N

770.84 Respiratory failure of newborn N
EXCLUDES *respiratory distress syndrome (769)*

● **770.85 Aspiration of postnatal stomach contents without respiratory symptoms** N
Aspiration of postnatal stomach contents NOS

● **770.86 Aspiration of postnatal stomach contents with respiratory symptoms** N
Aspiration of postnatal stomach contents with pneumonia
Aspiration of postnatal stomach contents with pneumonitis
Use additional code to identify any secondary pulmonary hypertension (416.8), if applicable

770.89 Other respiratory problems after birth N

770.9 Unspecified respiratory condition of fetus and newborn N

✓4th **771 Infections specific to the perinatal period**
INCLUDES infections acquired before or during birth or via the umbilicus ▶or during the first 28 days after birth◀
EXCLUDES *congenital pneumonia (770.0)*
congenital syphilis (090.0-090.9)
maternal infectious disease as a cause of mortality or morbidity in fetus or newborn, but fetus or newborn not manifesting the disease (760.2)
ophthalmia neonatorum due to gonococcus (098.40)
other infections not specifically classified to this category
AHA: N-D, '85, 4

771.0 Congenital rubella N
Congenital rubella pneumonitis

771.1 Congenital cytomegalovirus infection N
Congenital cytomegalic inclusion disease

771.2 Other congenital infections N
Congenital:
herpes simplex
listeriosis
malaria
Congenital:
toxoplasmosis
tuberculosis

771.3 Tetanus neonatorum N
Tetanus omphalitis
EXCLUDES *hypocalcemic tetany (775.4)*
DEF: Severe infection of central nervous system; due to exotoxin of tetanus bacillus from navel infection prompted by nonsterile technique during umbilical ligation.

771.4 Omphalitis of the newborn N
Infection:
navel cord
umbilical stump
EXCLUDES *tetanus omphalitis (771.3)*
DEF: Inflamed umbilicus.

771.5 Neonatal infective mastitis N
EXCLUDES *noninfective neonatal mastitis (778.7)*

771.6 Neonatal conjunctivitis and dacryocystitis N
Ophthalmia neonatorum NOS
EXCLUDES *ophthalmia neonatorum due to gonococcus (098.40)*

771.7 Neonatal Candida infection N
Neonatal moniliasis
Thrush in newborn

✓5th **771.8 Other infection specific to the perinatal period**
Use additional code to identify organism (041.00-041.9)
AHA: 4Q, '02, 66

771.81 Septicemia [sepsis] of newborn N

771.82 Urinary tract infection of newborn N

771.83 Bacteremia of newborn N

771.89 Other infections specific to the perinatal period N
Intra-amniotic infection of fetus NOS
Infection of newborn NOS

✓4th **772 Fetal and neonatal hemorrhage**
EXCLUDES *hematological disorders of fetus and newborn (776.0-776.9)*

772.0 Fetal blood loss N
Fetal blood loss from:
cut end of co-twin's cord
placenta
ruptured cord
vasa previa
Fetal exsanguination
Fetal hemorrhage into:
co-twin
mother's circulation

✓5th **772.1 Intraventricular hemorrhage**
Intraventricular hemorrhage from any perinatal cause
AHA: 4Q, '01, 49; 3Q, '92, 8; 4Q, '88, 8

772.10 Unspecified grade N

772.11 Grade I N
Bleeding into germinal matrix

772.12 Grade II N
Bleeding into ventricle

772.13 Grade III N
Bleeding with enlargement of ventricle
AHA: 4Q, '01, 51

772.14 Grade IV N
Bleeding into cerebral cortex

772.2 Subarachnoid hemorrhage N
Subarachnoid hemorrhage from any perinatal cause
EXCLUDES *subdural and cerebral hemorrhage (767.0)*

772.3 Umbilical hemorrhage after birth N
Slipped umbilical ligature

772.4 Gastrointestinal hemorrhage N
EXCLUDES *swallowed maternal blood (777.3)*

772.5 Adrenal hemorrhage N

772.6 Cutaneous hemorrhage N
Bruising, Ecchymoses, Petechiae, Superficial hematoma — in fetus or newborn

772.8 Other specified hemorrhage of fetus or newborn N
EXCLUDES *hemorrhagic disease of newborn (776.0)*
pulmonary hemorrhage (770.3)

772.9 Unspecified hemorrhage of newborn N

✓4th **773 Hemolytic disease of fetus or newborn, due to isoimmunization**
DEF: Hemolytic anemia of fetus or newborn due to maternal antibody formation against fetal erythrocytes; infant blood contains nonmaternal antigen.

773.0 Hemolytic disease due to Rh isoimmunization N
Anemia, Erythroblastosis (fetalis), Hemolytic disease (fetus) (newborn), Jaundice — due to RH: antibodies, isoimmunization, maternal/fetal incompatibility
Rh hemolytic disease
Rh isoimmunization

773.1 Hemolytic disease due to ABO isoimmunization N
ABO hemolytic disease
ABO isoimmunization
Anemia, Erythroblastosis (fetalis), Hemolytic disease (fetus) (newborn), Jaundice — due to ABO: antibodies, isoimmunization, maternal/fetal incompatibility
AHA: 3Q, '92, 8
DEF: Incompatible Rh fetal-maternal blood grouping; prematurely destroys red blood cells; detected by Coombs test.

773.2 Hemolytic disease due to other and unspecified isoimmunization N
Eythroblastosis (fetalis) (neonatorum) NOS
Hemolytic disease (fetus) (newborn) NOS
Jaundice or anemia due to other and unspecified blood-group incompatibility
AHA: 1Q, '94, 13

773.3 Hydrops fetalis due to isoimmunization N
Use additional code to identify type of isoimmunization (773.0-773.2)
DEF: Massive edema of entire body and severe anemia; may result in fetal death or stillbirth.

773.4 Kernicterus due to isoimmunization N
Use additional code to identify type of isoimmunization (773.0-773.2)
DEF: Complication of erythroblastosis fetalis associated with severe neural symptoms, high blood bilirubin levels and nerve cell destruction; results in bilirubin-pigmented gray matter of central nervous system.

773.5 Late anemia due to isoimmunization N

✓4th **774 Other perinatal jaundice**

774.0 Perinatal jaundice from hereditary hemolytic anemias N
Code first underlying disease (282.0-282.9)

774.1 Perinatal jaundice from other excessive hemolysis N
Fetal or neonatal jaundice from:
- bruising
- drugs or toxins transmitted from mother
- infection
- polycythemia
- swallowed maternal blood

Use additional code to identify cause
EXCLUDES *jaundice due to isoimmunization (773.0-773.2)*

774.2 Neonatal jaundice associated with preterm delivery N
Hyperbilirubinemia of prematurity
Jaundice due to delayed conjugation associated with preterm delivery
AHA: 3Q, '91, 21

✓5th **774.3 Neonatal jaundice due to delayed conjugation from other causes**

774.30 Neonatal jaundice due to delayed conjugation, cause unspecified N
DEF: Jaundice of newborn with abnormal bilirubin metabolism; causes excess accumulated unconjugated bilirubin in blood.

774.31 Neonatal jaundice due to delayed conjugation in diseases classified elsewhere N
Code first underlying diseases as:
- congenital hypothyroidism (243)
- Crigler-Najjar syndrome (277.4)
- Gilbert's syndrome (277.4)

774.39 Other N
Jaundice due to delayed conjugation from causes, such as:
- breast milk inhibitors
- delayed development of conjugating system

774.4 Perinatal jaundice due to hepatocellular damage N
Fetal or neonatal hepatitis
Giant cell hepatitis
Inspissated bile syndrome

774.5 Perinatal jaundice from other causes N
Code first underlying cause as:
- congenital obstruction of bile duct (751.61)
- galactosemia (271.1)
- Mucoviscidosis (277.00-277.09)

774.6 Unspecified fetal and neonatal jaundice N
Icterus neonatorum
Neonatal hyperbilirubinemia (transient)
Physiologic jaundice NOS in newborn
EXCLUDES *that in preterm infants (774.2)*
AHA: 1Q, '94, 13; 2Q, '89, 15

774.7 Kernicterus not due to isoimmunization N
Bilirubin encephalopathy
Kernicterus of newborn NOS
EXCLUDES *kernicterus due to isoimmunization (773.4)*

✓4th **775 Endocrine and metabolic disturbances specific to the fetus and newborn**
INCLUDES transitory endocrine and metabolic disturbances caused by the infant's response to maternal endocrine and metabolic factors, its removal from them, or its adjustment to extrauterine existence

775.0 Syndrome of "infant of a diabetic mother" N
Maternal diabetes mellitus affecting fetus or newborn (with hypoglycemia)
AHA: 1Q, '04, 7-8; 3Q, '91, 5

775.1 Neonatal diabetes mellitus N
Diabetes mellitus syndrome in newborn infant
AHA: 3Q, '91, 6

775.2 Neonatal myasthenia gravis N

775.3 Neonatal thyrotoxicosis N
Neonatal hyperthydroidism (transient)

775.4 Hypocalcemia and hypomagnesemia of newborn N
Cow's milk hypocalcemia
Hypocalcemic tetany, neonatal
Neonatal hypoparathyroidism
Phosphate-loading hypocalcemia

775.5 Other transitory neonatal electrolyte disturbances N
Dehydration, neonatal
AHA: ▶1Q, '05, 9◀

775.6 Neonatal hypoglycemia N
EXCLUDES *infant of mother with diabetes mellitus (775.0)*
AHA: 1Q, '94, 8

775.7 Late metabolic acidosis of newborn N

775.8 Other transitory neonatal endocrine and metabolic disturbances N
Amino-acid metabolic disorders described as transitory

775.9 Unspecified endocrine and metabolic disturbances specific to the fetus and newborn N

✓4th **776 Hematological disorders of fetus and newborn**
INCLUDES disorders specific to the fetus or newborn

776.0 Hemorrhagic disease of newborn N
Hemorrhagic diathesis of newborn
Vitamin K deficiency of newborn
EXCLUDES *fetal or neonatal hemorrhage (772.0-772.9)*

776.1 Transient neonatal thrombocytopenia N
Neonatal thrombocytopenia due to:
exchange transfusion
idiopathic maternal thrombocytopenia
isoimmunization
DEF: Temporary decrease in blood platelets of newborn.

776.2 Disseminated intravascular coagulation in newborn N
DEF: Disseminated intravascular coagulation of newborn: clotting disorder due to excess thromboplastic agents in blood as a result of disease or trauma; causes blood clotting within vessels and reduces available elements necessary for blood coagulation.

776.3 Other transient neonatal disorders of coagulation N
Transient coagulation defect, newborn

776.4 Polycythemia neonatorum N
Plethora of newborn
Polycythemia due to:
donor twin transfusion
Polycythemia due to:
maternal-fetal transfusion
DEF: Abnormal increase of total red blood cells of newborn.

776.5 Congenital anemia N
Anemia following fetal blood loss
EXCLUDES *anemia due to isoimmunization (773.0-773.2, 773.5)*
hereditary hemolytic anemias (282.0-282.9)

776.6 Anemia of prematurity N

776.7 Transient neonatal neutropenia N
Isoimmune neutropenia
Maternal transfer neutropenia
EXCLUDES *congenital neutropenia (nontransient) (288.0)*
DEF: Decreased neutrophilic leukocytes in blood of newborn.

776.8 Other specified transient hematological disorders N

776.9 Unspecified hematological disorder specific to fetus or newborn N

✓4th **777 Perinatal disorders of digestive system**
INCLUDES disorders specific to the fetus and newborn
EXCLUDES *intestinal obstruction classifiable to 560.0-560.9*

777.1 Meconium obstruction N
Congenital fecaliths
Delayed passage of meconium
Meconium ileus NOS
Meconium plug syndrome
EXCLUDES *meconium ileus in cystic fibrosis (277.01)*
DEF: Meconium blocked digestive tract of newborn.

777.2 Intestinal obstruction due to inspissated milk N

777.3 Hematemesis and melena due to swallowed maternal blood N
Swallowed blood syndrome in newborn
EXCLUDES *that not due to swallowed maternal blood (772.4)*

777.4 Transitory ileus of newborn N
EXCLUDES *Hirschsprung's disease (751.3)*

777.5 Necrotizing enterocolitis in fetus or newborn N
Pseudomembranous enterocolitis in newborn
DEF: Acute inflammation of small intestine due to pseudomembranous plaque over ulceration; may be due to aggressive antibiotic therapy.

777.6 Perinatal intestinal perforation N
Meconium peritonitis

777.8 Other specified perinatal disorders of digestive system N

777.9 Unspecified perinatal disorder of digestive system N

✓4th **778 Conditions involving the integument and temperature regulation of fetus and newborn**

778.0 Hydrops fetalis not due to isoimmunization N
Idiopathic hydrops
EXCLUDES *hydrops fetalis due to isoimmunization (773.3)*
DEF: Edema of entire body, unrelated to immune response.

778.1 Sclerema neonatorum N
Subcutaneous fat necrosis
DEF: Diffuse, rapidly progressing white, waxy, nonpitting hardening of tissue, usually of legs and feet, life-threatening; found in preterm or debilitated infants; unknown etiology.

778.2 Cold injury syndrome of newborn N

778.3 Other hypothermia of newborn N

778.4 Other disturbances of temperature regulation of newborn N
Dehydration fever in newborn
Environmentally-induced pyrexia
Hyperthermia in newborn
Transitory fever of newborn

778.5 Other and unspecified edema of newborn N
Edema neonatorum

778.6 Congenital hydrocele
Congenital hydrocele of tunica vaginalis

778.7 Breast engorgement in newborn N
Noninfective mastitis of newborn
EXCLUDES *infective mastitis of newborn (771.5)*

778.8 Other specified conditions involving the integument of fetus and newborn N
Urticaria neonatorum
EXCLUDES *impetigo neonatorum (684)*
pemphigus neonatorum (684)

778.9 Unspecified condition involving the integument and temperature regulation of fetus and newborn N

✓4th **779 Other and ill-defined conditions originating in the perinatal period**

779.0 Convulsions in newborn N
Fits } in newborn
Seizures }
AHA: N-D, '94, 11

779.1 Other and unspecified cerebral irritability in newborn N

779.2 Cerebral depression, coma, and other abnormal cerebral signs N
CNS dysfunction in newborn NOS

779.3 Feeding problems in newborn N
Regurgitation of food }
Slow feeding } in newborn
Vomiting }
AHA: 2Q, '89, 15

779.4 Drug reactions and intoxications specific to newborn N
Gray syndrome from chloramphenicol administration in newborn
EXCLUDES *fetal alcohol syndrome (760.71)*
reactions and intoxications from maternal opiates and tranquilizers (763.5)

779.5 Drug withdrawal syndrome in newborn N
Drug withdrawal syndrome in infant of dependent mother
EXCLUDES *fetal alcohol syndrome (760.71)*
AHA: 3Q, '94, 6

779.6 Termination of pregnancy (fetus) N
Fetal death due to:
induced abortion
termination of pregnancy
EXCLUDES *spontaneous abortion (fetus) (761.8)*

779.7 Periventricular leukomalacia
AHA: 4Q, '01, 50, 51

DEF: Necrosis of white matter adjacent to lateral ventricles with the formation of cysts; cause of PVL has not been firmly established, but thought to be related to inadequate blood flow in certain areas of the brain.

✓5th **779.8 Other specified conditions originating in the perinatal period**
AHA: 4Q, '02, 67; 1Q, '94, 15

779.81 Neonatal bradycardia N
EXCLUDES *abnormality in fetal heart rate or rhythm complicating labor and delivery (763.81-763.83)*
bradycardia due to birth asphyxia (768.5-768.9)

779.82 Neonatal tachycardia N
EXCLUDES *abnormality in fetal heart rate or rhythm complicating labor and delivery (763.81-763.83)*

779.83 Delayed separation of umbilical cord N
AHA: 4Q, '03, 71

● **779.84 Meconium staining** N
EXCLUDES *meconium aspiration (770.11, 770.12)*
meconium passage during delivery (763.84)

779.89 Other specified conditions originating in the perinatal period N
▶Use addtional code to specify condition◀
AHA: ▶1Q, '05, 9◀

779.9 Unspecified condition originating in the perinatal period N
Congenital debility NOS
Stillbirth NEC

16. SYMPTOMS, SIGNS, AND ILL-DEFINED CONDITIONS (780-799)

This section includes symptoms, signs, abnormal results of laboratory or other investigative procedures, and ill-defined conditions regarding which no diagnosis classifiable elsewhere is recorded.

Signs and symptoms that point rather definitely to a given diagnosis are assigned to some category in the preceding part of the classification. In general, categories 780-796 include the more ill-defined conditions and symptoms that point with perhaps equal suspicion to two or more diseases or to two or more systems of the body, and without the necessary study of the case to make a final diagnosis. Practically all categories in this group could be designated as "not otherwise specified," or as "unknown etiology," or as "transient." The Alphabetic Index should be consulted to determine which symptoms and signs are to be allocated here and which to more specific sections of the classification; the residual subcategories numbered .9 are provided for other relevant symptoms which cannot be allocated elsewhere in the classification.

The conditions and signs or symptoms included in categories 780-796 consist of: (a) cases for which no more specific diagnosis can be made even after all facts bearing on the case have been investigated; (b) signs or symptoms existing at the time of initial encounter that proved to be transient and whose causes could not be determined; (c) provisional diagnoses in a patient who failed to return for further investigation or care; (d) cases referred elsewhere for investigation or treatment before the diagnosis was made; (e) cases in which a more precise diagnosis was not available for any other reason; (f) certain symptoms which represent important problems in medical care and which it might be desired to classify in addition to a known cause.

SYMPTOMS (780-789)

AHA: 1Q, '91, 12; 2Q, '90, 3; 2Q, '90, 5; 2Q, '90, 15; M-A, '85, 3

✓4th **780 General symptoms**

✓5th **780.0 Alteration of consciousness**

EXCLUDES *coma:*
diabetic (250.2-250.3)
hepatic (572.2)
originating in the perinatal period (779.2)

AHA: 4Q, '92, 20

780.01 Coma

AHA: 3Q, '96, 16

DEF: State of unconsciousness from which the patient cannot be awakened.

780.02 Transient alteration of awareness

DEF: Temporary, recurring spells of reduced consciousness.

780.03 Persistent vegetative state

DEF: Persistent wakefulness without consciousness due to nonfunctioning cerebral cortex.

780.09 Other

Drowsiness
Semicoma
Somnolence
Stupor
Unconsciousness

780.1 Hallucinations

Hallucinations:
NOS
auditory
gustatory
olfactory
tactile

EXCLUDES *those associated with mental disorders, as functional psychoses (295.0-298.9)*
organic brain syndromes (290.0-294.9, 310.0-310.9)
visual hallucinations (368.16)

DEF: Perception of external stimulus in absence of stimulus; inability to distinguish between real and imagined.

780.2 Syncope and collapse

Blackout
Fainting
(Near) (Pre) syncope
Vasovagal attack

EXCLUDES *carotid sinus syncope (337.0)*
heat syncope (992.1)
neurocirculatory asthenia (306.2)
orthostatic hypotension (458.0)
shock NOS (785.50)

AHA: 1Q, '02, 6; 3Q, '00, 12; 3Q, '95, 14; N-D, '85, 12

DEF: Sudden unconsciousness due to reduced blood flow to brain.

✓5th **780.3 Convulsions**

EXCLUDES *convulsions:*
epileptic (345.10-345.91)
in newborn (779.0)

AHA: 2Q, '97, 8; 1Q, '97, 12; 3Q, '94, 9; 1Q, '93, 24; 4Q, '92, 23; N-D, '87, 12

DEF: Sudden, involuntary contractions of the muscles.

780.31 Febrile convulsions

Febrile seizure

AHA: 4Q, '97, 45

780.39 Other convulsions

Convulsive disorder NOS
Fit NOS
Seizure NOS

AHA: 4Q, '04, 51; 1Q, '03, 7; 2Q, '99, 17; 4Q, '98, 39

780.4 Dizziness and giddiness

Light-headedness
Vertigo NOS

EXCLUDES *Ménière's disease and other specified vertiginous syndromes (386.0-386.9)*

AHA: 2Q, '03, 11; 3Q, '00, 12; 2Q, '97, 9; 2Q, '91, 17

DEF: Whirling sensations in head with feeling of falling.

✓5th **780.5 Sleep disturbances**

EXCLUDES ▶*circadian rhythm sleep disorders (327.30-327.39)*
organic hypersomnia (327.10-327.19)
organic insomnia (327.00-327.09)
organic sleep apnea (327.20-327.29)
organic sleep related movement disorders (327.51-327.59)
parasomnias (327.40-327.49)◀
that of nonorganic origin (307.40-307.49)

▲ **780.51 Insomnia with sleep apnea, unspecified**

DEF: Transient cessation of breathing disturbing sleep.

▲ **780.52 Insomnia, unspecified**

DEF: Inability to maintain adequate sleep cycle.

▲ **780.53 Hypersomnia with sleep apnea, unspecified**

AHA: 1Q, '93, 28; N-D, '85, 4

DEF: Autonomic response inhibited during sleep; causes insufficient oxygen intake, acidosis and pulmonary hypertension.

▲ **780.54 Hypersomnia, unspecified**

DEF: Prolonged sleep cycle.

▲ **780.55 Disruptions of 24 hour sleep wake cycle, unspecified**

▲ **780.56 Dysfunctions associated with sleep stages or arousal from sleep**

▲ **780.57 Unspecified sleep apnea**

AHA: 1Q, '01, 6 ; 1Q, '97, 5; 1Q, '93, 28

▲ **780.58 Sleep related movement disorder, unspecified**

EXCLUDES *restless leg syndrome (333.99)*

AHA: 4Q, '04, 95

780.59 Other

Symptoms, Signs, and Ill-Defined Conditions 780–780.59

✓4th ✓5th Additional Digit Required · Unspecified Code · Other Specified Code · Manifestation Code · ▶◀ Revised Text · ● New Code · ▲ Revised Code Title

780.6 Fever

Chills with fever
Fever NOS
Fever of unknown origin (FUO)
Hyperpyrexia NOS
Pyrexia
Pyrexia of unknown origin

EXCLUDES *pyrexia of unknown origin (during):*
in newborn (778.4)
labor (659.2)
the puerperium (672)

AHA: 3Q, '00, 13; 4Q, '99, 26; 2Q, '91, 8

DEF: Elevated body temperature; no known cause.

✓5th **780.7 Malaise and fatigue**

EXCLUDES *debility, unspecified (799.3)*
fatigue (during):
combat (308.0-308.9)
heat (992.6)
pregnancy (646.8)
neurasthenia (300.5)
senile asthenia (797)

AHA: 4Q, '88, 12; M-A, '87, 8

DEF: Indefinite feeling of debility or lack of good health.

780.71 Chronic fatigue syndrome

AHA: 4Q, '98, 48

DEF: Persistent fatigue, symptoms include weak muscles, sore throat, lymphadenitis, headache, depression and mild fever; no known cause; also called chronic mononucleosis, benign myalgic encephalomyelitis, Iceland disease and neurosthenia.

780.79 Other malaise and fatigue

Asthenia NOS
Lethargy
Postviral (asthenic) syndrome
Tiredness

AHA: 4Q, '04, 78; 1Q, '00, 6; 4Q, '99, 26

DEF: Asthenia: any weakness, lack of strength or loss of energy, especially neuromuscular.
DEF: Lethargy: listlessness, drowsiness, stupor and apathy.
DEF: Postviral (asthenic) syndrome: listlessness, drowsiness, stupor and apathy; follows acute viral infection.
DEF: Tiredness: general exhaustion or fatigue.

780.8 Generalized hyperhidrosis

Diaphoresis
Excessive sweating
Secondary hyperhidrosis

EXCLUDES *focal (localized) (primary) (secondary) hyperhidrosis (705.21-705.22)*
Frey's syndrome (705.22)

DEF: Excessive sweating, appears as droplets on skin; generalized.

✓5th **780.9 Other general symptoms**

EXCLUDES *hypothermia:*
NOS (accidental) (991.6)
due to anesthesia (995.89)
of newborn (778.2-778.3)
memory disturbance as part of a pattern of mental disorder

AHA: 4Q, '02, 67; 4Q, '99, 10; 3Q, '93, 11; N-D, '85, 12

780.91 Fussy infant (baby) P

780.92 Excessive crying of infant (baby) P

EXCLUDES ▶*excessive crying of child, adolescent or adult (780.95)*◀

780.93 Memory loss

Amnesia (retrograde)
Memory loss NOS

EXCLUDES *mild memory disturbance due to organic brain damage (310.1)*
transient global amnesia (437.7)

AHA: 4Q, '03, 71

780.94 Early satiety

AHA: 4Q, '03, 72

DEF: The premature feeling of being full; mechanism of satiety is mutlifactorial.

● **780.95 Other excessive crying**

EXCLUDES *excessive crying of infant (baby) (780.92)*

780.99 Other general symptoms

Chill(s) NOS
Generalized pain
Hypothermia, not associated with low environmental temperature

AHA: 4Q, '03, 103

✓4th **781 Symptoms involving nervous and musculoskeletal systems**

EXCLUDES *depression NOS (311)*
disorders specifically relating to:
back (724.0-724.9)
hearing (388.0-389.9)
joint (718.0-719.9)
limb (729.0-729.9)
neck (723.0-723.9)
vision (368.0-369.9)
pain in limb (729.5)

781.0 Abnormal involuntary movements

Abnormal head movements
Fasciculation
Spasms NOS
Tremor NOS

EXCLUDES *abnormal reflex (796.1)*
chorea NOS (333.5)
infantile spasms (345.60-345.61)
spastic paralysis (342.1, 343.0-344.9)
specified movement disorders classifiable to 333 (333.0-333.9)
that of nonorganic origin (307.2-307.3)

781.1 Disturbances of sensation of smell and taste

Anosmia
Parageusia
Parosmia

DEF: Anosmia: loss of sense of smell due to organic factors, including loss of olfactory nerve conductivity, cerebral disease, nasal fossae formation and peripheral olfactory nerve diseases; can also be psychological disorder.

DEF: Parageusia: distorted sense of taste, or bad taste in mouth.

DEF: Parosmia: distorted sense of smell.

781.2 Abnormality of gait

Gait:
ataxic
paralytic
Gait:
spastic
staggering

EXCLUDES *ataxia:*
NOS (781.3)
locomotor (progressive) (094.0)
difficulty in walking (719.7)

AHA: ▶2Q, '04, 15◀

DEF: Abnormal, asymmetric gait.

781.3 Lack of coordination

Ataxia NOS
Muscular incoordination

EXCLUDES *ataxic gait (781.2)*
cerebellar ataxia (334.0-334.9)
difficulty in walking (719.7)
vertigo NOS (780.4)

AHA: 4Q, '04, 51; 3Q, '97, 12

781.4 Transient paralysis of limb

Monoplegia, transient NOS

EXCLUDES *paralysis (342.0-344.9)*

781.5 Clubbing of fingers

DEF: Enlarged soft tissue of distal fingers.

781.6 Meningismus
Dupré's syndrome
Meningism
AHA: 3Q, '00, 13; J-F, '87, 7
DEF: Condition with signs and symptoms that resemble meningeal irritation; it is associated with febrile illness and dehydration with no evidence of infection.

781.7 Tetany
Carpopedal spasm
EXCLUDES *tetanus neonatorum (771.3)*
tetany:
hysterical (300.11)
newborn (hypocalcemic) (775.4)
parathyroid (252.1)
psychogenic (306.0)
DEF: Nerve and muscle hyperexcitability; symptoms include muscle spasms, twitching, cramps, laryngospasm with inspiratory stridor, hyperreflexia and choreiform movements.

781.8 Neurologic neglect syndrome
Asomatognosia
Hemi-akinesia
Hemi-inattention
Hemispatial neglect
Left-sided neglect
Sensory extinction
Sensory neglect
Visuospatial neglect
AHA: 4Q, '94, 37

✓5th **781.9 Other symptoms involving nervous and musculoskeletal systems**
AHA: 4Q, '00, 45

781.91 Loss of height
EXCLUDES *osteoporosis (733.00-733.09)*

781.92 Abnormal posture

781.93 Ocular torticollis
AHA: 4Q, '02, 68
DEF: Abnormal head posture as a result of a contracted state of cervical muscles to correct a visual disturbance; either double vision or a visual field defect.

781.94 Facial weakness
Facial droop
EXCLUDES *facial weakness due to late effect of cerebrovascular accident (438.83)*
AHA: 4Q, '03, 72

781.99 Other symptoms involving nervous and musculoskeletal systems

✓4th **782 Symptoms involving skin and other integumentary tissue**
EXCLUDES *symptoms relating to breast (611.71-611.79)*

782.0 Disturbance of skin sensation
Anesthesia of skin
Burning or prickling sensation
Hyperesthesia
Hypoesthesia
Numbness
Paresthesia
Tingling

782.1 Rash and other nonspecific skin eruption
Exanthem
EXCLUDES *vesicular eruption (709.8)*

782.2 Localized superficial swelling, mass, or lump
Subcutaneous nodules
EXCLUDES *localized adiposity (278.1)*

782.3 Edema
Anasarca
Dropsy
Localized edema NOS
EXCLUDES *ascites (789.5)*
edema of:
newborn NOS (778.5)
pregnancy (642.0-642.9, 646.1)
fluid retention (276.6)
hydrops fetalis (773.3, 778.0)
hydrothorax (511.8)
nutritional edema (260, 262)
AHA: 2Q, '00, 18
DEF: Edema: excess fluid in intercellular body tissue.
DEF: Anasarca: massive edema in all body tissues.
DEF: Dropsy: serous fluid accumulated in body cavity or cellular tissue.
DEF: Localized edema: edema in specific body areas.

782.4 Jaundice, unspecified, not of newborn
Cholemia NOS
Icterus NOS
EXCLUDES *jaundice in newborn (774.0-774.7)*
due to isoimmunization (773.0-773.2, 773.4)
DEF: Bilirubin deposits of skin, causing yellow cast.

782.5 Cyanosis
EXCLUDES *newborn (770.83)*
DEF: Deficient oxygen of blood; causes blue cast to skin.

✓5th **782.6 Pallor and flushing**

782.61 Pallor

782.62 Flushing
Excessive blushing

782.7 Spontaneous ecchymoses
Petechiae
EXCLUDES *ecchymosis in fetus or newborn (772.6)*
purpura (287.0-287.9)
DEF: Hemorrhagic spots of skin; resemble freckles.

782.8 Changes in skin texture
Induration } of skin
Thickening } of skin

782.9 Other symptoms involving skin and integumentary tissues

✓4th **783 Symptoms concerning nutrition, metabolism, and development**

783.0 Anorexia
Loss of appetite
EXCLUDES *anorexia nervosa (307.1)*
loss of appetite of nonorganic origin (307.59)

783.1 Abnormal weight gain
EXCLUDES *excessive weight gain in pregnancy (646.1)*
obesity (278.00)
morbid (278.01)

✓5th **783.2 Abnormal loss of weight and underweight**
▶Use additional code to identify Body Mass Index (BMI), if known (V85.0)◀
AHA: 4Q, '00, 45

783.21 Loss of weight

783.22 Underweight

783.3 Feeding difficulties and mismanagement
Feeding problem (elderly) (infant)
EXCLUDES *feeding disturbance or problems:*
in newborn (779.3)
of nonorganic origin (307.50-307.59)
AHA: 3Q, '97, 12

✓5th **783.4 Lack of expected normal physiological development in childhood**
EXCLUDES *delay in sexual development and puberty (259.0)*
gonadal dysgenesis (758.6)
pituitary dwarfism (253.3)
slow fetal growth and fetal malnutrition (764.00-764.99)
specific delays in mental development (315.0-315.9)
AHA: 4Q, '00, 45; 3Q, '97, 4

783.40 Lack of normal physiological development, unspecified
Inadequate development
Lack of development

783.41 Failure to thrive P
Failure to gain weight
AHA: 1Q, '03, 12
DEF: Organic failure to thrive: acute or chronic illness that interferes with nutritional intake, absorption, metabolism excretion and energy requirements. Nonorganic FTT is symptom of neglect or abuse.

Symptoms, Signs, and Ill-Defined Conditions 781.6–783.41

✓4th ✓5th Additional Digit Required | Unspecified Code | Other Specified Code | Manifestation Code | ▶◀ Revised Text | ● New Code | ▲ Revised Code Title

783.42 Delayed milestones P
Late talker
Late walker

783.43 Short stature
Growth failure
Growth retardation
Lack of growth
Physical retardation

DEF: Constitutional short stature: stature inconsistent with chronological age. Genetic short stature is when skeletal maturation matches chronological age.

783.5 Polydipsia
Excessive thirst

783.6 Polyphagia
Excessive eating
Hyperalimentation NOS

EXCLUDES *disorders of eating of nonorganic origin (307.50-307.59)*

783.7 Adult failure to thrive A

783.9 Other symptoms concerning nutrition, metabolism, and development
Hypometabolism

EXCLUDES *abnormal basal metabolic rate (794.7)*
dehydration ▶(276.51)◀
other disorders of fluid, electrolyte, and acid-base balance (276.0-276.9)

AHA: 2Q, '04, 3

✓4th **784 Symptoms involving head and neck**

EXCLUDES *encephalopathy NOS (348.30)*
specific symptoms involving neck classifiable to 723 (723.0-723.9)

784.0 Headache
Facial pain
Pain in head NOS

EXCLUDES *atypical face pain (350.2)*
migraine (346.0-346.9)
tension headache (307.81)

AHA: 3Q, '00, 13; 1Q, '90, 4; 3Q, '92, 14

784.1 Throat pain

EXCLUDES *dysphagia (787.2)*
neck pain (723.1)
sore throat (462)
chronic (472.1)

784.2 Swelling, mass, or lump in head and neck
Space-occupying lesion, intracranial NOS

AHA: 1Q, '03, 8

784.3 Aphasia

EXCLUDES *developmental aphasia (315.31)*

AHA: 4Q, '04, 78; 4Q. '98, 87; 3Q, '97, 12

DEF: Inability to communicate through speech, written word, or sign language.

✓5th **784.4 Voice disturbance**

784.40 Voice disturbance, unspecified

784.41 Aphonia
Loss of voice

784.49 Other
Change in voice
Dysphonia
Hoarseness
Hypernasality
Hyponasality

784.5 Other speech disturbance
Dysarthria
Dysphasia
Slurred speech

EXCLUDES *stammering and stuttering (307.0)*
that of nonorganic origin (307.0, 307.9)

✓5th **784.6 Other symbolic dysfunction**

EXCLUDES *developmental learning delays (315.0-315.9)*

784.60 Symbolic dysfunction, unspecified

784.61 Alexia and dyslexia
Alexia (with agraphia)

DEF: Alexia: inability to understand written word due to central brain lesion.

DEF: Dyslexia: ability to recognize letters but inability to read, spell, and write words; genetic.

784.69 Other
Acalculia
Agnosia
Agraphia NOS
Apraxia

784.7 Epistaxis
Hemorrhage from nose
Nosebleed

AHA: 3Q, '04, 7

784.8 Hemorrhage from throat

EXCLUDES *hemoptysis (786.3)*

784.9 Other symptoms involving head and neck
Choking sensation
Halitosis
Mouth breathing
Sneezing

✓4th **785 Symptoms involving cardiovascular system**

EXCLUDES *heart failure NOS (428.9)*

785.0 Tachycardia, unspecified
Rapid heart beat

EXCLUDES *neonatal tachycardia (779.82)*
paroxysmal tachycardia (427.0-427.2)

AHA: 2Q, '03, 11

DEF: Excessively rapid heart rate.

785.1 Palpitations
Awareness of heart beat

EXCLUDES *specified dysrhythmias (427.0-427.9)*

785.2 Undiagnosed cardiac murmurs
Heart murmurs NOS

AHA: 4Q, '92, 16

785.3 Other abnormal heart sounds
Cardiac dullness, increased or decreased
Friction fremitus, cardiac
Precordial friction

785.4 Gangrene
Gangrene:
NOS
spreading cutaneous
Gangrenous cellulitis
Phagedena
Code first any associated underlying condition

EXCLUDES *gangrene of certain sites — see Alphabetic Index*
gangrene with atherosclerosis of the extremities (440.24)
gas gangrene (040.0)

AHA: 1Q, '04, 14; 3Q, '91, 12; 3Q, '90, 15; M-A, '86, 12

DEF: Gangrene: necrosis of skin tissue due to bacterial infection, diabetes, embolus and vascular supply loss.

DEF: Gangrenous cellulitis: group A streptococcal infection; begins with severe cellulitis, spreads to superficial and deep fascia; produces gangrene of underlying tissues.

✓5th **785.5 Shock without mention of trauma**

785.50 Shock, unspecified
Failure of peripheral circulation

AHA: 2Q, '96, 10

DEF: Peripheral circulatory failure due to heart insufficiencies.

785.51 Cardiogenic shock

DEF: Shock syndrome: associated with myocardial infarction, cardiac tamponade and massive pulmonary embolism; symptoms include mental torpor, reduced blood pressure, tachycardia, pallor and cold, clammy skin.

785.52 Septic shock
Shock:
endotoxic
gram-negative
Code first:
systemic inflammatory response syndrome due to infectious process with organ dysfunction (995.92)
systemic inflammatory response syndrome due to noninfectious process with organ dysfunction (995.94)

AHA: 4Q, '03, 73, 79

785.59 Other

Shock:
hypovolemic

EXCLUDES *shock (due to):*
anesthetic (995.4)
anaphylactic (995.0)
due to serum (999.4)
electric (994.8)
following abortion (639.5)
lightning (994.0)
obstetrical (669.1)
postoperative (998.0)
traumatic (958.4)

AHA: 2Q, '00, 3

785.6 Enlargement of lymph nodes

Lymphadenopathy "Swollen glands"

EXCLUDES *lymphadenitis (chronic) (289.1-289.3)*
acute (683)

785.9 Other symptoms involving cardiovascular system

Bruit (arterial) Weak pulse

✓4th **786 Symptoms involving respiratory system and other chest symptoms**

✓5th **786.0 Dyspnea and respiratory abnormalities**

786.00 Respiratory abnormality, unspecified

786.01 Hyperventilation

EXCLUDES *hyperventilation, psychogenic (306.1)*

DEF: Rapid breathing causes carbon dioxide loss from blood.

786.02 Orthopnea

DEF: Difficulty breathing except in upright position.

786.03 Apnea

EXCLUDES *apnea of newborn (770.81, 770.82)*
sleep apnea (780.51, 780.53, 780.57)

AHA: 4Q, '98, 50

DEF: Cessation of breathing.

786.04 Cheyne-Stokes respiration

AHA: 4Q, '98, 50

DEF: Rhythmic increase of depth and frequency of breathing with apnea; occurs in frontal lobe and diencephalic dysfunction.

786.05 Shortness of breath

AHA: 4Q, '99, 25; 1Q, '99, 6; 4Q, '98, 50

DEF: Inability to take in sufficient oxygen.

786.06 Tachypnea

EXCLUDES *transitory tachypnea of newborn (770.6)*

AHA: 4Q, '98, 50

DEF: Abnormal rapid respiratory rate; called hyperventilation.

786.07 Wheezing

EXCLUDES *asthma (493.00-493.92)*

AHA: 4Q, '98, 50

DEF: Stenosis of respiratory passageway; causes whistling sound; due to asthma, coryza, croup, emphysema, hay fever, edema, and pleural effusion.

786.09 Other

EXCLUDES *respiratory distress:*
following trauma and surgery (518.5)
newborn (770.89)
syndrome (newborn) (769)
adult (518.5)
respiratory failure (518.81, 518.83-518.84)
newborn (770.84)

AHA: 2Q, '98, 10; 1Q, '97, 7; 1Q, '90, 9

786.1 Stridor

EXCLUDES *congenital laryngeal stridor (748.3)*

DEF: Obstructed airway causes harsh sound.

786.2 Cough

EXCLUDES *cough:*
psychogenic (306.1)
smokers' (491.0)
with hemorrhage (786.3)

AHA: 4Q, '99, 26

786.3 Hemoptysis

Cough with hemorrhage
Pulmonary hemorrhage NOS

EXCLUDES *pulmonary hemorrhage of newborn (770.3)*

AHA: 4Q, '90, 26

DEF: Coughing up blood or blood-stained sputum.

786.4 Abnormal sputum

Abnormal:
amount, color, odor (of) sputum
Excessive

✓5th **786.5 Chest pain**

786.50 Chest pain, unspecified

AHA: 1Q, '03, 6; 1Q, '02, 4; 4Q, '99, 25

786.51 Precordial pain

DEF: Chest pain over heart and lower thorax.

786.52 Painful respiration

Pain: Pleurodynia
anterior chest wall
pleuritic

EXCLUDES *epidemic pleurodynia (074.1)*

AHA: N-D, '84, 17

786.59 Other

Discomfort, Pressure, Tightness in chest

EXCLUDES *pain in breast (611.71)*

AHA: 1Q, '02, 6

786.6 Swelling, mass, or lump in chest

EXCLUDES *lump in breast (611.72)*

786.7 Abnormal chest sounds

Abnormal percussion, chest Rales
Friction sounds, chest Tympany, chest

EXCLUDES *wheezing (786.07)*

786.8 Hiccough

EXCLUDES *psychogenic hiccough (306.1)*

786.9 Other symptoms involving respiratory system and chest

Breath-holding spell

✓4th **787 Symptoms involving digestive system**

EXCLUDES *constipation (564.00-564.09)*
pylorospasm (537.81)
congenital (750.5)

✓5th **787.0 Nausea and vomiting**

Emesis

EXCLUDES *hematemesis NOS (578.0)*
vomiting:
bilious, following gastrointestinal surgery (564.3)
cyclical (536.2)
psychogenic (306.4)
excessive, in pregnancy (643.0-643.9)
habit (536.2)
of newborn (779.3)
psychogenic NOS (307.54)

AHA: M-A, '85, 11

787.01 Nausea with vomiting
AHA: 1Q, '03, 5

787.02 Nausea alone
AHA: 3Q, '00, 12; 2Q, '97, 9

787.03 Vomiting alone

787.1 Heartburn
Pyrosis Waterbrash
EXCLUDES *dyspepsia or indigestion (536.8)*
AHA: 2Q, '01, 6

787.2 Dysphagia
Difficulty in swallowing
AHA: 4Q, '03, 103, 109; 2Q, '01, 4

787.3 Flatulence, eructation, and gas pain
Abdominal distention (gaseous)
Bloating
Tympanites (abdominal) (intestinal)
EXCLUDES *aerophagy (306.4)*
DEF: Flatulence: excess air or gas in intestine or stomach.
DEF: Eructation: belching, expelling gas through mouth.
DEF: Gas pain: gaseous pressure affecting gastrointestinal system.

787.4 Visible peristalsis
Hyperperistalsis
DEF: Increase in involuntary movements of intestines.

787.5 Abnormal bowel sounds
Absent bowel sounds
Hyperactive bowel sounds

787.6 Incontinence of feces
Encopresis NOS
Incontinence of sphincter ani
EXCLUDES *that of nonorganic origin (307.7)*
AHA: 1Q, '97, 9

787.7 Abnormal feces
Bulky stools
EXCLUDES *abnormal stool content (792.1)*
melena:
NOS (578.1)
newborn (772.4, 777.3)

✓5th **787.9 Other symptoms involving digestive system**
EXCLUDES *gastrointestinal hemorrhage (578.0-578.9)*
intestinal obstruction (560.0-560.9)
specific functional digestive disorders:
esophagus (530.0-530.9)
stomach and duodenum (536.0-536.9)
those not elsewhere classified (564.00-564.9)

787.91 Diarrhea
Diarrhea NOS
AHA: 4Q, '95, 54

787.99 Other
Change in bowel habits Tenesmus (rectal)
DEF: Tenesmus: painful, ineffective straining at the rectum with limited passage of fecal matter.

✓4th **788 Symptoms involving urinary system**
EXCLUDES *hematuria (599.7)*
nonspecific findings on examination of the urine (791.0-791.9)
small kidney of unknown cause (589.0-589.9)
uremia NOS (586)

788.0 Renal colic
Colic (recurrent) of: kidney
Colic (recurrent) of: ureter
AHA: 3Q, '04, 8
DEF: Kidney pain.

788.1 Dysuria
Painful urination Strangury

✓5th **788.2 Retention of urine**
EXCLUDES ▶ *urinary retention due to hyperplasia of prostate (600.0-600.9 with fifth-digit 1)*◀
DEF: Inability to void.

788.20 Retention of urine, unspecified
AHA: 2Q, '04, 18; 3Q, '03, 12-13; 1Q, '03, 6; 3Q, '96, 10

788.21 Incomplete bladder emptying

788.29 Other specified retention of urine

✓5th **788.3 Urinary incontinence**
Code, if applicable, any causal condition first, such as:
congenital ureterocele (753.23)
genital prolapse (618.00-618.9)
EXCLUDES *that of nonorganic origin (307.6)*
AHA: 4Q, '92, 22

788.30 Urinary incontinence, unspecified
Enuresis NOS

788.31 Urge incontinence
AHA: 1Q, '00, 19
DEF: Inability to control urination, upon urge to urinate.

788.32 Stress incontinence, male ♂
EXCLUDES *stress incontinence, female (625.6)*
DEF: Inability to control urination associated with weak sphincter in males.

788.33 Mixed incontinence, (male) (female)
Urge and stress
DEF: Urge, stress incontinence: involuntary discharge of urine due to anatomic displacement.

788.34 Incontinence without sensory awareness
DEF: Involuntary discharge of urine without sensory warning.

788.35 Post-void dribbling
DEF: Involuntary discharge of residual urine after voiding.

788.36 Nocturnal enuresis
DEF: Involuntary discharge of urine during the night.

788.37 Continuous leakage
DEF: Continuous, involuntary urine seepage.

788.38 Overflow incontinence
DEF: Leakage caused by pressure of retained urine in the bladder after the bladder has fully contracted due to weakened bladder muscles or an obstruction of the urethra.

788.39 Other urinary incontinence

✓5th **788.4 Frequency of urination and polyuria**

788.41 Urinary frequency
Frequency of micturition

788.42 Polyuria
DEF: Excessive urination.

788.43 Nocturia
DEF: Urination affecting sleep patterns.

788.5 Oliguria and anuria
Deficient secretion of urine
Suppression of urinary secretion
EXCLUDES *that complicating:*
abortion (634-638 with .3, 639.3)
ectopic or molar pregnancy (639.3)
pregnancy, childbirth, or the puerperium (642.0-642.9, 646.2)
DEF: Oliguria: diminished urinary secretion related to fluid intake.
DEF: Anuria: lack of urinary secretion due to renal failure or obstructed urinary tract.

✓5th **788.6 Other abnormality of urination**

788.61 Splitting of urinary stream
Intermittent urinary stream

788.62 Slowing of urinary stream
Weak stream

788.63 Urgency of urination
EXCLUDES *urge incontinence (788.31, 788.33)*
AHA: 4Q, '03, 74
DEF: Feeling of intense need to urinate; abrupt sensation of imminent urination.

N Newborn Age: 0 P Pediatric Age: 0-17 M Maternity Age: 12-55 A Adult Age: 15-124 MSP Medicare Secondary Payer

788.69 Other

788.7 Urethral discharge
Penile discharge
Urethrorrhea

788.8 Extravasation of urine
DEF: Leaking or infiltration of urine into tissues.

788.9 Other symptoms involving urinary system
Extrarenal uremia
Vesical:
pain
Vesical:
tenesmus
AHA: ▶1Q, '05, 12◀ 4Q, '88, 1

✓4th **789 Other symptoms involving abdomen and pelvis**
EXCLUDES *symptoms referable to genital organs:*
female (625.0-625.9)
male (607.0-608.9)
psychogenic (302.70-302.79)

The following fifth-digit subclassification is to be used for codes 789.0, 789.3, 789.4, 789.6:
0 unspecified site
1 right upper quadrant
2 left upper quadrant
3 right lower quadrant
4 left lower quadrant
5 periumbilic
6 epigastric
7 generalized
9 other specified site
Multiple sites

✓5th **789.0 Abdominal pain**
Colic:
NOS
infantile
Cramps, abdominal
EXCLUDES *renal colic (788.0)*
AHA: 1Q, '95, 3; For code 789.06: 1Q, '02, 5

789.1 Hepatomegaly
Enlargement of liver

789.2 Splenomegaly
Enlargement of spleen

✓5th **789.3 Abdominal or pelvic swelling, mass, or lump**
Diffuse or generalized swelling or mass:
abdominal NOS
umbilical
EXCLUDES *abdominal distention (gaseous) (787.3)*
ascites (789.5)

✓5th **789.4 Abdominal rigidity**

789.5 Ascites
Fluid in peritoneal cavity
AHA: 4Q, '89, 11
DEF: Serous fluid effusion and accumulation in abdominal cavity.

✓5th **789.6 Abdominal tenderness**
Rebound tenderness

789.9 Other symptoms involving abdomen and pelvis
Umbilical:
bleeding
Umbilical:
discharge

NONSPECIFIC ABNORMAL FINDINGS (790-796)

AHA: 2Q, '90, 16

✓4th **790 Nonspecific findings on examination of blood**
EXCLUDES *abnormality of:*
platelets (287.0-287.9)
thrombocytes (287.0-287.9)
white blood cells (288.0-288.9)

✓5th **790.0 Abnormality of red blood cells**
EXCLUDES *anemia:*
congenital (776.5)
newborn, due to isoimmunization (773.0-773.2, 773.5)
of premature infant (776.6)
other specified types (280.0-285.9)
hemoglobin disorders (282.5-282.7)
polycythemia:
familial (289.6)
neonatorum (776.4)
secondary (289.0)
vera (238.4)
AHA: 4Q, '00, 46

790.01 Precipitous drop in hematocrit
Drop in hematocrit

790.09 Other abnormality of red blood cells
Abnormal red cell morphology NOS
Abnormal red cell volume NOS
Anisocytosis
Poikilocytosis

790.1 Elevated sedimentation rate

✓5th **790.2 Abnormal glucose**
EXCLUDES *diabetes mellitus (250.00-250.93)*
dysmetabolic syndrome X (277.7)
gestational diabetes (648.8)
glycosuria (791.5)
hypoglycemia (251.2)
that complicating pregnancy, childbirth, or puerperium (648.8)
AHA: 4Q, '03, 74; 3Q, '91, 5

790.21 Impaired fasting glucose
Elevated fasting glucose

790.22 Impaired glucose tolerance test (oral)
Elevated glucose tolerance test

790.29 Other abnormal glucose
Abnormal glucose NOS
Abnormal non-fasting glucose
Pre-diabetes NOS

790.3 Excessive blood level of alcohol
Elevated blood-alcohol
AHA: S-O, '86, 3

790.4 Nonspecific elevation of levels of transaminase or lactic acid dehydrogenase [LDH]

790.5 Other nonspecific abnormal serum enzyme levels
Abnormal serum level of:
acid phosphatase
alkaline phosphatase
amylase
lipase
EXCLUDES *deficiency of circulating enzymes (277.6)*

790.6 Other abnormal blood chemistry
Abnormal blood level of:
cobalt
copper
iron
lithium
Abnormal blood level of:
magnesium
mineral
zinc
EXCLUDES *abnormality of electrolyte or acid-base balance (276.0-276.9)*
hypoglycemia NOS (251.2)
specific finding indicating abnormality of:
amino-acid transport and metabolism (270.0-270.9)
carbohydrate transport and metabolism (271.0-271.9)
lipid metabolism (272.0-272.9)
uremia NOS (586)
AHA: 4Q, '88, 1

790.7 Bacteremia
EXCLUDES *bacteremia of newborn (771.83)*
septicemia (038)
Use additional code to identify organism (041)
AHA: 2Q, '03, 7; 4Q, '93, 29; 3Q, '88, 12
DEF: Laboratory finding of bacteria in the blood in the absence of two or more signs of sepsis; transient in nature, progresses to septicemia with severe infectious process.

790.8 Viremia, unspecified
AHA: 4Q, '88, 10
DEF: Presence of a virus in the blood stream.

✓5th **790.9 Other nonspecific findings on examination of blood**
AHA: 4Q, '93, 29

790.91 Abnormal arterial blood gases

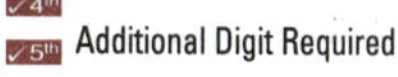
Additional Digit Required | Unspecified Code | Other Specified Code | Manifestation Code | ▶◀ Revised Text | ● New Code | ▲ Revised Code Title

790.92 Abnormal coagulation profile
Abnormal or prolonged:
bleeding time
coagulation time
partial thromboplastin time [PTT]
prothrombintime [PT]
EXCLUDES *coagulation (hemorrhagic) disorders (286.0-286.9)*

790.93 Elevated prostate specific antigen, (PSA) A ♂

790.94 Euthyroid sick syndrome
AHA: 4Q, '97, 45
DEF: Transient alteration of thyroid hormone metabolism due to nonthyroid illness or stress.

790.95 Elevated C-reactive protein (CRP)
DEF: Inflammation in an arterial wall results in elevated C-reactive protein (CRP) in the blood; CRP is a recognized risk factor in cardiovascular disease.

790.99 Other
AHA: 2Q, '03, 14

✓4th **791 Nonspecific findings on examination of urine**
EXCLUDES *hematuria NOS (599.7)*
specific findings indicating abnormality of:
amino-acid transport and metabolism (270.0-270.9)
carbohydrate transport and metabolism (271.0-271.9)

791.0 Proteinuria
Albuminuria
Bence-Jones proteinuria
EXCLUDES *postural proteinuria (593.6)*
that arising during pregnancy or the puerperium (642.0-642.9, 646.2)
AHA: 3Q, '91, 8
DEF: Excess protein in urine.

791.1 Chyluria
EXCLUDES *filarial (125.0-125.9)*
DEF: Excess chyle in urine.

791.2 Hemoglobinuria
DEF: Free hemoglobin in blood due to rapid hemolysis of red blood cells.

791.3 Myoglobinuria
DEF: Myoglobin (oxygen-transporting pigment) in urine.

791.4 Biliuria
DEF: Bile pigments in urine.

791.5 Glycosuria
EXCLUDES *renal glycosuria (271.4)*
DEF: Sugar in urine.

791.6 Acetonuria
Ketonuria
DEF: Excess acetone in urine.

791.7 Other cells and casts in urine

791.9 Other nonspecific findings on examination of urine
Crystalluria
Elevated urine levels of:
17-ketosteroids
catecholamines
indolacetic acid
Elevated urine levels of:
vanillylmandelic acid [VMA]
Melanuria
AHA: ▶1Q, '05, 12◀

✓4th **792 Nonspecific abnormal findings in other body substances**
EXCLUDES *that in chromosomal analysis (795.2)*

792.0 Cerebrospinal fluid

792.1 Stool contents
Abnormal stool color
Fat in stool
Mucus in stool
Occult stool
Pus in stool
EXCLUDES *blood in stool [melena] (578.1)*
newborn (772.4, 777.3)
AHA: 2Q, '92, 9

792.2 Semen ♂
Abnormal spermatozoa
EXCLUDES *azoospermia (606.0)*
oligospermia (606.1)

792.3 Amniotic fluid M ♀
AHA: N-D, '86, 4
DEF: Nonspecific abnormal findings in amniotic fluid.

792.4 Saliva
EXCLUDES *that in chromosomal analysis (795.2)*

792.5 Cloudy (hemodialysis) (peritoneal) dialysis effluent

792.9 Other nonspecific abnormal findings in body substances
Peritoneal fluid
Pleural fluid
Synovial fluid
Vaginal fluids

✓4th **793 Nonspecific abnormal findings on radiological and other examination of body structure**
INCLUDES nonspecific abnormal findings of:
thermography
ultrasound examination [echogram]
x-ray examination
EXCLUDES *abnormal results of function studies and radioisotope scans (794.0-794.9)*

793.0 Skull and head
EXCLUDES *nonspecific abnormal echoencephalogram (794.01)*

793.1 Lung field
Coin lesion } (of) lung
Shadow } (of) lung
DEF: Coin lesion of lung: coin-shaped, solitary pulmonary nodule.

793.2 Other intrathoracic organ
Abnormal:
echocardiogram
heart shadow
Abnormal:
ultrasound cardiogram
Mediastinal shift

793.3 Biliary tract
Nonvisualization of gallbladder

793.4 Gastrointestinal tract

793.5 Genitourinary organs
Filling defect:
bladder
kidney
Filling defect:
ureter
AHA: 4Q, '00, 46

793.6 Abdominal area, including retroperitoneum

793.7 Musculoskeletal system

✓5th **793.8 Breast**
AHA: 4Q, '01, 51

793.80 Abnormal mammogram, unspecified

793.81 Mammographic microcalcification
DEF: Calcium and cellular debris deposits in the breast that can't be felt but are detected on a mammogram; can be a sign of cancer, benign conditions, or changes in the breast tissue as a result of inflammation, injury, or obstructed duct.

793.89 Other abnormal findings on radiological examination of breast

793.9 Other
Abnormal:
placental finding by x-ray or ultrasound method
radiological findings in skin and subcutaneous tissue
EXCLUDES *abnormal finding by radioisotope localization of placenta (794.9)*

✓4th **794 Nonspecific abnormal results of function studies**
INCLUDES radioisotope:
scans
uptake studies
scintiphotography

✓5th **794.0 Brain and central nervous system**

794.00 Abnormal function study, unspecified

794.01 Abnormal echoencephalogram

794.02 Abnormal electroencephalogram [EEG]

N Newborn Age: 0 P Pediatric Age: 0-17 M Maternity Age: 12-55 A Adult Age: 15-124 MSP Medicare Secondary Payer

794.09 **Other**
Abnormal brain scan

✓5th **794.1 Peripheral nervous system and special senses**

794.10 **Abnormal response to nerve stimulation, unspecified**

794.11 **Abnormal retinal function studies**
Abnormal electroretinogram [ERG]

794.12 **Abnormal electro-oculogram [EOG]**

794.13 **Abnormal visually evoked potential**

794.14 **Abnormal oculomotor studies**

794.15 **Abnormal auditory function studies**
AHA: 1Q, '04, 15-16

794.16 **Abnormal vestibular function studies**

794.17 **Abnormal electromyogram [EMG]**
EXCLUDES *that of eye (794.14)*

794.19 **Other**

794.2 Pulmonary
Abnormal lung scan
Reduced:
ventilatory capacity
Reduced:
vital capacity

✓5th **794.3 Cardiovascular**

794.30 **Abnormal function study, unspecified**

794.31 **Abnormal electrocardiogram [ECG] [EKG]**
EXCLUDES ▶ *long QT syndrome (426.82)*◀

794.39 **Other**
Abnormal:
ballistocardiogram
phonocardiogram
Abnormal:
vectorcardiogram

794.4 Kidney
Abnormal renal function test

794.5 Thyroid
Abnormal thyroid:
scan
Abnormal thyroid:
uptake

794.6 Other endocrine function study

794.7 Basal metabolism
Abnormal basal metabolic rate [BMR]

794.8 Liver
Abnormal liver scan

794.9 Other
Bladder
Pancreas
Placenta
Spleen

✓4th **795 Other and nonspecific abnormal cytological, histological, immunological and DNA test findings**
EXCLUDES *nonspecific abnormalities of red blood cells (790.01-790.09)*

✓5th **795.0 Abnormal Papanicolaou smear of cervix and cervical HPV**
Abnormal thin preparation smear of cervix
Abnormal cervical cytology
EXCLUDES *carcinoma in-situ of cervix (233.1)*
cervical intraepithelial neoplasia I (CIN I) (622.11)
cervical intraepithelial neoplasia II (CIN II) (622.12)
cervical intraepithelial neoplasia III (CIN III) (233.1)
dysplasia (histologically confirmed) of cervix (uteri) NOS (622.10)
mild dysplasia (histologically confirmed) (622.11)
moderate dysplasia (histologically confirmed) (622.12)
severe dysplasia (histologically confirmed) (233.1)
AHA: 4Q, '02, 69

795.00 **Abnormal glandular Papanicolaou smear of cervix** ♀
Atypical endocervical cells NOS
Atypical endometrial cells NOS
Atypical glandular cells NOS

795.01 **Papanicolaou smear of cervix with atypical squamous cells of undetermined significance (ASC-US)** ♀

795.02 **Papanicolaou smear of cervix with atypical squamous cells cannot exclude high grade squamous intraepithelial lesion (ASC-H)** ♀

795.03 **Papanicolaou smear of cervix with low grade squamous intraepithelial lesion (LGSIL)** ♀

795.04 **Papanicolaou smear of cervix with high grade squamous intraepithelial lesion (HGSIL)** ♀
Cytologic evidence of carcinoma

795.05 **Cervical high risk human papillomavirus (HPV) DNA test positive** ♀

795.08 **Unsatisfactory smear** ♀
Inadequate sample

795.09 **Other abnormal Papanicolaou smear of cervix and cervical HPV** ♀
▶Cervical low risk human papillomavirus (HPV) DNA test positive◀
Use additional code for associated human papillomavirus (079.4)
EXCLUDES *encounter for Papanicolaou cervical smear to confirm findings of recent normal smear following initial abnormal smear (V72.32)*

795.1 Nonspecific abnormal Papanicolaou smear of other site

795.2 Nonspecific abnormal findings on chromosomal analysis
Abnormal karyotype

✓5th **795.3 Nonspecific positive culture findings**
Positive culture findings in:
nose
sputum
throat
wound
EXCLUDES *that of:*
blood (790.7-790.8)
urine (791.9)

795.31 **Nonspecific positive findings for anthrax**
Positive findings by nasal swab
AHA: 4Q, '02, 70

795.39 **Other nonspecific positive culture findings**

795.4 Other nonspecific abnormal histological findings

795.5 Nonspecific reaction to tuberculin skin test without active tuberculosis
Abnormal result of Mantoux test
PPD positive
Tuberculin (skin test):
positive
reactor

795.6 False positive serological test for syphilis
False positive Wassermann reaction

✓5th **795.7 Other nonspecific immunological findings**
EXCLUDES *isoimmunization, in pregnancy (656.1-656.2)*
affecting fetus or newborn (773.0-773.2)
AHA: 2Q, '93, 6

795.71 Nonspecific serologic evidence of human immunodeficiency virus [HIV]

Inclusive human immunodeficiency [HIV] test (adult) (infant)

Note: This code is ONLY to be used when a test finding is reported as nonspecific. Asymptomatic positive findings are coded to V08. If any HIV infection symptom or condition is present, see code 042. Negative findings are not coded.

EXCLUDES *acquired immunodeficiency syndrome [AIDS] (042)*
asymptomatic human immunodeficiency virus, [HIV] infection status (V08)
HIV infection, symptomatic (042)
human immunodeficiency virus [HIV] disease (042)
positive (status) NOS (V08)

AHA: 2Q, '04, 11; 1Q, '93, 21; 1Q, '93, 22; 2Q, '92, 11; J-A, '87, 24

795.79 Other and unspecified nonspecific immunological findings

Raised antibody titer
Raised level of immunoglobulins

✓4th **796 Other nonspecific abnormal findings**

796.0 Nonspecific abnormal toxicological findings

Abnormal levels of heavy metals or drugs in blood, urine, or other tissue

EXCLUDES *excessive blood level of alcohol (790.3)*

AHA: 1Q, '97, 16

796.1 Abnormal reflex

796.2 Elevated blood pressure reading without diagnosis of hypertension

Note: This category is to be used to record an episode of elevated blood pressure in a patient in whom no formal diagnosis of hypertension has been made, or as an incidental finding.

AHA: 2Q, '03, 11; 3Q, '90, 4; J-A, '84, 12

796.3 Nonspecific low blood pressure reading

796.4 Other abnormal clinical findings

AHA: 1Q, '97, 16

796.5 Abnormal finding on antenatal screening M ♀

AHA: 4Q, '97, 46

796.6 Abnormal findings on neonatal screening N

EXCLUDES *nonspecific serologic evidence of human immunodeficiency virus [HIV] (795.71)*

AHA: ▶4Q, '04, 99◀

796.9 Other

ILL-DEFINED AND UNKNOWN CAUSES OF MORBIDITY AND MORTALITY (797-799)

797 Senility without mention of psychosis

Old age
Senescence
Senile asthenia
Senile:
debility
exhaustion

EXCLUDES *senile psychoses (290.0-290.9)*

✓4th **798 Sudden death, cause unknown**

798.0 Sudden infant death syndrome P

Cot death
Crib death
Sudden death of nonspecific cause in infancy

DEF: Sudden Infant Death Syndrome (SIDS): death of infant under age one due to nonspecific cause.

798.1 Instantaneous death

798.2 Death occurring in less than 24 hours from onset of symptoms, not otherwise explained

Death known not to be violent or instantaneous, for which no cause could be discovered
Died without sign of disease

798.9 Unattended death

Death in circumstances where the body of the deceased was found and no cause could be discovered
Found dead

✓4th **799 Other ill-defined and unknown causes of morbidity and mortality**

DEF: Weakened organ functions due to complex chronic medical conditions.

▲ ✓5th **799.0 Asphyxia and hypoxemia**

EXCLUDES ▶*asphyxia and hypoxemia*◀ *(due to):*
carbon monoxide (986)
▶*hypercapnia (786.09)*◀
inhalation of food or foreign body (932-934.9)
newborn (768.0-768.9)
traumatic (994.7)

DEF: Lack of oxygen.

● **799.01 Asphyxia**

● **799.02 Hypoxemia**

799.1 Respiratory arrest

Cardiorespiratory failure

EXCLUDES *cardiac arrest (427.5)*
failure of peripheral circulation (785.50)
respiratory distress:
NOS (786.09)
acute (518.82)
following trauma and surgery (518.5)
newborn (770.89)
syndrome (newborn) (769)
adult (following trauma and surgery) (518.5)
other (518.82)
respiratory failure (518.81, 518.83-518.84)
newborn (770.84)
respiratory insufficiency (786.09)
acute (518.82)

799.2 Nervousness

"Nerves"

799.3 Debility, unspecified

EXCLUDES *asthenia (780.79)*
nervous debility (300.5)
neurasthenia (300.5)
senile asthenia (797)

799.4 Cachexia

Wasting disease

EXCLUDES *nutritional marasmus (261)*

AHA: 3Q, '90, 17

✓5th **799.8 Other ill-defined conditions**

799.81 Decreased libido A

Decreased sexual desire

EXCLUDES *psychosexual dysfunction with inhibited sexual desire (302.71)*

AHA: 4Q, '03, 75

799.89 Other ill-defined conditions

DEF: General ill health and poor nutrition.

799.9 Other unknown and unspecified cause

Undiagnosed disease, not specified as to site or system involved
Unknown cause of morbidity or mortality

AHA: 1Q, '98,.4; 1Q, '90, 20

N Newborn Age: 0 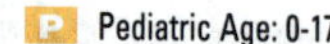 P Pediatric Age: 0-17 M Maternity Age: 12-55 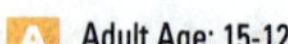 A Adult Age: 15-124 MSP Medicare Secondary Payer

17. INJURY AND POISONING (800-999)

Use E code(s) to identify the cause and intent of the injury or poisoning (E800-E999)

Note:

1. The principle of multiple coding of injuries should be followed wherever possible. Combination categories for multiple injuries are provided for use when there is insufficient detail as to the nature of the individual conditions, or for primary tabulation purposes when it is more convenient to record a single code; otherwise, the component injuries should be coded separately.

   Where multiple sites of injury are specified in the titles, the word "with" indicates involvement of both sites, and the word "and" indicates involvement of either or both sites. The word "finger" thumb.

2. Categories for "late effect" of injuries are to be found at 905-909.

FRACTURES (800-829)

EXCLUDES *malunion (733.81)*
nonunion (733.82)
pathological or spontaneous fracture (733.10-733.19)
stress fractures (733.93-733.95)

The terms "condyle," "coronoid process," "ramus," and "symphysis" indicate the portion of the bone fractured, not the name of the bone involved.

The descriptions "closed" and "open" used in the fourth-digit subdivisions include the following terms:

closed (with or without delayed healing):
comminuted
depressed
elevated
fissured
fracture NOS
greenstick
impacted
linear
simple
slipped epiphysis
spiral

open (with or without delayed healing):
compound
infected
missile
puncture
with foreign body

A fracture not indicated as closed or open should be classified as closed.

AHA: 4Q, '90, 26; 3Q, '90, 5; 3Q, '90, 13; 2Q, '90, 7; 2Q, '89, 15, S-O, '85, 3

FRACTURE OF SKULL (800-804)

The following fifth-digit subclassification is for use with the appropriate codes in categories 800, 801, 803, and 804:

0 unspecified state of consciousness
1 with no loss of consciousness
2 with brief [less than one hour] loss of consciousness
3 with moderate [1-24 hours] loss of consciousness
4 with prolonged [more than 24 hours] loss of consciousness and return to pre-existing conscious level
5 with prolonged [more than 24 hours] loss of consciousness, without return to pre-existing conscious level
Use fifth-digit 5 to designate when a patient is unconscious and dies before regaining consciousness, regardless of the duration of the loss of consciousness
6 with loss of consciousness of unspecified duration
9 with concussion, unspecified

✓4th **800 Fracture of vault of skull**
INCLUDES frontal bone
parietal bone

AHA: 4Q,'96, 36

DEF: Fracture of bone that forms skull dome and protects brain.

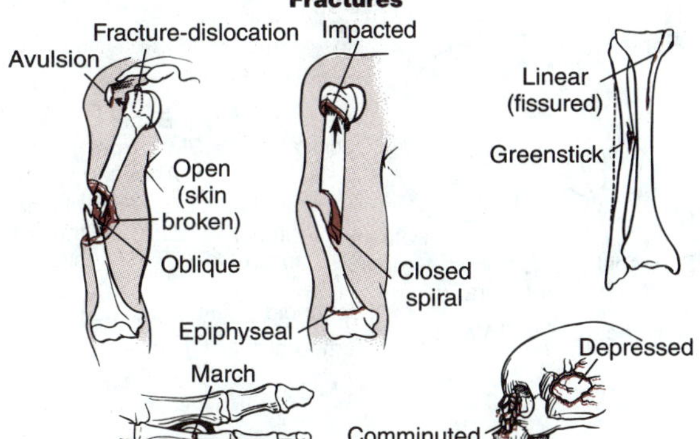

✓5th **800.0 Closed without mention of intracranial injury** MSP
✓5th **800.1 Closed with cerebral laceration and contusion** MSP
✓5th **800.2 Closed with subarachnoid, subdural, and extradural hemorrhage** MSP
✓5th **800.3 Closed with other and unspecified intracranial hemorrhage** MSP
✓5th **800.4 Closed with intracranial injury of other and unspecified nature** MSP
✓5th **800.5 Open without mention of intracranial injury** MSP
✓5th **800.6 Open with cerebral laceration and contusion** MSP
✓5th **800.7 Open with subarachnoid, subdural, and extradural hemorrhage** MSP
✓5th **800.8 Open with other and unspecified intracranial hemorrhage** MSP
✓5th **800.9 Open with intracranial injury of other and unspecified nature** MSP

✓4th **801 Fracture of base of skull**
INCLUDES fossa:
anterior
middle
posterior
occiput bone
orbital roof
sinus:
ethmoid
frontal
sphenoid bone
temporal bone

AHA: 4Q, '96, 36

DEF: Fracture of bone that forms skull floor.

✓5th **801.0 Closed without mention of intracranial injury** MSP
✓5th **801.1 Closed with cerebral laceration and contusion** MSP
✓5th **801.2 Closed with subarachnoid, subdural, and extradural hemorrhage** MSP
AHA: 4Q, '96, 36
✓5th **801.3 Closed with other and unspecified intracranial hemorrhage** MSP
✓5th **801.4 Closed with intracranial injury of other and unspecified nature** MSP
✓5th **801.5 Open without mention of intracranial injury** MSP
✓5th **801.6 Open with cerebral laceration and contusion** MSP
✓5th **801.7 Open with subarachnoid, subdural, and extradural hemorrhage** MSP
✓5th **801.8 Open with other and unspecified intracranial hemorrhage** MSP
✓5th **801.9 Open with intracranial injury of other and unspecified nature** MSP

✓4th **802 Fracture of face bones**
AHA: 4Q, '96, 36

802.0 Nasal bones, closed MSP

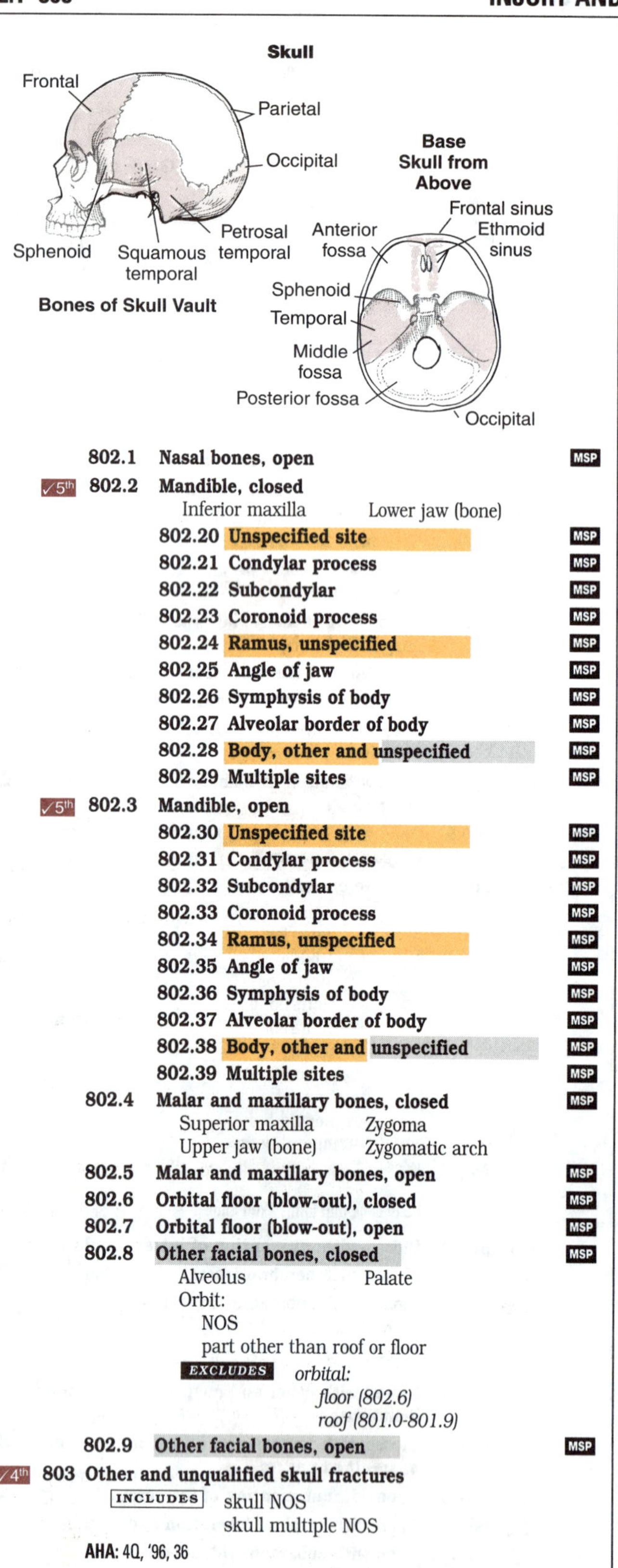

Facial Fractures
Frontal bone
Nasal bone
LeFort Fracture Types
Type III
Orbital floor
Zygomatic bone (malar) and arch
Type II
Type I
Maxilla
Subcondylar
Body
Angle
Symphysis
Parasymphysis
Common Fracture Sites of Mandible

802.1 **Nasal bones, open** MSP

✓5th 802.2 **Mandible, closed**
Inferior maxilla
Lower jaw (bone)

802.20 **Unspecified site** MSP
802.21 **Condylar process** MSP
802.22 **Subcondylar** MSP
802.23 **Coronoid process** MSP
802.24 **Ramus, unspecified** MSP
802.25 **Angle of jaw** MSP
802.26 **Symphysis of body** MSP
802.27 **Alveolar border of body** MSP
802.28 **Body, other and unspecified** MSP
802.29 **Multiple sites** MSP

✓5th 802.3 **Mandible, open**

802.30 **Unspecified site** MSP
802.31 **Condylar process** MSP
802.32 **Subcondylar** MSP
802.33 **Coronoid process** MSP
802.34 **Ramus, unspecified** MSP
802.35 **Angle of jaw** MSP
802.36 **Symphysis of body** MSP
802.37 **Alveolar border of body** MSP
802.38 **Body, other and unspecified** MSP
802.39 **Multiple sites** MSP

802.4 **Malar and maxillary bones, closed** MSP
Superior maxilla
Upper jaw (bone)
Zygoma
Zygomatic arch

802.5 **Malar and maxillary bones, open** MSP
802.6 **Orbital floor (blow-out), closed** MSP
802.7 **Orbital floor (blow-out), open** MSP
802.8 **Other facial bones, closed** MSP
Alveolus
Orbit:
NOS
part other than roof or floor
Palate

EXCLUDES *orbital:*
floor (802.6)
roof (801.0-801.9)

802.9 **Other facial bones, open** MSP

✓4th 803 **Other and unqualified skull fractures**

INCLUDES skull NOS
skull multiple NOS

AHA: 4Q, '96, 36

§ ✓5th 803.0 **Closed without mention of intracranial injury** MSP
§ ✓5th 803.1 **Closed with cerebral laceration and contusion** MSP
§ ✓5th 803.2 **Closed with subarachnoid, subdural, and extradural hemorrhage** MSP
§ ✓5th 803.3 **Closed with other and unspecified intracranial hemorrhage** MSP
§ ✓5th 803.4 **Closed with intracranial injury of other and unspecified nature** MSP
§ ✓5th 803.5 **Open without mention of intracranial injury** MSP
§ ✓5th 803.6 **Open with cerebral laceration and contusion** MSP
§ ✓5th 803.7 **Open with subarachnoid, subdural, and extradural hemorrhage** MSP
§ ✓5th 803.8 **Open with other and unspecified intracranial hemorrhage** MSP
§ ✓5th 803.9 **Open with intracranial injury of other and unspecified nature** MSP

✓4th 804 **Multiple fractures involving skull or face with other bones**

AHA: 4Q, '96, 36

§ ✓5th 804.0 **Closed without mention of intracranial injury** MSP
§ ✓5th 804.1 **Closed with cerebral laceration and contusion** MSP
§ ✓5th 804.2 **Closed with subarachnoid, subdural, and extradural hemorrhage** MSP
§ ✓5th 804.3 **Closed with other and unspecified intracranial hemorrhage** MSP
§ ✓5th 804.4 **Closed with intracranial injury of other and unspecified nature** MSP
§ ✓5th 804.5 **Open without mention of intracranial injury** MSP
§ ✓5th 804.6 **Open with cerebral laceration and contusion** MSP
§ ✓5th 804.7 **Open with subarachnoid, subdural, and extradural hemorrage** MSP
§ ✓5th 804.8 **Open with other and unspecified intracranial hemorrhage** MSP
§ ✓5th 804.9 **Open with intracranial injury of other and unspecified nature** MSP

FRACTURE OF NECK AND TRUNK (805-809)

✓4th 805 **Fracture of vertebral column without mention of spinal cord injury**

INCLUDES neural arch
spine
spinous process
transverse process
vertebra

The following fifth-digit subclassification is for use with codes 805.0-805.1:

0 **cervical vertebra, unspecified level**
1 **first cervical vertebra**
2 **second cervical vertebra**
3 **third cervical vertebra**
4 **fourth cervical vertebra**
5 **fifth cervical vertebra**
6 **sixth cervical vertebra**
7 **seventh cervical vertebra**
8 **multiple cervical vertebrae**

§ Requires fifth-digit. See beginning of section 800–804 for codes and definitions.

✓5th **805.0 Cervical, closed** MSP
Atlas Axis

✓5th **805.1 Cervical, open** MSP

805.2 Dorsal [thoracic], closed MSP

805.3 Dorsal [thoracic], open MSP

805.4 Lumbar, closed MSP
AHA: 4Q, '99, 12

805.5 Lumbar, open MSP

805.6 Sacrum and coccyx, closed MSP

805.7 Sacrum and coccyx, open MSP

805.8 Unspecified, closed MSP

805.9 Unspecified, open MSP

✓4th **806 Fracture of vertebral column with spinal cord injury**

INCLUDES any condition classifiable to 805 with:
- complete or incomplete transverse lesion (of cord)
- hematomyelia
- injury to:
  - cauda equina
  - nerve
- paralysis
- paraplegia
- quadriplegia
- spinal concussion

✓5th **806.0 Cervical, closed**

806.00 C_1-C_4 level with unspecified spinal cord injury MSP
Cervical region NOS with spinal cord injury NOS

806.01 C_1-C_4 level with complete lesion of cord MSP

806.02 C_1-C_4 level with anterior cord syndrome MSP

806.03 C_1-C_4 level with central cord syndrome MSP

806.04 C_1-C_4 level with other specified spinal cord injury MSP
C_1-C_4 level with:
- incomplete spinal cord lesion NOS
- posterior cord syndrome

806.05 C_5-C_7 level with unspecified spinal cord injury MSP

806.06 C_5-C_7 level with complete lesion of cord MSP

806.07 C_5-C_7 level with anterior cord syndrome MSP

806.08 C_5-C_7 level with central cord syndrome MSP

806.09 C_5-C_7 level with other specified spinal cord injury MSP
C_5-C_7 level with:
- incomplete spinal cord lesion NOS
- posterior cord syndrome

✓5th **806.1 Cervical, open**

806.10 C_1-C_4 level with unspecified spinal cord injury MSP

806.11 C_1-C_4 level with complete lesion of cord MSP

806.12 C_1-C_4 level with anterior cord syndrome MSP

806.13 C_1-C_4 level with central cord syndrome MSP

806.14 C_1-C_4 level with other specified spinal cord injury MSP
C_1-C_4 level with:
- incomplete spinal cord lesion NOS
- posterior cord syndrome

Vertebral Column

806.15 C_5-C_7 level with unspecified spinal cord injury MSP

806.16 C_5-C_7 level with complete lesion of cord MSP

806.17 C_5-C_7 level with anterior cord syndrome MSP

806.18 C_5-C_7 level with central cord syndrome MSP

806.19 C_5-C_7 level with other specified spinal cord injury MSP
C_5-C_7 level with:
- incomplete spinal cord lesion NOS
- posterior cord syndrome

✓5th **806.2 Dorsal [thoracic], closed**

806.20 T_1-T_6 level with unspecified spinal cord injury MSP
Thoracic region NOS with spinal cord injury NOS

806.21 T_1-T_6 level with complete lesion of cord MSP

806.22 T_1-T_6 level with anterior cord syndrome MSP

806.23 T_1-T_6 level with central cord syndrome MSP

806.24 T_1-T_6 level with other specified spinal cord injury MSP
T_1-T_6 level with:
- incomplete spinal cord lesion NOS
- posterior cord syndrome

806.25 T_7-T_{12} level with unspecified spinal cord injury MSP

806.26 T_7-T_{12} level with complete lesion of cord MSP

806.27 T_7-T_{12} level with anterior cord syndrome MSP

806.28 T_7-T_{12} level with central cord syndrome MSP

806.29 **T_7-T_{12} level with other specified spinal cord injury** MSP
T_7-T_{12} level with:
incomplete spinal cord lesion NOS
posterior cord syndrome

✓5th 806.3 **Dorsal [thoracic], open**

806.30 **T_1-T_6 level with unspecified spinal cord injury** MSP
806.31 **T_1-T_6 level with complete lesion of cord** MSP
806.32 **T_1-T_6 level with anterior cord syndrome** MSP
806.33 **T_1-T_6 level with central cord syndrome** MSP
806.34 **T_1-T_6 level with other specified spinal cord injury** MSP
T_1-T_6 level with:
incomplete spinal cord lesion NOS
posterior cord syndrome
806.35 **T_7-T_{12} level with unspecified spinal cord injury** MSP
806.36 **T_7-T_{12} level with complete lesion of cord** MSP
806.37 **T_7-T_{12} level with anterior cord syndrome** MSP
806.38 **T_7-T_{12} level with central cord syndrome** MSP
806.39 **T_7-T_{12} level with other specified spinal cord injury** MSP
T_7-T_{12} level with:
incomplete spinal cord lesion NOS
posterior cord syndrome

806.4 **Lumbar, closed** MSP
AHA: 4Q, '99, 11, 13

806.5 **Lumbar, open** MSP

✓5th 806.6 **Sacrum and coccyx, closed**

806.60 **With unspecified spinal cord injury** MSP
806.61 **With complete cauda equina lesion** MSP
806.62 **With other cauda equina injury** MSP
806.69 **With other spinal cord injury** MSP

✓5th 806.7 **Sacrum and coccyx, open**

806.70 **With unspecified spinal cord injury** MSP
806.71 **With complete cauda equina lesion** MSP
806.72 **With other cauda equina injury** MSP
806.79 **With other spinal cord injury** MSP

806.8 **Unspecified, closed** MSP
806.9 **Unspecified, open** MSP

✓4th **807 Fracture of rib(s), sternum, larynx, and trachea**

The following fifth-digit subclassification is for use with codes 807.0-807.1:

0 **rib(s), unspecified**
1 **one rib**
2 **two ribs**
3 **three ribs**
4 **four ribs**
5 **five ribs**
6 **six ribs**
7 **seven ribs**
8 **eight or more ribs**
9 **multiple ribs, unspecified**

✓5th 807.0 **Rib(s), closed** MSP
✓5th 807.1 **Rib(s), open** MSP
807.2 **Sternum, closed** MSP
DEF: Break in flat bone (breast bone) in anterior thorax.
807.3 **Sternum, open** MSP
DEF: Break, with open wound, in flat bone in mid anterior thorax.
807.4 **Flail chest** MSP
807.5 **Larynx and trachea, closed** MSP
Hyoid bone
Trachea
Thyroid cartilage
807.6 **Larynx and trachea, open** MSP

✓4th **808 Fracture of pelvis**

808.0 **Acetabulum, closed**
808.1 **Acetabulum, open**
808.2 **Pubis, closed**
808.3 **Pubis, open**

✓5th 808.4 **Other specified part, closed**

808.41 **Ilium**
808.42 **Ischium**
808.43 **Multiple pelvic fractures with disruption of pelvic circle**
808.49 **Other**
Innominate bone
Pelvic rim

✓5th 808.5 **Other specified part, open**

808.51 **Ilium**
808.52 **Ischium**
808.53 **Multiple pelvic fractures with disruption of pelvic circle**
808.59 **Other**

808.8 **Unspecified, closed**
808.9 **Unspecified, open**

✓4th **809 Ill-defined fractures of bones of trunk**

INCLUDES bones of trunk with other bones except those of skull and face
multiple bones of trunk

EXCLUDES *multiple fractures of:*
pelvic bones alone (808.0-808.9)
ribs alone (807.0-807.1, 807.4)
ribs or sternum with limb bones (819.0-819.1, 828.0-828.1)
skull or face with other bones (804.0-804.9)

809.0 **Fracture of bones of trunk, closed**
809.1 **Fracture of bones of trunk, open**

FRACTURE OF UPPER LIMB (810-819)

✓4th **810 Fracture of clavicle**

INCLUDES collar bone
interligamentous part of clavicle

The following fifth-digit subclassification is for use with category 810:

0 **unspecified part**
Clavicle NOS
1 **sternal end of clavicle**
2 **shaft of clavicle**
3 **acromial end of clavicle**

✓5th 810.0 **Closed** MSP
✓5th 810.1 **Open** MSP

Pelvis and Pelvic Fractures

Fractures Disrupting Pelvic Circle
Pelvic circle
Stable
Unstable (two-place fracture)
Iliac crest
Ilium
L5
Pelvic Bones
Anterior superior iliac spine
Sacrum
Ischial spine
Coccyx
Acetabulum
Pubis
Femur
Ischial tuberosity
Pubic symphysis
Acetabular Fractures
Posterior pillar
Transverse

✓4th 811 Fracture of scapula

INCLUDES shoulder blade

The following fifth-digit subclassification is for use with category 811:

- **0 unspecified part**
- **1 acromial process**
  - Acromion (process)
- **2 coracoid process**
- **3 glenoid cavity and neck of scapula**
- **9 other**

✓5th 811.0 Closed MSP

✓5th 811.1 Open MSP

✓4th 812 Fracture of humerus

✓5th 812.0 Upper end, closed

812.00 Upper end, unspecified part
Proximal end Shoulder

812.01 Surgical neck
Neck of humerus NOS

812.02 Anatomical neck

812.03 Greater tuberosity

812.09 Other
Head Upper epiphysis

✓5th 812.1 Upper end, open

812.10 Upper end, unspecified part

812.11 Surgical neck

812.12 Anatomical neck

812.13 Greater tuberosity

812.19 Other

✓5th 812.2 Shaft or unspecified part, closed

812.20 Unspecified part of humerus
Humerus NOS Upper arm NOS

812.21 Shaft of humerus
AHA: 3Q, '99, 14

✓5th 812.3 Shaft or unspecified part, open

812.30 Unspecified part of humerus

812.31 Shaft of humerus

✓5th 812.4 Lower end, closed
Distal end of humerus
Elbow

812.40 Lower end, unspecified part

812.41 Supracondylar fracture of humerus

812.42 Lateral condyle
External condyle

812.43 Medial condyle
Internal epicondyle

812.44 Condyle(s), unspecified
Articular process NOS
Lower epiphysis NOS

812.49 Other
Multiple fractures of lower end
Trochlea

Right Clavicle and Scapula, Anterior View

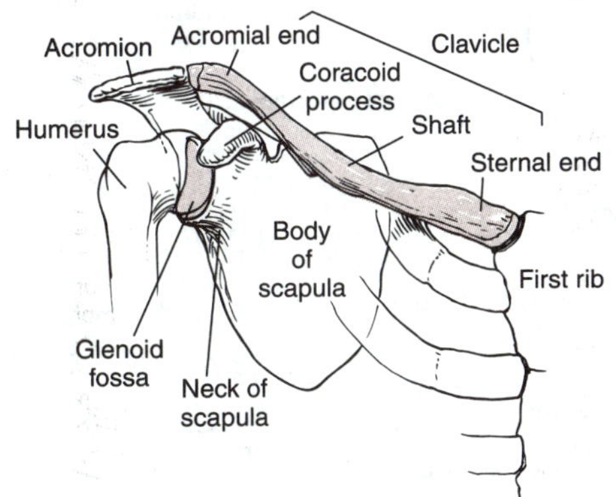

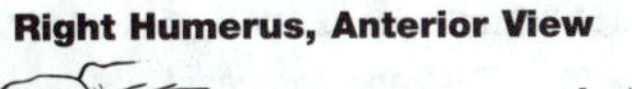
Right Humerus, Anterior View

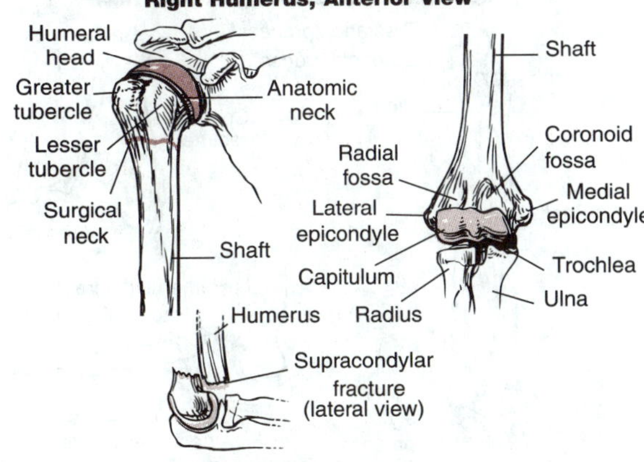

✓5th 812.5 Lower end, open

812.50 Lower end, unspecified part

812.51 Supracondylar fracture of humerus

812.52 Lateral condyle

812.53 Medial condyle

812.54 Condyle(s), unspecified

812.59 Other

✓4th 813 Fracture of radius and ulna

✓5th 813.0 Upper end, closed
Proximal end

813.00 Upper end of forearm, unspecified

813.01 Olecranon process of ulna

813.02 Coronoid process of ulna

813.03 Monteggia's fracture
DEF: Fracture near the head of the ulnar shaft, causing dislocation of the radial head.

813.04 Other and unspecified fractures of proximal end of ulna (alone)
Multiple fractures of ulna, upper end

813.05 Head of radius

813.06 Neck of radius

813.07 Other and unspecified fractures of proximal end of radius (alone)
Multiple fractures of radius, upper end

813.08 Radius with ulna, upper end [any part]

✓5th 813.1 Upper end, open

813.10 Upper end of forearm, unspecified

813.11 Olecranon process of ulna

813.12 Coronoid process of ulna

813.13 Monteggia's fracture

813.14 Other and unspecified fractures of proximal end of ulna (alone)

813.15 Head of radius

813.16 Neck of radius

813.17 Other and unspecified fractures of proximal end of radius (alone)

813.18 Radius with ulna, upper end [any part]

✓5th 813.2 Shaft, closed

813.20 Shaft, unspecified

813.21 Radius (alone)

813.22 Ulna (alone)

813.23 Radius with ulna

✓5th 813.3 Shaft, open

813.30 Shaft, unspecified

813.31 Radius (alone)

813.32 Ulna (alone)

813.33 Radius with ulna

✓5th 813.4 Lower end, closed
Distal end

813.40 Lower end of forearm, unspecified

Right Radius and Ulna, Anterior View

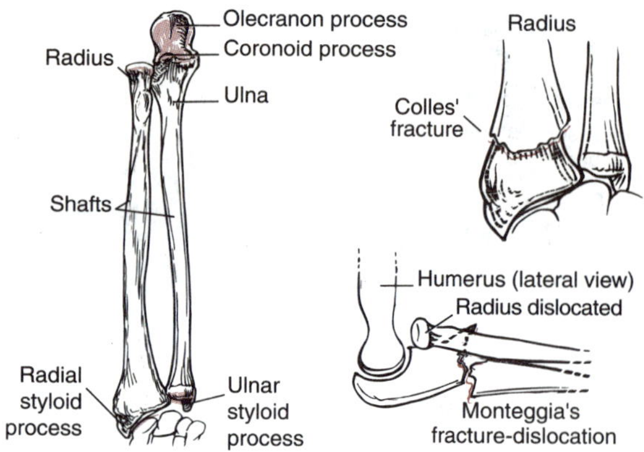

813.41 Colles' fracture
Smith's fracture
DEF: Break of lower end of radius; associated with backward movement of the radius lower section.

813.42 Other fractures of distal end of radius (alone)
Dupuytren's fracture, radius
Radius, lower end
DEF: Dupuytren's fracture: fracture and dislocation of the forearm; the fracture is of the radius above the wrist, and the dislocation is of the ulna at the lower end.

813.43 Distal end of ulna (alone)
Ulna: head, lower end
Ulna: lower epiphysis, styloid process

813.44 Radius with ulna, lower end

813.45 Torus fracture of radius
AHA: 4Q, '02, 70

✓5th **813.5 Lower end, open**
813.50 Lower end of forearm, unspecified
813.51 Colles' fracture
813.52 Other fractures of distal end of radius (alone)
813.53 Distal end of ulna (alone)
813.54 Radius with ulna, lower end

✓5th **813.8 Unspecified part, closed**
813.80 Forearm, unspecified
813.81 Radius (alone)
AHA: 2Q, '98, 19
813.82 Ulna (alone)
813.83 Radius with ulna

✓5th **813.9 Unspecified part, open**
813.90 Forearm, unspecified
813.91 Radius (alone)
813.92 Ulna (alone)
813.93 Radius with ulna

✓4th **814 Fracture of carpal bone(s)**
The following fifth-digit subclassification is for use with category 814:
0 carpal bone, unspecified
Wrist NOS
1 navicular [scaphoid] of wrist
2 lunate [semilunar] bone of wrist
3 triquetral [cuneiform] bone of wrist
4 pisiform
5 trapezium bone [larger multangular]
6 trapezoid bone [smaller multangular]
7 capitate bone [os magnum]
8 hamate [unciform] bone
9 other

✓5th **814.0 Closed**
✓5th **814.1 Open**

✓4th **815 Fracture of metacarpal bone(s)**
INCLUDES hand [except finger]
metacarpus
The following fifth-digit subclassification is for use with category 815:
0 metacarpal bone(s), site unspecified
1 base of thumb [first] metacarpal
Bennett's fracture
2 base of other metacarpal bone(s)
3 shaft of metacarpal bone(s)
4 neck of metacarpal bone(s)
9 multiple sites of metacarpus

✓5th **815.0 Closed**
✓5th **815.1 Open**

✓4th **816 Fracture of one or more phalanges of hand**
INCLUDES finger(s) thumb
The following fifth-digit subclassification is for use with category 816:
0 phalanx or phalanges, unspecified
1 middle or proximal phalanx or phalanges
2 distal phalanx or phalanges
3 multiple sites

✓5th **816.0 Closed**
✓5th **816.1 Open**
AHA: For code 816.12: 4Q, '03, 77

✓4th **817 Multiple fractures of hand bones**
INCLUDES metacarpal bone(s) with phalanx or phalanges of same hand
817.0 Closed
817.1 Open

✓4th **818 Ill-defined fractures of upper limb**
INCLUDES arm NOS
multiple bones of same upper limb
EXCLUDES *multiple fractures of:*
metacarpal bone(s) with phalanx or phalanges (817.0-817.1)
phalanges of hand alone (816.0-816.1)
radius with ulna (813.0-813.9)
818.0 Closed
818.1 Open

✓4th **819 Multiple fractures involving both upper limbs, and upper limb with rib(s) and sternum**
INCLUDES arm(s) with rib(s) or sternum
both arms [any bones]
819.0 Closed
819.1 Open

Hand Fractures

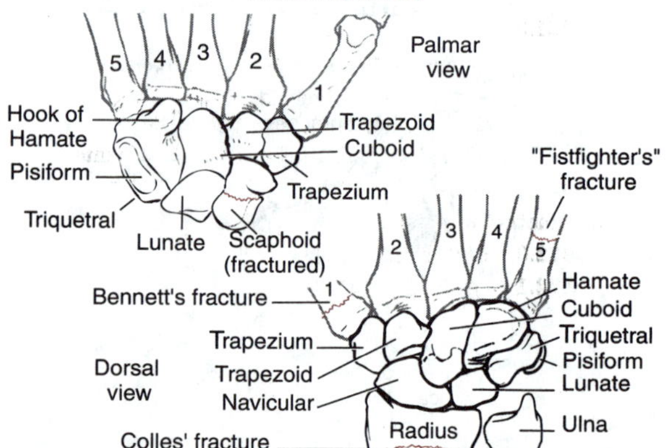

FRACTURE OF LOWER LIMB (820-829)

✓4th **820 Fracture of neck of femur**

✓5th **820.0 Transcervical fracture, closed**

820.00 Intracapsular section, unspecified

820.01 Epiphysis (separation) (upper)
Transepiphyseal

820.02 Midcervical section
Transcervical NOS
AHA: 3Q, '03, 12

820.03 Base of neck
Cervicotrochanteric section

820.09 Other
Head of femur Subcapital

✓5th **820.1 Transcervical fracture, open**

820.10 Intracapsular section, unspecified

820.11 Epiphysis (separation) (upper)

820.12 Midcervical section

820.13 Base of neck

820.19 Other

✓5th **820.2 Pertrochanteric fracture, closed**

820.20 Trochanteric section, unspecified
Trochanter: NOS, greater
Trochanter: lesser

820.21 Intertrochanteric section

820.22 Subtrochanteric section

✓5th **820.3 Pertrochanteric fracture, open**

820.30 Trochanteric section, unspecified

820.31 Intertrochanteric section

820.32 Subtrochanteric section

820.8 Unspecified part of neck of femur, closed
Hip NOS Neck of femur NOS

820.9 Unspecified part of neck of femur, open

✓4th **821 Fracture of other and unspecified parts of femur**

✓5th **821.0 Shaft or unspecified part, closed**

821.00 Unspecified part of femur
Thigh Upper leg
EXCLUDES *hip NOS (820.8)*

821.01 Shaft
AHA: 1Q, '99, 5

✓5th **821.1 Shaft or unspecified part, open**

821.10 Unspecified part of femur

821.11 Shaft

✓5th **821.2 Lower end, closed**
Distal end

821.20 Lower end, unspecified part

821.21 Condyle, femoral

821.22 Epiphysis, lower (separation)

821.23 Supracondylar fracture of femur
Multiple fractures of lower end

821.29 Other
Multiple fractures of lower end

✓5th **821.3 Lower end, open**

821.30 Lower end, unspecified part

821.31 Condyle, femoral

821.32 Epiphysis, lower (separation)

821.33 Supracondylar fracture of femur

821.39 Other

✓4th **822 Fracture of patella**

822.0 Closed

822.1 Open

Right Femur, Anterior View

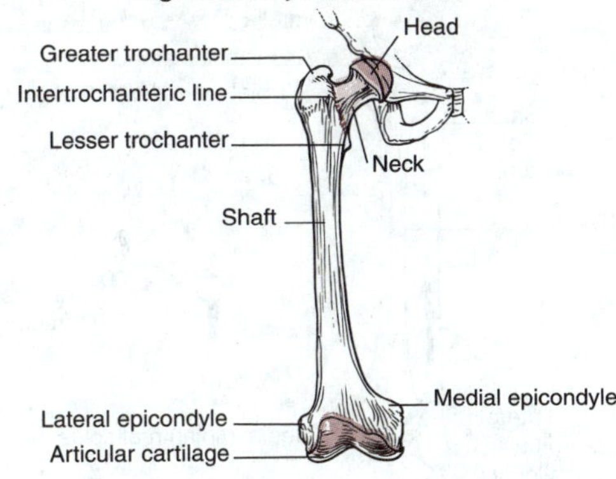

✓4th **823 Fracture of tibia and fibula**

EXCLUDES *Dupuytren's fracture (824.4-824.5)*
ankle (824.4-824.5)
radius (813.42, 813.52)
Pott's fracture (824.4-824.5)
that involving ankle (824.0-824.9)

The following fifth-digit subclassification is for use with category 823:
0 tibia alone
1 fibula alone
2 fibula with tibia

✓5th **823.0 Upper end, closed**
Head
Proximal end
Tibia: condyles, tuberosity

✓5th **823.1 Upper end, open**

✓5th **823.2 Shaft, closed**

✓5th **823.3 Shaft, open**

✓5th **823.4 Torus fracture**
DEF: A bone deformity in children, occurring commonly in the radius or ulna, in which the bone bends and buckles but does not fracture.
AHA: 4Q, '02, 70

✓5th **823.8 Unspecified part, closed**
Lower leg NOS
AHA: For code 823.82: 1Q, '97, 8

✓5th **823.9 Unspecified part, open**

✓4th **824 Fracture of ankle**

824.0 Medial malleolus, closed
Tibia involving: ankle
Tibia involving: malleolus
AHA: 1Q, '04, 9

824.1 Medial malleolus, open

824.2 Lateral malleolus, closed
Fibula involving: ankle
Fibula involving: malleolus
AHA: 2Q, '02, 3

Torus Fracture

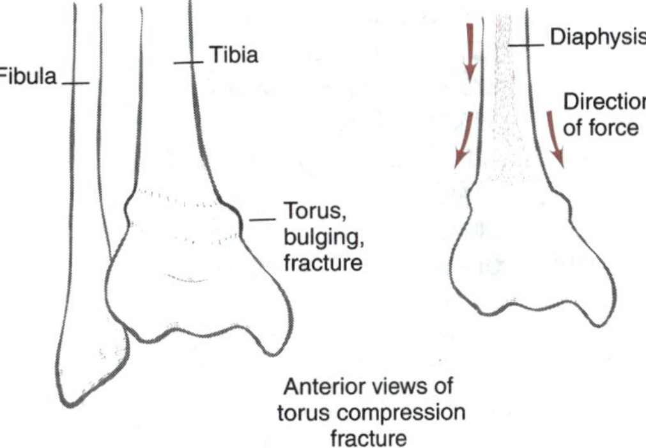

Right Tibia and Fibula, Anterior View

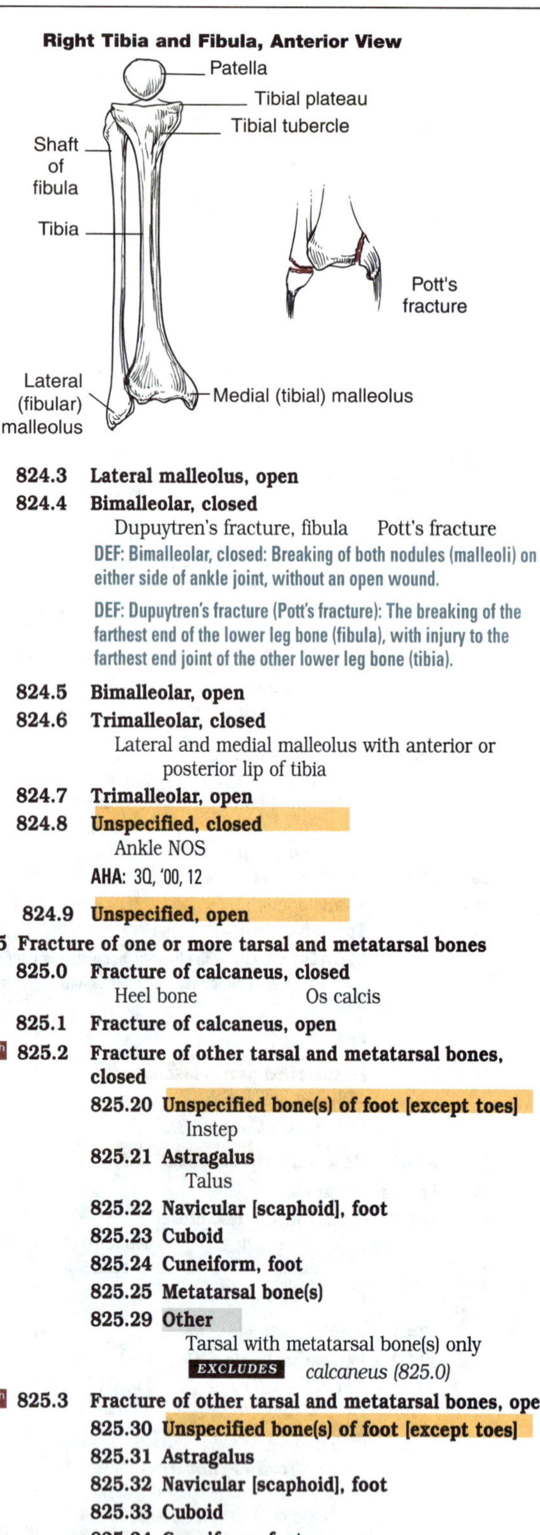

824.3 Lateral malleolus, open

824.4 Bimalleolar, closed

Dupuytren's fracture, fibula   Pott's fracture

DEF: Bimalleolar, closed: Breaking of both nodules (malleoli) on either side of ankle joint, without an open wound.

DEF: Dupuytren's fracture (Pott's fracture): The breaking of the farthest end of the lower leg bone (fibula), with injury to the farthest end joint of the other lower leg bone (tibia).

824.5 Bimalleolar, open

824.6 Trimalleolar, closed

Lateral and medial malleolus with anterior or posterior lip of tibia

824.7 Trimalleolar, open

824.8 Unspecified, closed

Ankle NOS

AHA: 3Q, '00, 12

824.9 Unspecified, open

✓4th **825 Fracture of one or more tarsal and metatarsal bones**

825.0 Fracture of calcaneus, closed

Heel bone   Os calcis

825.1 Fracture of calcaneus, open

✓5th **825.2 Fracture of other tarsal and metatarsal bones, closed**

825.20 Unspecified bone(s) of foot [except toes]

Instep

825.21 Astragalus

Talus

825.22 Navicular [scaphoid], foot

825.23 Cuboid

825.24 Cuneiform, foot

825.25 Metatarsal bone(s)

825.29 Other

Tarsal with metatarsal bone(s) only

EXCLUDES *calcaneus (825.0)*

✓5th **825.3 Fracture of other tarsal and metatarsal bones, open**

825.30 Unspecified bone(s) of foot [except toes]

825.31 Astragalus

825.32 Navicular [scaphoid], foot

825.33 Cuboid

825.34 Cuneiform, foot

825.35 Metatarsal bone(s)

825.39 Other

✓4th **826 Fracture of one or more phalanges of foot**

INCLUDES toe(s)

826.0 Closed

826.1 Open

Right Foot, Dorsal

Tarsals
Metatarsophalangeal joint
Cuneiform bones:
Intermediate
Medial
Lateral
Phalanges
Proximal
Distal
Medial
Astragalus (talus)
Navicular
Calcaneus
Cuboid
Metatarsals
1 2 3 4 5

✓4th **827 Other, multiple, and ill-defined fractures of lower limb**

INCLUDES leg NOS
multiple bones of same lower limb

EXCLUDES *multiple fractures of:*
ankle bones alone (824.4-824.9)
phalanges of foot alone (826.0-826.1)
tarsal with metatarsal bones (825.29, 825.39)
tibia with fibula (823.0-823.9 with fifth-digit 2)

827.0 Closed

827.1 Open

✓4th **828 Multiple fractures involving both lower limbs, lower with upper limb, and lower limb(s) with rib(s) and sternum**

INCLUDES arm(s) with leg(s) [any bones]
both legs [any bones]
leg(s) with rib(s) or sternum

828.0 Closed MSP

828.1 Open MSP

✓4th **829 Fracture of unspecified bones**

829.0 Unspecified bone, closed

829.1 Unspecified bone, open

DISLOCATION (830-839)

INCLUDES displacement
subluxation

EXCLUDES *congenital dislocation (754.0-755.8)*
pathological dislocation (718.2)
recurrent dislocation (718.3)

The descriptions "closed" and "open," used in the fourth-digit subdivisions, include the following terms:

closed:	open:
complete	compound
dislocation NOS	infected
partial	with foreign body
simple	
uncomplicated	

A dislocation not indicated as closed or open should be classified as closed.

AHA: 3Q, '90, 12

✓4th **830 Dislocation of jaw**

INCLUDES jaw (cartilage) (meniscus)
mandible
maxilla (inferior)
temporomandibular (joint)

830.0 Closed dislocation

830.1 Open dislocation

✓4th 831 Dislocation of shoulder

EXCLUDES *sternoclavicular joint (839.61, 839.71)*
sternum (839.61, 839.71)

The following fifth-digit subclassification is for use with category 831:
- **0 shoulder, unspecified**
  Humerus NOS
- **1 anterior dislocation of humerus**
- **2 posterior dislocation of humerus**
- **3 inferior dislocation of humerus**
- **4 acromioclavicular (joint)**
  Clavicle
- **9 other**
  Scapula

✓5th **831.0 Closed dislocation**

✓5th **831.1 Open dislocation**

✓4th 832 Dislocation of elbow

The following fifth-digit subclassification is for use with category 832:
- **0 elbow unspecified**
- **1 anterior dislocation of elbow**
- **2 posterior dislocation of elbow**
- **3 medial dislocation of elbow**
- **4 lateral dislocation of elbow**
- **9 other**

✓5th **832.0 Closed dislocation**

✓5th **832.1 Open dislocation**

✓4th 833 Dislocation of wrist

The following fifth-digit subclassification is for use with category 833:
- **0 wrist, unspecified part**
  Carpal (bone)
  Radius, distal end
- **1 radioulnar (joint), distal**
- **2 radiocarpal (joint)**
- **3 midcarpal (joint)**
- **4 carpometacarpal (joint)**
- **5 metacarpal (bone), proximal end**
- **9 other**
  Ulna, distal end

✓5th **833.0 Closed dislocation**

✓5th **833.1 Open dislocation**

✓4th 834 Dislocation of finger

INCLUDES finger(s)
phalanx of hand
thumb

The following fifth-digit subclassification is for use with category 834:
- **0 finger, unspecified part**
- **1 metacarpophalangeal (joint)**
  Metacarpal (bone), distal end
- **2 interphalangeal (joint), hand**

✓5th **834.0 Closed dislocation**

✓5th **834.1 Open dislocation**

✓4th 835 Dislocation of hip

The following fifth-digit subclassification is for use with category 835:
- **0 dislocation of hip, unspecified**
- **1 posterior dislocation**
- **2 obturator dislocation**
- **3 other anterior dislocation**

✓5th **835.0 Closed dislocation**

✓5th **835.1 Open dislocation**

✓4th 836 Dislocation of knee

EXCLUDES *dislocation of knee:*
old or pathological (718.2)
recurrent (718.3)
internal derangement of knee joint (717.0-717.5, 717.8-717.9)
old tear of cartilage or meniscus of knee (717.0-717.5, 717.8-717.9)

836.0 Tear of medial cartilage or meniscus of knee, current

Bucket handle tear: } current injury
NOS
medial meniscus

836.1 Tear of lateral cartilage or meniscus of knee, current

836.2 Other tear of cartilage or meniscus of knee, current

Tear of:
cartilage (semilunar) } current injury, not specified as medial or lateral
meniscus

836.3 Dislocation of patella, closed

836.4 Dislocation of patella, open

✓5th **836.5 Other dislocation of knee, closed**

836.50 Dislocation of knee, unspecified

836.51 Anterior dislocation of tibia, proximal end
Posterior dislocation of femur, distal end

836.52 Posterior dislocation of tibia, proximal end
Anterior dislocation of femur, distal end

836.53 Medial dislocation of tibia, proximal end

836.54 Lateral dislocation of tibia, proximal end

836.59 Other

✓5th **836.6 Other dislocation of knee, open**

836.60 Dislocation of knee, unspecified

836.61 Anterior dislocation of tibia, proximal end

836.62 Posterior dislocation of tibia, proximal end

836.63 Medial dislocation of tibia, proximal end

836.64 Lateral dislocation of tibia, proximal end

836.69 Other

✓4th 837 Dislocation of ankle

INCLUDES astragalus
fibula, distal end
navicular, foot
scaphoid, foot
tibia, distal end

837.0 Closed dislocation

837.1 Open dislocation

✓4th 838 Dislocation of foot

The following fifth-digit subclassification is for use with category 838:
- **0 foot, unspecified**
- **1 tarsal (bone), joint unspecified**
- **2 midtarsal (joint)**
- **3 tarsometatarsal (joint)**
- **4 metatarsal (bone), joint unspecified**
- **5 metatarsophalangeal (joint)**
- **6 interphalangeal (joint), foot**
- **9 other**
  Phalanx of foot
  Toe(s)

✓5th **838.0 Closed dislocation**

✓5th **838.1 Open dislocation**

✓4th 839 Other, multiple, and ill-defined dislocations

✓5th **839.0 Cervical vertebra, closed**

Cervical spine Neck

839.00 Cervical vertebra, unspecified MSP

839.01 First cervical vertebra MSP

839.02 **Second cervical vertebra** MSP
839.03 **Third cervical vertebra** MSP
839.04 **Fourth cervical vertebra** MSP
839.05 **Fifth cervical vertebra** MSP
839.06 **Sixth cervical vertebra** MSP
839.07 **Seventh cervical vertebra** MSP
839.08 **Multiple cervical vertebrae** MSP

✓5th 839.1 **Cervical vertebra, open**
839.10 **Cervical vertebra, unspecified** MSP
839.11 **First cervical vertebra** MSP
839.12 **Second cervical vertebra** MSP
839.13 **Third cervical vertebra** MSP
839.14 **Fourth cervical vertebra** MSP
839.15 **Fifth cervical vertebra** MSP
839.16 **Sixth cervical vertebra** MSP
839.17 **Seventh cervical vertebra** MSP
839.18 **Multiple cervical vertebrae** MSP

✓5th 839.2 **Thoracic and lumbar vertebra, closed**
839.20 **Lumbar vertebra** MSP
839.21 **Thoracic vertebra** MSP
Dorsal [thoracic] vertebra

✓5th 839.3 **Thoracic and lumbar vertebra, open**
839.30 **Lumbar vertebra** MSP
839.31 **Thoracic vertebra** MSP

✓5th 839.4 **Other vertebra, closed**
839.40 **Vertebra, unspecified site**
Spine NOS
839.41 **Coccyx**
839.42 **Sacrum**
Sacroiliac (joint)
839.49 **Other**

✓5th 839.5 **Other vertebra, open**
839.50 **Vertebra, unspecified site**
839.51 **Coccyx**
839.52 **Sacrum**
839.59 **Other**

✓5th 839.6 **Other location, closed**
839.61 **Sternum**
Sternoclavicular joint
839.69 **Other**
Pelvis

✓5th 839.7 **Other location, open**
839.71 **Sternum** MSP
839.79 **Other** MSP

839.8 **Multiple and ill-defined, closed** MSP
Arm
Back
Hand
Multiple locations, except fingers or toes alone
Other ill-defined locations
Unspecified location

839.9 **Multiple and ill-defined, open** MSP

SPRAINS AND STRAINS OF JOINTS AND ADJACENT MUSCLES (840-848)

INCLUDES avulsion, hemarthrosis, laceration, rupture, sprain, strain, tear of: joint capsule, ligament, muscle, tendon

EXCLUDES *laceration of tendon in open wounds (880-884 and 890-894 with .2)*

✓4th 840 **Sprains and strains of shoulder and upper arm**
840.0 **Acromioclavicular (joint) (ligament)**
840.1 **Coracoclavicular (ligament)**
840.2 **Coracohumeral (ligament)**
840.3 **Infraspinatus (muscle) (tendon)**
840.4 **Rotator cuff (capsule)**
EXCLUDES *complete rupture of rotator cuff, nontraumatic (727.61)*
840.5 **Subscapularis (muscle)**
840.6 **Supraspinatus (muscle) (tendon)**
840.7 **Superior glenoid labrum lesion**
SLAP lesion
AHA: 4Q,'01, 52

DEF: Detachment injury of the superior aspect of the glenoid labrum which is the ring of fibrocartilage attached to the rim of the glenoid cavity of the scapula.

840.8 **Other specified sites of shoulder and upper arm**
840.9 **Unspecified site of shoulder and upper arm**
Arm NOS
Shoulder NOS

✓4th 841 **Sprains and strains of elbow and forearm**
841.0 **Radial collateral ligament**
841.1 **Ulnar collateral ligament**
841.2 **Radiohumeral (joint)**
841.3 **Ulnohumeral (joint)**
841.8 **Other specified sites of elbow and forearm**
841.9 **Unspecified site of elbow and forearm**
Elbow NOS

✓4th 842 **Sprains and strains of wrist and hand**
✓5th 842.0 **Wrist**
842.00 **Unspecified site**
842.01 **Carpal (joint)**
842.02 **Radiocarpal (joint) (ligament)**
842.09 **Other**
Radioulnar joint, distal
✓5th 842.1 **Hand**
842.10 **Unspecified site**
842.11 **Carpometacarpal (joint)**
842.12 **Metacarpophalangeal (joint)**
842.13 **Interphalangeal (joint)**
842.19 **Other**
Midcarpal (joint)

✓4th 843 **Sprains and strains of hip and thigh**
843.0 **Iliofemoral (ligament)**
843.1 **Ischiocapsular (ligament)**
843.8 **Other specified sites of hip and thigh**
843.9 **Unspecified site of hip and thigh**
Hip NOS
Thigh NOS

✓4th 844 **Sprains and strains of knee and leg**
844.0 **Lateral collateral ligament of knee**
844.1 **Medial collateral ligament of knee**
844.2 **Cruciate ligament of knee**
844.3 **Tibiofibular (joint) (ligament), superior**
844.8 **Other specified sites of knee and leg**
844.9 **Unspecified site of knee and leg**
Knee NOS Leg NOS

✓4th 845 **Sprains and strains of ankle and foot**
✓5th 845.0 **Ankle**
845.00 **Unspecified site**
AHA: 2Q, '02, 3
845.01 **Deltoid (ligament), ankle**
Internal collateral (ligament), ankle
845.02 **Calcaneofibular (ligament)**
845.03 **Tibiofibular (ligament), distal**
AHA: 1Q, '04, 9
845.09 **Other**
Achilles tendon

✓5th **845.1 Foot**
845.10 Unspecified site
845.11 Tarsometatarsal (joint) (ligament)
845.12 Metatarsophalangeal (joint)
845.13 Interphalangeal (joint), toe
845.19 Other

✓4th **846 Sprains and strains of sacroiliac region**
846.0 Lumbosacral (joint) (ligament)
846.1 Sacroiliac ligament
846.2 Sacrospinatus (ligament)
846.3 Sacrotuberous (ligament)
846.8 Other specified sites of sacroiliac region
846.9 Unspecified site of sacroiliac region

✓4th **847 Sprains and strains of other and unspecified parts of back**
EXCLUDES *lumbosacral (846.0)*

847.0 Neck MSP
Anterior longitudinal (ligament), cervical
Atlanto-axial (joints)
Atlanto-occipital (joints)
Whiplash injury
EXCLUDES *neck injury NOS (959.0)*
thyroid region (848.2)

847.1 Thoracic
847.2 Lumbar
847.3 Sacrum
Sacrococcygeal (ligament)
847.4 Coccyx
847.9 Unspecified site of back
Back NOS

✓4th **848 Other and ill-defined sprains and strains**
848.0 Septal cartilage of nose
848.1 Jaw
Temporomandibular (joint) (ligament)
848.2 Thyroid region
Cricoarytenoid (joint) (ligament)
Cricothyroid (joint) (ligament)
Thyroid cartilage
848.3 Ribs
Chondrocostal (joint) } without mention of injury to sternum
Costal cartilage }

✓5th **848.4 Sternum**
848.40 Unspecified site
848.41 Sternoclavicular (joint) (ligament)
848.42 Chondrosternal (joint)
848.49 Other
Xiphoid cartilage

848.5 Pelvis
Symphysis pubis
EXCLUDES *that in childbirth (665.6)*

848.8 Other specified sites of sprains and strains
848.9 Unspecified site of sprain and strain

INTRACRANIAL INJURY, EXCLUDING THOSE WITH SKULL FRACTURE (850-854)

EXCLUDES *intracranial injury with skull fracture (800-801 and 803-804, except .0 and .5)*
open wound of head without intracranial injury (870.0-873.9)
skull fracture alone (800-801 and 803-804 with .0, .5)

The description "with open intracranial wound," used in the fourth-digit subdivisions, those specified as open or with mention of infection or foreign body.

The following fifth-digit subclassification is for use with categories 851-854:
0 unspecified state of consciousness
1 with no loss of consciousness
2 with brief [less than one hour] loss of consciousness
3 with moderate [1-24 hours] loss of consciousness
4 with prolonged [more than 24 hours] loss of consciousness and return to pre-existing conscious level
5 with prolonged [more than 24 hours] loss of consciousness,without return to pre-existing conscious level
Use fifth-digit 5 to designate when a patient is unconscious and dies before regaining consciousness, regardless of the duration of the loss of consciousness
6 with loss of consciousness of unspecified duration
9 with concussion, unspecified

AHA: 1Q, '93, 22

✓4th **850 Concussion**
INCLUDES commotio cerebri
EXCLUDES *concussion with:*
cerebral laceration or contusion (851.0-851.9)
cerebral hemorrhage (852-853)
head injury NOS (959.01)

AHA: 2Q, '96, 6; 4Q, '90, 24

850.0 With no loss of consciousness MSP
Concussion with mental confusion or disorientation, without loss of consciousness

✓5th **850.1 With brief loss of consciousness**
Loss of consciousness for less than one hour
AHA: 4Q, '03, 76; 1Q, '99, 10; 2Q, '92, 5

850.11 With loss of consciousness of 30 minutes or less MSP
850.12 With loss of consciousness from 31 to 59 minutes MSP

850.2 With moderate loss of consciousness MSP
Loss of consciousness for 1-24 hours
850.3 With prolonged loss of consciousness and return to pre-existing conscious level MSP
Loss of consciousness for more than 24 hours with complete recovery
850.4 With prolonged loss of consciousness, without return to pre-existing conscious level MSP
850.5 With loss of consciousness of unspecified duration MSP
850.9 Concussion, unspecified MSP

✓4th **851 Cerebral laceration and contusion**
AHA: 4Q, '96, 36; 1Q, '93, 22; 4Q, '90, 24

✓5th **851.0 Cortex (cerebral) contusion without mention of open intracranial wound** MSP
✓5th **851.1 Cortex (cerebral) contusion with open intracranial wound** MSP
AHA: 1Q, '92, 9

✓4th ✓5th Additional Digit Required | Unspecified Code | Other Specified Code | Manifestation Code | ►◄ Revised Text | ● New Code | ▲ Revised Code Title

§ ✓5th **851.2 Cortex (cerebral) laceration without mention of open intracranial wound** MSP

§ ✓5th **851.3 Cortex (cerebral) laceration with open intracranial wound** MSP

§ ✓5th **851.4 Cerebellar or brain stem contusion without mention of open intracranial wound** MSP

§ ✓5th **851.5 Cerebellar or brain stem contusion with open intracranial wound** MSP

§ ✓5th **851.6 Cerebellar or brain stem laceration without mention of open intracranial wound** MSP

§ ✓5th **851.7 Cerebellar or brain stem laceration with open intracranial wound** MSP

§ ✓5th **851.8 Other and unspecified cerebral laceration and contusion, without mention of open intracranial wound** MSP

Brain (membrane) NOS

AHA: 4Q, '96, 37

§ ✓5th **851.9 Other and unspecified cerebral laceration and contusion, with open intracranial wound** MSP

✓4th **852 Subarachnoid, subdural, and extradural hemorrhage, following injury**

EXCLUDES *cerebral contusion or laceration (with hemorrhage) (851.0-851.9)*

DEF: Bleeding from lining of brain; due to injury.

§ ✓5th **852.0 Subarachnoid hemorrhage following injury without mention of open intracranial wound** MSP

Middle meningeal hemorrhage following injury

§ ✓5th **852.1 Subarachnoid hemorrhage following injury with open intracranial wound** MSP

§ ✓5th **852.2 Subdural hemorrhage following injury without mention of open intracranialwound** MSP

AHA: 4Q, '96, 43

§ ✓5th **852.3 Subdural hemorrhage following injury with open intracranial wound** MSP

Brain

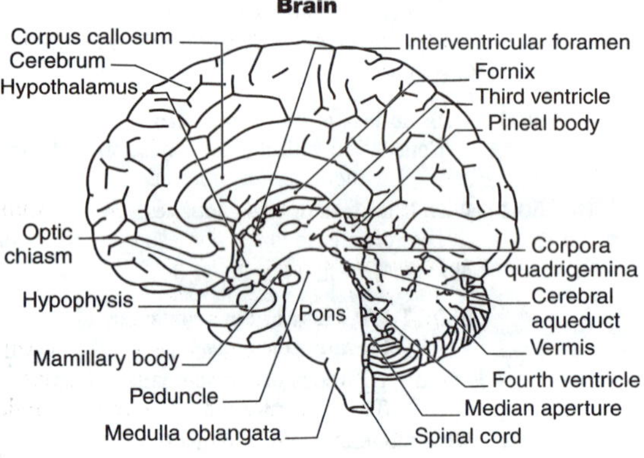

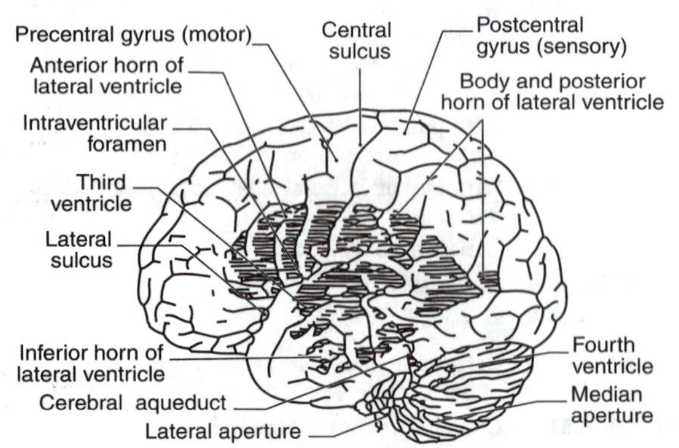

§ ✓5th **852.4 Extradural hemorrhage following injury without mention of open intracranial wound** MSP

Epidural hematoma following injury

§ ✓5th **852.5 Extradural hemorrhage following injury with open intracranial wound** MSP

✓4th **853 Other and unspecified intracranial hemorrhage following injury**

§ ✓5th **853.0 Without mention of open intracranial wound** MSP

Cerebral compression due to injury
Intracranial hematoma following injury
Traumatic cerebral hemorrhage

AHA: 3Q, '90, 14

§ ✓5th **853.1 With open intracranial wound** MSP

✓4th **854 Intracranial injury of other and unspecified nature**

INCLUDES brain injury NOS
cavernous sinus
intracranial injury

EXCLUDES *any condition classifiable to 850-853*
head injury NOS (959.01)

AHA: 1Q, '99, 10; 2Q, '92, 6

§ ✓5th **854.0 Without mention of open intracranial wound** MSP

§ ✓5th **854.1 With open intracranial wound** MSP

INTERNAL INJURY OF THORAX, ABDOMEN, AND PELVIS (860-869)

INCLUDES blast injuries, blunt trauma, bruise, concussion injuries (except cerebral), crushing, hematoma, laceration, puncture, tear, traumatic rupture } of internal organs

EXCLUDES *concussion NOS (850.0-850.9)*
flail chest (807.4)
foreign body entering through orifice (930.0-939.9)
injury to blood vessels (901.0-902.9)

The description "with open wound," used in the fourth-digit subdivisions, those with mention of infection or foreign body.

✓4th **860 Traumatic pneumothorax and hemothorax**

AHA: 2Q, '93, 4

DEF: Traumatic pneumothorax: air or gas leaking into pleural space of lung due to trauma.

DEF: Traumatic hemothorax: blood buildup in pleural space of lung due to trauma.

860.0 Pneumothorax without mention of open wound into thorax MSP

860.1 Pneumothorax with open wound into thorax MSP

860.2 Hemothorax without mention of open wound into thorax MSP

860.3 Hemothorax with open wound into thorax MSP

860.4 Pneumohemothorax without mention of open wound into thorax MSP

860.5 Pneumohemothorax with open wound into thorax MSP

✓4th **861 Injury to heart and lung**

EXCLUDES *injury to blood vessels of thorax (901.0-901.9)*

✓5th **861.0 Heart, without mention of open wound into thorax**

AHA: 1Q, '92, 9

§ Requires fifth-digit. See beginning of section 850–854 for codes and definitions.

861.00 Unspecified injury MSP
861.01 Contusion MSP
Cardiac contusion
Myocardial contusion
DEF: Bruising within the pericardium with no mention of open wound.
861.02 Laceration without penetration of heart chambers MSP
DEF: Tearing injury of heart tissue, without penetration of chambers; no open wound.
861.03 Laceration with penetration of heart chambers MSP

✓5th 861.1 Heart, with open wound into thorax
861.10 Unspecified injury MSP
861.11 Contusion MSP
861.12 Laceration without penetration of heart chambers MSP
861.13 Laceration with penetration of heart chambers MSP

✓5th 861.2 Lung, without mention of open wound into thorax
861.20 Unspecified injury MSP
861.21 Contusion MSP
DEF: Bruising of lung without mention of open wound.
861.22 Laceration MSP

✓5th 861.3 Lung, with open wound into thorax
861.30 Unspecified injury MSP
861.31 Contusion MSP
861.32 Laceration MSP

✓4th 862 Injury to other and unspecified intrathoracic organs
EXCLUDES *injury to blood vessels of thorax (901.0-901.9)*
862.0 Diaphragm, without mention of open wound into cavity
862.1 Diaphragm, with open wound into cavity
✓5th 862.2 Other specified intrathoracic organs, without mention of open wound into cavity
862.21 Bronchus
862.22 Esophagus
862.29 Other
Pleura Thymus gland
✓5th 862.3 Other specified intrathoracic organs, with open wound into cavity
862.31 Bronchus
862.32 Esophagus
862.39 Other
862.8 Multiple and unspecified intrathoracic organs, without mention of open wound into cavity MSP
Crushed chest
Multiple intrathoracic organs
862.9 Multiple and unspecified intrathoracic organs, with open wound into cavity

✓4th 863 Injury to gastrointestinal tract
EXCLUDES *anal sphincter laceration during delivery (664.2)*
bile duct (868.0-868.1 with fifth-digit 2)
gallbladder (868.0-868.1 with fifth-digit 2)
863.0 Stomach, without mention of open wound into cavity MSP
863.1 Stomach, with open wound into cavity MSP
✓5th 863.2 Small intestine, without mention of open wound into cavity
863.20 Small intestine, unspecified site MSP
863.21 Duodenum MSP
863.29 Other MSP
✓5th 863.3 Small intestine, with open wound into cavity
863.30 Small intestine, unspecified site MSP
863.31 Duodenum MSP
863.39 Other MSP
✓5th 863.4 Colon or rectum, without mention of open wound into cavity
863.40 Colon, unspecified site MSP
863.41 Ascending [right] colon MSP
863.42 Transverse colon MSP
863.43 Descending [left] colon MSP
863.44 Sigmoid colon MSP
863.45 Rectum MSP
863.46 Multiple sites in colon and rectum MSP
863.49 Other MSP
✓5th 863.5 Colon or rectum, with open wound into cavity
863.50 Colon, unspecified site MSP
863.51 Ascending [right] colon MSP
863.52 Transverse colon MSP
863.53 Descending [left] colon MSP
863.54 Sigmoid colon MSP
863.55 Rectum MSP
863.56 Multiple sites in colon and rectum MSP
863.59 Other MSP
✓5th 863.8 Other and unspecified gastrointestinal sites, without mention of open wound into cavity MSP
863.80 Gastrointestinal tract, unspecified site MSP
863.81 Pancreas, head MSP
863.82 Pancreas, body MSP
863.83 Pancreas, tail MSP
863.84 Pancreas, multiple and unspecified sites MSP
863.85 Appendix MSP
863.89 Other MSP
Intestine NOS
✓5th 863.9 Other and unspecified gastrointestinal sites, with open wound into cavity
863.90 Gastrointestinal tract, unspecified site MSP
863.91 Pancreas, head MSP
863.92 Pancreas, body MSP
863.93 Pancreas, tail MSP
863.94 Pancreas, multiple and unspecified sites MSP
863.95 Appendix MSP
863.99 Other MSP

✓4th 864 Injury to liver
The following fifth-digit subclassification is for use with category 864:
0 unspecified injury
1 hematoma and contusion
2 laceration, minor
Laceration involving capsule only, or without significant involvement of hepatic parenchyma [i.e., less than 1 cm deep]
3 laceration, moderate
Laceration involving parenchyma but without major disruption of parenchyma [i.e., less than 10 cm long and less than 3 cm deep]
4 laceration, major
Laceration with significant disruption of hepatic parenchyma [i.e., 10 cm long and 3 cm deep]
Multiple moderate lacerations, with or without hematoma
Stellate lacerations of liver
5 laceration, unspecified
9 other

✓5th 864.0 Without mention of open wound into cavity MSP
✓5th 864.1 With open wound into cavity MSP

✓4th **865 Injury to spleen**

The following fifth-digit subclassification is for use with category 865:

- 0 **unspecified injury**
- 1 **hematoma without rupture of capsule**
- 2 **capsular tears, without major disruption of parenchyma**
- 3 **laceration extending into parenchyma**
- 4 **massive parenchymal disruption**
- 9 **other**

✓5th **865.0 Without mention of open wound into cavity** MSP

✓5th **865.1 With open wound into cavity** MSP

✓4th **866 Injury to kidney**

The following fifth-digit subclassification is for use with category 866:

- 0 **unspecified injury**
- 1 **hematoma without rupture of capsule**
- 2 **laceration**
- 3 **complete disruption of kidney parenchyma**

✓5th **866.0 Without mention of open wound into cavity** MSP

✓5th **866.1 With open wound into cavity** MSP

✓4th **867 Injury to pelvic organs**

EXCLUDES *injury during delivery (664.0-665.9)*

867.0 Bladder and urethra, without mention of open wound into cavity MSP

AHA: N-D, '85, 15

867.1 Bladder and urethra, with open wound into cavity MSP

867.2 Ureter, without mention of open wound into cavity MSP

867.3 Ureter, with open wound into cavity MSP

867.4 Uterus, without mention of open wound into cavity ♀ MSP

867.5 Uterus, with open wound into cavity ♀ MSP

867.6 Other specified pelvic organs, without mention of open wound into cavity MSP

Fallopian tube
Ovary
Prostate
Seminal vesicle
Vas deferens

867.7 Other specified pelvic organs, with open wound into cavity MSP

867.8 Unspecified pelvic organ, without mention of open wound into cavity MSP

867.9 Unspecified pelvic organ, with open wound into cavity MSP

✓4th **868 Injury to other intra-abdominal organs**

The following fifth-digit subclassification is for use with category 868:

- 0 **unspecified intra-abdominal organ**
- 1 **adrenal gland**
- 2 **bile duct and gallbladder**
- 3 **peritoneum**
- 4 **retroperitoneum**
- 9 **other and multiple intra-abdominal organs**

✓5th **868.0 Without mention of open wound into cavity** MSP

✓5th **868.1 With open wound into cavity** MSP

✓4th **869 Internal injury to unspecified or ill-defined organs**

INCLUDES internal injury NOS
multiple internal injury NOS

869.0 Without mention of open wound into cavity MSP

869.1 With open wound into cavity MSP

AHA: 2Q, '89, 15

OPEN WOUND (870-897)

INCLUDES animal bite
avulsion
cut
laceration
puncture wound
traumatic amputation

EXCLUDES *burn (940.0-949.5)*
crushing (925-929.9)
puncture of internal organs (860.0-869.1)
superficial injury (910.0-919.9)
that incidental to:
dislocation (830.0-839.9)
fracture (800.0-829.1)
internal injury (860.0-869.1)
intracranial injury (851.0-854.1)

The description "complicated" used in the fourth-digit subdivisions includes those with mention of delayed healing, delayed treatment, foreign body, or infection.

Use additional code to identify infection

AHA: 4Q, '01, 52

OPEN WOUND OF HEAD, NECK, AND TRUNK (870-879)

✓4th **870 Open wound of ocular adnexa**

870.0 Laceration of skin of eyelid and periocular area

870.1 Laceration of eyelid, full-thickness, not involving lacrimal passages

870.2 Laceration of eyelid involving lacrimal passages

870.3 Penetrating wound of orbit, without mention of foreign body

870.4 Penetrating wound of orbit with foreign body

EXCLUDES *retained (old) foreign body in orbit (376.6)*

870.8 Other specified open wounds of ocular adnexa

870.9 Unspecified open wound of ocular adnexa

✓4th **871 Open wound of eyeball**

EXCLUDES *2nd cranial nerve [optic] injury (950.0-950.9)*
3rd cranial nerve [oculomotor] injury (951.0)

871.0 Ocular laceration without prolapse of intraocular tissue

AHA: 3Q, '96, 7

DEF: Tear in ocular tissue without displacing structures.

871.1 Ocular laceration with prolapse or exposure of intraocular tissue

871.2 Rupture of eye with partial loss of intraocular tissue

DEF: Forcible tearing of eyeball, with tissue loss.

871.3 Avulsion of eye

Traumatic enucleation

DEF: Traumatic extraction of eyeball from socket.

871.4 Unspecified laceration of eye

871.5 Penetration of eyeball with magnetic foreign body

EXCLUDES *retained (old) magnetic foreign body in globe (360.50-360.59)*

871.6 Penetration of eyeball with (nonmagnetic) foreign body

EXCLUDES *retained (old) (nonmagnetic) foreign body in globe (360.60-360.69)*

871.7 Unspecified ocular penetration

871.9 Unspecified open wound of eyeball

✓4th **872 Open wound of ear**

✓5th **872.0 External ear, without mention of complication**

872.00 External ear, unspecified site

872.01 Auricle, ear

Pinna

DEF: Open wound of fleshy, outer ear.

872.02 **Auditory canal**
DEF: Open wound of passage from external ear to eardrum.

✓5th 872.1 **External ear, complicated**
872.10 **External ear, unspecified site**
872.11 **Auricle, ear**
872.12 **Auditory canal**

✓5th 872.6 **Other specified parts of ear, without mention of complication**
872.61 **Ear drum**
Drumhead Tympanic membrane
872.62 **Ossicles**
872.63 **Eustachian tube**
DEF: Open wound of channel between nasopharynx and tympanic cavity.
872.64 **Cochlea**
DEF: Open wound of snail shell shaped tube of inner ear.
872.69 **Other and multiple sites**

✓5th 872.7 **Other specified parts of ear, complicated**
872.71 **Ear drum**
872.72 **Ossicles**
872.73 **Eustachian tube**
872.74 **Cochlea**
872.79 **Other and multiple sites**

872.8 **Ear, part unspecified, without mention of complication**
Ear NOS

872.9 **Ear, part unspecified, complicated**

✓4th 873 **Other open wound of head**
873.0 **Scalp, without mention of complication**
873.1 **Scalp, complicated**

✓5th 873.2 **Nose, without mention of complication**
873.20 **Nose, unspecified site**
873.21 **Nasal septum**
DEF: Open wound between nasal passages.
873.22 **Nasal cavity**
DEF: Open wound of nostrils.
873.23 **Nasal sinus**
DEF: Open wound of mucous-lined respiratory cavities.
873.29 **Multiple sites**

✓5th 873.3 **Nose, complicated**
873.30 **Nose, unspecified site**
873.31 **Nasal septum**
873.32 **Nasal cavity**
873.33 **Nasal sinus**
873.39 **Multiple sites**

✓5th 873.4 **Face, without mention of complication**
873.40 **Face, unspecified site**
873.41 **Cheek**
873.42 **Forehead**
Eyebrow
AHA: 4Q, '96, 43
873.43 **Lip**
873.44 **Jaw**
873.49 **Other and multiple sites**

✓5th 873.5 **Face, complicated**
873.50 **Face, unspecified site**
873.51 **Cheek**
873.52 **Forehead**
873.53 **Lip**
873.54 **Jaw**
873.59 **Other and multiple sites**

✓5th 873.6 **Internal structures of mouth, without mention of complication**
873.60 **Mouth, unspecified site**
873.61 **Buccal mucosa**
DEF: Open wound of inside of cheek.
873.62 **Gum (alveolar process)**
873.63 **Tooth (broken)**
AHA: 1Q, '04, 17
873.64 **Tongue and floor of mouth**
873.65 **Palate**
DEF: Open wound of roof of mouth.
873.69 **Other and multiple sites**

✓5th 873.7 **Internal structures of mouth, complicated**
873.70 **Mouth, unspecified site**
873.71 **Buccal mucosa**
873.72 **Gum (alveolar process)**
873.73 **Tooth (broken)**
AHA: 1Q, '04, 17
873.74 **Tongue and floor of mouth**
873.75 **Palate**
873.79 **Other and multiple sites**

873.8 **Other and unspecified open wound of head without mention of complication**
Head NOS

873.9 **Other and unspecified open wound of head, complicated**

✓4th 874 **Open wound of neck**

✓5th 874.0 **Larynx and trachea, without mention of complication**
874.00 **Larynx with trachea**
874.01 **Larynx**
874.02 **Trachea**

✓5th 874.1 **Larynx and trachea, complicated**
874.10 **Larynx with trachea**
874.11 **Larynx**
874.12 **Trachea**

874.2 **Thyroid gland, without mention of complication**
874.3 **Thyroid gland, complicated**
874.4 **Pharynx, without mention of complication**
Cervical esophagus
874.5 **Pharynx, complicated**
874.8 **Other and unspecified parts, without mention of complication**
Nape of neck Throat NOS
Supraclavicular region
874.9 **Other and unspecified parts, complicated**

✓4th 875 **Open wound of chest (wall)**
EXCLUDES *open wound into thoracic cavity (860.0-862.9)*
traumatic pneumothorax and hemothorax (860.1, 860.3, 860.5)
AHA: 3Q, '93, 17
875.0 **Without mention of complication**
875.1 **Complicated**

✓4th 876 **Open wound of back**
INCLUDES loin
lumbar region
EXCLUDES *open wound into thoracic cavity (860.0-862.9)*
traumatic pneumothorax and hemothorax (860.1, 860.3, 860.5)
876.0 **Without mention of complication**
876.1 **Complicated**

✓4th 877 **Open wound of buttock**
INCLUDES sacroiliac region
877.0 **Without mention of complication**
877.1 **Complicated**

✓4th **878 Open wound of genital organs (external), including traumatic amputation**

EXCLUDES *injury during delivery (664.0-665.9)*
internal genital organs (867.0-867.9)

878.0 Penis, without mention of complication ♂
878.1 Penis, complicated ♂
878.2 Scrotum and testes, without mention of complication ♂
878.3 Scrotum and testes, complicated ♂
878.4 Vulva, without mention of complication ♀
Labium (majus) (minus)
878.5 Vulva, complicated ♀
878.6 Vagina, without mention of complication ♀
878.7 Vagina, complicated ♀
878.8 Other and unspecified parts, without mention of complication
878.9 Other and unspecified parts, complicated

✓4th **879 Open wound of other and unspecified sites, except limbs**

879.0 Breast, without mention of complication
879.1 Breast, complicated
879.2 Abdominal wall, anterior, without mention of complication
Abdominal wall NOS
Epigastric region
Hypogastric region
Pubic region
Umbilical region
AHA: 2Q, '91, 22
879.3 Abdominal wall, anterior, complicated
879.4 Abdominal wall, lateral, without mention of complication
Flank
Groin
Hypochondrium
Iliac (region)
Inguinal region
879.5 Abdominal wall, lateral, complicated
879.6 Other and unspecified parts of trunk, without mention of complication
Pelvic region
Perineum
Trunk NOS
879.7 Other and unspecified parts of trunk, complicated
879.8 Open wound(s) (multiple) of unspecified site(s) without mention of complication
Multiple open wounds NOS
Open wound NOS
879.9 Open wound(s) (multiple) of unspecified site(s), complicated

OPEN WOUND OF UPPER LIMB (880-887)

AHA: N-D, '85, 5

✓4th **880 Open wound of shoulder and upper arm**

The following fifth-digit subclassification is for use with category 880:
0 shoulder region
1 scapular region
2 axillary region
3 upper arm
9 multiple sites

✓5th **880.0 Without mention of complication**
✓5th **880.1 Complicated**
✓5th **880.2 With tendon involvement**

✓4th **881 Open wound of elbow, forearm, and wrist**

The following fifth-digit subclassification is for use with category 881:
0 forearm
1 elbow
2 wrist

✓5th **881.0 Without mention of complication**
✓5th **881.1 Complicated**
✓5th **881.2 With tendon involvement**

✓4th **882 Open wound of hand except finger(s) alone**

882.0 Without mention of complication
882.1 Complicated
882.2 With tendon involvement

✓4th **883 Open wound of finger(s)**

INCLUDES fingernail
thumb (nail)

883.0 Without mention of complication
883.1 Complicated
883.2 With tendon involvement

✓4th **884 Multiple and unspecified open wound of upper limb**

INCLUDES arm NOS
multiple sites of one upper limb
upper limb NOS

884.0 Without mention of complication
884.1 Complicated
884.2 With tendon involvement

✓4th **885 Traumatic amputation of thumb (complete) (partial)**

INCLUDES thumb(s) (with finger(s) of either hand)

885.0 Without mention of complication
AHA: 1Q, '03, 7
885.1 Complicated

✓4th **886 Traumatic amputation of other finger(s) (complete) (partial)**

INCLUDES finger(s) of one or both hands, without mention of thumb(s)

886.0 Without mention of complication
886.1 Complicated

✓4th **887 Traumatic amputation of arm and hand (complete) (partial)**

887.0 Unilateral, below elbow, without mention of complication MSP
887.1 Unilateral, below elbow, complicated MSP
887.2 Unilateral, at or above elbow, without mention of complication MSP
887.3 Unilateral, at or above elbow, complicated MSP
887.4 Unilateral, level not specified, without mention of complication MSP
887.5 Unilateral, level not specified, complicated MSP
887.6 Bilateral [any level], without mention of complication MSP
One hand and other arm
887.7 Bilateral [any level], complicated MSP

OPEN WOUND OF LOWER LIMB (890-897)

AHA: N-D, '85, 5

✓4th **890 Open wound of hip and thigh**

890.0 Without mention of complication
890.1 Complicated
890.2 With tendon involvement

✓4th **891 Open wound of knee, leg [except thigh], and ankle**

INCLUDES leg NOS
multiple sites of leg, except thigh

EXCLUDES *that of thigh (890.0-890.2)*
with multiple sites of lower limb (894.0-894.2)

891.0 Without mention of complication
891.1 Complicated
891.2 With tendon involvement

✓4th **892 Open wound of foot except toe(s) alone**

INCLUDES heel

892.0 Without mention of complication
892.1 Complicated
892.2 With tendon involvement

✓4th **893 Open wound of toe(s)**

INCLUDES toenail

893.0 Without mention of complication

N Newborn Age: 0 | P Pediatric Age: 0-17 | M Maternity Age: 12-55 | A Adult Age: 15-124 | MSP Medicare Secondary Payer

893.1 Complicated
893.2 With tendon involvement

✓4th 894 **Multiple and unspecified open wound of lower limb**
INCLUDES lower limb NOS
multiple sites of one lower limb, with thigh
894.0 Without mention of complication
894.1 Complicated
894.2 With tendon involvement

✓4th 895 **Traumatic amputation of toe(s) (complete) (partial)**
INCLUDES toe(s) of one or both feet
895.0 Without mention of complication
895.1 Complicated

✓4th 896 **Traumatic amputation of foot (complete) (partial)**
896.0 Unilateral, without mention of complication MSP
896.1 Unilateral, complicated MSP
896.2 Bilateral, without mention of complication MSP
EXCLUDES *one foot and other leg (897.6-897.7)*
896.3 Bilateral, complicated MSP

✓4th 897 **Traumatic amputation of leg(s) (complete) (partial)**
897.0 Unilateral, below knee, without mention of complication MSP
897.1 Unilateral, below knee, complicated MSP
897.2 Unilateral, at or above knee, without mention of complication MSP
897.3 Unilateral, at or above knee, complicated MSP
897.4 Unilateral, level not specified, without mention of complication MSP
897.5 Unilateral, level not specified, complicated MSP
897.6 Bilateral [any level], without mention of complication MSP
One foot and other leg
897.7 Bilateral [any level], complicated MSP
AHA: 3Q, '90, 5

INJURY TO BLOOD VESSELS (900-904)

INCLUDES arterial hematoma, avulsion, cut, laceration, rupture, traumatic aneurysm or fistula (arteriovenous) } of blood vessel, secondary to other injuries e.g., fracture or open wound

EXCLUDES *accidental puncture or laceration during medical procedure (998.2)*
intracranial hemorrhage following injury (851.0-854.1)

AHA: 3Q, '90, 5

✓4th 900 **Injury to blood vessels of head and neck**
✓5th 900.0 Carotid artery
900.00 Carotid artery, unspecified MSP
900.01 Common carotid artery MSP
900.02 External carotid artery MSP
900.03 Internal carotid artery MSP
900.1 Internal jugular vein MSP
✓5th 900.8 Other specified blood vessels of head and neck
900.81 External jugular vein MSP
Jugular vein NOS
900.82 Multiple blood vessels of head and neck MSP
900.89 Other MSP
900.9 Unspecified blood vessel of head and neck MSP

✓4th 901 **Injury to blood vessels of thorax**
EXCLUDES *traumatic hemothorax (860.2-860.5)*
901.0 Thoracic aorta
901.1 Innominate and subclavian arteries
901.2 Superior vena cava
901.3 Innominate and subclavian veins
✓5th 901.4 Pulmonary blood vessels
901.40 Pulmonary vessel(s), unspecified
901.41 Pulmonary artery
901.42 Pulmonary vein
✓5th 901.8 Other specified blood vessels of thorax
901.81 Intercostal artery or vein
901.82 Internal mammary artery or vein
901.83 Multiple blood vessels of thorax
901.89 Other
Azygos vein
Hemiazygos vein
901.9 Unspecified blood vessel of thorax

✓4th 902 **Injury to blood vessels of abdomen and pelvis**
902.0 Abdominal aorta
✓5th 902.1 Inferior vena cava
902.10 Inferior vena cava, unspecified
902.11 Hepatic veins
902.19 Other
✓5th 902.2 Celiac and mesenteric arteries
902.20 Celiac and mesenteric arteries, unspecified
902.21 Gastric artery
902.22 Hepatic artery
902.23 Splenic artery
902.24 Other specified branches of celiac axis
902.25 Superior mesenteric artery (trunk)
902.26 Primary branches of superior mesenteric artery
Ileocolic artery
902.27 Inferior mesenteric artery
902.29 Other
✓5th 902.3 Portal and splenic veins
902.31 Superior mesenteric vein and primary subdivisions
Ileocolic vein
902.32 Inferior mesenteric vein
902.33 Portal vein
902.34 Splenic vein
902.39 Other
Cystic vein Gastric vein
✓5th 902.4 Renal blood vessels
902.40 Renal vessel(s), unspecified
902.41 Renal artery
902.42 Renal vein
902.49 Other
Suprarenal arteries
✓5th 902.5 Iliac blood vessels
902.50 Iliac vessel(s), unspecified
902.51 Hypogastric artery
902.52 Hypogastric vein
902.53 Iliac artery
902.54 Iliac vein
902.55 Uterine artery ♀
902.56 Uterine vein ♀
902.59 Other
✓5th 902.8 Other specified blood vessels of abdomen and pelvis
902.81 Ovarian artery ♀
902.82 Ovarian vein ♀
902.87 Multiple blood vessels of abdomen and pelvis
902.89 Other
902.9 Unspecified blood vessel of abdomen and pelvis

✓4th **903 Injury to blood vessels of upper extremity**

✓5th **903.0 Axillary blood vessels**

903.00 Axillary vessel(s), unspecified

903.01 Axillary artery

903.02 Axillary vein

903.1 Brachial blood vessels

903.2 Radial blood vessels

903.3 Ulnar blood vessels

903.4 Palmar artery

903.5 Digital blood vessels

903.8 Other specified blood vessels of upper extremity

Multiple blood vessels of upper extremity

903.9 Unspecified blood vessel of upper extremity

✓4th **904 Injury to blood vessels of lower extremity and unspecified sites**

904.0 Common femoral artery

Femoral artery above profunda origin

904.1 Superficial femoral artery

904.2 Femoral veins

904.3 Saphenous veins

Saphenous vein (greater) (lesser)

✓5th **904.4 Popliteal blood vessels**

904.40 Popliteal vessel(s), unspecified

904.41 Popliteal artery

904.42 Popliteal vein

✓5th **904.5 Tibial blood vessels**

904.50 Tibial vessel(s), unspecified

904.51 Anterior tibial artery

904.52 Anterior tibial vein

904.53 Posterior tibial artery

904.54 Posterior tibial vein

904.6 Deep plantar blood vessels

904.7 Other specified blood vessels of lower extremity

Multiple blood vessels of lower extremity

904.8 Unspecified blood vessel of lower extremity

904.9 Unspecified site

Injury to blood vessel NOS

LATE EFFECTS OF INJURIES, POISONINGS, TOXIC EFFECTS, AND OTHER EXTERNAL CAUSES (905-909)

Note: These categories are to be used to indicate conditions classifiable to 800-999 as the cause of late effects, which are themselves classified elsewhere. The "late effects" include those specified as such, or as sequelae, which may occur at any time after the acute injury.

✓4th **905 Late effects of musculoskeletal and connective tissue injuries**

AHA: 1Q, '95, 10; 2Q, '94, 3

905.0 Late effect of fracture of skull and face bones

Late effect of injury classifiable to 800-804

AHA: 3Q, '97, 12

905.1 Late effect of fracture of spine and trunk without mention of spinal cord lesion

Late effect of injury classifiable to 805, 807-809

905.2 Late effect of fracture of upper extremities

Late effect of injury classifiable to 810-819

905.3 Late effect of fracture of neck of femur

Late effect of injury classifiable to 820

905.4 Late effect of fracture of lower extremities

Late effect of injury classifiable to 821-827

905.5 Late effect of fracture of multiple and unspecified bones

Late effect of injury classifiable to 828-829

905.6 Late effect of dislocation

Late effect of injury classifiable to 830-839

905.7 Late effect of sprain and strain without mention of tendon injury

Late effect of injury classifiable to 840-848, except tendon injury

905.8 Late effect of tendon injury

Late effect of tendon injury due to:

open wound [injury classifiable to 880-884 with .2, 890-894 with .2]

sprain and strain [injury classifiable to 840-848]

AHA: 2Q, '89, 13; 2Q, '89, 15

905.9 Late effect of traumatic amputation

Late effect of injury classifiable to 885-887, 895-897

EXCLUDES *late amputation stump complication (997.60-997.69)*

✓4th **906 Late effects of injuries to skin and subcutaneous tissues**

906.0 Late effect of open wound of head, neck, and trunk

Late effect of injury classifiable to 870-879

906.1 Late effect of open wound of extremities without mention of tendon injury

Late effect of injury classifiable to 880-884, 890-894 except .2

906.2 Late effect of superficial injury

Late effect of injury classifiable to 910-919

906.3 Late effect of contusion

Late effect of injury classifiable to 920-924

906.4 Late effect of crushing

Late effect of injury classifiable to 925-929

906.5 Late effect of burn of eye, face, head, and neck

Late effect of injury classifiable to 940-941

AHA: ►4Q, '04, 76◄

906.6 Late effect of burn of wrist and hand

Late effect of injury classifiable to 944

AHA: 4Q, '94, 22

906.7 Late effect of burn of other extremities

Late effect of injury classifiable to 943 or 945

AHA: 4Q, '94, 22

906.8 Late effect of burns of other specified sites

Late effect of injury classifiable to 942, 946-947

AHA: 4Q, '94, 22

906.9 Late effect of burn of unspecified site

Late effect of injury classifiable to 948-949

AHA: 4Q, '94, 22

✓4th **907 Late effects of injuries to the nervous system**

907.0 Late effect of intracranial injury without mention of skull fracture

Late effect of injury classifiable to 850-854

AHA: 4Q, '03, 103; 3Q, '90, 14

907.1 Late effect of injury to cranial nerve

Late effect of injury classifiable to 950-951

907.2 Late effect of spinal cord injury

Late effect of injury classifiable to 806, 952

AHA: 4Q, '03, 103; 4Q, '98, 38

907.3 Late effect of injury to nerve root(s), spinal plexus(es), and other nerves of trunk

Late effect of injury classifiable to 953-954

907.4 Late effect of injury to peripheral nerve of shoulder girdle and upper limb

Late effect of injury classifiable to 955

907.5 Late effect of injury to peripheral nerve of pelvic girdle and lower limb

Late effect of injury classifiable to 956

907.9 Late effect of injury to other and unspecified nerve

Late effect of injury classifiable to 957

✓4th **908 Late effects of other and unspecified injuries**

908.0 Late effect of internal injury to chest

Late effect of injury classifiable to 860-862

908.1 Late effect of internal injury to intra-abdominal organs
Late effect of injury classifiable to 863-866, 868

908.2 Late effect of internal injury to other internal organs
Late effect of injury classifiable to 867 or 869

908.3 Late effect of injury to blood vessel of head, neck, and extremities
Late effect of injury classifiable to 900, 903-904

908.4 Late effect of injury to blood vessel of thorax, abdomen, and pelvis
Late effect of injury classifiable to 901-902

908.5 Late effect of foreign body in orifice
Late effect of injury classifiable to 930-939

908.6 Late effect of certain complications of trauma
Late effect of complications classifiable to 958

908.9 Late effect of unspecified injury
Late effect of injury classifiable to 959
AHA: 3Q, '00, 4

✓4th 909 Late effects of other and unspecified external causes

909.0 Late effect of poisoning due to drug, medicinal or biological substance
Late effect of conditions classifiable to 960-979
EXCLUDES *late effect of adverse effect of drug, medicinal or biological substance (909.5)*
AHA: 4Q, '03, 103

909.1 Late effect of toxic effects of nonmedical substances
Late effect of conditions classifiable to 980-989

909.2 Late effect of radiation
Late effect of conditions classifiable to 990

909.3 Late effect of complications of surgical and medical care
Late effect of conditions classifiable to 996-999
AHA: 1Q, '93, 29

909.4 Late effect of certain other external causes
Late effect of conditions classifiable to 991-994

909.5 Late effect of adverse effect of drug, medical or biological substance
EXCLUDES *late effect of poisoning due to drug, medical or biological substance (909.0)*
AHA: 4Q, '94, 48

909.9 Late effect of other and unspecified external causes

SUPERFICIAL INJURY (910-919)

EXCLUDES *burn (blisters) (940.0-949.5)*
contusion (920-924.9)
foreign body:
granuloma (728.82)
inadvertently left in operative wound (998.4)
residual in soft tissue (729.6)
insect bite, venomous (989.5)
open wound with incidental foreign body (870.0-897.7)

AHA: 2Q, '89, 15

✓4th 910 Superficial injury of face, neck, and scalp except eye
INCLUDES cheek
ear
gum
lip
nose
throat
EXCLUDES *eye and adnexa (918.0-918.9)*

910.0 Abrasion or friction burn without mention of infection
910.1 Abrasion or friction burn, infected
910.2 Blister without mention of infection
910.3 Blister, infected
910.4 Insect bite, nonvenomous, without mention of infection
910.5 Insect bite, nonvenomous, infected
910.6 Superficial foreign body (splinter) without major open wound and without mention of infection
910.7 Superficial foreign body (splinter) without major open wound, infected
910.8 Other and unspecified superficial injury of face, neck, and scalp without mention of infection
910.9 Other and unspecified superficial injury of face, neck, and scalp, infected

✓4th 911 Superficial injury of trunk
INCLUDES abdominal wall
anus
back
breast
buttock
mchest wall
flank
groin
interscapular region
labium (majus) (minus)
penis
perineum
scrotum
testis
vagina
vulva
EXCLUDES *hip (916.0-916.9)*
scapular region (912.0-912.9)

911.0 Abrasion or friction burn without mention of infection
AHA: 3Q, '01, 10
911.1 Abrasion or friction burn, infected
911.2 Blister without mention of infection
911.3 Blister, infected
911.4 Insect bite, nonvenomous, without mention of infection
911.5 Insect bite, nonvenomous, infected
911.6 Superficial foreign body (splinter) without major open wound and without mention of infection
911.7 Superficial foreign body (splinter) without major open wound, infected
911.8 Other and unspecified superficial injury of trunk without mention of infection
911.9 Other and unspecified superficial injury of trunk, infected

✓4th 912 Superficial injury of shoulder and upper arm
INCLUDES axilla
scapular region

912.0 Abrasion or friction burn without mention of infection
912.1 Abrasion or friction burn, infected
912.2 Blister without mention of infection
912.3 Blister, infected
912.4 Insect bite, nonvenomous, without mention of infection
912.5 Insect bite, nonvenomous, infected
912.6 Superficial foreign body (splinter) without major open wound and without mention of infection
912.7 Superficial foreign body (splinter) without major open wound, infected
912.8 Other and unspecified superficial injury of shoulder and upper arm without mention of infection
912.9 Other and unspecified superficial injury of shoulder and upper arm, infected

4th 913 Superficial injury of elbow, forearm, and wrist

- **913.0 Abrasion or friction burn without mention of infection**
- **913.1 Abrasion or friction burn, infected**
- **913.2 Blister without mention of infection**
- **913.3 Blister, infected**
- **913.4 Insect bite, nonvenomous, without mention of infection**
- **913.5 Insect bite, nonvenomous, infected**
- **913.6 Superficial foreign body (splinter) without major open wound and without mention of infection**
- **913.7 Superficial foreign body (splinter) without major open wound, infected**
- **913.8 Other and unspecified superficial injury of elbow, forearm, and wrist without mention of infection**
- **913.9 Other and unspecified superficial injury of elbow, forearm, and wrist, infected**

4th 914 Superficial injury of hand(s) except finger(s) alone

- **914.0 Abrasion or friction burn without mention of infection**
- **914.1 Abrasion or friction burn, infected**
- **914.2 Blister without mention of infection**
- **914.3 Blister, infected**
- **914.4 Insect bite, nonvenomous, without mention of infection**
- **914.5 Insect bite, nonvenomous, infected**
- **914.6 Superficial foreign body (splinter) without major open wound and without mention of infection**
- **914.7 Superficial foreign body (splinter) without major open wound, infected**
- **914.8 Other and unspecified superficial injury of hand without mention of infection**
- **914.9 Other and unspecified superficial injury of hand, infected**

4th 915 Superficial injury of finger(s)

INCLUDES fingernail
thumb (nail)

- **915.0 Abrasion or friction burn without mention of infection**
- **915.1 Abrasion or friction burn, infected**
- **915.2 Blister without mention of infection**
- **915.3 Blister, infected**
- **915.4 Insect bite, nonvenomous, without mention of infection**
- **915.5 Insect bite, nonvenomous, infected**
- **915.6 Superficial foreign body (splinter) without major open wound and without mention of infection**
- **915.7 Superficial foreign body (splinter) without major open wound, infected**
- **915.8 Other and unspecified superficial injury of fingers without mention of infection**
  AHA: 3Q, '01, 10
- **915.9 Other and unspecified superficial injury of fingers, infected**

4th 916 Superficial injury of hip, thigh, leg, and ankle

- **916.0 Abrasion or friction burn without mention of infection**
- **916.1 Abrasion or friction burn, infected**
- **916.2 Blister without mention of infection**
- **916.3 Blister, infected**
- **916.4 Insect bite, nonvenomous, without mention of infection**
- **916.5 Insect bite, nonvenomous, infected**
- **916.6 Superficial foreign body (splinter) without major open wound and without mention of infection**
- **916.7 Superficial foreign body (splinter) without major open wound, infected**
- **916.8 Other and unspecified superficial injury of hip, thigh, leg, and ankle without mention of infection**
- **916.9 Other and unspecified superficial injury of hip, thigh, leg, and ankle, infected**

4th 917 Superficial injury of foot and toe(s)

INCLUDES heel
toenail

- **917.0 Abrasion or friction burn without mention of infection**
- **917.1 Abrasion or friction burn, infected**
- **917.2 Blister without mention of infection**
- **917.3 Blister, infected**
- **917.4 Insect bite, nonvenomous, without mention of infection**
- **917.5 Insect bite, nonvenomous, infected**
- **917.6 Superficial foreign body (splinter) without major open wound and without mention of infection**
- **917.7 Superficial foreign body (splinter) without major open wound, infected**
- **917.8 Other and unspecified superficial injury of foot and toes without mention of infection**
  AHA: 1Q, '03, 13
- **917.9 Other and unspecified superficial injury of foot and toes, infected**
  AHA: 1Q, '03, 13

4th 918 Superficial injury of eye and adnexa

EXCLUDES *burn (940.0-940.9)*
foreign body on external eye (930.0-930.9)

- **918.0 Eyelids and periocular area**
  Abrasion
  Insect bite
  Superficial foreign body (splinter)
- **918.1 Cornea**
  Corneal abrasion
  Superficial laceration
  EXCLUDES *corneal injury due to contact lens (371.82)*
- **918.2 Conjunctiva**
- **918.9 Other and unspecified superficial injuries of eye**
  Eye (ball) NOS

4th 919 Superficial injury of other, multiple, and unspecified sites

EXCLUDES *multiple sites classifiable to the same three-digit category (910.0-918.9)*

- **919.0 Abrasion or friction burn without mention of infection**
- **919.1 Abrasion or friction burn, infected**
- **919.2 Blister without mention of infection**
- **919.3 Blister, infected**
- **919.4 Insect bite, nonvenomous, without mention of infection**
- **919.5 Insect bite, nonvenomous, infected**
- **919.6 Superficial foreign body (splinter) without major open wound and without mention of infection**
- **919.7 Superficial foreign body (splinter) without major open wound, infected**
- **919.8 Other and unspecified superficial injury without mention of infection**
- **919.9 Other and unspecified superficial injury, infected**

N Newborn Age: 0 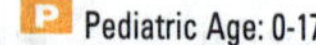 P Pediatric Age: 0-17 M Maternity Age: 12-55 A Adult Age: 15-124 MSP Medicare Secondary Payer

CONTUSION WITH INTACT SKIN SURFACE (920-924)

INCLUDES bruise, hematoma } without fracture or open wound

EXCLUDES *concussion (850.0-850.9)*
hemarthrosis (840.0-848.9)
internal organs (860.0-869.1)
that incidental to:
crushing injury (925-929.9)
dislocation (830.0-839.9)
fracture (800.0-829.1)
internal injury (860.0-869.1)
intracranial injury (850.0-854.1)
nerve injury (950.0-957.9)
open wound (870.0-897.7)

920 Contusion of face, scalp, and neck except eye(s)
Cheek
Ear (auricle)
Gum
Lip
Mandibular joint area
Nose
Throat

✓4th **921 Contusion of eye and adnexa**
921.0 Black eye, not otherwise specified
921.1 Contusion of eyelids and periocular area
921.2 Contusion of orbital tissues
921.3 Contusion of eyeball
AHA: J-A, '85, 16
921.9 Unspecified contusion of eye
Injury of eye NOS

✓4th **922 Contusion of trunk**
922.0 Breast
922.1 Chest wall
922.2 Abdominal wall
Flank
Groin
✓5th **922.3 Back**
AHA: 4Q, '96, 39
922.31 Back
EXCLUDES *interscapular region (922.33)*
922.32 Buttock
AHA: 3Q, '99, 14
922.33 Interscapular region
922.4 Genital organs
Labium (majus) (minus)
Penis
Perineum
Scrotum
Vulva
Vagina
Testis
922.8 Multiple sites of trunk
922.9 Unspecified part
Trunk NOS

✓4th **923 Contusion of upper limb**
✓5th **923.0 Shoulder and upper arm**
923.00 Shoulder region
923.01 Scapular region
923.02 Axillary region
923.03 Upper arm
923.09 Multiple sites
✓5th **923.1 Elbow and forearm**
923.10 Forearm
923.11 Elbow
✓5th **923.2 Wrist and hand(s), except finger(s) alone**
923.20 Hand(s)
923.21 Wrist
923.3 Finger
Fingernail
Thumb (nail)
923.8 Multiple sites of upper limb
923.9 Unspecified part of upper limb
Arm NOS

✓4th **924 Contusion of lower limb and of other and unspecified sites**
✓5th **924.0 Hip and thigh**
924.00 Thigh
924.01 Hip
✓5th **924.1 Knee and lower leg**
924.10 Lower leg
924.11 Knee
✓5th **924.2 Ankle and foot, excluding toe(s)**
924.20 Foot
Heel
924.21 Ankle
924.3 Toe
Toenail
924.4 Multiple sites of lower limb
924.5 Unspecified part of lower limb
Leg NOS
924.8 Multiple sites, not elsewhere classified
AHA: 1Q, '03, 7
924.9 Unspecified site

CRUSHING INJURY (925-929)

Use additional code to identify any associated injuries, such as:
fractures (800-829)
internal injuries (860.0-869.1)
intracranial injuries (850.0-854.1)

AHA: 4Q, '03, 77; 2Q, '93, 7

✓4th **925 Crushing injury of face, scalp, and neck**
Cheek
Ear
Larynx
Pharynx
Throat
925.1 Crushing injury of face and scalp MSP
Cheek
Ear
925.2 Crushing injury of neck MSP
Larynx
Pharynx
Throat

✓4th **926 Crushing injury of trunk**
926.0 External genitalia
Labium (majus) (minus)
Penis
Scrotum
Testis
Vulva
✓5th **926.1 Other specified sites**
926.11 Back
926.12 Buttock
926.19 Other
Breast
926.8 Multiple sites of trunk MSP
926.9 Unspecified site
Trunk NOS

✓4th **927 Crushing injury of upper limb**
✓5th **927.0 Shoulder and upper arm**
927.00 Shoulder region
927.01 Scapular region
927.02 Axillary region
927.03 Upper arm
927.09 Multiple sites
✓5th **927.1 Elbow and forearm**
927.10 Forearm
927.11 Elbow
✓5th **927.2 Wrist and hand(s), except finger(s) alone**
927.20 Hand(s)
927.21 Wrist
927.3 Finger(s)
AHA: 4Q, '03, 77
927.8 Multiple sites of upper limb
927.9 Unspecified site
Arm NOS

✓4th **928 Crushing injury of lower limb**

✓5th **928.0 Hip and thigh**

928.00 Thigh

928.01 Hip

✓5th **928.1 Knee and lower leg**

928.10 Lower leg

928.11 Knee

✓5th **928.2 Ankle and foot, excluding toe(s) alone**

928.20 Foot

Heel

928.21 Ankle

928.3 Toe(s)

928.8 Multiple sites of lower limb

928.9 Unspecified site

Leg NOS

✓4th **929 Crushing injury of multiple and unspecified sites**

929.0 Multiple sites, not elsewhere classified MSP

929.9 Unspecified site MSP

EFFECTS OF FOREIGN BODY ENTERING THROUGH ORIFICE (930-939)

EXCLUDES *foreign body:*
granuloma (728.82)
inadvertently left in operative wound (998.4, 998.7)
in open wound (800-839, 851-897)
residual in soft tissues (729.6)
superficial without major open wound (910-919 with .6 or .7)

✓4th **930 Foreign body on external eye**

EXCLUDES *foreign body in penetrating wound of:*
eyeball (871.5-871.6)
retained (old) (360.5-360.6)
ocular adnexa (870.4)
retained (old) (376.6)

930.0 Corneal foreign body

930.1 Foreign body in conjunctival sac

930.2 Foreign body in lacrimal punctum

930.8 Other and combined sites

930.9 Unspecified site

External eye NOS

931 Foreign body in ear

Auditory canal
Auricle

932 Foreign body in nose

Nasal sinus
Nostril

✓4th **933 Foreign body in pharynx and larynx**

933.0 Pharynx

Nasopharynx
Throat NOS

933.1 Larynx

Asphyxia due to foreign body
Choking due to:
food (regurgitated)
phlegm

✓4th **934 Foreign body in trachea, bronchus, and lung**

934.0 Trachea

934.1 Main bronchus

AHA: 3Q, '02, 18

934.8 Other specified parts

Bronchioles
Lung

934.9 Respiratory tree, unspecified

Inhalation of liquid or vomitus, lower respiratory tract NOS

✓4th **935 Foreign body in mouth, esophagus, and stomach**

935.0 Mouth

935.1 Esophagus

AHA: 1Q, '88, 13

935.2 Stomach

936 Foreign body in intestine and colon

937 Foreign body in anus and rectum

Rectosigmoid (junction)

938 Foreign body in digestive system, unspecified

Alimentary tract NOS
Swallowed foreign body

✓4th **939 Foreign body in genitourinary tract**

939.0 Bladder and urethra

939.1 Uterus, any part ♀

EXCLUDES *intrauterine contraceptive device:*
complications from (996.32, 996.65)
presence of (V45.51)

939.2 Vulva and vagina ♀

939.3 Penis ♂

939.9 Unspecified site

BURNS (940-949)

INCLUDES burns from:
electrical heating appliance
electricity
flame
hot object
lightning
radiation
chemical burns (external) (internal)
scalds

EXCLUDES *friction burns (910-919 with .0, .1)*
sunburn (692.71, 692.76-692.77)

AHA: 4Q, 94, 22; 2Q, '90, 7; 4Q, '88, 3; M-A, '86, 9

✓4th **940 Burn confined to eye and adnexa**

940.0 Chemical burn of eyelids and periocular area

940.1 Other burns of eyelids and periocular area

940.2 Alkaline chemical burn of cornea and conjunctival sac

940.3 Acid chemical burn of cornea and conjunctival sac

940.4 Other burn of cornea and conjunctival sac

940.5 Burn with resulting rupture and destruction of eyeball

940.9 Unspecified burn of eye and adnexa

✓4th **941 Burn of face, head, and neck**

EXCLUDES *mouth (947.0)*

The following fifth-digit subclassification is for use with category 941:

0 face and head, unspecified site
1 ear [any part]
2 eye (with other parts of face, head, and neck)
3 lip(s)
4 chin
5 nose (septum)
6 scalp [any part]
Temple (region)
7 forehead and cheek
8 neck
9 multiple sites [except with eye] of face, head, and neck

AHA: 4Q, '94, 22; M-A, '86, 9

✓5th **941.0 Unspecified degree**

Burns

Degrees of Burns

First (redness)
Second (blistering)
Third (fill thickness)
Deep Third (deep necrosis)
Eschar

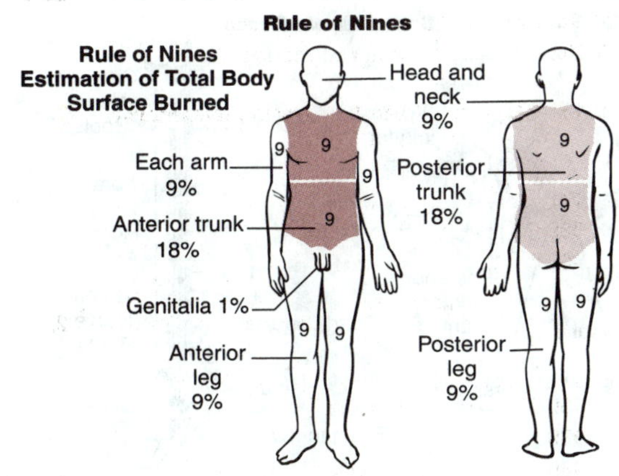

✓5th **941.1 Erythema [first degree]**

✓5th **941.2 Blisters, epidermal loss [second degree]**

✓5th **941.3 Full-thickness skin loss [third degree NOS]**

✓5th **941.4 Deep necrosis of underlying tissues [deep third degree] without mention of loss of a body part**

✓5th **941.5 Deep necrosis of underlying tissues [deep third degree] with loss of a body part**

✓4th **942 Burn of trunk**

EXCLUDES *scapular region (943.0-943.5 with fifth-digit 6)*

The following fifth-digit subclassification is for use with category 942:

- **0 trunk, unspecified site**
- **1 breast**
- **2 chest wall, excluding breast and nipple**
- **3 abdominal wall**
  - Flank
  - Groin
- **4 back [any part]**
  - Buttock
  - Interscapular region
- **5 genitalia**
  - Labium (majus) (minus)
  - Penis
  - Perineum
  - Scrotum
  - Testis
  - Vulva
- **9 other and multiple sites of trunk**

AHA: 4Q, '94, 22; M-A, '86, 9

✓5th **942.0 Unspecified degree**

✓5th **942.1 Erythema [first degree]**

✓5th **942.2 Blisters, epidermal loss [second degree]**

✓5th **942.3 Full-thickness skin loss [third degree NOS]**

✓5th **942.4 Deep necrosis of underlying tissues [deep third degree] without mention of loss of a body part**

✓5th **942.5 Deep necrosis of underlying tissues [deep third degree] with loss of a body part**

✓4th **943 Burn of upper limb, except wrist and hand**

The following fifth-digit subclassification is for use with category 943:

- **0 upper limb, unspecified site**
- **1 forearm**
- **2 elbow**
- **3 upper arm**
- **4 axilla**
- **5 shoulder**
- **6 scapular region**
- **9 multiple sites of upper limb, except wrist and hand**

AHA: 4Q, '94, 22; M-A, '86, 9

✓5th **943.0 Unspecified degree**

✓5th **943.1 Erythema [first degree]**

✓5th **943.2 Blisters, epidermal loss [second degree]**

✓5th **943.3 Full-thickness skin loss [third degree NOS]**

✓5th **943.4 Deep necrosis of underlying tissues [deep third degree] without mention of loss of a body part**

✓5th **943.5 Deep necrosis of underlying tissues [deep third degree] with loss of a body part**

✓4th **944 Burn of wrist(s) and hand(s)**

The following fifth-digit subclassification is for use with category 944:

- **0 hand, unspecified site**
- **1 single digit [finger (nail)] other than thumb**
- **2 thumb (nail)**
- **3 two or more digits, not including thumb**
- **4 two or more digits including thumb**
- **5 palm**
- **6 back of hand**
- **7 wrist**
- **8 multiple sites of wrist(s) and hand(s)**

✓5th **944.0 Unspecified degree**

✓5th **944.1 Erythema [first degree]**

✓5th **944.2 Blisters, epidermal loss [second degree]**

✓5th **944.3 Full-thickness skin loss [third degree NOS]**

✓5th **944.4 Deep necrosis of underlying tissues [deep third degree] without mention of loss of a body part**

✓5th **944.5 Deep necrosis of underlying tissues [deep third degree] with loss of a body part**

✓4th **945 Burn of lower limb(s)**

The following fifth-digit subclassification is for use with category 945:

- **0 lower limb [leg], unspecified site**
- **1 toe(s) (nail)**
- **2 foot**
- **3 ankle**
- **4 lower leg**
- **5 knee**
- **6 thigh [any part]**
- **9 multiple sites of lower limb(s)**

AHA: 4Q, '94, 22; M-A, '86, 9

✓5th **945.0 Unspecified degree**

✓5th **945.1 Erythema [first degree]**

✓5th **945.2 Blisters, epidermal loss [second degree]**

✓5th **945.3 Full-thickness skin loss [third degree NOS]**

✓5th **945.4 Deep necrosis of underlying tissues [deep third degree] without mention of loss of a body part**

✓5th **945.5 Deep necrosis of underlying tissues [deep third degree] with loss of a body part**

✓4th **946 Burns of multiple specified sites**

INCLUDES burns of sites classifiable to more than one three-digit category in 940-945

EXCLUDES *multiple burns NOS (949.0-949.5)*

AHA: 4Q, '94, 22; M-A, '86, 9

946.0 Unspecified degree

946.1 Erythema [first degree]

946.2 Blisters, epidermal loss [second degree]

946.3 Full-thickness skin loss [third degree NOS]

946.4 Deep necrosis of underlying tissues [deep third degree] without mention of loss of a body part

946.5 Deep necrosis of underlying tissues [deep third degree] with loss of a body part

✓4th **947 Burn of internal organs**

INCLUDES burns from chemical agents (ingested)

AHA: 4Q, '94, 22; M-A, '86, 9

947.0 Mouth and pharynx
- Gum
- Tongue

947.1 Larynx, trachea, and lung

947.2 Esophagus

947.3 Gastrointestinal tract
- Colon
- Rectum
- Small intestine
- Stomach

947.4 **Vagina and uterus** ♀

947.8 **Other specified sites**

947.9 **Unspecified site**

✓4th **948 Burns classified according to extent of body surface involved**

Note: This category is to be used when the site of the burn is unspecified, or with categories 940-947 when the site is specified.

EXCLUDES *sunburn (692.71, 692.76-692.77)*

The following fifth-digit subclassification is for use with category 948 to indicate the percent of body surface with third degree burn; valid digits are in [brackets] under each code:

0 less than 10 percent or unspecified
1 10-19%
2 20-29%
3 30-39%
4 40-49%
5 50-59%
6 60-69%
7 70-79%
8 80-89%
9 90% or more of body surface

AHA: 4Q, '94, 22; 4Q, '88, 3; M-A, '86, 9; N-D, '84, 13

✓5th 948.0 [0] **Burn [any degree] involving less than 10 percent of body surface**

✓5th 948.1 [0-1] **10-19 percent of body surface**

✓5th 948.2 [0-2] **20-29 percent of body surface**

✓5th 948.3 [0-3] **30-39 percent of body surface**

✓5th 948.4 [0-4] **40-49 percent of body surface**

✓5th 948.5 [0-5] **50-59 percent of body surface**

✓5th 948.6 [0-6] **60-69 percent of body surface**

✓5th 948.7 [0-7] **70-79 percent of body surface**

✓5th 948.8 [0-8] **80-89 percent of body surface**

✓5th 948.9 [0-9] **90 percent or more of body surface**

✓4th **949 Burn, unspecified**

INCLUDES burn NOS multiple burns NOS

EXCLUDES *burn of unspecified site but with statement of the extent of body surface involved (948.0-948.9)*

AHA: 4Q, '94, 22; M-A, '86, 9

949.0 **Unspecified degree**

949.1 **Erythema [first degree]**

949.2 **Blisters, epidermal loss [second degree]**

949.3 **Full-thickness skin loss [third degree NOS]**

949.4 **Deep necrosis of underlying tissues [deep third degree] without mention of loss of a body part**

949.5 **Deep necrosis of underlying tissues [deep third degree] with loss of a body part**

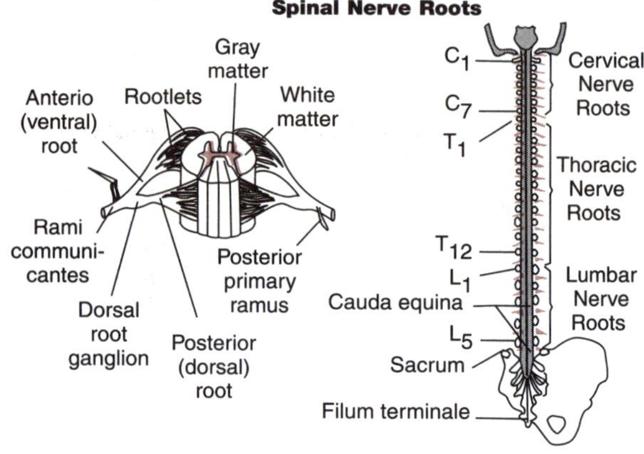

INJURY TO NERVES AND SPINAL CORD (950-957)

INCLUDES division of nerve
lesion in continuity (with open wound)
traumatic neuroma (with open wound)
traumatic transient paralysis (with open wound)

EXCLUDES *accidental puncture or laceration during medical procedure (998.2)*

✓4th **950 Injury to optic nerve and pathways**

950.0 **Optic nerve injury**
Second cranial nerve

950.1 **Injury to optic chiasm**

950.2 **Injury to optic pathways**

950.3 **Injury to visual cortex**

950.9 **Unspecified**
Traumatic blindness NOS

✓4th **951 Injury to other cranial nerve(s)**

951.0 **Injury to oculomotor nerve**
Third cranial nerve

951.1 **Injury to trochlear nerve**
Fourth cranial nerve

951.2 **Injury to trigeminal nerve**
Fifth cranial nerve

951.3 **Injury to abducens nerve**
Sixth cranial nerve

951.4 **Injury to facial nerve**
Seventh cranial nerve

951.5 **Injury to acoustic nerve**
Auditory nerve
Eighth cranial nerve
Traumatic deafness NOS

951.6 **Injury to accessory nerve**
Eleventh cranial nerve

951.7 **Injury to hypoglossal nerve**
Twelfth cranial nerve

951.8 **Injury to other specified cranial nerves**
Glossopharyngeal [9th cranial] nerve
Olfactory [1st cranial] nerve
Pneumogastric [10th cranial] nerve
Traumatic anosmia NOS
Vagus [10th cranial] nerve

951.9 **Injury to unspecified cranial nerve**

✓4th **952 Spinal cord injury without evidence of spinal bone injury**

✓5th 952.0 **Cervical**

952.00 **C_1-C_4 level with unspecified spinal cord injury**
Spinal cord injury, cervical region NOS

952.01 **C_1-C_4 level with complete lesion of spinal cord**

952.02 **C_1-C_4 level with anterior cord syndrome**

952.03 **C_1-C_4 level with central cord syndrome**

952.04 **C_1-C_4 level with other specified spinal cord injury**
Incomplete spinal cord lesion at C_1-C_4 level:
NOS
with posterior cord syndrome

952.05 **C_5-C_7 level with unspecified spinal cord injury**

952.06 **C_5-C_7 level with complete lesion of spinal cord**

952.07 **C_5-C_7 level with anterior cord syndrome**

952.08 **C_5-C_7 level with central cord syndrome**

952.09 **C_5-C_7 level with other specified spinal cord injury**
Incomplete spinal cord lesion at C_5-C_7 level:
NOS
with posterior cord syndrome

✓5th 952.1 **Dorsal [thoracic]**

952.10 **T_1-T_6 level with unspecified spinal cord injury**
Spinal cord injury, thoracic region NOS

952.11 **T_1-T_6 level with complete lesion of spinal cord**

952.12 **T_1-T_6 level with anterior cord syndrome**

952.13 **T_1-T_6 level with central cord syndrome**

952.14 **T_1-T_6 level with other specified spinal cord injury**
Incomplete spinal cord lesion at T_1-T_6 level:
NOS
with posterior cord syndrome

952.15 **T_7-T_{12} level with unspecified spinal cord injury**

952.16 **T_7-T_{12} level with complete lesion of spinal cord**

952.17 **T_7-T_{12} level with anterior cord syndrome**

952.18 **T_7-T_{12} level with central cord syndrome**

952.19 **T_7-T_{12} level with other specified spinal cord injury**
Incomplete spinal cord lesion at T_7-T_{12} level:
NOS
with posterior cord syndrome

952.2 **Lumbar**

952.3 **Sacral**

952.4 **Cauda equina**

952.8 **Multiple sites of spinal cord**

952.9 **Unspecified site of spinal cord**

✓4th **953 Injury to nerve roots and spinal plexus**

953.0 **Cervical root**

953.1 **Dorsal root**

953.2 **Lumbar root**

953.3 **Sacral root**

953.4 **Brachial plexus**

953.5 **Lumbosacral plexus**

953.8 **Multiple sites**

953.9 **Unspecified site**

✓4th **954 Injury to other nerve(s) of trunk, excluding shoulder and pelvic girdles**

954.0 **Cervical sympathetic**

954.1 **Other sympathetic**
Celiac ganglion or plexus
Inferior mesenteric plexus
Splanchnic nerve(s)
Stellate ganglion

954.8 **Other specified nerve(s) of trunk**

954.9 **Unspecified nerve of trunk**

✓4th **955 Injury to peripheral nerve(s) of shoulder girdle and upper limb**

955.0 **Axillary nerve**

955.1 **Median nerve**

955.2 **Ulnar nerve**

955.3 **Radial nerve**

955.4 **Musculocutaneous nerve**

955.5 **Cutaneous sensory nerve, upper limb**

955.6 **Digital nerve**

955.7 **Other specified nerve(s) of shoulder girdle and upper limb**

955.8 **Multiple nerves of shoulder girdle and upper limb**

955.9 **Unspecified nerve of shoulder girdle and upper limb**

✓4th **956 Injury to peripheral nerve(s) of pelvic girdle and lower limb**

956.0 **Sciatic nerve**

956.1 **Femoral nerve**

956.2 **Posterior tibial nerve**

956.3 **Peroneal nerve**

956.4 **Cutaneous sensory nerve, lower limb**

956.5 **Other specified nerve(s) of pelvic girdle and lower limb**

956.8 **Multiple nerves of pelvic girdle and lower limb**

956.9 **Unspecified nerve of pelvic girdle and lower limb**

✓4th **957 Injury to other and unspecified nerves**

957.0 **Superficial nerves of head and neck**

957.1 **Other specified nerve(s)**

957.8 **Multiple nerves in several parts**
Multiple nerve injury NOS

957.9 **Unspecified site**
Nerve injury NOS

CERTAIN TRAUMATIC COMPLICATIONS AND UNSPECIFIED INJURIES (958-959)

✓4th **958 Certain early complications of trauma**

EXCLUDES *adult respiratory distress syndrome (518.5)*
flail chest (807.4)
shock lung (518.5)
that occurring during or following medical procedures (996.0-999.9)

958.0 **Air embolism**
Pneumathemia
EXCLUDES *that complicating:*
abortion (634-638 with .6, 639.6)
ectopic or molar pregnancy (639.6)
pregnancy, childbirth, or the puerperium (673.0)

DEF: Arterial obstruction due to introduction of air bubbles into the veins following surgery or trauma.

958.1 **Fat embolism**
EXCLUDES *that complicating:*
abortion (634-638 with .6, 639.6)
pregnancy, childbirth, or the puerperium (673.8)

DEF: Arterial blockage due to the entrance of fat in circulatory system, after fracture of large bones or administration of corticosteroids.

958.2 **Secondary and recurrent hemorrhage**

958.3 **Posttraumatic wound infection, not elsewhere classified**
EXCLUDES *infected open wounds — code to complicated open wound of site*

AHA: 4Q, '01, 53; S-O, '85, 10

958.4 **Traumatic shock** MSP
Shock (immediate) (delayed) following injury
EXCLUDES *shock:*
anaphylactic (995.0)
due to serum (999.4)
anesthetic (995.4)
electric (994.8)
following abortion (639.5)
lightning (994.0)
nontraumatic NOS (785.50)
obstetric (669.1)
postoperative (998.0)

DEF: Shock, immediate or delayed following injury.

958.5 Traumatic anuria MSP
Crush syndrome
Renal failure following crushing
EXCLUDES *that due to a medical procedure (997.5)*
DEF: Complete suppression of urinary secretion by kidneys due to trauma.

958.6 Volkmann's ischemic contracture
Posttraumatic muscle contracture
DEF: Muscle deterioration due to loss of blood supply from injury or tourniquet; causes muscle contraction and results in inability to extend the muscles fully.

958.7 Traumatic subcutaneous emphysema
EXCLUDES *subcutaneous emphysema resulting from a procedure (998.81)*

958.8 Other early complications of trauma
AHA: 2Q, '92, 13
DEF: Compartmental syndrome is abnormal pressure in confined anatomical space, as in swollen muscle restricted by fascia.

✓4th **959 Injury, other and unspecified**
INCLUDES injury NOS
EXCLUDES *injury NOS of:*
blood vessels (900.0-904.9)
eye (921.0-921.9)
internal organs (860.0-869.1)
intracranial sites (854.0-854.1)
nerves (950.0-951.9, 953.0-957.9)
spinal cord (952.0-952.9)

✓5th **959.0 Head, face and neck**
959.01 Head injury, unspecified MSP
EXCLUDES *concussion (850.1-850.9)*
with head injury NOS (850.0-850.9)
head injury NOS with loss of consciousness (850.1-850.5)
specified injuries (850.0-854.1)
AHA: 4Q, '97, 46

959.09 Injury of face and neck MSP
Cheek
Ear
Eyebrow
Lip
Mouth
Nose
Throat
AHA: 4Q, '97, 46

✓5th **959.1 Trunk**
EXCLUDES *scapular region (959.2)*
AHA: 4Q, '03, 78; 1Q, '99, 10
959.11 Other injury of chest wall
959.12 Other injury of abdomen
959.13 Fracture of corpus cavernosum penis ♂
959.14 Other injury of external genitals
959.19 Other injury of other sites of trunk
Injury of trunk NOS

959.2 Shoulder and upper arm
Axilla
Scapular region

959.3 Elbow, forearm, and wrist
AHA: 1Q, '97, 8

959.4 Hand, except finger

959.5 Finger
Fingernail
Thumb (nail)

959.6 Hip and thigh
Upper leg

959.7 Knee, leg, ankle, and foot

959.8 Other specified sites, including multiple
EXCLUDES *multiple sites classifiable to the same four-digit category (959.0-959.7)*

959.9 Unspecified site

POISONING BY DRUGS, MEDICINAL AND BIOLOGICAL SUBSTANCES (960-979)

INCLUDES overdose of these substances
wrong substance given or taken in error
EXCLUDES *adverse effects ["hypersensitivity," "reaction," etc.] of correct substance properly administered. Such cases are to be classified according to the nature of the adverse effect, such as:*
adverse effect NOS (995.2)
allergic lymphadenitis (289.3)
aspirin gastritis (535.4)
blood disorders (280.0-289.9)
dermatitis:
contact (692.0-692.9)
due to ingestion (693.0-693.9)
nephropathy (583.9)
[The drug giving rise to the adverse effect may be identified by use of categories E930-E949.]
drug dependence (304.0-304.9)
drug reaction and poisoning affecting the newborn (760.0-779.9)
nondependent abuse of drugs (305.0-305.9)
pathological drug intoxication (292.2)

Use additional code to specify the effects of the poisoning
AHA: 2Q, '90, 11

✓4th **960 Poisoning by antibiotics**
EXCLUDES *antibiotics:*
ear, nose, and throat (976.6)
eye (976.5)
local (976.0)

960.0 Penicillins
Ampicillin
Carbenicillin
Cloxacillin
Penicillin G

960.1 Antifungal antibiotics
Amphotericin B
Griseofulvin
Nystatin
Trichomycin
EXCLUDES *preparations intended for topical use (976.0-976.9)*

960.2 Chloramphenicol group
Chloramphenicol
Thiamphenicol

960.3 Erythromycin and other macrolides
Oleandomycin
Spiramycin

960.4 Tetracycline group
Doxycycline
Minocycline
Oxytetracycline

960.5 Cephalosporin group
Cephalexin
Cephaloglycin
Cephaloridine
Cephalothin

960.6 Antimycobacterial antibiotics
Cycloserine
Kanamycin
Rifampin
Streptomycin

960.7 Antineoplastic antibiotics
Actinomycin such as:
Bleomycin
Cactinomycin
Dactinomycin
Daunorubicin
Mitomycin

960.8 Other specified antibiotics

960.9 Unspecified antibiotic

✓4th **961 Poisoning by other anti-infectives**
EXCLUDES *anti-infectives:*
ear, nose, and throat (976.6)
eye (976.5)
local (976.0)

961.0 Sulfonamides
Sulfadiazine
Sulfafurazole
Sulfamethoxazole

961.1 Arsenical anti-infectives

961.2 Heavy metal anti-infectives
Compounds of: antimony, bismuth
Compounds of: lead, mercury
EXCLUDES *mercurial diuretics (974.0)*

961.3 Quinoline and hydroxyquinoline derivatives
Chiniofon
Diiodohydroxyquin
EXCLUDES *antimalarial drugs (961.4)*

961.4 Antimalarials and drugs acting on other blood protozoa
Chloroquine
Cycloguanil
Primaquine
Proguanil [chloroguanide]
Pyrimethamine
Quinine

961.5 Other antiprotozoal drugs
Emetine

961.6 Anthelmintics
Hexylresorcinol
Piperazine
Thiabendazole

961.7 Antiviral drugs
Methisazone
EXCLUDES *amantadine (966.4)*
cytarabine (963.1)
idoxuridine (976.5)

961.8 Other antimycobacterial drugs
Ethambutol
Ethionamide
Isoniazid
Para-aminosalicylic acid derivatives
Sulfones

961.9 Other and unspecified anti-infectives
Flucytosine
Nitrofuran derivatives

✓4th **962 Poisoning by hormones and synthetic substitutes**
EXCLUDES *oxytocic hormones (975.0)*

962.0 Adrenal cortical steroids
Cortisone derivatives
Desoxycorticosterone derivatives
Fluorinated corticosteroids

962.1 Androgens and anabolic congeners
Methandriol
Nandrolone
Oxymetholone
Testosterone

962.2 Ovarian hormones and synthetic substitutes
Contraceptives, oral
Estrogens
Estrogens and progestogens, combined
Progestogens

962.3 Insulins and antidiabetic agents
Acetohexamide
Biguanide derivatives, oral
Chlorpropamide
Glucagon
Insulin
Phenformin
Sulfonylurea derivatives, oral
Tolbutamide
AHA: M-A, '85, 8

962.4 Anterior pituitary hormones
Corticotropin
Gonadotropin
Somatotropin [growth hormone]

962.5 Posterior pituitary hormones
Vasopressin
EXCLUDES *oxytocic hormones (975.0)*

962.6 Parathyroid and parathyroid derivatives

962.7 Thyroid and thyroid derivatives
Dextrothyroxin
Levothyroxine sodium
Liothyronine
Thyroglobulin

962.8 Antithyroid agents
Iodides
Thiouracil
Thiourea

962.9 Other and unspecified hormones and synthetic substitutes

✓4th **963 Poisoning by primarily systemic agents**

963.0 Antiallergic and antiemetic drugs
Antihistamines
Chlorpheniramine
Diphenhydramine
Diphenylpyraline
Thonzylamine
Tripelennamine
EXCLUDES *phenothiazine-based tranquilizers (969.1)*

963.1 Antineoplastic and immunosuppressive drugs
Azathioprine
Busulfan
Chlorambucil
Cyclophosphamide
Cytarabine
Fluorouracil
Mercaptopurine
thio-TEPA
EXCLUDES *antineoplastic antibiotics (960.7)*

963.2 Acidifying agents

963.3 Alkalizing agents

963.4 Enzymes, not elsewhere classified
Penicillinase

963.5 Vitamins, not elsewhere classified
Vitamin A
Vitamin D
EXCLUDES *nicotinic acid (972.2)*
vitamin K (964.3)

963.8 Other specified systemic agents
Heavy metal antagonists

963.9 Unspecified systemic agent

✓4th **964 Poisoning by agents primarily affecting blood constituents**

964.0 Iron and its compounds
Ferric salts
Ferrous sulfate and other ferrous salts

964.1 Liver preparations and other antianemic agents
Folic acid

964.2 Anticoagulants
Coumarin
Heparin
Phenindione
Warfarin sodium
AHA: 1Q, '94, 22

964.3 Vitamin K [phytonadione]

964.4 Fibrinolysis-affecting drugs
Aminocaproic acid
Streptodornase
Streptokinase
Urokinase

964.5 Anticoagulant antagonists and other coagulants
Hexadimethrine
Protamine sulfate

964.6 Gamma globulin

964.7 Natural blood and blood products
Blood plasma
Human fibrinogen
Packed red cells
Whole blood
EXCLUDES *transfusion reactions (999.4-999.8)*

964.8 Other specified agents affecting blood constituents
Macromolecular blood substitutes
Plasma expanders

964.9 Unspecified agent affecting blood constituents

✓4th **965 Poisoning by analgesics, antipyretics, and antirheumatics**
EXCLUDES *drug dependence (304.0-304.9)*
nondependent abuse (305.0-305.9)

✓5th **965.0 Opiates and related narcotics**

965.00 Opium (alkaloids), unspecified

965.01 Heroin
Diacetylmorphine

965.02 Methadone

965.09 Other
Codeine [methylmorphine]
Meperidine [pethidine]
Morphine

965.1 Salicylates
Acetylsalicylic acid [aspirin]
Salicylic acid salts
AHA: N-D, '94, 15

965.4 Aromatic analgesics, not elsewhere classified
Acetanilid
Paracetamol [acetaminophen]
Phenacetin [acetophenetidin]

965.5 Pyrazole derivatives
Aminophenazone [aminopyrine]
Phenylbutazone

5th **965.6 Antirheumatics [antiphlogistics]**
EXCLUDES *salicylates (965.1)*
steroids (962.0-962.9)

AHA: 4Q, '98, 50

965.61 Propionic acid derivatives
Fenoprofen
Flurbiprofen
Ibuprofen
Ketoprofen
Naproxen
Oxaprozin

AHA: 4Q, '98, 50

965.69 Other antirheumatics
Gold salts
Indomethacin

965.7 Other non-narcotic analgesics
Pyrabital

965.8 Other specified analgesics and antipyretics
Pentazocine

965.9 Unspecified analgesic and antipyretic

4th **966 Poisoning by anticonvulsants and anti-Parkinsonism drugs**

966.0 Oxazolidine derivatives
Paramethadione
Trimethadione

966.1 Hydantoin derivatives
Phenytoin

966.2 Succinimides
Ethosuximide
Phensuximide

966.3 Other and unspecified anticonvulsants
Primidone
EXCLUDES *barbiturates (967.0)*
sulfonamides (961.0)

966.4 Anti-Parkinsonism drugs
Amantadine
Ethopropazine [profenamine]
Levodopa [L-dopa]

4th **967 Poisoning by sedatives and hypnotics**
EXCLUDES *drug dependence (304.0-304.9)*
nondependent abuse (305.0-305.9)

967.0 Barbiturates
Amobarbital [amylobarbitone]
Barbital [barbitone]
Butabarbital [butabarbitone]
Pentobarbital [pentobarbitone]
Phenobarbital [phenobarbitone]
Secobarbital [quinalbarbitone]
EXCLUDES *thiobarbiturate anesthetics (968.3)*

967.1 Chloral hydrate group

967.2 Paraldehyde

967.3 Bromine compounds
Bromide
Carbromal (derivatives)

967.4 Methaqualone compounds

967.5 Glutethimide group

967.6 Mixed sedatives, not elsewhere classified

967.8 Other sedatives and hypnotics

967.9 Unspecified sedative or hypnotic
Sleeping:
drug, pill, tablet } NOS

4th **968 Poisoning by other central nervous system depressants and anesthetics**
EXCLUDES *drug dependence (304.0-304.9)*
nondependent abuse (305.0-305.9)

968.0 Central nervous system muscle-tone depressants
Chlorphenesin (carbamate)
Methocarbamol
Mephenesin

968.1 Halothane

968.2 Other gaseous anesthetics
Ether
Halogenated hydrocarbon derivatives, except halothane
Nitrous oxide

968.3 Intravenous anesthetics
Ketamine
Methohexital [methohexitone]
Thiobarbiturates, such as thiopental sodium

968.4 Other and unspecified general anesthetics

968.5 Surface [topical] and infiltration anesthetics
Cocaine
Procaine
Lidocaine [lignocaine]
Tetracaine

AHA: 1Q, '93, 25

968.6 Peripheral nerve- and plexus-blocking anesthetics

968.7 Spinal anesthetics

968.9 Other and unspecified local anesthetics

4th **969 Poisoning by psychotropic agents**
EXCLUDES *drug dependence (304.0-304.9)*
nondependent abuse (305.0-305.9)

969.0 Antidepressants
Amitriptyline
Imipramine
Monoamine oxidase [MAO] inhibitors

969.1 Phenothiazine-based tranquilizers
Chlorpromazine
Prochlorperazine
Fluphenazine
Promazine

969.2 Butyrophenone-based tranquilizers
Haloperidol
Trifluperidol
Spiperone

969.3 Other antipsychotics, neuroleptics, and major tranquilizers

969.4 Benzodiazepine-based tranquilizers
Chlordiazepoxide
Lorazepam
Diazepam
Medazepam
Flurazepam
Nitrazepam

969.5 Other tranquilizers
Hydroxyzine
Meprobamate

969.6 Psychodysleptics [hallucinogens]
Cannabis (derivatives)
Mescaline
Lysergide [LSD]
Psilocin
Marihuana (derivatives)
Psilocybin

969.7 Psychostimulants
Amphetamine
Caffeine
EXCLUDES *central appetite depressants (977.0)*

AHA: 2Q, '03, 11

969.8 Other specified psychotropic agents

969.9 Unspecified psychotropic agent

4th **970 Poisoning by central nervous system stimulants**

970.0 Analeptics
Lobeline
Nikethamide

970.1 Opiate antagonists
Levallorphan
Naloxone
Nalorphine

970.8 Other specified central nervous system stimulants

AHA: ▶1Q, '05, 6◀

970.9 Unspecified central nervous system stimulant

4th **971 Poisoning by drugs primarily affecting the autonomic nervous system**

971.0 Parasympathomimetics [cholinergics]
Acetylcholine
Pilocarpine
Anticholinesterase:
organophosphorus
reversible

971.1 **Parasympatholytics [anticholinergics and antimuscarinics] and spasmolytics**
Atropine
Homatropine
Hyoscine [scopolamine]
Quaternary ammonium derivatives
EXCLUDES *papaverine (972.5)*

971.2 **Sympathomimetics [adrenergics]**
Epinephrine [adrenalin]
Levarterenol [noradrenalin]

971.3 **Sympatholytics [antiadrenergics]**
Phenoxybenzamine
Tolazolinehydrochloride

971.9 **Unspecified drug primarily affecting autonomic nervous system**

4th 972 **Poisoning by agents primarily affecting the cardiovascular system**

972.0 **Cardiac rhythm regulators**
Practolol
Procainamide
Propranolol
Quinidine
EXCLUDES *lidocaine (968.5)*

972.1 **Cardiotonic glycosides and drugs of similar action**
Digitalis glycosides
Digoxin
Strophanthins

972.2 **Antilipemic and antiarteriosclerotic drugs**
Clofibrate
Nicotinic acid derivatives

972.3 **Ganglion-blocking agents**
Pentamethonium bromide

972.4 **Coronary vasodilators**
Dipyridamole
Nitrates [nitroglycerin]
Nitrites

972.5 **Other vasodilators**
Cyclandelate
Diazoxide
Papaverine
EXCLUDES *nicotinic acid (972.2)*

972.6 **Other antihypertensive agents**
Clonidine
Guanethidine
Rauwolfia alkaloids
Reserpine

972.7 **Antivaricose drugs, including sclerosing agents**
Sodium morrhuate
Zinc salts

972.8 **Capillary-active drugs**
Adrenochrome derivatives
Metaraminol

972.9 **Other and unspecified agents primarily affecting the cardiovascular system**

4th 973 **Poisoning by agents primarily affecting the gastrointestinal system**

973.0 **Antacids and antigastric secretion drugs**
Aluminum hydroxide
Magnesium trisilicate
AHA: 1Q, '03, 19

973.1 **Irritant cathartics**
Bisacodyl
Castor oil
Phenolphthalein

973.2 **Emollient cathartics**
Dioctyl sulfosuccinates

973.3 **Other cathartics, including intestinal atonia drugs**
Magnesium sulfate

973.4 **Digestants**
Pancreatin
Papain
Pepsin

973.5 **Antidiarrheal drugs**
Kaolin
Pectin
EXCLUDES *anti-infectives (960.0-961.9)*

973.6 **Emetics**

973.8 **Other specified agents primarily affecting the gastrointestinal system**

973.9 **Unspecified agent primarily affecting the gastrointestinal system**

4th 974 **Poisoning by water, mineral, and uric acid metabolism drugs**

974.0 **Mercurial diuretics**
Chlormerodrin
Mercaptomerin
Mersalyl

974.1 **Purine derivative diuretics**
Theobromine
Theophylline
EXCLUDES *aminophylline [theophylline ethylenediamine] (975.7)*
caffeine (969.7)

974.2 **Carbonic acid anhydrase inhibitors**
Acetazolamide

974.3 **Saluretics**
Benzothiadiazides
Chlorothiazide group

974.4 **Other diuretics**
Ethacrynic acid
Furosemide

974.5 **Electrolytic, caloric, and water-balance agents**

974.6 **Other mineral salts, not elsewhere classified**

974.7 **Uric acid metabolism drugs**
Allopurinol
Colchicine
Probenecid

4th 975 **Poisoning by agents primarily acting on the smooth and skeletal muscles and respiratory system**

975.0 **Oxytocic agents**
Ergot alkaloids
Oxytocin
Prostaglandins

975.1 **Smooth muscle relaxants**
Adiphenine
Metaproterenol [orciprenaline]
EXCLUDES *papaverine (972.5)*

975.2 **Skeletal muscle relaxants**

975.3 **Other and unspecified drugs acting on muscles**

975.4 **Antitussives**
Dextromethorphan
Pipazethate

975.5 **Expectorants**
Acetylcysteine
Guaifenesin
Terpin hydrate

975.6 **Anti-common cold drugs**

975.7 **Antiasthmatics**
Aminophylline [theophylline ethylenediamine]

975.8 **Other and unspecified respiratory drugs**

4th 976 **Poisoning by agents primarily affecting skin and mucous membrane, ophthalmological, otorhinolaryngological, and dental drugs**

976.0 **Local anti-infectives and anti-inflammatory drugs**

976.1 **Antipruritics**

976.2 **Local astringents and local detergents**

976.3 **Emollients, demulcents, and protectants**

976.4 **Keratolytics, keratoplastics, other hair treatment drugs and preparations**

976.5 **Eye anti-infectives and other eye drugs**
Idoxuridine

976.6 **Anti-infectives and other drugs and preparations for ear, nose, and throat**

976.7 **Dental drugs topically applied**
EXCLUDES *anti-infectives (976.0)*
local anesthetics (968.5)

976.8 **Other agents primarily affecting skin and mucous membrane**
Spermicides [vaginal contraceptives]

976.9 **Unspecified agent primarily affecting skin and mucous membrane**

4th 977 **Poisoning by other and unspecified drugs and medicinal substances**

977.0 **Dietetics**
Central appetite depressants

977.1 **Lipotropic drugs**

977.2 **Antidotes and chelating agents, not elsewhere classified**

977.3 **Alcohol deterrents**

977.4 **Pharmaceutical excipients**
Pharmaceutical adjuncts

977.8 **Other specified drugs and medicinal substances**
Contrast media used for diagnostic x-ray procedures
Diagnostic agents and kits

977.9 **Unspecified drug or medicinal substance**

✓4th **978 Poisoning by bacterial vaccines**

978.0 **BCG**

978.1 **Typhoid and paratyphoid**

978.2 **Cholera**

978.3 **Plague**

978.4 **Tetanus**

978.5 **Diphtheria**

978.6 **Pertussis vaccine, including combinations with a pertussis component**

978.8 **Other and unspecified bacterial vaccines**

978.9 **Mixed bacterial vaccines, except combinations with a pertussis component**

✓4th **979 Poisoning by other vaccines and biological substances**

EXCLUDES *gamma globulin (964.6)*

979.0 **Smallpox vaccine**

979.1 **Rabies vaccine**

979.2 **Typhus vaccine**

979.3 **Yellow fever vaccine**

979.4 **Measles vaccine**

979.5 **Poliomyelitis vaccine**

979.6 **Other and unspecified viral and rickettsial vaccines**
Mumps vaccine

979.7 **Mixed viral-rickettsial and bacterial vaccines, except combinations with a pertussis component**

EXCLUDES *combinations with a pertussis component (978.6)*

979.9 **Other and unspecified vaccines and biological substances**

TOXIC EFFECTS OF SUBSTANCES CHIEFLY NONMEDICINAL AS TO SOURCE (980-989)

EXCLUDES *burns from chemical agents (ingested) (947.0-947.9)*
localized toxic effects indexed elsewhere (001.0-799.9)
respiratory conditions due to external agents (506.0-508.9)

Use additional code to specify the nature of the toxic effect

✓4th **980 Toxic effect of alcohol**

980.0 **Ethyl alcohol**
Denatured alcohol
Grain alcohol
Ethanol
Use additional code to identify any associated:
acute alcohol intoxication (305.0)
in alcoholism (303.0)
drunkenness (simple) (305.0)
pathological (291.4)
AHA: 3Q, '96, 16

980.1 **Methyl alcohol**
Methanol
Wood alcohol

980.2 **Isopropyl alcohol**
Dimethyl carbinol
Rubbing alcohol
Isopropanol

980.3 **Fusel oil**
Alcohol:
amyl
butyl
Alcohol:
propyl

980.8 **Other specified alcohols**

980.9 **Unspecified alcohol**

981 Toxic effect of petroleum products
Benzine
Gasoline
Kerosene
Paraffin wax
Petroleum:
ether
naphtha
spirit

✓4th **982 Toxic effect of solvents other than petroleum-based**

982.0 **Benzene and homologues**

982.1 **Carbon tetrachloride**

982.2 **Carbon disulfide**
Carbon bisulfide

982.3 **Other chlorinated hydrocarbon solvents**
Tetrachloroethylene
Trichloroethylene

EXCLUDES *chlorinated hydrocarbon preparations other than solvents (989.2)*

982.4 **Nitroglycol**

982.8 **Other nonpetroleum-based solvents**
Acetone

✓4th **983 Toxic effect of corrosive aromatics, acids, and caustic alkalis**

983.0 **Corrosive aromatics**
Carbolic acid or phenol
Cresol

983.1 **Acids**
Acid:
hydrochloric
nitric
Acid:
sulfuric

983.2 **Caustic alkalis**
Lye
Potassium hydroxide
Sodium hydroxide

983.9 **Caustic, unspecified**

✓4th **984 Toxic effect of lead and its compounds (including fumes)**

INCLUDES that from all sources except medicinal substances

984.0 **Inorganic lead compounds**
Lead dioxide
Lead salts

984.1 **Organic lead compounds**
Lead acetate
Tetraethyl lead

984.8 **Other lead compounds**

984.9 **Unspecified lead compound**

✓4th **985 Toxic effect of other metals**

INCLUDES that from all sources except medicinal substances

985.0 **Mercury and its compounds**
Minamata disease

985.1 **Arsenic and its compounds**

985.2 **Manganese and its compounds**

985.3 **Beryllium and its compounds**

985.4 **Antimony and its compounds**

985.5 **Cadmium and its compounds**

985.6 **Chromium**

985.8 **Other specified metals**
Brass fumes
Copper salts
Iron compounds
Nickel compounds
AHA: 1Q, '88, 5

985.9 **Unspecified metal**

986 Toxic effect of carbon monoxide
Carbon monoxide from any source

✓4th **987 Toxic effect of other gases, fumes, or vapors**

987.0 **Liquefied petroleum gases**
Butane
Propane

987.1 **Other hydrocarbon gas**

987.2 **Nitrogen oxides**
Nitrogen dioxide
Nitrous fumes

987.3 **Sulfur dioxide**

987.4 **Freon**
Dichloromonofluoromethane

987.5 **Lacrimogenic gas**
Bromobenzyl cyanide
Chloroacetophenone
Ethyliodoacetate

987.6 **Chlorine gas**

987.7 **Hydrocyanic acid gas**

987.8 **Other specified gases, fumes, or vapors**
Phosgene
Polyester fumes

987.9 **Unspecified gas, fume, or vapor**

N Newborn Age: 0 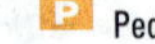 Pediatric Age: 0-17 M Maternity Age: 12-55 A Adult Age: 15-124 MSP Medicare Secondary Payer

✓4th **988 Toxic effect of noxious substances eaten as food**

EXCLUDES *allergic reaction to food, such as:*
gastroenteritis (558.3)
rash (692.5, 693.1)
food poisoning (bacterial) (005.0-005.9)
toxic effects of food contaminants, such as:
aflatoxin and other mycotoxin (989.7)
mercury (985.0)

988.0 Fish and shellfish

988.1 Mushrooms

988.2 Berries and other plants

988.8 Other specified noxious substances eaten as food

988.9 Unspecified noxious substance eaten as food

✓4th **989 Toxic effect of other substances, chiefly nonmedicinal as to source**

989.0 Hydrocyanic acid and cyanides
Potassium cyanide
Sodium cyanide
EXCLUDES *gas and fumes (987.7)*

989.1 Strychnine and salts

989.2 Chlorinated hydrocarbons
Aldrin
DDT
Chlordane
Dieldrin
EXCLUDES *chlorinated hydrocarbon solvents (982.0-982.3)*

989.3 Organophosphate and carbamate
Carbaryl
Parathion
Dichlorvos
Phorate
Malathion
Phosdrin

989.4 Other pesticides, not elsewhere classified
Mixtures of insecticides

989.5 Venom
Bites of venomous snakes, lizards, and spiders
Tick paralysis

989.6 Soaps and detergents

989.7 Aflatoxin and other mycotoxin [food contaminants]

✓5th **989.8 Other substances, chiefly nonmedicinal as to source**
AHA: 4Q, '95, 60

989.81 Asbestos
EXCLUDES *asbestosis (501)*
exposure to asbestos (V15.84)

989.82 Latex

989.83 Silicone
EXCLUDES *silicone used in medical devices, implants and grafts (996.00-996.79)*

989.84 Tobacco

989.89 Other

989.9 Unspecified substance, chiefly nonmedicinal as to source

OTHER AND UNSPECIFIED EFFECTS OF EXTERNAL CAUSES (990-995)

990 Effects of radiation, unspecified
Complication of:
phototherapy
radiation therapy
Radiation sickness
EXCLUDES *specified adverse effects of radiation. Such conditions are to be classified according to the nature of the adverse effect, as:*
burns (940.0-949.5)
dermatitis (692.7-692.8)
leukemia (204.0-208.9)
pneumonia (508.0)
sunburn (692.71, 692.76-692.77)
[The type of radiation giving rise to the adverse effect may be identified by use of the E codes.]

✓4th **991 Effects of reduced temperature**

991.0 Frostbite of face

991.1 Frostbite of hand

991.2 Frostbite of foot

991.3 Frostbite of other and unspecified sites

991.4 Immersion foot
Trench foot
DEF: Paresthesia, edema, blotchy cyanosis of foot, the skin is soft (macerated), pale and wrinkled, and the sole is swollen with surface ridging and following sustained immersion in water.

991.5 Chilblains
Erythema pernio
Perniosis
DEF: Red, swollen, itchy skin; follows damp cold exposure; also associated with pruritus and a burning feeling, in hands, feet, ears, and face in children, legs and toes in women, and hands and fingers in men.

991.6 Hypothermia
Hypothermia (accidental)
EXCLUDES *hypothermia following anesthesia (995.89)*
hypothermia not associated with low environmental temperature (780.99)
DEF: Reduced body temperature due to low environmental temperatures.

991.8 Other specified effects of reduced temperature

991.9 Unspecified effect of reduced temperature
Effects of freezing or excessive cold NOS

✓4th **992 Effects of heat and light**
EXCLUDES *burns (940.0-949.5)*
diseases of sweat glands due to heat (705.0-705.9)
malignant hyperpyrexia following anesthesia (995.86)
sunburn (692.71, 692.76-692.77)

992.0 Heat stroke and sunstroke
Heat apoplexy
Siriasis
Heat pyrexia
Thermoplegia
Ictus solaris
DEF: Headache, vertigo, cramps and elevated body temperature due to high environmental temperatures.

992.1 Heat syncope
Heat collapse

992.2 Heat cramps

992.3 Heat exhaustion, anhydrotic
Heat prostration due to water depletion
EXCLUDES *that associated with salt depletion (992.4)*

992.4 Heat exhaustion due to salt depletion
Heat prostration due to salt (and water) depletion

992.5 Heat exhaustion, unspecified
Heat prostration NOS

992.6 Heat fatigue, transient

992.7 Heat edema
DEF: Fluid retention due to high environmental temperatures.

992.8 Other specified heat effects

992.9 Unspecified

✓4th **993 Effects of air pressure**

993.0 Barotrauma, otitic
Aero-otitis media
Effects of high altitude on ears
DEF: Ringing ears, deafness, pain and vertigo due to air pressure changes.

993.1 Barotrauma, sinus
Aerosinusitis
Effects of high altitude on sinuses

993.2 Other and unspecified effects of high altitude
Alpine sickness
Hypobaropathy
Andes disease
Mountain sickness
Anoxia due to high altitude
AHA: 3Q, '88, 4

993.3 Caisson disease
Bends
Compressed-air disease
Decompression sickness
Divers' palsy or paralysis
DEF: Rapid reduction in air pressure while breathing compressed air; symptoms include skin lesions, joint pains, respiratory and neurological problems.

993.4 Effects of air pressure caused by explosion

993.8 Other specified effects of air pressure

993.9 Unspecified effect of air pressure

✓4th 994 Effects of other external causes
EXCLUDES *certain adverse effects not elsewhere classified (995.0-995.8)*

994.0 Effects of lightning
Shock from lightning
Struck by lightning NOS
EXCLUDES *burns (940.0-949.5)*

994.1 Drowning and nonfatal submersion
Bathing cramp
Immersion
AHA: 3Q, '88, 4

994.2 Effects of hunger
Deprivation of food
Starvation

994.3 Effects of thirst
Deprivation of water

994.4 Exhaustion due to exposure

994.5 Exhaustion due to excessive exertion
Overexertion

994.6 Motion sickness
Air sickness
Seasickness
Travel sickness

994.7 Asphyxiation and strangulation
Suffocation (by):
- bedclothes
- cave-in
- constriction
- mechanical

Suffocation (by):
- plastic bag
- pressure
- strangulation

EXCLUDES *asphyxia from:*
- *carbon monoxide (986)*
- *inhalation of food or foreign body (932-934.9)*
- *other gases, fumes, and vapors (987.0-987.9)*

994.8 Electrocution and nonfatal effects of electric current
Shock from electric current
EXCLUDES *electric burns (940.0-949.5)*

994.9 Other effects of external causes
Effects of:
- abnormal gravitational [G] forces or states
- weightlessness

✓4th 995 Certain adverse effects not elsewhere classified
EXCLUDES *complications of surgical and medical care (996.0-999.9)*

995.0 Other anaphylactic shock
Allergic shock, Anaphylactic reaction, Anaphylaxis — NOS or due to adverse effect of correct medicinal substance properly administered

Use additional E code to identify external cause, such as:
- adverse effects of correct medicinal substance properly administered [E930-E949]

EXCLUDES *anaphylactic reaction to serum (999.4)*
anaphylactic shock due to adverse food reaction (995.60-995.69)

AHA: 4Q, '93, 30

DEF: Immediate sensitivity response after exposure to specific antigen; results in life-threatening respiratory distress; usually followed by vascular collapse, shock, urticaria, angioedema and pruritus.

995.1 Angioneurotic edema
Giant urticaria
EXCLUDES *urticaria:*
- *due to serum (999.5)*
- *other specified (698.2, 708.0-708.9, 757.33)*

DEF: Circulatory response of deep dermis, subcutaneous or submucosal tissues; causes localized edema and wheals.

995.2 Unspecified adverse effect of drug, medicinal and biological substance
Adverse effect, Allergic reaction, Hypersensitivity, Idiosyncrasy — (due) to correct medicinal substance properly administered

Drug:
- hypersensitivity NOS

Drug:
- reaction NOS

EXCLUDES *pathological drug intoxication (292.2)*

AHA: 2Q, '97, 12; 3Q, '95, 13; 3Q, '92, 16

995.3 Allergy, unspecified
Allergic reaction NOS
Hypersensitivity NOS
Idiosyncrasy NOS
EXCLUDES *allergic reaction NOS to correct medicinal substance properly administered (995.2)*
specific types of allergic reaction, such as:
- *allergic diarrhea (558.3)*
- *dermatitis (691.0-693.9)*
- *hayfever (477.0-477.9)*

995.4 Shock due to anesthesia
Shock due to anesthesia in which the correct substance was properly administered
EXCLUDES *complications of anesthesia in labor or delivery (668.0-668.9)*
overdose or wrong substance given (968.0-969.9)
postoperative shock NOS (998.0)
specified adverse effects of anesthesia classified elsewhere, such as:
- *anoxic brain damage (348.1)*
- *hepatitis (070.0-070.9), etc.*

unspecified adverse effect of anesthesia (995.2)

✓5th 995.5 Child maltreatment syndrome
Use additional code(s), if applicable, to identify any associated injuries
Use additional E code to identify:
- nature of abuse (E960-E968)
- perpetrator (E967.0-E967.9)

AHA: 1Q, '98, 11

995.50 Child abuse, unspecified P

995.51 Child emotional/psychological abuse P
AHA: 4Q, '96, 38, 40

995.52 Child neglect (nutritional) P
AHA: 4Q, '96, 38, 40

995.53 Child sexual abuse P
AHA: 4Q, '96, 39, 40

995.54 Child physical abuse P
Battered baby or child syndrome
EXCLUDES *shaken infant syndrome (995.55)*
AHA: 3Q, '99, 14; 4Q, '96, 39, 40

995.55 Shaken infant syndrome P
Use additional code(s) to identify any associated injuries
AHA: 4Q, '96, 40, 43

995.59 Other child abuse and neglect P
Multiple forms of abuse

✓5th **995.6 Anaphylactic shock due to adverse food reaction**
Anaphylactic shock due to nonpoisonous foods
AHA: 4Q, '93, 30

995.60 Due to unspecified food
995.61 Due to peanuts
995.62 Due to crustaceans
995.63 Due to fruits and vegetables
995.64 Due to tree nuts and seeds
995.65 Due to fish
995.66 Due to food additives
995.67 Due to milk products
995.68 Due to eggs
995.69 Due to other specified food

995.7 Other adverse food reactions, not elsewhere classified
Use additional code to identify the type of reaction, such as:
hives (708.0)
wheezing (786.07)

EXCLUDES *anaphylactic shock due to adverse food reaction (995.60-995.69)*
asthma (493.0, 493.9)
dermatitis due to food (693.1)
in contact with the skin (692.5)
gastroenteritis and colitis due to food (558.3)
rhinitis due to food (477.1)

✓5th **995.8 Other specified adverse effects, not elsewhere classified**

995.80 Adult maltreatment, unspecified A
Abused person NOS
Use additional code to identify:
any associated injury
perpetrator (E967.0-E967.9)
AHA: 4Q, '96, 41, 43

995.81 Adult physical abuse A
Battered:
person syndrome NEC
man
spouse
woman
Use additional code to identify:
any association injury
nature of abuse (E960-E968)
perpetrator (E967.0-E967.9)
AHA: 4Q, '96, 42, 43

995.82 Adult emotional/psychological abuse A
Use additional E code to identify perpetrator (E967.0-E967.9)

995.83 Adult sexual abuse A
Use additional code to identify:
any associated injury
perpetrator (E967.0-E967.9)

995.84 Adult neglect (nutritional) A
Use addition code to identify:
intent of neglect (E904.0, E968.4)
perpetrator (E967.0-E967.9)

995.85 Other adult abuse and neglect A
Multiple forms of abuse and neglect
Use additional code to identify:
any associated injury
intent of neglect (E904.0, E968.4)
nature of abuse (E960-E968)
perpetrator (E967.0-E967.9)

995.86 Malignant hyperthermia
Malignant hyperpyrexia due to anesthesia
AHA: 4Q, '98, 51

995.89 Other
Hypothermia due to anesthesia
AHA: 2Q, '04, 18; 3Q, '03, 12

✓5th **995.9 Systemic inflammatory response syndrome (SIRS)**
Code first underlying systemic infection
AHA: 2Q, '04, 16; 4Q, '02, 71

DEF: Clinical response to infection or trauma that can trigger an acute inflammatory reaction and progresses to coagulation, impaired fibrinolysis, and organ failure; manifested by two or more of the following symptoms: fever, tachycardia, tachypnea, leukocytosis or leukopenia.

995.90 Systemic inflammatory response syndrome, unspecified
SIRS NOS

995.91 Systemic inflammatory response syndrome due to infectious process without organ dysfunction
Sepsis
AHA: 2Q, '04, 16; 4Q, '03, 79

995.92 Systemic inflammatory response syndrome due to infectious process with organ dysfunction
Severe sepsis
Use additional code to specify organ dysfunction, such as:
acute renal failure (584.5-584.9)
acute respiratory failure (518.81)
critical illness myopathy (359.81)
critical illness polyneuropathy (357.82)
encephalopathy (348.31)
hepatic failure (570)
septic shock (785.52)
AHA: ►1Q, '05, 7;◄ 2Q, '04, 16; 4Q, '03, 73, 79

995.93 Systemic inflammatory response syndrome due to noninfectious process without organ dysfunction

995.94 Systemic inflammatory response syndrome due to noninfectious process with organ dysfunction
Use additional code to specify organ dysfunction, such as:
acute renal failure (584.5-584.9)
acute respiratory failure (518.81)
critical illness myopathy (359.81)
critical illness polyneuropathy (357.82)
encephalopathy (348.31)
hepatic failure (570)
septic shock (785.52)
AHA: 4Q, '03, 79

Continuum of Illness Due to Infection

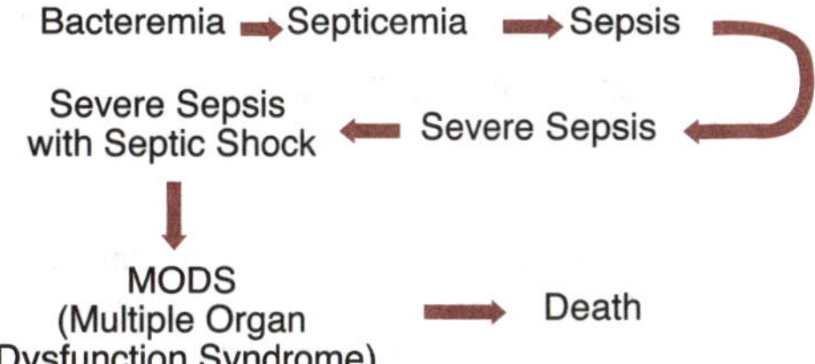

COMPLICATIONS OF SURGICAL AND MEDICAL CARE, NOT ELSEWHERE CLASSIFIED (996-999)

EXCLUDES *adverse effects of medicinal agents (001.0-799.9, 995.0-995.8)*
burns from local applications and irradiation (940.0-949.5)
complications of:
conditions for which the procedure was performed
surgical procedures during abortion, labor, and delivery (630-676.9)
poisoning and toxic effects of drugs and chemicals (960.0-989.9)
postoperative conditions in which no complications are present, such as:
artificial opening status (V44.0-V44.9)
closure of external stoma (V55.0-V55.9)
fitting of prosthetic device (V52.0-V52.9)
specified complications classified elsewhere
anesthetic shock (995.4)
electrolyte imbalance (276.0-276.9)
postlaminectomy syndrome (722.80-722.83)
postmastectomy lymphedema syndrome (457.0)
postoperative psychosis (293.0-293.9)
any other condition classified elsewhere in the Alphabetic Index when described as due to a procedure

✓4th **996 Complications peculiar to certain specified procedures**

INCLUDES complications, not elsewhere classified, in the use of artificial substitutes [e.g., Dacron, metal, Silastic, Teflon] or natural sources [e.g., bone] involving:
anastomosis (internal)
graft (bypass) (patch)
implant
internal device:
catheter
electronic
fixation
prosthetic
reimplant
transplant

EXCLUDES *accidental puncture or laceration during procedure (998.2)*
complications of internal anastomosis of:
gastrointestinal tract (997.4)
urinary tract (997.5)
▶*mechanical complication of respirator (V46.14)*◀
other specified complications classified elsewhere, such as:
hemolytic anemia (283.1)
functional cardiac disturbances (429.4)
serum hepatitis (070.2-070.3)

AHA: 1Q, '94, 3

✓5th **996.0 Mechanical complication of cardiac device, implant, and graft**

Breakdown (mechanical)
Displacement
Leakage
Obstruction, mechanical
Perforation
Protrusion

AHA: 2Q, '93, 9

996.00 Unspecified device, implant, and graft MSP

996.01 Due to cardiac pacemaker (electrode) MSP

AHA: 2Q, '99, 11

996.02 Due to heart valve prosthesis MSP

996.03 Due to coronary bypass graft MSP

EXCLUDES *atherosclerosis of graft (414.02, 414.03)*
embolism [occlusion NOS] [thrombus] of graft (996.72)

AHA: 2Q, '95, 17; N-D, '86, 5

996.04 Due to automatic implantable cardiac defibrillator

996.09 Other MSP

AHA: 2Q, '93, 9

996.1 Mechanical complication of other vascular device, implant, and graft MSP

femoral-popliteal bypass graft
Mechanical complications involving:
aortic (bifurcation) graft (replacement)
arteriovenous: dialysis catheter, fistula, shunt — surgically created
balloon (counterpulsation) device, intra-aortic
carotid artery bypass graft
umbrella device, vena cava

EXCLUDES *atherosclerosis of biological graft (440.30-440.32)*
embolism [occlusion NOS] [thrombus] of (biological) (synthetic) graft (996.74)
peritoneal dialysis catheter (996.56)

AHA: 1Q, '02, 13; 1Q, '95, 3

996.2 Mechanical complication of nervous system device, implant, and graft MSP

Mechanical complications involving:
dorsal column stimulator
electrodes implanted in brain [brain "pacemaker"]
peripheral nerve graft
ventricular (communicating) shunt

AHA: 2Q, '99, 4; S-O, '87, 10

✓5th **996.3 Mechanical complication of genitourinary device, implant, and graft**

AHA: 3Q, '01, 13; S-O, '85, 3

996.30 Unspecified device, implant, and graft MSP

996.31 Due to urethral [indwelling] catheter MSP

996.32 Due to intrauterine contraceptive device ♀ MSP

996.39 Other MSP

Cystostomy catheter
Prosthetic reconstruction of vas deferens
Repair (graft) of ureter without mention of resection

EXCLUDES *complications due to:*
external stoma of urinary tract (997.5)
internal anastomosis of urinary tract (997.5)

✓5th **996.4 Mechanical complication of internal orthopedic device, implant, and graft**

Mechanical complications involving:
external (fixation) device utilizing internal screw(s), pin(s) or other methods of fixation
grafts of bone, cartilage, muscle, or tendon
internal (fixation) device such as nail, plate, rod, etc.

▶Use additional code to identify prosthetic joint with mechanical complication (V43.60-V43.69)◀

EXCLUDES *complications of external orthopedic device, such as:*
pressure ulcer due to cast (707.00-707.09)

AHA: 2Q, '99, 10; 2Q, '98, 19; 2Q, '96, 11; 3Q, '95, 16; N-D, '85, 11

● **996.40 Unspecified mechanical complication of internal orthopedic device, implant, and graft**

● **996.41 Mechanical loosening of prosthetic joint**

Aseptic loosening

● **996.42 Dislocation of prosthetic joint**

Instability of prosthetic joint
Subluxation of prosthetic joint

● **996.43 Prosthetic joint implant failure**

Breakage (fracture) of prosthetic joint

● **996.44 Peri-prosthetic fracture around prosthetic joint**

● **996.45 Peri-prosthetic osteolysis**

● **996.46 Articular bearing surface wear of prosthetic joint**

● **996.47 Other mechanical complication of prosthetic joint implant**
Mechanical complication of prosthetic joint NOS

● **996.49 Other mechanical complication of other internal orthopedic device, implant, and graft**
EXCLUDES *mechanical complication of prosthetic joint implant (996.41-996.47)*

✓5th **996.5 Mechanical complication of other specified prosthetic device, implant, and graft**
Mechanical complications involving:
prosthetic implant in:
bile duct
breast
prosthetic implant in:
chin
orbit of eye
nonabsorbable surgical material NOS
other graft, implant, and internal device, not elsewhere classified
AHA: 1Q, '98, 11

996.51 Due to corneal graft

996.52 Due to graft of other tissue, not elsewhere classified
Skin graft failure or rejection
EXCLUDES *failure of artificial skin graft (996.55)*
failure of decellularized allodermis (996.55)
sloughing of temporary skin allografts or xenografts (pigskin)—omit code
AHA: 1Q, '96, 10

996.53 Due to ocular lens prosthesis
EXCLUDES *contact lenses—code to condition*
AHA: 1Q, '00, 9

996.54 Due to breast prosthesis
Breast capsule (prosthesis)
Mammary implant
AHA: 2Q, '98, 14; 3Q, '92, 4

996.55 Due to artificial skin graft and decellularized allodermis
Dislodgement
Displacement
Failure
Non-adherence
Poor incorporation
Shearing
AHA: 4Q, '98, 52

996.56 Due to peritoneal dialysis catheter
EXCLUDES *mechanical complication of arteriovenous dialysis catheter (996.1)*
AHA: 4Q, '98, 54

996.57 Due to insulin pump
AHA: 4Q, '03, 81-82

996.59 Due to other implant and internal device, not elsewhere classified
Nonabsorbable surgical material NOS
Prosthetic implant in:
bile duct
chin
orbit of eye
AHA: 2Q, '99, 13; 3Q, '94, 7

✓5th **996.6 Infection and inflammatory reaction due to internal prosthetic device, implant, and graft**
Infection (causing obstruction)
Inflammation
} due to (presence of) any device, implant, and graft classifiable to 996.0-996.5

Use additional code to identify specified infections
AHA: 2Q, '89, 16; J-F, '87, 14

996.60 Due to unspecified device, implant, and graft

996.61 Due to cardiac device, implant, and graft
Cardiac pacemaker or defibrillator:
electrode(s), lead(s)
pulse generator
subcutaneous pocket
Coronary artery bypass graft
Heart valve prosthesis

996.62 Due to other vascular device, implant and graft
Arterial graft
Arteriovenous fistula or shunt
Infusion pump
Vascular catheter (arterial) (dialysis) (venous)
AHA: 2Q, '04, 16; 1Q, '04, 5; 4Q, '03, 107, 111; 2Q, '03, 7; 2Q, '94, 13

996.63 Due to nervous system device, implant and graft
Electrodes implanted in brain
Peripheral nerve graft
Spinal canal catheter
Ventricular (communicating) shunt (catheter)

996.64 Due to indwelling urinary catheter
Use additional code to identify specified infections, such as:
Cystitis (595.0-595.9)
Sepsis (038.0-038.9)
AHA: 3Q, '93, 6

996.65 Due to other genitourinary device, implant and graft
Intrauterine contraceptive device
AHA: 1Q, '00, 15

996.66 Due to internal joint prosthesis
▶Use additional code to identify infected prosthetic joint (V43.60-V43.69)◀
AHA: 2Q, '91, 18

996.67 Due to other internal orthopedic device implant and graft
Bone growth stimulator (electrode)
Internal fixation device (pin) (rod) (screw)

996.68 Due to peritoneal dialysis catheter
Exit-site infection or inflammation
AHA: 4Q, '98, 54

996.69 Due to other internal prosthetic device, implant and graft
Breast prosthesis
Ocular lens prosthesis
Prosthetic orbital implant
AHA: 4Q, '03, 108; 4Q, '98, 52

✓5th **996.7 Other complications of internal (biological) (synthetic) prosthetic device, implant, and graft**
Complication NOS
occlusion NOS
Embolism
Fibrosis
Hemorrhage
Pain
Stenosis
Thrombus
} due to (presence of) any device, implant, and graft classifiable to 996.0-996.5

EXCLUDES *transplant rejection (996.8)*
AHA: 1Q, '89, 9; N-D, '86, 5

996.70 Due to unspecified device, implant, and graft

996.71 Due to heart valve prosthesis

996.72 Due to other cardiac device, implant, and graft
Cardiac pacemaker or defibrillator:
electrode(s), lead(s)
subcutaneous pocket
Coronary artery bypass (graft)
EXCLUDES *occlusion due to atherosclerosis (414.02-414.06)*
AHA: 3Q, '01, 20

996.73 Due to renal dialysis device, implant, and graft
AHA: 2Q, '91, 18

996.74 Due to other vascular device, implant, and graft
EXCLUDES *occlusion of biological graft due to atherosclerosis (440.30-440.32)*
AHA: 1Q, '03, 16, 17

996.75 Due to nervous system device, implant, and graft

996.76 Due to genitourinary device, implant, and graft
AHA: 1Q, '00, 15

996.77 Due to internal joint prosthesis

996.78 Due to other internal orthopedic device, implant, and graft
AHA: 2Q, '03, 14

996.79 Due to other internal prosthetic device, implant, and graft
AHA: ▶2Q, '04, 7;◀ 1Q,'01, 8; 3Q, '95, 14; 3Q, '92, 4

✓5th **996.8 Complications of transplanted organ**
Transplant failure or rejection
Use additional code to identify nature of complication, such as:
Cytomegalovirus (CMV) infection (078.5)
AHA: 3Q, '01, 12; 3Q, '93, 3, 4; 2Q, '93, 11; 1Q, '93, 24

996.80 Transplanted organ, unspecified

996.81 Kidney
AHA: 3Q. '03, 16; 3Q, '98, 6, 7; 3Q, '94, 8; 2Q, '94, 9; 1Q, '93, 24

996.82 Liver
AHA: 3Q. '03, 17; 3Q, '98, 3, 4

996.83 Heart
AHA: 3Q. '03, 16; 4Q, '02, 53; 3Q, '98, 5

996.84 Lung
AHA: 2Q. '03, 12; 3Q, '98, 5

996.85 Bone marrow
Graft-versus-host disease (acute) (chronic)
AHA: 4Q, '90, 4

996.86 Pancreas

996.87 Intestine

996.89 Other specified transplanted organ
AHA: 3Q, '94, 5

✓5th **996.9 Complications of reattached extremity or body part**

996.90 Unspecified extremity

996.91 Forearm

996.92 Hand

996.93 Finger(s)

996.94 Upper extremity, other and unspecified

996.95 Foot and toe(s)

996.96 Lower extremity, other and unspecified

996.99 Other specified body part

✓4th **997 Complications affecting specified body systems, not elsewhere classified**
Use additional code to identify complications
EXCLUDES *the listed conditions when specified as:*
causing shock (998.0)
complications of:
anesthesia:
adverse effect (001.0-799.9, 995.0-995.8)
in labor or delivery (668.0-668.9)
poisoning (968.0-969.9)
implanted device or graft (996.0-996.9)
obstetrical procedures (669.0-669.4)
reattached extremity (996.90-996.96)
transplanted organ (996.80-996.89)
AHA: 1Q, '94, 4; 1Q, '93, 26

✓5th **997.0 Nervous system complications**

997.00 Nervous system complication, unspecified

997.01 Central nervous system complication
Anoxic brain damage
Cerebral hypoxia
EXCLUDES *cerebrovascular hemorrhage or infarction (997.02)*

997.02 Iatrogenic cerebrovascular infarction or hemorrhage
Postoperative stroke
AHA: ▶2Q, '04, 8;◀ 4Q, '95, 57

997.09 Other nervous system complications

997.1 Cardiac complications
Cardiac:
arrest
insufficiency
Cardiorespiratory failure
Heart failure
} during or resulting from a procedure
EXCLUDES *the listed conditions as long-term effects of cardiac surgery or due to the presence of cardiac prosthetic device (429.4)*
AHA: 2Q, '02, 12

997.2 Peripheral vascular complications
Phlebitis or thrombophlebitis during or resulting from a procedure
EXCLUDES *the listed conditions due to:*
implant or catheter device (996.62)
infusion, perfusion, or transfusion (999.2)
complications affecting blood vessels (997.71-997.79)
AHA: 1Q, '03, 6; 3Q, '02, 24-26

997.3 Respiratory complications
Mendelson's syndrome
Pneumonia (aspiration)
} resulting from a procedure
EXCLUDES *iatrogenic [postoperative] pneumothorax (512.1)*
iatrogenic pulmonary embolism (415.11)
Mendelson's syndrome in labor and delivery (668.0)
specified complications classified elsewhere, such as:
adult respiratory distress syndrome (518.5)
pulmonary edema, postoperative (518.4)
respiratory insufficiency, acute, postoperative (518.5)
shock lung (518.5)
tracheostomy complications (519.00-519.09)
AHA: 1Q, '97, 10; 2Q, '93, 3; 2Q, '93, 9; 4Q, '90, 25
DEF: Mendelson's syndrome: acid pneumonitis due to aspiration of gastric acids, may occur after anesthesia or sedation.

997.4 Digestive system complications
Complications of:
intestinal (internal) anastomosis and bypass, not elsewhere classified, except that involving urinary tract
Hepatic failure
Hepatorenal syndrome
Intestinal obstruction NOS
} specified as due to a procedure
EXCLUDES *gastrostomy complications (536.40-536.49)*
specified gastrointestinal complications classified elsewhere, such as:
blind loop syndrome (579.2)
colostomy and enterostomy complications (569.60-569.69)
gastrojejunal ulcer (534.0-534.9)
infection of esophagostomy (530.86)
infection of external stoma (569.61)
mechanical complication of esophagostomy (530.87)
pelvic peritoneal adhesions, female (614.6)
peritoneal adhesions (568.0)
peritoneal adhesions with obstruction (560.81)
postcholecystectomy syndrome (576.0)
postgastric surgery syndromes (564.2)
vomiting following gastrointestinal surgery (564.3)
AHA: 2Q, '01, 4-6; 3Q, '99, 4; 2Q, '99, 14; 3Q, '97, 7; 1Q, '97, 11; 2Q, '95, 7; 1Q, '93, 26; 3Q, '92, 15; 2Q, '89, 15; 1Q, '88, 14

997.5 Urinary complications
Complications of:
external stoma of urinary tract
internal anastomosis and bypass of urinary tract, including that involving intestinal tract
Oliguria or anuria
Renal:
failure (acute)
insufficiency (acute)
Tubular necrosis (acute)
} specified as due to procedure

EXCLUDES *specified complications classified elsewhere, such as:*
postoperative stricture of:
ureter (593.3)
urethra (598.2)

AHA: 3Q, '03, 13; 3Q '96, 10, 15; 4Q, '95, 73; 1Q, '92, 13; 2Q, '89, 16; M-A, '87, 10; S-O, '85, 3

✓5th **997.6 Amputation stump complication**
EXCLUDES *admission for treatment for a current traumatic amputation — code to complicated traumatic amputation*
phantom limb (syndrome) (353.6)

AHA: 4Q, '95, 82

997.60 Unspecified complication

997.61 Neuroma of amputation stump
DEF: Hyperplasia generated nerve cell mass following amputation.

997.62 Infection (chronic)
Use additional code to identify organism
AHA: ►1Q, '05, 14;◄ 4Q, '96, 46

997.69 Other
AHA: ►1Q, '05, 15◄

✓5th **997.7 Vascular complications of other vessels**
EXCLUDES *peripheral vascular complications (997.2)*

997.71 Vascular complications of mesenteric artery
AHA: 4Q, '01, 53

997.72 Vascular complications of renal artery

997.79 Vascular complications of other vessels

✓5th **997.9 Complications affecting other specified body systems, not elsewhere classified**
EXCLUDES *specified complications classified elsewhere, such as:*
broad ligament laceration syndrome (620.6)
postartificial menopause syndrome (627.4)
postoperative stricture of vagina (623.2)

997.91 Hypertension
EXCLUDES *essential hypertension (401.0-401.9)*
AHA: 4Q, '95, 57

997.99 Other
Vitreous touch syndrome
AHA: 2Q, '94, 12; 1Q, '94, 17
DEF: Vitreous touch syndrome: vitreous protruding through pupil and attaches to corneal epithelium; causes aqueous fluid in vitreous body; marked by corneal edema, loss of lucidity; complication of cataract surgery.

✓4th **998 Other complications of procedures, not elsewhere classified**
AHA: 1Q, '94, 4

998.0 Postoperative shock
Collapse NOS
Shock (endotoxic) (hypovolemic) (septic)
} during or resulting from a surgical procedure

EXCLUDES *shock:*
anaphylactic due to serum (999.4)
anesthetic (995.4)
electric (994.8)
following abortion (639.5)
obstetric (669.1)
traumatic (958.4)

✓5th **998.1 Hemorrhage or hematoma or seroma complicating a procedure**
EXCLUDES *hemorrhage, hematoma, or seroma:*
complicating cesarean section or puerperal perineal wound (674.3)

998.11 Hemorrhage complicating a procedure
AHA: 3Q, '03, 13; 1Q, '03, 4; 4Q, '97, 52; 1Q, '97, 10

998.12 Hematoma complicating a procedure
AHA: 1Q, '03, 6; 3Q, '02, 24, 26

998.13 Seroma complicating a procedure
AHA: 4Q, '96, 46; 1Q, '93, 26; 2Q, '92, 15; S-O, '87, 8

998.2 Accidental puncture or laceration during a procedure
Accidental perforation by catheter or other instrument during a procedure on:
blood vessel
nerve
organ

EXCLUDES *iatrogenic [postoperative] pneumothorax (512.1)*
puncture or laceration caused by implanted device intentionally left in operation wound (996.0-996.5)
specified complications classified elsewhere, such as:
broad ligament laceration syndrome (620.6)
trauma from instruments during delivery (664.0-665.9)

AHA: 3Q, '02, 24, 26; 3Q, '94, 6; 3Q, '90, 17; 3Q, '90, 18

✓5th **998.3 Disruption of operation wound**
Dehiscence
Rupture
} of operation wound

EXCLUDES *disruption of:*
cesarean wound (674.1)
perineal wound, puerperal (674.2)

AHA: 4Q, '02, 73; 1Q, '93, 19

998.31 Disruption of internal operation wound

998.32 Disruption of external operation wound
Disruption of operation wound NOS
AHA: ►1Q, '05, 11;◄ 4Q, '03, 104, 106

998.4 Foreign body accidentally left during a procedure
Adhesions
Obstruction
Perforation
} due to foreign body accidentally left in operative wound or body cavity during a procedure

EXCLUDES *obstruction or perforation caused by implanted device intentionally left in body (996.0-996.5)*

AHA: 1Q, '89, 9

✓5th **998.5 Postoperative infection**
EXCLUDES *infection due to:*
implanted device (996.60-996.69)
infusion, perfusion, or transfusion (999.3)
postoperative obstetrical wound infection (674.3)

998.51 Infected postoperative seroma
Use additional code to identify organism
AHA: 4Q, '96, 46

998.59 Other postoperative infection
Abscess:
intra-abdominal
stitch
subphrenic
wound
Septicemia
} postoperative

Use additional code to identify infection
AHA: 4Q, '04, 76; 4Q, '03, 104, 106-107; 3Q, '98, 3; 3Q, '95, 5; 2Q, '95, 7; 3Q, '94, 6; 1Q, '93, 19; J-F, '87, 14

998.6 Persistent postoperative fistula

AHA: J-F, '87, 14

998.7 Acute reaction to foreign substance accidentally left during a procedure

Peritonitis: aseptic
Peritonitis: chemical

✓5th **998.8 Other specified complications of procedures, not elsewhere classified**

AHA: 4Q, '94, 46; 1Q, '89, 9

998.81 Emphysema (subcutaneous) (surgical) resulting from a procedure

998.82 Cataract fragments in eye following cataract surgery

998.83 Non-healing surgical wound

AHA: 4Q, '96, 47

998.89 Other specified complications

AHA: 3Q, '99, 13; 2Q, '98, 16

998.9 Unspecified complication of procedure, not elsewhere classified

Postoperative complication NOS

EXCLUDES *complication NOS of obstetrical, surgery or procedure (669.4)*

AHA: 4Q, '93, 37

✓4th **999 Complications of medical care, not elsewhere classified**

INCLUDES complications, not elsewhere classified, of:
- dialysis (hemodialysis) (peritoneal) (renal)
- extracorporeal circulation
- hyperalimentation therapy
- immunization
- infusion
- inhalation therapy
- injection
- inoculation
- perfusion
- transfusion
- vaccination
- ventilation therapy

EXCLUDES *specified complications classified elsewhere such as:*
- *complications of implanted device (996.0-996.9)*
- *contact dermatitis due to drugs (692.3)*
- *dementia dialysis (294.8)*
  - *transient (293.9)*
- *dialysis disequilibrium syndrome (276.0-276.9)*
- *poisoning and toxic effects of drugs and chemicals (960.0-989.9)*
- *postvaccinal encephalitis (323.5)*
- *water and electrolyte imbalance (276.0-276.9)*

999.0 Generalized vaccinia

DEF: Skin eruption, self-limiting; follows vaccination; due to transient viremia with virus localized in skin.

999.1 Air embolism

Air embolism to any site following infusion, perfusion, or transfusion

EXCLUDES *embolism specified as:*
- *complicating:*
  - *abortion (634-638 with .6, 639.6)*
  - *ectopic or molar pregnancy (639.6)*
  - *pregnancy, childbirth, or the puerperium (673.0)*
- *due to implanted device (996.7)*
- *traumatic (958.0)*

999.2 Other vascular complications

Phlebitis / Thromboembolism / Thrombophlebitis } following infusion, perfusion, or transfusion

EXCLUDES *the listed conditions when specified as:*
- *due to implanted device (996.61-996.62. 996.72-996.74)*
- *postoperative NOS (997.2, 997.71-997.79)*

AHA: 2Q, '97, 5

999.3 Other infection

Infection / Sepsis / Septicemia } following infusion, injection, transfusion, or vaccination

EXCLUDES *the listed conditions when specified as:*
- *due to implanted device (996.60-996.69)*
- *postoperative NOS (998.51-998.59)*

AHA: 2Q, '01, 11, 12; 2Q, '97, 5; J-F, '87, 14

999.4 Anaphylactic shock due to serum

EXCLUDES *shock:*
- *allergic NOS (995.0)*
- *anaphylactic:*
  - *NOS (995.0)*
  - *due to drugs and chemicals (995.0)*

DEF: Life-threatening hypersensitivity to foreign serum; causes respiratory distress, vascular collapse, and shock.

999.5 Other serum reaction

Intoxication by serum
Protein sickness
Serum rash
Serum sickness
Urticaria due to serum

EXCLUDES *serum hepatitis (070.2-070.3)*

DEF: Serum sickness: Hypersensitivity to foreign serum; causes fever, hives, swelling, and lymphadenopathy.

999.6 ABO incompatibility reaction

Incompatible blood transfusion
Reaction to blood group incompatibility in infusion or transfusion

999.7 Rh incompatibility reaction

Reactions due to Rh factor in infusion or transfusion

999.8 Other transfusion reaction

Septic shock due to transfusion
Transfusion reaction NOS

EXCLUDES *postoperative shock (998.0)*

AHA: 3Q, '00, 9

999.9 Other and unspecified complications of medical care, not elsewhere classified

Complications, not elsewhere classified, of:
electroshock / inhalation / ultrasound / ventilation } therapy

Unspecified misadventure of medical care

EXCLUDES *unspecified complication of:*
- *phototherapy (990)*
- *radiation therapy (990)*

AHA: 1Q, '03, 19; 2Q, '97, 5

SUPPLEMENTARY CLASSIFICATION OF FACTORS INFLUENCING HEALTH STATUS AND CONTACT WITH HEALTH SERVICES ▶(V01-V85)◀

This classification is provided to deal with occasions when circumstances other than a disease or injury classifiable to categories 001-999 (the main part of ICD) are recorded as "diagnoses" or "problems." This can arise mainly in three ways:

a) When a person who is not currently sick encounters the health services for some specific purpose, such as to act as a donor of an organ or tissue, to receive prophylactic vaccination, or to discuss a problem which is in itself not a disease or injury. This will be a fairly rare occurrence among hospital inpatients, but will be relatively more common among hospital outpatients and patients of family practitioners, health clinics, etc.

b) When a person with a known disease or injury, whether it is current or resolving, encounters the health care system for a specific treatment of that disease or injury (e.g., dialysis for renal disease; chemotherapy for malignancy; cast change).

c) When some circumstance or problem is present which influences the person's health status but is not in itself a current illness or injury. Such factors may be elicited during population surveys, when the person may or may not be currently sick, or be recorded as an additional factor to be borne in mind when the person is receiving care for some current illness or injury classifiable to categories 001-999.

In the latter circumstances the V code should be used only as a supplementary code and should not be the one selected for use in primary, single cause tabulations. Examples of these circumstances are a personal history of certain diseases, or a person with an artificial heart valve in situ.

AHA: J-F, '87, 8

PERSONS WITH POTENTIAL HEALTH HAZARDS RELATED TO COMMUNICABLE DISEASES (V01-V06)

EXCLUDES *family history of infectious and parasitic diseases (V18.8)*
personal history of infectious and parasitic diseases (V12.0)

✓4th **V01 Contact with or exposure to communicable diseases**

V01.0 Cholera
Conditions classifiable to 001

V01.1 Tuberculosis
Conditions classifiable to 010-018

V01.2 Poliomyelitis
Conditions classifiable to 045

V01.3 Smallpox
Conditions classifiable to 050

V01.4 Rubella
Conditions classifiable to 056

V01.5 Rabies
Conditions classifiable to 071

V01.6 Venereal diseases
Conditions classifiable to 090-099

✓5th **V01.7 Other viral diseases**
Conditions classifiable to 042-078 and V08, except as above
AHA: 2Q, '92, 11

V01.71 Varicella

V01.79 Other viral diseases

✓5th **V01.8 Other communicable diseases**
Conditions classifiable to 001-136, except as above
AHA: J-A, '87, 24

V01.81 Anthrax
AHA: 4Q, '02, 70, 78

V01.82 Exposure to SARS-associated coronavirus
AHA: 4Q, '03, 46-47

V01.83 Escherichia coli (E. coli)

V01.84 Meningococcus

V01.89 Other communicable diseases

V01.9 Unspecified communicable disease

✓4th **V02 Carrier or suspected carrier of infectious diseases**
AHA: 3Q, '95, 18; 3Q, '94, 4

V02.0 Cholera

V02.1 Typhoid

V02.2 Amebiasis

V02.3 Other gastrointestinal pathogens

V02.4 Diphtheria

✓5th **V02.5 Other specified bacterial diseases**

V02.51 Group B streptococcus
AHA: 1Q, '02, 14; 4Q, '98, 56

V02.52 Other streptococcus

V02.59 Other specified bacterial diseases
Meningococcal Staphylococcal

✓5th **V02.6 Viral hepatitis**
Hepatitis Australian-antigen [HAA] [SH] carrier
Serum hepatitis carrier

V02.60 Viral hepatitis carrier, unspecified
AHA: 4Q, '97, 47

V02.61 Hepatitis B carrier
AHA: 4Q, '97, 47

V02.62 Hepatitis C carrier
AHA: 4Q, '97, 47

V02.69 Other viral hepatitis carrier
AHA: 4Q, '97, 47

V02.7 Gonorrhea

V02.8 Other venereal diseases

V02.9 Other specified infectious organism
AHA: 3Q, '95, 18; 1Q, '93, 22; J-A, '87, 24

✓4th **V03 Need for prophylactic vaccination and inoculation against bacterial diseases**

EXCLUDES ▶*vaccination not carried out (V64.00-V64.09)*◀
vaccines against combinations of diseases (V06.0-V06.9)

V03.0 Cholera alone

V03.1 Typhoid-paratyphoid alone [TAB]

V03.2 Tuberculosis [BCG]

V03.3 Plague

V03.4 Tularemia

V03.5 Diphtheria alone

V03.6 Pertussis alone

V03.7 Tetanus toxoid alone

✓5th **V03.8 Other specified vaccinations against single bacterial diseases**

V03.81 Hemophilus influenza, type B [Hib]

V03.82 Streptococcus pneumoniae [pneumococcus]

V03.89 Other specified vaccination
AHA: 2Q, '00, 9

V03.9 Unspecified single bacterial disease

✓4th **V04 Need for prophylactic vaccination and inoculation against certain viral diseases**

EXCLUDES *vaccines against combinations of diseases (V06.0-V06.9)*

V04.0 Poliomyelitis

V04.1 Smallpox

V04.2 Measles alone

V04.3 Rubella alone

V04.4 Yellow fever

V04.5 Rabies

V04.6 Mumps alone

V04.7 Common cold

✓5th **V04.8 Other viral diseases**
AHA: 4Q, '03, 83

V04.81 Influenza

V04.82 Respiratory syncytial virus (RSV)

V04.89 Other viral diseases

Additional Digit Required | Unspecified Code | Other Specified Code | Manifestation Code | ▶◀ Revised Text | ● New Code | ▲ Revised Code Title

4th V05 Need for other prophylactic vaccination and inoculation against single diseases

EXCLUDES *vaccines against combinations of diseases (V06.0-V06.9)*

V05.0 Arthropod-borne viral encephalitis

V05.1 Other arthropod-borne viral diseases

V05.2 Leishmaniasis

V05.3 Viral hepatitis

V05.4 Varicella

Chickenpox

V05.8 Other specified disease

AHA: 1Q, '01, 4; 3Q, '91, 20

V05.9 Unspecified single disease

4th V06 Need for prophylactic vaccination and inoculation against combinations of diseases

Note: Use additional single vaccination codes from categories V03-V05 to identify any vaccinations not included in a combination code.

V06.0 Cholera with typhoid-paratyphoid [cholera+TAB]

V06.1 Diphtheria-tetanus-pertussis, combined [DTP] [DTaP]

AHA: 4Q, '03, 83; 3Q, '98, 13

V06.2 Diphtheria-tetanus-pertussis with typhoid-paratyphoid [DTP+TAB]

V06.3 Diphtheria-tetanus-pertussis with poliomyelitis [DTP+polio]

V06.4 Measles-mumps-rubella [MMR]

V06.5 Tetanus-diphtheria [Td] [DT]

AHA: 4Q, '03, 83

V06.6 Streptococcus pneumoniae [pneumococcus] and influenza

V06.8 Other combinations

EXCLUDES *multiple single vaccination codes (V03.0-V05.9)*

AHA: 1Q, '94, 19

V06.9 Unspecified combined vaccine

PERSONS WITH NEED FOR ISOLATION, OTHER POTENTIAL HEALTH HAZARDS AND PROPHYLACTIC MEASURES (V07-V09)

4th V07 Need for isolation and other prophylactic measures

EXCLUDES *prophylactic organ removal (V50.41-V50.49)*

V07.0 Isolation

Admission to protect the individual from his surroundings or for isolation of individual after contact with infectious diseases

V07.1 Desensitization to allergens

V07.2 Prophylactic immunotherapy

Administration of:
antivenin
immune sera [gamma globulin]

Administration of:
RhoGAM
tetanus antitoxin

5th V07.3 Other prophylactic chemotherapy

V07.31 Prophylactic fluoride administration

V07.39 Other prophylactic chemotherapy

EXCLUDES *maintenance chemotherapy following disease ▶(V58.12)◀*

V07.4 Hormone replacement therapy (postmenopausal) ♀

V07.8 Other specified prophylactic measure

AHA: 1Q, '92, 11

V07.9 Unspecified prophylactic measure

V08 Asymptomatic human immunodeficiency virus [HIV] infection status

HIV positive NOS

Note: This code is ONLY to be used when NO HIV infection symptoms or conditions are present. If any HIV infection symptoms or conditions are present, see code 042.

EXCLUDES *AIDS (042)*
human immunodeficiency virus [HIV] disease (042)
exposure to HIV (V01.79)
nonspecific serologic evidence of HIV (795.71)
symptomatic human immunodeficiency virus [HIV] infection (042)

AHA: 2Q, '04, 11; 2Q, '99, 8; 3Q, '95, 18

4th V09 Infection with drug-resistant microorganisms

Note: This category is intended for use as an additional code for infectious conditions classified elsewhere to indicate the presence of drug-resistance of the infectious organism.

AHA: 3Q, '94, 4; 4Q, '93, 22

V09.0 Infection with microorganisms resistant to penicillins SDx

Methicillin-resistant staphylococcus aureus (MRSA)

AHA: 4Q, '03, 104, 106

V09.1 Infection with microorganisms resistant to cephalosporins and other B-lactam antibiotics SDx

V09.2 Infection with microorganisms resistant to macrolides SDx

V09.3 Infection with microorganisms resistant to tetracyclines SDx

V09.4 Infection with microorganisms resistant to aminoglycosides SDx

5th V09.5 Infection with microorganisms resistant to quinolones and fluoroquinolones

V09.50 Without mention of resistance to multiple quinolones and fluoroquinoles SDx

V09.51 With resistance to multiple quinolones and fluoroquinoles SDx

V09.6 Infection with microorganisms resistant to sulfonamides SDx

5th V09.7 Infection with microorganisms resistant to other specified antimycobacterial agents

EXCLUDES *Amikacin (V09.4)*
Kanamycin (V09.4)
Streptomycin [SM] (V09.4)

V09.70 Without mention of resistance to multiple antimycobacterial agents SDx

V09.71 With resistance to multiple antimycobacterial agents SDx

5th V09.8 Infection with microorganisms resistant to other specified drugs

Vancomycin (glycopeptide) intermediate staphylococcus aureus (VISA/GISA)
Vancomycin (glycopeptide) resistant enterococcus (VRE)
Vancomycin (glycopeptide) resistant staphylococcus aureus (VRSA/GRSA)

V09.80 Without mention of resistance to multiple drugs SDx

V09.81 With resistance to multiple drugs SDx

5th V09.9 Infection with drug-resistant microorganisms, unspecified

Drug resistance, NOS

V09.90 Without mention of multiple drug resistance SDx

V09.91 With multiple drug resistance SDx

Multiple drug resistance NOS

PERSONS WITH POTENTIAL HEALTH HAZARDS RELATED TO PERSONAL AND FAMILY HISTORY

EXCLUDES *obstetric patients where the possibility that the fetus might be affected is the reason for observation or management during pregnancy (655.0-655.9)*

AHA: J-F, '87, 1

4th **V10 Personal history of malignant neoplasm**
AHA: 4Q, '02, 80; 4Q, '98, 69; 1Q, '95, 4; 3Q, '92, 5; M-J, '85, 10; 2Q, '90, 9

5th **V10.0 Gastrointestinal tract**
History of conditions classifiable to 140-159
- **V10.00 Gastrointestinal tract, unspecified**
- **V10.01 Tongue**
- **V10.02 Other and unspecified oral cavity and pharynx**
- **V10.03 Esophagus**
- **V10.04 Stomach**
- **V10.05 Large intestine**
  AHA: 3Q, '99, 7; 1Q, '95, 4
- **V10.06 Rectum, rectosigmoid junction, and anus**
- **V10.07 Liver**
- **V10.09 Other**
  AHA: 4Q, '03, 111

5th **V10.1 Trachea, bronchus, and lung**
History of conditions classifiable to 162
- **V10.11 Bronchus and lung**
- **V10.12 Trachea**

5th **V10.2 Other respiratory and intrathoracic organs**
History of conditions classifiable to 160, 161, 163-165
- **V10.20 Respiratory organ, unspecified**
- **V10.21 Larynx**
  AHA: 4Q, '03, 108, 110
- **V10.22 Nasal cavities, middle ear, and accessory sinuses**
- **V10.29 Other**

V10.3 Breast
History of conditions classifiable to 174 and 175
AHA: 2Q. '03, 5; 4Q, '01, 66; 4Q, '98, 65; 4Q, '97, 50; 1Q, '91, 16; 1Q, '90, 21

5th **V10.4 Genital organs**
History of conditions classifiable to 179-187
- **V10.40 Female genital organ, unspecified** ♀
- **V10.41 Cervix uteri** ♀
- **V10.42 Other parts of uterus** ♀
- **V10.43 Ovary** ♀
- **V10.44 Other female genital organs** ♀
- **V10.45 Male genital organ, unspecified** ♂
- **V10.46 Prostate** ♂
- **V10.47 Testis** ♂
- **V10.48 Epididymis** ♂
- **V10.49 Other male genital organs** ♂

5th **V10.5 Urinary organs**
History of conditions classifiable to 188 and 189
- **V10.50 Urinary organ, unspecified**
- **V10.51 Bladder**
- **V10.52 Kidney**
  EXCLUDES *renal pelvis (V10.53)*
  AHA: 2Q, '04, 4
- **V10.53 Renal pelvis**
  AHA: 4Q, '01, 55
- **V10.59 Other**

5th **V10.6 Leukemia**
Conditions classifiable to 204-208
EXCLUDES *leukemia in remission (204-208)*
AHA: 2Q, '92, 13; 4Q, '91, 26; 4Q, '90, 3
- **V10.60 Leukemia, unspecified**
- **V10.61 Lymphoid leukemia**
- **V10.62 Myeloid leukemia**
- **V10.63 Monocytic leukemia**
- **V10.69 Other**

5th **V10.7 Other lymphatic and hematopoietic neoplasms**
Conditions classifiable to 200-203
EXCLUDES *listed conditions in 200-203 in remission*
AHA: M-J, '85, 18
- **V10.71 Lymphosarcoma and reticulosarcoma**
- **V10.72 Hodgkin's disease**
- **V10.79 Other**

5th **V10.8 Personal history of malignant neoplasm of other sites**
History of conditions classifiable to 170-173, 190-195
- **V10.81 Bone**
  AHA: 2Q, '03, 13
- **V10.82 Malignant melanoma of skin**
- **V10.83 Other malignant neoplasm of skin**
- **V10.84 Eye**
- **V10.85 Brain**
  AHA: 1Q, '01, 6
- **V10.86 Other parts of nervous system**
  EXCLUDES *peripheral sympathetic, and parasympathetic nerves (V10.89)*
- **V10.87 Thyroid**
- **V10.88 Other endocrine glands and related structures**
- **V10.89 Other**

V10.9 Unspecified personal history of malignant neoplasm

4th **V11 Personal history of mental disorder**

V11.0 Schizophrenia
EXCLUDES *that in remission (295.0-295.9 with fifth-digit 5)*

V11.1 Affective disorders
Personal history of manic-depressive psychosis
EXCLUDES *that in remission (296.0-296.6 with fifth-digit 5, 6)*

V11.2 Neurosis

V11.3 Alcoholism

V11.8 Other mental disorders

V11.9 Unspecified mental disorder

4th **V12 Personal history of certain other diseases**
AHA: 3Q, '92, 11

5th **V12.0 Infectious and parasitic diseases**
EXCLUDES ▶ *personal history of infectious diseases specific to a body system*◀
- **V12.00 Unspecified infectious and parasitic disease**
- **V12.01 Tuberculosis**
- **V12.02 Poliomyelitis**
- **V12.03 Malaria**
- **V12.09 Other**

V12.1 Nutritional deficiency

V12.2 Endocrine, metabolic, and immunity disorders
EXCLUDES *history of allergy (V14.0-V14.9, V15.01-V15.09)*

V12.3 Diseases of blood and blood-forming organs

5th **V12.4 Disorders of nervous system and sense organs**
- **V12.40 Unspecified disorder of nervous system and sense organs**
- **V12.41 Benign neoplasm of the brain**
  AHA: 4Q, '97, 48
- ● **V12.42 Infections of the central nervous system**
  Encephalitis   Meningitis
- **V12.49 Other disorders of nervous system and sense organs**
  AHA: 4Q, '98, 59

4th 5th Additional Digit Required | Unspecified Code | Other Specified Code | Manifestation Code | ▶◀ Revised Text | ● New Code | ▲ Revised Code Title

✓5th **V12.5 Diseases of circulatory system**
EXCLUDES *old myocardial infarction (412)*
postmyocardial infarction syndrome (411.0)
AHA: 4Q, '95, 61
V12.50 Unspecified circulatory disease
V12.51 Venous thrombosis and embolism
Pulmonary embolism
AHA: 4Q, '03, 108; 1Q, '02, 15
V12.52 Thrombophlebitis
V12.59 Other
AHA: 4Q, '99, 4; 4Q, '98, 88; 4Q, '97, 37

✓5th **V12.6 Diseases of respiratory system**
EXCLUDES ▶ *tuberculosis (V12.01)*◀
● **V12.60 Unspecified disease of respiratory system**
● **V12.61 Pneumonia (recurrent)**
● **V12.69 Other diseases of respiratory system**

✓5th **V12.7 Diseases of digestive system**
AHA: 1Q, '95, 3; 2Q, '89, 16
V12.70 Unspecified digestive disease
V12.71 Peptic ulcer disease
V12.72 Colonic polyps
AHA: 3Q, '02, 15
V12.79 Other

✓4th **V13 Personal history of other diseases**

✓5th **V13.0 Disorders of urinary system**
V13.00 Unspecified urinary disorder
V13.01 Urinary calculi
● **V13.02 Urinary (tract) infection**
● **V13.03 Nephrotic syndrome**
V13.09 Other

V13.1 Trophoblastic disease ♀
EXCLUDES *supervision during a current pregnancy (V23.1)*

✓5th **V13.2 Other genital system and obstetric disorders**
EXCLUDES *supervision during a current pregnancy of a woman with poor obstetric history (V23.0-V23.9)*
habitual aborter (646.3)
without current pregnancy (629.9)
V13.21 Personal history of pre-term labor ♀
EXCLUDES *current pregnancy with history of pre-term labor (V23.41)*
AHA: 4Q, '02, 78
V13.29 Other genital system and obstetric disorders ♀

V13.3 Diseases of skin and subcutaneous tissue
V13.4 Arthritis
V13.5 Other musculoskeletal disorders

✓5th **V13.6 Congenital malformations**
AHA: 4Q, '98, 63
V13.61 Hypospadias SDx ♂
V13.69 Other congenital malformations
AHA: 1Q, '04, 16

V13.7 Perinatal problems
EXCLUDES *low birth weight status (V21.30-V21.35)*
V13.8 Other specified diseases
V13.9 Unspecified disease

✓4th **V14 Personal history of allergy to medicinal agents**
V14.0 Penicillin SDx
V14.1 Other antibiotic agent SDx
V14.2 Sulfonamides SDx
V14.3 Other anti-infective agent SDx
V14.4 Anesthetic agent SDx
V14.5 Narcotic agent SDx
V14.6 Analgesic agent SDx
V14.7 Serum or vaccine SDx
V14.8 Other specified medicinal agents SDx
V14.9 Unspecified medicinal agent SDx

✓4th **V15 Other personal history presenting hazards to health**

✓5th **V15.0 Allergy, other than to medicinal agents**
EXCLUDES *allergy to food substance used as base for medicinal agent (V14.0-V14.9)*
AHA: 4Q, '00, 42, 49
V15.01 Allergy to peanuts SDx
V15.02 Allergy to milk products SDx
EXCLUDES *lactose intolerance (271.3)*
AHA: 1Q, '03, 12
V15.03 Allergy to eggs SDx
V15.04 Allergy to seafood SDx
Seafood (octopus) (squid) ink
Shellfish
V15.05 Allergy to other foods SDx
Food additives
Nuts other than peanuts
V15.06 Allergy to insects SDx
Bugs
Spiders
Insect bites and stings
V15.07 Allergy to latex SDx
Latex sensitivity
V15.08 Allergy to radiographic dye SDx
Contrast media used for diagnostic x-ray procedures
V15.09 Other allergy, other than to medicinal agents SDx

V15.1 Surgery to heart and great vessels SDx
EXCLUDES *replacement by transplant or other means (V42.1-V42.2, V43.2-V43.4)*
AHA: 1Q, '04, 16

V15.2 Surgery to other major organs SDx
EXCLUDES *replacement by transplant or other means (V42.0-V43.8)*

V15.3 Irradiation SDx
Previous exposure to therapeutic or other ionizing radiation

✓5th **V15.4 Psychological trauma**
EXCLUDES *history of condition classifiable to 290-316 (V11.0-V11.9)*
V15.41 History of physical abuse SDx
Rape
AHA: 3Q, '99, 15
V15.42 History of emotional abuse SDx
Neglect
AHA: 3Q, '99, 15
V15.49 Other SDx
AHA: 3Q, '99, 15

V15.5 Injury SDx
V15.6 Poisoning SDx
V15.7 Contraception
EXCLUDES *current contraceptive management (V25.0-V25.4)*
presence of intrauterine contraceptive device as incidental finding (V45.5)

✓5th **V15.8 Other specified personal history presenting hazards to health**
AHA: 4Q, '95, 62
V15.81 Noncompliance with medical treatment SDx
AHA: 2Q, '03, 7; 2Q, '01, 11; 12, 13; 2Q '99, 17; 2Q, '97, 11; 1Q, '97, 12; 3Q, '96, 9

V15.82 History of tobacco use SDx
EXCLUDES *tobacco dependence (305.1)*
V15.84 Exposure to asbestos SDx
V15.85 Exposure to potentially hazardous body fluids SDx
V15.86 Exposure to lead SDx
V15.87 History of extracorporeal membrane oxygenation [ECMO] SDx
AHA: 4Q, '03, 84
● V15.88 History of fall SDx
At risk for falling
V15.89 Other SDx
AHA: 1Q, '90, 21; N-D, '84, 12

V15.9 Unspecified personal history presenting hazards to health SDx

✓4th **V16 Family history of malignant neoplasm**
V16.0 Gastrointestinal tract
Family history of condition classifiable to 140-159
AHA: 1Q, '99, 4
V16.1 Trachea, bronchus, and lung
Family history of condition classifiable to 162
V16.2 Other respiratory and intrathoracic organs
Family history of condition classifiable to 160-161, 163-165
V16.3 Breast
Family history of condition classifiable to 174
AHA: 4Q, '04, 107; 2Q, '03, 4; 2Q, '00, 8; 1Q, '92, 11
✓5th V16.4 Genital organs
Family history of condition classifiable to 179-187
AHA: 4Q, '97, 48
V16.40 Genital organ, unspecified
V16.41 Ovary
V16.42 Prostate
V16.43 Testis
V16.49 Other
✓5th V16.5 Urinary organs
Family history of condition classifiable to 189
V16.51 Kidney
V16.59 Other
V16.6 Leukemia
Family history of condition classifiable to 204-208
V16.7 Other lymphatic and hematopoietic neoplasms
Family history of condition classifiable to 200-203
V16.8 Other specified malignant neoplasm
Family history of other condition classifiable to 140-199
V16.9 Unspecified malignant neoplasm

✓4th **V17 Family history of certain chronic disabling diseases**
V17.0 Psychiatric condition
EXCLUDES *family history of mental retardation (V18.4)*
V17.1 Stroke (cerebrovascular)
V17.2 Other neurological diseases
Epilepsy
Huntington's chorea
V17.3 Ischemic heart disease
V17.4 Other cardiovascular diseases
AHA: 1Q, '04, 6
V17.5 Asthma
V17.6 Other chronic respiratory conditions
V17.7 Arthritis
✓5th V17.8 Other musculoskeletal diseases
● V17.81 Osteoporosis
● V17.89 Other musculoskeletal diseases

✓4th **V18 Family history of certain other specific conditions**
V18.0 Diabetes mellitus
AHA: 1Q, '04, 8
V18.1 Other endocrine and metabolic diseases
V18.2 Anemia
V18.3 Other blood disorders
V18.4 Mental retardation
V18.5 Digestive disorders
✓5th V18.6 Kidney diseases
V18.61 Polycystic kidney
V18.69 Other kidney diseases
V18.7 Other genitourinary diseases
V18.8 Infectious and parasitic diseases
● V18.9 Genetic disease carrier

✓4th **V19 Family history of other conditions**
V19.0 Blindness or visual loss
V19.1 Other eye disorders
V19.2 Deafness or hearing loss
V19.3 Other ear disorders
V19.4 Skin conditions
V19.5 Congenital anomalies
V19.6 Allergic disorders
V19.7 Consanguinity
V19.8 Other condition

PERSONS ENCOUNTERING HEALTH SERVICES IN CIRCUMSTANCES RELATED TO REPRODUCTION AND DEVELOPMENT (V20-V29)

✓4th **V20 Health supervision of infant or child**
V20.0 Foundling PDx P
V20.1 Other healthy infant or child receiving care PDx P
Medical or nursing care supervision of healthy infant in cases of:
maternal illness, physical or psychiatric
socioeconomic adverse condition at home
too many children at home preventing or interfering with normal care
AHA: 1Q, '00, 25; 3Q, '89, 14
V20.2 Routine infant or child health check PDx P
Developmental testing of infant or child
Immunizations appropriate for age
Routine vision and hearing testing
Use additional code(s) to identify:
special screening examination(s) performed (V73.0-V82.9)
EXCLUDES *special screening for developmental handicaps (V79.3)*
AHA: 1Q, '04, 15

✓4th **V21 Constitutional states in development**
V21.0 Period of rapid growth in childhood SDx
V21.1 Puberty SDx
V21.2 Other adolescence SDx
✓5th V21.3 Low birth weight status
EXCLUDES *history of perinatal problems (V13.7)*
AHA: 4Q, '00, 51
V21.30 Low birth weight status, unspecified SDx
V21.31 Low birth weight status, less than 500 grams SDx
V21.32 Low birth weight status, 500-999 grams SDx
V21.33 Low birth weight status, 1000-1499 grams SDx
V21.34 Low birth weight status, 1500-1999 grams SDx
V21.35 Low birth weight status, 2000-2500 grams SDx
V21.8 Other specified constitutional states in development SDx
V21.9 Unspecified constitutional state in development SDx

✓4th ✓5th Additional Digit Required | Unspecified Code | Other Specified Code | Manifestation Code | ▶◀ Revised Text | ● New Code | ▲ Revised Code Title

✓4th **V22 Normal pregnancy**

EXCLUDES *pregnancy examination or test, pregnancy unconfirmed (V72.40)*

V22.0 Supervision of normal first pregnancy PDx ♀
AHA: 3Q, '99, 16

V22.1 Supervision of other normal pregnancy PDx ♀
AHA: 3Q, '99, 16

V22.2 Pregnant state, incidental SDx ♀
Pregnant state NOS

✓4th **V23 Supervision of high-risk pregnancy**
AHA: 1Q, 90, 10

V23.0 Pregnancy with history of infertility M ♀

V23.1 Pregnancy with history of trophoblastic disease M ♀
Pregnancy with history of:
hydatidiform mole
vesicular mole
EXCLUDES *that without current pregnancy (V13.1)*

V23.2 Pregnancy with history of abortion M ♀
Pregnancy with history of conditions classifiable to 634-638
EXCLUDES *habitual aborter:*
care during pregnancy (646.3)
that without current pregnancy (629.9)

V23.3 Grand multiparity M ♀
EXCLUDES *care in relation to labor and delivery (659.4)*
that without current pregnancy (V61.5)

✓5th **V23.4 Pregnancy with other poor obstetric history**
Pregnancy with history of other conditions classifiable to 630-676

V23.41 Pregnancy with history of pre-term labor M ♀
AHA: 4Q, '02, 79

V23.49 Pregnancy with other poor obstetric history M ♀

V23.5 Pregnancy with other poor reproductive history M ♀
Pregnancy with history of stillbirth or neonatal death

V23.7 Insufficient prenatal care M ♀
History of little or no prenatal care

✓5th **V23.8 Other high-risk pregnancy**
AHA: 4Q, '98, 56, 63

V23.81 Elderly primigravida M ♀
First pregnancy in a woman who will be 35 years of age or older at expected date of delivery
EXCLUDES *elderly primigravida complicating pregnancy (659.5)*

V23.82 Elderly multigravida M ♀
Second or more pregnancy in a woman who will be 35 years of age or older at expected date of delivery
EXCLUDES *elderly multigravida complicating pregnancy (659.6)*

V23.83 Young primigravida M ♀
First pregnancy in a female less than 16 years old at expected date of delivery
EXCLUDES *young primigravida complicating pregnancy (659.8)*

V23.84 Young multigravida M ♀
Second or more pregnancy in a female less than 16 years old at expected date of delivery
EXCLUDES *young multigravida complicating pregnancy (659.8)*

V23.89 Other high-risk pregnancy M ♀

V23.9 Unspecified high-risk pregnancy M ♀

✓4th **V24 Postpartum care and examination**

V24.0 Immediately after delivery PDx M ♀
Care and observation in uncomplicated cases

V24.1 Lactating mother PDx ♀
Supervision of lactation

V24.2 Routine postpartum follow-up PDx ♀

✓4th **V25 Encounter for contraceptive management**
AHA: 4Q, '92, 24

✓5th **V25.0 General counseling and advice**

V25.01 Prescription of oral contraceptives ♀

V25.02 Initiation of other contraceptive measures
Fitting of diaphragm
Prescription of foams, creams, or other agents
AHA: 3Q, '97, 7

V25.03 Encounter for emergency contraceptive counseling and prescription
Encounter for postcoital contraceptive counseling and prescription
AHA: 4Q, '03, 84

V25.09 Other
Family planning advice

V25.1 Insertion of intrauterine contraceptive device ♀

V25.2 Sterilization
Admission for interruption of fallopian tubes or vas deferens

V25.3 Menstrual extraction ♀
Menstrual regulation

✓5th **V25.4 Surveillance of previously prescribed contraceptive methods**
Checking, reinsertion, or removal of contraceptive device
Repeat prescription for contraceptive method
Routine examination in connection with contraceptive maintenance
EXCLUDES *presence of intrauterine contraceptive device as incidental finding (V45.5)*

V25.40 Contraceptive surveillance, unspecified

V25.41 Contraceptive pill ♀

V25.42 Intrauterine contraceptive device ♀
Checking, reinsertion, or removal of intrauterine device

V25.43 Implantable subdermal contraceptive ♀

V25.49 Other contraceptive method
AHA: 3Q, '97, 7

V25.5 Insertion of implantable subdermal contraceptive ♀
AHA: 3Q, '92, 9

V25.8 Other specified contraceptive management
Postvasectomy sperm count
EXCLUDES *sperm count following sterilization reversal (V26.22)*
sperm count for fertility testing (V26.21)
AHA: 3Q, '96, 9

V25.9 Unspecified contraceptive management

✓4th **V26 Procreative management**

V26.0 Tuboplasty or vasoplasty after previous sterilization
AHA: 2Q, '95, 10

V26.1 Artificial insemination ♀

✓5th **V26.2 Investigation and testing**
EXCLUDES *postvasectomy sperm count (V25.8)*
AHA: 4Q, '00, 56

V26.21 Fertility testing
Fallopian insufflation
Sperm count for fertility testing
EXCLUDES *genetic counseling and testing ▶(V26.31-V26.33)◀*

V26.22 **Aftercare following sterilization reversal**
Fallopian insufflation following sterilization reversal
Sperm count following sterilization reversal

V26.29 **Other investigation and testing**
AHA: 2Q, '96, 9; N-D, '85, 15

✓5th V26.3 **Genetic counseling and testing**
EXCLUDES *fertility testing (V26.21)*

● V26.31 **Testing for genetic disease carrier status**
● V26.32 **Other genetic testing**
● V26.33 **Genetic counseling**

V26.4 **General counseling and advice**

✓5th V26.5 **Sterilization status**

V26.51 **Tubal ligation status** SDx ♀
EXCLUDES *infertility not due to previous tubal ligation (628.0-628.9)*

V26.52 **Vasectomy status** SDx ♂

V26.8 **Other specified procreative management**
V26.9 **Unspecified procreative management**

✓4th V27 **Outcome of delivery**
Note: This category is intended for the coding of the outcome of delivery on the mother's record.
AHA: 2Q, '91, 16

V27.0 **Single liveborn** M SDx ♀
AHA: 2Q, '03, 9; 2Q, '02, 10; 1Q, '01, 10; 3Q, '00, 5; 4Q, '98, 77; 4Q, '95, 59; 1Q, '92, 9

V27.1 **Single stillborn** M SDx ♀
V27.2 **Twins, both liveborn** M SDx ♀
V27.3 **Twins, one liveborn and one stillborn** M SDx ♀
V27.4 **Twins, both stillborn** M SDx ♀
V27.5 **Other multiple birth, all liveborn** M SDx ♀
V27.6 **Other multiple birth, some liveborn** M SDx ♀
V27.7 **Other multiple birth, all stillborn** M SDx ♀
V27.9 **Unspecified outcome of delivery** M SDx ♀
Single birth } outcome to infant
Multiple birth } unspecified

✓4th V28 **Antenatal screening**
EXCLUDES *abnormal findings on screening — code to findings*
routine prenatal care (V22.0-V23.9)
AHA: 1Q, '04, 11

V28.0 **Screening for chromosomal anomalies by amniocentesis** M ♀
V28.1 **Screening for raised alpha-fetoprotein levels in amniotic fluid** M ♀
V28.2 **Other screening based on amniocentesis** M ♀
V28.3 **Screening for malformation using ultrasonics** ♀
V28.4 **Screening for fetal growth retardation using ultrasonics** ♀
V28.5 **Screening for isoimmunization** ♀
V28.6 **Screening for Streptococcus B** M ♀
AHA: 4Q, '97, 46

V28.8 **Other specified antenatal screening** ♀
AHA: 3Q, '99, 16

V28.9 **Unspecified antenatal screening** ♀

✓4th V29 **Observation and evaluation of newborns and infants for suspected condition not found**
Note: This category is to be used for newborns, within the neonatal period, (the first 28 days of life) who are suspected of having an abnormal condition resulting from exposure from the mother or the birth process, but without signs or symptoms, and, which after examination and observation, is found not to exist.
AHA: 1Q, '00, 25; 4Q, '94, 47; 1Q, '94, 9; 4Q, '92, 21

[1] V29.0 **Observation for suspected infectious condition** N PDx
AHA: 1Q, '01, 10

[1] V29.1 **Observation for suspected neurological condition** N PDx

[1] V29.2 **Observation for suspected respiratory condition** N PDx

[1] V29.3 **Observation for suspected genetic or metabolic condition** N PDx
AHA: 4Q, '98, 59, 68

[1] V29.8 **Observation for other specified suspected condition** N PDx
AHA: 2Q, '03, 15

[1] V29.9 **Observation for unspecified suspected condition** N PDx
AHA: 1Q, '02, 6

LIVEBORN INFANTS ACCORDING TO TYPE OF BIRTH (V30-V39)

Note: These categories are intended for the coding of liveborn infants who are consuming health care [e.g., crib or bassinet occupancy].

The following fourth-digit subdivisions are for use with categories V30-V39:
✓5th **0 Born in hospital** N
1 Born before admission to hospital N
2 Born outside hospital and not hospitalized

The following two fifth-digits are for use with the fourth-digit .0, Born in hospital:
0 delivered without mention of cesarean delivery
1 delivered by cesarean delivery

AHA: 1Q, '01, 10

✓4th V30 **Single liveborn** PDx
AHA: 2Q, '03, 9; 4Q, '98, 46, 59; 1Q, '94, 9 ; For code V30.00: 1Q, '04, 8, 16; 4Q, '03, 68

✓4th V31 **Twin, mate liveborn** PDx
AHA: 3Q, '92, 10

✓4th V32 **Twin, mate stillborn** PDx
✓4th V33 **Twin, unspecified** PDx
✓4th V34 **Other multiple, mates all liveborn** PDx
✓4th V35 **Other multiple, mates all stillborn** PDx
✓4th V36 **Other multiple, mates live- and stillborn** PDx
✓4th V37 **Other multiple, unspecified** PDx
✓4th V39 **Unspecified** PDx

PERSONS WITH A CONDITION INFLUENCING THEIR HEALTH STATUS (V40-V49)

Note: These categories are intended for use when these conditions are recorded as "diagnoses" or "problems."

✓4th V40 **Mental and behavioral problems**
V40.0 **Problems with learning**
V40.1 **Problems with communication [including speech]**
V40.2 **Other mental problems**
V40.3 **Other behavioral problems**
V40.9 **Unspecified mental or behavioral problem**

✓4th V41 **Problems with special senses and other special functions**
V41.0 **Problems with sight**
V41.1 **Other eye problems**
V41.2 **Problems with hearing**
V41.3 **Other ear problems**
V41.4 **Problems with voice production**
V41.5 **Problems with smell and taste**

[1] A code from the V30–V39 series may be sequenced before the V29 on the newborn medical record.

✓4th ✓5th Additional Digit Required   Unspecified Code   Other Specified Code   Manifestation Code   ▶◀ Revised Text   ● New Code   ▲ Revised Code Title

V41.6 **Problems with swallowing and mastication**

V41.7 **Problems with sexual function**

EXCLUDES *marital problems (V61.10)*
psychosexual disorders (302.0-302.9)

V41.8 **Other problems with special functions**

V41.9 **Unspecified problem with special functions**

✓4th **V42 Organ or tissue replaced by transplant**

INCLUDES homologous or heterologous (animal) (human) transplant organ status

AHA: 3Q, '98, 3, 4

V42.0 **Kidney** SDx
AHA: 1Q, '03, 10; 3Q, '01, 12

V42.1 **Heart** SDx
AHA: 3Q, '03, 16; 3Q, '01, 13

V42.2 **Heart valve** SDx

V42.3 **Skin** SDx

V42.4 **Bone** SDx

V42.5 **Cornea** SDx

V42.6 **Lung** SDx

V42.7 **Liver** SDx

✓5th V42.8 **Other specified organ or tissue**
AHA: 4Q, '98, 64; 4Q, '97, 49

V42.81 **Bone marrow** SDx

V42.82 **Peripheral stem cells** SDx

V42.83 **Pancreas** SDx
AHA: 1Q, '03, 10; 2Q, '01, 16

V42.84 **Intestines** SDx
AHA: 4Q, '00, 48, 50

V42.89 **Other** SDx

V42.9 **Unspecified organ or tissue** SDx

✓4th **V43 Organ or tissue replaced by other means**

INCLUDES organ or tissue assisted by other means
replacement of organ by:
artificial device
mechanical device
prosthesis

EXCLUDES *cardiac pacemaker in situ (V45.01)*
fitting and adjustment of prosthetic device (V52.0-V52.9)
renal dialysis status (V45.1)

V43.0 **Eye globe** SDx

V43.1 **Lens** SDx
Pseudophakos
AHA: 4Q, '98, 65

✓5th V43.2 **Heart**
Fully implantable artificial heart
Heart assist device
AHA: 4Q, '03, 85

V43.21 **Heart assist device** SDx

V43.22 **Fully implantable artificial heart**

V43.3 **Heart valve** SDx
AHA: 3Q, '02, 13, 14

V43.4 **Blood vessel** SDx

V43.5 **Bladder** SDx

✓5th V43.6 **Joint**

V43.60 **Unspecified joint** SDx

V43.61 **Shoulder** SDx

V43.62 **Elbow** SDx

V43.63 **Wrist** SDx

V43.64 **Hip** SDx
AHA: 2Q, '04, 15

V43.65 **Knee** SDx

V43.66 **Ankle** SDx

V43.69 **Other** SDx

V43.7 **Limb** SDx

✓5th V43.8 **Other organ or tissue**

V43.81 **Larynx** SDx
AHA: 4Q, '95, 55

V43.82 **Breast** SDx
AHA: 4Q, '95, 55

V43.83 **Artificial skin** SDx

V43.89 **Other** SDx

✓4th **V44 Artificial opening status**

EXCLUDES *artificial openings requiring attention or management (V55.0-V55.9)*

V44.0 **Tracheostomy** SDx
AHA: 4Q, '03, 103, 107, 111; 1Q, '01, 6

V44.1 **Gastrostomy** SDx
AHA: 4Q, '03, 103, 107-108, 110; 1Q, '01, 12; 3Q, '97, 12; 1Q, '93, 26

V44.2 **Ileostomy** SDx

V44.3 **Colostomy** SDx
AHA: 4Q, '03, 110

V44.4 **Other artificial opening of gastrointestinal tract** SDx

✓5th V44.5 **Cystostomy**

V44.50 **Cystostomy, unspecified** SDx

V44.51 **Cutaneous-vesicostomy** SDx

V44.52 **Appendico-vesicostomy** SDx

V44.59 **Other cystostomy** SDx

V44.6 **Other artificial opening of urinary tract** SDx
Nephrostomy
Urethrostomy
Ureterostomy

V44.7 **Artificial vagina** SDx

V44.8 **Other artificial opening status** SDx

V44.9 **Unspecified artificial opening status** SDx

✓4th **V45 Other postprocedural states**

EXCLUDES *aftercare management (V51-V58.9)*
malfunction or other complication — code to condition

AHA: 4Q, '03, 85

✓5th V45.0 **Cardiac device in situ**

EXCLUDES *artificial heart (V43.22)*
heart assist device (V43.21)

V45.00 **Unspecified cardiac device** SDx

V45.01 **Cardiac pacemaker** SDx

V45.02 **Automatic implantable cardiac defibrillator** SDx

V45.09 **Other specified cardiac device** SDx
Carotid sinus pacemaker in situ

V45.1 **Renal dialysis status** SDx
▶Hemodialysis status◀
Patient requiring intermittent renal dialysis
▶Peritoneal dialysis status◀
Presence of arterial-venous shunt (for dialysis)

EXCLUDES *admission for dialysis treatment or session (V56.0)*

AHA: 1Q, '04, 22-23; 2Q, '03, 7; 2Q, '01, 12, 13

V45.2 **Presence of cerebrospinal fluid drainage device** SDx
Cerebral ventricle (communicating) shunt, valve, or device in situ

EXCLUDES *malfunction (996.2)*

AHA: 4Q, '03, 106

V45.3 **Intestinal bypass or anastomosis status** SDx

V45.4 **Arthrodesis status** SDx
AHA: N-D, '84, 18

✓5th V45.5 **Presence of contraceptive device**

EXCLUDES *checking, reinsertion, or removal of device (V25.42)*
complication from device (996.32)
insertion of device (V25.1)

V45.51 **Intrauterine contraceptive device** SDx ♀

V45.52 **Subdermal contraceptive implant** SDx

V45.59 **Other** SDx

✓5th **V45.6 States following surgery of eye and adnexa**
Cataract extraction
Filtering bleb
Surgical eyelid adhesion
} state following eye surgery

EXCLUDES *aphakia (379.31)*
artificial eye globe (V43.0)

AHA: 4Q, '98, 65; 4Q, '97, 49

V45.61 Cataract extraction status SDx
Use additional code for associated artificial lens status (V43.1)

V45.69 Other states following surgery of eye and adnexa SDx
AHA: 2Q, '01, 16; 1Q, '98, 10; 4Q, '97, 19

✓5th **V45.7 Acquired absence of organ**
AHA: 4Q, '98, 65; 4Q, '97, 50

V45.71 Acquired absence of breast
AHA: 4Q, '01, 66; 4Q, '97, 50

V45.72 Acquired absence of intestine (large) (small)

V45.73 Acquired absence of kidney

V45.74 Other parts of urinary tract
Bladder
AHA: 4Q, '00, 51

V45.75 Stomach
AHA: 4Q, '00, 51

V45.76 Lung
AHA: 4Q, '00, 51

V45.77 Genital organs
EXCLUDES *female genital mutilation status (629.20-629.23)*
AHA: 1Q, '03, 13, 14; 4Q, '00, 51

V45.78 Eye
AHA: 4Q, '00, 51

V45.79 Other acquired absence of organ
AHA: 4Q, '00, 51

✓5th **V45.8 Other postprocedural status**

V45.81 Aortocoronary bypass status SDx
AHA: 4Q, '03, 105; 3Q, '01, 15; 3Q, '97, 16

V45.82 Percutaneous transluminal coronary angioplasty status SDx

V45.83 Breast implant removal status SDx
AHA: 4Q, '95, 55

V45.84 Dental restoration status SDx
Dental crowns status
Dental fillings status
AHA: 4Q, '01, 54

V45.85 Insulin pump status SDx

V45.89 Other SDx
Presence of neuropacemaker or other electronic device
EXCLUDES *artificial heart valve in situ (V43.3)*
vascular prosthesis in situ (V43.4)
AHA: 1Q, '95, 11

✓4th **V46 Other dependence on machines**

V46.0 Aspirator SDx

▲ ✓5th **V46.1 Respirator [Ventilator]**
Iron lung
AHA: 4Q, '03, 103; 1Q, '01, 12; J-F, '87, 7 3

V46.11 Dependence on respirator, status SDx
AHA: 4Q, '04, 100

V46.12 Encounter for respirator dependence during power failure PDx
AHA: 4Q, '04, 100

● **V46.13 Encounter for weaning from respirator [ventilator]**

● **V46.14 Mechanical complication of respirator [ventilator]**
Mechanical failure of respirator [ventilator]

V46.2 Supplemental oxygen SDx
Long-term oxygen therapy
AHA: 4Q, '03, 108; 4Q, '02, 79

V46.8 Other enabling machines SDx
Hyperbaric chamber
Possum [Patient-Operated-Selector-Mechanism]
EXCLUDES *cardiac pacemaker (V45.0)*
kidney dialysis machine (V45.1)

V46.9 Unspecified machine dependence SDx

✓4th **V47 Other problems with internal organs**

V47.0 Deficiencies of internal organs

V47.1 Mechanical and motor problems with internal organs

V47.2 Other cardiorespiratory problems
Cardiovascular exercise intolerance with pain (with):
at rest
less than ordinary activity
ordinary activity

V47.3 Other digestive problems

V47.4 Other urinary problems

V47.5 Other genital problems

V47.9 Unspecified

✓4th **V48 Problems with head, neck, and trunk**

V48.0 Deficiencies of head
EXCLUDES *deficiencies of ears, eyelids, and nose (V48.8)*

V48.1 Deficiencies of neck and trunk

V48.2 Mechanical and motor problems with head

V48.3 Mechanical and motor problems with neck and trunk

V48.4 Sensory problem with head

V48.5 Sensory problem with neck and trunk

V48.6 Disfigurements of head

V48.7 Disfigurements of neck and trunk

V48.8 Other problems with head, neck, and trunk

V48.9 Unspecified problem with head, neck, or trunk

✓4th **V49 Other conditions influencing health status**

V49.0 Deficiencies of limbs

V49.1 Mechanical problems with limbs

V49.2 Motor problems with limbs

V49.3 Sensory problems with limbs

V49.4 Disfigurements of limbs

V49.5 Other problems of limbs

✓5th **V49.6 Upper limb amputation status**
AHA: 4Q, '98, 42; 4Q, '94, 39

V49.60 Unspecified level SDx

V49.61 Thumb SDx

V49.62 Other finger(s) SDx

V49.63 Hand SDx

V49.64 Wrist SDx
Disarticulation of wrist

V49.65 Below elbow SDx

V49.66 Above elbow SDx
Disarticulation of elbow

V49.67 Shoulder SDx
Disarticulation of shoulder

✓5th **V49.7 Lower limb amputation status**
AHA: 4Q, '98, 42; 4Q, '94, 39

V49.70 Unspecified level SDx

V49.71 Great toe SDx

V49.72 Other toe(s) SDx

V49.73 Foot SDx

V49.74 **Ankle** SDx
Disarticulation of ankle

V49.75 **Below knee** SDx

V49.76 **Above knee** SDx
Disarticulation of knee

V49.77 **Hip** SDx
Disarticulation of hip

✓5th **V49.8 Other specified conditions influencing health status**
AHA: 4Q, '00, 51

V49.81 **Asymptomatic postmenopausal status (age-related) (natural)** A ♀
EXCLUDES *menopausal and premenopausal disorders (627.0-627.9)*
postsurgical menopause (256.2)
premature menopause (256.31)
symptomatic menopause (627.0-627.9)
AHA: 4Q, '02, 79; 4Q, '00, 54

V49.82 **Dental sealant status** SDx
AHA: 4Q, '01, 54

V49.83 **Awaiting organ transplant status** SDx

● V49.84 **Bed confinement status**

V49.89 **Other specified conditions influencing health status**

V49.9 Unspecified

PERSONS ENCOUNTERING HEALTH SERVICES FOR SPECIFIC PROCEDURES AND AFTERCARE (V50-V59)

Note: Categories V51-V58 are intended for use to indicate a reason for care in patients who may have already been treated for some disease or injury not now present, or who are receiving care to consolidate the treatment, to deal with residual states, or to prevent recurrence.

EXCLUDES *follow-up examination for medical surveillance following treatment (V67.0-V67.9)*

✓4th **V50 Elective surgery for purposes other than remedying health states**

V50.0 Hair transplant

V50.1 Other plastic surgery for unacceptable cosmetic appearance
Breast augmentation or reduction
Face-lift
EXCLUDES *plastic surgery following healed injury or operation (V51)*

V50.2 Routine or ritual circumcision ♂
Circumcision in the absence of significant medical indication

V50.3 Ear piercing

✓5th **V50.4 Prophylactic organ removal**
EXCLUDES *organ donations (V59.0-V59.9)*
therapeutic organ removal — code to condition
AHA: 4Q, '94, 44

V50.41 **Breast**
AHA: 4Q, '04, 107

V50.42 **Ovary** ♀

V50.49 **Other**

V50.8 Other

V50.9 Unspecified

V51 Aftercare involving the use of plastic surgery SDx
Plastic surgery following healed injury or operation
EXCLUDES *cosmetic plastic surgery (V50.1)*
plastic surgery as treatment for current injury — code to condition
repair of scarred tissue — code to scar

✓4th **V52 Fitting and adjustment of prosthetic device and implant**
INCLUDES removal of device
EXCLUDES *malfunction or complication of prosthetic device (996.0-996.7)*
status only, without need for care (V43.0-V43.8)
AHA: 4Q, '95, 55 ; 1Q, '90, 7

V52.0 Artificial arm (complete) (partial)

V52.1 Artificial leg (complete) (partial)

V52.2 Artificial eye

V52.3 Dental prosthetic device

V52.4 Breast prosthesis and implant ♀
EXCLUDES *admission for implant insertion (V50.1)*
AHA: 4Q, '95, 80, 81

V52.8 Other specified prosthetic device
AHA: 2Q, '02, 12, 16

V52.9 Unspecified prosthetic device

✓4th **V53 Fitting and adjustment of other device**
INCLUDES removal of device
replacement of device
EXCLUDES *status only, without need for care (V45.0-V45.8)*

✓5th **V53.0 Devices related to nervous system and special senses**
AHA: 4Q, '98, 66; 4Q, '97, 51

V53.01 **Fitting and adjustment of cerebral ventricular (communicating) shunt**
AHA: 4Q, '97, 51

V53.02 **Neuropacemaker (brain) (peripheral nerve) (spinal cord)**

V53.09 **Fitting and adjustment of other devices related to nervous system and special senses**
Auditory substitution device
Visual substitution device
AHA: 2Q '99, 4

V53.1 Spectacles and contact lenses

V53.2 Hearing aid

✓5th **V53.3 Cardiac device**
Reprogramming
AHA: 3Q, '92, 3; 1Q, '90, 7; M-J, '87, 8 ; N-D, '84, 18

V53.31 **Cardiac pacemaker**
EXCLUDES *mechanical complication of cardiac pacemaker (996.01)*
AHA: 1Q, '02, 3

V53.32 **Automatic implantable cardiac defibrillator**

V53.39 **Other cardiac device**

V53.4 Orthodontic devices

V53.5 Other intestinal appliance
EXCLUDES *colostomy (V55.3)*
ileostomy (V55.2)
other artificial opening of digestive tract (V55.4)

V53.6 Urinary devices
Urinary catheter
EXCLUDES *cystostomy (V55.5)*
nephrostomy (V55.6)
ureterostomy (V55.6)
urethrostomy (V55.6)

V53.7 Orthopedic devices
Orthopedic:
brace
cast
Orthopedic:
corset
shoes
EXCLUDES *other orthopedic aftercare (V54)*

V53.8 Wheelchair

✓5th **V53.9 Other and unspecified device**
AHA: 2Q, '03, 6

V53.90 **Unspecified device**

V53.91 **Fitting and adjustment of insulin pump**
Insulin pump titration

V53.99 **Other device**

✓4th **V54 Other orthopedic aftercare**

EXCLUDES *fitting and adjustment of orthopedic devices (V53.7)*
malfunction of internal orthopedic device ►(996.40-996.49)◄
other complication of nonmechanical nature (996.60-996.79)

AHA: 3Q, '95, 3

✓5th **V54.0 Aftercare involving internal fixation device**

EXCLUDES *malfunction of internal orthopedic device ►(996.40-996.49)◄*
other complication of nonmechanical nature (996.60-996.79)
removal of external fixation device (V54.89)

AHA: 4Q, '03, 87

V54.01 Encounter for removal of internal fixation device

V54.02 Encounter for lengthening/adjustment of growth rod

V54.09 Other aftercare involving internal fixation device

✓5th **V54.1 Aftercare for healing traumatic fracture**

AHA: 4Q, '02, 80

V54.10 Aftercare for healing traumatic fracture of arm, unspecified

V54.11 Aftercare for healing traumatic fracture of upper arm

V54.12 Aftercare for healing traumatic fracture of lower arm

V54.13 Aftercare for healing traumatic fracture of hip

AHA: 4Q, '03, 103, 105; 2Q, '03, 16

V54.14 Aftercare for healing traumatic fracture of leg, unspecified

V54.15 Aftercare for healing traumatic fracture of upper leg

EXCLUDES *aftercare for healing traumatic fracture of hip (V54.13)*

V54.16 Aftercare for healing traumatic fracture of lower leg

V54.17 Aftercare for healing traumatic fracture of vertebrae

V54.19 Aftercare for healing traumatic fracture of other bone

AHA: ►1Q, '05, 13◄ 4Q, '02, 80

✓5th **V54.2 Aftercare for healing pathologic fracture**

AHA: 4Q, '02, 80

V54.20 Aftercare for healing pathologic fracture of arm, unspecified

V54.21 Aftercare for healing pathologic fracture of upper arm

V54.22 Aftercare for healing pathologic fracture of lower arm

V54.23 Aftercare for healing pathologic fracture of hip

V54.24 Aftercare for healing pathologic fracture of leg, unspecified

V54.25 Aftercare for healing pathologic fracture of upper leg

EXCLUDES *aftercare for healing pathologic fracture of hip (V54.23)*

V54.26 Aftercare for healing pathologic fracture of lower leg

V54.27 Aftercare for healing pathologic fracture of vertebrae

AHA: 4Q, '03, 108

V54.29 Aftercare for healing pathologic fracture of other bone

AHA: 4Q, '02, 80

✓5th **V54.8 Other orthopedic aftercare**

AHA: 3Q, '01, 19; 4Q, '99, 5

V54.81 Aftercare following joint replacement

Use additional code to identify joint replacement site (V43.60-V43.69)

AHA: 2Q, '04, 15; 4Q, '02, 80

V54.89 Other orthopedic aftercare

Aftercare for healing fracture NOS

V54.9 Unspecified orthopedic aftercare

✓4th **V55 Attention to artificial openings**

INCLUDES adjustment or repositioning of catheter
closure
passage of sounds or bougies
reforming
removal or replacement of catheter
toilet or cleansing

EXCLUDES *complications of external stoma (519.00-519.09, 569.60-569.69, 997.4, 997.5)*
status only, without need for care (V44.0-V44.9)

V55.0 Tracheostomy

V55.1 Gastrostomy

AHA: 4Q, '99, 9; 3Q, '97, 7, 8; 1Q, '96, 14; 3Q, '95, 13

V55.2 Ileostomy

V55.3 Colostomy

AHA: 3Q, '97, 9

V55.4 Other artificial opening of digestive tract

AHA: 1Q, '03, 10

V55.5 Cystostomy

V55.6 Other artificial opening of urinary tract

Nephrostomy
Urethrostomy
Ureterostomy

V55.7 Artificial vagina

V55.8 Other specified artificial opening

V55.9 Unspecified artificial opening

✓4th **V56 Encounter for dialysis and dialysis catheter care**

Use additional code to identify the associated condition

EXCLUDES *dialysis preparation — code to condition*

AHA: 4Q, '98, 66; 1Q, '93, 29

V56.0 Extracorporeal dialysis PDx

Dialysis (renal) NOS

EXCLUDES *dialysis status (V45.1)*

AHA: 1Q, '04, 23; 4Q, '00, 40; 3Q, '98, 6; 2Q, '98, 20

V56.1 Fitting and adjustment of extracorporeal dialysis catheter

Removal or replacement of catheter
Toilet or cleansing
Use additional code for any concurrent extracorporeal dialysis (V56.0)

AHA: 2Q, '98, 20

V56.2 Fitting and adjustment of peritoneal dialysis catheter

Use additional code for any concurrent peritoneal dialysis (V56.8)

AHA: 4Q, '98, 55

✓5th **V56.3 Encounter for adequacy testing for dialysis**

AHA: 4Q, '00, 55

V56.31 Encounter for adequacy testing for hemodialysis

V56.32 Encounter for adequacy testing for peritoneal dialysis

Peritoneal equilibration test

V56.8 Other dialysis

Peritoneal dialysis

AHA: 4Q, '98, 55

✓4th V57 Care involving use of rehabilitation procedures
Use additional code to identify underlying condition
AHA: 1Q, '02, 19; 3Q, '97, 12; 1Q, '90, 6; S-O, '86, 3

V57.0 Breathing exercises

V57.1 Other physical therapy
Therapeutic and remedial exercises, except breathing
AHA: 2Q, '04, 15; 4Q, '02, 56; 4Q, '99, 5

✓5th V57.2 Occupational therapy and vocational rehabilitation

V57.21 Encounter for occupational therapy
AHA: 4Q, '99, 7

V57.22 Encounter for vocational therapy

V57.3 Speech therapy
AHA: 4Q, '97, 36

V57.4 Orthoptic training

✓5th V57.8 Other specified rehabilitation procedure

V57.81 Orthotic training
Gait training in the use of artificial limbs

V57.89 Other
Multiple training or therapy
AHA: 4Q, '03, 105-106, 108; 2Q, '03, 16; 1Q, '02, 16; 3Q, '01, 21; 3Q, '97, 11, 12; S-O, '86, 4

V57.9 Unspecified rehabilitation procedure

✓4th V58 Encounter for other and unspecified procedures and aftercare
EXCLUDES *convalescence and palliative care (V66)*

V58.0 Radiotherapy PDx
Encounter or admission for radiotherapy
EXCLUDES *encounter for radioactive implant — code to condition*
radioactive iodine therapy — code to condition
AHA: 3Q, '92, 5; 2Q, '90, 7; J-F, '87, 13

▲ **✓5th V58.1 Encounter for antineoplastic chemotherapy and immunotherapy**
Encounter or admission for chemotherapy
EXCLUDES ▶ *chemotherapy and immunotherapy for nonneoplastic conditions — code to condition*◀
prophylactic chemotherapy against disease which has never been present (V03.0-V07.9)
AHA: 1Q, '04, 13; 2Q, '03, 16; 3Q, '93, 4; 2Q, '92, 6; 2Q, '91, 17; 2Q, '90, 7; S-O, '84, 5

● **V58.11 Encounter for antineoplastic chemotherapy** PDx

● **V58.12 Encounter for antineoplastic immunotherapy** PDx

V58.2 Blood transfusion, without reported diagnosis

V58.3 Attention to surgical dressings and sutures
Change of dressings
Removal of sutures

✓5th V58.4 Other aftercare following surgery
EXCLUDES *aftercare following sterilization reversal surgery (V26.22)*
attention to artificial openings (V55.0-V55.9)
orthopedic aftercare (V54.0-V54.9)
Note: Codes from this subcategory should be used in conjunction with other aftercare codes to fully identify the reason for the aftercare encounter
AHA: 4Q, '99, 9; N-D, '87, 9

V58.41 Encounter for planned postoperative wound closure
EXCLUDES *disruption of operative wound (998.3)*
AHA: 4Q, '99, 15

V58.42 Aftercare following surgery for neoplasm
Conditions classifiable to 140-239
AHA: 4Q, '02, 80

V58.43 Aftercare following surgery for injury and trauma
Conditions classifiable to 800-999
EXCLUDES *aftercare for healing traumatic fracture (V54.10-V54.19)*
AHA: 4Q, '02, 80

V58.44 Aftercare following organ transplant
Use additional code to identify the organ transplanted (V42.0-V42.9)
AHA: 4Q, '04, 101

V58.49 Other specified aftercare following surgery
AHA: 1Q, '96, 8, 9

V58.5 Orthodontics
EXCLUDES *fitting and adjustment of orthodontic device (V53.4)*

✓5th V58.6 Long-term (current) drug use
EXCLUDES *drug abuse (305.00-305.93)*
drug dependence (304.00-304.93)
hormone replacement therapy (postmenopausal) (V07.4)
AHA: 4Q, '03, 85; 4Q, '02, 84; 3Q, '02, 15; 4Q, '95, 61

V58.61 Long-term (current) use of anticoagulants
EXCLUDES *long-term (current) use of aspirin (V58.66)*
AHA: 3Q, '04, 7; 4Q, '03, 108; 3Q, '02, 13-16; 1Q, '02, 15, 16

V58.62 Long-term (current) use of antibiotics
AHA: 4Q, '98, 59

V58.63 Long-term (current) use of antiplatelets/antithrombotics
EXCLUDES *long-term (current) use of aspirin (V58.66)*

V58.64 Long-term (current) use of non-steroidal anti-inflammatories (NSAID)
EXCLUDES *long-term (current) use of aspirin (V58.66)*

V58.65 Long-term (current) use of steroids

V58.66 Long-term (current) use of aspirin
AHA: 4Q, '04, 102

V58.67 Long-term (current) use of insulin
AHA: 4Q, '04, 55-56, 103

V58.69 Long-term (current) use of other medications
High-risk medications
AHA: 2Q, '04, 10; 1Q, '03, 11; 2Q, '00, 8; 3Q, '99, 13; 2Q, '99, 17; 1Q, '97, 12; 2Q, '96, 7

✓5th V58.7 Aftercare following surgery to specified body systems, not elsewhere classified
Note: Codes from this subcategory should be used in conjunction with other aftercare codes to fully identify the reason for the aftercare encounter
EXCLUDES *aftercare following organ transplant (V58.44)*
aftercare following surgery for neoplasm (V58.42)
AHA: 4Q, '03, 104; 4Q, '02, 80

V58.71 Aftercare following surgery of the sense organs, NEC
Conditions classifiable to 360-379, 380-389

V58.72 Aftercare following surgery of the nervous system, NEC
Conditions classifiable to 320-359
EXCLUDES *aftercare following surgery of the sense organs, NEC (V58.71)*

V58.73 Aftercare following surgery of the circulatory system, NEC
Conditions classifiable to 390-459
AHA: 4Q, '03, 105

V58.74 Aftercare following surgery of the respiratory system, NEC
Conditions classifiable to 460-519

V58.75 Aftercare following surgery of the teeth, oral cavity and digestive system, NEC
Conditions classifiable to 520-579

V58.76 Aftercare following surgery of the genitourinary system, NEC
Conditions classifiable to 580-629
EXCLUDES *aftercare following sterilization reversal (V26.22)*
AHA: ▶1Q, '05, 11-12◀

V58.77 Aftercare following surgery of the skin and subcutaneous tissue, NEC
Conditions classifiable to 680-709

V58.78 Aftercare following surgery of the musculoskeletal system, NEC
Conditions classifiable to 710-739

5th **V58.8 Other specified procedures and aftercare**
AHA: 4Q, '94, 45; 2Q, '94, 8

V58.81 Fitting and adjustment of vascular catheter
Removal or replacement of catheter
Toilet or cleansing
EXCLUDES *complication of renal dialysis (996.73)*
complication of vascular catheter (996.74)
dialysis preparation — code to condition
encounter for dialysis (V56.0-V56.8)
fitting and adjustment of dialysis catheter (V56.1)

V58.82 Fitting and adjustment of nonvascular catheter, NEC
Removal or replacement of catheter
Toilet or cleansing
EXCLUDES *fitting and adjustment of peritoneal dialysis catheter (V56.2)*
fitting and adjustment of urinary catheter (V53.6)

V58.83 Encounter for therapeutic drug monitoring
Use additional code for any associated long-term (current) drug use (V58.61-V58.69)
EXCLUDES *blood-drug testing for medico-legal reasons (V70.4)*
AHA: 2Q, '04, 10; 1Q, '04, 13; 4Q, '03, 85; 4Q, '02, 84; 3Q, '02, 13-16
DEF: Drug monitoring: Measurement of the level of a specific drug in the body or measurement of a specific function to assess effectiveness of a drug.

V58.89 Other specified aftercare
AHA: 4Q, '98, 59

V58.9 Unspecified aftercare

4th **V59 Donors**
EXCLUDES *examination of potential donor (V70.8)*
self-donation of organ or tissue — code to condition
AHA: 4Q, '95, 62; 1Q, '90, 10; N-D, '84, 8

5th **V59.0 Blood**
V59.01 Whole blood PDx
V59.02 Stem cells PDx
V59.09 Other PDx

V59.1 Skin PDx
V59.2 Bone PDx
V59.3 Bone marrow PDx
V59.4 Kidney PDx
V59.5 Cornea PDx
V59.6 Liver PDx

● 5th **V59.7 Egg (oocyte) (ovum)**
V59.70 Egg (oocyte) (ovum) donor, unspecified PDx
● **V59.71 Egg (oocyte) (ovum) donor, under age 35, anonymous recipient** PDx
Egg donor, under age 35 NOS
● **V59.72 Egg (oocyte) (ovum) donor, under age 35, designated reci pient** PDx
● **V59.73 Egg (oocyte) (ovum) donor, age 35 and over, anonymous recipient** PDx
Egg donor, age 35 and over NOS
● **V59.74 Egg (oocyte) (ovum) donor, age 35 and over, designated recipient** PDx

V59.8 Other specified organ or tissue PDx
AHA: 3Q, '02, 20

V59.9 Unspecified organ or tissue PDx

PERSONS ENCOUNTERING HEALTH SERVICES IN OTHER CIRCUMSTANCES (V60-V69)

4th **V60 Housing, household, and economic circumstances**

V60.0 Lack of housing SDx
Hobos
Social migrants
Tramps
Transients
Vagabonds

V60.1 Inadequate housing SDx
Lack of heating
Restriction of space
Technical defects in home preventing adequate care

V60.2 Inadequate material resources SDx
Economic problem
Poverty NOS

V60.3 Person living alone SDx

V60.4 No other household member able to render care SDx
Person requiring care (has) (is):
family member too handicapped, ill, or otherwise unsuited to render care
partner temporarily away from home
temporarily away from usual place of abode
EXCLUDES *holiday relief care (V60.5)*

V60.5 Holiday relief care SDx
Provision of health care facilities to a person normally cared for at home, to enable relatives to take a vacation

V60.6 Person living in residential institution SDx
Boarding school resident

V60.8 Other specified housing or economic circumstances SDx

V60.9 Unspecified housing or economic circumstances SDx

4th **V61 Other family circumstances**
INCLUDES when these circumstances or fear of them, affecting the person directly involved or others, are mentioned as the reason, justified or not, for seeking or receiving medical advice or care
AHA: 1Q, '90, 9

V61.0 Family disruption
Divorce
Estrangement

5th **V61.1 Counseling for marital and partner problems**
EXCLUDES *problems related to:*
psychosexual disorders (302.0-302.9)
sexual function (V41.7)

V61.10 Counseling for marital and partner problems, unspecified
Marital conflict
▶Marital relationship problem◀
Partner conflict
▶Partner relationship problem◀

V61.11 Counseling for victim of spousal and partner abuse
EXCLUDES *encounter for treatment of current injuries due to abuse (995.80-995.85)*

V61.12 Counseling for perpetrator of spousal and partner abuse

4th 5th Additional Digit Required · Unspecified Code · Other Specified Code · Manifestation Code · ▶◀ Revised Text · ● New Code · ▲ Revised Code Title

✓5th **V61.2 Parent-child problems**

V61.20 Counseling for parent-child problem, unspecified
Concern about behavior of child
Parent-child conflict
▶Parent-child relationship problem◀

V61.21 Counseling for victim of child abuse
Child battering
Child neglect
EXCLUDES *current injuries due to abuse (995.50-995.59)*

V61.22 Counseling for perpetrator of parental child abuse
EXCLUDES *counseling for non-parental abuser (V62.83)*

V61.29 Other
Problem concerning adopted or foster child
AHA: 3Q, '99, 16

V61.3 Problems with aged parents or in-laws

✓5th **V61.4 Health problems within family**

V61.41 Alcoholism in family

V61.49 Other
Care of / Presence of } sick or handicapped person in family or household

V61.5 Multiparity

V61.6 Illegitimacy or illegitimate pregnancy M♀

V61.7 Other unwanted pregnancy M♀

V61.8 Other specified family circumstances
Problems with family members NEC
▶Sibling relationship problem◀

V61.9 Unspecified family circumstance

✓4th **V62 Other psychosocial circumstances**
INCLUDES those circumstances or fear of them, affecting the person directly involved or others, mentioned as the reason, justified or not, for seeking or receiving medical advice or care
EXCLUDES *previous psychological trauma (V15.41-V15.49)*

▲ **V62.0 Unemployment** SDx
EXCLUDES *circumstances when main problem is economic inadequacy or poverty (V60.2)*

V62.1 Adverse effects of work environment SDx

V62.2 Other occupational circumstances or maladjustment SDx
Career choice problem
Dissatisfaction with employment
▶Occupational problem◀

V62.3 Educational circumstances SDx
▶Academic problem◀
Dissatisfaction with school environment
Educational handicap

V62.4 Social maladjustment SDx
▶Acculturation problem◀
Cultural deprivation
Political, religious, or sex discrimination
Social:
- isolation
- persecution

V62.5 Legal circumstances SDx
Imprisonment
Legal investigation
Litigation
Prosecution

V62.6 Refusal of treatment for reasons of religion or conscience SDx

✓5th **V62.8 Other psychological or physical stress, not elsewhere classified**

V62.81 Interpersonal problems, not elsewhere classified SDx
▶Relational problem NOS◀

V62.82 Bereavement, uncomplicated SDx
EXCLUDES *bereavement as adjustment reaction (309.0)*

V62.83 Counseling for perpetrator of physical/sexual abuse SDx
EXCLUDES *counseling for perpetrator of parental child abuse (V61.22)*
counseling for perpetrator of spousal and partner abuse (V61.12)

● **V62.84 Suicidal ideation** SDx
EXCLUDES *suicidal tendencies (300.9)*

V62.89 Other SDx
▶Borderline intellectual functioning◀
Life circumstance problems
Phase of life problems
▶Religious or spiritual problem◀

V62.9 Unspecified psychosocial circumstance SDx

✓4th **V63 Unavailability of other medical facilities for care**
AHA: 1Q, '91, 21

V63.0 Residence remote from hospital or other health care facility

V63.1 Medical services in home not available
EXCLUDES *no other household member able to render care (V60.4)*
AHA: 4Q, '01, 67; 1Q, '01, 12

V63.2 Person awaiting admission to adequate facility elsewhere

V63.8 Other specified reasons for unavailability of medical facilities
Person on waiting list undergoing social agency investigation

V63.9 Unspecified reason for unavailability of medical facilities

✓4th **V64 Persons encountering health services for specific procedures, not carried out**

✓5th **V64.0 Vaccination not carried out**

● **V64.00 Vaccination not carried out, unspecified reason** SDx

● **V64.01 Vaccination not carried out because of acute illness** SDx

● **V64.02 Vaccination not carried out because of chronic illness or condition** SDx

● **V64.03 Vaccination not carried out because of immune compromised state** SDx

● **V64.04 Vaccination not carried out because of allergy to vaccine or component** SDx

● **V64.05 Vaccination not carried out because of caregiver refusal** SDx

● **V64.06 Vaccination not carried out because of patient refusal** SDx

● **V64.07 Vaccination not carried out for religious reasons** SDx

● **V64.08 Vaccination not carried out because patient had disease being vaccinated against** SDx

● **V64.09 Vaccination not carried out for other reason** SDx

V64.1 Surgical or other procedure not carried out because of contraindication SDx

V64.2 Surgical or other procedure not carried out because of patient's decision SDx
AHA: 2Q, '01, 8

V64.3 Procedure not carried out for other reasons SDx

✓5th **V64.4 Closed surgical procedure converted to open procedure**
AHA: 4Q, '03, 87; 4Q, '98, 68; 4Q, '97, 52

V64.41 Laparoscopic surgical procedure converted to open procedure SDx

N Newborn Age: 0 | P Pediatric Age: 0-17 | M Maternity Age: 12-55 | A Adult Age: 15-124 | MSP Medicare Secondary Payer
SDx Secondary Diagnosis | PDx Primary Diagnosis

V64.42 **Thoracoscopic surgical procedure converted to open procedure** SDx

V64.43 **Arthroscopic surgical procedure converted to open procedure** SDx

V65 Other persons seeking consultation (4th)

V65.0 **Healthy person accompanying sick person**
Boarder

V65.1 **Person consulting on behalf of another person** (5th)
Advice or treatment for nonattending third party
EXCLUDES *concern (normal) about sick person in family (V61.41-V61.49)*
AHA: 4Q, '03, 84

V65.11 **Pediatric pre-birth visit for expectant mother** M ♀

V65.19 **Other person consulting on behalf of another person**

V65.2 **Person feigning illness**
Malingerer
Peregrinating patient
AHA: 3Q, '99, 20

V65.3 **Dietary surveillance and counseling**
Dietary surveillance and counseling (in):
NOS
colitis
diabetes mellitus
food allergies or intolerance
gastritis
hypercholesterolemia
hypoglycemia
obesity

V65.4 **Other counseling, not elsewhere classified** (5th)
Health:
advice
education
instruction
EXCLUDES *counseling (for):*
contraception (V25.40-V25.49)
genetic ▶(V26.31-V26.33)◀
on behalf of third party (V65.11-V65.19)
procreative management (V26.4)

V65.40 **Counseling NOS**

V65.41 **Exercise counseling**

V65.42 **Counseling on substance use and abuse**

V65.43 **Counseling on injury prevention**

V65.44 **Human immunodeficiency virus [HIV] counseling**

V65.45 **Counseling on other sexually transmitted diseases**

V65.46 **Encounter for insulin pump training**

V65.49 **Other specified counseling**
AHA: 2Q, '00, 8

V65.5 **Person with feared complaint in whom no diagnosis was made**
Feared condition not demonstrated
Problem was normal state
"Worried well"

V65.8 **Other reasons for seeking consultation**
EXCLUDES *specified symptoms*
AHA: 3Q, '92, 4

V65.9 **Unspecified reason for consultation**

V66 Convalescence and palliative care (4th)

V66.0 **Following surgery** PDx

V66.1 **Following radiotherapy** PDx

V66.2 **Following chemotherapy** PDx

V66.3 **Following psychotherapy and other treatment for mental disorder** PDx

V66.4 **Following treatment of fracture** PDx

V66.5 **Following other treatment** PDx

V66.6 **Following combined treatment** PDx

V66.7 **Encounter for palliative care** SDx
End-of-life care
Hospice care
Terminal care
Code first underlying disease
AHA: 4Q, '03, 107; 1Q, '98, 11; 4Q, '96, 47, 48

V66.9 **Unspecified convalescence** PDx
AHA: 4Q, '99, 8

V67 Follow-up examination (4th)
INCLUDES surveillance only following completed treatment
EXCLUDES *surveillance of contraception (V25.40-V25.49)*
AHA: 2Q, '03, 5; 4Q, '94, 48

V67.0 **Following surgery** (5th)
AHA: 4Q, '00, 56; 4Q, '98, 69; 4Q, '97, 50; 2Q, '95, 8;1Q, '95, 4; 3Q, '92, 11

V67.00 **Following surgery, unspecified**

V67.01 **Follow-up vaginal pap smear** ♀
Vaginal pap-smear, status-post hysterectomy for malignant condition
Use additional code to identify:
acquired absence of uterus (V45.77)
personal history of malignant neoplasm (V10.40-V10.44)
EXCLUDES *vaginal pap smear status-post hysterectomy for non-malignant condition (V76.47)*

V67.09 **Following other surgery**
EXCLUDES *sperm count following sterilization reversal (V26.22)*
sperm count for fertility testing (V26.21)
AHA: 3Q, '03, 16; 3Q, '02, 15

V67.1 **Following radiotherapy**

V67.2 **Following chemotherapy**
Cancer chemotherapy follow-up

V67.3 **Following psychotherapy and other treatment for mental disorder**

V67.4 **Following treatment of healed fracture**
EXCLUDES *current (healing) fracture aftercare (V54.0-V54.9)*
AHA: 1Q, '90, 7

V67.5 **Following other treatment** (5th)

V67.51 **Following completed treatment with high-risk medications, not elsewhere classified**
EXCLUDES *long-term (current) drug use (V58.61-V58.69)*
AHA: 1Q, '99, 5, 6; 4Q, '95, 61 ; 1Q, '90, 18

V67.59 **Other**

V67.6 **Following combined treatment**

V67.9 **Unspecified follow-up examination**

V68 Encounters for administrative purposes (4th)

V68.0 **Issue of medical certificates** PDx
Issue of medical certificate of:
cause of death
fitness
incapacity
EXCLUDES *encounter for general medical examination (V70.0-V70.9)*

V68.1 **Issue of repeat prescriptions** PDx
Issue of repeat prescription for:
appliance
glasses
medications
EXCLUDES *repeat prescription for contraceptives (V25.41-V25.49)*

V68.2 **Request for expert evidence** PDx

✓5th V68.8 **Other specified administrative purpose**

V68.81 **Referral of patient without examination or treatment** PDx

V68.89 **Other** PDx

V68.9 **Unspecified administrative purpose** PDx

✓4th **V69 Problems related to lifestyle**

AHA: 4Q, '94, 48

V69.0 **Lack of physical exercise**

V69.1 **Inappropriate diet and eating habits**

EXCLUDES *anorexia nervosa (307.1)*
bulimia (783.6)
malnutrition and other nutritional deficiencies (260-269.9)
other and unspecified eating disorders (307.50-307.59)

V69.2 **High-risk sexual behavior**

V69.3 **Gambling and betting**

EXCLUDES *pathological gambling (312.31)*

V69.4 **Lack of adequate sleep**

Sleep deprivation

EXCLUDES *insomnia (780.52)*

● V69.5 **Behavioral insomnia of childhood**

V69.8 **Other problems related to lifestyle**

Self-damaging behavior

V69.9 **Problem related to lifestyle, unspecified**

PERSONS WITHOUT REPORTED DIAGNOSIS ENCOUNTERED DURING EXAMINATION AND INVESTIGATION OF INDIVIDUALS AND POPULATIONS ▶(V70-V85)◀

Note: Nonspecific abnormal findings disclosed at the time of these examinations are classifiable to categories 790-796.

✓4th **V70 General medical examination**

Use additional code(s) to identify any special screening examination(s) performed (V73.0-V82.9)

V70.0 **Routine general medical examination at a health care facility** PDx

Health checkup

EXCLUDES *health checkup of infant or child (V20.2)*
▶*pre-procedural general physical examination (V72.83)*◀

V70.1 **General psychiatric examination, requested by the authority** PDx

V70.2 **General psychiatric examination, other and unspecified** PDx

V70.3 **Other medical examination for administrative purposes** PDx

General medical examination for:
admission to old age home
adoption
camp
driving license
immigration and naturalization
insurance certification
marriage
prison
school admission
sports competition

EXCLUDES *attendance for issue of medical certificates (V68.0)*
pre-employment screening (V70.5)

AHA: 1Q, '90, 6

V70.4 **Examination for medicolegal reasons** PDx

Blood-alcohol tests
Blood-drug tests
Paternity testing

EXCLUDES *examination and observation following:*
accidents (V71.3, V71.4)
assault (V71.6)
rape (V71.5)

V70.5 **Health examination of defined subpopulations** PDx

Armed forces personnel
Inhabitants of institutions
Occupational health examinations
Pre-employment screening
Preschool children
Prisoners
Prostitutes
Refugees
School children
Students

V70.6 **Health examination in population surveys** PDx

EXCLUDES *special screening (V73.0-V82.9)*

V70.7 **Examination of participant in clinical trial**

Examination of participant or control in clinical research

AHA: 4Q, '01, 55

V70.8 **Other specified general medical examinations** PDx

Examination of potential donor of organ or tissue

V70.9 **Unspecified general medical examination** PDx

✓4th **V71 Observation and evaluation for suspected conditions not found**

INCLUDES This category is to be used when persons without a diagnosis are suspected of having an abnormal condition, without signs or symptoms, which requires study, but after examination and observation, is found not to exist. This category is also for use for administrative and legal observation status.

AHA: 4Q, '94, 47; 2Q, '90, 5; M-A, '87, 1

✓5th V71.0 **Observation for suspected mental condition**

V71.01 **Adult antisocial behavior** A PDx

Dyssocial behavior or gang activity in adult without manifest psychiatric disorder

V71.02 **Childhood or adolescent antisocial behavior** PDx

Dyssocial behavior or gang activity in child or adolescent without manifest psychiatric disorder

V71.09 **Other suspected mental condition** PDx

V71.1 **Observation for suspected malignant neoplasm** PDx

V71.2 **Observation for suspected tuberculosis** PDx

V71.3 **Observation following accident at work** PDx

V71.4 **Observation following other accident** PDx

Examination of individual involved in motor vehicle traffic accident

V71.5 **Observation following alleged rape or seduction** PDx

Examination of victim or culprit

V71.6 **Observation following other inflicted injury** PDx

Examination of victim or culprit

V71.7 **Observation for suspected cardiovascular disease** PDx

AHA: 1Q, '04, 6; 3Q, '90, 10; S-O, '87, 10

✓5th V71.8 **Observation and evaluation for other specified suspected conditions**

AHA: 4Q, '00, 54 ; 1Q, '90, 19

V71.81 **Abuse and neglect** PDx

EXCLUDES *adult abuse and neglect (995.80-995.85)*
child abuse and neglect (995.50-995.59)

AHA: 4Q, '00, 55

V71.82 **Observation and evaluation for suspected exposure to anthrax** PDx

AHA: 4Q, '02, 70, 85

V71.83 **Observation and evaluation for suspected exposure to other biological agent** PDx

AHA: 4Q, '03, 47

V71.89 **Other specified suspected conditions** PDx

AHA: 2Q, '03, 15

V71.9 Observation for unspecified suspected condition PDx
AHA: 1Q, '02, 6

✓4th **V72 Special investigations and examinations**
INCLUDES routine examination of specific system
EXCLUDES *general medical examination (V70.0-V70.4)*
general screening examination of defined population groups (V70.5, V70.6, V70.7)
routine examination of infant or child (V20.2)
Use additional code(s) to identify any special screening examination(s) performed (V73.0-V82.9)

V72.0 Examination of eyes and vision PDx
AHA: 1Q, '04, 15

V72.1 Examination of ears and hearing PDx
AHA: 1Q, '04, 15

V72.2 Dental examination PDx

✓5th **V72.3 Gynecological examination**
EXCLUDES *cervical Papanicolaou smear without general gynecological examination (V76.2)*
routine examination in contraceptive management (V25.40-V25.49)

V72.31 Routine gynecological examination PDx ♀
General gynecological examination with or without Papanicolaou cervical smear
Pelvic examination (annual) (periodic)
Use additional code to identify routine vaginal Papanicolaou smear (V76.47)

V72.32 Encounter for Papanicolaou cervical smear to confirm findings of recent normal smear following initial abnormal smear PDx ♀

✓5th **V72.4 Pregnancy examination or test**

V72.40 Pregnancy examination or test, pregnancy unconfirmed PDx ♀
Possible pregnancy, not (yet) confirmed

V72.41 Pregnancy examination or test, negative result PDx ♀

● **V72.42 Pregnancy examination or test, positive result** PDx ♀

V72.5 Radiological examination, not elsewhere classified
Routine chest x-ray
EXCLUDES *examination for suspected tuberculosis (V71.2)*
AHA: 1Q, '90, 19

V72.6 Laboratory examination
EXCLUDES *that for suspected disorder (V71.0-V71.9)*
AHA: 1Q, '90, 22

V72.7 Diagnostic skin and sensitization tests PDx
Allergy tests
Skin tests for hypersensitivity
EXCLUDES *diagnostic skin tests for bacterial diseases (V74.0-V74.9)*

✓5th **V72.8 Other specified examinations**

V72.81 Pre-operative cardiovascular examination PDx
▶Pre-procedural cardiovascular examination◀

V72.82 Pre-operative respiratory examination PDx
▶Pre-procedural respiratory examination◀
AHA: 3Q, '96, 14

V72.83 Other specified pre-operative examination PDx
▶Other pre-procedural examination
Pre-procedural general physical examination◀
EXCLUDES ▶ *routine general medical examination (V70.0)*◀
AHA: 3Q, '96, 14

V72.84 Pre-operative examination, unspecified PDx
▶Pre-procedural examination, unspecified◀

V72.85 Other specified examination PDx
AHA: 1Q, '04, 12

● **V72.86 Encounter for blood typing** PDx

V72.9 Unspecified examination PDx

✓4th **V73 Special screening examination for viral and chlamydial diseases**
AHA: 1Q, '04, 11

V73.0 Poliomyelitis
V73.1 Smallpox
V73.2 Measles
V73.3 Rubella
V73.4 Yellow fever
V73.5 Other arthropod-borne viral diseases
Dengue fever
Hemorrhagic fever
Viral encephalitis:
mosquito-borne
tick-borne

V73.6 Trachoma

✓5th **V73.8 Other specified viral and chlamydial diseases**
V73.88 Other specified chlamydial diseases
V73.89 Other specified viral diseases

✓5th **V73.9 Unspecified viral and chlamydial disease**
V73.98 Unspecified chlamydial disease
V73.99 Unspecified viral disease

✓4th **V74 Special screening examination for bacterial and spirochetal diseases**
INCLUDES diagnostic skin tests for these diseases
AHA: 1Q, '04, 11

V74.0 Cholera
V74.1 Pulmonary tuberculosis
V74.2 Leprosy [Hansen's disease]
V74.3 Diphtheria
V74.4 Bacterial conjunctivitis
V74.5 Venereal disease
V74.6 Yaws
V74.8 Other specified bacterial and spirochetal diseases
Brucellosis
Leptospirosis
Plague
Tetanus
Whooping cough

V74.9 Unspecified bacterial and spirochetal disease

✓4th **V75 Special screening examination for other infectious diseases**
AHA: 1Q, '04, 11

V75.0 Rickettsial diseases
V75.1 Malaria
V75.2 Leishmaniasis
V75.3 Trypanosomiasis
Chagas' disease
Sleeping sickness
V75.4 Mycotic infections
V75.5 Schistosomiasis
V75.6 Filariasis
V75.7 Intestinal helminthiasis
V75.8 Other specified parasitic infections
V75.9 Unspecified infectious disease

✓4th **V76 Special screening for malignant neoplasms**
AHA: 1Q, '04, 11

V76.0 Respiratory organs

✓5th **V76.1 Breast**
AHA: 4Q, '98, 67

V76.10 Breast screening, unspecified

V76.11 Screening mammogram for high-risk patient ♀
AHA: 2Q, '03, 4

V76.12 Other screening mammogram
AHA: 2Q, '03, 3-4

V76.19 Other screening breast examination

V76.2 Cervix ♀
Routine cervical Papanicolaou smear
EXCLUDES *that as part of a general gynecological examination (V72.31)*

V76.3 Bladder

✓5th **V76.4 Other sites**

V76.41 Rectum
V76.42 Oral cavity
V76.43 Skin
V76.44 Prostate ♂
V76.45 Testis ♂
V76.46 Ovary ♀
AHA: 4Q, '00, 52

V76.47 Vagina ♀
Vaginal pap smear status-post hysterectomy for non-malignant condition
Use additional code to identify acquired absence of uterus (V45.77)
EXCLUDES *vaginal pap smear status-post hysterectomy for malignant condition (V67.01)*
AHA: 4Q, '00, 52

V76.49 Other sites
AHA: 1Q, '99, 4

✓5th **V76.5 Intestine**
AHA: 4Q, '00, 52

V76.50 Intestine, unspecified
V76.51 Colon
EXCLUDES *rectum (V76.41)*
AHA: 4Q, '01, 56

V76.52 Small intestine

✓5th **V76.8 Other neoplasm**
AHA: 4Q, '00, 52

V76.81 Nervous system
V76.89 Other neoplasm

V76.9 Unspecified

✓4th **V77 Special screening for endocrine, nutritional, metabolic, and immunity disorders**
AHA: 1Q, '04, 11

V77.0 Thyroid disorders
V77.1 Diabetes mellitus
V77.2 Malnutrition
V77.3 Phenylketonuria [PKU]
V77.4 Galactosemia
V77.5 Gout
V77.6 Cystic fibrosis
Screening for mucoviscidosis
V77.7 Other inborn errors of metabolism
V77.8 Obesity

✓5th **V77.9 Other and unspecified endocrine, nutritional, metabolic, and immunity disorders**
AHA: 4Q, '00, 53

V77.91 Screening for lipoid disorders
Screening cholesterol level
Screening for hypercholesterolemia
Screening for hyperlipidemia
V77.99 Other and unspecified endocrine, nutritional, metabolic, and immunity disorders

✓4th **V78 Special screening for disorders of blood and blood-forming organs**
AHA: 1Q, '04, 11

V78.0 Iron deficiency anemia
V78.1 Other and unspecified deficiency anemia
V78.2 Sickle cell disease or trait
V78.3 Other hemoglobinopathies
V78.8 Other disorders of blood and blood-forming organs
V78.9 Unspecified disorder of blood and blood-forming organs

✓4th **V79 Special screening for mental disorders and developmental handicaps**
AHA: 1Q, '04, 11

V79.0 Depression
V79.1 Alcoholism
V79.2 Mental retardation
V79.3 Developmental handicaps in early childhood
V79.8 Other specified mental disorders and developmental handicaps
V79.9 Unspecified mental disorder and developmental handicap

✓4th **V80 Special screening for neurological, eye, and ear diseases**
AHA: 1Q, '04, 11

V80.0 Neurological conditions
V80.1 Glaucoma
V80.2 Other eye conditions
Screening for:
cataract
congenital anomaly of eye
senile macular lesions
EXCLUDES *general vision examination (V72.0)*
V80.3 Ear diseases
EXCLUDES *general hearing examination (V72.1)*

✓4th **V81 Special screening for cardiovascular, respiratory, and genitourinary diseases**
AHA: 1Q, '04, 11

V81.0 Ischemic heart disease
V81.1 Hypertension
V81.2 Other and unspecified cardiovascular conditions
V81.3 Chronic bronchitis and emphysema
V81.4 Other and unspecified respiratory conditions
EXCLUDES *screening for:*
lung neoplasm (V76.0)
pulmonary tuberculosis (V74.1)
V81.5 Nephropathy
Screening for asymptomatic bacteriuria
V81.6 Other and unspecified genitourinary conditions

✓4th **V82 Special screening for other conditions**
AHA: 1Q, '04, 11

V82.0 Skin conditions
V82.1 Rheumatoid arthritis
V82.2 Other rheumatic disorders
V82.3 Congenital dislocation of hip
V82.4 Maternal postnatal screening for chromosomal anomalies ♀
EXCLUDES *antenatal screening by amniocentesis (V28.0)*
V82.5 Chemical poisoning and other contamination
Screening for:
heavy metal poisoning
ingestion of radioactive substance
poisoning from contaminated water supply
radiation exposure

V82.6 Multiphasic screening

✓5th **V82.8 Other specified conditions**

AHA: 4Q, '00, 53

V82.81 Osteoporosis

Use additional code to identify:
hormone replacement therapy (postmenopausal) status (V07.4)
postmenopausal (age-related) (natural) status (V49.81)

AHA: 4Q, '00, 54

V82.89 Other specified conditions

V82.9 Unspecified condition

✓4th **V83 Genetic carrier status**

AHA: 4Q, '02, 79; 4Q, '01, 54

✓5th **V83.0 Hemophilia A carrier**

V83.01 Asymptomatic hemophilia A carrier

V83.02 Symptomatic hemophilia A carrier

✓5th **V83.8 Other genetic carrier status**

V83.81 Cystic fibrosis gene carrier

V83.89 Other genetic carrier status

✓4th **V84 Genetic susceptibility to disease**

INCLUDES confirmed abnormal gene

Use additional code, if applicable, for any associated family history of the disease (V16-V19)

AHA: 4Q, '04, 106

✓5th **V84.0 Genetic susceptibility to malignant neoplasm**

Code first, if applicable, any current malignant neoplasms (140.0-195.8, 200.0-208.9, 230.0-234.9)

Use additional code, if applicable, for any personal history of malignant neoplasm (V10.0-V10.9)

V84.01 Genetic susceptibility to malignant neoplasm of breast SDx

AHA: 4Q, '04, 107

V84.02 Genetic susceptibility to malignant neoplasm of ovary SDx ♀

V84.03 Genetic susceptibility to malignant neoplasm of prostate SDx ♂

V84.04 Genetic susceptibility to malignant neoplasm of endometrium SDx ♀

V84.09 Genetic susceptibility to other malignant neoplasm SDx

V84.8 Genetic susceptibility to other disease SDx

● ✓4th **V85 Body Mass Index**

Kilograms per meters squared

Note: BMI adult codes are for use for persons over 20 years old

● **V85.0 Body Mass Index less than 19, adult** SDx

● **V85.1 Body Mass Index between 19-24, adult** SDx

● ✓5th **V85.2 Body Mass Index between 25-29, adult** SDx

● **V85.21 Body Mass Index 25.0-25.9, adult** SDx

● **V85.22 Body Mass Index 26.0-26.9, adult** SDx

● **V85.23 Body Mass Index 27.0-27.9, adult** SDx

● **V85.24 Body Mass Index 28.0-28.9, adult** SDx

● **V85.25 Body Mass Index 29.0-29.9, adult** SDx

● ✓5th **V85.3 Body Mass Index between 30-39, adult**

● **V85.30 Body Mass Index 30.0-30.9, adult** SDx

● **V85.31 Body Mass Index 31.0-31.9, adult** SDx

● **V85.32 Body Mass Index 32.0-32.9, adult** SDx

● **V85.33 Body Mass Index 33.0-33.9, adult** SDx

● **V85.34 Body Mass Index 34.0-34.9, adult** SDx

● **V85.35 Body Mass Index 35.0-35.9, adult** SDx

● **V85.36 Body Mass Index 36.0-36.9, adult** SDx

● **V85.37 Body Mass Index 37.0-37.9, adult** SDx

● **V85.38 Body Mass Index 38.0-38.9, adult** SDx

● **V85.39 Body Mass Index 39.0-39.9, adult** SDx

● **V85.4 Body Mass Index 40 and over, adult** SDx

SUPPLEMENTARY CLASSIFICATION OF EXTERNAL CAUSES OF INJURY AND POISONING (E800-E999)

This section is provided to permit the classification of environmental events, circumstances, and conditions as the cause of injury, poisoning, and other adverse effects. Where a code from this section is applicable, it is intended that it shall be used in addition to a code from one of the main chapters of ICD-9-CM, indicating the nature of the condition. Certain other conditions which may be stated to be due to external causes are classified in Chapters 1 to 16 of ICD-9-CM. For these, the "E" code classification should be used as an additional code for more detailed analysis.

Machinery accidents [other than those connected with transport] are classifiable to category E919, in which the fourth-digit allows a broad classification of the type of machinery involved. If a more detailed classification of type of machinery is required, it is suggested that the "Classification of Industrial Accidents according to Agency," prepared by the International Labor Office, be used in addition. This is reproduced in Appendix D for optional use.

Categories for "late effects" of accidents and other external causes are to be found at E929, E959, E969, E977, E989, and E999.

DEFINITIONS AND EXAMPLES RELATED TO TRANSPORT ACCIDENTS

(a) A **transport accident** (E800-E848) is any accident involving a device designed primarily for, or being used at the time primarily for, conveying persons or goods from one place to another.

INCLUDES accidents involving:
- aircraft and spacecraft (E840-E845)
- watercraft (E830-E838)
- motor vehicle (E810-E825)
- railway (E800-E807)
- other road vehicles (E826-E829)

In classifying accidents which involve more than one kind of transport, the above order of precedence of transport accidents should be used.

Accidents involving agricultural and construction machines, such as tractors, cranes, and bulldozers, are regarded as transport accidents only when these vehicles are under their own power on a highway [otherwise the vehicles are regarded as machinery]. Vehicles which can travel on land or water, such as hovercraft and other amphibious vehicles, are regarded as watercraft when on the water, as motor vehicles when on the highway, and as off-road motor vehicles when on land, but off the highway.

EXCLUDES *accidents:*
- *in sports which involve the use of transport but where the transport vehicle itself was not involved in the accident*
- *involving vehicles which are part of industrial equipment used entirely on industrial premises*
- *occurring during transportation but unrelated to the hazards associated with the means of transportation [e.g., injuries received in a fight on board ship; transport vehicle involved in a cataclysm such as an earthquake]*
- *to persons engaged in the maintenance or repair of transport equipment or vehicle not in motion, unlesss injured by another vehicle in motion*

(b) A **railway accident** is a transport accident involving a railway train or other railway vehicle operated on rails, whether in motion or not.

EXCLUDES *accidents:*
- *in repair shops*
- *in roundhouse or on turntable*
- *on railway premises but not involving a train or other railway vehicle*

(c) A **railway train** or **railway vehicle** is any device with or without cars coupled to it, desiged for traffic on a railway.

INCLUDES interurban:
- electric car, streetcar } (operated chiefly on its own right-of-way, not open to other traffic)

railway train, any power [diesel] [electric] [steam]
- funicular
- monorail or two-rail
- subterranean or elevated

other vehicle designed to run on a railway track

EXCLUDES *interurban electric cars [streetcars] specified to be operating on a right-of-way that forms part of the public street or highway [definition (n)]*

(d) A **railway** or **railroad** is a right-of-way designed for traffic on rails, which is used by carriages or wagons transporting passengers or freight, and by other rolling stock, and which is not open to other public vehicular traffic.

(e) A **motor vehicle accident** is a transport accident involving a motor vehicle. It is defined as a motor vehicle traffic accident or as a motor vehicle nontraffic accident according to whether the accident occurs on a public highway or elsewhere.

EXCLUDES *injury or damage due to cataclysm*
injury or damage while a motor vehicle, not under its own power, is being loaded on, or unloaded from, another conveyance

(f) A **motor vehicle traffic accident** is any motor vehicle accident occurring on a public highway [i.e., originating, terminating, or involving a vehicle partially on the highway]. A motor vehicle accident is assumed to have occurred on the highway unless another place is specified, except in the case of accidents involving only off-road motor vehicles which are classified as nontraffic accidents unless the contrary is stated.

(g) A **motor vehicle nontraffic accident** is any motor vehicle accident which occurs entirely in any place other than a public highway.

(h) A **public highway [trafficway]** or **street** is the entire width between property lines [or other boundary lines] of every way or place, of which any part is open to the use of the public for purposes of vehicular traffic as a matter of right or custom. A **roadway** is that part of the public highway designed, improved, and ordinarily used, for vehicular travel.

INCLUDES approaches (public) to:
- docks
- public building
- station

EXCLUDES *driveway (private)*
parking lot
ramp
roads in:
- *airfield*
- *farm*
- *industrial premises*
- *mine*
- *private grounds*
- *quarry*

(i) A **motor vehicle** is any mechanically or electrically powered device, not operated on rails, upon which any person or property may be transported or drawn upon a highway. Any object such as a trailer, coaster, sled, or wagon being towed by a motor vehicle is considerd a part of the motor vehicle.

INCLUDES automobile [any type]
bus
construction machinery, farm and industrial machinery, steam roller, tractor, army tank, highway grader, or similar vehicle on wheels or treads, while in transport under own power
fire engine (motorized)
motorcycle
motorized bicycle [moped] or scooter
trolley bus not operating on rails
truck
van

EXCLUDES *devices used solely to move persons or materials within the confines of a building and its premises, such as:*
building elevator
coal car in mine
electric baggage or mail truck used solely within a railroad station
electric truck used solely within an industrial plant
moving overhead crane

(j) A **motorcycle** is a two-wheeled motor vehicle having one or two riding saddles and sometimes having a third wheel for the support of a sidecar. The sidecar is considered part of the motorcycle.

INCLUDES motorized:
bicycle [moped]
scooter
tricycle

(k) An **off-road motor vehicle** is a motor vehicle of special design, to enable it to negotiate rough or soft terrain or snow. Examples of special design are high construction, special wheels and tires, driven by treads, or support on a cushion of air.

INCLUDES all terrain vehicle [ATV]
army tank
hovercraft, on land or swamp
snowmobile

(l) A **driver** of a motor vehicle is the occupant of the motor vehicle operating it or intending to operate it. A **motorcyclist** is the driver of a motorcycle. Other authorized occupants of a motor vehicle are **passengers**.

(m) An **other road vehicle** is any device, except a motor vehicle, in, on, or by which any person or property may be transported on a highway.

INCLUDES animal carrying a person or goods
animal-drawn vehicles
animal harnessed to conveyance
bicycle [pedal cycle]
streetcar
tricycle (pedal)

EXCLUDES *pedestrian conveyance [definition (q)]*

(n) A **streetcar** is a device designed and used primarily for transporting persons within a municipality, running on rails, usually subject to normal traffic control signals, and operated principally on a right-of-way that forms part of the traffic way. A trailer being towed by a streetcar is considered a part of the streetcar.

INCLUDES interurban or intraurban electric or streetcar, when specified to be operating on a street or public highway
tram (car)
trolley (car)

(o) A **pedal cycle** is any road transport vehicle operated solely by pedals.

INCLUDES bicycle
pedal cycle
tricycle

EXCLUDES *motorized bicycle [definition (i)]*

(p) A **pedal cyclist** is any person riding on a pedal cycle or in a sidecar attached to such a vehicle.

(q) A **pedestrian conveyance** is any human powered device by which a pedestrian may move other than by walking or by which a walking person may move another pedestrian.

INCLUDES baby carriage
coaster wagon
ice skates
perambulator
pushcart
pushchair
roller skates
scooter
skateboard
skis
sled
wheelchair

(r) A **pedestrian** is any person involved in an accident who was not at the time of the accident riding in or on a motor vehicle, railroad train, streetcar, animal-drawn or other vehicle, or on a bicycle or animal.

INCLUDES person:
changing tire of vehicle
in or operating a pedestrian conveyance
making adjustment to motor of vehicle
on foot

(s) A **watercraft** is any device for transporting passengers or goods on the water.

(t) A **small boat** is any watercraft propelled by paddle, oars, or small motor, with a passenger capacity of less than ten.

INCLUDES boat NOS
canoe
coble
dinghy
punt
raft
rowboat
rowing shell
scull
skiff
small motorboat

EXCLUDES *barge*
lifeboat (used after abandoning ship)
raft (anchored) being used as a diving platform
yacht

(u) An **aircraft** is any device for transporting passengers or goods in the air.

INCLUDES airplane [any type]
balloon
bomber
dirigible
glider (hang)
military aircraft
parachute

(v) A **commercial transport aircraft** is any device for collective passenger or freight transportation by air, whether run on commercial lines for profit or by government authorities, with the exception of military craft.

RAILWAY ACCIDENTS (E800-E807)

Note: For definitions of railway accident and related terms see definitions (a) to (d).

EXCLUDES *accidents involving railway train and:*
aircraft (E840.0-E845.9)
motor vehicle (E810.0-E825.9)
watercraft (E830.0-E838.9)

The following fourth-digit subdivisions are for use with categories E800-E807 to identify the injured person:

.0 Railway employee
Any person who by virtue of his employment in connection with a railway, whether by the railway company or not, is at increased risk of involvement in a railway accident, such as:
catering staff of train
driver
guard
porter
postal staff on train
railway fireman
shunter
sleeping car attendant

.1 Passenger on railway
Any authorized person traveling on a train, except a railway employee.
EXCLUDES *intending passenger waiting at station (.8)*
unauthorized rider on railway vehicle (.8)

.2 Pedestrian
See definition (r)

.3 Pedal cyclist
See definition (p)

.8 Other specified person
Intending passenger or bystander waiting at station
Unauthorized rider on railway vehicle

.9 Unspecified person

4th E800 Railway accident involving collision with rolling stock
INCLUDES collision between railway trains or railway vehicles, any kind
collision NOS on railway
derailment with antecedent collision with rolling stock or NOS

4th E801 Railway accident involving collision with other object
INCLUDES collision of railway train with:
buffers
fallen tree on railway
gates
platform
rock on railway
streetcar
other nonmotor vehicle
other object
EXCLUDES *collision with:*
aircraft (E840.0-E842.9)
motor vehicle (E810.0-E810.9, E820.0-E822.9)

4th E802 Railway accident involving derailment without antecedent collision

4th E803 Railway accident involving explosion, fire, or burning
EXCLUDES *explosion or fire, with antecedent derailment (E802.0-E802.9)*
explosion or fire, with mention of antecedent collision (E800.0-E801.9)

4th E804 Fall in, on, or from railway train
INCLUDES fall while alighting from or boarding railway train
EXCLUDES *fall related to collision, derailment, or explosion of railway train (E800.0-E803.9)*

4th E805 Hit by rolling stock
INCLUDES crushed, injured, killed, knocked down, run over } by railway train or part
EXCLUDES *pedestrian hit by object set in motion by railway train (E806.0-E806.9)*

4th E806 Other specified railway accident
INCLUDES hit by object falling in railway train
injured by door or window on railway train
nonmotor road vehicle or pedestrian hit by object set in motion by railway train
railway train hit by falling:
earth NOS
rock
tree
other object
EXCLUDES *railway accident due to cataclysm (E908-E909)*

4th E807 Railway accident of unspecified nature
INCLUDES found dead, injured } on railway right-of-way NOS
railway accident NOS

MOTOR VEHICLE TRAFFIC ACCIDENTS (E810-E819)

Note: For definitions of motor vehicle traffic accident, and related terms, see definitions (e) to (k).

EXCLUDES *accidents involving motor vehicle and aircraft (E840.0-E845.9)*

The following fourth-digit subdivisions are for use with categories E810-E819 to identify the injured person:

.0 Driver of motor vehicle other than motorcycle
See definition (1)

.1 Passenger in motor vehicle other than motorcycle
See definition (1)

.2 Motorcyclist
See definition (1)

.3 Passenger on motorcycle
See definition (1)

.4 Occupant of streetcar

.5 Rider of animal; occupant of animal-drawn vehicle

.6 Pedal cyclist
See definition (p)

.7 Pedestrian
See definition (r)

.8 Other specified person
Occupant of vehicle other than above
Person in railway train involved in accident
Unauthorized rider of motor vehicle

.9 Unspecified person

4th E810 Motor vehicle traffic accident involving collision with train
EXCLUDES *motor vehicle collision with object set in motion by railway train (E815.0-E815.9)*
railway train hit by object set in motion by motor vehicle (E818.0-E818.9)

4th E811 Motor vehicle traffic accident involving re-entrant collision with another motor vehicle
INCLUDES collision between motor vehicle which accidentally leaves the roadway then re-enters the same roadway, or the opposite roadway on a divided highway, and another motor vehicle
EXCLUDES *collision on the same roadway when none of the motor vehicles involved have left and re-entered the highway (E812.0-E812.9)*

§ ✓4th **E812 Other motor vehicle traffic accident involving collision with motor vehicle**

INCLUDES collision with another motor vehicle parked, stopped, stalled, disabled, or abandoned on the highway
motor vehicle collision NOS

EXCLUDES *collision with object set in motion by another motor vehicle (E815.0-E815.9)*
re-entrant collision with another motor vehicle (E811.0-E811.9)

§ ✓4th **E813 Motor vehicle traffic accident involving collision with other vehicle**

INCLUDES collision between motor vehicle, any kind, and:
other road (nonmotor transport) vehicle, such as:
animal carrying a person
animal-drawn vehicle
pedal cycle
streetcar

EXCLUDES *collision with:*
object set in motion by nonmotor road vehicle (E815.0-E815.9)
pedestrian (E814.0-E814.9)
nonmotor road vehicle hit by object set in motion by motor vehicle (E818.0-E818.9)

§ ✓4th **E814 Motor vehicle traffic accident involving collision with pedestrian**

INCLUDES collision between motor vehicle, any kind, and pedestrian
pedestrian dragged, hit, or run over by motor vehicle, any kind

EXCLUDES *pedestrian hit by object set in motion by motor vehicle (E818.0-E818.9)*

§ ✓4th **E815 Other motor vehicle traffic accident involving collision on the highway**

INCLUDES collision (due to loss of control) (on highway) between motor vehicle, any kind, and:
abutment (bridge) (overpass)
animal (herded) (unattended)
fallen stone, traffic sign, tree, utility pole
guard rail or boundary fence
interhighway divider
landslide (not moving)
object set in motion by railway train or road vehicle (motor) (nonmotor)
object thrown in front of motor vehicle
other object, fixed, movable, or moving
safety island
temporary traffic sign or marker
wall of cut made for road

EXCLUDES *collision with:*
any object off the highway (resulting from loss of control) (E816.0-E816.9)
any object which normally would have been off the highway and is not stated to have been on it (E816.0-E816.9)
motor vehicle parked, stopped, stalled, disabled, or abandoned on highway (E812.0-E812.9)
moving landslide (E909)
motor vehicle hit by object:
set in motion by railway train or road vehicle (motor) (nonmotor) (E818.0-E818.9)
thrown into or on vehicle (E818.0-E818.9)

§ ✓4th **E816 Motor vehicle traffic accident due to loss of control, without collision on the highway**

INCLUDES motor vehicle:
failing to make curve
going out of control (due to):
blowout
burst tire
driver falling asleep
driver inattention
excessive speed
failure of mechanical part
} and:
coliding with object off the highway
overturning
stopping abruptly off the highway

EXCLUDES *collision on highway following loss of control (E810.0-E815.9)*
loss of control of motor vehicle following collision on the highway (E810.0-E815.9)

§ ✓4th **E817 Noncollision motor vehicle traffic accident while boarding or alighting**

INCLUDES fall down stairs of motor bus
fall from car in street
injured by moving part of the vehicle
trapped by door of motor bus
} while boarding or alighting

§ ✓4th **E818 Other noncollision motor vehicle traffic accident**

INCLUDES accidental poisoning from exhaust gas generated by
breakage of any part of
explosion of any part of
fall, jump, or being accidentally pushed from
fire starting in
hit by object thrown into or on
injured by being thrown against some part of, or object in
injury from moving part of
object falling in or on
object thrown on
} motor vehicle while in motion

collision of railway train or road vehicle except motor vehicle, with object set in motion by motor vehicle
motor vehicle hit by object set in motion by railway train or road vehicle (motor) (nonmotor)
pedestrian, railway train, or road vehicle (motor) (nonmotor) hit by object set in motion by motor vehicle

EXCLUDES *collision between motor vehicle and:*
object set in motion by railway train or road vehicle (motor) (nonmotor) (E815.0-E815.9)
object thrown towards the motor vehicle (E815.0-E815.9)
person overcome by carbon monoxide generated by stationary motor vehicle off the roadway with motor running (E868.2)

§ ✓4th **E819 Motor vehicle traffic accident of unspecified nature**

INCLUDES motor vehicle traffic accident NOS
traffic accident NOS

§ Requires fourth-digit. See beginning of section E810-E819 for codes and definitions.

MOTOR VEHICLE NONTRAFFIC ACCIDENTS (E820-E825)

Note: For definitions of motor vehicle nontraffic accident and related terms see definition (a) to (k).

INCLUDES accidents involving motor vehicles being used in recreational or sporting activities off the highway
collision and noncollision motor vehicle accidents occurring entirely off the highway

EXCLUDES *accidents involving motor vehicle and:*
aircraft (E840.0-E845.9)
watercraft (E830.0-E838.9)
accidents, not on the public highway, involving agricultural and construction machinery but not involving another motor vehicle (E919.0, E919.2, E919.7)

The following fourth-digit subdivisions are for use with categories E820-E825 to identify the injured person:

.0 Driver of motor vehicle other than motorcycle
See definition (l)

.1 Passenger in motor vehicle other than motorcycle
See definition (l)

.2 Motorcyclist
See definition (l)

.3 Passenger on motorcycle
See definition (l)

.4 Occupant of streetcar

.5 Rider of animal; occupant of animal-drawn vehicle

.6 Pedal cyclist
See definition (p)

.7 Pedestrian
See definition (r)

.8 Other specified person
Occupant of vehicle other than above
Person on railway train involved in accident
Unauthorized rider of motor vehicle

.9 Unspecified person

E820 Nontraffic accident involving motor-driven snow vehicle

INCLUDES breakage of part of / fall from / hit by / overturning of / run over or dragged by } motor-driven snow vehicle (not on public highway)

collision of motor-driven snow vehicle with:
animal (being ridden) (-drawn vehicle)
another off-road motor vehicle
other motor vehicle, not on public highway
railway train
other object, fixed or movable
injury caused by rough landing of motor-driven snow vehicle (after leaving ground on rough terrain)

EXCLUDES *accident on the public highway involving motor driven snow vehicle (E810.0-E819.9)*

E821 Nontraffic accident involving other off-road motor vehicle

INCLUDES breakage of part of / fall from / hit by / overturning of / run over or dragged by / thrown against some part of or object in } off-road motor vehicle, except snow vehicle (not on public highway)

collision with:
animal (being ridden) (-drawn vehicle)
another off-road motor vehicle, except snow vehicle
other motor vehicle, not on public highway
other object, fixed or movable

EXCLUDES *accident on public highway involving off-road motor vehicle (E810.0-E819.9)*
collision between motor driven snow vehicle and other off-road motor vehicle (E820.0-E820.9)
hovercraft accident on water (E830.0-E838.9)

E822 Other motor vehicle nontraffic accident involving collision with moving object

INCLUDES collision, not on public highway, between motor vehicle, except off-road motor vehicle and:
animal
nonmotor vehicle
other motor vehicle, except off-road motor vehicle
pedestrian
railway train
other moving object

EXCLUDES *collision with:*
motor-driven snow vehicle (E820.0-E820.9)
other off-road motor vehicle (E821.0-E821.9)

E823 Other motor vehicle nontraffic accident involving collision with stationary object

INCLUDES collision, not on public highway, between motor vehicle, except off-road motor vehicle, and any object, fixed or movable, but not in motion

E824 Other motor vehicle nontraffic accident while boarding and alighting

INCLUDES fall / injury from moving part of motor vehicle / trapped by door of motor vehicle } while boarding or alighting from motor vehicle, except off-road motor vehicle, not on public highway

Fourth-digit Required · Revised Text · New Code · Revised Code Title

§ **✓4th E825 Other motor vehicle nontraffic accident of other and unspecified nature**

INCLUDES accidental poisoning from carbon monoxide generated by } motor vehicle while in motion, not on public highway
breakage of any part of
explosion of any part of
fall, jump, or being accidentally pushed from
fire starting in
hit by object thrown into, towards, or on
injured by being thrown against some part of, or object in
injury from moving part of
object falling in or on

motor vehicle nontraffic accident NOS

EXCLUDES *fall from or in stationary motor vehicle (E884.9, E885.9)*
overcome by carbon monoxide or exhaust gas generated by stationary motor vehicle off the roadway with motor running (E868.2)
struck by falling object from or in stationary motor vehicle (E916)

OTHER ROAD VEHICLE ACCIDENTS (E826-E829)

Note: Other road vehicle accidents are transport accidents involving road vehicles other than motor vehicles. For definitions of other road vehicle and related terms see definitions (m) to (o).

INCLUDES accidents involving other road vehicles being used in recreational or sporting activities

EXCLUDES *collision of other road vehicle [any] with:*
aircraft (E840.0-E845.9)
motor vehicle (E813.0-E813.9, E820.0-E822.9)
railway train (E801.0-E801.9)

The following fourth-digit subdivisions are for use with categories E826-E829 to identify the injured person.

.0 Pedestrian
See definition (r)
.1 Pedal cyclist
See definition (p)
.2 Rider of animal
.3 Occupant of animal-drawn vehicle
.4 Occupant of streetcar
.8 Other specified person
.9 Unspecified person

✓4th E826 Pedal cycle accident

[0-9]

INCLUDES breakage of any part of pedal cycle
collision between pedal cycle and:
animal (being ridden) (herded) (unattended)
another pedal cycle
any pedestrian
nonmotor road vehicle
other object, fixed, movable, or moving, not set in motion by motor vehicle, railway train, or aircraft
entanglement in wheel of pedal cycle
fall from pedal cycle
hit by object falling or thrown on the pedal cycle
pedal cycle accident NOS
pedal cycle overturned

✓4th E827 Animal-drawn vehicle accident

[0,2-4,8,9]

INCLUDES breakage of any part of vehicle
collision between animal-drawn vehicle and:
animal (being ridden) (herded) (unattended)
nonmotor road vehicle, except pedal cycle
pedestrian, pedestrian conveyance, or pedestrian vehicle
other object, fixed, movable, or moving, not set in motion by motor vehicle, railway train, or aircraft
fall from } animal-drawn vehicle
knocked down by
overturning of
run over by
thrown from

EXCLUDES *collision of animal-drawn vehicle with pedal cycle (E826.0-E826.9)*

✓4th E828 Accident involving animal being ridden

[0,2,4,8,9]

INCLUDES collision between animal being ridden and:
another animal
nonmotor road vehicle, except pedal cycle, and animal-drawn vehicle
pedestrian, pedestrian conveyance, or pedestrian vehicle
other object, fixed, movable, or moving, not set in motion by motor vehicle, railway train, or aircraft
fall from } animal being ridden
knocked down by
thrown from
trampled by
ridden animal stumbled and fell

EXCLUDES *collision of animal being ridden with:*
animal-drawn vehicle (E827.0-E827.9)
pedal cycle (E826.0-E826.9)

✓4th E829 Other road vehicle accidents

[0,4,8,9]

INCLUDES accident while boarding or alighting from } streetcar nonmotor road vehicle not classifiable to E826-E828
blow from object in
breakage of any part of
caught in door of-
derailment of
fall in, on, or from
fire in

collision between streetcar or nonmotor road vehicle, except as in E826-E828, and:
animal (not being ridden)
another nonmotor road vehicle not classifiable to E826-E828
pedestrian
other object, fixed, movable, or moving, not set in motion by motor vehicle, railway train, or aircraft
nonmotor road vehicle accident NOS
streetcar accident NOS

EXCLUDES *collision with:*
animal being ridden (E828.0-E828.9)
animal-drawn vehicle (E827.0-E827.9)
pedal cycle (E826.0-E826.9)

§ Requires fourth-digit. Valid digits are in [brackets] under each code. See beginning of section E820-E825 for codes and definitions.

4th Fourth-digit Required ▶◀ Revised Text ● New Code ▲ Revised Code Title

WATER TRANSPORT ACCIDENTS (E830-E838)

Note: For definitions of water transport accident and related terms see definitions (a), (s), and (t).

INCLUDES watercraft accidents in the course of recreational activities

EXCLUDES *accidents involving both aircraft, including objects set in motion by aircraft, and watercraft (E840.0-E845.9)*

The following fourth-digit subdivisions are for use with categories E830-E838 to identify the injured person:

.0 Occupant of small boat, unpowered

.1 Occupant of small boat, powered

See definition (t)

EXCLUDES *water skier (.4)*

.2 Occupant of other watercraft — crew

Persons:
- engaged in operation of watercraft
- providing passenger services [cabin attendants, ship's physician, catering personnel]
- working on ship during voyage in other capacity [musician in band, operators of shops and beauty parlors]

.3 Occupant of other watercraft — other than crew

Passenger

Occupant of lifeboat, other than crew, after abandoning ship

.4 Water skier

.5 Swimmer

.6 Dockers, stevedores

Longshoreman employed on the dock in loading and unloading ships

.8 Other specified person

Immigration and custom officials on board ship

Person:
- accompanying passenger or member of crew visiting boat

Pilot (guiding ship into port)

.9 Unspecified person

4th E830 Accident to watercraft causing submersion

INCLUDES submersion and drowning due to:
- boat overturning
- boat submerging
- falling or jumping from burning ship
- falling or jumping from crushed watercraft
- ship sinking
- other accident to watercraft

4th E831 Accident to watercraft causing other injury

INCLUDES any injury, except submersion and drowning, as a result of an accident to watercraft
- burned while ship on fire
- crushed between ships in collision
- crushed by lifeboat after abandoning ship
- fall due to collision or other accident to watercraft
- hit by falling object due to accident to watercraft
- injured in watercraft accident involving collision
- struck by boat or part thereof after fall or jump from damaged boat

EXCLUDES *burns from localized fire or explosion on board ship (E837.0-E837.9)*

4th E832 Other accidental submersion or drowning in water transport accident

INCLUDES submersion or drowning as a result of an accident other than accident to the watercraft, such as:
- fall:
  - from gangplank
  - from ship
  - overboard
- thrown overboard by motion of ship
- washed overboard

EXCLUDES *submersion or drowning of swimmer or diver who voluntarily jumps from boat not involved in an accident (E910.0-E910.9)*

4th E833 Fall on stairs or ladders in water transport

EXCLUDES *fall due to accident to watercraft (E831.0-E831.9)*

4th E834 Other fall from one level to another in water transport

EXCLUDES *fall due to accident to watercraft (E831.0-E831.9)*

4th E835 Other and unspecified fall in water transport

EXCLUDES *fall due to accident to watercraft (E831.0-E831.9)*

4th E836 Machinery accident in water transport

INCLUDES injuries in water transport caused by:
- deck machinery
- engine room machinery
- galley machinery
- laundry machinery
- loading machinery

4th E837 Explosion, fire, or burning in watercraft

INCLUDES explosion of boiler on steamship
- localized fire on ship

EXCLUDES *burning ship (due to collision or explosion) resulting in:*
- *submersion or drowning (E830.0-E830.9)*
- *other injury (E831.0-E831.9)*

4th E838 Other and unspecified water transport accident

INCLUDES accidental poisoning by gases or fumes on ship
- atomic power plant malfunction in watercraft
- crushed between ship and stationary object [wharf]
- crushed between ships without accident to watercraft
- crushed by falling object on ship or while loading or unloading
- hit by boat while water skiing
- struck by boat or part thereof (after fall from boat)
- watercraft accident NOS

4th Fourth-digit Required ▶◀ Revised Text ● New Code ▲ Revised Code Title

AIR AND SPACE TRANSPORT ACCIDENTS (E840-E845)

Note: For definition of aircraft and related terms see definitions (u) and (v).

The following fourth-digit subdivisions are for use with categories E840-E845 to identify the injured person. Valid fourth digits are in [brackets] under codes E842-E845.

.0 Occupant of spacecraft

.1 Occupant of military aircraft, any

Crew in military aircraft [air force] [army] [national guard] [navy]
Passenger (civilian) (military) in military aircraft [air force] [army] [national guard] [navy]
Troops in military aircraft [air force] [army] [national guard] [navy]

EXCLUDES *occupants of aircraft operated under jurisdiction of police departments (.5)*
parachutist (.7)

.2 Crew of commercial aircraft (powered) in surface to surface transport

.3 Other occupant of commercial aircraft (powered) in surface to surface transport

Flight personnel:
not part of crew
on familiarization flight
Passenger on aircraft (powered) NOS

.4 Occupant of commercial aircraft (powered) in surface to air transport

Occupant [crew] [passenger] of aircraft (powered) engaged in activities, such as:
aerial spraying (crops) (fire retardants)
air drops of emergency supplies
air drops of parachutists, except from military craft
crop dusting
lowering of construction material [bridge or telephone pole]
sky writing

.5 Occupant of other powered aircraft

Occupant [crew][passenger] of aircraft [powered] engaged in activities, such as:
aerobatic flying
aircraft racing
rescue operation
storm surveillance
traffic surveillance
Occupant of private plane NOS

.6 Occupant of unpowered aircraft, except parachutist

Occupant of aircraft classifiable to E842

.7 Parachutist (military) (other)

Person making voluntary descent

EXCLUDES *person making descent after accident to aircraft (.1-.6)*

.8 Ground crew, airline employee

Persons employed at airfields (civil) (military) or launching pads, not occupants of aircraft

.9 Other person

✓4th E840 Accident to powered aircraft at takeoff or landing

INCLUDES
collision of aircraft with any object, fixed, movable, or moving } while taking off or landing
crash } while taking off or landing
explosion on aircraft } while taking off or landing
fire on aircraft } while taking off or landing
forced landing } while taking off or landing

✓4th E841 Accident to powered aircraft, other and unspecified

INCLUDES
aircraft accident NOS
aircraft crash or wreck NOS
any accident to powered aircraft while in transit or when not specified whether in transit, taking off, or landing
collision of aircraft with another aircraft, bird, or any object, while in transit
explosion on aircraft while in transit
fire on aircraft while in transit

✓4th E842 Accident to unpowered aircraft

[6-9] INCLUDES
any accident, except collision with powered aircraft, to:
balloon
glider
hang glider
kite carrying a person
hit by object falling from unpowered aircraft

✓4th E843 Fall in, on, or from aircraft

[0-9] INCLUDES
accident in boarding or alighting from aircraft, any kind
fall in, on, or from aircraft [any kind], while in transit, taking off, or landing, except when as a result of an accident to aircraft

✓4th E844 Other specified air transport accidents

[0-9] INCLUDES
hit by:
aircraft
object falling from aircraft } without accident to aircraft
injury by or from:
machinery on aircraft } without accident to aircraft
rotating propeller } without accident to aircraft
voluntary parachute descent } without accident to aircraft
poisoning by carbon monoxide from aircraft while in transit } without accident to aircraft
sucked into jet
any accident involving other transport vehicle (motor) (nonmotor) due to being hit by object set in motion by aircraft (powered)

EXCLUDES *air sickness (E903)*
effects of:
high altitude (E902.0-E902.1)
pressure change (E902.0-E902.1)
injury in parachute descent due to accident to aircraft (E840.0-E842-9)

✓4th E845 Accident involving spacecraft

[0,8,9] INCLUDES launching pad accident
EXCLUDES *effects of weightlessness in spacecraft (E928.0)*

VEHICLE ACCIDENTS NOT ELSEWHERE CLASSIFIABLE (E846-E848)

E846 Accidents involving powered vehicles used solely within the buildings and premises of industrial or commercial establishment

Accident to, on, or involving:
- battery powered airport passenger vehicle
- battery powered trucks (baggage) (mail)
- coal car in mine
- logging car
- self propelled truck, industrial
- station baggage truck (powered)
- tram, truck, or tub (powered) in mine or quarry

Collision with:
- pedestrian
- other vehicle or object within premises

Explosion of / Fall from / Overturning of / Struck by } powered vehicle, industrial or commercial

EXCLUDES *accidental poisoning by exhaust gas from vehicle not elsewhere classifiable (E868.2)*
injury by crane, lift (fork), or elevator (E919.2)

E847 Accidents involving cable cars not running on rails

Accident to, on, or involving:
- cable car, not on rails
- ski chair-lift
- ski-lift with gondola
- téléférique

Breakage of cable

Caught or dragged by / Fall or jump from / Object thrown from or in } cable car, not on rails

E848 Accidents involving other vehicles, not elsewhere classifiable

Accident to, on, or involving:
- ice yacht
- land yacht
- nonmotor, nonroad vehicle NOS

✓4th ***E849 Place of occurrence***

The following category is for use to denote the place where the injury or poisoning occurred.

E849.0 Home

Apartment
Boarding house
Farm house
Home premises
House (residential)
Noninstitutional place of residence
Private:
- *driveway*
- *garage*
- *garden*
- *home*
- *walk*

Swimming pool in private house or garden
Yard of home

EXCLUDES *home under construction but not yet occupied (E849.3)*
institutional place of residence (E849.7)

E849.1 Farm

Farm:
- *buildings*
- *land under cultivation*

EXCLUDES *farm house and home premises of farm (E849.0)*

E849.2 Mine and quarry

Gravel pit
Sand pit
Tunnel under construction

E849.3 Industrial place and premises

Building under construction
Dockyard
Dry dock
Factory
- *building*
- *premises*

Garage (place of work)
Industrial yard
Loading platform (factory) (store)
Plant, industrial
Railway yard
Shop (place of work)
Warehouse
Workhouse

E849.4 Place for recreation and sport

Amusement park
Baseball field
Basketball court
Beach resort
Cricket ground
Fives court
Football field
Golf course
Gymnasium
Hockey field
Holiday camp
Ice palace
Lake resort
Mountain resort
Playground, including school playground
Public park
Racecourse
Resort NOS
Riding school
Rifle range
Seashore resort
Skating rink
Sports palace
Stadium
Swimming pool, public
Tennis court
Vacation resort

EXCLUDES *that in private house or garden (E849.0)*

E849.5 Street and highway

E849.6 Public building

Building (including adjacent grounds) used by the general public or by a particular group of the public, such as:
- *airport*
- *bank*
- *café*
- *casino*
- *church*
- *cinema*
- *clubhouse*
- *courthouse*
- *dance hall*
- *garage building (for car storage)*
- *hotel*
- *market (grocery or other commodity)*
- *movie house*
- *music hall*
- *nightclub*
- *office*
- *office building*
- *opera house*
- *post office*
- *public hall*
- *radio broadcasting station*
- *restaurant*
- *school (state) (public) (private)*
- *shop, commercial*
- *station (bus) (railway)*
- *store*
- *theater*

EXCLUDES *home garage (E849.0)*
industrial building or workplace (E849.3)

E849.7 Residential institution

Children's home
Dormitory
Hospital
Jail
Old people's home
Orphanage
Prison
Reform school

E849.8 Other specified places

Beach NOS
Canal
Caravan site NOS
Derelict house
Desert
Dock
Forest
Harbor
Hill
Lake NOS
Mountain
Parking lot
Parking place
Pond or pool (natural)
Prairie
Public place NOS
Railway line
Reservoir
River
Sea
Seashore NOS
Stream
Swamp
Trailer court
Woods

E849.9 Unspecified place

ACCIDENTAL POISONING BY DRUGS, MEDICINAL SUBSTANCES, AND BIOLOGICALS (E850-E858)

INCLUDES accidental overdose of drug, wrong drug given or taken in error, and drug taken inadvertently
accidents in the use of drugs and biologicals in medical and surgical procedures

EXCLUDES *administration with suicidal or homicidal intent or intent to harm, or in circumstances classifiable to E980-E989 (E950.0-E950.5, E962.0, E980.0-E980.5)*
correct drug properly administered in therapeutic or prophylactic dosage, as the cause of adverse effect (E930.0-E949.9)

See Alphabetic Index for more complete list of specific drugs to be classified under the fourth-digit subdivisions.
The American Hospital Formulary numbers can be used to classify new drugs listed by the American Hospital Formulary Service (AHFS). See Appendix C.

✓4th **E850 Accidental poisoning by analgesics, antipyretics, and antirheumatics**

E850.0 Heroin
Diacetylmorphine

E850.1 Methadone

E850.2 Other opiates and related narcotics
Codeine [methylmorphine]
Meperidine [pethidine]
Morphine
Opium (alkaloids)

E850.3 Salicylates
Acetylsalicylic acid [aspirin]
Amino derivatives of salicylic acid
Salicylic acid salts

E850.4 Aromatic analgesics, not elsewhere classified
Acetanilid
Paracetamol [acetaminophen]
Phenacetin [acetophenetidin]

E850.5 Pyrazole derivatives
Aminophenazone [amidopyrine]
Phenylbutazone

E850.6 Antirheumatics [antiphlogistics]
Gold salts
Indomethacin
EXCLUDES *salicylates (E850.3)*
steroids (E858.0)

E850.7 Other non-narcotic analgesics
Pyrabital

E850.8 Other specified analgesics and antipyretics
Pentazocine

E850.9 Unspecified analgesic or antipyretic

E851 Accidental poisoning by barbiturates
Amobarbital [amylobarbitone]
Barbital [barbitone]
Butabarbital [butabarbitone]
Pentobarbital [pentobarbitone]
Phenobarbital [phenobarbitone]
Secobarbital [quinalbarbitone]
EXCLUDES *thiobarbiturates (E855.1)*

✓4th **E852 Accidental poisoning by other sedatives and hypnotics**

E852.0 Chloral hydrate group

E852.1 Paraldehyde

E852.2 Bromine compounds
Bromides
Carbromal (derivatives)

E852.3 Methaqualone compounds

E852.4 Glutethimide group

E852.5 Mixed sedatives, not elsewhere classified

E852.8 Other specified sedatives and hypnotics

E852.9 Unspecified sedative or hypnotic
Sleeping:
drug } NOS
pill } NOS
tablet } NOS

✓4th **E853 Accidental poisoning by tranquilizers**

E853.0 Phenothiazine-based tranquilizers
Chlorpromazine
Fluphenazine
Prochlorperazine
Promazine

E853.1 Butyrophenone-based tranquilizers
Haloperidol
Spiperone
Trifluperidol

E853.2 Benzodiazepine-based tranquilizers
Chlordiazepoxide
Diazepam
Flurazepam
Lorazepam
Medazepam
Nitrazepam

E853.8 Other specified tranquilizers
Hydroxyzine
Meprobamate

E853.9 Unspecified tranquilizer

✓4th **E854 Accidental poisoning by other psychotropic agents**

E854.0 Antidepressants
Amitriptyline
Imipramine
Monoamine oxidase [MAO] inhibitors

E854.1 Psychodysleptics [hallucinogens]
Cannabis derivatives
Lysergide [LSD]
Marihuana (derivatives)
Mescaline
Psilocin
Psilocybin

E854.2 Psychostimulants
Amphetamine
Caffeine
EXCLUDES *central appetite depressants (E858.8)*

E854.3 Central nervous system stimulants
Analeptics
Opiate antagonists

E854.8 Other psychotropic agents

✓4th **E855 Accidental poisoning by other drugs acting on central and autonomic nervous system**

E855.0 Anticonvulsant and anti-Parkinsonism drugs
Amantadine
Hydantoin derivatives
Levodopa [L-dopa]
Oxazolidine derivatives [paramethadione] [trimethadione]
Succinimides

E855.1 Other central nervous system depressants
Ether
Gaseous anesthetics
Halogenated hydrocarbon derivatives
Intravenous anesthetics
Thiobarbiturates, such as thiopental sodium

E855.2 Local anesthetics
Cocaine
Lidocaine [lignocaine]
Procaine
Tetracaine

E855.3 Parasympathomimetics [cholinergics]
Acetylcholine
Anticholinesterase:
organophosphorus
reversible
Pilocarpine

E855.4 Parasympatholytics [anticholinergics and antimuscarinics] and spasmolytics
Atropine
Homatropine
Hyoscine [scopolamine]
Quaternary ammonium derivatives

E855.5 Sympathomimetics [adrenergics]
Epinephrine [adrenalin]
Levarterenol [noradrenalin]

E855.6 Sympatholytics [antiadrenergics]
Phenoxybenzamine
Tolazoline hydrochloride

E855.8 Other specified drugs acting on central and autonomic nervous systems

E855.9 Unspecified drug acting on central and autonomic nervous systems

E856 Accidental poisoning by antibiotics

E857 Accidental poisoning by other anti-infectives

✓4th **E858 Accidental poisoning by other drugs**

E858.0 Hormones and synthetic substitutes

E858.1 Primarily systemic agents

E858.2 Agents primarily affecting blood constituents

E858.3 Agents primarily affecting cardiovascular system

E858.4 Agents primarily affecting gastrointestinal system

E858.5 Water, mineral, and uric acid metabolism drugs

E858.6 Agents primarily acting on the smooth and skeletal muscles and respiratory system

E858.7 Agents primarily affecting skin and mucous membrane, ophthalmological, otorhinolaryngological, and dental drugs

E858.8 Other specified drugs
Central appetite depressants

E858.9 Unspecified drug

ACCIDENTAL POISONING BY OTHER SOLID AND LIQUID SUBSTANCES, GASES, AND VAPORS (E860-E869)

Note: Categories in this section are intended primarily to indicate the external cause of poisoning states classifiable to 980-989. They may also be used to indicate external causes of localized effects classifiable to 001-799.

✓4th E860 Accidental poisoning by alcohol, not elsewhere classified

E860.0 Alcoholic beverages
Alcohol in preparations intended for consumption

E860.1 Other and unspecified ethyl alcohol and its products
Denatured alcohol
Ethanol NOS
Grain alcohol NOS
Methylated spirit

E860.2 Methyl alcohol
Methanol
Wood alcohol

E860.3 Isopropyl alcohol
Dimethyl carbinol
Isopropanol
Rubbing alcohol subsitute
Secondary propyl alcohol

E860.4 Fusel oil
Alcohol:
amyl
butyl
propyl

E860.8 Other specified alcohols

E860.9 Unspecified alcohol

✓4th E861 Accidental poisoning by cleansing and polishing agents, disinfectants, paints, and varnishes

E861.0 Synthetic detergents and shampoos

E861.1 Soap products

E861.2 Polishes

E861.3 Other cleansing and polishing agents
Scouring powders

E861.4 Disinfectants
Household and other disinfectants not ordinarily used on the person
EXCLUDES *carbolic acid or phenol (E864.0)*

E861.5 Lead paints

E861.6 Other paints and varnishes
Lacquers
Oil colors
Paints, other than lead
White washes

E861.9 Unspecified

✓4th E862 Accidental poisoning by petroleum products, other solvents and their vapors, not elsewhere classified

E862.0 Petroleum solvents
Petroleum:
ether
benzine
naphtha

E862.1 Petroleum fuels and cleaners
Antiknock additives to petroleum fuels
Gas oils
Gasoline or petrol
Kerosene
EXCLUDES *kerosene insecticides (E863.4)*

E862.2 Lubricating oils

E862.3 Petroleum solids
Paraffin wax

E862.4 Other specified solvents
Benzene

E862.9 Unspecified solvent

✓4th E863 Accidental poisoning by agricultural and horticultural chemical and pharmaceutical preparations other than plant foods and fertilizers
EXCLUDES *plant foods and fertilizers (E866.5)*

E863.0 Insecticides of organochlorine compounds
Benzene hexachloride
Chlordane
DDT
Dieldrin
Endrine
Toxaphene

E863.1 Insecticides of organophosphorus compounds
Demeton
Diazinon
Dichlorvos
Malathion
Methyl parathion
Parathion
Phenylsulphthion
Phorate
Phosdrin

E863.2 Carbamates
Aldicarb
Carbaryl
Propoxur

E863.3 Mixtures of insecticides

E863.4 Other and unspecified insecticides
Kerosene insecticides

E863.5 Herbicides
2, 4-Dichlorophenoxyacetic acid [2, 4-D]
2, 4, 5-Trichlorophenoxyacetic acid [2, 4, 5-T]
Chlorates
Diquat
Mixtures of plant foods and fertilizers with herbicides
Paraquat

E863.6 Fungicides
Organic mercurials (used in seed dressing)
Pentachlorophenols

E863.7 Rodenticides
Fluoroacetates
Squill and derivatives
Thallium
Warfarin
Zinc phosphide

E863.8 Fumigants
Cyanides
Methyl bromide
Phosphine

E863.9 Other and unspecified

✓4th E864 Accidental poisoning by corrosives and caustics, not elsewhere classified
EXCLUDES *those as components of disinfectants (E861.4)*

E864.0 Corrosive aromatics
Carbolic acid or phenol

E864.1 Acids
Acid:
hydrochloric
nitric
sulfuric

E864.2 Caustic alkalis
Lye

E864.3 Other specified corrosives and caustics

E864.4 Unspecified corrosives and caustics

✓4th E865 Accidental poisoning from poisonous foodstuffs and poisonous plants
INCLUDES any meat, fish, or shellfish
plants, berries, and fungi eaten as, or in mistake for, food, or by a child
EXCLUDES *anaphylactic shock due to adverse food reaction (995.60-995.69)*
food poisoning (bacterial) (005.0-005.9)
poisoning and toxic reactions to venomous plants (E905.6-E905.7)

E865.0 Meat

E865.1 Shellfish

E865.2 Other fish

E865.3 Berries and seeds

E865.4 Other specified plants

E865.5 Mushrooms and other fungi

E865.8 Other specified foods

E865.9 Unspecified foodstuff or poisonous plant

✓4th Fourth-digit Required ▶◀ Revised Text ● New Code ▲ Revised Code Title

E866 Accidental poisoning by other and unspecified solid and liquid substances

EXCLUDES *these substances as a component of:*
medicines (E850.0-E858.9)
paints (E861.5-E861.6)
pesticides (E863.0-E863.9)
petroleum fuels (E862.1)

E866.0 Lead and its compounds and fumes

E866.1 Mercury and its compounds and fumes

E866.2 Antimony and its compounds and fumes

E866.3 Arsenic and its compounds and fumes

E866.4 Other metals and their compounds and fumes

Beryllium (compounds)
Brass fumes
Cadmium (compounds)
Copper salts
Iron (compounds)
Manganese (compounds)
Nickel (compounds)
Thallium (compounds)

E866.5 Plant foods and fertilizers

EXCLUDES *mixtures with herbicides (E863.5)*

E866.6 Glues and adhesives

E866.7 Cosmetics

E866.8 Other specified solid or liquid substances

E866.9 Unspecified solid or liquid substance

E867 Accidental poisoning by gas distributed by pipeline

Carbon monoxide from incomplete combustion of piped gas
Coal gas NOS
Liquefied petroleum gas distributed through pipes (pure or mixed with air)
Piped gas (natural) (manufactured)

E868 Accidental poisoning by other utility gas and other carbon monoxide

E868.0 Liquefied petroleum gas distributed in mobile containers

Butane
Liquefied hydrocarbon gas NOS
Propane
} or carbon monoxide from incomplete conbustion of these gases

E868.1 Other and unspecified utility gas

Acetylene
Gas NOS used for lighting, heating, or cooking
Water gas
} or carbon monoxide from incomplete conbustion of these gases

E868.2 Motor vehicle exhaust gas

Exhaust gas from:
farm tractor, not in transit
gas engine
motor pump
motor vehicle, not in transit
any type of combustion engine not in watercraft

EXCLUDES *poisoning by carbon monoxide from:*
aircraft while in transit (E844.0-E844.9)
motor vehicle while in transit (E818.0-E818.9)
watercraft whether or not in transit (E838.0-E838.9)

E868.3 Carbon monoxide from incomplete combustion of other domestic fuels

Carbon monoxide from incomplete combustion of:
coal
coke
kerosene
wood
} in domestic stove or fireplace

EXCLUDES *carbon monoxide from smoke and fumes due to conflagration (E890.0-E893.9)*

E868.8 Carbon monoxide from other sources

Carbon monoxide from:
blast furnace gas
incomplete combustion of fuels in industrial use
kiln vapor

E868.9 Unspecified carbon monoxide

E869 Accidental poisoning by other gases and vapors

EXCLUDES *effects of gases used as anesthetics (E855.1, E938.2)*
fumes from heavy metals (E866.0-E866.4)
smoke and fumes due to conflagration or explosion (E890.0-E899)

E869.0 Nitrogen oxides

E869.1 Sulfur dioxide

E869.2 Freon

E869.3 Lacrimogenic gas [tear gas]

Bromobenzyl cyanide
Chloroacetophenone
Ethyliodoacetate

E869.4 Second-hand tobacco smoke

E869.8 Other specified gases and vapors

Chlorine
Hydrocyanic acid gas

E869.9 Unspecified gases and vapors

MISADVENTURES TO PATIENTS DURING SURGICAL AND MEDICAL CARE (E870-E876)

EXCLUDES *accidental overdose of drug and wrong drug given in error (E850.0-E858.9)*
surgical and medical procedures as the cause of abnormal reaction by the patient, without mention of misadventure at the time of procedure (E878.0-E879.9)

E870 Accidental cut, puncture, perforation, or hemorrhage during medical care

E870.0 Surgical operation

E870.1 Infusion or transfusion

E870.2 Kidney dialysis or other perfusion

E870.3 Injection or vaccination

E870.4 Endoscopic examination

E870.5 Aspiration of fluid or tissue, puncture, and catheterization

Abdominal paracentesis
Aspirating needle biopsy
Blood sampling
Lumbar puncture
Thoracentesis

EXCLUDES *heart catheterization (E870.6)*

E870.6 Heart catheterization

E870.7 Administration of enema

E870.8 Other specified medical care

E870.9 Unspecified medical care

E871 Foreign object left in body during procedure

E871.0 Surgical operation

E871.1 Infusion or transfusion

E871.2 Kidney dialysis or other perfusion

E871.3 Injection or vaccination

E871.4 Endoscopic examination

E871.5 Aspiration of fluid or tissue, puncture, and catheterization

Abdominal paracentesis
Aspiration needle biopsy
Blood sampling
Lumbar puncture
Thoracentesis

EXCLUDES *heart catheterization (E871.6)*

E871.6 Heart catheterization

E871.7 Removal of catheter or packing

E871.8 Other specified procedures

E871.9 Unspecified procedure

E872 Failure of sterile precautions during procedure

E872.0 Surgical operation

E872.1 Infusion or transfusion

E872.2 Kidney dialysis and other perfusion

E872.3 Injection or vaccination

E872.4 Endoscopic examination

E872.5 Aspiration of fluid or tissue, puncture, and catheterization

Abdominal paracentesis
Aspiration needle biopsy
Blood sampling
Lumbar puncture
Thoracentesis

EXCLUDES *heart catheterization (E872.6)*

4th Fourth-digit Required ▶◀ Revised Text ● New Code ▲ Revised Code Title

E872.6 Heart catheterization

E872.8 Other specified procedures

E872.9 Unspecified procedure

✓4th E873 Failure in dosage

EXCLUDES *accidental overdose of drug, medicinal or biological substance (E850.0-E858.9)*

E873.0 Excessive amount of blood or other fluid during transfusion or infusion

E873.1 Incorrect dilution of fluid during infusion

E873.2 Overdose of radiation in therapy

E873.3 Inadvertent exposure of patient to radiation during medical care

E873.4 Failure in dosage in electroshock or insulin-shock therapy

E873.5 Inappropriate [too hot or too cold] temperature in local application and packing

E873.6 Nonadministration of necessary drug or medicinal substance

E873.8 Other specified failure in dosage

E873.9 Unspecified failure in dosage

✓4th E874 Mechanical failure of instrument or apparatus during procedure

E874.0 Surgical operation

E874.1 Infusion and transfusion

Air in system

E874.2 Kidney dialysis and other perfusion

E874.3 Endoscopic examination

E874.4 Aspiration of fluid or tissue, puncture, and catheterization

Abdominal paracentesis
Aspiration needle biopsy
Blood sampling
Lumbar puncture
Thoracentesis

EXCLUDES *heart catheterization (E874.5)*

E874.5 Heart catheterization

E874.8 Other specified procedures

E874.9 Unspecified procedure

✓4th E875 Contaminated or infected blood, other fluid, drug, or biological substance

INCLUDES presence of:
bacterial pyrogens
endotoxin-producing bacteria
serum hepatitis-producing agent

E875.0 Contaminated substance transfused or infused

E875.1 Contaminated substance injected or used for vaccination

E875.2 Contaminated drug or biological substance administered by other means

E875.8 Other

E875.9 Unspecified

✓4th E876 Other and unspecified misadventures during medical care

E876.0 Mismatched blood in transfusion

E876.1 Wrong fluid in infusion

E876.2 Failure in suture and ligature during surgical operation

E876.3 Endotracheal tube wrongly placed during anesthetic procedure

E876.4 Failure to introduce or to remove other tube or instrument

EXCLUDES *foreign object left in body during procedure (E871.0-E871.9)*

E876.5 Performance of inappropriate operation

E876.8 Other specified misadventures during medical care

Performance of inappropriate treatment NEC

E876.9 Unspecified misadventure during medical care

SURGICAL AND MEDICAL PROCEDURES AS THE CAUSE OF ABNORMAL REACTION OF PATIENT OR LATER COMPLICATION, WITHOUT MENTION OF MISADVENTURE AT THE TIME OF PROCEDURE (E878-E879)

INCLUDES procedures as the cause of abnormal reaction, such as:
displacement or malfunction of prosthetic device
hepatorenal failure, postoperative
malfunction of external stoma
postoperative intestinal obstruction
rejection of transplanted organ

EXCLUDES *anesthetic management properly carried out as the cause of adverse effect (E937.0-E938.9)*
infusion and transfusion, without mention of misadventure in the technique of procedure (E930.0-E949.9)

✓4th E878 Surgical operation and other surgical procedures as the cause of abnormal reaction of patient, or of later complication, without mention of misadventure at the time of operation

E878.0 Surgical operation with transplant of whole organ

Transplantation of:
heart
kidney
Transplantation of:
liver

E878.1 Surgical operation with implant of artificial internal device

Cardiac pacemaker
Electrodes implanted in brain
Heart valve prosthesis
Internal orthopedic device

E878.2 Surgical operation with anastomosis, bypass, or graft, with natural or artificial tissues used as implant

Anastomosis:
arteriovenous
gastrojejunal
Graft of blood vessel, tendon, or skin

EXCLUDES *external stoma (E878.3)*

E878.3 Surgical operation with formation of external stoma

Colostomy
Cystostomy
Duodenostomy
Gastrostomy
Ureterostomy

E878.4 Other restorative surgery

E878.5 Amputation of limb(s)

E878.6 Removal of other organ (partial) (total)

E878.8 Other specified surgical operations and procedures

E878.9 Unspecified surgical operations and procedures

✓4th E879 Other procedures, without mention of misadventure at the time of procedure, as the cause of abnormal reaction of patient, or of later complication

E879.0 Cardiac catheterization

E879.1 Kidney dialysis

E879.2 Radiological procedure and radiotherapy

EXCLUDES *radio-opaque dyes for diagnostic x-ray procedures (E947.8)*

E879.3 Shock therapy

Electroshock therapy
Insulin-shock therapy

E879.4 Aspiration of fluid

Lumbar puncture
Thoracentesis

E879.5 Insertion of gastric or duodenal sound

E879.6 Urinary catheterization

E879.7 Blood sampling

E879.8 Other specified procedures

Blood transfusion

E879.9 Unspecified procedure

ACCIDENTAL FALLS (E880-E888)

EXCLUDES *falls (in or from):*
burning building (E890.8, E891.8)
into fire (E890.0-E899)
into water (with submersion or drowning) (E910.0-E910.9)
machinery (in operation) (E919.0-E919.9)
on edged, pointed, or sharp object (E920.0-E920.9)
transport vehicle (E800.0-E845.9)
vehicle not elsewhere classifiable (E846-E848)

E880 Fall on or from stairs or steps (4th)
E880.0 Escalator
E880.1 Fall on or from sidewalk curb
EXCLUDES *fall from moving sidewalk (E885.9)*
E880.9 Other stairs or steps

E881 Fall on or from ladders or scaffolding (4th)
E881.0 Fall from ladder
E881.1 Fall from scaffolding

E882 Fall from or out of building or other structure
Fall from:
balcony
bridge
building
flagpole
tower
turret
viaduct
wall
window
Fall through roof
EXCLUDES *collapse of a building or structure (E916)*
fall or jump from burning building (E890.8, E891.8)

E883 Fall into hole or other opening in surface (4th)
INCLUDES fall into:
cavity
dock
hole
pit
quarry
shaft
swimming pool
tank
well
EXCLUDES *fall into water NOS (E910.9)*
that resulting in drowning or submersion without mention of injury (E910.0-E910.9)
E883.0 Accident from diving or jumping into water [swimming pool]
Strike or hit:
against bottom when jumping or diving into water
wall or board of swimming pool
water surface
EXCLUDES *diving with insufficient air supply (E913.2)*
effects of air pressure from diving (E902.2)
E883.1 Accidental fall into well
E883.2 Accidental fall into storm drain or manhole
E883.9 Fall into other hole or other opening in surface

E884 Other fall from one level to another (4th)
E884.0 Fall from playground equipment
EXCLUDES *recreational machinery (E919.8)*
E884.1 Fall from cliff
E884.2 Fall from chair
E884.3 Fall from wheelchair
E884.4 Fall from bed
E884.5 Fall from other furniture
E884.6 Fall from commode
Toilet
E884.9 Other fall from one level to another
Fall from:
embankment
haystack
stationary vehicle
tree

E885 Fall on same level from slipping, tripping, or stumbling (4th)
E885.0 Fall from (nonmotorized) scooter
E885.1 Fall from roller skates
In-line skates
E885.2 Fall from skateboard
E885.3 Fall from skis
E885.4 Fall from snowboard
E885.9 Fall from other slipping, tripping, or stumbling
Fall on moving sidewalk

E886 Fall on same level from collision, pushing, or shoving, by or with other person (4th)
EXCLUDES *crushed or pushed by a crowd or human stampede (E917.1, E917.6)*
E886.0 In sports
Tackles in sports
EXCLUDES *kicked, stepped on, struck by object, in sports (E917.0, E917.5)*
E886.9 Other and unspecified
Fall from collision of pedestrian (conveyance) with another pedestrian (conveyance)

E887 Fracture, cause unspecified

E888 Other and unspecified fall (4th)
Accidental fall NOS
Fall on same level NOS
E888.0 Fall resulting in striking against sharp object
Use additional external cause code to identify object (E920)
E888.1 Fall resulting in striking against other object
E888.8 Other fall
E888.9 Unspecified fall
Fall NOS

ACCIDENTS CAUSED BY FIRE AND FLAMES (E890-E899)

INCLUDES asphyxia or poisoning due to conflagration or ignition
burning by fire
secondary fires resulting from explosion
EXCLUDES *arson (E968.0)*
fire in or on:
machinery (in operation) (E919.0-E919.9)
transport vehicle other than stationary vehicle (E800.0-E845.9)
vehicle not elsewhere classifiable (E846-E848)

E890 Conflagration in private dwelling (4th)
INCLUDES conflagration in:
apartment
boarding house
camping place
caravan
farmhouse
house
lodging house
mobile home
private garage
rooming house
tenement
conflagration originating from sources classifiable to E893-E898 in the above buildings
E890.0 Explosion caused by conflagration
E890.1 Fumes from combustion of polyvinylchloride [PVC] and similar material in conflagration
E890.2 Other smoke and fumes from conflagration
Carbon monoxide, Fumes NOS, Smoke NOS } from conflagration in private building
E890.3 Burning caused by conflagration
E890.8 Other accident resulting from conflagration
Collapse of, Fall from, Hit by object falling from, Jump from } burning private building
E890.9 Unspecified accident resulting from conflagration in private dwelling

4th Fourth-digit Required ⧓ Revised Text ● New Code ▲ Revised Code Title

✓4th E891 Conflagration in other and unspecified building or structure

Conflagration in:
- barn
- church
- convalescent and other residential home
- dormitory of educational institution
- factory
- farm outbuildings
- hospital
- hotel
- school
- store
- theater

Conflagration originating from sources classifiable to E893-E898, in the above buildings

E891.0 Explosion caused by conflagration

E891.1 Fumes from combustion of polyvinylchloride [PVC] and similar material in conflagration

E891.2 Other smoke and fumes from conflagration

Carbon monoxide, Fumes NOS, Smoke NOS } from conflagration in building or structure

E891.3 Burning caused by conflagration

E891.8 Other accident resulting from conflagration

Collapse of, Fall from, Hit by object falling from, Jump from } burning building or structure

E891.9 Unspecified accident resulting from conflagration of other and unspecified building or structure

E892 Conflagration not in building or structure

Fire (uncontrolled) (in) (of):
- forest
- grass
- hay
- lumber
- mine
- prairie
- transport vehicle [any], except while in transit
- tunnel

✓4th E893 Accident caused by ignition of clothing

EXCLUDES *ignition of clothing:*
from highly inflammable material (E894)
with conflagration (E890.0-E892)

E893.0 From controlled fire in private dwelling

Ignition of clothing from:
normal fire (charcoal) (coal) (electric) (gas) (wood) in: brazier, fireplace, furnace, stove } in private dwelling (as listed in E890)

E893.1 From controlled fire in other building or structure

Ignition of clothing from:
normal fire (charcoal) (coal) (electric) (gas) (wood) in: brazier, fireplace, furnace, stove } in other building or structure (as listed in E81)

E893.2 From controlled fire not in building or structure

Ignition of clothing from:
- bonfire (controlled)
- brazier fire (controlled), not in building or structure
- trash fire (controlled)

EXCLUDES *conflagration not in building (E892)*
trash fire out of control (E892)

E893.8 From other specified sources

Ignition of clothing from:
- blowlamp
- blowtorch
- burning bedspread
- candle
- cigar
- cigarette
- lighter
- matches
- pipe
- welding torch

E893.9 Unspecified source

Ignition of clothing (from controlled fire NOS) (in building NOS) NOS

E894 Ignition of highly inflammable material

Ignition of:
benzine, gasoline, fat, kerosene, paraffin, petrol } (with ignition of clothing)

EXCLUDES *ignition of highly inflammable material with:*
conflagration (E890.0-E892)
explosion (E923.0-E923.9)

E895 Accident caused by controlled fire in private dwelling

Burning by (flame of) normal fire (charcoal) (coal) (electric) (gas) (wood) in: brazier, fireplace, furnace, stove } in private dwelling (as listed in E890)

EXCLUDES *burning by hot objects not producing fire or flames (E924.0-E924.9)*
ignition of clothing from these sources (E893.0)
poisoning by carbon monoxide from incomplete combustion of fuel (E867-E868.9)
that with conflagration (E890.0-E890.9)

E896 Accident caused by controlled fire in other and unspecified building or structure

Burning by (flame of) normal fire (charcoal) (coal) (electric) (gas) (wood) in:
brazier, fireplace, furnace, stove } in other building or structure (as listed in E891)

EXCLUDES *burning by hot objects not producing fire or flames (E924.0-E924.9)*
ignition of clothing from these sources (E893.1)
poisoning by carbon monoxide from incomplete combustion of fuel (E867-E868.9)
that with conflagration (E891.0-E891.9)

E897 Accident caused by controlled fire not in building or structure

Burns from flame of:
bonfire, brazier fire, not in building or structure, trash fire } controlled

EXCLUDES *ignition of clothing from these sources (E893.2)*
trash fire out of control (E892)
that with conflagration (E892)

✓4th E898 Accident caused by other specified fire and flames

EXCLUDES *conflagration (E890.0-E892)*
that with ignition of:
clothing (E893.0-E893.9)
highly inflammable material (E894)

E898.0 Burning bedclothes

Bed set on fire NOS

E898.1 Other

Burning by:
- blowlamp
- blowtorch
- candle
- cigar
- cigarette
- fire in room NOS
- lamp
- lighter
- matches
- pipe
- welding torch

E899 Accident caused by unspecified fire

Burning NOS

ACCIDENTS DUE TO NATURAL AND ENVIRONMENTAL FACTORS (E900-E909)

✓4th E900 Excessive heat

E900.0 Due to weather conditions

Excessive heat as the external cause of:
- ictus solaris
- siriasis
- sunstroke

E900.1 Of man-made origin
Heat (in):
boiler room
drying room
factory
furnace room
Heat (in):
generated in transport vehicle
kitchen

E900.9 Of unspecified origin

E901 Excessive cold

E901.0 Due to weather conditions
Excessive cold as the cause of:
chilblains NOS
immersion foot

E901.1 Of man-made origin
Contact with or inhalation of:
dry ice
liquid air
liquid hydrogen
liquid nitrogen
Prolonged exposure in:
deep freeze unit
refrigerator

E901.8 Other specified origin

E901.9 Of unspecified origin

E902 High and low air pressure and changes in air pressure

E902.0 Residence or prolonged visit at high altitude
Residence or prolonged visit at high altitude as the cause of:
Acosta syndrome
Alpine sickness
altitude sickness
Andes disease
anoxia, hypoxia
barotitis, barodontalgia, barosinusitis, otitic barotrauma
hypobarism, hypobaropathy
mountain sickness
range disease

E902.1 In aircraft
Sudden change in air pressure in aircraft during ascent or descent as the cause of:
aeroneurosis
aviators' disease

E902.2 Due to diving
High air pressure from rapid descent in water
Reduction in atmospheric pressure while surfacing from deep water diving
} as the cause of:
caisson disease
divers' disease
divers' palsy or paralysis

E902.8 Due to other specified causes
Reduction in atmospheric pressure whilesurfacing from underground

E902.9 Unspecified cause

E903 Travel and motion

E904 Hunger, thirst, exposure, and neglect
EXCLUDES *any condition resulting from homicidal intent (E968.0-E968.9)*
hunger, thirst, and exposure resulting from accidents connected with transport (E800.0-E848)

E904.0 Abandonment or neglect of infants and helpless persons
Exposure to weather conditions
Hunger or thirst
} resulting from abandonment or neglect

Desertion of newborn
Inattention at or after birth
Lack of care (helpless person) (infant)
EXCLUDES *criminal [purposeful] neglect (E968.4)*

E904.1 Lack of food
Lack of food as the cause of:
inanition
insufficient nourishment
starvation
EXCLUDES *hunger resulting from abandonment or neglect (E904.0)*

E904.2 Lack of water
Lack of water as the cause of:
dehydration
inanition
EXCLUDES *dehydration due to acute fluid loss ▶(276.51)◀*

E904.3 Exposure (to weather conditions), not elsewhere classifiable
Exposure NOS
Humidity
Struck by hailstones
EXCLUDES *struck by lightning (E907)*

E904.9 Privation, unqualified
Destitution

E905 Venomous animals and plants as the cause of poisoning and toxic reactions
INCLUDES chemical released by animal
insects
release of venom through fangs, hairs, spines, tentacles, and other venom apparatus
EXCLUDES *eating of poisonous animals or plants (E865.0-E865.9)*

E905.0 Venomous snakes and lizards
Cobra
Copperhead snake
Coral snake
Fer de lance
Gila monster
Krait
Mamba
Rattlesnake
Sea snake
Snake (venomous)
Viper
Water moccasin
EXCLUDES *bites of snakes and lizards known to be nonvenomous (E906.2)*

E905.1 Venomous spiders
Black widow spider
Brown spider
Tarantula (venomous)

E905.2 Scorpion

E905.3 Hornets, wasps, and bees
Yellow jacket

E905.4 Centipede and venomous millipede (tropical)

E905.5 Other venomous arthropods
Sting of:
ant
Sting of:
caterpillar

E905.6 Venomous marine animals and plants
Puncture by sea urchin spine
Sting of:
coral
jelly fish
nematocysts
Sting of:
sea anemone
sea cucumber
other marine animal or plant
EXCLUDES *bites and other injuries caused by nonvenomous marine animal (E906.2-E906.8)*
bite of sea snake (venomous) (E905.0)

E905.7 Poisoning and toxic reactions caused by other plants
Injection of poisons or toxins into or through skin by plant thorns, spines, or other mechanisms
EXCLUDES *puncture wound NOS by plant thorns or spines (E920.8)*

E905.8 Other specified

E905.9 Unspecified
Sting NOS
Venomous bite NOS

E906 Other injury caused by animals
EXCLUDES *poisoning and toxic reactions caused by venomous animals and insects (E905.0-E905.9)*
road vehicle accident involving animals (E827.0-E828.9)
tripping or falling over an animal (E885.9)

Fourth-digit Required ▶◀ Revised Text ● New Code ▲ Revised Code Title

E906.0 Dog bite

E906.1 Rat bite

E906.2 Bite of nonvenomous snakes and lizards

E906.3 Bite of other animal except arthropod

Cats
Moray eel
Rodents, except rats
Shark

E906.4 Bite of nonvenomous arthropod

Insect bite NOS

E906.5 Bite by unspecified animal

Animal bite NOS

E906.8 Other specified injury caused by animal

Butted by animal
Fallen on by horse or other animal, not being ridden
Gored by animal
Implantation of quills of porcupine
Pecked by bird
Run over by animal, not being ridden
Stepped on by animal, not being ridden

EXCLUDES *injury by animal being ridden (E828.0-E828.9)*

E906.9 Unspecified injury caused by animal

E907 Lightning

EXCLUDES *injury from:*
fall of tree or other object caused by lightning (E916)
fire caused by lightning (E890.0-E892)

4th **E908 Cataclysmic storms, and floods resulting from storms**

EXCLUDES *collapse of dam or man-made structure causing flood (E909.3)*

E908.0 Hurricane

Storm surge
"Tidal wave" caused by storm action
Typhoon

E908.1 Tornado

Cyclone
Twisters

E908.2 Floods

Torrential rainfall
Flash flood

EXCLUDES *collapse of dam or man-made structure causing flood (E909.3)*

E908.3 Blizzard (snow) (ice)

E908.4 Dust storm

E908.8 Other cataclysmic storms

E908.9 Unspecified cataclysmic storms, and floods resulting from storms

Storm NOS

4th **E909 Cataclysmic earth surface movements and eruptions**

E909.0 Earthquakes

E909.1 Volcanic eruptions

Burns from lava
Ash inhalation

E909.2 Avalanche, landslide, or mudslide

E909.3 Collapse of dam or man-made structure

E909.4 Tidalwave caused by earthquake

Tidalwave NOS
Tsunami

EXCLUDES *tidalwave caused by tropical storm (E908.0)*

E909.8 Other cataclysmic earth surface movements and eruptions

E909.9 Unspecified cataclysmic earth surface movements and eruptions

ACCIDENTS CAUSED BY SUBMERSION, SUFFOCATION, AND FOREIGN BODIES (E910-E915)

4th **E910 Accidental drowning and submersion**

INCLUDES immersion
swimmers' cramp

EXCLUDES *diving accident (NOS) (resulting in injury except drowning) (E883.0)*
diving with insufficient air supply (E913.2)
drowning and submersion due to:
cataclysm (E908-E909)
machinery accident (E919.0-E919.9)
transport accident (E800.0-E845.9)
effect of high and low air pressure (E902.2)
injury from striking against objects while in running water (E917.2)

E910.0 While water-skiing

Fall from water skis with submersion or drowning

EXCLUDES *accident to water-skier involving a watercraft and resulting in submersion or other injury (E830.4, E831.4)*

E910.1 While engaged in other sport or recreational activity with diving equipment

Scuba diving NOS
Skin diving NOS
Underwater spear fishing NOS

E910.2 While engaged in other sport or recreational activity without diving equipment

Fishing or hunting, except from boat or with diving equipment
Ice skating
Playing in water
Surfboarding
Swimming NOS
Voluntarily jumping from boat, not involved in accident, for swim NOS
Wading in water

EXCLUDES *jumping into water to rescue another person (E910.3)*

E910.3 While swimming or diving for purposes other than recreation or sport

Marine salvage
Pearl diving
Placement of fishing nets
Rescue (attempt) of another person
Underwater construction or repairs
} (with diving equipment)

E910.4 In bathtub

E910.8 Other accidental drowning or submersion

Drowning in:
quenching tank
Drowning in:
swimming pool

E910.9 Unspecified accidental drowning or submersion

Accidental fall into water NOS
Drowning NOS

E911 Inhalation and ingestion of food causing obstruction of respiratory tract or suffocation

Aspiration and inhalation of food [any] (into respiratory tract) NOS

Asphyxia by
Choked on
Suffocation by
} food [including bone, seed in food, regurgitated food]

Compression of trachea
Interruption of respiration
Obstruction of respiration
} by food lodged in esophagus

Obstruction of pharynx by food (bolus)

EXCLUDES *injury, except asphyxia and obstruction of respiratory passage, caused by food (E915)*
obstruction of esophagus by food without mention of asphyxia or obstruction of respiratory passage (E915)

E912 Inhalation and ingestion of other object causing obstruction of respiratory tract or suffocation

Aspiration and inhalation of foreign body except food (into respiratory tract) NOS
Foreign object [bean] [marble] in nose
Obstruction of pharynx by foreign body
Compression, Interruption of respiration, Obstruction of respiration } by foreign body in esophagus

EXCLUDES *injury, except asphyxia and obstruction of respiratory passage, caused by foreign body (E915)*
obstruction of esophagus by foreign body without mention of asphyxia or obstruction in respiratory passage (E915)

✓4th **E913 Accidental mechanical suffocation**

EXCLUDES *mechanical suffocation from or by:*
accidental inhalation or ingestion of:
food (E911)
foreign object (E912)
cataclysm (E908-E909)
explosion (E921.0-E921.9, E923.0-E923.9)
machinery accident (E919.0-E919.9)

E913.0 In bed or cradle

EXCLUDES *suffocation by plastic bag (E913.1)*

E913.1 By plastic bag

E913.2 Due to lack of air (in closed place)

Accidentally closed up in refrigerator or other airtight enclosed space
Diving with insufficient air supply

EXCLUDES *suffocation by plastic bag (E913.1)*

E913.3 By falling earth or other substance

Cave-in NOS

EXCLUDES *cave-in caused by cataclysmic earth surface movements and eruptions (E909)*
struck by cave-in without asphyxiation or suffocation (E916)

E913.8 Other specified means

Accidental hanging, except in bed or cradle

E913.9 Unspecified means

Asphyxia, mechanical NOS
Suffocation NOS
Strangulation NOS

E914 Foreign body accidentally entering eye and adnexa

EXCLUDES *corrosive liquid (E924.1)*

E915 Foreign body accidentally entering other orifice

EXCLUDES *aspiration and inhalation of foreign body, any, (into respiratory tract) NOS (E911-E912)*

OTHER ACCIDENTS (E916-E928)

E916 Struck accidentally by falling object

Collapse of building, except on fire
Falling:
rock
snowslide NOS
stone
tree
Object falling from:
machine, not in operation
stationary vehicle

Code first:
collapse of building on fire (E890.0-E891.9)
falling object in:
cataclysm (E908-E909)
machinery accidents (E919.0-E919.9)
transport accidents (E800.0-E845.9)
vehicle accidents not elsewhere classifiable (E846-E848)
object set in motion by:
explosion (E921.0-E921.9, E923.0-E923.9)
firearm (E922.0-E922.9)
projected object (E917.0-E917.9)

✓4th **E917 Striking against or struck accidentally by objects or persons**

INCLUDES bumping into or against, colliding with, kicking against, stepping on, struck by } object (moving) (projected) (stationary), pedestrian conveyance, person

EXCLUDES *fall from:*
collision with another person, except when caused by a crowd (E886.0-E886.9)
stumbling over object (E885.9)
fall resulting in striking against object (E888.0, E888.1)
injury caused by:
assault (E960.0-E960.1, E967.0-E967.9)
cutting or piercing instrument (E920.0-E920.9)
explosion (E921.0-E921.9, E923.0-E923.9)
firearm (E922.0-E922.9)
machinery (E919.0-E919.9)
transport vehicle (E800.0-E845.9)
vehicle not elsewhere classifiable (E846-E848)

E917.0 In sports without subsequent fall

Kicked or stepped on during game (football) (rugby)
Struck by hit or thrown ball
Struck by hockey stick or puck

E917.1 Caused by a crowd, by collective fear or panic without subsequent fall

Crushed, Pushed, Stepped on } by crowd or human stampede

E917.2 In running water without subsequent fall

EXCLUDES *drowning or submersion (E910.0-E910.9)*
that in sports (E917.0, E917.5)

E917.3 Furniture without subsequent fall

EXCLUDES *fall from furniture (E884.2, E884.4-E884.5)*

E917.4 Other stationary object without subsequent fall

Bath tub
Fence
Lamp-post

E917.5 Object in sports with subsequent fall

Knocked down while boxing

E917.6 Caused by a crowd, by collective fear or panic with subsequent fall

E917.7 Furniture with subsequent fall

EXCLUDES *fall from furniture (E884.2, E884.4-E884.5)*

E917.8 Other stationary object with subsequent fall

Bath tub
Fence
Lamp-post

E917.9 Other striking against with or without subsequent fall

E918 Caught accidentally in or between objects

Caught, crushed, jammed, or pinched in or between moving or stationary objects, such as:
escalator
folding object
hand tools, appliances, or implements
sliding door and door frame
under packing crate
washing machine wringer

EXCLUDES *injury caused by:*
cutting or piercing instrument (E920.0-E920.9)
machinery (E919.0-E919.9)
transport vehicle (E800.0-E845.9)
vehicle not elsewhere classifiable (E846-E848)
struck accidentally by:
falling object (E916)
object (moving) (projected) (E917.0-E917.9)

✓4th E919 Accidents caused by machinery

INCLUDES burned by | caught in (moving parts of) | collapse of | crushed by | cut or pierced by | drowning or submersion caused by | explosion of, on, in | fall from or into moving part of | fire starting in or on | mechanical suffocation caused by | object falling from, on, in motion by | overturning of | pinned under | run over by | struck by | thrown from } machinery (accident)

caught between machinery and other object
machinery accident NOS

EXCLUDES *accidents involving machinery, not in operation (E884.9, E916-E918)*
injury caused by:
electric current in connection with machinery (E925.0-E925.9)
escalator (E880.0, E918)
explosion of pressure vessel in connection with machinery (E921.0-E921.9)
moving sidewalk (E885.9)
powered hand tools, appliances, and implements (E916-E918, E920.0-E921.9, E923.0-E926.9)
transport vehicle accidents involving machinery (E800.0-E848)
poisoning by carbon monoxide generated by machine (E868.8)

E919.0 Agricultural machines

Animal-powered agricultural machine
Combine
Derrick, hay
Farm machinery NOS
Farm tractor
Harvester
Hay mower or rake
Reaper
Thresher

EXCLUDES *that in transport under own power on the highway (E810.0-E819.9)*
that being towed by another vehicle on the highway (E810.0-E819.9, E827.0-E827.9, E829.0-E829.9)
that involved in accident classifiable to E820-E829 (E820.0-E829.9)

E919.1 Mining and earth-drilling machinery

Bore or drill (land) (seabed)
Shaft hoist
Shaft lift
Under-cutter

EXCLUDES *coal car, tram, truck, and tub in mine (E846)*

E919.2 Lifting machines and appliances

Chain hoist | Crane | Derrick | Elevator (building) (grain) | Forklift truck | Lift | Pulley block | Winch } except in agricultural or mining operations

EXCLUDES *that being towed by another vehicle on the highway (E810.0-E819.9, E827.0-E827.9, E829.0-829.9)*
that in transport under own power on the highway (E810.0-E819.9)
that involved in accident classifiable to E820-E829 (E820.0-E829.9)

E919.3 Metalworking machines

Abrasive wheel
Forging machine
Lathe
Mechanical shears
Metal:
drilling machine
milling machine
power press
rolling-mill
sawing machine

E919.4 Woodworking and forming machines

Band saw
Bench saw
Circular saw
Molding machine
Overhead plane
Powered saw
Radial saw
Sander

EXCLUDES *hand saw (E920.1)*

E919.5 Prime movers, except electrical motors

Gas turbine
Internal combustion engine
Steam engine
Water driven turbine

EXCLUDES *that being towed by other vehicle on the highway (E810.0-E819.9, E827.0-E827.9, E829.0-E829.9)*
that in transport under own power on the highway (E810.0-E819.9)

E919.6 Transmission machinery

Transmission:
belt
cable
chain
gear
Transmission:
pinion
pulley
shaft

E919.7 Earth moving, scraping, and other excavating machines

Bulldozer
Road scraper
Steam shovel

EXCLUDES *that being towed by other vehicle on the highway (E810.0-E819.9, E827.0-E827.9, E829.0-E829.9)*
that in transport under own power on the highway (E810.0-E819.9)

E919.8 Other specified machinery

Machines for manufacture of:
clothing
foodstuffs and beverages
paper
Printing machine
Recreational machinery
Spinning, weaving, and textile machines

E919.9 Unspecified machinery

✓4th E920 Accidents caused by cutting and piercing instruments or objects

INCLUDES accidental injury (by) } object: edged | pointed | sharp

E920.0 Powered lawn mower

E920.1 Other powered hand tools

Any powered hand tool [compressed air] [electric] [explosive cartridge] [hydraulic power], such as:
drill
hand saw
hedge clipper
rivet gun
snow blower
staple gun

EXCLUDES *band saw (E919.4)*
bench saw (E919.4)

E920.2 Powered household appliances and implements

Blender
Electric:
beater or mixer
can opener
Electric:
fan
knife
sewing machine
Garbage disposal appliance

E920.3 Knives, swords, and daggers

E920.4 Other hand tools and implements

Axe
Can opener NOS
Chisel
Fork
Hand saw
Hoe
Ice pick
Needle (sewing)
Paper cutter
Pitchfork
Rake
Scissors
Screwdriver
Sewing machine, not powered
Shovel

E920.5 Hypodermic needle

Contaminated needle
Needle stick

E920.8 Other specified cutting and piercing instruments or objects

Arrow
Broken glass
Dart
Edge of stiff paper
Lathe turnings
Nail
Plant thorn
Splinter
Tin can lid

EXCLUDES *animal spines or quills (E906.8)*
flying glass due to explosion (E921.0-E923.9)

E920.9 Unspecified cutting and piercing instrument or object

✓4th **E921 Accident caused by explosion of pressure vessel**

INCLUDES accidental explosion of pressure vessels, whether or not part of machinery

EXCLUDES *explosion of pressure vessel on transport vehicle (E800.0-E845.9)*

E921.0 Boilers

E921.1 Gas cylinders

Air tank
Pressure gas tank

E921.8 Other specified pressure vessels

Aerosol can
Automobile tire
Pressure cooker

E921.9 Unspecified pressure vessel

✓4th **E922 Accident caused by firearm, and air gun missile**

E922.0 Handgun

Pistol
Revolver

EXCLUDES *Verey pistol (E922.8)*

E922.1 Shotgun (automatic)

E922.2 Hunting rifle

E922.3 Military firearms

Army rifle
Machine gun

E922.4 Air gun

BB gun
Pellet gun

E922.5 Paintball gun

E922.8 Other specified firearm missile

Verey pistol [flare]

E922.9 Unspecified firearm missile

Gunshot wound NOS
Shot NOS

✓4th **E923 Accident caused by explosive material**

INCLUDES flash burns and other injuries resulting from explosion of explosive material
ignition of highly explosive material with explosion

EXCLUDES *explosion:*
in or on machinery (E919.0-E919.9)
on any transport vehicle, except stationary motor vehicle (E800.0-E848)
with conflagration (E890.0, E891.0,E892)
secondary fires resulting from explosion (E890.0-E899)

E923.0 Fireworks

E923.1 Blasting materials

Blasting cap
Detonator
Dynamite
Explosive [any] used in blasting operations

E923.2 Explosive gases

Acetylene
Butane
Coal gas
Explosion in mine NOS
Fire damp
Gasoline fumes
Methane
Propane

E923.8 Other explosive materials

Bomb
Explosive missile
Grenade
Mine
Shell
Torpedo
Explosion in munitions:
dump
factory

E923.9 Unspecified explosive material

Explosion NOS

✓4th **E924 Accident caused by hot substance or object, caustic or corrosive material, and steam**

EXCLUDES *burning NOS (E899)*
chemical burn resulting from swallowing a corrosive substance (E860.0-E864.4)
fire caused by these substances and objects (E890.0-E894)
radiation burns (E926.0-E926.9)
therapeutic misadventures (E870.0-E876.9)

E924.0 Hot liquids and vapors, including steam

Burning or scalding by:
boiling water
hot or boiling liquids not primarily caustic or corrosive
liquid metal
steam
other hot vapor

EXCLUDES *hot (boiling) tap water (E924.2)*

E924.1 Caustic and corrosive substances

Burning by:
acid [any kind]
ammonia
caustic oven cleaner or other substance

Burning by:
corrosive substance
lye
vitriol

E924.2 Hot (boiling) tap water

E924.8 Other

Burning by:
heat from electric heating appliance
hot object NOS
light bulb
steam pipe

E924.9 Unspecified

✓4th **E925 Accident caused by electric current**

INCLUDES electric current from exposed wire, faulty appliance, high voltage cable, live rail, or open electric socket as the cause of:
burn
cardiac fibrillation
convulsion
electric shock
electrocution
puncture wound
respiratory paralysis

EXCLUDES *burn by heat from electrical appliance (E924.8)*
lightning (E907)

E925.0 Domestic wiring and appliances

E925.1 Electric power generating plants, distribution stations, transmission lines

Broken power line

E925.2 Industrial wiring, appliances, and electrical machinery

Conductors
Control apparatus
Electrical equipment and machinery
Transformers

E925.8 Other electric current

Wiring and appliances in or on:
farm [not farmhouse]
outdoors
public building
residential institutions
schools

E925.9 Unspecified electric current
Burns or other injury from electric current NOS
Electric shock NOS
Electrocution NOS

✓4th E926 Exposure to radiation

EXCLUDES *abnormal reaction to or complication of treatment without mention of misadventure (E879.2)*
atomic power plant malfunction in water transport (E838.0-E838.9)
misadventure to patient in surgical and medical procedures (E873.2-E873.3)
use of radiation in war operations (E996-E997.9)

E926.0 Radiofrequency radiation
Overexposure to: microwave radiation, radar radiation, radiofrequency, radiofrequency radiation [any] } from: high-powered radio and television transmitters; industrial radiofrequency induction heaters; radar installations

E926.1 Infrared heaters and lamps
Exposure to infrared radiation from heaters and lamps as the cause of:
blistering
burning
charring
inflammatory change

EXCLUDES *physical contact with heater or lamp (E924.8)*

E926.2 Visible and ultraviolet light sources
Arc lamps
Black light sources
Electrical welding arc
Oxygas welding torch
Sun rays
Tanning bed

EXCLUDES *excessive heat from these sources (E900.1-E900.9)*

E926.3 X-rays and other electromagnetic ionizing radiation
Gamma rays
X-rays (hard) (soft)

E926.4 Lasers

E926.5 Radioactive isotopes
Radiobiologicals
Radiopharmaceuticals

E926.8 Other specified radiation
Artificially accelerated beams of ionized particles generated by:
betatrons
synchrotrons

E926.9 Unspecified radiation
Radiation NOS

E927 Overexertion and strenuous movements
Excessive physical exercise
Overexertion (from):
lifting
pulling
pushing
Strenuous movements in:
recreational activities
other activities

✓4th E928 Other and unspecified environmental and accidental causes

E928.0 Prolonged stay in weightless environment
Weightlessness in spacecraft (simulator)

E928.1 Exposure to noise
Noise (pollution)
Sound waves
Supersonic waves

E928.2 Vibration

E928.3 Human bite

E928.4 External constriction caused by hair

E928.5 External constriction caused by other object

E928.8 Other

E928.9 Unspecified accident
Accident NOS, Blow NOS, Casualty (not due to war), Decapitation } stated as accidentally inflicted

Knocked down, Killed, Injury [any part of body, or unspecified], Mangled, Wound } stated as accidentally inflicted, but not otherwise specified

EXCLUDES *fracture, cause unspecified (E887)*
injuries undetermined whether accidentally or purposely inflicted (E980.0-E989)

LATE EFFECTS OF ACCIDENTAL INJURY (E929)

Note: This category is to be used to indicate accidental injury as the cause of death or disability from late effects, which are themselves classifiable elsewhere. The "late effects" include conditions reported as such, or as sequelae which may occur at any time after the attempted suicide or self-inflicted injury.

✓4th E929 Late effects of accidental injury

EXCLUDES *late effects of:*
surgical and medical procedures (E870.0-E879.9)
therapeutic use of drugs and medicines (E930.0-E949.9)

E929.0 Late effects of motor vehicle accident
Late effects of accidents classifiable to E810-E825

E929.1 Late effects of other transport accident
Late effects of accidents classifiable to E800-E807, E826-E838, E840-E848

E929.2 Late effects of accidental poisoning
Late effects of accidents classifiable to E850-E858, E860-E869

E929.3 Late effects of accidental fall
Late effects of accidents classifiable to E880-E888

E929.4 Late effects of accident caused by fire
Late effects of accidents classifiable to E890-E899

E929.5 Late effects of accident due to natural and environmental factors
Late effects of accidents classifiable to E900-E909

E929.8 Late effects of other accidents
Late effects of accidents classifiable to E910-E928.8

E929.9 Late effects of unspecified accident
Late effects of accidents classifiable to E928.9

DRUGS, MEDICINAL AND BIOLOGICAL SUBSTANCES CAUSING ADVERSE EFFECTS IN THERAPEUTIC USE (E930-E949)

INCLUDES correct drug properly administered in therapeutic or prophylactic dosage, as the cause of any adverse effect including allergic or hypersensitivity reactions

EXCLUDES *accidental overdose of drug and wrong drug given or taken in error (E850.0-E858.9)*
accidents in the technique of administration of drug or biological substance, such as accidental puncture during injection, or contamination of drug (E870.0-E876.9)
administration with suicidal or homicidal intent or intent to harm, or in circumstances classifiable to E980-E989 (E950.0-E950.5, E962.0, E980.0-E980.5)

See Alphabetic Index for more complete list of specific drugs to be classified under the fourth-digit subdivisions. The American Hospital Formulary numbers can be used to classify new drugs listed by the American Hospital Formulary Service (AHFS). See Appendix C.

✓4th E930 Antibiotics

EXCLUDES *that used as eye, ear, nose, and throat [ENT], and local anti-infectives (E946.0-E946.9)*

E930.0 Penicillins
Natural
Synthetic
Semisynthetic, such as:
ampicillin
cloxacillin
nafcillin
oxacillin

E930.1 Antifungal antibiotics
Amphotericin B
Griseofulvin
Hachimycin [trichomycin]
Nystatin

E930.2 Chloramphenicol group
Chloramphenicol
Thiamphenicol

E930.3 Erythromycin and other macrolides
Oleandomycin
Spiramycin

E930.4 Tetracycline group
Doxycycline
Minocycline
Oxytetracycline

E930.5 Cephalosporin group
Cephalexin
Cephaloglycin
Cephaloridine
Cephalothin

E930.6 Antimycobacterial antibiotics
Cycloserine
Kanamycin
Rifampin
Streptomycin

E930.7 Antineoplastic antibiotics
Actinomycins, such as:
Bleomycin
Cactinomycin
Dactinomycin
Daunorubicin
Mitomycin
EXCLUDES *other antineoplastic drugs (E933.1)*

E930.8 Other specified antibiotics

E930.9 Unspecified antibiotic

4th E931 Other anti-infectives
EXCLUDES *ENT, and local anti-infectives (E946.0-E946.9)*

E931.0 Sulfonamides
Sulfadiazine
Sulfafurazole
Sulfamethoxazole

E931.1 Arsenical anti-infectives

E931.2 Heavy metal anti-infectives
Compounds of:
antimony
bismuth
lead
mercury
EXCLUDES *mercurial diuretics (E944.0)*

E931.3 Quinoline and hydroxyquinoline derivatives
Chiniofon
Diiodohydroxyquin
EXCLUDES *antimalarial drugs (E931.4)*

E931.4 Antimalarials and drugs acting on other blood protozoa
Chloroquine phosphate
Cycloguanil
Primaquine
Proguanil [chloroguanide]
Pyrimethamine
Quinine (sulphate)

E931.5 Other antiprotozoal drugs
Emetine

E931.6 Anthelmintics
Hexylresorcinol
Male fern oleoresin
Piperazine
Thiabendazole

E931.7 Antiviral drugs
Methisazone
EXCLUDES *amantadine (E936.4)*
cytarabine (E933.1)
idoxuridine (E946.5)

E931.8 Other antimycobacterial drugs
Ethambutol
Ethionamide
Isoniazid
Para-aminosalicylic acid derivatives
Sulfones

E931.9 Other and unspecified anti-infectives
Flucytosine
Nitrofuranderivatives

4th E932 Hormones and synthetic substitutes

E932.0 Adrenal cortical steroids
Cortisone derivatives
Desoxycorticosterone derivatives
Fluorinated corticosteroid

E932.1 Androgens and anabolic congeners
Nandrolone phenpropionate
Oxymetholone
Testosterone and preparations

E932.2 Ovarian hormones and synthetic substitutes
Contraceptives, oral
Estrogens
Estrogens and progestogens combined
Progestogens

E932.3 Insulins and antidiabetic agents
Acetohexamide
Biguanide derivatives, oral
Chlorpropamide
Glucagon
Insulin
Phenformin
Sulfonylurea derivatives, oral
Tolbutamide
EXCLUDES *adverse effect of insulin administered for shock therapy (E879.3)*

E932.4 Anterior pituitary hormones
Corticotropin
Gonadotropin
Somatotropin [growth hormone]

E932.5 Posterior pituitary hormones
Vasopressin
EXCLUDES *oxytocic agents (E945.0)*

E932.6 Parathyroid and parathyroid derivatives

E932.7 Thyroid and thyroid derivatives
Dextrothyroxine
Levothyroxine sodium
Liothyronine
Thyroglobulin

E932.8 Antithyroid agents
Iodides
Thiouracil
Thiourea

E932.9 Other and unspecified hormones and synthetic substitutes

4th E933 Primarily systemic agents

E933.0 Antiallergic and antiemetic drugs
Antihistamines
Chlorpheniramine
Diphenhydramine
Diphenylpyraline
Thonzylamine
Tripelennamine
EXCLUDES *phenothiazine-based tranquilizers (E939.1)*

E933.1 Antineoplastic and immunosuppressive drugs
Azathioprine
Busulfan
Chlorambucil
Cyclophosphamide
Cytarabine
Fluorouracil
Mechlorethamine hydrochloride
Mercaptopurine
Triethylenethiophosphoramide [thio-TEPA]
EXCLUDES *antineoplastic antibiotics (E930.7)*

E933.2 Acidifying agents

E933.3 Alkalizing agents

E933.4 Enzymes, not elsewhere classified
Penicillinase

E933.5 Vitamins, not elsewhere classified
Vitamin A
Vitamin D
EXCLUDES *nicotinic acid (E942.2)*
vitamin K (E934.3)

E933.8 Other systemic agents, not elsewhere classified
Heavy metal antagonists

E933.9 Unspecified systemic agent

4th E934 Agents primarily affecting blood constituents

E934.0 Iron and its compounds
Ferric salts
Ferrous sulphate and other ferrous salts

E934.1 Liver preparations and other antianemic agents
Folic acid

E934.2 Anticoagulants
Coumarin
Heparin
Phenindione
Prothrombin synthesis inhibitor
Warfarin sodium

E934.3 Vitamin K [phytonadione]

E934.4 Fibrinolysis-affecting drugs
Aminocaproic acid
Streptodornase
Streptokinase
Urokinase

E934.5 Anticoagulant antagonists and other coagulants
Hexadimethrine bromide
Protamine sulfate

E934.6 Gamma globulin

E934.7 Natural blood and blood products
Blood plasma
Human fibrinogen
Packed red cells
Whole blood

E934.8 Other agents affecting blood constituents
Macromolecular blood substitutes

E934.9 Unspecified agent affecting blood constituents

✓4th **E935 Analgesics, antipyretics, and antirheumatics**

E935.0 Heroin
Diacetylmorphine

E935.1 Methadone

E935.2 Other opiates and related narcotics
Codeine [methylmorphine]
Meperidine [pethidine]
Morphine
Opium (alkaloids)

E935.3 Salicylates
Acetylsalicylic acid [aspirin]
Amino derivatives of salicylic acid
Salicylic acid salts

E935.4 Aromatic analgesics, not elsewhere classified
Acetanilid
Paracetamol [acetaminophen]
Phenacetin [acetophenetidin]

E935.5 Pyrazole derivatives
Aminophenazone [aminopyrine]
Phenylbutazone

E935.6 Antirheumatics [antiphlogistics]
Gold salts
Indomethacin

EXCLUDES *salicylates (E935.3)*
steroids (E932.0)

E935.7 Other non-narcotic analgesics
Pyrabital

E935.8 Other specified analgesics and antipyretics
Pentazocine

E935.9 Unspecified analgesic and antipyretic

✓4th **E936 Anticonvulsants and anti-Parkinsonism drugs**

E936.0 Oxazolidine derivatives
Paramethadione
Trimethadione

E936.1 Hydantoin derivatives
Phenytoin

E936.2 Succinimides
Ethosuximide
Phensuximide

E936.3 Other and unspecified anticonvulsants
Beclamide
Primidone

E936.4 Anti-Parkinsonism drugs
Amantadine
Ethopropazine [profenamine]
Levodopa [L-dopa]

✓4th **E937 Sedatives and hypnotics**

E937.0 Barbiturates
Amobarbital [amylobarbitone]
Barbital [barbitone]
Butabarbital [butabarbitone]
Pentobarbital [pentobarbitone]
Phenobarbital [phenobarbitone]
Secobarbital [quinalbarbitone]

EXCLUDES *thiobarbiturates (E938.3)*

E937.1 Chloral hydrate group

E937.2 Paraldehyde

E937.3 Bromine compounds
Bromide
Carbromal (derivatives)

E937.4 Methaqualone compounds

E937.5 Glutethimide group

E937.6 Mixed sedatives, not elsewhere classified

E937.8 Other sedatives and hypnotics

E937.9 Unspecified
Sleeping:
drug, pill, tablet } NOS

✓4th **E938 Other central nervous system depressants and anesthetics**

E938.0 Central nervous system muscle-tone depressants
Chlorphenesin (carbamate)
Mephenesin
Methocarbamol

E938.1 Halothane

E938.2 Other gaseous anesthetics
Ether
Halogenated hydrocarbon derivatives, except halothane
Nitrous oxide

E938.3 Intravenous anesthetics
Ketamine
Methohexital [methohexitone]
Thiobarbiturates, such as thiopental sodium

E938.4 Other and unspecified general anesthetics

E938.5 Surface and infiltration anesthetics
Cocaine
Lidocaine [lignocaine]
Procaine
Tetracaine

E938.6 Peripheral nerve- and plexus-blocking anesthetics

E938.7 Spinal anesthetics

E938.9 Other and unspecified local anesthetics

✓4th **E939 Psychotropic agents**

E939.0 Antidepressants
Amitriptyline
Imipramine
Monoamine oxidase [MAO] inhibitors

E939.1 Phenothiazine-based tranquilizers
Chlorpromazine
Fluphenazine
Phenothiazine
Prochlorperazine
Promazine

E939.2 Butyrophenone-based tranquilizers
Haloperidol
Spiperone
Trifluperidol

E939.3 Other antipsychotics, neuroleptics, and major tranquilizers

E939.4 Benzodiazepine-based tranquilizers
Chlordiazepoxide
Diazepam
Flurazepam
Lorazepam
Medazepam
Nitrazepam

E939.5 Other tranquilizers
Hydroxyzine
Meprobamate

E939.6 Psychodysleptics [hallucinogens]
Cannabis (derivatives)
Lysergide [LSD]
Marihuana (derivatives)
Mescaline
Psilocin
Psilocybin

E939.7 Psychostimulants
Amphetamine
Caffeine

EXCLUDES *central appetite depressants (E947.0)*

E939.8 Other psychotropic agents

E939.9 Unspecified psychotropic agent

✓4th **E940 Central nervous system stimulants**

E940.0 Analeptics
Lobeline
Nikethamide

E940.1 Opiate antagonists
Levallorphan
Nalorphine
Naloxone

E940.8 Other specified central nervous system stimulants

E940.9 Unspecified central nervous system stimulant

✓4th **E941 Drugs primarily affecting the autonomic nervous system**

E941.0 Parasympathomimetics [cholinergics]
Acetylcholine
Anticholinesterase:
organophosphorus
reversible
Pilocarpine

✓4th Fourth-digit Required ▶◀ Revised Text ● New Code ▲ Revised Code Title

E941.1 Parasympatholytics [anticholinergics and antimuscarinics] and spasmolytics
Atropine
Homatropine
Hyoscine [scopolamine]
Quaternary ammonium derivatives
EXCLUDES *papaverine (E942.5)*

E941.2 Sympathomimetics [adrenergics]
Epinephrine [adrenalin]
Levarterenol [noradrenalin]

E941.3 Sympatholytics [antiadrenergics]
Phenoxybenzamine
Tolazolinehydrochloride

E941.9 Unspecified drug primarily affecting the autonomic nervous system

4th E942 Agents primarily affecting the cardiovascular system

E942.0 Cardiac rhythm regulators
Practolol
Procainamide
Propranolol
Quinidine

E942.1 Cardiotonic glycosides and drugs of similar action
Digitalis glycosides
Digoxin
Strophanthins

E942.2 Antilipemic and antiarteriosclerotic drugs
Cholestyramine
Clofibrate
Nicotinic acid derivatives
Sitosterols
EXCLUDES *dextrothyroxine (E932.7)*

E942.3 Ganglion-blocking agents
Pentamethonium bromide

E942.4 Coronary vasodilators
Dipyridamole
Nitrates [nitroglycerin]
Nitrites
Prenylamine

E942.5 Other vasodilators
Cyclandelate
Diazoxide
Hydralazine
Papaverine

E942.6 Other antihypertensive agents
Clonidine
Guanethidine
Rauwolfia alkaloids
Reserpine

E942.7 Antivaricose drugs, including sclerosing agents
Monoethanolamine
Zinc salts

E942.8 Capillary-active drugs
Adrenochrome derivatives
Bioflavonoids
Metaraminol

E942.9 Other and unspecified agents primarily affecting the cardiovascular system

4th E943 Agents primarily affecting gastrointestinal system

E943.0 Antacids and antigastric secretion drugs
Aluminum hydroxide
Magnesium trisilicate

E943.1 Irritant cathartics
Bisacodyl
Castor oil
Phenolphthalein

E943.2 Emollient cathartics
Sodium dioctyl sulfosuccinate

E943.3 Other cathartics, including intestinal atonia drugs
Magnesium sulfate

E943.4 Digestants
Pancreatin
Papain
Pepsin

E943.5 Antidiarrheal drugs
Bismuth subcarbonate
Kaolin
Pectin
EXCLUDES *anti-infectives (E930.0-E931.9)*

E943.6 Emetics

E943.8 Other specified agents primarily affecting the gastrointestinal system

E943.9 Unspecified agent primarily affecting the gastrointestinal system

4th E944 Water, mineral, and uric acid metabolism drugs

E944.0 Mercurial diuretics
Chlormerodrin
Mercaptomerin
Mercurophylline
Mersalyl

E944.1 Purine derivative diuretics
Theobromine
Theophylline
EXCLUDES *aminophylline [theophylline ethylenediamine] (E945.7)*

E944.2 Carbonic acid anhydrase inhibitors
Acetazolamide

E944.3 Saluretics
Benzothiadiazides
Chlorothiazide group

E944.4 Other diuretics
Ethacrynic acid
Furosemide

E944.5 Electrolytic, caloric, and water-balance agents

E944.6 Other mineral salts, not elsewhere classified

E944.7 Uric acid metabolism drugs
Cinchophen and congeners
Colchicine
Phenoquin
Probenecid

4th E945 Agents primarily acting on the smooth and skeletal muscles and respiratory system

E945.0 Oxytocic agents
Ergot alkaloids
Prostaglandins

E945.1 Smooth muscle relaxants
Adiphenine
Metaproterenol [orciprenaline]
EXCLUDES *papaverine (E942.5)*

E945.2 Skeletal muscle relaxants
Alcuronium chloride
Suxamethonium chloride

E945.3 Other and unspecified drugs acting on muscles

E945.4 Antitussives
Dextromethorphan
Pipazethate hydrochloride

E945.5 Expectorants
Acetylcysteine
Cocillana
Guaifenesin [glyceryl guaiacolate]
Ipecacuanha
Terpin hydrate

E945.6 Anti-common cold drugs

E945.7 Antiasthmatics
Aminophylline [theophylline ethylenediamine]

E945.8 Other and unspecified respiratory drugs

4th E946 Agents primarily affecting skin and mucous membrane, ophthalmological, otorhinolaryngological, and dental drugs

E946.0 Local anti-infectives and anti-inflammatory drugs

E946.1 Antipruritics

E946.2 Local astringents and local detergents

E946.3 Emollients, demulcents, and protectants

E946.4 Keratolytics, kerstoplastics, other hair treatment drugs and preparations

E946.5 Eye anti-infectives and other eye drugs
Idoxuridine

E946.6 Anti-infectives and other drugs and preparations for ear, nose, and throat

E946.7 Dental drugs topically applied

E946.8 Other agents primarily affecting skin and mucous membrane
Spermicides

E946.9 Unspecified agent primarily affecting skin and mucous membrane

4th E947 Other and unspecified drugs and medicinal substances

E947.0 Dietetics

E947.1 Lipotropic drugs

E947.2 Antidotes and chelating agents, not elsewhere classified

E947.3 Alcohol deterrents

E947.4 Pharmaceutical excipients

E947.8 Other drugs and medicinal substances
Contrast media used for diagnostic x-ray procedures
Diagnostic agents and kits

E947.9 Unspecified drug or medicinal substance

4th E948 Bacterial vaccines

E948.0 BCG vaccine

E948.1 Typhoid and paratyphoid
E948.2 Cholera
E948.3 Plague
E948.4 Tetanus
E948.5 Diphtheria
E948.6 Pertussis vaccine, including combinations with a pertussis component
E948.8 Other and unspecified bacterial vaccines
E948.9 Mixed bacterial vaccines, except combinations with a pertussis component

✓4th **E949 Other vaccines and biological substances**
EXCLUDES *gamma globulin (E934.6)*
E949.0 Smallpox vaccine
E949.1 Rabies vaccine
E949.2 Typhus vaccine
E949.3 Yellow fever vaccine
E949.4 Measles vaccine
E949.5 Poliomyelitis vaccine
E949.6 Other and unspecified viral and rickettsial vaccines
Mumps vaccine
E949.7 Mixed viral-rickettsial and bacterial vaccines, except combinations with a pertussis component
EXCLUDES *combinations with a pertussis component (E948.6)*
E949.9 Other and unspecified vaccines and biological substances

SUICIDE AND SELF-INFLICTED INJURY (E950-E959)

INCLUDES injuries in suicide and attempted suicide
self-inflicted injuries specified as intentional

✓4th **E950 Suicide and self-inflicted poisoning by solid or liquid substances**
E950.0 Analgesics, antipyretics, and antirheumatics
E950.1 Barbiturates
E950.2 Other sedatives and hypnotics
E950.3 Tranquilizers and other psychotropic agents
E950.4 Other specified drugs and medicinal substances
E950.5 Unspecified drug or medicinal substance
E950.6 Agricultural and horticultural chemical and pharmaceutical preparations other than plant foods and fertilizers
E950.7 Corrosive and caustic substances
Suicide and self-inflicted poisoning by substances classifiable to E864
E950.8 Arsenic and its compounds
E950.9 Other and unspecified solid and liquid substances

✓4th **E951 Suicide and self-inflicted poisoning by gases in domestic use**
E951.0 Gas distributed by pipeline
E951.1 Liquefied petroleum gas distributed in mobile containers
E951.8 Other utility gas

✓4th **E952 Suicide and self-inflicted poisoning by other gases and vapors**
E952.0 Motor vehicle exhaust gas
E952.1 Other carbon monoxide
E952.8 Other specified gases and vapors
E952.9 Unspecified gases and vapors

✓4th **E953 Suicide and self-inflicted injury by hanging, strangulation, and suffocation**
E953.0 Hanging
E953.1 Suffocation by plastic bag
E953.8 Other specified means
E953.9 Unspecified means

E954 Suicide and self-inflicted injury by submersion [drowning]

✓4th **E955 Suicide and self-inflicted injury by firearms, air guns and explosives**
E955.0 Handgun
E955.1 Shotgun
E955.2 Hunting rifle
E955.3 Military firearms
E955.4 Other and unspecified firearm
Gunshot NOS Shot NOS
E955.5 Explosives
E955.6 Air gun
BB gun Pellet gun
E955.7 Paintball gun
E955.9 Unspecified

E956 Suicide and self-inflicted injury by cutting and piercing instrument

✓4th **E957 Suicide and self-inflicted injuries by jumping from high place**
E957.0 Residential premises
E957.1 Other man-made structures
E957.2 Natural sites
E957.9 Unspecified

✓4th **E958 Suicide and self-inflicted injury by other and unspecified means**
E958.0 Jumping or lying before moving object
E958.1 Burns, fire
E958.2 Scald
E958.3 Extremes of cold
E958.4 Electrocution
E958.5 Crashing of motor vehicle
E958.6 Crashing of aircraft
E958.7 Caustic substances, except poisoning
EXCLUDES *poisoning by caustic substance (E950.7)*
E958.8 Other specified means
E958.9 Unspecified means

E959 Late effects of self-inflicted injury
Note: This category is to be used to indicate circumstances classifiable to E950-E958 as the cause of death or disability from late effects, which are themselves classifiable elsewhere. The "late effects" include conditions reported as such, or as sequelae which may occur at any time after the attempted suicide or self-inflicted injury.

HOMICIDE AND INJURY PURPOSELY INFLICTED BY OTHER PERSONS (E960-E969)

INCLUDES injuries inflicted by another person with intent to injure or kill, by any means
EXCLUDES *injuries due to:*
legal intervention (E970-E978)
operations of war (E990-E999)
terrorism (E979)

✓4th **E960 Fight, brawl, rape**
E960.0 Unarmed fight or brawl
Beatings NOS
Brawl or fight with hands, fists, feet
Injured or killed in fight NOS
EXCLUDES *homicidal:*
injury by weapons (E965.0-E966, E969)
strangulation (E963)
submersion (E964)
E960.1 Rape

E961 Assault by corrosive or caustic substance, except poisoning
Injury or death purposely caused by corrosive or caustic substance, such as:
acid [any]
corrosive substance
vitriol
EXCLUDES *burns from hot liquid (E968.3)*
chemical burns from swallowing a corrosive substance (E962.0-E962.9)

✓4th E962 Assault by poisoning

E962.0 Drugs and medicinal substances
Homicidal poisoning by any drug or medicinal substance

E962.1 Other solid and liquid substances

E962.2 Other gases and vapors

E962.9 Unspecified poisoning

E963 Assault by hanging and strangulation
Homicidal (attempt):
garrotting or ligature
hanging
Homicidal (attempt):
strangulation
suffocation

E964 Assault by submersion [drowning]

✓4th E965 Assault by firearms and explosives

E965.0 Handgun
Pistol
Revolver

E965.1 Shotgun

E965.2 Hunting rifle

E965.3 Military firearms

E965.4 Other and unspecified firearm

E965.5 Antipersonnel bomb

E965.6 Gasoline bomb

E965.7 Letter bomb

E965.8 Other specified explosive
Bomb NOS (placed in):
car
house
Dynamite

E965.9 Unspecified explosive

E966 Assault by cutting and piercing instrument
Assassination (attempt), homicide (attempt) by any instrument classifiable under E920
Homicidal:
cut
puncture
stab
Stabbed
} any part of body

✓4th E967 Perpetrator of child and adult abuse
Note: Selection of the correct perpetrator code is based on the relationship between the perpetrator and the victim

E967.0 By father, stepfather, or boyfriend
Male partner of child's parent or guardian

E967.1 By other specified person

E967.2 By mother, stepmother, or girlfriend
Female partner of child's parent or guardian

E967.3 By spouse or partner
Abuse of spouse or partner by ex-spouse or ex-partner

E967.4 By child

E967.5 By sibling

E967.6 By grandparent

E967.7 By other relative

E967.8 By non-related caregiver

E967.9 By unspecified person

✓4th E968 Assault by other and unspecified means

E968.0 Fire
Arson
Homicidal burns NOS
EXCLUDES *burns from hot liquid (E968.3)*

E968.1 Pushing from a high place

E968.2 Striking by blunt or thrown object

E968.3 Hot liquid
Homicidal burns by scalding

E968.4 Criminal neglect
Abandonment of child, infant, or other helpless person with intent to injure or kill

E968.5 Transport vehicle
Being struck by other vehicle or run down with intent to injure
Pushed in front of, thrown from, or dragged by moving vehicle with intent to injure

E968.6 Air gun
BB gun
Pellet gun

E968.7 Human bite

E968.8 Other specified means

E968.9 Unspecified means
Assassination (attempt) NOS
Homicidal (attempt):
injury NOS
wound NOS
Manslaughter (nonaccidental)
Murder (attempt) NOS
Violence, non-accidental

E969 Late effects of injury purposely inflicted by other person
Note: This category is to be used to indicate circumstances classifiable to E960-E968 as the cause of death or disability from late effects, which are themselves classifiable elsewhere. The "late effects" include conditions reported as such, or as sequelae which may occur at any time after injury purposely inflicted by another person.

LEGAL INTERVENTION (E970-E978)

INCLUDES injuries inflicted by the police or other law-enforcing agents, including military on duty, in the course of arresting or attempting to arrest lawbreakers, suppressing disturbances, maintaining order, and other legal action
legal execution

EXCLUDES *injuries caused by civil insurrections (E990.0-E999)*

E970 Injury due to legal intervention by firearms
Gunshot wound
Injury by:
machine gun
revolver
Injury by:
rifle pellet or rubber bullet
shot NOS

E971 Injury due to legal intervention by explosives
Injury by:
dynamite
explosive shell
Injury by:
grenade
mortar bomb

E972 Injury due to legal intervention by gas
Asphyxiation by gas
Injury by tear gas
Poisoning by gas

E973 Injury due to legal intervention by blunt object
Hit, struck by:
baton (nightstick)
blunt object
Hit, struck by:
stave

E974 Injury due to legal intervention by cutting and piercing instrument
Cut
Incised wound
Injured by bayonet
Stab wound

E975 Injury due to legal intervention by other specified means
Blow
Manhandling

E976 Injury due to legal intervention by unspecified means

E977 Late effects of injuries due to legal intervention
Note: This category is to be used to indicate circumstances classifiable to E970-E976 as the cause of death or disability from late effects, which are themselves classifiable elsewhere. The "late effects" include conditions reported as such, or as sequelae, which may occur at any time after the injury due to legal intervention.

E978 Legal execution
All executions performed at the behest of the judiciary or ruling authority [whether permanent or temporary] as:
asphyxiation by gas
beheading, decapitation (by guillotine)
capital punishment
electrocution
hanging
poisoning
shooting
other specified means

✓4th Fourth-digit Required ▶◀ Revised Text ● New Code ▲ Revised Code Title

TERRORISM (E979)

✓4th E979 Terrorism

Injuries resulting from the unlawful use of force or violence against persons or property to intimidate or coerce a Government, the civilian population, or any segment thereof, in furtherance of political or social objective

E979.0 Terrorism involving explosion of marine weapons
- Depth-charge
- Marine mine
- Mine NOS, at sea or in harbour
- Sea-based artillery shell
- Torpedo
- Underwater blast

E979.1 Terrorism involving destruction of aircraft
- Aircraft used as a weapon
- Aircraft:
  - burned
  - exploded
  - shot down
- Crushed by falling aircraft

E979.2 Terrorism involving other explosions and fragments
- Antipersonnel bomb (fragments)
- Blast NOS
- Explosion (of):
  - artillery shell
  - breech-block
  - cannon block
  - mortar bomb
  - munitions being used in terrorism
  - NOS
- Fragments from:
  - artillery shell
  - bomb
  - grenade
  - guided missile
  - land-mine
  - rocket
  - shell
  - shrapnel
- Mine NOS

E979.3 Terrorism involving fires, conflagration and hot substances
- Burning building or structure:
  - collapse of
  - fall from
  - hit by falling object in
  - jump from
- Conflagration NOS
- Fire (causing):
  - Asphyxia
  - Burns
  - NOS
  - Other injury
- Melting of fittings and furniture in burning
- Petrol bomb
- Smouldering building or structure

E979.4 Terrorism involving firearms
- Bullet:
  - carbine
  - machine gun
  - pistol
  - rifle
  - rubber (rifle)
- Pellets (shotgun)

E979.5 Terrorism involving nuclear weapons
- Blast effects
- Exposure to ionizing radiation from nuclear weapon
- Fireball effects
- Heat from nuclear weapon
- Other direct and secondary effects of nuclear weapons

E979.6 Terrorism involving biological weapons
- Anthrax
- Cholera
- Smallpox

E979.7 Terrorism involving chemical weapons
- Gases, fumes, chemicals
- Hydrogen cyanide
- Phosgene
- Sarin

E979.8 Terrorism involving other means
- Drowning and submersion
- Lasers
- Piercing or stabbing instruments
- Terrorism NOS

E979.9 Terrorism, secondary effects

Note: This code is for use to identify conditions occurring subsequent to a terrorist attack not those that are due to the initial terrorist act

EXCLUDES *late effect of terrorist attack (E999.1)*

INJURY UNDETERMINED WHETHER ACCIDENTALLY OR PURPOSELY INFLICTED (E980-E989)

Note: Categories E980-E989 are for use when it is unspecified or it cannot be determined whether the injuries are accidental (unintentional), suicide (attempted), or assault.

✓4th E980 Poisoning by solid or liquid substances, undetermined whether accidentally or purposely inflicted

E980.0 Analgesics, antipyretics, and antirheumatics

E980.1 Barbiturates

E980.2 Other sedatives and hypnotics

E980.3 Tranquilizers and other psychotropic agents

E980.4 Other specified drugs and medicinal substances

E980.5 Unspecified drug or medicinal substance

E980.6 Corrosive and caustic substances

Poisoning, undetermined whether accidental or purposeful, by substances classifiable to E864

E980.7 Agricultural and horticultural chemical and pharmaceutical preparations other than plant foods and fertilizers

E980.8 Arsenic and its compounds

E980.9 Other and unspecified solid and liquid substances

✓4th E981 Poisoning by gases in domestic use, undetermined whether accidentally or purposely inflicted

E981.0 Gas distributed by pipeline

E981.1 Liquefied petroleum gas distributed in mobile containers

E981.8 Other utility gas

✓4th E982 Poisoning by other gases, undetermined whether accidentally or purposely inflicted

E982.0 Motor vehicle exhaust gas

E982.1 Other carbon monoxide

E982.8 Other specified gases and vapors

E982.9 Unspecified gases and vapors

✓4th E983 Hanging, strangulation, or suffocation, undetermined whether accidentally or purposely inflicted

E983.0 Hanging

E983.1 Suffocation by plastic bag

E983.8 Other specified means

E983.9 Unspecified means

E984 Submersion [drowning], undetermined whether accidentally or purposely inflicted

✓4th E985 Injury by firearms, air guns and explosives, undetermined whether accidentally or purposely inflicted

E985.0 Handgun

E985.1 Shotgun

E985.2 Hunting rifle

E985.3 Military firearms

E985.4 Other and unspecified firearm

E985.5 Explosives

E985.6 Air gun

BB gun   Pellet gun

E985.7 Paintball gun

✓4th Fourth-digit Required ⧓ Revised Text ● New Code ▲ Revised Code Title

E986 Injury by cutting and piercing instruments, undetermined whether accidentally or purposely inflicted

✓4th **E987 Falling from high place, undetermined whether accidentally or purposely inflicted**

E987.0 Residential premises

E987.1 Other man-made structures

E987.2 Natural sites

E987.9 Unspecified site

✓4th **E988 Injury by other and unspecified means, undetermined whether accidentally or purposely inflicted**

E988.0 Jumping or lying before moving object

E988.1 Burns, fire

E988.2 Scald

E988.3 Extremes of cold

E988.4 Electrocution

E988.5 Crashing of motor vehicle

E988.6 Crashing of aircraft

E988.7 Caustic substances, except poisoning

E988.8 Other specified means

E988.9 Unspecified means

E989 Late effects of injury, undetermined whether accidentally or purposely inflicted

Note: This category is to be used to indicate circumstances classifiable to E980-E988 as the cause of death or disability from late effects, which are themselves classifiable elsewhere. The "late effects" include conditions reported as such, or as sequelae, which may occur at any time after injury, undetermined whether accidentally or purposely inflicted.

INJURY RESULTING FROM OPERATIONS OF WAR (E990-E999)

INCLUDES injuries to military personnel and civilians caused by war and civil insurrections and occurring during the time of war and insurrection

EXCLUDES *accidents during training of military personnel manufacture of war material and transport, unless attributable to enemy action*

✓4th **E990 Injury due to war operations by fires and conflagrations**

INCLUDES asphyxia, burns, or other injury originating from fire caused by a fire-producing device or indirectly by any conventional weapon

E990.0 From gasoline bomb

E990.9 From other and unspecified source

✓4th **E991 Injury due to war operations by bullets and fragments**

E991.0 Rubber bullets (rifle)

E991.1 Pellets (rifle)

E991.2 Other bullets

Bullet [any, except rubber bullets and pellets]
- carbine
- machine gun
- pistol
- rifle
- shotgun

E991.3 Antipersonnel bomb (fragments)

E991.9 Other and unspecified fragments

Fragments from:
- artillery shell
- bombs, except anti-personnel
- grenade
- guided missile

Fragments from:
- land mine
- rockets
- shell

Shrapnel

E992 Injury due to war operations by explosion of marine weapons

Depth charge
Marine mines
Mine NOS, at sea or in harbor
Sea-based artillery shell
Torpedo
Underwater blast

E993 Injury due to war operations by other explosion

Accidental explosion of munitions being used in war
Accidental explosion of own weapons
Air blast NOS
Blast NOS
Explosion NOS

Explosion of:
- artillery shell
- breech block
- cannon block
- mortar bomb

Injury by weapon burst

E994 Injury due to war operations by destruction of aircraft

Airplane:
- burned
- exploded

Airplane:
- shot down

Crushed by falling airplane

E995 Injury due to war operations by other and unspecified forms of conventional warfare

Battle wounds
Bayonet injury
Drowned in war operations

E996 Injury due to war operations by nuclear weapons

Blast effects
Exposure to ionizing radiation from nuclear weapons
Fireball effects
Heat
Other direct and secondary effects of nuclear weapons

✓4th **E997 Injury due to war operations by other forms of unconventional warfare**

E997.0 Lasers

E997.1 Biological warfare

E997.2 Gases, fumes, and chemicals

E997.8 Other specified forms of unconventional warfare

E997.9 Unspecified form of unconventional warfare

E998 Injury due to war operations but occurring after cessation of hostilities

Injuries due to operations of war but occurring after cessation of hostilities by any means classifiable under E990-E997

Injuries by explosion of bombs or mines placed in the course of operations of war, if the explosion occurred after cessation of hostilities

✓4th **E999 Late effect of injury due to war operations and terrorism**

Note: This category is to be used to indicate circumstances classifiable to E979, E990-E998 as the cause of death or disability from late effects, which are themselves classifiable elsewhere. The "late effects" include conditions reported as such, or as sequelae, which may occur at any time after the injury, resulting from operations of war or terrorism

E999.0 Late effect of injury due to war operations

E999.1 Late effect of injury due to terrorism

Official ICD-9-CM Government Appendixes

MORPHOLOGY OF NEOPLASMS

The World Health Organization has published an adaptation of the International Classification of Diseases for oncology (ICD-O). It contains a coded nomenclature for the morphology of neoplasms, which is reproduced here for those who wish to use it in conjunction with Chapter 2 of the International Classification of Diseases, 9th Revision, Clinical Modification.

The morphology code numbers consist of five digits; the first four identify the histological type of the neoplasm and the fifth indicates its behavior. The one-digit behavior code is as follows:

- /0 Benign
- /1 Uncertain whether benign or malignant
  Borderline malignancy
- /2 Carcinoma in situ
  Intraepithelial
  Noninfiltrating
  Noninvasive
- /3 Malignant, primary site
- /6 Malignant, metastatic site
  Secondary site
- /9 Malignant, uncertain whether primary or metastatic site

In the nomenclature below, the morphology code numbers include the behavior code appropriate to the histological type of neoplasm, but this behavior code should be changed if other reported information makes this necessary. For example, "chordoma (M9370/3)" is assumed to be malignant; the term "benign chordoma" should be coded M9370/0. Similarly, "superficial spreading adenocarcinoma (M8143/3)" described as "noninvasive" should be coded M8143/2 and "melanoma (M8720/3)" described as "secondary" should be coded M8720/6.

The following table shows the correspondence between the morphology code and the different sections of Chapter 2:

Morphology Code Histology/Behavior		ICD-9-CM Chapter 2	
Any	0	210-229	Benign neoplasms
M8000-M8004	1	239	Neoplasms of unspecified nature
M8010+	1	235-238	Neoplasms of uncertain behavior
Any	2	230-234	Carcinoma in situ
Any	3	140-195 200-208	Malignant neoplasms, stated or presumed to be primary
Any	6	196-198	Malignant neoplasms, stated or presumed to be secondary

The ICD-O behavior digit /9 is inapplicable in an ICD context, since all malignant neoplasms are presumed to be primary (/3) or secondary (/6) according to other information on the medical record.

Only the first-listed term of the full ICD-O morphology nomenclature appears against each code number in the list below. The ICD-9-CM Alphabetical Index (Volume 2), however, includes all the ICD-O synonyms as well as a number of other morphological names still likely to be encountered on medical records but omitted from ICD-O as outdated or otherwise undesirable.

A coding difficulty sometimes arises where a morphological diagnosis contains two qualifying adjectives that have different code numbers. An example is "transitional cell epidermoid carcinoma." "Transitional cell carcinoma NOS" is M8120/3 and "epidermoid carcinoma NOS" is M8070/3. In such circumstances, the higher number (M8120/3 in this example) should be used, as it is usually more specific.

CODED NOMENCLATURE FOR MORPHOLOGY OF NEOPLASMS

M800 Neoplasms NOS

M8000/0 *Neoplasm, benign*
M8000/1 *Neoplasm, uncertain whether benign or malignant*
M8000/3 *Neoplasm, malignant*
M8000/6 *Neoplasm, metastatic*
M8000/9 *Neoplasm, malignant, uncertain whether primary or metastatic*
M8001/0 *Tumor cells, benign*
M8001/1 *Tumor cells, uncertain whether benign or malignant*
M8001/3 *Tumor cells, malignant*
M8002/3 *Malignant tumor, small cell type*
M8003/3 *Malignant tumor, giant cell type*
M8004/3 *Malignant tumor, fusiform cell type*

M801-M804 Epithelial neoplasms NOS

M8010/0 *Epithelial tumor, benign*
M8010/2 *Carcinoma in situ NOS*
M8010/3 *Carcinoma NOS*
M8010/6 *Carcinoma, metastatic NOS*
M8010/9 *Carcinomatosis*
M8011/0 *Epithelioma, benign*
M8011/3 *Epithelioma, malignant*
M8012/3 *Large cell carcinoma NOS*
M8020/3 *Carcinoma, undifferentiated type NOS*
M8021/3 *Carcinoma, anaplastic type NOS*
M8022/3 *Pleomorphic carcinoma*
M8030/3 *Giant cell and spindle cell carcinoma*
M8031/3 *Giant cell carcinoma*
M8032/3 *Spindle cell carcinoma*
M8033/3 *Pseudosarcomatous carcinoma*
M8034/3 *Polygonal cell carcinoma*
M8035/3 *Spheroidal cell carcinoma*
M8040/1 *Tumorlet*
M8041/3 *Small cell carcinoma NOS*
M8042/3 *Oat cell carcinoma*
M8043/3 *Small cell carcinoma, fusiform cell type*

M805-M808 Papillary and squamous cell neoplasms

M8050/0 *Papilloma NOS (except Papilloma of urinary bladder M8120/1)*
M8050/2 *Papillary carcinoma in situ*
M8050/3 *Papillary carcinoma NOS*
M8051/0 *Verrucous papilloma*
M8051/3 *Verrucous carcinoma NOS*
M8052/0 *Squamous cell papilloma*
M8052/3 *Papillary squamous cell carcinoma*
M8053/0 *Inverted papilloma*
M8060/0 *Papillomatosis NOS*
M8070/2 *Squamous cell carcinoma in situ NOS*
M8070/3 *Squamous cell carcinoma NOS*
M8070/6 *Squamous cell carcinoma, metastatic NOS*
M8071/3 *Squamous cell carcinoma, keratinizing type NOS*
M8072/3 *Squamous cell carcinoma, large cell, nonkeratinizing type*
M8073/3 *Squamous cell carcinoma, small cell, nonkeratinizing type*
M8074/3 *Squamous cell carcinoma, spindle cell type*
M8075/3 *Adenoid squamous cell carcinoma*
M8076/2 *Squamous cell carcinoma in situ with questionable stromal invasion*
M8076/3 *Squamous cell carcinoma, microinvasive*
M8080/2 *Queyrat's erythroplasia*
M8081/2 *Bowen's disease*
M8082/3 *Lymphoepithelial carcinoma*

M809-M811 Basal cell neoplasms

M8090/1 *Basal cell tumor*
M8090/3 *Basal cell carcinoma NOS*
M8091/3 *Multicentric basal cell carcinoma*
M8092/3 *Basal cell carcinoma, morphea type*
M8093/3 *Basal cell carcinoma, fibroepithelial type*
M8094/3 *Basosquamous carcinoma*
M8095/3 *Metatypical carcinoma*
M8096/0 *Intraepidermal epithelioma of Jadassohn*
M8100/0 *Trichoepithelioma*
M8101/0 *Trichofolliculoma*
M8102/0 *Tricholemmoma*
M8110/0 *Pilomatrixoma*

M812-M813 Transitional cell papillomas and carcinomas

M8120/0 *Transitional cell papilloma NOS*
M8120/1 *Urothelial papilloma*
M8120/2 *Transitional cell carcinoma in situ*
M8120/3 *Transitional cell carcinoma NOS*
M8121/0 *Schneiderian papilloma*
M8121/1 *Transitional cell papilloma, inverted type*
M8121/3 *Schneiderian carcinoma*
M8122/3 *Transitional cell carcinoma, spindle cell type*
M8123/3 *Basaloid carcinoma*
M8124/3 *Cloacogenic carcinoma*
M8130/3 *Papillary transitional cell carcinoma*

M814-M838 Adenomas and adenocarcinomas

M8140/0 *Adenoma NOS*
M8140/1 *Bronchial adenoma NOS*
M8140/2 *Adenocarcinoma in situ*
M8140/3 *Adenocarcinoma NOS*
M8140/6 *Adenocarcinoma, metastatic NOS*
M8141/3 *Scirrhous adenocarcinoma*
M8142/3 *Linitis plastica*
M8143/3 *Superficial spreading adenocarcinoma*
M8144/3 *Adenocarcinoma, intestinal type*
M8145/3 *Carcinoma, diffuse type*
M8146/0 *Monomorphic adenoma*
M8147/0 *Basal cell adenoma*
M8150/0 *Islet cell adenoma*
M8150/3 *Islet cell carcinoma*
M8151/0 *Insulinoma NOS*
M8151/3 *Insulinoma, malignant*
M8152/0 *Glucagonoma NOS*
M8152/3 *Glucagonoma, malignant*
M8153/1 *Gastrinoma NOS*

M8153/3 *Gastrinoma, malignant*
M8154/3 *Mixed islet cell and exocrine adenocarcinoma*
M8160/0 *Bile duct adenoma*
M8160/3 *Cholangiocarcinoma*
M8161/0 *Bile duct cystadenoma*
M8161/3 *Bile duct cystadenocarcinoma*
M8170/0 *Liver cell adenoma*
M8170/3 *Hepatocellular carcinoma NOS*
M8180/0 *Hepatocholangioma, benign*
M8180/3 *Combined hepatocellular carcinoma and cholangiocarcinoma*
M8190/0 *Trabecular adenoma*
M8190/3 *Trabecular adenocarcinoma*
M8191/0 *Embryonal adenoma*
M8200/0 *Eccrine dermal cylindroma*
M8200/3 *Adenoid cystic carcinoma*
M8201/3 *Cribriform carcinoma*
M8210/0 *Adenomatous polyp NOS*
M8210/3 *Adenocarcinoma in adenomatous polyp*
M8211/0 *Tubular adenoma NOS*
M8211/3 *Tubular adenocarcinoma*
M8220/0 *Adenomatous polyposis coli*
M8220/3 *Adenocarcinoma in adenomatous polyposis coli*
M8221/0 *Multiple adenomatous polyps*
M8230/3 *Solid carcinoma NOS*
M8231/3 *Carcinoma simplex*
M8240/1 *Carcinoid tumor NOS*
M8240/3 *Carcinoid tumor, malignant*
M8241/1 *Carcinoid tumor, argentaffin NOS*
M8241/3 *Carcinoid tumor, argentaffin, malignant*
M8242/1 *Carcinoid tumor, nonargentaffin NOS*
M8242/3 *Carcinoid tumor, nonargentaffin, malignant*
M8243/3 *Mucocarcinoid tumor, malignant*
M8244/3 *Composite carcinoid*
M8250/1 *Pulmonary adenomatosis*
M8250/3 *Bronchiolo-alveolar adenocarcinoma*
M8251/0 *Alveolar adenoma*
M8251/3 *Alveolar adenocarcinoma*
M8260/0 *Papillary adenoma NOS*
M8260/3 *Papillary adenocarcinoma NOS*
M8261/1 *Villous adenoma NOS*
M8261/3 *Adenocarcinoma in villous adenoma*
M8262/3 *Villous adenocarcinoma*
M8263/0 *Tubulovillous adenoma*
M8270/0 *Chromophobe adenoma*
M8270/3 *Chromophobe carcinoma*
M8280/0 *Acidophil adenoma*
M8280/3 *Acidophil carcinoma*
M8281/0 *Mixed acidophil-basophil adenoma*
M8281/3 *Mixed acidophil-basophil carcinoma*
M8290/0 *Oxyphilic adenoma*
M8290/3 *Oxyphilic adenocarcinoma*
M8300/0 *Basophil adenoma*
M8300/3 *Basophil carcinoma*
M8310/0 *Clear cell adenoma*
M8310/3 *Clear cell adenocarcinoma NOS*
M8311/1 *Hypernephroid tumor*
M8312/3 *Renal cell carcinoma*
M8313/0 *Clear cell adenofibroma*
M8320/3 *Granular cell carcinoma*
M8321/0 *Chief cell adenoma*
M8322/0 *Water-clear cell adenoma*
M8322/3 *Water-clear cell adenocarcinoma*
M8323/0 *Mixed cell adenoma*
M8323/3 *Mixed cell adenocarcinoma*
M8324/0 *Lipoadenoma*
M8330/0 *Follicular adenoma*
M8330/3 *Follicular adenocarcinoma NOS*
M8331/3 *Follicular adenocarcinoma, well differentiated type*
M8332/3 *Follicular adenocarcinoma, trabecular type*
M8333/0 *Microfollicular adenoma*
M8334/0 *Macrofollicular adenoma*
M8340/3 *Papillary and follicular adenocarcinoma*
M8350/3 *Nonencapsulated sclerosing carcinoma*
M8360/1 *Multiple endocrine adenomas*
M8361/1 *Juxtaglomerular tumor*
M8370/0 *Adrenal cortical adenoma NOS*
M8370/3 *Adrenal cortical carcinoma*
M8371/0 *Adrenal cortical adenoma, compact cell type*
M8372/0 *Adrenal cortical adenoma, heavily pigmented variant*
M8373/0 *Adrenal cortical adenoma, clear cell type*
M8374/0 *Adrenal cortical adenoma, glomerulosa cell type*
M8375/0 *Adrenal cortical adenoma, mixed cell type*
M8380/0 *Endometrioid adenoma NOS*
M8380/1 *Endometrioid adenoma, borderline malignancy*
M8380/3 *Endometrioid carcinoma*
M8381/0 *Endometrioid adenofibroma NOS*
M8381/1 *Endometrioid adenofibroma, borderline malignancy*
M8381/3 *Endometrioid adenofibroma, malignant*

M839-M842 Adnexal and skin appendage neoplasms

M8390/0 *Skin appendage adenoma*
M8390/3 *Skin appendage carcinoma*
M8400/0 *Sweat gland adenoma*
M8400/1 *Sweat gland tumor NOS*
M8400/3 *Sweat gland adenocarcinoma*
M8401/0 *Apocrine adenoma*
M8401/3 *Apocrine adenocarcinoma*
M8402/0 *Eccrine acrospiroma*
M8403/0 *Eccrine spiradenoma*
M8404/0 *Hidrocystoma*
M8405/0 *Papillary hydradenoma*
M8406/0 *Papillary syringadenoma*
M8407/0 *Syringoma NOS*
M8410/0 *Sebaceous adenoma*
M8410/3 *Sebaceous adenocarcinoma*
M8420/0 *Ceruminous adenoma*
M8420/3 *Ceruminous adenocarcinoma*

M843 Mucoepidermoid neoplasms

M8430/1 *Mucoepidermoid tumor*
M8430/3 *Mucoepidermoid carcinoma*

M844-M849 Cystic, mucinous, and serous neoplasms

M8440/0 *Cystadenoma NOS*
M8440/3 *Cystadenocarcinoma NOS*
M8441/0 *Serous cystadenoma NOS*
M8441/1 *Serous cystadenoma, borderline malignancy*
M8441/3 *Serous cystadenocarcinoma NOS*
M8450/0 *Papillary cystadenoma NOS*
M8450/1 *Papillary cystadenoma, borderline malignancy*
M8450/3 *Papillary cystadenocarcinoma NOS*
M8460/0 *Papillary serous cystadenoma NOS*
M8460/1 *Papillary serous cystadenoma, borderline malignancy*
M8460/3 *Papillary serous cystadenocarcinoma*
M8461/0 *Serous surface papilloma NOS*
M8461/1 *Serous surface papilloma, borderline malignancy*
M8461/3 *Serous surface papillary carcinoma*
M8470/0 *Mucinous cystadenoma NOS*
M8470/1 *Mucinous cystadenoma, borderline malignancy*
M8470/3 *Mucinous cystadenocarcinoma NOS*
M8471/0 *Papillary mucinous cystadenoma NOS*
M8471/1 *Papillary mucinous cystadenoma, borderline malignancy*
M8471/3 *Papillary mucinous cystadenocarcinoma*
M8480/0 *Mucinous adenoma*
M8480/3 *Mucinous adenocarcinoma*
M8480/6 *Pseudomyxoma peritonei*
M8481/3 *Mucin-producing adenocarcinoma*
M8490/3 *Signet ring cell carcinoma*
M8490/6 *Metastatic signet ring cell carcinoma*

M850-M854 Ductal, lobular, and medullary neoplasms

M8500/2 *Intraductal carcinoma, noninfiltrating NOS*
M8500/3 *Infiltrating duct carcinoma*
M8501/2 *Comedocarcinoma, noninfiltrating*
M8501/3 *Comedocarcinoma NOS*
M8502/3 *Juvenile carcinoma of the breast*
M8503/0 *Intraductal papilloma*
M8503/2 *Noninfiltrating intraductal papillary adenocarcinoma*
M8504/0 *Intracystic papillary adenoma*
M8504/2 *Noninfiltrating intracystic carcinoma*
M8505/0 *Intraductal papillomatosis NOS*
M8506/0 *Subareolar duct papillomatosis*
M8510/3 *Medullary carcinoma NOS*
M8511/3 *Medullary carcinoma with amyloid stroma*
M8512/3 *Medullary carcinoma with lymphoid stroma*
M8520/2 *Lobular carcinoma in situ*
M8520/3 *Lobular carcinoma NOS*
M8521/3 *Infiltrating ductular carcinoma*
M8530/3 *Inflammatory carcinoma*
M8540/3 *Paget's disease, mammary*
M8541/3 *Paget's disease and infiltrating duct carcinoma of breast*
M8542/3 *Paget's disease, extramammary (except Paget's disease of bone)*

M855 Acinar cell neoplasms

M8550/0 *Acinar cell adenoma*
M8550/1 *Acinar cell tumor*
M8550/3 *Acinar cell carcinoma*

M856-M858 Complex epithelial neoplasms

M8560/3 *Adenosquamous carcinoma*
M8561/0 *Adenolymphoma*
M8570/3 *Adenocarcinoma with squamous metaplasia*
M8571/3 *Adenocarcinoma with cartilaginous and osseous metaplasia*
M8572/3 *Adenocarcinoma with spindle cell metaplasia*
M8573/3 *Adenocarcinoma with apocrine metaplasia*
M8580/0 *Thymoma, benign*
M8580/3 *Thymoma, malignant*

M859-M867 Specialized gonadal neoplasms

M8590/1 *Sex cord-stromal tumor*
M8600/0 *Thecoma NOS*
M8600/3 *Theca cell carcinoma*
M8610/0 *Luteoma NOS*
M8620/1 *Granulosa cell tumor NOS*
M8620/3 *Granulosa cell tumor, malignant*
M8621/1 *Granulosa cell-theca cell tumor*
M8630/0 *Androblastoma, benign*
M8630/1 *Androblastoma NOS*
M8630/3 *Androblastoma, malignant*
M8631/0 *Sertoli-Leydig cell tumor*
M8632/1 *Gynandroblastoma*
M8640/0 *Tubular androblastoma NOS*
M8640/3 *Sertoli cell carcinoma*
M8641/0 *Tubular androblastoma with lipid storage*

M8650/0 *Leydig cell tumor, benign*
M8650/1 *Leydig cell tumor NOS*
M8650/3 *Leydig cell tumor, malignant*
M8660/0 *Hilar cell tumor*
M8670/0 *Lipid cell tumor of ovary*
M8671/0 *Adrenal rest tumor*
M868-M871 Paragangliomas and glomus tumors
M8680/1 *Paraganglioma NOS*
M8680/3 *Paraganglioma, malignant*
M8681/1 *Sympathetic paraganglioma*
M8682/1 *Parasympathetic paraganglioma*
M8690/1 *Glomus jugulare tumor*
M8691/1 *Aortic body tumor*
M8692/1 *Carotid body tumor*
M8693/1 *Extra-adrenal paraganglioma NOS*
M8693/3 *Extra-adrenal paraganglioma, malignant*
M8700/0 *Pheochromocytoma NOS*
M8700/3 *Pheochromocytoma, malignant*
M8710/3 *Glomangiosarcoma*
M8711/0 *Glomus tumor*
M8712/0 *Glomangioma*
M872-M879 Nevi and melanomas
M8720/0 *Pigmented nevus NOS*
M8720/3 *Malignant melanoma NOS*
M8721/3 *Nodular melanoma*
M8722/0 *Balloon cell nevus*
M8722/3 *Balloon cell melanoma*
M8723/0 *Halo nevus*
M8724/0 *Fibrous papule of the nose*
M8725/0 *Neuronevus*
M8726/0 *Magnocellular nevus*
M8730/0 *Nonpigmented nevus*
M8730/3 *Amelanotic melanoma*
M8740/0 *Junctional nevus*
M8740/3 *Malignant melanoma in junctional nevus*
M8741/2 *Precancerous melanosis NOS*
M8741/3 *Malignant melanoma in precancerous melanosis*
M8742/2 *Hutchinson's melanotic freckle*
M8742/3 *Malignant melanoma in Hutchinson's melanotic freckle*
M8743/3 *Superficial spreading melanoma*
M8750/0 *Intradermal nevus*
M8760/0 *Compound nevus*
M8761/1 *Giant pigmented nevus*
M8761/3 *Malignant melanoma in giant pigmented nevus*
M8770/0 *Epithelioid and spindle cell nevus*
M8771/3 *Epithelioid cell melanoma*
M8772/3 *Spindle cell melanoma NOS*
M8773/3 *Spindle cell melanoma, type A*
M8774/3 *Spindle cell melanoma, type B*
M8775/3 *Mixed epithelioid and spindle cell melanoma*
M8780/0 *Blue nevus NOS*
M8780/3 *Blue nevus, malignant*
M8790/0 *Cellular blue nevus*
M880 Soft tissue tumors and sarcomas NOS
M8800/0 *Soft tissue tumor, benign*
M8800/3 *Sarcoma NOS*
M8800/9 *Sarcomatosis NOS*
M8801/3 *Spindle cell sarcoma*
M8802/3 *Giant cell sarcoma (except of bone M9250/3)*
M8803/3 *Small cell sarcoma*
M8804/3 *Epithelioid cell sarcoma*
M881-M883 Fibromatous neoplasms
M8810/0 *Fibroma NOS*
M8810/3 *Fibrosarcoma NOS*
M8811/0 *Fibromyxoma*
M8811/3 *Fibromyxosarcoma*
M8812/0 *Periosteal fibroma*
M8812/3 *Periosteal fibrosarcoma*
M8813/0 *Fascial fibroma*
M8813/3 *Fascial fibrosarcoma*
M8814/3 *Infantile fibrosarcoma*
M8820/0 *Elastofibroma*
M8821/1 *Aggressive fibromatosis*
M8822/1 *Abdominal fibromatosis*
M8823/1 *Desmoplastic fibroma*
M8830/0 *Fibrous histiocytoma NOS*
M8830/1 *Atypical fibrous histiocytoma*
M8830/3 *Fibrous histiocytoma, malignant*
M8831/0 *Fibroxanthoma NOS*
M8831/1 *Atypical fibroxanthoma*
M8831/3 *Fibroxanthoma, malignant*
M8832/0 *Dermatofibroma NOS*
M8832/1 *Dermatofibroma protuberans*
M8832/3 *Dermatofibrosarcoma NOS*
M884 Myxomatous neoplasms
M8840/0 *Myxoma NOS*
M8840/3 *Myxosarcoma*
M885-M888 Lipomatous neoplasms
M8850/0 *Lipoma NOS*
M8850/3 *Liposarcoma NOS*
M8851/0 *Fibrolipoma*
M8851/3 *Liposarcoma, well differentiated type*
M8852/0 *Fibromyxolipoma*
M8852/3 *Myxoid liposarcoma*
M8853/3 *Round cell liposarcoma*
M8854/3 *Pleomorphic liposarcoma*
M8855/3 *Mixed type liposarcoma*
M8856/0 *Intramuscular lipoma*
M8857/0 *Spindle cell lipoma*
M8860/0 *Angiomyolipoma*
M8860/3 *Angiomyoliposarcoma*
M8861/0 *Angiolipoma NOS*
M8861/1 *Angiolipoma, infiltrating*
M8870/0 *Myelolipoma*
M8880/0 *Hibernoma*
M8881/0 *Lipoblastomatosis*
M889-M892 Myomatous neoplasms
M8890/0 *Leiomyoma NOS*
M8890/1 *Intravascular leiomyomatosis*
M8890/3 *Leiomyosarcoma NOS*
M8891/1 *Epithelioid leiomyoma*
M8891/3 *Epithelioid leiomyosarcoma*
M8892/1 *Cellular leiomyoma*
M8893/0 *Bizarre leiomyoma*
M8894/0 *Angiomyoma*
M8894/3 *Angiomyosarcoma*
M8895/0 *Myoma*
M8895/3 *Myosarcoma*
M8900/0 *Rhabdomyoma NOS*
M8900/3 *Rhabdomyosarcoma NOS*
M8901/3 *Pleomorphic rhabdomyosarcoma*
M8902/3 *Mixed type rhabdomyosarcoma*
M8903/0 *Fetal rhabdomyoma*
M8904/0 *Adult rhabdomyoma*
M8910/3 *Embryonal rhabdomyosarcoma*
M8920/3 *Alveolar rhabdomyosarcoma*
M893-M899 Complex mixed and stromal neoplasms
M8930/3 *Endometrial stromal sarcoma*
M8931/1 *Endolymphatic stromal myosis*
M8932/0 *Adenomyoma*
M8940/0 *Pleomorphic adenoma*
M8940/3 *Mixed tumor, malignant NOS*
M8950/3 *Mullerian mixed tumor*
M8951/3 *Mesodermal mixed tumor*
M8960/1 *Mesoblastic nephroma*
M8960/3 *Nephroblastoma NOS*
M8961/3 *Epithelial nephroblastoma*
M8962/3 *Mesenchymal nephroblastoma*
M8970/3 *Hepatoblastoma*
M8980/3 *Carcinosarcoma NOS*
M8981/3 *Carcinosarcoma, embryonal type*
M8982/0 *Myoepithelioma*
M8990/0 *Mesenchymoma, benign*
M8990/1 *Mesenchymoma NOS*
M8990/3 *Mesenchymoma, malignant*
M8991/3 *Embryonal sarcoma*
M900-M903 Fibroepithelial neoplasms
M9000/0 *Brenner tumor NOS*
M9000/1 *Brenner tumor, borderline malignancy*
M9000/3 *Brenner tumor, malignant*
M9010/0 *Fibroadenoma NOS*
M9011/0 *Intracanalicular fibroadenoma NOS*
M9012/0 *Pericanalicular fibroadenoma*
M9013/0 *Adenofibroma NOS*
M9014/0 *Serous adenofibroma*
M9015/0 *Mucinous adenofibroma*
M9020/0 *Cellular intracanalicular fibroadenoma*
M9020/1 *Cystosarcoma phyllodes NOS*
M9020/3 *Cystosarcoma phyllodes, malignant*
M9030/0 *Juvenile fibroadenoma*
M904 Synovial neoplasms
M9040/0 *Synovioma, benign*
M9040/3 *Synovial sarcoma NOS*
M9041/3 *Synovial sarcoma, spindle cell type*
M9042/3 *Synovial sarcoma, epithelioid cell type*
M9043/3 *Synovial sarcoma, biphasic type*
M9044/3 *Clear cell sarcoma of tendons and aponeuroses*
M905 Mesothelial neoplasms
M9050/0 *Mesothelioma, benign*
M9050/3 *Mesothelioma, malignant*
M9051/0 *Fibrous mesothelioma, benign*
M9051/3 *Fibrous mesothelioma, malignant*
M9052/0 *Epithelioid mesothelioma, benign*
M9052/3 *Epithelioid mesothelioma, malignant*
M9053/0 *Mesothelioma, biphasic type, benign*
M9053/3 *Mesothelioma, biphasic type, malignant*
M9054/0 *Adenomatoid tumor NOS*
M906-M909 Germ cell neoplasms
M9060/3 *Dysgerminoma*
M9061/3 *Seminoma NOS*
M9062/3 *Seminoma, anaplastic type*
M9063/3 *Spermatocytic seminoma*
M9064/3 *Germinoma*
M9070/3 *Embryonal carcinoma NOS*
M9071/3 *Endodermal sinus tumor*
M9072/3 *Polyembryoma*
M9073/1 *Gonadoblastoma*
M9080/0 *Teratoma, benign*
M9080/1 *Teratoma NOS*
M9080/3 *Teratoma, malignant NOS*
M9081/3 *Teratocarcinoma*
M9082/3 *Malignant teratoma, undifferentiated type*
M9083/3 *Malignant teratoma, intermediate type*
M9084/0 *Dermoid cyst*
M9084/3 *Dermoid cyst with malignant transformation*
M9090/0 *Struma ovarii NOS*
M9090/3 *Struma ovarii, malignant*
M9091/1 *Strumal carcinoid*
M910 Trophoblastic neoplasms
M9100/0 *Hydatidiform mole NOS*
M9100/1 *Invasive hydatidiform mole*
M9100/3 *Choriocarcinoma*
M9101/3 *Choriocarcinoma combined with teratoma*
M9102/3 *Malignant teratoma, trophoblastic*
M911 Mesonephromas
M9110/0 *Mesonephroma, benign*
M9110/1 *Mesonephric tumor*
M9110/3 *Mesonephroma, malignant*
M9111/1 *Endosalpingioma*

M912-M916 Blood vessel tumors
M9120/0 *Hemangioma NOS*
M9120/3 *Hemangiosarcoma*
M9121/0 *Cavernous hemangioma*
M9122/0 *Venous hemangioma*
M9123/0 *Racemose hemangioma*
M9124/3 *Kupffer cell sarcoma*
M9130/0 *Hemangioendothelioma, benign*
M9130/1 *Hemangioendothelioma NOS*
M9130/3 *Hemangioendothelioma, malignant*
M9131/0 *Capillary hemangioma*
M9132/0 *Intramuscular hemangioma*
M9140/3 *Kaposi's sarcoma*
M9141/0 *Angiokeratoma*
M9142/0 *Verrucous keratotic hemangioma*
M9150/0 *Hemangiopericytoma, benign*
M9150/1 *Hemangiopericytoma NOS*
M9150/3 *Hemangiopericytoma, malignant*
M9160/0 *Angiofibroma NOS*
M9161/1 *Hemangioblastoma*

M917 Lymphatic vessel tumors
M9170/0 *Lymphangioma NOS*
M9170/3 *Lymphangiosarcoma*
M9171/0 *Capillary lymphangioma*
M9172/0 *Cavernous lymphangioma*
M9173/0 *Cystic lymphangioma*
M9174/0 *Lymphangiomyoma*
M9174/1 *Lymphangiomyomatosis*
M9175/0 *Hemolymphangioma*

M918-M920 Osteomas and osteosarcomas
M9180/0 *Osteoma NOS*
M9180/3 *Osteosarcoma NOS*
M9181/3 *Chondroblastic osteosarcoma*
M9182/3 *Fibroblastic osteosarcoma*
M9183/3 *Telangiectatic osteosarcoma*
M9184/3 *Osteosarcoma in Paget's disease of bone*
M9190/3 *Juxtacortical osteosarcoma*
M9191/0 *Osteoid osteoma NOS*
M9200/0 *Osteoblastoma*

M921-M924 Chondromatous neoplasms
M9210/0 *Osteochondroma*
M9210/1 *Osteochondromatosis NOS*
M9220/0 *Chondroma NOS*
M9220/1 *Chondromatosis NOS*
M9220/3 *Chondrosarcoma NOS*
M9221/0 *Juxtacortical chondroma*
M9221/3 *Juxtacortical chondrosarcoma*
M9230/0 *Chondroblastoma NOS*
M9230/3 *Chondroblastoma, malignant*
M9240/3 *Mesenchymal chondrosarcoma*
M9241/0 *Chondromyxoid fibroma*

M925 Giant cell tumors
M9250/1 *Giant cell tumor of bone NOS*
M9250/3 *Giant cell tumor of bone, malignant*
M9251/1 *Giant cell tumor of soft parts NOS*
M9251/3 *Malignant giant cell tumor of soft parts*

M926 Miscellaneous bone tumors
M9260/3 *Ewing's sarcoma*
M9261/3 *Adamantinoma of long bones*
M9262/0 *Ossifying fibroma*

M927-M934 Odontogenic tumors
M9270/0 *Odontogenic tumor, benign*
M9270/1 *Odontogenic tumor NOS*
M9270/3 *Odontogenic tumor, malignant*
M9271/0 *Dentinoma*
M9272/0 *Cementoma NOS*
M9273/0 *Cementoblastoma, benign*
M9274/0 *Cementifying fibroma*
M9275/0 *Gigantiform cementoma*
M9280/0 *Odontoma NOS*
M9281/0 *Compound odontoma*
M9282/0 *Complex odontoma*
M9290/0 *Ameloblastic fibro-odontoma*
M9290/3 *Ameloblastic odontosarcoma*
M9300/0 *Adenomatoid odontogenic tumor*
M9301/0 *Calcifying odontogenic cyst*
M9310/0 *Ameloblastoma NOS*
M9310/3 *Ameloblastoma, malignant*
M9311/0 *Odontoameloblastoma*
M9312/0 *Squamous odontogenic tumor*
M9320/0 *Odontogenic myxoma*
M9321/0 *Odontogenic fibroma NOS*
M9330/0 *Ameloblastic fibroma*
M9330/3 *Ameloblastic fibrosarcoma*
M9340/0 *Calcifying epithelial odontogenic tumor*

M935-M937 Miscellaneous tumors
M9350/1 *Craniopharyngioma*
M9360/1 *Pinealoma*
M9361/1 *Pineocytoma*
M9362/3 *Pineoblastoma*
M9363/0 *Melanotic neuroectodermal tumor*
M9370/3 *Chordoma*

M938-M948 Gliomas
M9380/3 *Glioma, malignant*
M9381/3 *Gliomatosis cerebri*
M9382/3 *Mixed glioma*
M9383/1 *Subependymal glioma*
M9384/1 *Subependymal giant cell astrocytoma*
M9390/0 *Choroid plexus papilloma NOS*
M9390/3 *Choroid plexus papilloma, malignant*
M9391/3 *Ependymoma NOS*
M9392/3 *Ependymoma, anaplastic type*
M9393/1 *Papillary ependymoma*
M9394/1 *Myxopapillary ependymoma*
M9400/3 *Astrocytoma NOS*
M9401/3 *Astrocytoma, anaplastic type*
M9410/3 *Protoplasmic astrocytoma*
M9411/3 *Gemistocytic astrocytoma*
M9420/3 *Fibrillary astrocytoma*
M9421/3 *Pilocytic astrocytoma*
M9422/3 *Spongioblastoma NOS*
M9423/3 *Spongioblastoma polare*
M9430/3 *Astroblastoma*
M9440/3 *Glioblastoma NOS*
M9441/3 *Giant cell glioblastoma*
M9442/3 *Glioblastoma with sarcomatous component*
M9443/3 *Primitive polar spongioblastoma*
M9450/3 *Oligodendroglioma NOS*
M9451/3 *Oligodendroglioma, anaplastic type*
M9460/3 *Oligodendroblastoma*
M9470/3 *Medulloblastoma NOS*
M9471/3 *Desmoplastic medulloblastoma*
M9472/3 *Medullomyoblastoma*
M9480/3 *Cerebellar sarcoma NOS*
M9481/3 *Monstrocellular sarcoma*

M949-M952 Neuroepitheliomatous neoplasms
M9490/0 *Ganglioneuroma*
M9490/3 *Ganglioneuroblastoma*
M9491/0 *Ganglioneuromatosis*
M9500/3 *Neuroblastoma NOS*
M9501/3 *Medulloepithelioma NOS*
M9502/3 *Teratoid medulloepithelioma*
M9503/3 *Neuroepithelioma NOS*
M9504/3 *Spongioneuroblastoma*
M9505/1 *Ganglioglioma*
M9506/0 *Neurocytoma*
M9507/0 *Pacinian tumor*
M9510/3 *Retinoblastoma NOS*
M9511/3 *Retinoblastoma, differentiated type*
M9512/3 *Retinoblastoma, undifferentiated type*
M9520/3 *Olfactory neurogenic tumor*
M9521/3 *Esthesioneurocytoma*
M9522/3 *Esthesioneuroblastoma*
M9523/3 *Esthesioneuroepithelioma*

M953 Meningiomas
M9530/0 *Meningioma NOS*
M9530/1 *Meningiomatosis NOS*
M9530/3 *Meningioma, malignant*
M9531/0 *Meningotheliomatous meningioma*
M9532/0 *Fibrous meningioma*
M9533/0 *Psammomatous meningioma*
M9534/0 *Angiomatous meningioma*
M9535/0 *Hemangioblastic meningioma*
M9536/0 *Hemangiopericytic meningioma*
M9537/0 *Transitional meningioma*
M9538/1 *Papillary meningioma*
M9539/3 *Meningeal sarcomatosis*

M954-M957 Nerve sheath tumor
M9540/0 *Neurofibroma NOS*
M9540/1 *Neurofibromatosis NOS*
M9540/3 *Neurofibrosarcoma*
M9541/0 *Melanotic neurofibroma*
M9550/0 *Plexiform neurofibroma*
M9560/0 *Neurilemmoma NOS*
M9560/1 *Neurinomatosis*
M9560/3 *Neurilemmoma, malignant*
M9570/0 *Neuroma NOS*

M958 Granular cell tumors and alveolar soft part sarcoma
M9580/0 *Granular cell tumor NOS*
M9580/3 *Granular cell tumor, malignant*
M9581/3 *Alveolar soft part sarcoma*

M959-M963 Lymphomas, NOS or diffuse
M9590/0 *Lymphomatous tumor, benign*
M9590/3 *Malignant lymphoma NOS*
M9591/3 *Malignant lymphoma, non Hodgkin's type*
M9600/3 *Malignant lymphoma, undifferentiated cell type NOS*
M9601/3 *Malignant lymphoma, stem cell type*
M9602/3 *Malignant lymphoma, convoluted cell type NOS*
M9610/3 *Lymphosarcoma NOS*
M9611/3 *Malignant lymphoma, lymphoplasmacytoid type*
M9612/3 *Malignant lymphoma, immunoblastic type*
M9613/3 *Malignant lymphoma, mixed lymphocytic-histiocytic NOS*
M9614/3 *Malignant lymphoma, centroblastic-centrocytic, diffuse*
M9615/3 *Malignant lymphoma, follicular center cell NOS*
M9620/3 *Malignant lymphoma, lymphocytic, well differentiated NOS*
M9621/3 *Malignant lymphoma, lymphocytic, intermediate differentiation NOS*
M9622/3 *Malignant lymphoma, centrocytic*
M9623/3 *Malignant lymphoma, follicular center cell, cleaved NOS*
M9630/3 *Malignant lymphoma, lymphocytic, poorly differentiated NOS*
M9631/3 *Prolymphocytic lymphosarcoma*
M9632/3 *Malignant lymphoma, centroblastic type NOS*
M9633/3 *Malignant lymphoma, follicular center cell, noncleaved NOS*

M964 Reticulosarcomas
M9640/3 *Reticulosarcoma NOS*
M9641/3 *Reticulosarcoma, pleomorphic cell type*
M9642/3 *Reticulosarcoma, nodular*

M965-M966 Hodgkin's disease
M9650/3 *Hodgkin's disease NOS*
M9651/3 *Hodgkin's disease, lymphocytic predominance*
M9652/3 *Hodgkin's disease, mixed cellularity*
M9653/3 *Hodgkin's disease, lymphocytic depletion NOS*
M9654/3 *Hodgkin's disease, lymphocytic depletion, diffuse fibrosis*
M9655/3 *Hodgkin's disease, lymphocytic depletion, reticular type*

M9656/3 *Hodgkin's disease, nodular sclerosis NOS*
M9657/3 *Hodgkin's disease, nodular sclerosis, cellular phase*
M9660/3 *Hodgkin's paragranuloma*
M9661/3 *Hodgkin's granuloma*
M9662/3 *Hodgkin's sarcoma*

M969 Lymphomas, nodular or follicular
M9690/3 *Malignant lymphoma, nodular NOS*
M9691/3 *Malignant lymphoma, mixed lymphocytic-histiocytic, nodular*
M9692/3 *Malignant lymphoma, centroblastic-centrocytic, follicular*
M9693/3 *Malignant lymphoma, lymphocytic, well differentiated, nodular*
M9694/3 *Malignant lymphoma, lymphocytic, intermediate differentiation, nodular*
M9695/3 *Malignant lymphoma, follicular center cell, cleaved, follicular*
M9696/3 *Malignant lymphoma, lymphocytic, poorly differentiated, nodular*
M9697/3 *Malignant lymphoma, centroblastic type, follicular*
M9698/3 *Malignant lymphoma, follicular center cell, noncleaved, follicular*

M970 Mycosis fungoides
M9700/3 *Mycosis fungoides*
M9701/3 *Sezary's disease*

M971-M972 Miscellaneous reticuloendothelial neoplasms
M9710/3 *Microglioma*
M9720/3 *Malignant histiocytosis*
M9721/3 *Histiocytic medullary reticulosis*
M9722/3 *Letterer-Siwe's disease*

M973 Plasma cell tumors
M9730/3 *Plasma cell myeloma*
M9731/0 *Plasma cell tumor, benign*
M9731/1 *Plasmacytoma NOS*
M9731/3 *Plasma cell tumor, malignant*

M974 Mast cell tumors
M9740/1 *Mastocytoma NOS*
M9740/3 *Mast cell sarcoma*
M9741/3 *Malignant mastocytosis*

M975 Burkitt's tumor
M9750/3 *Burkitt's tumor*

M980-M994 Leukemias

M980 Leukemias NOS
M9800/3 *Leukemia NOS*
M9801/3 *Acute leukemia NOS*
M9802/3 *Subacute leukemia NOS*
M9803/3 *Chronic leukemia NOS*
M9804/3 *Aleukemic leukemia NOS*

M981 Compound leukemias
M9810/3 *Compound leukemia*

M982 Lymphoid leukemias
M9820/3 *Lymphoid leukemia NOS*
M9821/3 *Acute lymphoid leukemia*
M9822/3 *Subacute lymphoid leukemia*
M9823/3 *Chronic lymphoid leukemia*
M9824/3 *Aleukemic lymphoid leukemia*
M9825/3 *Prolymphocytic leukemia*

M983 Plasma cell leukemias
M9830/3 *Plasma cell leukemia*

M984 Erythroleukemias
M9840/3 *Erythroleukemia*
M9841/3 *Acute erythremia*
M9842/3 *Chronic erythremia*

M985 Lymphosarcoma cell leukemias
M9850/3 *Lymphosarcoma cell leukemia*

M986 Myeloid leukemias
M9860/3 *Myeloid leukemia NOS*
M9861/3 *Acute myeloid leukemia*
M9862/3 *Subacute myeloid leukemia*
M9863/3 *Chronic myeloid leukemia*
M9864/3 *Aleukemic myeloid leukemia*
M9865/3 *Neutrophilic leukemia*
M9866/3 *Acute promyelocytic leukemia*

M987 Basophilic leukemias
M9870/3 *Basophilic leukemia*

M988 Eosinophilic leukemias
M9880/3 *Eosinophilic leukemia*

M989 Monocytic leukemias
M9890/3 *Monocytic leukemia NOS*
M9891/3 *Acute monocytic leukemia*
M9892/3 *Subacute monocytic leukemia*
M9893/3 *Chronic monocytic leukemia*
M9894/3 *Aleukemic monocytic leukemia*

M990-M994 Miscellaneous leukemias
M9900/3 *Mast cell leukemia*
M9910/3 *Megakaryocytic leukemia*
M9920/3 *Megakaryocytic myelosis*
M9930/3 *Myeloid sarcoma*
M9940/3 *Hairy cell leukemia*

M995-M997 Miscellaneous myeloproliferative and lymphoproliferative disorders
M9950/1 *Polycythemia vera*
M9951/1 *Acute panmyelosis*
M9960/1 *Chronic myeloproliferative disease*
M9961/1 *Myelosclerosis with myeloid metaplasia*
M9962/1 *Idiopathic thrombocythemia*
M9970/1 *Chronic lymphoproliferative disease*

Appendix B was officially deleted October 1, 2004

CLASSIFICATION OF DRUGS BY AMERICAN HOSPITAL FORMULARY SERVICE LIST NUMBER AND THEIR ICD-9-CM EQUIVALENTS

The coding of adverse effects of drugs is keyed to the continually revised Hospital Formulary of the American Hospital Formulary Service (AHFS) published under the direction of the American Society of Hospital Pharmacists.

The following section gives the ICD-9-CM diagnosis code for each AHFS list.

	AHFS* List	ICD-9-CM Diagnosis Code
4:00	ANTIHISTAMINE DRUGS	963.0
8:00	ANTI-INFECTIVE AGENTS	
8:04	Amebacides	961.5
	hydroxyquinoline derivatives	961.3
	arsenical anti-infectives	961.1
8:08	Anthelmintics	961.6
	quinoline derivatives	961.3
8:12.04	Antifungal Antibiotics	960.1
	nonantibiotics	961.9
8:12.06	Cephalosporins	960.5
8:12.08	Chloramphenicol	960.2
8:12.12	The Erythromycins	960.3
8:12.16	The Penicillins	960.0
8:12.20	The Streptomycins	960.6
8:12.24	The Tetracyclines	960.4
8:12.28	Other Antibiotics	960.8
	antimycobacterial antibiotics	960.6
	macrolides	960.3
8:16	Antituberculars	961.8
	antibiotics	960.6
8:18	Antivirals	961.7
8:20	Plasmodicides (antimalarials)	961.4
8:24	Sulfonamides	961.0
8:26	The Sulfones	961.8
8:28	Treponemicides	961.2
8:32	Trichomonacides	961.5
	hydroxyquinoline derivatives	961.3
	nitrofuran derivatives	961.9
8:36	Urinary Germicides	961.9
	quinoline derivatives	961.3
8:40	Other Anti-Infectives	961.9
10:00	ANTINEOPLASTIC AGENTS	963.1
	antibiotics	960.7
	progestogens	962.2
12:00	AUTONOMIC DRUGS	
12:04	Parasympathomimetic (Cholinergic) Agents	971.0
12:08	Parasympatholytic (Cholinergic Blocking) Agents	971.1
12:12	Sympathomimetic (Adrenergic) Agents	971.2
12:16	Sympatholytic (Adrenergic Blocking) Agents	971.3
12:20	Skeletal Muscle Relaxants	975.2
	central nervous system muscle-tone depressants	968.0
16:00	BLOOD DERIVATIVES	964.7
20:00	BLOOD FORMATION AND COAGULATION	
20:04	Antianemia Drugs	964.1
20:04.04	Iron Preparations	964.0
20:04.08	Liver and Stomach Preparations	964.1
20:12.04	Anticoagulants	964.2
20:12.08	Antiheparin Agents	964.5
20:12.12	Coagulants	964.5
20.12.16	Hemostatics	964.5
	capillary-active drugs	972.8
	fibrinolysis-affecting agents	964.4
	natural products	964.7
24:00	CARDIOVASCULAR DRUGS	
24:04	Cardiac Drugs	972.9
	cardiotonic agents	972.1
	rhythm regulators	972.0
24:06	Antilipemic Agents	972.2
	thyroid derivatives	962.7
24:08	Hypotensive Agents	972.6
	adrenergic blocking agents	971.3
	ganglion-blocking agents	972.3
	vasodilators	972.5
24:12	Vasodilating Agents	972.5
	coronary	972.4
	nicotinic acid derivatives	972.2
24:16	Sclerosing Agents	972.7
28:00	CENTRAL NERVOUS SYSTEM DRUGS	
28:04	General Anesthetics	968.4
	gaseous anesthetics	968.2
	halothane	968.1
	intravenous anesthetics	968.3
28:08	Analgesics and Antipyretics	965.9
	antirheumatics	965.61-965.69
	aromatic analgesics	965.4
	non-narcotics NEC	965.7
	opium alkaloids	965.00
	heroin	965.01
	methadone	965.02
	specified type NEC	965.09
	pyrazole derivatives	965.5
	salicylates	965.1
	specified type NEC	965.8
28:10	Narcotic Antagonists	970.1
28:12	Anticonvulsants	966.3
	barbiturates	967.0
	benzodiazepine-based tranquilizers	969.4
	bromides	967.3
	hydantoin derivatives	966.1
	oxazolidine derivative	966.0
	succinimides	966.2
28:16.04	Antidepressants	969.0
28:16.08	Tranquilizers	969.5
	benzodiazepine-based	969.4
	butyrophenone-based	969.2
	major NEC	969.3
	phenothiazine-based	969.1
28:16.12	Other Psychotherapeutic Agents	969.8
28:20	Respiratory and Cerebral Stimulants	970.9
	analeptics	970.0
	anorexigenic agents	977.0
	psychostimulants	969.7
	specified type NEC	970.8
28:24	Sedatives and Hypnotics	967.9
	barbiturates	967.0
	benzodiazepine-based tranquilizers	969.4
	chloral hydrate group	967.1
	glutethamide group	967.5
	intravenous anesthetics	968.3
	methaqualone	967.4
	paraldehyde	967.2
	phenothiazine-based tranquilizers	969.1
	specified type NEC	967.8
	thiobarbiturates	968.3
	tranquilizer NEC	969.5
36:00	DIAGNOSTIC AGENTS	977.8
40:00	ELECTROLYTE, CALORIC, AND WATER BALANCE AGENTS NEC	974.5
40:04	Acidifying Agents	963.2
40:08	Alkalinizing Agents	963.3
40:10	Ammonia Detoxicants	974.5
40:12	Replacement Solutions NEC	974.5
	plasma volume expanders	964.8
40:16	Sodium-Removing Resins	974.5
40:18	Potassium-Removing Resins	974.5
40:20	Caloric Agents	974.5
40:24	Salt and Sugar Substitutes	974.5
40:28	Diuretics NEC	974.4
	carbonic acid anhydrase inhibitors	974.2
	mercurials	974.0
	purine derivatives	974.1
	saluretics	974.3
40:36	Irrigating Solutions	974.5
40:40	Uricosuric Agents	974.7
44:00	ENZYMES NEC	963.4
	fibrinolysis-affecting agents	964.4
	gastric agents	973.4

	AHFS* List	ICD-9-CM Diagnosis Code
48:00	EXPECTORANTS AND COUGH PREPARATIONS	
	antihistamine agents	963.0
	antitussives	975.4
	codeine derivatives	965.09
	expectorants	975.5
	narcotic agents NEC	965.09
52:00	EYE, EAR, NOSE, AND THROAT PREPARATIONS	
52:04	Anti-Infectives	
	ENT	976.6
	ophthalmic	976.5
52:04.04	Antibiotics	
	ENT	976.6
	ophthalmic	976.5
52:04.06	Antivirals	
	ENT	976.6
	ophthalmic	976.5
52:04.08	Sulfonamides	
	ENT	976.6
	ophthalmic	976.5
52:04.12	Miscellaneous Anti-Infectives	
	ENT	976.6
	ophthalmic	976.5
52:08	Anti-Inflammatory Agents	
	ENT	976.6
	ophthalmic	976.5
52:10	Carbonic Anhydrase Inhibitors	974.2
52:12	Contact Lens Solutions	976.5
52:16	Local Anesthetics	968.5
52:20	Miotics	971.0
52:24	Mydriatics	
	adrenergics	971.2
	anticholinergics	971.1
	antimuscarinics	971.1
	parasympatholytics	971.1
	spasmolytics	971.1
	sympathomimetics	971.2
52:28	Mouth Washes and Gargles	976.6
52:32	Vasoconstrictors	971.2
52:36	Unclassified Agents	
	ENT	976.6
	ophthalmic	976.5
56:00	GASTROINTESTINAL DRUGS	
56:04	Antacids and Absorbents	973.0
56:08	Anti-Diarrhea Agents	973.5
56:10	Antiflatulents	973.8
56:12	Cathartics NEC	973.3
	emollients	973.2
	irritants	973.1
56:16	Digestants	973.4
56:20	Emetics and Antiemetics	
	antiemetics	963.0
	emetics	973.6
56:24	Lipotropic Agents	977.1
60:00	GOLD COMPOUNDS	965.69
64:00	HEAVY METAL ANTAGONISTS	963.8
68:00	HORMONES AND SYNTHETIC SUBSTITUTES	
68:04	Adrenals	962.0
68:08	Androgens	962.1
68:12	Contraceptives	962.2
68:16	Estrogens	962.2
68:18	Gonadotropins	962.4
68:20	Insulins and Antidiabetic Agents	962.3
68:20.08	Insulins	962.3
68:24	Parathyroid	962.6
68:28	Pituitary	
	anterior	962.4
	posterior	962.5
68:32	Progestogens	962.2
68:34	Other Corpus Luteum Hormones	962.2
68:36	Thyroid and Antithyroid	
	antithyroid	962.8
	thyroid	962.7

	AHFS* List	ICD-9-CM Diagnosis Code
72:00	LOCAL ANESTHETICS NEC	968.9
	topical (surface) agents	968.5
	infiltrating agents (intradermal) (subcutaneous) (submucosal)	968.5
	nerve blocking agents (peripheral) (plexus) (regional)	968.6
	spinal	968.7
76:00	OXYTOCICS	975.0
78:00	RADIOACTIVE AGENTS	990
80:00	SERUMS, TOXOIDS, AND VACCINES	
80:04	Serums	979.9
	immune globulin (gamma) (human)	964.6
80:08	Toxoids NEC	978.8
	diphtheria	978.5
	and tetanus	978.9
	with pertussis component	978.6
	tetanus	978.4
	and diphtheria	978.9
	with pertussis component	978.6
80:12	Vaccines NEC	979.9
	bacterial NEC	978.8
	with	
	other bacterial component	978.9
	pertussis component	978.6
	viral and rickettsial component	979.7
	rickettsial NEC	979.6
	with	
	bacterial component	979.7
	pertussis component	978.6
	viral component	979.7
	viral NEC	979.6
	with	
	bacterial component	979.7
	pertussis component	978.6
	rickettsial component	979.7
84:00	SKIN AND MUCOUS MEMBRANE PREPARATIONS	
84:04	Anti-Infectives	976.0
84:04.04	Antibiotics	976.0
84:04.08	Fungicides	976.0
84:04.12	Scabicides and Pediculicides	976.0
84:04.16	Miscellaneous Local Anti-Infectives	976.0
84:06	Anti-Inflammatory Agents	976.0
84:08	Antipruritics and Local Anesthetics	
	antipruritics	976.1
	local anesthetics	968.5
84:12	Astringents	976.2
84:16	Cell Stimulants and Proliferants	976.8
84:20	Detergents	976.2
84:24	Emollients, Demulcents, and Protectants	976.3
84:28	Keratolytic Agents	976.4
84:32	Keratoplastic Agents	976.4
84:36	Miscellaneous Agents	976.8
86:00	SPASMOLYTIC AGENTS	975.1
	antiasthmatics	975.7
	papaverine	972.5
	theophyllin	974.1
88:00	VITAMINS	
88:04	Vitamin A	963.5
88:08	Vitamin B Complex	963.5
	hematopoietic vitamin	964.1
	nicotinic acid derivatives	972.2
88:12	Vitamin C	963.5
88:16	Vitamin D	963.5
88:20	Vitamin E	963.5
88:24	Vitamin K Activity	964.3
88:28	Multivitamin Preparations	963.5
92:00	UNCLASSIFIED THERAPEUTIC AGENTS	977.8

* American Hospital Formulary Service

CLASSIFICATION OF INDUSTRIAL ACCIDENTS ACCORDING TO AGENCY
Annex B to the Resolution concerning Statistics of Employment Injuries adopted by the Tenth International Conference of Labor Statisticians on 12 October 1962

1 MACHINES

11 **Prime-Movers, except Electrical Motors**
111 *Steam engines*
112 *Internal combustion engines*
119 *Others*
12 **Transmission Machinery**
121 *Transmission shafts*
122 *Transmission belts, cables, pulleys, pinions, chains, gears*
129 *Others*
13 **Metalworking Machines**
131 *Power presses*
132 *Lathes*
133 *Milling machines*
134 *Abrasive wheels*
135 *Mechanical shears*
136 *Forging machines*
137 *Rolling-mills*
139 *Others*
14 **Wood and Assimilated Machines**
141 *Circular saws*
142 *Other saws*
143 *Molding machines*
144 *Overhand planes*
149 *Others*
15 **Agricultural Machines**
151 *Reapers (including combine reapers)*
152 *Threshers*
159 *Others*
16 **Mining Machinery**
161 *Under-cutters*
169 *Others*
19 **Other Machines Not Elsewhere Classified**
191 *Earth-moving machines, excavating and scraping machines, except means of transport*
192 *Spinning, weaving and other textile machines*
193 *Machines for the manufacture of foodstuffs and beverages*
194 *Machines for the manufacture of paper*
195 *Printing machines*
199 *Others*

2 MEANS OF TRANSPORT AND LIFTING EQUIPMENT

21 **Lifting Machines and Appliances**
211 *Cranes*
212 *Lifts and elevators*
213 *Winches*
214 *Pulley blocks*
219 *Others*
22 **Means of Rail Transport**
221 *Inter-urban railways*
222 *Rail transport in mines, tunnels, quarries, industrial establishments, docks, etc.*
229 *Others*
23 **Other Wheeled Means of Transport, Excluding Rail Transport**
231 *Tractors*
232 *Lorries*
233 *Trucks*
234 *Motor vehicles, not elsewhere classified*
235 *Animal-drawn vehicles*
236 *Hand-drawn vehicles*
239 *Others*
24 **Means of Air Transport**
25 **Means of Water Transport**
251 *Motorized means of water transport*
252 *Non-motorized means of water transport*
26 **Other Means of Transport**
261 *Cable-cars*
262 *Mechanical conveyors, except cable-cars*
269 *Others*

3 OTHER EQUIPMENT

31 **Pressure Vessels**
311 *Boilers*
312 *Pressurized containers*
313 *Pressurized piping and accessories*
314 *Gas cylinders*
315 *Caissons, diving equipment*
319 *Others*
32 **Furnaces, Ovens, Kilns**
321 *Blast furnaces*
322 *Refining furnaces*
323 *Other furnaces*
324 *Kilns*
325 *Ovens*
33 **Refrigerating Plants**
34 **Electrical Installations, Including Electric Motors, but Excluding Electric Hand Tools**
341 *Rotating machines*
342 *Conductors*
343 *Transformers*
344 *Control apparatus*
349 *Others*
35 **Electric Hand Tools**
36 **Tools, Implements, and Appliances, Except Electric Hand Tools**
361 *Power-driven hand tools, except electric hand tools*
362 *Hand tools, not power-driven*
369 *Others*
37 **Ladders, Mobile Ramps**
38 **Scaffolding**
39 **Other Equipment, Not Elsewhere Classified**

4 MATERIALS, SUBSTANCES AND RADIATIONS

41 **Explosives**
42 **Dusts, Gases, Liquids and Chemicals, Excluding Explosives**
421 *Dusts*
422 *Gases, vapors, fumes*
423 *Liquids, not elsewhere classified*
424 *Chemicals, not elsewhere classified*
43 **Flying Fragments**
44 **Radiations**
441 *Ionizing radiations*
449 *Others*
49 **Other Materials and Substances Not Elsewhere Classified**

5 WORKING ENVIRONMENT

51 **Outdoor**
511 *Weather*
512 *Traffic and working surfaces*
513 *Water*
519 *Others*
52 **Indoor**
521 *Floors*
522 *Confined quarters*
523 *Stairs*
524 *Other traffic and working surfaces*
525 *Floor openings and wall openings*
526 *Environmental factors (lighting, ventilation, temperature, noise, etc.)*
529 *Others*
53 **Underground**
531 *Roofs and faces of mine roads and tunnels, etc.*
532 *Floors of mine roads and tunnels, etc.*
533 *Working-faces of mines, tunnels, etc.*
534 *Mine shafts*
535 *Fire*
536 *Water*
539 *Others*

6 OTHER AGENCIES, NOT ELSEWHERE CLASSIFIED

61 **Animals**
611 *Live animals*
612 *Animal products*
69 **Other Agencies, Not Elsewhere Classified**

7 AGENCIES NOT CLASSIFIED FOR LACK OF SUFFICIENT DATA

LIST OF THREE-DIGIT CATEGORIES

1. INFECTIOUS AND PARASITIC DISEASES

Intestinal infectious diseases (001-009)

001 Cholera
002 Typhoid and paratyphoid fevers
003 Other salmonella infections
004 Shigellosis
005 Other food poisoning (bacterial)
006 Amebiasis
007 Other protozoal intestinal diseases
008 Intestinal infections due to other organisms
009 Ill-defined intestinal infections

Tuberculosis (010-018)

010 Primary tuberculous infection
011 Pulmonary tuberculosis
012 Other respiratory tuberculosis
013 Tuberculosis of meninges and central nervous system
014 Tuberculosis of intestines, peritoneum, and mesenteric glands
015 Tuberculosis of bones and joints
016 Tuberculosis of genitourinary system
017 Tuberculosis of other organs
018 Miliary tuberculosis

Zoonotic bacterial diseases (020-027)

020 Plague
021 Tularemia
022 Anthrax
023 Brucellosis
024 Glanders
025 Melioidosis
026 Rat-bite fever
027 Other zoonotic bacterial diseases

Other bacterial diseases (030-042)

030 Leprosy
031 Diseases due to other mycobacteria
032 Diphtheria
033 Whooping cough
034 Streptococcal sore throat and scarlatina
035 Erysipelas
036 Meningococcal infection
037 Tetanus
038 Septicemia
039 Actinomycotic infections
040 Other bacterial diseases
041 Bacterial infection in conditions classified elsewhere and of unspecified site

Human immunodeficiency virus (042)

042 Human immunodeficiency virus [HIV] disease

Poliomyelitis and other non-arthropod-borne viral diseases of central nervous system (045-049)

045 Acute poliomyelitis
046 Slow virus infection of central nervous system
047 Meningitis due to enterovirus
048 Other enterovirus diseases of central nervous system
049 Other non-arthropod-borne viral diseases of central nervous system

Viral diseases accompanied by exanthem (050-057)

050 Smallpox
051 Cowpox and paravaccinia
052 Chickenpox
053 Herpes zoster
054 Herpes simplex
055 Measles
056 Rubella
057 Other viral exanthemata

Arthropod-borne viral diseases (060-066)

060 Yellow fever
061 Dengue
062 Mosquito-borne viral encephalitis
063 Tick-borne viral encephalitis
064 Viral encephalitis transmitted by other and unspecified arthropods
065 Arthropod-borne hemorrhagic fever
066 Other arthropod-borne viral diseases

Other diseases due to viruses and Chlamydiae (070-079)

070 Viral hepatitis
071 Rabies
072 Mumps
073 Ornithosis
074 Specific diseases due to Coxsackievirus
075 Infectious mononucleosis
076 Trachoma
077 Other diseases of conjunctiva due to viruses and Chlamydiae
078 Other diseases due to viruses and Chlamydiae
079 Viral infection in conditions classified elsewhere and of unspecified site

Rickettsioses and other arthropod-borne diseases (080-088)

080 Louse-borne [epidemic] typhus
081 Other typhus
082 Tick-borne rickettsioses
083 Other rickettsioses
084 Malaria
085 Leishmaniasis
086 Trypanosomiasis
087 Relapsing fever
088 Other arthropod-borne diseases

Syphilis and other venereal diseases (090-099)

090 Congenital syphilis
091 Early syphilis, symptomatic
092 Early syphilis, latent
093 Cardiovascular syphilis
094 Neurosyphilis
095 Other forms of late syphilis, with symptoms
096 Late syphilis, latent
097 Other and unspecified syphilis
098 Gonococcal infections
099 Other venereal diseases

Other spirochetal diseases (100-104)

100 Leptospirosis
101 Vincent's angina
102 Yaws
103 Pinta
104 Other spirochetal infection

Mycoses (110-118)

110 Dermatophytosis
111 Dermatomycosis, other and unspecified
112 Candidiasis
114 Coccidioidomycosis
115 Histoplasmosis
116 Blastomycotic infection
117 Other mycoses
118 Opportunistic mycoses

Helminthiases (120-129)

120 Schistosomiasis [bilharziasis]
121 Other trematode infections
122 Echinococcosis
123 Other cestode infection
124 Trichinosis
125 Filarial infection and dracontiasis
126 Ancylostomiasis and necatoriasis
127 Other intestinal helminthiases
128 Other and unspecified helminthiases
129 Intestinal parasitism, unspecified

Other infectious and parasitic diseases (130-136)

130 Toxoplasmosis
131 Trichomoniasis
132 Pediculosis and phthirus infestation
133 Acariasis
134 Other infestation
135 Sarcoidosis
136 Other and unspecified infectious and parasitic diseases

Late effects of infectious and parasitic diseases (137-139)

137 Late effects of tuberculosis
138 Late effects of acute poliomyelitis
139 Late effects of other infectious and parasitic diseases

2. NEOPLASMS

Malignant neoplasm of lip, oral cavity, and pharynx (140-149)

140 Malignant neoplasm of lip
141 Malignant neoplasm of tongue
142 Malignant neoplasm of major salivary glands
143 Malignant neoplasm of gum
144 Malignant neoplasm of floor of mouth
145 Malignant neoplasm of other and unspecified parts of mouth
146 Malignant neoplasm of oropharynx
147 Malignant neoplasm of nasopharynx
148 Malignant neoplasm of hypopharynx
149 Malignant neoplasm of other and ill-defined sites within the lip, oral cavity, and pharynx

Malignant neoplasm of digestive organs and peritoneum (150-159)

150 Malignant neoplasm of esophagus
151 Malignant neoplasm of stomach
152 Malignant neoplasm of small intestine, including duodenum
153 Malignant neoplasm of colon
154 Malignant neoplasm of rectum, rectosigmoid junction, and anus
155 Malignant neoplasm of liver and intrahepatic bile ducts
156 Malignant neoplasm of gallbladder and extrahepatic bile ducts
157 Malignant neoplasm of pancreas
158 Malignant neoplasm of retroperitoneum and peritoneum
159 Malignant neoplasm of other and ill-defined sites within the digestive organs and peritoneum

Malignant neoplasm of respiratory and intrathoracic organs (160-165)

160 Malignant neoplasm of nasal cavities, middle ear, and accessory sinuses
161 Malignant neoplasm of larynx
162 Malignant neoplasm of trachea, bronchus, and lung
163 Malignant neoplasm of pleura
164 Malignant neoplasm of thymus, heart, and mediastinum
165 Malignant neoplasm of other and ill-defined sites within the respiratory system and intrathoracic organs

Malignant neoplasm of bone, connective tissue, skin, and breast (170-176)

170 Malignant neoplasm of bone and articular cartilage
171 Malignant neoplasm of connective and other soft tissue
172 Malignant melanoma of skin
173 Other malignant neoplasm of skin
174 Malignant neoplasm of female breast
175 Malignant neoplasm of male breast
176 Kaposi's sarcoma

Malignant neoplasm of genitourinary organs (179-189)

179 Malignant neoplasm of uterus, part unspecified
180 Malignant neoplasm of cervix uteri
181 Malignant neoplasm of placenta
182 Malignant neoplasm of body of uterus
183 Malignant neoplasm of ovary and other uterine adnexa
184 Malignant neoplasm of other and unspecified female genital organs
185 Malignant neoplasm of prostate

186 Malignant neoplasm of testis
187 Malignant neoplasm of penis and other male genital organs
188 Malignant neoplasm of bladder
189 Malignant neoplasm of kidney and other unspecified urinary organs

Malignant neoplasm of other and unspecified sites (190-199)

190 Malignant neoplasm of eye
191 Malignant neoplasm of brain
192 Malignant neoplasm of other and unspecified parts of nervous system
193 Malignant neoplasm of thyroid gland
194 Malignant neoplasm of other endocrine glands and related structures
195 Malignant neoplasm of other and ill-defined sites
196 Secondary and unspecified malignant neoplasm of lymph nodes
197 Secondary malignant neoplasm of respiratory and digestive systems
198 Secondary malignant neoplasm of other specified sites
199 Malignant neoplasm without specification of site

Malignant neoplasm of lymphatic and hematopoietic tissue (200-208)

200 Lymphosarcoma and reticulosarcoma
201 Hodgkin's disease
202 Other malignant neoplasm of lymphoid and histiocytic tissue
203 Multiple myeloma and immunoproliferative neoplasms
204 Lymphoid leukemia
205 Myeloid leukemia
206 Monocytic leukemia
207 Other specified leukemia
208 Leukemia of unspecified cell type

Benign neoplasms (210-229)

210 Benign neoplasm of lip, oral cavity, and pharynx
211 Benign neoplasm of other parts of digestive system
212 Benign neoplasm of respiratory and intrathoracic organs
213 Benign neoplasm of bone and articular cartilage
214 Lipoma
215 Other benign neoplasm of connective and other soft tissue
216 Benign neoplasm of skin
217 Benign neoplasm of breast
218 Uterine leiomyoma
219 Other benign neoplasm of uterus
220 Benign neoplasm of ovary
221 Benign neoplasm of other female genital organs
222 Benign neoplasm of male genital organs
223 Benign neoplasm of kidney and other urinary organs
224 Benign neoplasm of eye
225 Benign neoplasm of brain and other parts of nervous system
226 Benign neoplasm of thyroid gland
227 Benign neoplasm of other endocrine glands and related structures
228 Hemangioma and lymphangioma, any site
229 Benign neoplasm of other and unspecified sites

Carcinoma in situ (230-234)

230 Carcinoma in situ of digestive organs
231 Carcinoma in situ of respiratory system
232 Carcinoma in situ of skin
233 Carcinoma in situ of breast and genitourinary system
234 Carcinoma in situ of other and unspecified sites

Neoplasms of uncertain behavior (235-238)

235 Neoplasm of uncertain behavior of digestive and respiratory systems
236 Neoplasm of uncertain behavior of genitourinary organs
237 Neoplasm of uncertain behavior of endocrine glands and nervous system
238 Neoplasm of uncertain behavior of other and unspecified sites and tissues

Neoplasms of unspecified nature (239)

239 Neoplasm of unspecified nature

3. ENDOCRINE, NUTRITIONAL AND METABOLIC DISEASES, AND IMMUNITY DISORDERS

Disorders of thyroid gland (240-246)

240 Simple and unspecified goiter
241 Nontoxic nodular goiter
242 Thyrotoxicosis with or without goiter
243 Congenital hypothyroidism
244 Acquired hypothyroidism
245 Thyroiditis
246 Other disorders of thyroid

Diseases of other endocrine glands (250-259)

250 Diabetes mellitus
251 Other disorders of pancreatic internal secretion
252 Disorders of parathyroid gland
253 Disorders of the pituitary gland and its hypothalamic control
254 Diseases of thymus gland
255 Disorders of adrenal glands
256 Ovarian dysfunction
257 Testicular dysfunction
258 Polyglandular dysfunction and related disorders
259 Other endocrine disorders

Nutritional deficiencies (260-269)

260 Kwashiorkor
261 Nutritional marasmus
262 Other severe protein-calorie malnutrition
263 Other and unspecified protein-calorie malnutrition
264 Vitamin A deficiency
265 Thiamine and niacin deficiency states
266 Deficiency of B-complex components
267 Ascorbic acid deficiency
268 Vitamin D deficiency
269 Other nutritional deficiencies

Other metabolic disorders and immunity disorders (270-279)

270 Disorders of amino-acid transport and metabolism
271 Disorders of carbohydrate transport and metabolism
272 Disorders of lipoid metabolism
273 Disorders of plasma protein metabolism
274 Gout
275 Disorders of mineral metabolism
276 Disorders of fluid, electrolyte, and acid-base balance
277 Other and unspecified disorders of metabolism
278 Overweight, obesity and other hyperalimentation
279 Disorders involving the immune mechanism

4. DISEASES OF BLOOD AND BLOOD-FORMING ORGANS (280-289)

280 Iron deficiency anemias
281 Other deficiency anemias
282 Hereditary hemolytic anemias
283 Acquired hemolytic anemias
284 Aplastic anemia
285 Other and unspecified anemias
286 Coagulation defects
287 Purpura and other hemorrhagic conditions
288 Diseases of white blood cells
289 Other diseases of blood and blood-forming organs

5. MENTAL DISORDERS

Organic psychotic conditions (290-294)

290 Senile and presenile organic psychotic conditions
291 Alcoholic psychoses
292 Drug psychoses
293 Transient organic psychotic conditions
294 Other organic psychotic conditions (chronic)

Other psychoses (295-299)

295 Schizophrenic psychoses
296 Affective psychoses
297 Paranoid states
298 Other nonorganic psychoses
299 Psychoses with origin specific to childhood

Neurotic disorders, personality disorders, and other nonpsychotic mental disorders (300-316)

300 Neurotic disorders
301 Personality disorders
302 Sexual deviations and disorders
303 Alcohol dependence syndrome
304 Drug dependence
305 Nondependent abuse of drugs
306 Physiological malfunction arising from mental factors
307 Special symptoms or syndromes, not elsewhere classified
308 Acute reaction to stress
309 Adjustment reaction
310 Specific nonpsychotic mental disorders following organic brain damage
311 Depressive disorder, not elsewhere classified
312 Disturbance of conduct, not elsewhere classified
313 Disturbance of emotions specific to childhood and adolescence
314 Hyperkinetic syndrome of childhood
315 Specific delays in development
316 Psychic factors associated with diseases classified elsewhere

Mental retardation (317-319)

317 Mild mental retardation
318 Other specified mental retardation
319 Unspecified mental retardation

6. DISEASES OF THE NERVOUS SYSTEM AND SENSE ORGANS

Inflammatory diseases of the central nervous system (320-326)

320 Bacterial meningitis
321 Meningitis due to other organisms
322 Meningitis of unspecified cause
323 Encephalitis, myelitis, and encephalomyelitis
324 Intracranial and intraspinal abscess
325 Phlebitis and thrombophlebitis of intracranial venous sinuses
326 Late effects of intracranial abscess or pyogenic infection

Organic Sleep Disorders (327)

327 Organic sleep disorders

Hereditary and degenerative diseases of the central nervous system (330-337)

330 Cerebral degenerations usually manifest in childhood
331 Other cerebral degenerations
332 Parkinson's disease
333 Other extrapyramidal diseases and abnormal movement disorders
334 Spinocerebellar disease
335 Anterior horn cell disease
336 Other diseases of spinal cord
337 Disorders of the autonomic nervous system

Other disorders of the central nervous system (340-349)

340 Multiple sclerosis
341 Other demyelinating diseases of central nervous system
342 Hemiplegia and hemiparesis
343 Infantile cerebral palsy
344 Other paralytic syndromes
345 Epilepsy
346 Migraine
347 Cataplexy and narcolepsy
348 Other conditions of brain
349 Other and unspecified disorders of the nervous system

Disorders of the peripheral nervous system (350-359)

350 Trigeminal nerve disorders
351 Facial nerve disorders
352 Disorders of other cranial nerves
353 Nerve root and plexus disorders
354 Mononeuritis of upper limb and mononeuritis multiplex
355 Mononeuritis of lower limb
356 Hereditary and idiopathic peripheral neuropathy
357 Inflammatory and toxic neuropathy
358 Myoneural disorders
359 Muscular dystrophies and other myopathies

Disorders of the eye and adnexa (360-379)

360 Disorders of the globe
361 Retinal detachments and defects
362 Other retinal disorders
363 Chorioretinal inflammations and scars and other disorders of choroid
364 Disorders of iris and ciliary body
365 Glaucoma
366 Cataract
367 Disorders of refraction and accommodation
368 Visual disturbances
369 Blindness and low vision
370 Keratitis
371 Corneal opacity and other disorders of cornea
372 Disorders of conjunctiva
373 Inflammation of eyelids
374 Other disorders of eyelids
375 Disorders of lacrimal system
376 Disorders of the orbit
377 Disorders of optic nerve and visual pathways
378 Strabismus and other disorders of binocular eye movements
379 Other disorders of eye

Diseases of the ear and mastoid process (380-389)

380 Disorders of external ear
381 Nonsuppurative otitis media and Eustachian tube disorders
382 Suppurative and unspecified otitis media
383 Mastoiditis and related conditions
384 Other disorders of tympanic membrane
385 Other disorders of middle ear and mastoid
386 Vertiginous syndromes and other disorders of vestibular system
387 Otosclerosis
388 Other disorders of ear
389 Hearing loss

7. DISEASES OF THE CIRCULATORY SYSTEM

Acute rheumatic fever (390-392)

390 Rheumatic fever without mention of heart involvement
391 Rheumatic fever with heart involvement
392 Rheumatic chorea

Chronic rheumatic heart disease (393-398)

393 Chronic rheumatic pericarditis
394 Diseases of mitral valve
395 Diseases of aortic valve
396 Diseases of mitral and aortic valves
397 Diseases of other endocardial structures
398 Other rheumatic heart disease

Hypertensive disease (401-405)

401 Essential hypertension
402 Hypertensive heart disease
403 Hypertensive kidney disease
404 Hypertensive heart and kidney disease
405 Secondary hypertension

Ischemic heart disease (410-414)

410 Acute myocardial infarction
411 Other acute and subacute form of ischemic heart disease
412 Old myocardial infarction
413 Angina pectoris
414 Other forms of chronic ischemic heart disease

Diseases of pulmonary circulation (415-417)

415 Acute pulmonary heart disease
416 Chronic pulmonary heart disease
417 Other diseases of pulmonary circulation

Other forms of heart disease (420-429)

420 Acute pericarditis
421 Acute and subacute endocarditis
422 Acute myocarditis
423 Other diseases of pericardium
424 Other diseases of endocardium
425 Cardiomyopathy
426 Conduction disorders
427 Cardiac dysrhythmias
428 Heart failure
429 Ill-defined descriptions and complications of heart disease

Cerebrovascular disease (430-438)

430 Subarachnoid hemorrhage
431 Intracerebral hemorrhage
432 Other and unspecified intracranial hemorrhage
433 Occlusion and stenosis of precerebral arteries
434 Occlusion of cerebral arteries
435 Transient cerebral ischemia
436 Acute but ill-defined cerebrovascular disease
437 Other and ill-defined cerebrovascular disease
438 Late effects of cerebrovascular disease

Diseases of arteries, arterioles, and capillaries (440-448)

440 Atherosclerosis
441 Aortic aneurysm and dissection
442 Other aneurysm
443 Other peripheral vascular disease
444 Arterial embolism and thrombosis
445 Atheroembolism
446 Polyarteritis nodosa and allied conditions
447 Other disorders of arteries and arterioles
448 Diseases of capillaries

Diseases of veins and lymphatics, and other diseases of circulatory system (451-459)

451 Phlebitis and thrombophlebitis
452 Portal vein thrombosis
453 Other venous embolism and thrombosis
454 Varicose veins of lower extremities
455 Hemorrhoids
456 Varicose veins of other sites
457 Noninfective disorders of lymphatic channels
458 Hypotension
459 Other disorders of circulatory system

8. DISEASES OF THE RESPIRATORY SYSTEM

Acute respiratory infections (460-466)

460 Acute nasopharyngitis [common cold]
461 Acute sinusitis
462 Acute pharyngitis
463 Acute tonsillitis
464 Acute laryngitis and tracheitis
465 Acute upper respiratory infections of multiple or unspecified sites
466 Acute bronchitis and bronchiolitis

Other diseases of upper respiratory tract (470-478)

470 Deviated nasal septum
471 Nasal polyps
472 Chronic pharyngitis and nasopharyngitis
473 Chronic sinusitis
474 Chronic disease of tonsils and adenoids
475 Peritonsillar abscess
476 Chronic laryngitis and laryngotracheitis
477 Allergic rhinitis
478 Other diseases of upper respiratory tract

Pneumonia and influenza (480-487)

480 Viral pneumonia
481 Pneumococcal pneumonia [Streptococcus pneumoniae pneumonia]
482 Other bacterial pneumonia
483 Pneumonia due to other specified organism
484 Pneumonia in infectious diseases classified elsewhere
485 Bronchopneumonia, organism unspecified
486 Pneumonia, organism unspecified
487 Influenza

Chronic obstructive pulmonary disease and allied conditions (490-496)

490 Bronchitis, not specified as acute or chronic
491 Chronic bronchitis
492 Emphysema
493 Asthma
494 Bronchiectasis
495 Extrinsic allergic alveolitis
496 Chronic airways obstruction, not elsewhere classified

Pneumoconioses and other lung diseases due to external agents (500-508)

500 Coal workers' pneumoconiosis
501 Asbestosis
502 Pneumoconiosis due to other silica or silicates
503 Pneumoconiosis due to other inorganic dust
504 Pneumopathy due to inhalation of other dust
505 Pneumoconiosis, unspecified
506 Respiratory conditions due to chemical fumes and vapors
507 Pneumonitis due to solids and liquids
508 Respiratory conditions due to other and unspecified external agents

Other diseases of respiratory system (510-519)

510 Empyema
511 Pleurisy
512 Pneumothorax
513 Abscess of lung and mediastinum
514 Pulmonary congestion and hypostasis
515 Postinflammatory pulmonary fibrosis
516 Other alveolar and parietoalveolar pneumopathy
517 Lung involvement in conditions classified elsewhere
518 Other diseases of lung
519 Other diseases of respiratory system

9. DISEASES OF THE DIGESTIVE SYSTEM

Diseases of oral cavity, salivary glands, and jaws (520-529)

520 Disorders of tooth development and eruption
521 Diseases of hard tissues of teeth
522 Diseases of pulp and periapical tissues
523 Gingival and periodontal diseases
524 Dentofacial anomalies, including malocclusion
525 Other diseases and conditions of the teeth and supporting structures
526 Diseases of the jaws
527 Diseases of the salivary glands

528 Diseases of the oral soft tissues, excluding lesions specific for gingiva and tongue
529 Diseases and other conditions of the tongue

Diseases of esophagus, stomach, and duodenum (530-537)
530 Diseases of esophagus
531 Gastric ulcer
532 Duodenal ulcer
533 Peptic ulcer, site unspecified
534 Gastrojejunal ulcer
535 Gastritis and duodenitis
536 Disorders of function of stomach
537 Other disorders of stomach and duodenum

Appendicitis (540-543)
540 Acute appendicitis
541 Appendicitis, unqualified
542 Other appendicitis
543 Other diseases of appendix

Hernia of abdominal cavity (550-553)
550 Inguinal hernia
551 Other hernia of abdominal cavity, with gangrene
552 Other hernia of abdominal cavity, with obstruction, but without mention of gangrene
553 Other hernia of abdominal cavity without mention of obstruction or gangrene

Noninfective enteritis and colitis (555-558)
555 Regional enteritis
556 Ulcerative colitis
557 Vascular insufficiency of intestine
558 Other noninfective gastroenteritis and colitis

Other diseases of intestines and peritoneum (560-569)
560 Intestinal obstruction without mention of hernia
562 Diverticula of intestine
564 Functional digestive disorders, not elsewhere classified
565 Anal fissure and fistula
566 Abscess of anal and rectal regions
567 Peritonitis and retroperitoneal infections
568 Other disorders of peritoneum
569 Other disorders of intestine

Other diseases of digestive system (570-579)
570 Acute and subacute necrosis of liver
571 Chronic liver disease and cirrhosis
572 Liver abscess and sequelae of chronic liver disease
573 Other disorders of liver
574 Cholelithiasis
575 Other disorders of gallbladder
576 Other disorders of biliary tract
577 Diseases of pancreas
578 Gastrointestinal hemorrhage
579 Intestinal malabsorption

10. DISEASES OF THE GENITOURINARY SYSTEM

Nephritis, nephrotic syndrome, and nephrosis (580-589)
580 Acute glomerulonephritis
581 Nephrotic syndrome
582 Chronic glomerulonephritis
583 Nephritis and nephropathy, not specified as acute or chronic
584 Acute renal failure
585 Chronic kidney disease (CKD)
586 Renal failure, unspecified
587 Renal sclerosis, unspecified
588 Disorders resulting from impaired renal function
589 Small kidney of unknown cause

Other diseases of urinary system (590-599)
590 Infections of kidney
591 Hydronephrosis
592 Calculus of kidney and ureter
593 Other disorders of kidney and ureter
594 Calculus of lower urinary tract
595 Cystitis
596 Other disorders of bladder
597 Urethritis, not sexually transmitted, and urethral syndrome
598 Urethral stricture
599 Other disorders of urethra and urinary tract

Diseases of male genital organs (600-608)
600 Hyperplasia of prostate
601 Inflammatory diseases of prostate
602 Other disorders of prostate
603 Hydrocele
604 Orchitis and epididymitis
605 Redundant prepuce and phimosis
606 Infertility, male
607 Disorders of penis
608 Other disorders of male genital organs

Disorders of breast (610-611)
610 Benign mammary dysplasias
611 Other disorders of breast

Inflammatory disease of female pelvic organs (614-616)
614 Inflammatory disease of ovary, fallopian tube, pelvic cellular tissue, and peritoneum
615 Inflammatory diseases of uterus, except cervix
616 Inflammatory disease of cervix, vagina, and vulva

Other disorders of female genital tract (617-629)
617 Endometriosis
618 Genital prolapse
619 Fistula involving female genital tract
620 Noninflammatory disorders of ovary, fallopian tube, and broad ligament
621 Disorders of uterus, not elsewhere classified
622 Noninflammatory disorders of cervix
623 Noninflammatory disorders of vagina
624 Noninflammatory disorders of vulva and perineum
625 Pain and other symptoms associated with female genital organs
626 Disorders of menstruation and other abnormal bleeding from female genital tract
627 Menopausal and postmenopausal disorders
628 Infertility, female
629 Other disorders of female genital organs

11. COMPLICATIONS OF PREGNANCY, CHILDBIRTH AND THE PUERPERIUM

Ectopic and molar pregnancy and other pregnancy with abortive outcome (630-639)
630 Hydatidiform mole
631 Other abnormal product of conception
632 Missed abortion
633 Ectopic pregnancy
634 Spontaneous abortion
635 Legally induced abortion
636 Illegally induced abortion
637 Unspecified abortion
638 Failed attempted abortion
639 Complications following abortion and ectopic and molar pregnancies

Complications mainly related to pregnancy (640-648)
640 Hemorrhage in early pregnancy
641 Antepartum hemorrhage, abruptio placentae, and placenta previa
642 Hypertension complicating pregnancy, childbirth, and the puerperium
643 Excessive vomiting in pregnancy
644 Early or threatened labor
645 Prolonged pregnancy
646 Other complications of pregnancy, not elsewhere classified
647 Infective and parasitic conditions in the mother classifiable elsewhere but complicating pregnancy, childbirth, and the puerperium
648 Other current conditions in the mother classifiable elsewhere but complicating pregnancy, childbirth, and the puerperium

Normal delivery, and other indications for care in pregnancy, labor, and delivery (650-659)
650 Normal delivery
651 Multiple gestation
652 Malposition and malpresentation of fetus
653 Disproportion
654 Abnormality of organs and soft tissues of pelvis
655 Known or suspected fetal abnormality affecting management of mother
656 Other fetal and placental problems affecting management of mother
657 Polyhydramnios
658 Other problems associated with amniotic cavity and membranes
659 Other indications for care or intervention related to labor and delivery and not elsewhere classified

Complications occurring mainly in the course of labor and delivery (660-669)
660 Obstructed labor
661 Abnormality of forces of labor
662 Long labor
663 Umbilical cord complications
664 Trauma to perineum and vulva during delivery
665 Other obstetrical trauma
666 Postpartum hemorrhage
667 Retained placenta or membranes, without hemorrhage
668 Complications of the administration of anesthetic or other sedation in labor and delivery
669 Other complications of labor and delivery, not elsewhere classified

Complications of the puerperium (670-677)
670 Major puerperal infection
671 Venous complications in pregnancy and the puerperium
672 Pyrexia of unknown origin during the puerperium
673 Obstetrical pulmonary embolism
674 Other and unspecified complications of the puerperium, not elsewhere classified
675 Infections of the breast and nipple associated with childbirth
676 Other disorders of the breast associated with childbirth, and disorders of lactation
677 Late effect of complication of pregnancy, childbirth, and the puerperium

12. DISEASES OF THE SKIN AND SUBCUTANEOUS TISSUE

Infections of skin and subcutaneous tissue (680-686)
680 Carbuncle and furuncle
681 Cellulitis and abscess of finger and toe
682 Other cellulitis and abscess
683 Acute lymphadenitis
684 Impetigo
685 Pilonidal cyst
686 Other local infections of skin and subcutaneous tissue

Other inflammatory conditions of skin and subcutaneous tissue (690-698)
690 Erythematosquamous dermatosis
691 Atopic dermatitis and related conditions
692 Contact dermatitis and other eczema
693 Dermatitis due to substances taken internally
694 Bullous dermatoses
695 Erythematous conditions
696 Psoriasis and similar disorders
697 Lichen
698 Pruritus and related conditions

Other diseases of skin and subcutaneous tissue (700-709)
700 Corns and callosities
701 Other hypertrophic and atrophic conditions of skin
702 Other dermatoses
703 Diseases of nail
704 Diseases of hair and hair follicles
705 Disorders of sweat glands
706 Diseases of sebaceous glands
707 Chronic ulcer of skin
708 Urticaria
709 Other disorders of skin and subcutaneous tissue

13. DISEASES OF THE MUSCULOSKELETAL SYSTEM AND CONNECTIVE TISSUE

Arthropathies and related disorders (710-719)
710 Diffuse diseases of connective tissue
711 Arthropathy associated with infections
712 Crystal arthropathies
713 Arthropathy associated with other disorders classified elsewhere
714 Rheumatoid arthritis and other inflammatory polyarthropathies
715 Osteoarthrosis and allied disorders
716 Other and unspecified arthropathies
717 Internal derangement of knee
718 Other derangement of joint
719 Other and unspecified disorder of joint

Dorsopathies (720-724)
720 Ankylosing spondylitis and other inflammatory spondylopathies
721 Spondylosis and allied disorders
722 Intervertebral disc disorders
723 Other disorders of cervical region
724 Other and unspecified disorders of back

Rheumatism, excluding the back (725-729)
725 Polymyalgia rheumatica
726 Peripheral enthesopathies and allied syndromes
727 Other disorders of synovium, tendon, and bursa
728 Disorders of muscle, ligament, and fascia
729 Other disorders of soft tissues

Osteopathies, chondropathies, and acquired musculoskeletal deformities (730-739)
730 Osteomyelitis, periostitis, and other infections involving bone
731 Osteitis deformans and osteopathies associated with other disorders classified elsewhere
732 Osteochondropathies
733 Other disorders of bone and cartilage
734 Flat foot
735 Acquired deformities of toe
736 Other acquired deformities of limbs
737 Curvature of spine
738 Other acquired deformity
739 Nonallopathic lesions, not elsewhere classified

14. CONGENITAL ANOMALIES

740 Anencephalus and similar anomalies
741 Spina bifida
742 Other congenital anomalies of nervous system
743 Congenital anomalies of eye
744 Congenital anomalies of ear, face, and neck
745 Bulbus cordis anomalies and anomalies of cardiac septal closure
746 Other congenital anomalies of heart
747 Other congenital anomalies of circulatory system
748 Congenital anomalies of respiratory system
749 Cleft palate and cleft lip
750 Other congenital anomalies of upper alimentary tract
751 Other congenital anomalies of digestive system
752 Congenital anomalies of genital organs
753 Congenital anomalies of urinary system
754 Certain congenital musculoskeletal deformities
755 Other congenital anomalies of limbs
756 Other congenital musculoskeletal anomalies
757 Congenital anomalies of the integument
758 Chromosomal anomalies
759 Other and unspecified congenital anomalies

15. CERTAIN CONDITIONS ORIGINATING IN THE PERINATAL PERIOD

Maternal causes of perinatal morbidity and mortality (760-763)
760 Fetus or newborn affected by maternal conditions which may be unrelated to present pregnancy
761 Fetus or newborn affected by maternal complications of pregnancy
762 Fetus or newborn affected by complications of placenta, cord, and membranes
763 Fetus or newborn affected by other complications of labor and delivery

Other conditions originating in the perinatal period (764-779)
764 Slow fetal growth and fetal malnutrition
765 Disorders relating to short gestation and unspecified low birthweight
766 Disorders relating to long gestation and high birthweight
767 Birth trauma
768 Intrauterine hypoxia and birth asphyxia
769 Respiratory distress syndrome
770 Other respiratory conditions of fetus and newborn
771 Infections specific to the perinatal period
772 Fetal and neonatal hemorrhage
773 Hemolytic disease of fetus or newborn, due to isoimmunization
774 Other perinatal jaundice
775 Endocrine and metabolic disturbances specific to the fetus and newborn
776 Hematological disorders of fetus and newborn
777 Perinatal disorders of digestive system
778 Conditions involving the integument and temperature regulation of fetus and newborn
779 Other and ill-defined conditions originating in the perinatal period

16. SYMPTOMS, SIGNS, AND ILL-DEFINED CONDITIONS

Symptoms (780-789)
780 General symptoms
781 Symptoms involving nervous and musculoskeletal systems
782 Symptoms involving skin and other integumentary tissue
783 Symptoms concerning nutrition, metabolism, and development
784 Symptoms involving head and neck
785 Symptoms involving cardiovascular system
786 Symptoms involving respiratory system and other chest symptoms
787 Symptoms involving digestive system
788 Symptoms involving urinary system
789 Other symptoms involving abdomen and pelvis

Nonspecific abnormal findings (790-796)
790 Nonspecific findings on examination of blood
791 Nonspecific findings on examination of urine
792 Nonspecific abnormal findings in other body substances
793 Nonspecific abnormal findings on radiological and other examination of body structure
794 Nonspecific abnormal results of function studies
795 Nonspecific abnormal histological and immunological findings
796 Other nonspecific abnormal findings

Ill-defined and unknown causes of morbidity and mortality (797-799)
797 Senility without mention of psychosis
798 Sudden death, cause unknown
799 Other ill-defined and unknown causes of morbidity and mortality

17. INJURY AND POISONING

Fracture of skull (800-804)
800 Fracture of vault of skull
801 Fracture of base of skull
802 Fracture of face bones
803 Other and unqualified skull fractures
804 Multiple fractures involving skull or face with other bones

Fracture of spine and trunk (805-809)
805 Fracture of vertebral column without mention of spinal cord lesion
806 Fracture of vertebral column with spinal cord lesion
807 Fracture of rib(s), sternum, larynx, and trachea
808 Fracture of pelvis
809 Ill-defined fractures of bones of trunk

Fracture of upper limb (810-819)
810 Fracture of clavicle
811 Fracture of scapula
812 Fracture of humerus
813 Fracture of radius and ulna
814 Fracture of carpal bone(s)
815 Fracture of metacarpal bone(s)
816 Fracture of one or more phalanges of hand
817 Multiple fractures of hand bones
818 Ill-defined fractures of upper limb
819 Multiple fractures involving both upper limbs, and upper limb with rib(s) and sternum

Fracture of lower limb (820-829)
820 Fracture of neck of femur
821 Fracture of other and unspecified parts of femur
822 Fracture of patella
823 Fracture of tibia and fibula
824 Fracture of ankle
825 Fracture of one or more tarsal and metatarsal bones
826 Fracture of one or more phalanges of foot
827 Other, multiple, and ill-defined fractures of lower limb
828 Multiple fractures involving both lower limbs, lower with upper limb, and lower limb(s) with rib(s) and sternum
829 Fracture of unspecified bones

Dislocation (830-839)
830 Dislocation of jaw
831 Dislocation of shoulder
832 Dislocation of elbow
833 Dislocation of wrist
834 Dislocation of finger
835 Dislocation of hip
836 Dislocation of knee
837 Dislocation of ankle
838 Dislocation of foot
839 Other, multiple, and ill-defined dislocations

Sprains and strains of joints and adjacent muscles (840-848)
840 Sprains and strains of shoulder and upper arm
841 Sprains and strains of elbow and forearm
842 Sprains and strains of wrist and hand
843 Sprains and strains of hip and thigh
844 Sprains and strains of knee and leg
845 Sprains and strains of ankle and foot
846 Sprains and strains of sacroiliac region
847 Sprains and strains of other and unspecified parts of back

848 Other and ill-defined sprains and strains

Intracranial injury, excluding those with skull fracture (850-854)

850 Concussion
851 Cerebral laceration and contusion
852 Subarachnoid, subdural, and extradural hemorrhage, following injury
853 Other and unspecified intracranial hemorrhage following injury
854 Intracranial injury of other and unspecified nature

Internal injury of chest, abdomen, and pelvis (860-869)

860 Traumatic pneumothorax and hemothorax
861 Injury to heart and lung
862 Injury to other and unspecified intrathoracic organs
863 Injury to gastrointestinal tract
864 Injury to liver
865 Injury to spleen
866 Injury to kidney
867 Injury to pelvic organs
868 Injury to other intra-abdominal organs
869 Internal injury to unspecified or ill-defined organs

Open wound of head, neck, and trunk (870-879)

870 Open wound of ocular adnexa
871 Open wound of eyeball
872 Open wound of ear
873 Other open wound of head
874 Open wound of neck
875 Open wound of chest (wall)
876 Open wound of back
877 Open wound of buttock
878 Open wound of genital organs (external), including traumatic amputation
879 Open wound of other and unspecified sites, except limbs

Open wound of upper limb (880-887)

880 Open wound of shoulder and upper arm
881 Open wound of elbow, forearm, and wrist
882 Open wound of hand except finger(s) alone
883 Open wound of finger(s)
884 Multiple and unspecified open wound of upper limb
885 Traumatic amputation of thumb (complete) (partial)
886 Traumatic amputation of other finger(s) (complete) (partial)
887 Traumatic amputation of arm and hand (complete) (partial)

Open wound of lower limb (890-897)

890 Open wound of hip and thigh
891 Open wound of knee, leg [except thigh], and ankle
892 Open wound of foot except toe(s) alone
893 Open wound of toe(s)
894 Multiple and unspecified open wound of lower limb
895 Traumatic amputation of toe(s) (complete) (partial)
896 Traumatic amputation of foot (complete) (partial)
897 Traumatic amputation of leg(s) (complete) (partial)

Injury to blood vessels (900-904)

900 Injury to blood vessels of head and neck
901 Injury to blood vessels of thorax
902 Injury to blood vessels of abdomen and pelvis
903 Injury to blood vessels of upper extremity
904 Injury to blood vessels of lower extremity and unspecified sites

Late effects of injuries, poisonings, toxic effects, and other external causes (905-909)

905 Late effects of musculoskeletal and connective tissue injuries
906 Late effects of injuries to skin and subcutaneous tissues
907 Late effects of injuries to the nervous system
908 Late effects of other and unspecified injuries
909 Late effects of other and unspecified external causes

Superficial injury (910-919)

910 Superficial injury of face, neck, and scalp except eye
911 Superficial injury of trunk
912 Superficial injury of shoulder and upper arm
913 Superficial injury of elbow, forearm, and wrist
914 Superficial injury of hand(s) except finger(s) alone
915 Superficial injury of finger(s)
916 Superficial injury of hip, thigh, leg, and ankle
917 Superficial injury of foot and toe(s)
918 Superficial injury of eye and adnexa
919 Superficial injury of other, multiple, and unspecified sites

Contusion with intact skin surface (920-924)

920 Contusion of face, scalp, and neck except eye(s)
921 Contusion of eye and adnexa
922 Contusion of trunk
923 Contusion of upper limb
924 Contusion of lower limb and of other and unspecified sites

Crushing injury (925-929)

925 Crushing injury of face, scalp, and neck
926 Crushing injury of trunk
927 Crushing injury of upper limb
928 Crushing injury of lower limb
929 Crushing injury of multiple and unspecified sites

Effects of foreign body entering through orifice (930-939)

930 Foreign body on external eye
931 Foreign body in ear
932 Foreign body in nose
933 Foreign body in pharynx and larynx
934 Foreign body in trachea, bronchus, and lung
935 Foreign body in mouth, esophagus, and stomach
936 Foreign body in intestine and colon
937 Foreign body in anus and rectum
938 Foreign body in digestive system, unspecified
939 Foreign body in genitourinary tract

Burns (940-949)

940 Burn confined to eye and adnexa
941 Burn of face, head, and neck
942 Burn of trunk
943 Burn of upper limb, except wrist and hand
944 Burn of wrist(s) and hand(s)
945 Burn of lower limb(s)
946 Burns of multiple specified sites
947 Burn of internal organs
948 Burns classified according to extent of body surface involved
949 Burn, unspecified

Injury to nerves and spinal cord (950-957)

950 Injury to optic nerve and pathways
951 Injury to other cranial nerve(s)
952 Spinal cord injury without evidence of spinal bone injury
953 Injury to nerve roots and spinal plexus
954 Injury to other nerve(s) of trunk excluding shoulder and pelvic girdles
955 Injury to peripheral nerve(s) of shoulder girdle and upper limb
956 Injury to peripheral nerve(s) of pelvic girdle and lower limb
957 Injury to other and unspecified nerves

Certain traumatic complications and unspecified injuries (958-959)

958 Certain early complications of trauma
959 Injury, other and unspecified

Poisoning by drugs, medicinals and biological substances (960-979)

960 Poisoning by antibiotics
961 Poisoning by other anti-infectives
962 Poisoning by hormones and synthetic substitutes
963 Poisoning by primarily systemic agents
964 Poisoning by agents primarily affecting blood constituents
965 Poisoning by analgesics, antipyretics, and antirheumatics
966 Poisoning by anticonvulsants and anti-Parkinsonism drugs
967 Poisoning by sedatives and hypnotics
968 Poisoning by other central nervous system depressants and anesthetics
969 Poisoning by psychotropic agents
970 Poisoning by central nervous system stimulants
971 Poisoning by drugs primarily affecting the autonomic nervous system
972 Poisoning by agents primarily affecting the cardiovascular system
973 Poisoning by agents primarily affecting the gastrointestinal system
974 Poisoning by water, mineral, and uric acid metabolism drugs
975 Poisoning by agents primarily acting on the smooth and skeletal muscles and respiratory system
976 Poisoning by agents primarily affecting skin and mucous membrane, ophthalmological, otorhinolaryngological, and dental drugs
977 Poisoning by other and unspecified drugs and medicinals
978 Poisoning by bacterial vaccines
979 Poisoning by other vaccines and biological substances

Toxic effects of substances chiefly nonmedicinal as to source (980-989)

980 Toxic effect of alcohol
981 Toxic effect of petroleum products
982 Toxic effect of solvents other than petroleum-based
983 Toxic effect of corrosive aromatics, acids, and caustic alkalis
984 Toxic effect of lead and its compounds (including fumes)
985 Toxic effect of other metals
986 Toxic effect of carbon monoxide
987 Toxic effect of other gases, fumes, or vapors
988 Toxic effect of noxious substances eaten as food
989 Toxic effect of other substances, chiefly nonmedicinal as to source

Other and unspecified effects of external causes (990-995)

990 Effects of radiation, unspecified
991 Effects of reduced temperature
992 Effects of heat and light
993 Effects of air pressure
994 Effects of other external causes
995 Certain adverse effects, not elsewhere classified

Complications of surgical and medical care, not elsewhere classified (996-999)

996 Complications peculiar to certain specified procedures
997 Complications affecting specified body systems, not elsewhere classified
998 Other complications of procedures, not elsewhere classified
999 Complications of medical care, not elsewhere classified

SUPPLEMENTARY CLASSIFICATION OF FACTORS INFLUENCING HEALTH STATUS AND CONTACT WITH HEALTH SERVICES

Persons with potential health hazards related to communicable diseases (V01-V09)

V01 Contact with or exposure to communicable diseases
V02 Carrier or suspected carrier of infectious diseases
V03 Need for prophylactic vaccination and inoculation against bacterial diseases
V04 Need for prophylactic vaccination and inoculation against certain viral diseases
V05 Need for other prophylactic vaccination and inoculation against single diseases
V06 Need for prophylactic vaccination and inoculation against combinations of diseases
V07 Need for isolation and other prophylactic measures
V08 Asymptomatic human immunodeficiency virus [HIV] infection status
V09 Infection with drug-resistant microorganisms

Persons with potential health hazards related to personal and family history (V10-V19)

V10 Personal history of malignant neoplasm
V11 Personal history of mental disorder
V12 Personal history of certain other diseases
V13 Personal history of other diseases
V14 Personal history of allergy to medicinal agents
V15 Other personal history presenting hazards to health
V16 Family history of malignant neoplasm
V17 Family history of certain chronic disabling diseases
V18 Family history of certain other specific conditions
V19 Family history of other conditions

Persons encountering health services in circumstances related to reproduction and development (V20-V29)

V20 Health supervision of infant or child
V21 Constitutional states in development
V22 Normal pregnancy
V23 Supervision of high-risk pregnancy
V24 Postpartum care and examination
V25 Encounter for contraceptive management
V26 Procreative management
V27 Outcome of delivery
V28 Antenatal screening
V29 Observation and evaluation of newborns and infants for suspected condition not found

Liveborn infants according to type of birth (V30-V39)

V30 Single liveborn
V31 Twin, mate liveborn
V32 Twin, mate stillborn
V33 Twin, unspecified
V34 Other multiple, mates all liveborn
V35 Other multiple, mates all stillborn
V36 Other multiple, mates live- and stillborn
V37 Other multiple, unspecified
V39 Unspecified

Persons with a condition influencing their health status (V40-V49)

V40 Mental and behavioral problems
V41 Problems with special senses and other special functions
V42 Organ or tissue replaced by transplant
V43 Organ or tissue replaced by other means
V44 Artificial opening status
V45 Other postprocedural states
V46 Other dependence on machines
V47 Other problems with internal organs
V48 Problems with head, neck, and trunk
V49 Problems with limbs and other problems

Persons encountering health services for specific procedures and aftercare (V50-V59)

V50 Elective surgery for purposes other than remedying health states
V51 Aftercare involving the use of plastic surgery
V52 Fitting and adjustment of prosthetic device
V53 Fitting and adjustment of other device
V54 Other orthopedic aftercare
V55 Attention to artificial openings
V56 Encounter for dialysis and dialysis catheter care
V57 Care involving use of rehabilitation procedures
V58 Encounter for other and unspecified procedures and aftercare
V59 Donors

Persons encountering health services in other circumstances (V60-V69)

V60 Housing, household, and economic circumstances
V61 Other family circumstances
V62 Other psychosocial circumstances
V63 Unavailability of other medical facilities for care
V64 Persons encountering health services for specific procedures, not carried out
V65 Other persons seeking consultation
V66 Convalescence and palliative care
V67 Follow-up examination
V68 Encounters for administrative purposes
V69 Problems related to lifestyle

Persons without reported diagnosis encountered during examination and investigation of individuals and populations (V70-V85)

V70 General medical examination
V71 Observation and evaluation for suspected conditions not found
V72 Special investigations and examinations
V73 Special screening examination for viral and chlamydial diseases
V74 Special screening examination for bacterial and spirochetal diseases
V75 Special screening examination for other infectious diseases
V76 Special screening for malignant neoplasms
V77 Special screening for endocrine, nutritional, metabolic, and immunity disorders
V78 Special screening for disorders of blood and blood-forming organs
V79 Special screening for mental disorders and developmental handicaps
V80 Special screening for neurological, eye, and ear diseases
V81 Special screening for cardiovascular, respiratory, and genitourinary diseases
V82 Special screening for other conditions
V83 Genetic carrier status
V84 Genetic susceptibility to disease
V85 Body Mass Index

SUPPLEMENTARY CLASSIFICATION OF EXTERNAL CAUSES OF INJURY AND POISONING

Railway accidents (E800-E807)

E800 Railway accident involving collision with rolling stock
E801 Railway accident involving collision with other object
E802 Railway accident involving derailment without antecedent collision
E803 Railway accident involving explosion, fire, or burning
E804 Fall in, on, or from railway train
E805 Hit by rolling stock
E806 Other specified railway accident
E807 Railway accident of unspecified nature

Motor vehicle traffic accidents (E810-E819)

E810 Motor vehicle traffic accident involving collision with train
E811 Motor vehicle traffic accident involving re-entrant collision with another motor vehicle
E812 Other motor vehicle traffic accident involving collision with another motor vehicle
E813 Motor vehicle traffic accident involving collision with other vehicle
E814 Motor vehicle traffic accident involving collision with pedestrian
E815 Other motor vehicle traffic accident involving collision on the highway
E816 Motor vehicle traffic accident due to loss of control, without collision on the highway
E817 Noncollision motor vehicle traffic accident while boarding or alighting
E818 Other noncollision motor vehicle traffic accident
E819 Motor vehicle traffic accident of unspecified nature

Motor vehicle nontraffic accidents (E820-E825)

E820 Nontraffic accident involving motor-driven snow vehicle
E821 Nontraffic accident involving other off-road motor vehicle
E822 Other motor vehicle nontraffic accident involving collision with moving object
E823 Other motor vehicle nontraffic accident involving collision with stationary object
E824 Other motor vehicle nontraffic accident while boarding and alighting
E825 Other motor vehicle nontraffic accident of other and unspecified nature

Other road vehicle accidents (E826-E829)

E826 Pedal cycle accident
E827 Animal-drawn vehicle accident
E828 Accident involving animal being ridden
E829 Other road vehicle accidents

Water transport accidents (E830-E838)

E830 Accident to watercraft causing submersion
E831 Accident to watercraft causing other injury
E832 Other accidental submersion or drowning in water transport accident
E833 Fall on stairs or ladders in water transport
E834 Other fall from one level to another in water transport
E835 Other and unspecified fall in water transport
E836 Machinery accident in water transport
E837 Explosion, fire, or burning in watercraft
E838 Other and unspecified water transport accident

Air and space transport accidents (E840-E845)

E840 Accident to powered aircraft at takeoff or landing
E841 Accident to powered aircraft, other and unspecified
E842 Accident to unpowered aircraft
E843 Fall in, on, or from aircraft
E844 Other specified air transport accidents
E845 Accident involving spacecraft

Vehicle accidents, not elsewhere classifiable (E846-E849)

E846 Accidents involving powered vehicles used solely within the buildings and premises of an industrial or commercial establishment
E847 Accidents involving cable cars not running on rails
E848 Accidents involving other vehicles, not elsewhere classifiable
E849 Place of occurrence

Accidental poisoning by drugs, medicinal substances, and biologicals (E850-E858)

E850 Accidental poisoning by analgesics, antipyretics, and antirheumatics
E851 Accidental poisoning by barbiturates
E852 Accidental poisoning by other sedatives and hypnotics
E853 Accidental poisoning by tranquilizers

E854 Accidental poisoning by other psychotropic agents
E855 Accidental poisoning by other drugs acting on central and autonomic nervous systems
E856 Accidental poisoning by antibiotics
E857 Accidental poisoning by anti-infectives
E858 Accidental poisoning by other drugs

Accidental poisoning by other solid and liquid substances, gases, and vapors (E860-E869)
E860 Accidental poisoning by alcohol, not elsewhere classified
E861 Accidental poisoning by cleansing and polishing agents, disinfectants, paints, and varnishes
E862 Accidental poisoning by petroleum products, other solvents and their vapors, not elsewhere classified
E863 Accidental poisoning by agricultural and horticultural chemical and pharmaceutical preparations other than plant foods and fertilizers
E864 Accidental poisoning by corrosives and caustics, not elsewhere classified
E865 Accidental poisoning from poisonous foodstuffs and poisonous plants
E866 Accidental poisoning by other and unspecified solid and liquid substances
E867 Accidental poisoning by gas distributed by pipeline
E868 Accidental poisoning by other utility gas and other carbon monoxide
E869 Accidental poisoning by other gases and vapors

Misadventures to patients during surgical and medical care (E870-E876)
E870 Accidental cut, puncture, perforation, or hemorrhage during medical care
E871 Foreign object left in body during procedure
E872 Failure of sterile precautions during procedure
E873 Failure in dosage
E874 Mechanical failure of instrument or apparatus during procedure
E875 Contaminated or infected blood, other fluid, drug, or biological substance
E876 Other and unspecified misadventures during medical care

Surgical and medical procedures as the cause of abnormal reaction of patient or later complication, without mention of misadventure at the time of procedure (E878-E879)
E878 Surgical operation and other surgical procedures as the cause of abnormal reaction of patient, or of later complication, without mention of misadventure at the time of operation
E879 Other procedures, without mention of misadventure at the time of procedure, as the cause of abnormal reaction of patient, or of later complication

Accidental falls (E880-E888)
E880 Fall on or from stairs or steps
E881 Fall on or from ladders or scaffolding
E882 Fall from or out of building or other structure
E883 Fall into hole or other opening in surface
E884 Other fall from one level to another
E885 Fall on same level from slipping, tripping, or stumbling
E886 Fall on same level from collision, pushing or shoving, by or with other person
E887 Fracture, cause unspecified
E888 Other and unspecified fall

Accidents caused by fire and flames (E890-E899)
E890 Conflagration in private dwelling
E891 Conflagration in other and unspecified building or structure
E892 Conflagration not in building or structure
E893 Accident caused by ignition of clothing
E894 Ignition of highly inflammable material
E895 Accident caused by controlled fire in private dwelling
E896 Accident caused by controlled fire in other and unspecified building or structure
E897 Accident caused by controlled fire not in building or structure
E898 Accident caused by other specified fire and flames
E899 Accident caused by unspecified fire

Accidents due to natural and environmental factors (E900-E909)
E900 Excessive heat
E901 Excessive cold
E902 High and low air pressure and changes in air pressure
E903 Travel and motion
E904 Hunger, thirst, exposure, and neglect
E905 Venomous animals and plants as the cause of poisoning and toxic reactions
E906 Other injury caused by animals
E907 Lightning
E908 Cataclysmic storms, and floods resulting from storms
E909 Cataclysmic earth surface movements and eruptions

Accidents caused by submersion, suffocation, and foreign bodies (E910-E915)
E910 Accidental drowning and submersion
E911 Inhalation and ingestion of food causing obstruction of respiratory tract or suffocation
E912 Inhalation and ingestion of other object causing obstruction of respiratory tract or suffocation
E913 Accidental mechanical suffocation
E914 Foreign body accidentally entering eye and adnexa
E915 Foreign body accidentally entering other orifice

Other accidents (E916-E928)
E916 Struck accidentally by falling object
E917 Striking against or struck accidentally by objects or persons
E918 Caught accidentally in or between objects
E919 Accidents caused by machinery
E920 Accidents caused by cutting and piercing instruments or objects
E921 Accident caused by explosion of pressure vessel
E922 Accident caused by firearm missile
E923 Accident caused by explosive material
E924 Accident caused by hot substance or object, caustic or corrosive material, and steam
E925 Accident caused by electric current
E926 Exposure to radiation
E927 Overexertion and strenuous movements
E928 Other and unspecified environmental and accidental causes

Late effects of accidental injury (E929)
E929 Late effects of accidental injury

Drugs, medicinal and biological substances causing adverse effects in therapeutic use (E930-E949)
E930 Antibiotics
E931 Other anti-infectives
E932 Hormones and synthetic substitutes
E933 Primarily systemic agents
E934 Agents primarily affecting blood constituents
E935 Analgesics, antipyretics, and antirheumatics
E936 Anticonvulsants and anti-Parkinsonism drugs
E937 Sedatives and hypnotics
E938 Other central nervous system depressants and anesthetics
E939 Psychotropic agents
E940 Central nervous system stimulants
E941 Drugs primarily affecting the autonomic nervous system
E942 Agents primarily affecting the cardiovascular system
E943 Agents primarily affecting gastrointestinal system
E944 Water, mineral, and uric acid metabolism drugs
E945 Agents primarily acting on the smooth and skeletal muscles and respiratory system
E946 Agents primarily affecting skin and mucous membrane, ophthalmological, otorhinolaryngological, and dental drugs
E947 Other and unspecified drugs and medicinal substances
E948 Bacterial vaccines
E949 Other vaccines and biological substances

Suicide and self-inflicted injury (E950-E959)
E950 Suicide and self-inflicted poisoning by solid or liquid substances
E951 Suicide and self-inflicted poisoning by gases in domestic use
E952 Suicide and self-inflicted poisoning by other gases and vapors
E953 Suicide and self-inflicted injury by hanging, strangulation, and suffocation
E954 Suicide and self-inflicted injury by submersion [drowning]
E955 Suicide and self-inflicted injury by firearms and explosives
E956 Suicide and self-inflicted injury by cutting and piercing instruments
E957 Suicide and self-inflicted injuries by jumping from high place
E958 Suicide and self-inflicted injury by other and unspecified means
E959 Late effects of self-inflicted injury

Homicide and injury purposely inflicted by other persons (E960-E969)
E960 Fight, brawl, and rape
E961 Assault by corrosive or caustic substance, except poisoning
E962 Assault by poisoning
E963 Assault by hanging and strangulation
E964 Assault by submersion [drowning]
E965 Assault by firearms and explosives
E966 Assault by cutting and piercing instrument
E967 Child and adult battering and other maltreatment
E968 Assault by other and unspecified means
E969 Late effects of injury purposely inflicted by other person

Legal intervention (E970-E978)
E970 Injury due to legal intervention by firearms
E971 Injury due to legal intervention by explosives
E972 Injury due to legal intervention by gas
E973 Injury due to legal intervention by blunt object
E974 Injury due to legal intervention by cutting and piercing instruments
E975 Injury due to legal intervention by other specified means
E976 Injury due to legal intervention by unspecified means
E977 Late effects of injuries due to legal intervention
E978 Legal execution

Terrorism (E979)
E979 Terrorism

Injury undetermined whether accidentally or purposely inflicted (E980-E989)
E980 Poisoning by solid or liquid substances, undetermined whether accidentally or purposely inflicted

E981 Poisoning by gases in domestic use, undetermined whether accidentally or purposely inflicted
E982 Poisoning by other gases, undetermined whether accidentally or purposely inflicted
E983 Hanging, strangulation, or suffocation, undetermined whether accidentally or purposely inflicted
E984 Submersion [drowning], undetermined whether accidentally or purposely inflicted
E985 Injury by firearms and explosives, undetermined whether accidentally or purposely inflicted
E986 Injury by cutting and piercing instruments, undetermined whether accidentally or purposely inflicted
E987 Falling from high place, undetermined whether accidentally or purposely inflicted
E988 Injury by other and unspecified means, undetermined whether accidentally or purposely inflicted
E989 Late effects of injury, undetermined whether accidentally or purposely inflicted

Injury resulting from operations of war (E990-E999)

E990 Injury due to war operations by fires and conflagrations
E991 Injury due to war operations by bullets and fragments
E992 Injury due to war operations by explosion of marine weapons
E993 Injury due to war operations by other explosion
E994 Injury due to war operations by destruction of aircraft
E995 Injury due to war operations by other and unspecified forms of conventional warfare
E996 Injury due to war operations by nuclear weapons
E997 Injury due to war operations by other forms of unconventional warfare
E998 Injury due to war operations but occurring after cessation of hostilities
E999 Late effects of injury due to war operations